Readings in
Developmental
Neurobiology

Readings in Developmental Neurobiology

Edited by

PAUL H. PATTERSON

Department of Neurobiology
Harvard Medical School

DALE PURVES

Department of Physiology
and Biophysics
Washington University
School of Medicine

Cold Spring Harbor Laboratory
1982

Readings in Developmental Neurobiology

Other titles in the Neurosciences
available from Cold Spring Harbor Laboratory

Cold Spring Harbor Reports in the Neurosciences
   Volume 1 · Molluscan Nerve Cells: From Biophysics to Behavior
   Volume 2 · Monoclonal Antibodies to Neural Antigens
Neurobiology of the Leech

Library of Congress Cataloging in Publication Data
Main entry under title:

Readings in Developmental Neurobiology
   1. Developmental neurology--Addresses,
essays, lectures. I. Patterson, Paul H.
II. Purves, Dale. [DNLM: 1. Nervous system--
Embryology--Collected works. WL 101 R287]
QP363.5.R4   591.3'3   81-68892
ISBN 0-87969-144-1   AACR2

Front cover: The development of the neural basis for birdsong and its sexual dimorphism is discussed in Section 12.
Illustrated here are a singing canary, a male's song displayed
in a spectrogram, and male and female neurons from an area
of the brain involved in song production (adapted from
Nottebohm and Nottebohm, *J. Comp. Physiol. A* 108: 171
[1976]; Gurney, *J. Neurosci.* 1: 658 [1981]). Bird photograph
courtesy of Dr. Peter R. Marler.

All Cold Spring Harbor Laboratory publications are avail-
able through booksellers or may be ordered directly from
Cold Spring Harbor Laboratory, Box 100, Cold Spring
Harbor, New York 11724.   SAN 203-6185

Contents

v

vi

Preface

Putting together a reprint collection of this sort is beset by a number of difficulties. The most significant of these for us was the need to make relatively arbitrary decisions about which papers to include or exclude. We would have preferred to reprint many additional papers, but given the economics of publishing, this was simply not possible. Somewhat reluctantly, we chose to focus on more recent papers, although a number of older papers are included. Thus, the average age of the papers reprinted here is only a few years. This decision was based on the fact that developmental neurobiology is changing so rapidly and fundamentally that a judicious account could not be given without a majority of recent papers. We sought to remedy this imbalance in several ways. First, we have written brief reviews to introduce each of the thirteen sections. These reviews attempt to put the topic of each section into conceptual and historical perspective, and they are accompanied by fairly extensive (but by no means complete) bibliographies that will lead readers to other important, often older, papers. Second, we have reprinted a few papers that are primarily historical accounts of events in developmental neurobiology. Third, we have favored papers for inclusion that give a scholarly and lucid account of their precedents.

A second decision, also arbitrary to some degree, was to sample as broadly as possible without recourse to reviews, even if this meant omitting important papers that should otherwise have been included. As a rule, there are only one or two papers from any single investigator's laboratory, although by rights a half-dozen papers from each of several laboratories could easily have been selected. Again, our aim was to provide reasonably full coverage of current approaches within the space allotted.

We began working on this collection at the suggestion, and with the encouragement, of Jim Watson. The subject matter, and its arrangement, is based largely on the topics covered in our biennial course at Cold Spring Harbor Laboratory. We are therefore especially grateful for the information and opinions provided by the visiting lecturers in the course: David Bentley, Darwin Berg, Ira Black, Jeremy Brockes, Max Cowan, Mike Dennis, Steve Easter, Doug Fambrough, David Hubel, Kevin Hunt, Lionel Jaffe, Lynn Landmesser, Peter Lawrence, Nicole Le Douarin, Eduardo Macagno, Fernando Nottebohm, Martha Constantine-Paton, Pasko Rakic, Josh Sanes, and Nick Spitzer. Some of these individuals kindly provided more specific advice on early drafts of the section introductions. The two of us take full responsibility, however, for the many prejudices exposed in this volume.

Dale Purves
Paul Patterson
Cold Spring Harbor
July 1981

Readings in Developmental Neurobiology

Section 1
Early Events in Neural Development: Proliferation of Nerve and Glial Cells

Hamburger, V. 1980. S. Ramón y Cajal, R.G. Harrison, and the beginnings of neuroembryology. *Perspect. Biol. Med. 23:*600–616.

Rakic, P. 1974. Neurons in rhesus monkey visual cortex: Systematic relation between time of origin and eventual disposition. *Science 183:*425–427.

Levitt, P., M.L. Cooper, and P. Rakic. 1981. Coexistence of neuronal and glial precursor cells in the cerebral ventricular zone of the fetal monkey: An ultrastructural immunoperoxidase analysis. *J. Neurosci. 1:*27–39.

To discuss the specific problems that must be solved by the developing nervous system, it is useful to have some knowledge of the overall sequence of development and the terms used to describe major developmental structures and events. This task is beyond the scope of what we can cover here; nonetheless, it may help many readers to begin with a brief summary of the general scheme of neural development.

In both vertebrates and invertebrates, fertilization is followed by a period of cell division that produces a ball of cells, which, in turn, becomes hollowed out to form the blastula. This usually takes place with relatively little increase in the size of the zygote and is thus more a partitioning than growth. The next step in embryogenesis, again common to most animals, is known as gastrulation. At a particular point on the surface of the blastula an indentation forms (the blastopore), and a portion of the cellular sphere begins to invaginate. The result of gastrulation is a three-layered structure surrounding a central cavity that is open to the outside through the blastopore. The embryo in the gastrula stage then has an outside (the ectoderm), a middle (the mesoderm), and an inner cellular layer (the endoderm); it also has a front and a back (identified by the position of the blastopore in amphibians or the primitive streak in birds and mammals) and bilateral symmetry. It is at this stage in development that the formation of the nervous system proper begins.

In vertebrate embryos the earliest sign of the formation of the nervous system is the appearance of a dorsal groove running along the outside or ectodermal surface of the gastrula. The formation of this groove (a process called neurulation) proceeds caudally from the blastopore or its equivalent in birds and mammals. As the neural groove widens, ectoderm heaps up along its margins to form a platelike structure on the dorsal surface of the embryo, with distinct edges called the neural folds (Fig. 1). Beginning anteriorly, the neural folds fuse to form the neural tube; a widening of the anterior end of the tube is the first visible sign of the development of the primitive brain. Most, but not all, of the cells that ultimately form the brain and spinal cord are derived from the neural tube.

The peripheral nervous system, in contrast, originates from the neural crest. This group of cells, which also arises from the ectoderm, forms a band running the length of the neural plate just at the dorsolateral border of the neural folds. As the neural tube closes, the crest becomes distinct, lying just dorsal and lateral to it (see Fig. 1). Crest cells give rise to the spinal and autonomic ganglia, to the glial cells of the peripheral nervous system, and to a variety of nonneural tissues such as melanocytes, chromaffin cells of the adrenal medulla, and other tissues. Because of its accessibility, the neural crest figures heavily in many of the studies described in subsequent sections.

A final source of neural tissue, in addition to neural tube and neural crest, is the epidermal placodes that arise from separate thickenings of the ectoderm of the head region. There are five such thickenings in vertebrates; along with the neural crest, these thickenings give rise to the sensory ganglia of the cranial nerves.

As might be imagined, the mechanisms underlying these earliest events in the development of the nervous system are poorly understood. Among the major questions that concerned early neuroembryologists were the following: What triggers the nervous system to form and to become regionally diversified? What controls neuronal proliferation? and How do neurons migrate to appropriate positions? (See Detwiler 1936; Spemann 1938; Ramón y Cajal 1911, 1960.) In the remainder of this section we consider some aspects of neuronal proliferation; in the following two sections we discuss neuronal migration and differentiation. Some of the history of the people and ideas in this field is given in the paper by **Hamburger 1980** (see also Hamburger 1981), which, incidentally, introduces a number

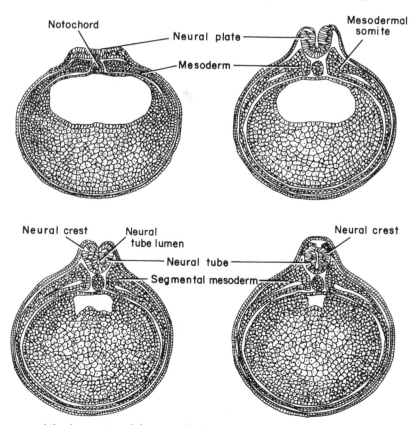

Figure 1.   *Diagram of the formation of the neural tube and neural crest from the neural plate in a vertebrate (amphibian) embryo. Cross-sections are from successive developmental stages (Saunders 1970).*

of additional themes, such as axon outgrowth and neurotrophism, that are taken up in subsequent sections.

Perhaps the first recognized principle of nerve cell proliferation was that cell division among the precursors of the central nervous system in the developing neural tube is limited to a population of cells that forms a columnar epithelium at its luminal or ventricular surface. Some early neuroembryologists, His (1887) in particular, imagined that there was a special subpopulation of these epithelial cells that gave rise to neurons, with supporting (glial) cells arising from a separate population of deeper cells; the present view is that all of the cells of this epithelium undergo a characteristic kind of mitosis to give rise to neurons and supporting cells (Sauer 1935; see also Cowan 1978).

In general, cells that ultimately form the neurons of the brain and spinal cord do not migrate away from the ventricular zone until they have finished dividing. The neural crest cells that give rise to peripheral ganglia, on the other hand, continue to divide as they migrate. Furthermore, some cells that give rise to central nervous system structures such as the cerebellar cortex

and the dentate gyrus of the hippocampus arise from precursor cells that migrate away from the ventricular zone and set up new proliferative zones (see Cowan 1978). Thus, proliferation appears to be drawn out in many instances and is compatible with other developmental events, such as migration.

Within any particular zone of the developing nervous system, cell proliferation shows a characteristic spatiotemporal pattern: there are both a rostral-to-caudal sequence and a ventral-to-dorsal sequence of maturation. An important result of this latter gradient is that the motor system is born, differentiates, and becomes functional before the sensory system (see Hamburger 1977). Another general point is that each subpopulation of neurons in a given region tends to finish dividing during a limited and well-defined period. The time of last division is referred to as the cell's birthday and can be determined with the technique of thymidine autoradiography (Sidman 1970). This method is the basis of a number of important studies. It has been found, for example, that neurons in a given cortical layer tend to have similar birthdays, thus enabling an analysis of the way in which the lamination of the cortex occurs (**Rakic 1974**).

Much debate over the years has centered on the question of how neurons and glia are actually generated in proliferative zones (see, for example, His 1887, 1889; Schaper 1897; Sauer 1935; Fujita 1964). Do these two major components of the nervous system arise from a common stem cell? If so, at what point in development do these two lineages diverge? Although these questions remain unanswered, modern techniques have made it possible to explore them in increasingly precise ways. For example, a glial-specific marker (glial fibrillary acidic protein) is present only in some proliferating cells of the ventricular and subventricular zones (Levitt and Rakic 1980; **Levitt, Cooper,** and **Rakic 1981**). Thus, glial and neuronal cell lines can already be distinguished at the peak of neurogenesis, before postmitotic migration occurs. The definition of a number of other cell-type-specific markers (see Raff et al. 1979) promises much additional information of this sort (see also Section 10).

Despite such recent advances, it is fair to say that the initiation and control of neuronal proliferation (as the control of the proliferation of other cell types) is not yet understood.

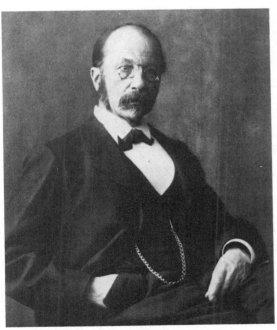

Wilhelm His, who, together with Santiago Ramón y Cajal, is considered by many the founder of modern neuroembryology.

References

Cowan, W.M. 1978. Aspects of neural development. *Int. Rev. Physiol. 17:* 149–191.

Detwiler, S.R. 1936. *Neuroembryology. An experimental study.* MacMillan, New York.

Fujita, S. 1964. The matrix cell and cytogenesis in the developing central nervous system. *J. Comp. Neurol. 120:* 37–42.

Hamburger, V. 1977. The developmental history of the motor neuron. *Neurosci. Res. Program Bull.* (Suppl.) *15:* 1–37.

———. 1980. S. Ramón y Cajal, R.G. Harrison, and the beginnings of neuroembryology. *Perspect. Biol. Med. 23:* 600–616.

———. 1981. Historical landmarks in neurogenesis. *Trends Neurosci. 4:* 151–155.

His, W. 1887. Die Entwicklung der ersten Nervenbahnen beim menschlichen Embryo: Uebersichtliche Darstellung. *Arch. Anat. Physiol. Lpz. Anat. Abt. 92:* 368–378.

———. 1889. Die Neuroblasten und deren Entstehung im embryonalen *Mark. Abh. Kgl. Sachs. Ges. Wiss. Math. Phys. Kl. 15:* 313–372.

Levitt, P. and P. Rakic. 1980. Immunoperoxidase localization of glial fibrillary acidic protein in radial glial cells and astrocytes of the developing rhesus monkey brain. *J. Comp. Neurol. 193:* 815–846.

Levitt, P., M.L. Cooper, and P. Rakic. 1981. Coexistence of neuronal and glial precursor cells in the cerebral ventricular zone of the fetal monkey: An ultrastructural immunoperoxidase analysis. *J. Neurosci. 1:* 27–39.

Raff, M.C., K.L. Fields, S.-I. Hakamori, R. Mirsky, R.M. Pruss, and J. Winter. 1979. Cell-type-specific markers for distinguishing and studying neurons and major classes of glial cells in culture. *Brain Res. 174:* 283–308.

Rakic, P. 1974. Neurons in rhesus monkey visual cortex: Systematic relation between time of origin and eventual disposition. *Science 183:* 425–427.

Ramón y Cajal, S. 1911. *Histologie du système nerveux de l'homme et des vertébrés,* vol. 1. A. Maloine, Paris. Reprinted by Consejo Superior de Investigaciones Cientificas, Instituto Ramón y Cajal, Madrid, 1955.

———. 1960. *Studies in vertebrate neurogenesis.* (Translation of the 1929 edition by L. Guth.) C.C. Thomas, Springfield, Illinois.

Sauer, F.C. 1935. Mitosis in the neural tube. *J. Comp. Neurol. 62:* 377–405.

Saunders, J.W. 1970. *Patterns and principles of animal development.* MacMillan, New York.

Schaper, A. 1897. The earliest differentiation in the central nervous system of vertebrates. *Science 5:* 430–431.

Sidman, R.L. 1970. Autoradiographic methods and principles for study of the nervous system with [³H]thymidine. In *Contemporary research methods in neuroanatomy* (ed. W.J.H. Nauta and S.O.E. Ebbesson), pp. 252–274. Springer-Verlag, Berlin.

Reprinted from Perspect. Biol. Med., Vol. 23, pp. 600–616. 1980

S. RAMÓN Y CAJAL, R. G. HARRISON, AND THE BEGINNINGS OF NEUROEMBRYOLOGY

*VIKTOR HAMBURGER**

Santiago Ramón y Cajal (1852–1934)

It is rare that the birth date of a branch of science can be determined rather precisely. The beginnings of modern developmental neurobiology can be traced to the eighties of the last century and to two eminent men: the German embryologist and anatomist Wilhelm His (1831–1904) and the Spanish neurologist Santiago Ramón y Cajal (1852–1934). Of course, the development of the nervous system had been studied before, but the foundations of our present view were laid by these men during the years 1886–1890.

Since our focus will be on Ramón y Cajal, he should be introduced briefly to nonneurologists. I rank him among the leading biologists of the last century, a peer to Darwin, Carl Ernst von Baer, Pasteur, Johannes Müller, von Helmholtz. He is the founder of modern neurology, which is also the basis of neurophysiology, neuropathology, and physiological psychology. Almost singlehandedly, he unraveled the design of the central nervous system of the vertebrates and man and traced its structure to the most intricate details. Some of his drawings, all of which bear the stamp of his originality, may still be found in modern textbooks, testifying to the amazing accuracy of his observations. His monumental *Histologie du système nerveux de l'homme et des vertébrés* (1904) is still a standard work.

The combination of extraordinary conceptual insight and observational power which characterizes his genius were displayed right at the beginning of his work, around 1887 and 1888, in a breakthrough which liberated neurology from a fallacy that had hindered all progress and at the same time set it on the right track. The then-prevailing conception of the structure of the nervous system was embodied in the reticular theory. It envisaged the nervous system as a syncytial network of nerve

*Professor emeritus, Department of Biology, Washington University, St. Louis, Missouri 63130.

fibers which were continuous with each other; the cell bodies were considered as trophic elements, at the intersection of the web. The fatal flaw of this theory is obvious: it obviates the establishment of specific pathways and connections, which are the necessary prerequisites of integrated function. Cajal revolutionized the concept of the nervous system by asserting—and demonstrating—that nerve fibers are not continuous but contiguous, that they possess terminal structures which contact other nerve cells but do not fuse with them. The contacts are now called "synapses." The hypothesis of contiguity had been proposed independently, then unknown to Cajal, by two German investigators, A. Forel and W. His. But, as Cajal points out, their hypothesis, based largely on inferences, does not take us much farther than the reticular theory as long as the possibility of diffuseness of contacts is not ruled out. He states: "To settle the question [of contiguity vs. continuity] definitely, it was necessary to demonstrate clearly, precisely, and indisputably the final ramifications of the central nerve fibers, which no one had seen, and to determine which parts of the cells made the imagined contacts" [1, pp. 337–338]. The momentous discovery of the synapse was made in 1888. During an investigation of the structure of the cerebellum of birds, he observed that terminal branches of the axons of the so-called stellate cells "applied closely to the bodies of the cells of Purkinje about which they form a kind of complicated nests or baskets" [1, p. 330]. Other synapses of different types were observed in rapid succession, and synaptic contact was recognized as a basic phenomenon. Ironically, Cajal's success in demonstrating synapses was based on the method of chrome-silver impregnation of nerve fibers which had been introduced by the Italian neurologist C. Golgi, the major proponent of the reticular theory. The same method, later improved by Cajal himself, enabled him to identify specific nerve centers and specific connections of nerve centers on a large scale.

The idea that individual nerve cells, or neurons, are the basic units of the structure of the nervous system and that axons and dendrites are parts of the neuron became known as the *neuron theory*. For many years it was pitted againt the reticular theory.

But why did Cajal turn to embryos? This was done by deliberate design. His motive is told best in his own words.

. . . the great enigma in the organization of the brain was the way in which the nervous ramifications ended and in which the neurons were mutually connected. Repeating a simile already used, it was a case of finding out how the roots and branches of these trees in the gray matter terminate, in that forest so dense that, by a refinement of complexity, there are no spaces in it, so that the trunks, branches, and leaves touch everywhere.

Two methods come to mind for investigating adequately the true form of the elements in this inextricable thicket. The most natural and simple apparently,

6

but really the most difficult, consists of exploring the full-grown forest intrepidly, clearing the ground of shrubs and parasitic plants, and eventually isolating each species of tree, as well from its parasites as from its relatives. Such was the approach employed in neurology by most authors. . . . Such tactics, however, are inappropriate for the elucidation of the problem proposed, by reason of the enormous length and extraordinary luxuriance of the nervous ramifications, which inevitably appear mutilated and almost indecipherable in each section.

The second path open to reason is what, in biological terms, is designated the ontogenetic or embryological method. Since the full grown forest turns out to be impenetrable and indefinable, why not revert to the study of the young wood, in the nursery stage, as we might say? Such was the very simple idea which inspired my repeated trials of the silver method upon embryos of birds and mammals. If the stage of development is well chosen, or, more specifically, if the method is applied before the appearance of the myelin sheaths upon the axons (these forming an almost insuperable obstacle to the reaction), the nerve cells, which are still relatively small, stand out complete in each section; the terminal ramifications of the axis cylinder are depicted with the utmost clearness and perfectly free; the pericellular nests, that is the interneuronal articulations, appear simple, gradually acquiring intricacy and extension; in sum, the fundamental plan of the histological composition of the gray matter rises before our eyes with admirable clarity and precision. As a crowning piece of good fortune, the chrome silver reaction which is so incomplete and uncertain in the adult, gives in embryos splendid colourations, singularly extensive and constant. . . .

Realizing that I had discovered a rich field, I proceeded to take advantage of it, dedicating myself to work, no longer merely with earnesteness, but with fury. In proportion as new facts appeared in my preparations, ideas boiled up and jostled each other in my mind. A fever for publication devoured me. [1, pp. 323–25]

His "fever for publications" produced 12 papers and monographs in 1889 and 16 in 1890, his most productive years. Very soon, what began as a "strategic subterfuge" became an endeavour in its own right, with intriguing problems of its own.

In 1890, Cajal was successful in obtaining splendid silver impregnations of the spinal cord of early (2½-day) chick embryos [2]. They showed the early stages of differentiation of an embryonic neuron, or neuroblast; that is, cell bodies with a short outgrowth which was identified as the incipient axon. It terminated in a club-shaped thickening with short spikes. The latter were recognized later as filamentous pseudopodia. Cajal designated the terminal structure as the "growth cone." As was stated, the neuron theory asserted that the axon is part of the neuron. The discovery of the mode of origin of the axon was the categorical affirmation of this aspect of the neuron theory. Cajal observed that neuroblasts are polarized in the sense that the site of the outgrowth of dendrites is opposite to that of the axons, and he established the general rule that dendrites differentiate later than the axon. He found the clearest demonstration of neuroblast polarity in the earliest differentiation stages of spinal ganglion neuroblasts: they are at first bipolar, with two outgrowths at opposite ends of the cell. These extensions fuse later at their bases to form the single sensory fiber. The recognition of structural polarity later on became the basis of the theory of physiological polarity. But of all his observations in the field of neurogenesis, Cajal was most intrigued by the growth cone. We shall return to this point later.

To appreciate the fundamental importance of these discoveries, one has to place them in their historical setting. The axon outgrowth theory had two formidable rivals: *the cell chain theory* of Schwann postulated that nerve fibers are produced by chains of Schwann cells which connect the nervous system with the peripheral organs. The nerve fibers are considered as products of these cells which fuse with each other and with the neuroblasts. More widely accepted was the *plasmodesm theory* of Hensen and Held. It was based on the ubiquity of protoplasmic bridges, or plasmodesms, resulting from incomplete cell divisions. In the original version of Hensen [3], some plasmodesms would be transformed into nerve fibers by functional validation. In the more sophisticated version of Held [4], an approach to the His-Cajal notion of axon outgrowth is evident. According to Held, the axon is built by two components. One is *neurofibrillar* material spun out by neuroblasts (demonstrable in Held's silver-impregnated material and distinguished by him from the protoplasmic outgrowth described by His and Cajal). The neurofibrils penetrate into plasmodesms, and these intraplasmatic neurofibrils are then transformed into nerve fibers by utilization and incorporation of plasmodesm material. Ramón y Cajal fought all his life battles on two fronts: for contiguity and against continuity in the structure of the nervous system; and for protoplasmic outgrowth, against cell chains and plasmodesms, in the origin of the nerve fiber.

During the crucial years in his career, from 1887 to 1892, Cajal was professor of histology in Barcelona. In this provincial place, he was remote from the mainstream of scientific research and not aware of the work of Wilhelm His, one of the leading German anatomists and embryologists of that time. In 1886 and 1889 [5, 6], His had given a very detailed account of the development of the spinal cord, first in human embryos and then in other vertebrate embryos. He had described the transformation of the neural epithelium into mantle and marginal velum. The neuroblasts were derived from mitotic cells at the inner lining of the central canal. Erroneously, he considered these proliferating "germinal cells" as a special strain of neuroblast precursors, and he derived ependymal layer and glia from the neural epithelium. We know now that the "germinal cells" are merely the mitotic phase of neuroepithelial cells which give rise to both neurons and glia. He coined the terms "neuroblast" and "dendrites." He was the first to describe the transformation of the postmitotic cell into a neuroblast and the formation of axon and dendrites as protoplasmic outgrowths from the neuroblast. Earlier than Cajal, he described the migration of neuroblasts to the periphery, where they form the mantle. He also noticed the originally bipolar configuration of the spinal ganglion cell.

In 1886 he stated the neuron theory very concisely: "I consider it as an established principle that each nerve fiber emerges as an outgrowth from a single cell. This is its genetic, trophic and functional center. All other connections of fibers are either indirect or secondary" [5, p. 513]. This statement includes implicitly the concept of contiguity as against a network.

Cajal did not learn of these findings until 1890, when His sent him copies of his work. From then on, Cajal gives His full credit for his discoveries, but he states explicitly that his own discoveries were made independently of those of His. He adds: "This coincidence in thought on the part of the leading workers in the field, without any oral or written collaboration, constitutes the best moral encouragement and the strongest guarantee of the validity of the adopted interpretation" [7, p. 6].

Yet it is the merit of Cajal to have realized fully the dynamic implications of the outgrowth theory. In this he went far beyond His. I shall turn to this aspect and omit any further references to his substantial contributions to the development of many structures, such as retina, cerebellum, spinal cord, optic tectum [8]. The silver-impregnation method had permitted Cajal the observation of the growth cone which was not discernible in the material of His, treated with ordinary stains. Cajal describes it as a swelling with spiny extensions, sometimes triangular or lamellar, and ramified. In his treatise on histology he gives the following interpretation: "From the functional point of view the growth cone may be regarded as a sort of club or battering ram, endowed with exquisite chemical sensitivity, with rapid ameboid movements, and with certain impulsive force, thanks to which it is able to proceed forward and overcome obstacles met in its way, forcing cellular interstices until it arrives at its destination" [9, p. 599]. In this quotation, two points deserve attention: the uniquely dynamic interpretation of the static microscope slide picture; and the clear visualization of problems of pathfinding which are implicit in the outgrowth theory. Sherrington has an interesting comment on the first point:

A trait very noticeable in him was that in describing what the microscope showed he spoke habitually as though it were a living scene. This was perhaps the more striking because not only were his preparations all dead and fixed, but they were to appearance roughly made and rudely treated—no cover-glass and as many as half a dozen tiny scraps of tissue set in one large blob of balsam and left to dry, the curved and sometimes slightly wrinkled surface of the balsam creating a difficulty for microphotography. He was an accomplished photographer but, so

9

far as I know, he never practiced microphotography. Such scanty illustrations as he vouchsafed for the preparations he demonstrated were a few slight, rapid sketches of points taken here and there—depicted, however, by a master's hand.

The intense anthropomorphism of his descriptions of what the preparations showed was at first startling to accept. He treated the microscopic scene as though it were alive and were inhabited by beings which felt and did and hoped and tried even as we do. It was personification of natural forces as unlimited as that of Goethe's *Faust,* Part 2. A nerve-cell by its emergent fibre "groped to find another"! We must, if we would enter adequately into Cajal's thought in this field, suppose his entrance, through his microscope, into a world populated by tiny beings actuated by motives and strivings and satisfactions not very remotely different from our own. He would envisage the sperm-cells as activated by a sort of passionate urge in their rivalry for penetration into the ovum-cell. Listening to him I asked myself how far this capacity for anthropomorphizing might not contribute to his success as an investigator. I never met anyone else in whom it was so marked. [10, pp. xiii–xiv]

Indeed, the climbing fibers climbed and the synapses were "protoplasmic kisses, . . . the final ecstasy of an epic love story" [1, p. 373]. Cajal's dynamic view was all-pervasive. For instance, it led him to postulate the polarization of impulse conduction, based solely on morphological data.

As to the second point, his immense intellectual analytical power equals his power of observation. In fact, both are two facets of his creative genius. Whatever he observed took on a meaning transcending the microscope picture. There are few problems on our present-day mind on which he did not reflect at one occasion or another. I shall elaborate on one example, his theory of neurotropism, which deals with the problem of how nerves find their way to their targets. This problem does not exist in the cell chain and plasmodesm theories. Cajal became aware of it when he discovered the growth cone. In his monograph on the retina he mentions for the first time a solution that had occurred to him, in terms of a chemical attraction of the growth cone by substances produced by the target structures (chemotropism):

How does the mechanical development of the nerve fibers occur, and wherein lies that marvelous power which enables the nerve fibers from very distant cells to make contact directly with certain other nerve cells or the mesoderm or ectoderm without going astray or taking a roundabout course?

His has concerned himself with this important question and is of the following opinion: The axis cylinder of the neuroblasts, whether in the medulla or in the mesoderm, always follows the path of least resistance. That resistance is offered by bone, cartilage, connective tissue, etc. which are found along the route of growing nerves. This accounts for the major part of the phenomenon.

Without wanting to deny the importance of such a mechanical influence, especially in the growth of the nerve fibers from the retina to the brain and vice versa, I believe that one could also think of processes like the phenomenon called Pfeffer's chemotaxis, whose influences on the leukocytes was established by Massart and Bordet, Gabritschewsky, Buchner, and Metchnikoff. . . .

10

If a chemotaxic sensitivity in the neuroblasts is assumed, then it must be supposed that these cells are capable of amoeboid movement and are responsive to certain substances secreted by cells of the epithelium or mesoderm. The processes of the neuroblasts become oriented by chemical stimulation, and move toward the secretion products of certain cells. [11, p. 146]

The discoveries of plant physiologists concerning tropisms (chemotropism, geotropisms, etc.) and taxies figured prominently in contemporary thought. Taxies refer to directed movements of cells and organisms, and tropisms to directed outgrowth of parts, such as roots. Cajal refers specifically to the German plant physiologist W. Pfeffer, who among many other discoveries had described the attraction of sperm in mosses by malate produced by the ovary. Chemotaxis was suggested to Cajal for the first time when he observed the migration of granule cells from the superficial layer in the embryonic cerebellum to deeper layers [8, p. 291]. But the notion of chemotropism came to fruition only a decade later in the context of nerve regeneration.

A brief discourse on the status of nerve regeneration at the time when Cajal became active in this field (around 1905) is necessary. In the middle of the nineteenth century, Waller had discovered the degeneration of the distal stump, if regeneration after transection is prevented; and the central stump was recognized as the necessary "trophic center." It was also known that in the case of regeneration, Schwann cells in the distal stump proliferate and penetrate the scar between proximal and distal stump. Cajal encountered here again the unsettled controversy between those who, beginning with Waller and Ranvier, postulated that the regenerated nerve is an outgrowth from the proximal stump, and the adherents of the Schwann cell chain and plasmodesm theories who brought forth the same arguments as in nerve fiber origin in the embryo. In fact, the first decade of this century is marked by a remarkable revival of the old erroneous theories, combined with renewed attacks on the axon outgrowth theory, even in the face of Harrison's tissue culture experiment of 1907 (see, for instance, the treatise of Held [4]). Cajal, applying his silver-impregnation method, had no difficulty in finding growth cones both in the proximal stump and in later stages in the distal stump, thus bringing regeneration in line with axon production in the embryo. I omit again numerous other original findings by Cajal on nerve regeneration. I may mention the observation that, after nerve constriction, strings of beads are formed in the region proximal to the ligature. They were then rediscovered by Weiss and Hiscoe [12] and interpreted correctly as indication of axoplasmic flow.

In the meantime, the chemotropism theory had gotten a foothold in neurogenesis; and since, at the turn of the century, there were no methods available for testing it in the embryo, experimentation was carried out on regenerating nerves. Forssman [13], one of the experimenters in this field, believed that degenerating axons and Schwann sheath produced a chemotropic agent. He coined the term "neurotropism," which was adopted by Cajal, though he believed that Schwann cells (Buengner bands) rather than degenerating material generate the tropic agent. A representative example of this type of experiment is the following, done by Cajal (fig. 1): The sciatic nerve of a kitten was split longitudinally. One half was transected once, the other half was transected at the same level and also at a more proximal level. In the latter half, the nerve sector between the two cuts degenerated. Six days after the operation, a strong bridge of nerve fibers connected the distalmost cut ends. They originated in the half that had been cut only at that level, and entered the degenerating tubes of the other half, where they grew in proximal direction. This and numerous similar experiments by Cajal, Tello, Forssman, and others were interpreted as evidence for neurotropism (see [14]). However, as was pointed out later by Weiss and others, they can be explained in a different way, that is, in terms of original random outgrowth of fibers in all directions, and survival of those which happened to grow in the direction of the other stump. In fact, at the right distal stump in figure 1, fibers do grow out in all directions.

At this point, I wish to follow the theoretical reflections of Cajal, which, though purely speculative, have a bearing on very recent developments. The simplistic statement of neurotropism in 1892, quoted above, was superseded by a very sophisticated version in 1913 [15]. He recognized three basic conditions for successful regeneration: "The nervous reunion of the peripheral stump and restoration, without physio-

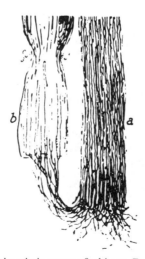

FIG. 1.—Nerve regeneration in sciatic nerve of a kitten. For details see text (from [15, p. 317]).

12

logical errors, of the terminal nerve structures, are the combined effect of three conditions: the neurotropic action of the sheath of Schwann and terminal structures; the mechanical guidance of the sprouts along the old sheaths; and, finally, the superproduction of fibres, in order to insure the arrival of some of them at the peripheral motor or sensory regions.—Of all these conditions the most essential, especially as regards the reconstruction of the terminal apparatus, is the trophism or neurotropism of the peripheral stump, motor plates, and sensory structures" [15, p. 371]. The strange juxtaposition of "trophism and neurotropism" will be commented on presently.

Furthermore, he distinguishes between general neurotropic action on the part of the peripheral stump, guiding nerve fibers toward the target, and specific action guaranteeing the appropriate connection with specific target structures: "The orienting chemical stimuli are probably, so far as their selective power is concerned, both generic and specific.— The attractive substance elaborated by the embryonic connective cells and by the cells of Schwann of the peripheral stump have a generic character, acting without distinction on all sprouts; while the attractive substances given out by the spindles of Kühne, motor plates, cutaneous sensory structures, etc., have a specific character, acting only on certain functional categories of regenerated axons" [15, p. 371]. Apart from neurotropism, his distinction between pathfinding toward the target and specificity of synaptic connections is now generally accepted. His notion of an overproduction of fibers, to insure the safe arrival of some of them at the target, in the earlier quotation has a very modern ring. In fact, he suggests that in synaptogenesis unsuccessful fibers and branches atrophy and unsuccessful neurons disappear, thus anticipating the phenomenon of naturally occurring neuronal death.

There is no doubt that, at first, many imperfect connections are formed, and that many duplications and errors of distribution occur. But these incongruences are progressively corrected, up to a certain point, by two parallel methods of rectification. One of these occurs in the periphery, and is the atrophy through disuse of superfluous and parasitic ramifications, in combination with the growth of congruent sprouts. The other occurs in the ganglia and spinal centres; by this there would be a selection, due to the atrophy of certain collaterals and the progressive disappearance of disconnected or useless neurones, of the sensory-motor fibres capable of being useful. [15, p. 279]

He even anticipates our present idea of a process of competition (for a synaptic site, or for a trophic agent) which figures prominently in our search for the explanation of naturally occurring neuronal death. ". . . It is only those expansions which are able to establish useful relations with afferent nerve fibres which survive in this contest for space and con-

608 | *Viktor Hamburger · S. Ramón y Cajal and R. G. Harrison*

13

nections. In nervous regeneration this process of hyperformation is repeated" [15, p. 278].

I was particularly intrigued by the refinement of the original notion of attraction at a distance. In his later view, the distal stump (and, more specifically, the Buengner bands) would release an agent whose function is to stimulate metabolism and assimilation in the sprouting axon growth cones. What I regard as a novel conceptualization is the combination of the idea of a trophic action with *tropism*—that is, directional growth—to which I had called attention in an earlier quotation. The following paragraph clarifies what he has in mind: "The neurotropic stimulus acts as a ferment or enzyme, provoking protoplasmic assimilation. . . . While in the present state of knowledge we cannot penetrate the mechanism of the neurotropic action, an analysis of all the facts of nervous reunion known to us suggest the hypothesis that the orienting agent of the sprouts does not operate through attraction, as many have supposed, but by creating a region that is favourable, eminently trophic, and stimulative of the assimilation and growth of the newly-formed axons" [15, p. 372]. In other words, he envisages the production, by the target, of a trophic agent which stimulates growth in the growth cone and then, so to speak, nurses the axon along toward the target. I shall come back to this point presently.

Ingenious as it was, the neurotropism theory has not fared well in recent decades. It is true that not very extensive efforts have been made to test it and that practically all experiments, both in vivo and in vitro, to that effect have given negative results. Admittedly, the regeneration experiments of Cajal, Forssman, and others are not conclusive, as I have pointed out above. But the negative results of Weiss and others are not a final verdict either. When such efforts are unsuccessful, one can always raise the question of whether the experimental design was sufficiently subtle. Anyway, neurotropism has been pronounced dead as recently as 1976 [16].

As it happened, the deceased was resurrected in the same book by R. Levi-Montalcini [17]. She had discovered a case of neurotropism in the central nervous system. In order to test the claim of Swedish investigators that transected axons of monoaminergic neurons in the brain stem of young rodents can be stimulated to sprouting by Nerve Growth Factor (NGF), a nerve-growth-stimulating protein, she injected NGF into the medulla of newborn rats, near the locus coeruleus. She observed a conspicuous enlargement of the sympathetic chain ganglia on the side of injection and a massive invasion of sympathetic fibers through dorsal roots to the site of injection (fig. 2). Histofluorescence treatment demonstrated the passage of these fibers in the dorsal funiculus. They did not innervate any particular structure and disappeared when NGF injection was discontinued.

14

Of particular interest is her interpretation of this phenomenon which, mutatis mutandis, comes remarkably close to what Cajal had envisaged to be a tropic-trophic mechanism. I quote from a recent publication: "The entrance of sympathetic nerves into the CNS of neonatal rodents injected intracerebrally with NGF should however not be regarded as evidence of an attraction at a distance produced by the high NGF concentration gradient in the neural tube of the experimental mice and rats." (One remembers Cajal's statement that "the orienting agent does not operate through attraction as many have supposed.") "The direct access of NGF to the sympathetic ganglia through the motor and sensory roots is clearly indicated by the hypertrophic and hyperplastic effects elicited by the intracerebral NGF treatment. The same roots which served as transport channels and are presumably imbued with NGF provide in turn most convenient routes for the sympathetic fibers which engage in these paths and . . . gain in this way entrance into the

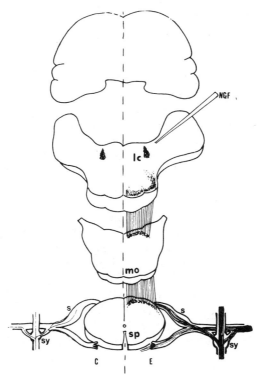

Fig. 2.—Chemotropic attraction of sympathetic fiber bundles to NGF injected intracerebrally into neonatal rats (from [17, p. 244]). *C* = control side, *E* = experimental side, *lc* = locus coeruleus; *mo* = medulla oblongata, *s* = sensory ganglia; *sp* = spinal cord; *sy* = sympathetic ganglia.

610 | *Viktor Hamburger · S. Ramón y Cajal and R. G. Harrison*

CNS. . . . The axonal tip of the fibers moves along gradients of diffusion of *trophic and tropic* factors released by end organs. . . . Neurotropism would assist, rather than determining the course of nerve fibers toward their correct destination" [18, pp. 79–80]. The linkage of the words "trophic and tropic" by Cajal in 1913 and Levi-Montalcini in 1978 is startling; one is reminded again of what Cajal had to say of independent discoveries. What was envisaged by Cajal, by pure reflection, namely that a growth promoting agent, released by the target, imbues the intervening tissue and guides the growing tip of the axon along to its source, seems now to be demonstrated in a controlled experiment. NGF has long been established as a trophic agent. If a tropic function can be added, then the revival of Cajal's idea that trophic and tropic may be two sides of the same coin could become an important new model in modern developmental neurobiology. Indeed, it is very difficult to be original in neurogenesis with Cajal looking over one's shoulder.

Ross Granville Harrison (1870–1959)

Harrison's major contribution to biology in general and to neuroembryology in particular is the invention of the tissue culture method. It will be remembered that in his classical experiment he isolated pieces of the neural tube of a frog embryo and reared it in frog's lymph, in a depression slide. What links this experiment directly with Ramón y Cajal is the fact that it was motivated by the same concerns which preoccupied Cajal: to find a direct test for the axon outgrowth theory. Of equal importance is another major contribution of Harrison: Almost single-handedly, he introduced the analytical experiment, that is, microsurgery on the embryo, as a tool for the exploration of neurogenetic problems. These two achievements would have been sufficient to rank him among the leading experimental biologists of the first half of the century. If one adds the solution of another fundamental problem, the origin of axial polarization and bilateral symmetry in vertebrates by ingenious experiments, then it is hard to understand that he did not share the Nobel Prize with Spemann, in 1935, as had been expected. In fact, he was proposed twice: first in 1914, but the prizes were suspended on account of the war, and then again in 1933. According to the official account of the Nobel Committee, in a special committee in 1933 "opinions diverged, and in view of the rather limited value of the method and the age of the discovery, an award could not be recommended" [19, p. 259]. What was actually of limited value was the judgment of the committee, and not Harrison's achievements.

I knew Harrison well. He was a frequent summer visitor in the laboratory of his friend H. Spemann, in Freiburg, where I took my Ph.D. and then advanced to an instructorship. After a vacation in the Swiss moun-

16

tains, he would occasionally spend a few weeks in Freiburg. Since the interest of Spemann in the nervous system ended with the closure of the neural tube and that of Harrison began at that stage, I got more help in my neuroembryological work from him than from Spemann.

Communication with Harrison was easy. He spoke German fluently, he had spent several pre- and postdoctoral years in Bonn, where he obtained an M.D. in 1899; he had published some of his early papers in German, he had a German wife—in short, he was at home in Germany. He was informal, unassuming, soft-spoken, and reserved; he had a good sense of humor. And he had an amiable human trait, the capacity for procrastination.

Harrison had been a graduate student in one of the best graduate schools for zoology of that time, at the Johns Hopkins University. W. K. Brooks was outstanding in embryology and remarkable for the number of prominent men who were his students. Among Harrison's fellow graduate students were T. H. Morgan and E. G. Conklin. He obtained his Ph.D. in 1894 and became then a staff member in the Anatomy Department under F. P. Mall, who was well known as a human embryologist. In 1907 he was called to Yale, and soon its Zoology Department became one of the most prominent in the country. Yale and Freiburg shared the reputation of being the leading centers of experimental embryology. For his students, most of whom became his friends, Harrison was "the Chief." He was influential in raising the standard of excellence at Yale, both in the sciences and in the medical school. For many years, he was the managing editor of the *Journal of Experimental Zoology*, the most prestigious in its field. He was not particularly enthusiastic about teaching or administration. Most administrative chores were handled by his student, later colleague, and successor, J. S. Nicholas. Harrison's due place was in the research laboratory.

One of Harrison's first experiments was based on an experiment of a young German anatomist, G. Born. In 1894, Born had discovered by chance that parts of frog embryos when cut apart could be healed together again. Taking advantage of this extraordinary healing power, he had been able to fuse parts of embryos of different genera, such as frog and toad. This method of "xenoplastic" combinations, made possible by the absence of immunological barriers in embryos, was used widely by Harrison and Spemann. Harrison was the first to apply this kind of experimentation on the embryo to neurogenetic problems. In one of his earliest experiments, he employed the method of Born to demonstrate the mode of origin of the lateral line sense organs of aquatic vertebrates. These are sensors for water perturbations; they are evenly spaced in several rows in the head and along the trunk and tail. Each sense organ consists of sensory hair cells and supporting cells; those of the head are innervated by a branch of the facial nerve and those of the trunk and tail by a branch of the vagus nerve. Harrison ingeniously took advantage of species differences in pigmentation. He fused the darkly pigmented head of an early embryo of *Rana sylvatica* with the body of a lightly pigmented *R. palustris* embryo. He observed in the living composite tadpole the step-by-step deposition of dark spots, identified as embryonic lateral line sense organs, from tissue that emerged from the dark head and moved in several rows down the yellowish trunk and tail. He had thus uncovered a peculiar, unique long-range migration of cell clusters that followed prespecified paths, as was shown by variants of the experiment [20].

The major contributions of Harrison to experimental neurogenesis were motivated by the controversy between the axon outgrowth theory of His-Cajal and the cell chain and plasmodesm theories of the origin of the nerve fiber. In the first decade of this century, when Harrison became active, the plasmodesm theory had regained ground, and even support for Schwann's cell chain theory had not subsided completely. Harrison had become convinced of the correctness of the outgrowth theory in his earlier work on neuroblast differentiation in the salmon embryo and, like Cajal, he set out to put the competing theories to a test. It was clear to him that the best histological techniques could not solve the problem, so he took the crucial step of applying the powerful tool of experimentation to its solution.

First, he took on the relatively easier task. He addressed the question, Is nerve fiber formation dependent on Schwann cells? Assuming that the Schwann cells originate in the neural crest, he removed the dorsal part of the neural tube and the adjacent neural crest, in early tail bud stages of frog embryos. He found that in the tadpole normal ventral roots and motor nerve fibers had developed which were naked and devoid of any cellular companions. Hence, the independence of nerve fiber formation from Schwann cells was proven. Furthermore, the then controversial question of the origin of Schwann cells was settled in favor of the neural crest, at least for frog embryos. These experiments date back to 1904 and 1906 [21].

Harrison turned next to the problem of the role of protoplasmic bridges in nerve fiber formation. We remember the claim of Hensen that the substance of plasmodesms is actually incorporated in the formation of nerve fibers. As was mentioned, this theory had been revived by Held and others, and the opinion of leaders in the field was divided. Experiments by the German anatomist H. Braus, in which limb transplantations were used for the first time to address neurological questions, had been interpreted by the author in support of the plasmodesm theory [22]. In the spring of 1906, Harrison repeated the experiments; and his findings, which I shall not describe in detail, led him to a rejection of the claim of Braus [23]. Two points deserve mentioning. First, this was Har-

18

rison's first experience in the transplantation of limb primordia, an experiment which was to preoccupy him in his later work devoted to problems of regulation and determination of laterality. Second, Braus had found that the nerves in the limb transplants formed a normal pattern. This was to be expected if plasmodesms in the limb are transformed into nerves. But in Harrison's reinterpretation of limb innervation in terms of the axon outgrowth theory, the fact that ingrowing nerves from any source form a typical limb pattern can be interpreted only in one way: "that the structures contained within the limb must have a very important directive action upon the developing nerve fibers, in that they determine their mode of distribution" [23, p. 276]. The contribution of the limb structures to pathfinding and patterning of their innervation is basic to an understanding of directional nerve outgrowth.

Yet, Harrison realized clearly "that in all of the first experiments the nerve fibers had developed in surroundings composed of living organized tissues, and that the possibility of the latter contributing organized material to the nerve elements stood in the way of rigorous proof of the view that the nerve fiber was entirely the product of the nerve center. The really crucial experiment remained to be performed, and that was to test the power of the nerve centers to form nerve fibers within some foreign medium which could not by any possibility be suspected of contributing organized protoplasma to them" [24, p. 790]. At another point, he said: "In order to reach a final settlement of this question, it thus became necessary to devise a method by which to test the ability of a nerve fiber to grow outside the body of the embryo, where it would be independent of protoplasmic bridges" [25, p. 402].

The decisive step had been taken in 1907. Pieces of neural tube of frog embryos, prior to nerve outgrowth, were grown in a hanging drop of frog's lymph. The outgrowth of individual fibers and their growth cones was observed under the microscope; the rate of growth was determined, and the important fact was established that nerves require a solid substrate for extension. Thus the plasmodesms, or, for that matter, any microscopic or submicroscopic materials in the embryo, are assigned their proper role: they serve for guidance but do not contribute materially to the formation of the nerve fiber.

It is clear that the design of the tissue culture method was the logical final step on the long road toward the solution of the problem of the origin of the axon. The immediate purpose was the crucial test of the plasmodesm theory. But, as the title of the detailed report of the tissue culture experiments in 1910 [24] indicates, the emphasis is shifted immediately from the critical to a positive aspect. The phenomenon of "the outgrowth of the nerve fiber as a mode of protoplasmic movement" is placed in the center of the scene. This, we remember, was a key element in Cajal's appraisal of the growth cone. Harrison states "the primary factor, protoplasmic movement, must be regarded as definitely established and it will have to form the basis of any adequate theory of nerve development. The chief claim to progress that the present work has is that it has taken this factor out of the realm of inference and placed it upon the secure foundation of direct observation." And he goes a step further and fits this discovery in a broader frame of reference: "the first manifestations of activity observable in the differentiating nerve cell are of the same fundamental nature as those found not only in other embryonic cells but also in the protoplasm of the widest variety of organisms" [24, p. 840]. Thus, the tradition of Cajal's dynamic view of the growth cone was continued and it became a reality. The later discovery of axoplasmic transport [12] follows the same tradition.

It may seem strange that while the tissue culture method opened up a new field of knowledge and became an indispensable tool in a very broad range of biological endeavors, Harrison himself never made use of it again. The answer suggests itself to those who knew Harrison. The method was designed by him to solve a specific problem—which it did. The time was not ripe for analysis of protoplasmic movement in depth. He became intrigued by other fundamental problems and turned to their solution. His primary concerns were the basic theoretical issues in embryology and *not* the exploitation of what he called a technique. He made decisive contributions to the analysis of a key phenomenon in animal development, the "morphogenetic field" [26] and, as was stated earlier, he solved one of the most difficult problems in embryology, the origin of bilateral symmetry, which is a basic morphological attribute of vertebrates [27]. This led him to the consideration of the polarization of the three main axes, rostro-caudal, dorso-ventral, medio-lateral, in terms of molecular repeat patterns of protein molecules. He actually went to Leeds, to the laboratory of the great biophysicist V. T. Astbury, and they published jointly a paper on X-ray diffraction pictures of embryonic materials [28], a premature step in the direction of molecular embryology. The fact that this enterprise was doomed to failure at that time is less important than the insight it gives in the train of thought of a truly great scientist who was far ahead of his time. His later achievements fully justify the abandonment of his gifted brainchild that was born in 1907 and is still very much alive and thriving.

REFERENCES

1. S. RAMÓN Y CAJAL. Recollections of my life. Trans. E. HORNE-CRAIGIE. Philadelphia: American Philosophical Society, 1937.
2. S. RAMÓN Y CAJAL. Anat. Anz., **5**:609, 1890.
3. V. HENSEN. 1903. Die Entwicklungsmechanik der Nervenbahnen im Embryo der Säugetiere. Kiel and Leipzig: Lipsius & Tischer, 1903.

20

4. HELD. Die Entwicklung des Nervengewebes bei den Wirbeltieren. Leipzig: Barth, 1909.
5. W. HIS. Abhandl. Kgl. Sächs. Gesellsch. D. Wiss., **13**:479, 1886.
6. W. HIS. Arch. Anat. Entwicklungsgesch., **10**:249, 1889.
7. S. RAMÓN Y CAJAL. Neuron theory or reticular theory? Trans. M. U. PURKISS and C. A. Fox. Madrid: Instituto "Ramón y Cajal," 1954.
8. S. RAMÓN Y CAJAL. Studies on vertebrate neurogenesis. Trans. L. GUTH. 1929. Reprint. Springfield, Ill.: Thomas, 1960.
9. S. RAMÓN Y CAJAL. Histologie du système nerveux de l'homme et des vertébrés. Madrid: Instituto "Ramòn y Cajal," 1909.
10. C. SHERRINGTON. *In:* D. F. CANON. Explorer of the human brain: the life of S. Ramón y Cajal, p. xiii. New York: Schuman, 1949.
11. S. RAMÓN Y CAJAL. The structure of the retina. Trans. THORPE and GLICK. Springfield, Ill.: Thomas, 1972.
12. P. WEISS and H. B. HISCOE. J. Exp. Zool., **107**:315, 1948.
13. J. FORSSMAN. Beitr. Z. Pathol. Anat. Allg. Pathol., **24**:56, 1898; **27**:407, 1900.
14. J. F. TELLO. Gegenwärtige Anschauungen über den Neurotropismus. Vorträge und Aufsätze über Entwicklungsmechanik der Organismen 33. Ed. W. ROUX. Berlin: Springer Verlag, 1923.
15. S. RAMÓN Y CAJAL. Degeneration and regeneration of the nervous system. Trans. R. MAY. 1928. Reprint. New York: Hafner, 1968.
16. P. WEISS. *In:* M. A. CORNER and E. F. SCHWAB (eds.). Brain research, p. 11. New York: Elsevier, 1976.
17. R. LEVI-MONTALCINI. *in:* CORNER and SCHWAB (eds.), [16], p. 235.
18. M. G. M. CHEN, J. S. CHEN, and R. LEVI-MONTALCINI. Arch. Ital. Biol., **116**:53, 1978.
19. NOBEL COMMITTEE (eds.). Nobel, the man and his prizes. New York: Elsevier, 1962.
20. R. G. HARRISON. Arch. Mikr. Anat., **63**:65, 1903.
21. R. G. HARRISON. J. Comp. Neurol., **37**:123, 1924.
22. H. BRAUS. Anat. Anz., **25**:433, 1905.
23. R. G. HARRISON. J. Exp. Zool., **4**:239, 1907.
24. R. G. HARRISON. J. Exp. Zool., **9**:787, 1910.
25. R. G. HARRISON. Anat. Rec., **2**:385, 1908.
26. R. G. HARRISON. J. Exp. Zool., **25**:413, 1918.
27. R. G. HARRISON. J. Exp. Zool., **32**:1, 1921.
28. R. G. HARRISON, W. T. ASTBURY, and K. M. RUDALL. J. Exp. Zool., **85**:339, 1940.

21

Reprinted from Science, Vol. 183, pp. 425–427. 1974

Neurons in Rhesus Monkey Visual Cortex: Systematic Relation between Time of Origin and Eventual Disposition

Abstract. *Autoradiographic evidence after injection of tritiated thymidine indicates that cell position in the laminae of the monkey visual cortex is systematically related to time of cell orgin. The earliest-formed neurons, destined for the deepest stratum, arise at about embryonic day 45, and the last ones, destined for the outermost cell stratum, form at about day 102; cells of intervening layers are generated at intervening times. No neocortical neurons are produced in the last two prenatal months or after birth. Compared to cortical neurons in rodents, those in the monkey arise earlier, and the "inside-out" relation of cell position to time of origin is more rigid.*

Morphological and physiological studies of the visual cortex in the monkey have increased our understanding of the organizational properties of the cerebral cortex in general (*1*). It is important to determine how such a complex and ordered system develops. Almost 100 years ago, it was demonstrated with the use of the Golgi method that cellular development of the mammalian cerebral cortex follows a consistent pattern, with large pyramidal neurons of the lower layers taking a laminar position and differentiating earlier than neurons destined to be situated more superficially (*2*). More recently, it was shown by autoradiography with [³H]thymidine ([³H]dT) that the deeper cortical neurons in rodents are generated earlier than the more superficial neurons (*3*). In addition, these studies provided direct evidence that cortical neurons originate in proliferative zones close to the ventricular surface and migrate to the cortical plate only after final division of the precursor cells.

It is essential to establish whether the neocortex in primates develops according to the same principle as in rodents and to determine the time span during which cortical neurons are generated in a slowly developing gyrencephalic brain similar to that of man. In addition, important questions concern the generation and migration rates of cortical neurons, the relation between laminar position and neuronal type with reference to time of cell genesis, and the possible interaction of young neurons with each other and with the specific afferents with which they will make synaptic contacts.

Several properties of the primary visual cortex (area 17) of the rhesus monkey make it a suitable model for study of these problems. The horizontal stratification of neurons into separate layers in this species is more precise than in most mammals, and area 17 can be distinguished from adjacent areas at relatively early embryonic stages. The large size of monkey fetuses allows adequate fixation for electron microscopy by vascular perfusion (*4*), and the protracted span of development increases the resolution of temporal sequences in neurogenesis (*5*). The present demonstration of the time of neuron origin for each of the six cortical layers is a

first step in the more detailed analysis of neocortical cell genesis in primates.

Ten pregnant monkeys weighing 6 to 10 kg were each injected once intravenously with [³H]dT (5 or 10 mc per kilogram of body weight) at 40, 45, 54, 62, 70, 80, 90, 102, 120, and 140 days of gestation. Females were caged with males from day 11 to 15 following onset of estrus, and the time of conception was estimated on the assumption that ovulation occurred on day 12. Pregnancy in the rhesus monkey lasts 165 days. All fetuses were delivered normally and killed 2 to 5 months after birth (the "juvenile" period, when most cortical cells have attained their final position). Two additional monkeys were injected 2 and 18 days after birth, respectively, and killed 3 months after birth. All brains were processed for autoradiography (*5, 6*). With the aid of a Zeiss microscope equipped with a drawing tube, the positions of heavily labeled neurons were recorded within a strip of visual cortex approximately 10 mm long situated in the depth of the calcarine fissure between the two arrows in Fig. 1A. Only heavily labeled cells are considered to have had their "birthday" on the day of [³H]dT injection (*5, 6*). [In the interpretation of autoradiographic data, the term "birthday" is empirically defined as the last day on which nuclear DNA is replicated in a given cell line (*6*).] The minimum number of grains for classification of cells as "heavily labeled" was arbitrarily determined for each specimen as half of the grain count neurons with maximum radioactivity. Brodman's nomenclature of layers was adopted (*7*).

No heavily labeled neurons were seen in the visual cortex of the 3-month-old monkey that had been exposed to [³H]-

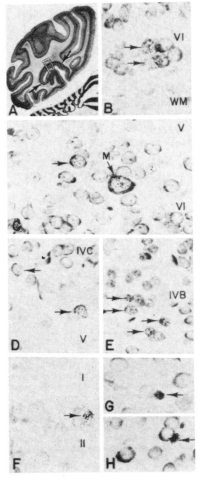

Fig. 1. (A) Coronal section of the occipital lobe of a 3-month-old monkey. The two arrows indicate a strip of visual cortex about 10 mm long in the depth of the calcarine fissure, for which the time of neuron origin was analyzed in this study. The area in the rectangle is enlarged on the left side of Fig. 2. The 30-μm section was stained with cresyl violet (× 1.2). (B to H) Autoradiograms of the visual cortex in juvenile monkeys that had been injected with [³H]dT at various embryonic (E) days: E45 (B), E62 (C), E70 (D), E80 (E), E102 (F and G), and E120 (H). Roman numerals indicate cortical layers according to Brodman's classification (*7*). Arrows point to heavily labeled cells; *M*, solitary pyramid of Meynert; *WM*, white matter (× 650).

dT on embryonic day 40 (E40). However, a few lightly labeled neurons, located exclusively in the deepest part of the cortex, were found in more than 50 sections examined. Since heavily labeled cells were found elsewhere in the brain, these lightly labeled cells were probably the products of several cell divisions subsequent to the time of injection and it is unlikely that any visual cortical neurons were born at E40.

The first heavily labeled neurons were detected in the monkey injected at E45. They were localized in a narrow zone in the deeper portion of layer VI (Figs. 1B and 2A). Scattered neurons in the white matter below layer VI were also labeled in this specimen. In most fields, a number of lightly labeled cells were detected superficial to the heavily labeled cells, an indication that cells generated later take up more external positions. This was confirmed by the finding that heavily labeled neurons in the animal injected at E54 were located somewhat more superficially, although still within layer VI (Fig. 2B). The majority of neurons generated at E62 were later situated in the upper two-thirds of layer VI, while some were localized in layer V (Figs. 1C and 2C). Cells with axons passing from area 17 to the midbrain, the so-called giant solitary pyramidal neurons of Meynert (8) which are situated in layers V and VI in the rhesus monkey (Fig. 1C), were also labeled by injection at E26.

At E70, the number of labeled neurons per unit length of visual cortex reached a maximum (Fig. 2). Injection at this stage labeled mainly neurons that later were located in layer V, and also many cells in layer IVC (Figs. 1D and 2D). Neurons generated at E80 became distributed over the entire width of layer IV, with the highest concentration in layer IVB (Figs. 1E and 2E); a few radioactive cells were situated in layer III. Injection at E90 labeled neurons in both layers III and II (Fig. 2F).

By E102, almost all neurons in the visual cortex had been born, since few neurons (less than 1 in 10^6) at the border between layer II and the cell-sparse layer I were labeled in the 3-month-old monkey that had been injected on E102 (Figs. 1F and 2G). However, in this specimen, some small nuclei situated mainly in the deeper half of the cortex were radioactive; these were classified as glia on the basis of small nuclear size, absence of Nissl substance, and satellite position with respect to neurons (Fig. 1G). This correlates with the time of appearance of numerous astrocytes in the depth of the fetal monkey visual cortex as assessed by the Golgi method (9). Injections at E120, later during gestation, or after birth did not label neurons of the visual cortex. However, numerous glial (Fig. 1H) and endothelial cells were labeled in the cortex in these specimens.

The neurons in the plexiform layer I were not labeled in any of the specimens studied. These neurons either were generated before E40, or they arose during a relatively brief interval between the ages sampled by injection of [³H]dT in this series of animals.

As shown in Fig. 2, the position of heavily labeled neurons in the juvenile monkey visual cortex is correlated with the time of cell origin in the fetus; cells destined for deep cortical positions are generated first, and more superficial ones at progressively later times. Thus, most of the neurons of layer VI are born between E40 and E60, neurons in layer V between E60 and E70, those in layer IV between E70 and E80, and those in layers III and II between E80 and E100. These data pertain only to the time of cell origin and do not define

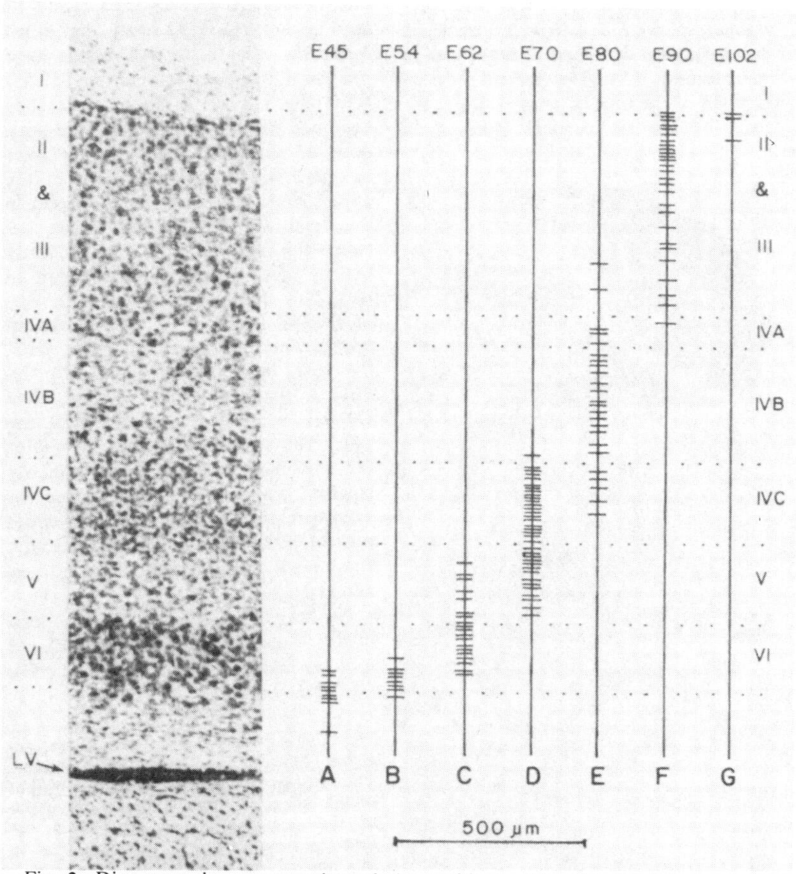

Fig. 2. Diagrammatic representation of the positions of heavily labeled neurons in the visual cortex of juvenile animals that had been injected with [H³]dT at various days of gestation (indicated at the top of each vertical line). On the left is a photomicrograph of a 30-μm cresyl violet–stained section photographed at the same magnification used for plotting labeled neurons with the drawing tube. Horizontal markers on each vertical line except G indicate positions of all heavily labeled neurons encountered in a randomly selected strip (2.5 mm long) of the calcarine cortex. The three labeled neurons represented in G were found only after examination of 80 areas of calcarine cortex, each 2.5 mm long, in 40 autoradiograms of a single specimen. Roman numerals indicate cortical layers according to Brodman's classification (7); LV, obliterated posterior horn of the lateral ventricle.

23

when the cells actually attained their final positions.

This study establishes that neurons generated on a day early in development eventually occupy a relatively narrow zone of the mature cortex, while those generated on a later day are eventually distributed over a somewhat wider zone; also, neurons born 8 to 10 days apart overlap somewhat in position along the radial axis (Fig. 2). One reason for the wide distribution of cells generated simultaneously may be differences in rates of migration. Slower-moving neurons might reach the cortex when it had increased several hundred micrometers in thickness by the addition of neurons that were generated later but had migrated faster. Within a population of simultaneously labeled cells, the slower-moving neurons would presumably take more superficial positions than the faster-moving ones. Indeed, initial examination of monkey embryos killed at shorter intervals after injection of [³H]dT suggests that some labeled neurons reach the outer border of the cortical plate in less than 3 days, whereas others labeled simultaneously take 7 or more days to reach a comparable destination (10). Variations in the length of the cell generation cycle also could influence eventual neuron position in the cortex, as might differences in the detailed aspects of cell interaction during migration (11).

Autoradiographic results in the brain of this primate corroborate in general the "inside-out" pattern of cell disposition described for rodents (3). Initial observations suggest that cells in other cortical areas in the monkey behave similarly, although on slightly different time schedules (10). Comparison of the data in Fig. 2 with studies in mice (12) shows that simultaneously generated neurons in the monkey eventually become confined to relatively narrow strata of the cortex; that is, the "inside-out" principle is more rigidly followed in the monkey. This may be the developmental basis for the sharper boundaries of cortical layers in the visual cortex of adult primates.

The monkey neocortex acquires its full complement of neurons at relatively early stages of gestation. The last cortical neurons are generated close to birth in mice and rats, and cortical genesis continues for a few days after birth in the hamster (3). In contrast, the last neurons destined for the primary visual cortex are generated around E100 in the monkey, that is, about 2 months before birth. It is probable that other primates, including man, also acquire a full complement of neocortical neurons well before birth.

PASKO RAKIC

Department of Neuropathology,
Harvard Medical School, and
Department of Neuroscience,
Children's Hospital Medical
Center, Boston, Massachusetts 02115

References and Notes

1. D. H. Hubel and T. N. Wiesel, *J. Physiol.* (*Lond.*) **195**, 215 (1968); *Nature* (*Lond.*) **225**, 41 1970); *J. Comp. Neurol.* **146**, 421 (1972); F. Valverde, *Int. J. Neurosci.* **1**, 181 (1971); J. S. Lund, *J. Comp. Neurol.* **147**, 455 (1973); S. LeVay, *ibid.* **150**, 53 (1973).
2. W. Vignal, *Arch. Physiol. Norm. Pathol.* **2**, 338 (1888); S. Ramón y Cajal, *Cellule* **7**, 125 (1893); A. Kölliker, *Handbuch der Gewebelehre des Menschen* (Engelmann, Leipzig, 1896); M. Stefanowska, *Trav. Lab. Invest.* **2**, 1 (1898).
3. J. B. Angevine and R. L. Sidman, *Nature* (*Lond.*) **192**, 766 (1961); M. Berry and A. W. Rogers, *J. Anat.* **99**, 691 (1965); S. P. Hicks and C. J. D'Amato, *Anat. Rec.* **160**, 619 (1968); M. Shimada and J. Langman, *J. Comp. Neurol.* **139**, 227 (1970).
4. P. Rakic, *J. Comp. Neurol.* **145**, 61 (1972).
5. ———, *ibid.* **147**, 523 (1973).
6. R. L. Sidman, in *Contemporary Research Methods in Neuroanatomy,* W. J. H. Nauta and S. O. E. Ebbeson, Eds. (Springer-Verlag, Berlin, 1970), pp. 252–274.
7. K. Brodman, *J. Psychol. Neurol.* **4**, 177 (1905).
8. T. Meynert, in *Handbuch der Lehre von den Geweben des Menschen und der Thiere,* S. Striker, Ed. (Engelmann, Leipzig, 1871), pp. 694–808; W. E. Le Gros Clark, *J. Anat.* **76**, 369 (1942).
9. D. E. Schmechel and P. Rakic, *Anat. Rec.* **175**, 436 (1973).
10. P. Rakic, unpublished observations.
11. R. L. Sidman and P. Rakic, *Brain Res.* **62**, 1 (1973).
12. V. S. Caviness, Jr., and R. L. Sidman, *J. Comp. Neurol.* **148**, 141 (1973).
13. Supported by PHS grant NS09081. I am grateful to T. C. Jones and F. Garcia of the New England Regional Primate Research Center, Southboro, Massachusetts, for making available timed pregnancies used in this study.

4 September 1973; revised 15 October 1973 ∎

The Journal of Neuroscience
Vol. 1, No. 1, pp. 27–39
January 1981

COEXISTENCE OF NEURONAL AND GLIAL PRECURSOR CELLS IN THE CEREBRAL VENTRICULAR ZONE OF THE FETAL MONKEY: AN ULTRASTRUCTURAL IMMUNOPEROXIDASE ANALYSIS[1]

PAT LEVITT, MICHAEL LEE COOPER, AND PASKO RAKIC

Section of Neuroanatomy, Yale University School of Medicine, New Haven, Connecticut 06510

Abstract

The cytological composition of the proliferative zones in the fetal monkey occipital lobe was examined at the light and electron microscopic levels by immunoperoxidase localization of glial fibrillary acid protein (GFA), a protein that is present in astrocytes and radial glial cells but not neurons. During the peak of neurogenesis at embryonic day 80, two distinct classes of proliferative cells, GFA-positive and GFA-negative, are intermixed in the ventricular and subventricular zones. Both cell types are readily recognized in different phases of the mitotic cycle along the ventricular surface. The results indicate that, contrary to prevailing views, (1) glial and neuronal cell lines coexist within the fetal proliferative zones and (2) the onset of glial phenotypic expression occurs prior to the last cell division.

All neurons, with few exceptions, are generated near the surface of the embryonic cerebral ventricles at sites far from their ultimate positions in the adult mammalian brain (see Sidman and Rakic, 1973; Rakic, 1975a for reviews). Glial cell proliferation is thought to occur at sites distant to the ventricles, although the glioblast must originate from the neuroepithelium at some time (Jacobson, 1978). The uncertainty concerning the developmental stage at which glial and neuronal cell lines diverge in the proliferative zone has been a persistent problem in neuroembryology for almost a century. From his classic observations on the embryonic ventricular zone,[2] His (1889) suggested that the proliferative zone is composed of two cell lines, one that gives rise to neurons (*Keimzellen* or "germinal cells") and the other that produces glia or glioblasts ("spongioblasts"). Examination of similar histological material induced Schaper (1897a, b) to propose that the ventricular zone is comprised of a single, homogeneous, mitotically active cell population which produces "indifferent" cells that migrate into the intermediate (mantle) zone to give rise to both neurons and glial cells. This hypothesis was supported by Sauer (1935), who showed that His's two cell classes simply represent different phases of the mitotic cycle of the same cell type.

More recently, autoradiographic data obtained from studies using pulse and/or cumulative [³H]thymidine (³H-TdR) labeling of ventricular zone cells have also been interpreted as supporting the view that the ventricular zone contains a homogeneous population of dividing cells (Fujita, 1963; Sidman et al., 1959). These results, taken in conjunction with studies using ³H-TdR to determine the time of cell origin, have indicated to many investigators that the glial cells in a given structure are usually generated only after neuronal production ceases (e.g., Angevine, 1970; Berry and Rogers, 1965; Fujita, 1965; Hicks and D'Amato, 1968; see Jacobson, 1978 for review) and have led to the widely held view that the ventricular zone may be comprised of only a single precursor cell population. According to Fujita (1963, 1966), this lone precursor (or "matrix") cell first gives rise to neurons; only later, after the completion of neurogenesis, is it supposed to switch to glial production and then finally transform into a mature ependymal cell. Fujita's formulation is representative of the prevailing view (e.g., see Boulder Committee, 1970; Jacobson, 1978).

Contrary to this notion, detailed quantitative analysis of the cell proliferation cycle in the telencephalon raises the possibility that the ventricular zone in young rodents consists of at least two cell populations with different generation times (Gracheva, 1969; Waechter and Jaensch, 1972). Furthermore, studies using Golgi and electron microscopic methods have indicated that glial cells, particularly radial glial cells and Bergmann glial cells, exist during late stages of neurogenesis (Rakic,

[1] This research was supported by United States Public Health Service Grants NS14841 and EY02503. We are grateful to Ms. Katherine Riley for technical assistance. The secretarial assistance of Ms. Elizabeth Thomas and Mrs. Mary Interrante is appreciated. The antibody directed against glial fibrillary acidic protein was generously provided by Dr. L. F. Eng. We thank Drs. K. Herrup, J. Dekker, P. Goldman-Rackic, and D. Kankel for their comments concerning this manuscript.

[2] When describing the principal embryonic zones of the central nervous system, the nomenclature suggested by the Boulder Committee (1970) will be used. Under this terminology, two proliferative zones, the *ventricular* and *subventricular* zones, correspond to the germinal matrix zones of His (1889).

1971, 1972; Schmechel and Rakic, 1979). More recently, immunocytochemical staining for the specific glial fibrillary acid protein (GFA) (Bignami et al., 1972; Eng, 1980; Eng and Bigbee, 1978; Eng et al., 1971; Ludwin et al., 1976) provided more direct evidence of the presence of radial glial cells during early periods of neurogenesis in the human cerebrum (Antanitus et al., 1976; Choi and Lapham, 1978) and in all major subdivisions of the fetal monkey central nervous system (Levitt and Rakic, 1980). This method showed that the number of radial glial cells increases during periods of peak neuronal proliferation and subsides only after neuronal migration ceases (Levitt and Rakic, 1980). Thus, it has become increasingly evident that neuronal and glial proliferative precursor cells must coexist at relatively early stages of brain development. However, light microscopic studies cannot determine conclusively whether both neurons and glial cells arise from a single mitotically active cell population, as suggested by Schaper (1897a, b), or whether there exist two distinct classes of proliferative cells in the ventricular and subventricular zones, as advocated by His (1889). In addition, previous electron microscopic studies failed to display ultrastructural features that would permit classification of the dividing cells into multiple classes (Fujita and Fujita, 1963, 1964; Stensaas and Stensaas, 1968).

The present study is the first use of electron microscopy in conjunction with a sensitive immunohistochemical technique (Sternberger, 1979) in the fetal brain. The combination of these techniques for the localization of GFA has allowed, for the first time, the direct determination of whether two classes of proliferative cells exist in the ventricular zone during the peak of neurogenesis in the cerebral wall.

Materials and Methods

Rhesus monkeys (*Macaca mulatta*) of 80 and 123 embryonic (E) days were used for this ultrastructural immunohistochemical study. These ages represent, respectively, the period of peak neurogenesis and the period by which all neurons have been generated in the occipital lobe (Rakic, 1974). In addition, sections from two fetal monkeys of approximately the same ages were prepared for light microscopic immunohistochemistry (Levitt and Rakic, 1980). The gestational period of the rhesus monkey is about 165 days. Animals were bred and pregnancies were dated as previously described (Rakic, 1973).

Anti-GFA immunoperoxidase staining of the occipital lobe was performed for light and electron microscopic localization of glial cells. The embryos at each age were perfused transcardially with a 1.25% formaldehyde, 1.0% glutaraldehyde phosphate-buffered fixative (pH 7.4). The brains were then immersed in the fixative for 24 hr at 4°C prior to dissection of the occipital lobes. One lobe was processed for polyester wax embedding (Sidman et al., 1961) and subsequent antibody staining using the peroxidase-antiperoxidase (PAP) technique as previously described (Levitt and Rakic, 1980). The other occipital lobe was used for GFA localization at the ultrastructural level. Coronal 20- to 30-μm-thick sections of this lobe were cut using a vibratome (Oxford Instruments); then, the sections were rinsed overnight at 4°C in a phosphate-buffered saline solution (PBS) prior to exposure to the antibody. During the first incubation, sections were bathed for 7 hr at room temperature in a 1:150 dilution of rabbit antibody directed against GFA (Eng and Rubinstein, 1978; the antibody was supplied by Dr. L. F. Eng, Veterans Administration Hospital, Palo Alto, CA), followed by a 5-hr incubation at 4°C. The antibody was prepared in PBS containing normal swine serum, diluted 1:20. (In order to preserve ultrastructural quality, our methodology did not include detergent in the incubation steps.) The tissue next was rinsed five times with cold PBS over a 1-hr period and then washed overnight in PBS at 4°C. Control sections were processed as noted above, substituting normal rabbit serum for the primary antibody. The following day, the sections were allowed to warm to room temperature, rinsed twice with PBS, and then incubated for 5 hr at room temperature in a 1:50 dilution of horseradish peroxidase (HRP)-linked swine anti-rabbit immunoglobulin G (Dako), followed by an additional 5 hr at 4°C. Next, the tissue was rinsed as described for the first incubation. Finally, the HRP was visualized with the 3,3'-diaminobenzidine reaction. The vibratome sections were mounted in a glycerol:PBS solution (3:1), examined and photographed light microscopically, and then processed for electron microscopic analysis.

For electron microscopy, the tissue was trimmed into 3- to 4-mm-wide segments which spanned the entire width of the occipital cerebral wall, from the ventricular to the pial surfaces. Following a 30-min rinse in 0.1 M phosphate buffer, the tissue was osmicated (2% OsO_4, 60 min), briefly stained *en bloc* with uranyl acetate (15 to 30 min), dehydrated in a graded series of alcohols and propylene oxide, and finally embedded in a 1:1 mixture of Epon 812 and Araldite 8005. The sections were flat mounted on plastic coverslips which, in turn, were glued to plastic blocks. Then, the tissue blocks were trimmed into pyramids containing the proliferative and intermediate zones. Thick plastic sections (0.5 to 1.0 μm) were collected, counterstained lightly with toluidine blue, and examined to determine the distribution and number of mitotic figures lining the ventricular surface. Next, silver thin sections were collected on Formvar-coated grids and examined with a JEOL 100A electron microscope. These thin sections were not counterstained with either uranyl acetate or lead citrate in order to improve the contrast between the HRP reaction product and the surrounding unlabeled tissue.

GFA-positive cells situated in the proliferative zones were identified in over 300 micrographs printed at magnifications ranging from × 2,000 to × 75,000. Each mitotic figure identified in the thick plastic sections was also localized ultrastructurally for final determination of the presence or absence of GFA staining. The sensitivity and specificity of the GFA antibody and the immunohistochemical methods utilized here for the localization of glial cells are well documented (Eng and Kosec, 1974; Levitt and Rakic, 1980; Ludwin et al., 1976). There is little doubt concerning the specificity of GFA as a major constituent of astroglial filaments (Bignami et al., 1972; Bignami and Dahl, 1974; Eng, 1980; Eng and Bigbee, 1978; Eng and Kosec, 1974). In the results presented below, the ultrastructural localization of the immuno-

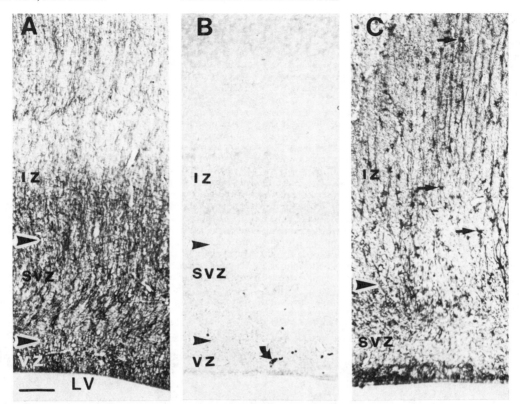

Figure 1.[3] Immunoperoxidase localization of GFA-positive glial cells in uncounterstained 25-µm vibratome sections of the occipital lobe. *Horizontal arrowheads* indicate the approximate boundaries between the primary embryonic zones. Lateral cerebral ventricle is at the bottom of the figures. *Marker bar* = 150 µm. *A,* Cerebral wall of occipital lobe of 80-day-old monkey fetus (E80) shows dense array of positively stained radial glial cells and their elongated fibers. The glial shafts extend from the cell somata, situated within the ventricular and subventricular zones, through the intermediate zone and enter the developing cortical plate, which lies above the area encompassed by the photograph. *B,* An adjacent section, used as a control, was processed identically to that illustrated in *A* except that normal rabbit serum was substituted for the GFA antibody. No glial cells or their fibers are stained in this preparation. The small dark spots (*curved arrow*) in the ventricular zone are red blood cells whose hemoglobin has endogenous peroxidase-like activity. *C,* As in younger specimens, the cerebral wall in a 123-day-old monkey fetus contains densely staining radial glial fibers. In addition, there are numerous transitional profiles representing radial glial cells transforming into mature astrocytes (*arrows*), which are situated predominantly in the intermediate zone. Differentiated astrocytes are conspicuously absent at E80 (*A*). Also, note the decrease in the number of radial fibers, particularly in the proliferative zones, compared to the E80 specimen (*A*).

peroxidase reaction product within the embryonic glial cells correlates closely with previous electron microscopic characterizations in mature astrocytes (Maunoury et al., 1979; Schachner et al., 1977).

Results

The proliferative zones of the occipital lobe in the rhesus monkey fetuses at both E80 and E123 contain a large number of cells stained positively for GFA intermixed with cells containing no reaction product (Fig. 1).

---

[3] The abbreviations used on the figures are: C, chromatin; Cy, cytoplasm; IZ, intermediate zone; LV, lateral cerebral ventricle; N, nucleus; SVZ, subventricular zone; VZ, ventricular zone.

As reported previously (Levitt and Rakic, 1980), the only morphologically differentiated cells which contain the fine brown HRP reaction product are glial in nature. There is no immunoperoxidase staining in the control material (Fig. 1*B*) or in any neuronal elements in either the E80 or E123 specimens.

Light microscopic examination. At E80, the cerebral occipital wall contains denser GFA staining than at E123 or any other stage previously examined (Levitt and Rakic, 1980). The reaction product at E80 is located mostly in radial glial cells, the perikarya of which are situated within the ventricular and subventricular zones (Fig. 1). The GFA-positive radial glial processes course in a palisade-like fashion through the intermediate zone and developing cortical plate to terminate in conical endfeet along the pial surface. As is evident in the 25-μm vibratome sections, large numbers of the radial glial processes run in dense fascicles from the proliferative zones into the intermediate zone, where the fascicles usually split into single processes prior to entering the developing cortical plate. Fibrous and protoplasmic astrocytes are not evident in the occipital lobe at this embryonic age.

The number of positively stained radial glial fibers seems to decrease by E123, although some areas of the occipital lobe still contain an abundance of densely stained radial processes (Fig. 1C). Many of the GFA-positive perikarya of radial glial cells are located now in the subventricular zone, and a large number of their elongated processes still traverse the expanded width of the cerebral wall to terminate at the pial surface. In addition to the radial glial cells, positively stained, morphologically differentiated astrocytes are situated in the intermediate zone and cortex at E123 (Fig. 1C). However, the ventricular zone in most regions of the occipital lobe at this stage has been depleted of proliferative germinal cells and contains only maturing ependymal cells and some radial glial cell somata. As expected, the specialized ependymal cells do not stain positively for GFA (Eng, 1980). Neuronal proliferation in the monkey occipital lobe has ceased by E123 (Rakic, 1974, 1975b), so that all

dividing cells remaining in the subventricular zone at this age are presumably glial. Indeed, most cells in this zone are positively stained with the immunoperoxidase method at E123 (Fig. 1).

The light microscopic observations of the ventricular and subventricular zones at E80 indicate the presence of two cell populations. GFA-positive cell somata lie at varying distances from the ventricular surface. Intermingled among these is a population of cells that does not stain positively and thus is presumed to contain the neuronal precursor population. A crucial question is whether or not the two cell classes are determined developmentally before or after final cell division.

During the peak of neurogenesis at E80, there is considerable cell proliferation at the ventricular surface, which contains many mitotic figures. At the light microscopic level, a number of these dividing cells appear to have a thin cytoplasmic rim containing the HRP reaction product, while in the others, the cytoplasm seems to be unlabeled (Fig. 2). This finding raises the possibility that two distinct mitotically active cell populations exist within the ventricular zone. Thus, two distinct precursor cell types (glial and neuronal) may proliferate side by side. Light microscopic examination of the immunoperoxidase labeling does not provide sufficient resolution to answer this question because it could be argued that

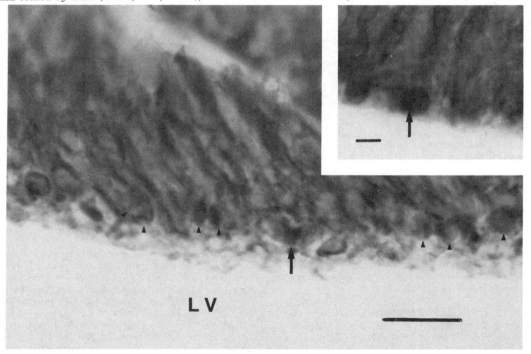

Figure 2. Vericolor photomicrograph of cresyl violet counterstained 8-μm-thick polyester wax embedded section. Numerous mitotic figures (*arrowheads*) are situated along the ventricular surface of the occipital lobe in an 80-day-old monkey fetus. The *arrowheads* on the *far left* point to GFA-negative mitotic cells which lie under a GFA-positive process. Two adjacent daughter cells are positively stained (*arrow*). At higher magnification (*inset*), a dividing cell in metaphase (*arrow*) contains the brown HRP reaction product. Although it appears here that the positive HRP staining is in the cytoplasm, it is not possible at the light microscopic level to exclude the possibility that the product lies within a glial process which surrounds the dividing cell. *Marker bar = 20 μm. Inset marker bar = 5 μm.*

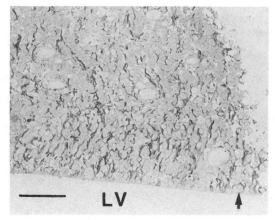

Figure 3. Numerous radial glial fibers are densely stained for GFA in a 0.5-μm-thick plastic section through the cerebral wall of the E80 specimen. The positively labeled processes penetrate the ventricular and subventricular zones in a wavy, but approximately parallel fashion. The *arrow* indicates an uncounterstained cell that is outlined by a dense cytoplasmic rim of HRP reaction product. Counterstaining with toluidine blue shows that this cell is in the anaphase stage of its mitotic cycle (see also Fig. 8). *Marker bar = 50 μm.*

the apparently positively stained mitotic cells at the ventricular surface only represent basal processes of postmitotic glial cells wrapping around the somata of the dividing neuronal precursors (Fig. 2). Thus, analysis at the ultrastructural level is essential in order to determine the location of the HRP reaction product within ventricular zone cells.

Electron microscopic examination. A thorough inspection of the ventricular surface in the 0.5-μm-thick plastic sections permits a somewhat more detailed characterization of the cells stained positively for GFA (Fig. 3). The cytoplasmic rim of each mitotically active cell is either clearly stained or completely unstained by the antibody-HRP complex (Figs. 7 and 8 *insets*). The light counterstaining of the 0.5-μm-thick sections with toluidine blue enables clear visualization of the mitotic figure in each cell in addition to the HRP reaction product. Of the 15 mitotic cells examined in the thick sections of the E80 specimen, approximately 60% were labeled by the GFA antibody. Following their identification in the thick sections, these mitotic cells were examined in thin sections under the electron microscope.

Ultrastructural examination of the E80 specimen at low power reveals a number of positively stained cell bodies and their processes throughout the ventricular zones (Fig. 4). Although the staining is occasionally pale (probably due to either detergent omission or less GFA), each cell can easily be classified as either GFA-positive or GFA-negative. The cell perikarya are situated at varying distances from the ventricular surface, many in the DNA-synthesizing region at the outer edge of the ventricular zone. Distal processes containing the HRP product can usually be followed for only a short distance in a single ultrathin section. Basal processes arising from both

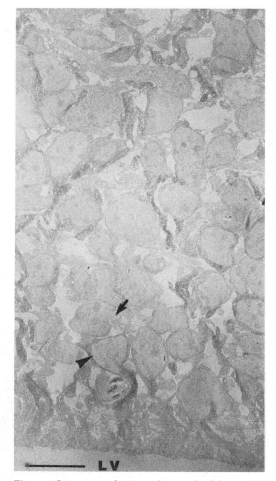

Figure 4. Low power electron micrograph of the ventricular and subventricular zones of the monkey occipital lobe at E80. Labeled cells (*arrowhead*) are distinguished readily from GFA-negative cells (*arrow*). This preparation reveals the heterogeneity of cells in the proliferative zones. The GFA-positive basal processes of the glial cells are intermingled with unstained cells of the ventricular and subventricular zones. In this and all subsequent electron micrographs, lead citrate and uranyl acetate counterstaining of the ultrathin sections has been omitted (see "Materials and Methods"). Thus, contrast of the electron micrographs is low compared to that in routinely counterstained sections. Counterstaining was omitted to render more visible the HRP reaction product located in GFA-positive cells. *Marker bar = 10 μm.*

labeled and unlabeled cells can often be traced directly to their termination in the form of an end-foot along the ventricular surface. Commonly, GFA-positive and -negative endings alternate at this surface (Fig. 5). Such a regular pattern of labeled and unlabeled cells present at this embryonic age corroborates previous light microscopic observations that indicated that GFA-positive processes run between columns of unlabeled ventricular zone cells (Levitt and Rakic, 1980; see also Fig. 2). The labeled and unlabeled processes are in intimate contact with each other at the ventricular surface; desmosomes are prevalent, joining stained with unstained fibers (Fig. 5). Both types of endings contain an abundance of clear, large vacuoles, mitochondria, and cilia projecting into the ventricular cavity.

Electron microscopic examination reveals that, in addition to the GFA-positive cells located at varying depths throughout the ventricular zone at E80, a number of the mitotic cells situated along the ventricular surface contain HRP reaction product in their cytoplasm. Again, there is a clear distinction between the cytoplasm of stained and unstained cells in different phases of mitosis (Figs. 6 to 8). The mitotic cells lack long proximal processes, consistent with the idea that precursor cells round up while undergoing cell division (Stensaas and Stensaas, 1968; Seymour and Berry, 1975). Both labeled and unlabeled mitotic cells contain the typical organelles observed

in proliferative cells of the central nervous system (Fujita and Fujita, 1963, 1964; Stensaas and Stensaas, 1968). Previous investigators noted that it is not possible to distinguish whether there is more than one class of mitotically active cells on the basis of the usual ultrastructural criteria. Thus, there is no obvious ultrastructural difference between the labeled and unlabeled cell types apart from the presence or absence of the antibody staining reaction product (Figs. 6 to 8). Within the cytoplasm of stained cells, the label was distributed evenly as a ring around the entire circumference of the mitotic figure (Figs. 6 and 8). Therefore, after division, both daughter cells presumably contain an approximately equal amount of the GFA. This is supported by the observation that obvious daughter cells are both stained (cf., Fig. 2).

The typical, rather globular HRP reaction product is located mainly on fibrillary structures in the labeled radial processes, on the cytoplasmic surface of the plasma

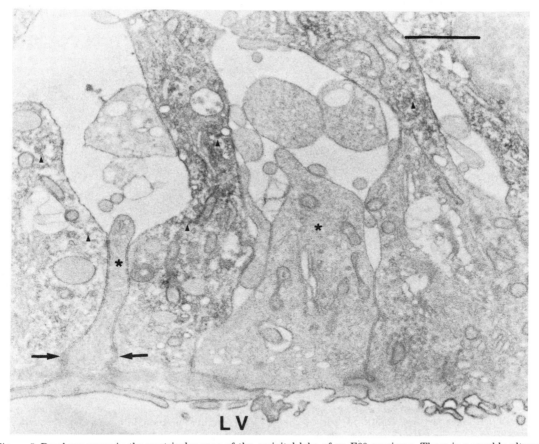

Figure 5. Basal processes in the ventricular zone of the occipital lobe of an E80 specimen. There is a roughly alternating pattern of GFA-negative (*) and GFA-positive processes (*arrowheads*) that terminate along the ventricular surface. Desmosomal junctions (*arrows*) are formed between both types of processes. All the basal processes appear to contain an identical complement of organelles, including mitochondria and large, clear vacuoles. Typical projecting cilia are commonly visible along the surface of the lateral ventricle in both labeled and unlabeled cells. *Marker bar* = 1 μm.

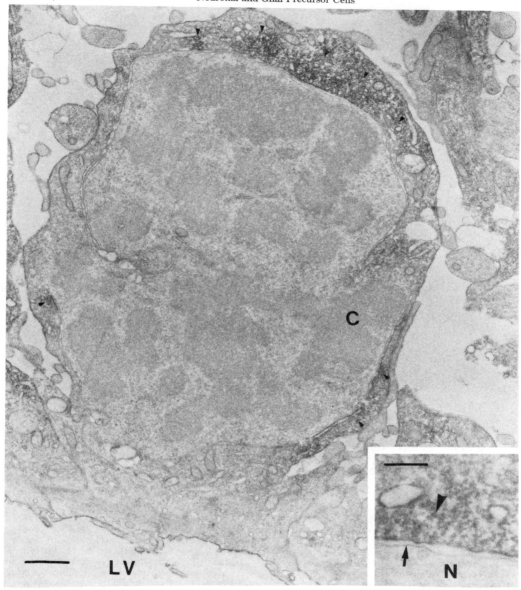

Figure 6. A dividing cell in late prophase situated at the ventricular surface of the occipital lobe in the E80 monkey. Even in this uncounterstained section, the clumped chromatin is evident in the nucleus, which during this mitotic phase still remains separated from the cytoplasm by a nuclear envelope (*inset, arrow*). The *arrowheads* denote the HRP reaction product, indicative of GFA-positive staining. The dense, globular reaction product (*arrowhead*) is seen more clearly at higher power in the *inset*. *Marker bar = 1 μm. Inset marker bar = 0.2 μm.*

membrane, outside mitochondrial membranes, and diffusely throughout the cytoplasm (Figs. 5, 6, and 8). The inner compartments of the Golgi complex, endoplasmic reticulum, mitochondria, and the cell nucleus are totally devoid of reaction product (Figs. 5, 6, and 8). This pattern of labeling is typical of the ultrastructural localization of GFA (Eng and Bigbee, 1978; Maunoury et al., 1979;

Schachner et al., 1977). The present study was not designed to precisely localize GFA within cytoplasmic organelles or to determine the site of its synthesis. The localization of the antigen-antibody binding site depends upon many factors, including fixation, antibody access to different tissue compartments, and staining parameters. Thus, it is difficult with our methodology to define pre-

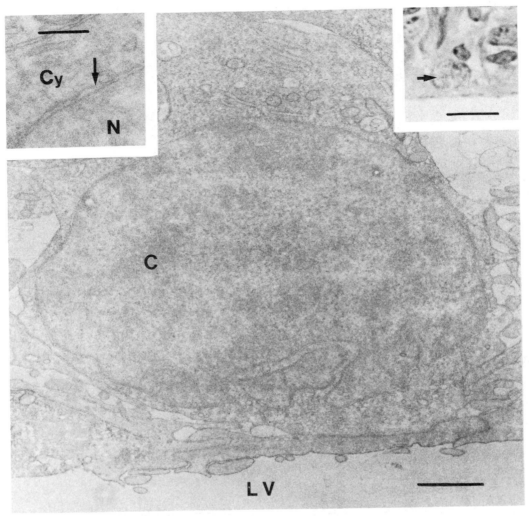

Figure 7. A GFA-negative cell in early prophase is situated in the ventricular zone of the occipital lobe in the E80 specimen. The lightly clumped chromatin in the cell nucleus is characteristic of this mitotic phase; this feature is visible more readily in the 0.5-μm-thick plastic section (*arrow, right inset*) of the same cell. Note the lack of any HRP reaction product in the cytoplasm in this mitotic cell at both the light and ultrastructural levels. The absence of any GFA staining in the cytoplasm is more evident at higher power (*left inset*). The nuclear envelope (*arrow*), normally present in prophase, separates the nucleus from the cytoplasm. Note that the nucleus and cytoplasm show identical contrast due to lack of the HRP reaction product and the omission of the lead citrate and uranyl acetate counterstaining. *Marker bar = 1 μm. Right inset marker bar = 10 μm. Left inset marker bar = 0.2 μm.*

cisely the normal intracellular sites of GFA. However, for our purposes, the simple identification of the positively and negatively staining cells is sufficient.

Discussion

The present immunocytochemical study provides new insights into two major issues in developmental neurobiology. First, we have demonstrated the heterogeneity of the proliferative zones during the peak period of neurogenesis in the rhesus monkey occipital lobe by showing the coexistence of mitotically active neuronal and glial precursor cells. Secondly, we have shown that the two cell lines begin to diverge prior to completion of final cell division. These results stand in contrast to the widely held views that neurogenesis precedes gliogenesis and that the ventricular zone is composed of a single cell type during neurogenesis (see Boulder Committee, 1970; Jacobson, 1978 for review).

GFA as a specific marker of developing glial cells. The GFA antigen was selected as a marker for glial cell

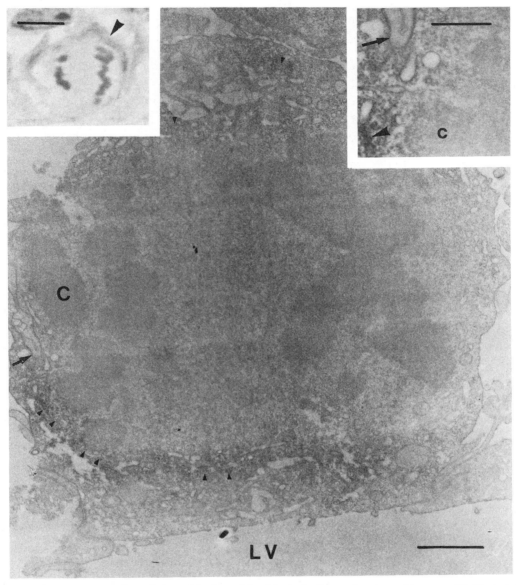

Figure 8. A GFA-positive dividing cell situated in the occipital lobe in the E80 monkey fetus; this same cell is illustrated in the 0.5-μm section in Figure 3. Distinct chromatids (*C*), characteristic of anaphase, are evident in both the light (*left inset*) and ultrastructural views. A densely labeled cytoplasmic rim (*arrowhead*) surrounding the nucleus is prominent in the 0.5-μm-thick plastic section (*left inset*). The HRP reaction product is evident also throughout the cytoplasm (*arrowheads*) at the ultrastructural level. An unstained mitochondrion (*arrow*), and the typical HRP reaction product (*arrowhead*), characteristic of anti-GFA immunoperoxidase staining, are visible more clearly at higher magnification (*right inset*). The nuclear envelope has disintegrated by this phase of the mitotic cycle. In spite of this, the GFA reaction product remains at the periphery of the perikaryon and does not intermix with the nuclear material. *Marker bar = 1 μm. Left inset marker bar = 5 μm. Right inset marker bar = 0.4 μm.*

differentiation during brain development only after careful consideration. This structural protein is well documented as a specific component of astroglial filaments that are present in protoplasmic and fibrillary astrocytes as well as in radial and Bergmann glial cells (see Eng,

1980 for review). The GFA protein is found neither in non-nervous tissues nor in either developing or mature oligodendrocytes and neurons. Furthermore, it should be emphasized that those proliferating cell populations of the central nervous system that can be identified readily as consisting of purely neuronal precursors, such as the external granule cells of the cerebellum or the granule cells of the hippocampal dentate gyrus, do not stain positively for GFA (Bignami and Dahl, 1973; Levitt and Rakic, 1980). Taken together, all available data support the contention that GFA is a specific, stable gene product of glial cells of astrocytic lineage and that it is not normally expressed in any other cell classes.

Although several other macromolecules such as non-neuronal enolase (NNE; EC 4.2.1.11) and S-100 protein have been utilized as glial cell markers in the adult brain (Cicero et al., 1970; Ludwin et al., 1976; Schmechel et al., 1978), the case for their usefulness as differentiation antigens during development is less convincing. For example, NNE or its hybrid form has been detected in mature cerebellar stellate and basket neurons, in non-glial brain tissues such as choroid plexus and ependymal cells, and even in non-brain tissue such as liver (Schmechel et al., 1980). Thus, this protein cannot be considered as a specific gene product of glial cells, since several other cell types, including developing neurons, express NNE (Schmechel et al., 1980). The S-100 protein is a highly soluble macromolecule that presents considerable difficulties in its use as a glial differentiation marker in the developing brain. This protein has been found in both neurons and glial cells using a variety of fixation and staining methods, and controversy still exists as to whether its localization is truly specific to glial cells (cf., Varon and Somjen, 1979). The protein is localized only to glial cells in brains that are extremely well fixed. However, S-100 protein is found in both glial and neuronal elements when the tissue is fixed only moderately or inadequately (Eng and Bigbee, 1978; Hartman et al., 1977). The presence of S-100 protein in neurons may be due to intercellular transfer of this protein, and such a problem would be especially acute in tightly packed regions such as the embryonic ventricular zone, which in any event is difficult to fix well. These problems concerning the utilization of S-100 protein raise questions about its suitability for use (as in DeVitry et al., 1980) in determining cell lineages in developing brain. Therefore, given the available data, it seems that GFA best meets rigorous criteria for use as a specific glial differentiation marker.

Heterogeneity of the cerebral proliferative zones. As noted in the introduction, His (1889) proposed that the germinal epithelium of the cerebral wall consists of two precursor cell classes, one neuronal and the other glial (Fig. 9A). Furthermore, he thought that glial cells are organized in the form of a multinuclear syncytium. Subsequently, an opposing view was elaborated by Schaper (1897a, b), who considered the ventricular zone to be composed of a single precursor cell type giving rise to indifferent cells (Fig. 9B). The idea of a homogeneous ventricular zone gained support from Sauer's (1935) demonstration that ventricular zone cells with different shapes and nuclear locations simply represent various phases of the cell mitotic cycle, from detailed ultrastructural examinations in chick embryos (Fujita, 1966; Fujita and Fujita, 1963, 1964), and from studies by Fujita (1963) and Sidman et al. (1959) that showed that all cells in the proliferative zone could be labeled by ³H-TdR. Furthermore, investigations of the time of cell origin with this

autoradiographic technique were interpreted by many investigators to show that, in general, neurons of the vertebrate central nervous system are generated prior to glial cells (see the introduction). For example, Fujita (1963, 1966) proposed that the germinal cells first give rise to neurons and that later, after cessation of neuronal production, these proliferative cells undergo some undefined changes to become glial precursor cells (Fig. 9C).

There are at least two problems in the interpretation of ³H-TdR autoradiographic labeling after either short or long survival times. First, labeling of all ventricular cells with cumulative administration of ³H-TdR does not necessarily imply a homogeneous cell population. Rather, it indicates only that all cells in this zone are synthesizing DNA during this period. Secondly, embryonic glial cells may have prolonged periods of cell division, resulting in the dilution of the ³H-TdR label to an undetectable level in the mature brain. Thus, the ³H-TdR technique is not adequate to determine the onset of differentiation of glial cells during the development of a given structure.

The first indication that neuronal and glial cell lines coexist in the embryonic brain was provided by descriptions of radial glial cells. This class of glial cells was described in the spinal cord by the Golgi impregnation method at the end of the last century (Golgi, 1885; Ramón y Cajal, 1890; Retzius, 1894). Because radial glial cells are present and increase in number along with neurons prior to and during the peak of corticogenesis (Levitt and Rakic, 1980; Rakic, 1972, 1974, 1975b; Schmechel and Rakic, 1979), the precursors for these cell types theoretically must be present concomitantly (Fig. 9D). However, prior to this report, the actual location and coexistence of the two precursor cell types had never been established.

The use of an immunological probe in the present study reveals for the first time the heterogeneous character of the ventricular zone by demonstrating the presence of two distinct mitotically active cell types (GFA-positive and GFA-negative) (Figs. 6 to 8). Therefore, although His's (1889) description of a cellular syncytium proved to be wrong, his concept that two classes of proliferative cells coexist in the ventricular zone, one giving rise to neurons and the other to glia, gains support by the present immunocytochemical study (Fig. 9D).

Onset of glial phenotypic expression as indicated by the presence of GFA. Our results demonstrate the presence of at least two mitotically active precursor cell types in the embryonic ventricular zone. The localization of a differentiation antigen, GFA, in cells that are actively dividing and synthesizing DNA also indicates that proliferative cells are committed to their specific lineage prior to final mitosis. Thus, the onset of expression of a specific cell phenotype is not rigidly linked to *final* mitosis. This concept has been documented for the processes of erythropoiesis and chondrogenesis (see Caplan and Ordahl, 1978; Marks et al., 1978; Rutter et al., 1973 for reviews). Likewise, in the developing sympathetic nervous system, mitotically active cells that are destined to become sympathetic neurons contain the specific enzymes which are involved in the synthesis of the neurotransmitter norepinephrine (Cohen, 1974; Rothman et al., 1978).

It should be emphasized that the present results do not resolve the questions of whether and at what stage a

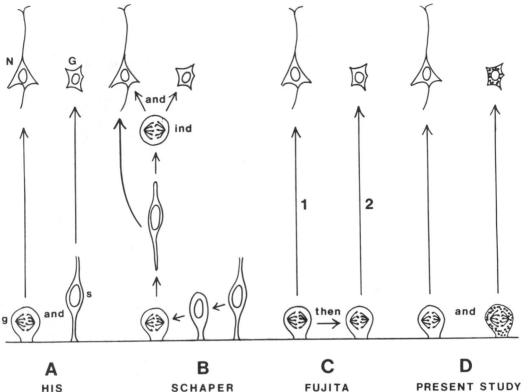

Figure 9. A schematic diagram summarizing in a simplified manner previous theories of the origin of neuronal and glial cell lines (A, B, and C) in comparison to the scheme suggested by the results of the present study (D). A, His (1889) distinguished two types of cells in the germinal matrix (now called ventricular) zone lining the surface of the embryonic ventricles (represented by the *horizontal line*). The first type is the rounded "germinal cell" (*g*), which contains a mitotic nucleus in proximity to the ventricular surface. The second is the columnar "spongioblast" (*s*), with a nucleus that can lie at various distances from the ventricle. His believed that the "germinal cells" give rise to neurons (*N*), whereas the "spongioblasts," which he held to form a syncytium, give rise to glia (*G*). Thus, His proposed that separate and different neuronal and glial precursor lines coexist in the ventricular zone. B, Schaper (1897a, b) considered that His's two cell types actually represented different phases of a single type of cell; this was confirmed later by Sauer's (1935) study. Furthermore, Schaper suggested that the mitotically active cells of the ventricular zone are indifferent cells (i.e., not yet determined as either glial or neuronal). He supposed these cells to give origin to migrating cells which move into the overlying intermediate (mantle) zone, where they yield either neurons directly or both neurons and glia after further divisions as indifferent (*IND*) cells. Schaper's theory, therefore, supported the homogeneity of the ventricular zone. C, Tritiated thymidine autoradiographic evidence led to Fujita's (1963) scheme, which also emphasizes the homogeneity of the ventricular zone. According to Fujita, the dividing cell population in the ventricular zone first gives rise to neurons (*1*); then, after neurogenesis ceases, this same dividing population changes proliferative programs and begins to produce glial cells (*2*). Thus, Fujita suggested that at any given time, the proliferative population is homogeneous and composed of cells which first give rise to neurons and only later to glia. D, In the present study, we have demonstrated that both GFA-positive (*stippled*) and GFA-negative mitotic cells coexist in the ventricular zone at the time of peak neurogenesis during midgestation in the monkey occipital lobe. Therefore, the labeled cells already possess a glial differentiation marker and accordingly may be a committed glial precursor cell line. The data point to the coexistence of distinct neuronal and glial precursors in the ventricular zone, implying that the proliferative cell population is heterogeneous in its composition.

single, indifferent germinal cell gives rise to both glial and neuronal precursor types. Neither do we address the issue of whether all or only some astrocytes pass through the stage of radial glial cell phenotype. Finally, we do not know whether the unlabeled cells consist of multiple cell classes, including some "indifferent" cells. Therefore, although our data demonstrate clearly that at E80, there already exist distinct neuronal and glial precursors in the ventricular zone of the monkey occipital lobe, the details

of the lineage relationships between these cells remain unclear. However, as noted above, the fact that cellular populations that are known to contain proliferating neuronal percursors, such as those which produce the hippocampal and cerebellar granule cells, do not express detectable levels of GFA indicates that transient expression of this marker by neuronal precursor cell lines is unlikely. Given the early coexistence (by E47) of neurons and differentiated radial glial cells in the cerebral wall of monkey embryos (Levitt and Rakic, 1980), we favor the hypothesis that neuronal and glial lines maintain separate identities from the time that neurogenesis is initiated in a given structure (Fig. 9*D*). However, we cannot rule out the possibility that some glial precursor cells arise from dividing cells which had at some point generated neurons. Even at E80, we are certain only that many of the unlabeled cells in the ventricular zone represent a neuronal precursor line which eventually forms layer III of the visual cortex (Rakic, 1974). Theoretically, a fraction of the unlabeled cells could be either indifferent cells yielding both neuronal and glial precursors or cells which have ceased producing neurons and subsequently changed over to glial production without having yet expressed GFA. These two possibilities seem to be unlikely; to test them, one would need glial markers that are present in the proliferative cell population at ages before the first neurons are generated.

The present study demonstrates that the precursor cell population of the ventricular zone contains at least two cell types. In the future, the use of immunocytochemistry may provide a means for subdividing the germinal population into even more than two classes and for a precise spatial separation of the proliferative zone into areas that produce neurons destined for specific cytoarchitectonic fields. The possibility of detecting cell classes by immunocytochemical techniques will also provide new criteria for defining the onset of cell differentiation that cannot be attained by conventional morphological changes alone.

References

Angevine, J. B., Jr. (1970) Critical cellular events in the shaping of neural centers. In *The Neurosciences: Second Study Program,* F. O. Schmitt, ed., pp. 62–72, Rockefeller University Press, New York.

Antanitus, D. S., B. H. Choi, and L. W. Lapham (1976) The demonstration of glial fibrillary acidic protein in the cerebrum of the human fetus by indirect immunofluorescence. Brain Res. *103:* 613–616.

Berry, M., and A. W. Rogers (1965) The migration of neuroblasts in the developing cerebral cortex. J. Anat. *99:* 691–709.

Bignami, A., and D. Dahl (1973) Differentiation of astrocytes in the cerebellar cortex and the pyramidal tracts of the newborn rat. An immunofluorescence study with antibodies to a protein specific to astrocytes. Brain Res. *49:* 393–402.

Bignami, A., and D. Dahl (1974) Astrocyte-specific protein and neuroglial differentiation. An immunofluorescence study with antibodies to the glial fibrillary acidic protein. J. Comp. Neurol. *153:* 27–38.

Bignami, A., L. F. Eng, D. Dahl, and C. T. Uyeda (1972) Localization of the glial fibrillary acidic protein in astrocytes by immunofluorescence. Brain Res. *43:* 429–435.

Boulder Committee (1970) Embryonic vertebrate central nervous system: Revised terminology. Anat. Rec. *166:* 257–261.

Caplan, A. T., and C. P. Ordahl (1978) Irreversible gene repression model for control of development. Science *201:* 120–130.

Choi, B. H., and L. W. Lapham (1978) Radial glia in the human fetal cerebrum: A combined Golgi immunofluorescent and electron microscopic study. Brain Res. *148:* 295–311.

Cicero, T. J., W. M. Cowan, B. W. Moore, and V. Suntzeff (1970) The cellular localization of the two brain-specific proteins, S-100 and 14-3-2. Brain Res. *18:* 25–34.

Cohen, A. (1974) DNA synthesis and cell division in differentiating avian adrenergic neuroblasts. In *Wenner-Gren Center*

International Symposium Series. Vol. 22: *Dynamics of Degeneration and Growth of Neurons,* K. Fuxe, L. Olson, and Y. Zotterman, eds., pp. 359–370, Pergamon Press, Oxford.

DeVitry, F., R. Picart, C. Jacque, L. Legault, P. Dupouey, and A. Tixier-Vidal (1980) Presumptive common precursor for neuronal and glial cell lineages in mouse hypothalamus. Proc. Natl. Acad. Sci. U. S. A. *77:* 4165–4169.

Eng, L. F. (1980) The glial fibrillary acidic (GFA) protein. In *Proteins of the Nervous System,* R. Bradshaw and D. Schneider, eds., pp. 85–117, Raven Press, New York.

Eng, L. F., and J. W. Bigbee (1978) Immunochemistry of nervous system-specific proteins. In *Advances in Neurochemistry,* B. W. Agranoff and M. H. Aprison, eds., Vol. 3, pp. 43–98, Plenum Publishing Corp., New York.

Eng, L. F., and J. C. Kosec (1974) Light and electron microscopic localization of the glial fibrillary acidic protein and S-100 protein by immunoenzymatic techniques. Trans. Am. Soc. Neurochem. *5:* 160.

Eng, L. F., and L. J. Rubinstein (1978) Contribution of immunohistochemistry to diagnostic problems of human cerebral tumors. J. Histochem. Cytochem. *26:* 513–522.

Eng, L. F., J. J. Vanderhaeghen, A. Bignami, and B. Gerstl (1971) An acidic protein isolated from fibrous astrocytes. Brain Res. *28:* 351–354.

Fujita, S. (1963) The matrix cell and cytogenesis in the developing central nervous system. J. Comp. Neurol. *120:* 37–42.

Fujita, S. (1965) An autoradiographic study on the origin and fate of the subpial glioblasts in the embryonic chick spinal cord. J. Comp. Neurol. *124:* 51–60.

Fujita, S. (1966) Application of light and electron microscopic autoradiography to the study of cytogenesis of the forebrain. In *Evolution of the Forebrain,* R. Hassler and H. Stephan, eds., pp. 180–196, Plenum Press, New York.

Fujita, H., and S. Fujita (1963) Electron microscopic studies on neuroblast differentiation in the central nervous system of domestic fowl. Z. Zellforsch. Mikrosk. Anat. *60:* 463–478.

Fujita, H., and S. Fujita (1964) Electron microscopic studies on the differentiation of the ependymal cells and the glioblast in the spinal cord of domestic fowl. Z. Zellforsch. Mikrosk. Anat. *64:* 262–272.

Golgi, G. (1885) Sulla fina anatomia degli organi centrali del sistema nervoso. Republished in: Oper Omnia Hoepli, Milan (1903) 397–536.

Gracheva, N. D. (1969) Autoradiography of DNA synthesis in estimation of proliferative activity of rat brain subependymal cells. Tsitologiia *11:* 1521–1527.

Hartman, B. K., M. Cimino, B. W. Moore, and H. C. Agrawal (1977) Immunohistochemical localization of brain specific proteins during development. Trans. Am. Soc. Neurochem. *8:* 66.

Hicks, S. P., and C. J. D'Amato (1968) Cell migrations to the isocortex in the rat. Anat. Rec. *160:* 619–634.

His, W. (1889) Die Neuroblasten und deren Entstehung im embryonal Marke. Abh. Math. Phys. Cl. Kgl. Sach. Ges. Wiss. *15:* 313–372.

Jacobson, M. (1978) *Developmental Neurobiology,* Plenum Press, New York.

Levitt, P., and P. Rakic (1980) Immunoperoxidase localization of glial fibrillary acidic protein in radial glial cells and astrocytes of the developing rhesus monkey brain. J. Comp. Neurol. *193:* 417–448.

Ludwin, S. K., J. C. Kosek, and L. F. Eng (1976) The topographical distribution of S-100 and GFA proteins in the adult rat brain: An immunohistochemical study using horseradish peroxidase-labeled antibodies. J. Comp. Neurol. *165:* 197–208.

Marks, P. A., R. A. Rifkind, M. Terada, R. C. Reuben, Y. Gazitt, and E. Fibach (1978) Erythropoiesis—Normal erythropoiesis in induced erythroleukemia differentiation. In *Hematopoietic*

Cell Differentiation. ICN-UCLA Symposia on Molecular and Cellular Biology, D. W. Golde, M. J. Cline, D. Metcalf, and C. F. Fox, eds., Vol. 10, pp. 25–35, Academic Press, New York.

Maunoury, R., C. Daumas-Duport, C. Fontaine, and C. Vedrenne (1979) Ultrastructural localization of glial fibrillary acidic protein (GFAP) in human glioma culture by immunoperoxidase method. Brain Res. 170: 392–398.

Rakic, P. (1971) Neuron-glia relationship during granule cell migration in developing cerebellar cortex. A Golgi and electron microscopic study in macacus rhesus. J. Comp. Neurol. 141: 283–312.

Rakic, P. (1972) Mode of cell migration to the superficial layers of fetal monkey neocortex. J. Comp. Neurol. 145: 61–84.

Rakic, P. (1973) Kinetics of proliferation and latency between final cell division and onset of differentiation of the cerebellar stellate and basket neurons. J. Comp. Neurol. 147: 523–546.

Rakic, P. (1974) Neurons in rhesus monkey visual cortex: Systematic relation between time of origin and eventual disposition. Science 183: 425–427.

Rakic, P. (1975a) Cell migration and neuronal ectopias in the brain. In Birth Defects: Original Series, D. Bergsma, ed., Vol. 9, pp. 95–129, Liss, New York.

Rakic, P. (1975b) Timing of major ontogenetic events in the visual cortex of the rhesus monkey. In Brain Mechanisms in Mental Retardation, N. A. Buchwald and M. Brazier, eds., pp. 3–40, Academic Press, New York.

Ramón y Cajal, S. (1890) Sur l'origine et les ramifications des fibres nerveuses de la moelle embryonnaire. Anat. Anz. 5: 85–95; 111–119.

Retzius, G. (1894) Die Neuroglia des Gehirns beim Menschen und bei Säugentiere. Biol. Unters. 6: 1–24.

Rothman, T. P., M. D. Gershon, and H. Holtzer (1978) The relationship of cell division to the acquisition of adrenergic characteristics by developing sympathetic ganglion cell precursors. Dev. Biol. 65: 322–341.

Rutter, W. J., R. L. Pictet, and P. W. Morris (1973) Toward molecular mechanisms of developmental processes. Annu. Rev. Biochem. 42: 601–646.

Sauer, F. C. (1935) Mitosis in the neural tube. J. Comp. Neurol. 62: 377–405.

Schachner, M., E. T. Hedley-Whyte, D. W. Hsu, G. Schoonmaker, and A. Bignami (1977) Ultrastructural localization of glial fibrillary acidic protein in mouse cerebellum by immunoperoxidase labeling. J. Cell Biol. 75: 67–73.

Schaper, A. (1897a) Die fruhesten Differenzierungsvorgänger im Centralnervensystem. Arch. Entw.-Mech. Org. 5: 81–132.

Schaper, A. (1897b) The earliest differentiation in the central nervous system of vertebrates. Science 5: 430–431.

Schmechel, D. E., and P. Rakic (1979) A Golgi study of radial glial cells in developing monkey telencephalon: Morphogenesis and transformation into astrocytes. Anat. Embryol. (Berl.) 156: 115–152.

Schmechel, D. E., P. J. Marangos, A. P. Zis, M. Brightman, and F. K. Goodwin (1978) The brain enolases as specific markers of neuronal and glial cells. Science 199: 313–315.

Schmechel, D. E., M. W. Brightman, and P. J. Marangos (1980) Neurons switch from non-neuronal enolase to neuron-specific enolase during differentiation. Brain Res. 190: 195–214.

Seymour, R. M., and M. Berry (1975) Scanning and transmission electron microscope studies of interkinetic nuclear migration in the cerebral vesicles of the rat. J. Comp. Neurol. 160: 105–126.

Sidman, R. L., and P. Rakic (1973) Neuronal migration, with special reference to developing human brain: A review. Brain Res. 62: 1–35.

Sidman, R. L., I. L. Miale, and N. Feder (1959) Cell proliferation in the primitive ependymal zone: An autoradiographic study of histogenesis in the nervous system. Exp. Neurol. 1: 322–333.

Sidman, R. L., P. A. Mottla, and N. Feder (1961) Improved polyester wax embedding for histology. Stain Technol. 36: 279–284.

Stensaas, L. J., and S. S. Stensaas (1968) An electron microscope study of cells in the matrix and intermediate laminae of the cerebral hemisphere of the 45mm rabbit embryo. Z. Zellforsch. Mikrosk. Anat. 91: 341–365.

Sternberger, L. A. (1979) Immunocytochemistry, John Wiley and Sons, New York.

Varon, S. S., and G. G. Somjen (1979) Neuron-glia interactions. Neurosci. Res. Program Bull. 17: 47–65.

von Waechter, R., and B. Jaensch (1972) Generation times of the matrix cells during embryonic development: An autoradiographic study in rats. Brain Res. 46: 235–250.

Section 2
Neuronal Migration
and Positional Information

Rakic, P. 1972. Mode of cell migration to the superficial layers of fetal monkey neocortex. *J. Comp. Neurol.* *145:*61–84.

Noden, D.M. 1975. An analysis of the migratory behavior of avian cephalic neural crest cells. *Dev. Biol.* *42:*106–130.

Crick, F.H.C. and P.A. Lawrence. 1975. Compartments and polyclones in insect development. *Science 189:* 340–347.

Lawrence, P.A. 1978. Compartments and the insect nervous system. *Zoon 6:*157–160.

During the time that neuronal precursors divide and differentiate, they must attain (or maintain) appropriate positions relative to other cells in order to facilitate later events in development, such as axon outgrowth and the formation of synaptic connections. Often this involves migration over long distances through a variety of environments. Since many cell types must solve the problem of attaining an appropriate position, developing neurons may use the same migratory mechanisms used by nonneuronal cells. In accord with this idea, many embryonic cell types (including neuronal precursors) have prominent ruffled membranes and filopodia and contain filamentous cytoplasmic protein systems considered to be important for cell motility (Bray and Gilbert 1981).

How do developing neurons know where to migrate and when to stop? Some classes of neurons, such as those in the developing mammalian cortex, appear to move along the surface of a particular nonneuronal cell type, the radial (or Bergmann) glia (**Rakic** 1971a,b, **1972**). Several aspects of these glial elements suggest a role in neuronal migration. First, they have an orientation appropriate for radially migrating neurons, and they extend from the ventricular surface to the pial surface of the developing cortex. Second, they are present throughout the developing central nervous system at the appropriate times (Levitt and Rakic 1980); indeed, in many areas of cortex the radial glia are transitory elements and disappear after the period of migration is over, possibly becoming astrocytes (Ramón y Cajal 1911; Levitt and Rakic 1980). Third, migrating neurons are intimately associated with the processes of radial glial cells (Rakic 1971b, 1972; Rakic et al. 1974). The only experimental evidence for a necessary relationship between radial glia and the appropriate migration of cortical neurons, however, comes from observa-

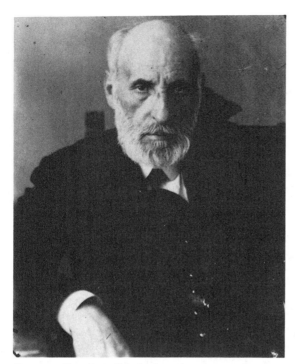

Santiago Ramón y Cajal, whose heroic contributions influenced nearly every aspect of developmental neurobiology.

tions on a mutant mouse (Weaver) in which disordered radial glia are associated with a failure of granule cells to migrate to their correct locations in the cerebellum (Rakic and Sidman 1973a,b; see, however, Goldowitz and Mullen 1980; Sotelo and Rio 1980). If radial glia are guides for early migration in the cortex, there must also be other cues in the local environment to signal different classes of neurons to stop at the appropriate cortical layer.

The migration of neuronal precursors from the neural crest is different from migration in the central nervous system in that crest cells travel long distances through embryonic mesenchyme to their final destinations. Moreover, some crest cells continue to divide during the early stages of neuronal differentiation, when migration has ceased (Cohen 1974; Rothman et al. 1978). That the embryonic environment through which crest cells move influences the pattern of their migration was suggested by the early experiments of Weston (Weston 1963; Weston and Butler 1966). Subsequently, it has been shown that a crest cell population that normally shows a pattern of migration characteristic of its axial level can, when transplanted to a new axial level, adopt a

different migratory pattern typical of the new site (**Noden 1975**). These patterns were deduced by examining the locations of crest cells in the process of migration. As discussed in the next section, similar conclusions have been derived from experiments that analyzed the distribution of crest cell derivatives in their final locations after migration had ended.

The environment through which crest cells move consists of other cells (see, for instance, LeDouarin and Teillet 1973), as well as cell-free regions of extracellular matrix material (Pratt et al. 1975; Pintar 1978) which gradually change in both composition and morphology during development (Derby 1978; Tosney 1978; Löfberg et al. 1980). This matrix is known to include fibronectin (Newgreen and Thiery 1980) and glycosaminoglycans such as hyaluronic acid, a molecule that may be especially important for migratory pathways (Toole 1976). Further information about the molecular composition of the migratory environment will obviously be useful in designing experiments to test the basis of guidance during migration.

The problem of how specific migration patterns are achieved in molecular terms leads to a broader question. Is there an overall scheme of positional information in the developing embryo which tells both neural and nonneural cells where to go, or is migration governed simply by local cues and mechanical guides? (See also Section 4.)

Although this question remains open, several observations in studies of both invertebrates and vertebrates suggest that the developing embryo does have information that enables cells to interpret their position. One body of evidence is provided by the compartmentalization of insect development (Garcia-Bellido et al. 1973, 1979; Garcia-Bellido 1975; **Crick** and **Lawrence 1975**; Lawrence and Morata 1976). The paper by Crick and Lawrence (1975) provides a lucid summary of the basic ideas of compartmental development and a brief paper by **Lawrence (1978)** draws attention to the relevance of compartmentalization to neural development. The adult *Drosophila* arises from 19 isolated groups of cells that are formed in the embryo but serve little or no function during larval life. Each of these imaginal disks, as they are called, differentiates during metamorphosis and gives rise to a particular part of the adult. Because they are both anatomically distinct and accessible, imag-

40

inal disks can be manipulated in various ways. It is possible, for example, to irradiate a larval fly so as to produce in an imaginal disk a mutant cell whose descendants are phenotypically different in the adult (commonly used markers are abnormal wing hairs and cell color). The descendants of such a mutant cell (or indeed any cell) are called a clone. The striking result of such experiments is that clones of sufficient size form a regular border in a structure such as the wing, as if the dividing cells were strictly prohibited from mixing with cells occupying other positions. These findings gave rise to the idea of the developmental compartment, defined as a region to which a clone of cells is restricted, even though the borders present no obvious anatomical boundary. Each compartment, then, is made up of a set of clones (called a polyclone) that represents the surviving descendants of a small group of founder cells, which appear to have held some positional quality in common. Indeed, some genes in *Drosophila* are concerned with the development of entire compartments, since they affect all of the structures within a compartment, but not similar structures in adjacent compartments (Garcia-Bellido 1975; Morata and Lawrence 1975). Morata and Lawrence (1975) have suggested that the function of such "selector genes" may be to label the founder cells of the clones that make up a compartment so as to prevent mixing with the clones of other compartments. Some evidence suggesting a similar compartmentalization of development in the vertebrate nervous system has also been presented (Hirose and Jacobson 1979; Jacobson and Hirose 1981), but the interpretation is disputed (see Cooke 1980).

A rather different series of experiments on the imaginal disks of *Drosophila* has also provided evidence for a general scheme of positional information during development (French et al. 1976). If a fragment of an imaginal disk is transplanted from a larva to an adult host, the disk heals and grows. When the fragment is transplanted back into a larva, it differentiates as the host undergoes metamorphosis. In general, the disks so treated produce either their normal derivative or a portion of the appropriate adult part plus its mirror-image duplicate. An analysis of these results (see French et al. 1976; Bryant et al. 1978; Bryant et al. 1981), together with related observations on limb regeneration in both invertebrates and vertebrates, has led French, Bryant, and Bryant to suggest what they have called the polar-coordinate model of positional information. In this model, each cell in the imaginal disk (or in a limb capable of regeneration) is labeled with circumferential and radial (or proximodistal) positional values; cells are thus envisioned as assessing their places in the animal by means of local interactions with neighboring cells. The operation of a few relatively simple rules within this scheme appears to account for a remarkably large number of otherwise puzzling results. The general idea underlying these rules is that the division of a cell continues to be stimulated until the cell finds itself among other cells with appropriate (similar) positional values. In another class of models, position is read out according to distance from the source of a morphogen which diffuses toward a sink. The best known of these is the "French flag" model (see Wolpert 1969, 1978).

In addition to migration, other phenomena peculiar to the development of the nervous system, such as axon outgrowth and selective synapse formation, may make use of a general scheme of information about position (see Sections 4, 9, 10, and 12). A common mechanism of instruction may thus operate in these diverse situations in which cells pay attention to some positional quality of their neighbors.

References

Bray, D. and D. Gilbert. 1981. Cytoskeletal elements in neurons. *Annu. Rev. Neurosci. 4:* 505–523.

Bryant, P.J., S.V. Bryant, and V. French. 1978. Biological regeneration and pattern formation. *Sci. Am. 237:* 66–81.

Bryant, S.V., V. French, and P.J. Bryant. 1981. Distal regeneration and symmetry. *Science 212:* 993–1002.

Cohen, A.M. 1974. DNA synthesis and cell division in differentiating avian adrenergic neuroblasts. In *Dynamics of degeneration and growth in neurons* (ed. K. Fuxe et al.), pp. 359–370. Pergamon Press, New York.

Cooke, J. 1980. Clones and compartments in the vertebrate central nervous system—A valid approach to the development of the neural plate? *Trends Neurosci. 3:* 100.

Crick, F.H.C. and P.A. Lawrence. 1975. Compartments and polyclones in insect development. *Science 189:* 340–347.

Derby, M.A. 1978. Analysis of glycosaminoglycans within the extracellular environments encountered by migrating neural crest cells. *Dev. Biol. 66:* 321–336.

French, V., P.J. Bryant, and S.V. Bryant. 1976. Pattern regulation in epimorphic fields. *Science 193:* 969–981.

Garcia-Bellido, A. 1975. Genetic control of wing disc development in *Drosophila. CIBA Found. Symp. 29:* 161–182.

Garcia-Bellido, A., P.A. Lawrence, and G. Morata. 1979. Compartments in animal development. *Sci. Am. 241:* 102–110.

Garcia-Bellido, A., P. Ripoll, and G. Morata. 1973. Developmental compartmentalization in the wing disk of *Drosophila. Nat. New Biol. 245:* 251–253.

Goldowitz, D. and R.J. Mullen. 1980. Weaver mutant granule cell defect expressed in chimeric mice. *Soc. Neurosci. Abstr. 6:* 743.

Hirose, G. and M. Jacobson. 1979. Clonal organization of the central nervous system of the frog. I. Clones stemming from individual blastomeres of the 16-cell and earlier stages. *Dev. Biol. 71:* 191–202.

Jacobson, M. and G. Hirose. 1981. Clonal organization of the central nervous system of the frog. II. Clones stemming from individual blastomeres of the 32- and 64-cell stages. *J. Neurosci. 1:* 271–284.

Lawrence, P.A. 1978. Compartments and the insect nervous system. *Zoon 6:* 157–160.

Lawrence, P.A. and G. Morata. 1976. The compartment hypothesis. In *Insect development, 8th Symposium of the Royal Entomological Society* (ed. P.A. Lawrence), pp. 132–149. Blackwell, London.

LeDouarin, N.M. and M.-A. Teillet. 1973. The migration of neural crest cells to the wall of the digestive tract in avian embryo. *J. Embryol. Exp. Morphol. 30:* 31–48.

Levitt, P. and P. Rakic. 1980. Immunoperoxidase localization of glial acidic protein in radial glial cells and astrocytes of the developing rhesus monkey brain. *J. Comp. Neurol. 193:* 815–846.

Löfberg, J., K. Ahlfors, and C. Fällström. 1980. Neural crest cell migration in relation to extracellular matrix organization in the embryonic axolotl trunk. *Dev. Biol. 75:* 148–167.

Morata, G. and P.A. Lawrence. 1975. Control of compartment development by the *engrailed* gene in *Drosophila. Nature 255:* 614–617.

Newgreen, D. and J.-P. Thiery. 1980. Fibronectin in early avian embryo. Synthesis and distribution along the migratory pathway of neural crest cells. *Cell Tissue Res. 211:* 269–291.

Noden, D.M. 1975. An analysis of the migratory behavior of avian cephalic neural crest cells. *Dev. Biol. 42:* 106–130.

Pintar, J.E. 1978. Distribution and synthesis of glycosaminoglycans during quail neural crest morphogenesis. *Dev. Biol. 67:* 444–464.

Pratt, R.M., M.A. Larsen, and M.C. Johnston. 1975. Migration of cranial neural crest cells in a cell-free hyaluronate-rich matrix. *Dev. Biol. 44:* 298–305.

Rakic, P. 1971a. Guidance of neurons migrating to the fetal monkey neocortex. *Brain Res. 33:* 471–476.

———. 1971b. Neuron-glia relationship during granule cell migration in developing cerebellar cortex. A Golgi and electron microscopic study in *Macacus rhesus. J. Comp. Neurol. 141:* 283–312.

———. 1972. Mode of cell migration to the superficial layers of fetal monkey neocortex. *J. Comp. Neurol. 145:* 61–84.

Rakic, P. and R.L. Sidman. 1973a. Weaver mutant mouse cerebellum: Defective neuronal migration secondary to specific abnormality of Bergmann glia. *Proc. Natl. Acad. Sci. 70:* 240–244.

———. 1973b. Sequence of developmental abnormalities leading to granule cell deficit in cerebellar cortex of Weaver mutant mice. *J. Comp. Neurol. 152:* 103–132.

Rakic, P., L.J. Stensas, E.P. Sayre, and R.L. Sidman. 1974. Computer-aided three-dimensional reconstruction and quantitative analysis of cells from serial electron microscopic montages of foetal monkey brain. *Nature 250:* 31–34.

Ramón y Cajal, S. 1911. *Histologie du système nerveaux de l'homme et des vertébrés,* vol. 1. A. Maloine, Paris. Reprinted by Consejo Superior de Investigaciones Cientificas, Instituto Ramón y Cajal, Madrid, 1955.

Rothman, T.P., M.D. Gershon, and H. Holtzer. 1978. The relationship of cell division to the acquisition of adrenergic characteristics by developing sympathetic ganglion cell precursors. *Dev. Biol. 65:* 322–341.

Sotelo, C. and J.P. Rio. 1980. Cerebellar malformation obtained in rats by early postnatal treatment with 6-aminonicotinamide. Role of neuron-glia interactions in cerebellar development. *Neuroscience 5:* 1737–1759.

Toole, B.P. 1976. Morphogenetic role of glycosaminoglycans (acid mucopolysaccharides) in brain and other tissues. In *Neuronal recognition* (ed. S.H. Barondes), pp. 275–329. Plenum Press, New York.

Tosney, K.W. 1978. The early migration of neural crest cells in the trunk region of the avian embryo: An electron microscopic study. *Dev. Biol. 62:* 317–333.

Weston, J.A. 1963. A radioautographic analysis of the migration and localization of trunk neural crest cells in the chick. *Dev. Biol. 6:* 279–310.

Weston, J.A. and S.L. Butler. 1966. Temporal factors affecting localization of neural crest cells in the chicken embryo. *Dev. Biol. 14:* 246–266.

Wolpert, L. 1969. Positional information and the spatial pattern of cellular differentiation. *J. Theor. Biol. 25:* 1–47.

———. 1978. Pattern formation in biological development. *Sci. Am. 239:* 154–164.

Reprinted from J. Comp. Neurol., Vol. 145, pp. 61–84. 1972

Mode of Cell Migration to the Superficial Layers of Fetal Monkey Neocortex [1]

PASKO RAKIC

Department of Neuropathology, Harvard Medical School, Boston, Massachusetts 02115

ABSTRACT   Golgi and electronmicroscopic methods were used to define the shapes and intercellular relationships of cells migrating from their sites of origin near the ventricular surface across the intermediate zone to the superficial neocortical layers of the parietooccipital region in the brains of 75- to 97-day monkey fetuses. After mitotic division in either ventricular or subventricular zones, the cells enter the intermediate zone and assume an elongated bipolar form oriented toward the cortical plate. The leading processes, 50 to 70 μ long, are irregular cytoplasmic cylinders containing prominent Golgi apparatus, mitochondria, microtubules, ribosomal rosettes, immature endoplasmic reticulum and occasional centrioles. They usually terminate in several attenuated expansions, the longest one oriented toward the cortical plate. The trailing processes are more slender, relatively uniform in caliber and display few organelles.

Throughout the 3500 μ pathway across the intermediate zone the migrating cells are apposed to elongated, radially oriented, immature glial processes which span the full thickness of the cerebral wall. Most of the perikarya of these glial cells in the younger specimens lie in the ventricular or subventricular zones, but in older fetuses of this series many are found in the intermediate zone. The main characteristics of these fibers are: elongated cylindrical form containing numerous microtubules; electronlucent cytoplasmic matrix; short lamellate expansions protruding at right angles from the segment of the fiber which runs through the intermediate zone; and terminal endfeet joined at the pial surface to form a continuous sheet coated externally with basement membrane. It is suggested that glial radial fibers provide guidelines for cell migration through the complex mixture of closely packed cell processes and cell bodies that compose the developing cerebral wall. Strong surface affinity between radial fiber and migrating cell is suggested in regions where both follow precisely the same curving course from subventricular to intermediate zones and also in areas where large extracellular spaces separate other cells and processes but in which migrating cells and radial fibers remain closely paired nonetheless. Specific affinity between them is implied in the failure of migrating cells to follow any of the myriad differently-oriented processes they encounter. Several generations of postmitotic cells appear to migrate along the same radial fiber, a developmental mechanism that would allow for the vertical cell columns of adult neocortex.

The classical hypothesis that neocortex is formed by outward movement of postmitotic cells generated in proliferative zones close to the ventricular surface (Vignal, 1888; Ramón y Cajal, 1891; Kölliker, 1896; His, '04) was based on observation of numerous mitotic figures in the ventricular zone (terminology recommended by the Boulder Committee, '70), their absence in the developing cortical plate itself, and the presence of bipolar cells oriented in the intermediate zone so as to suggest migration. Thymidine-H³ autoradiography has provided further evidence for this hypothesis. In rodents, cells synthesizing DNA at the time of exposure to thymidine-H³ undergo final division in

[1] Supported by research grant 5-R01-NS09081 from the National Institute of Neurological Diseases and Stroke, National Institutes of Health (USA).

the ventricular zone and their daughter cells can be detected as labeled neurons in neocortex (Angevine and Sidman, '61; Berry and Rogers, '65; Hicks and D'Amato, '68; Shimada and Langman, '70). These studies demonstrated further that cells are not passively displaced to the periphery by cells subsequently generated, but rather, many late-forming cells take up final positions external to their predecessors and constitute progressively more superficial layers of the cortex.

An unsolved problem concerns how the postmitotic cells, particularly at late stages of cortical development, pass virtually in a straight line first through an intermediate zone composed of fibers in several orientations and then through a deep cortical zone already packed with maturing neurons. One hypothesis holds that neurons do not actually migrate, but instead, simply translocate their nuclei from ventricular zone to cortical plate within attenuated cytoplasmic cylinders attached to both inner and outer surfaces of the thickening brain wall (Berry and Rogers, '65; Morest, '70). An alternative mechanism is considered in the present study. Cells are migratory, and move outward along processes of other cells which traverse the entire thickness of the cerebral wall. Such a mechanism has been demonstrated recently by electronmicroscopic analysis of granule cell migration from the external granular layer to the (internal) granular layer in the developing cerebellum. In this case the migrating cells lie directly apposed to radially-oriented Bergmann glial fibers during the entire course of their movement across the molecular layer (Rakic, '71a). It was suggested that this neuron-glia relationship both guides and facilitates the migration of young granule cells, especially at late developmental stages when the molecular layer is more than 250 μ wide and already contains well-established synaptic contacts. In addition, it has been shown that cells destined to reach the cerebral neocortex at late developmental stages must complete even longer trajectories and are similarly apposed to radially oriented glial fibers which appear to provide the guidance for their movement (Rakic, '71b,c).

The present report deals in more detail with the structure and intercellular relationships of such migrating cells as observed in Golgi and electronmicroscopic preparations. The reasons for studying migration in this particular late-forming cell population in primate material are that (a) the number of cells and complexity of their ramifications in the superficial layers increase in the evolutionary scale and reach a peak in primates (Hines, '34; Poliakov, '66); (b) these cells follow very long trajectories and in the large primate brain bypass numerous cells and processes on the way to their final destination, so that the mechanism for their migration might differ from that for early-formed neurons or even possibly for neurons in species with smaller brains; and (c) delineation of features characteristic of primates might contribute more directly than studies in rodents to an understanding of some salient developmental anomalies in man. In addition there is a practical, technical advantage, in that the size of monkey fetuses in the midgestational period, when the cell population in question migrates, is large and permits fixation by vascular perfusion for electron microscopy.

MATERIALS AND METHODS

Six *Macacus rhesus* monkeys pregnant for 75, 80, 81, 87, 95, and 97 days respectively (gestation in this species lasts 165–167 days) were used. The fetuses were removed by hysterotomy and while still in contact with the anesthetized mother via the umbilical cord, or immediately after separation, were perfused through the left side of the heart with the aid of a nitrogen-driven pump. The fixative was a gluteraldehyde-formaldehyde mixture (Karnovsky, '65) buffered to pH 7.4 with 0.1 M phosphate buffer to which 0.02% trinitrocresol was added. Quarter-strength fixative at 35°C was used for the first 15 minutes of perfusion, followed by half-strength fixative at room temperature during the next 10 to 20 minutes. Further procedures for processing the tissue were described previously (Rakic, '71a).

Particular attention was given to the dissection and orientation of the tissue blocks for electron microscopy. The exact orientation of the the migratory pathway in the cerebral hemishpere at the parieto-occipital junction was previously determined in Golgi preparations of fetal brains at similar ages, and blocks of tissue through the full thickness of the cerebral wall were dissected as nearly as possible parallel to the longitudinal axis of the migrating cells (fig. 1). Plastic sections through the entire block face (A in fig. 1) were cut at a thickness of 1 μ in order to verify and to adjust more precisely the angle of orientation. Only then was the specimen divided into four to six smaller cubes. Each was separately remounted either parallel (for example, a in fig. 1) or transverse (for example, b in fig. 1) to the axis of cell migration. A three-dimensional reconstruction of cell images was obtained by alternating

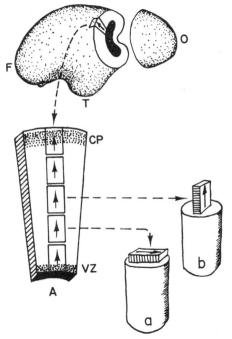

Fig. 1 The position of the dissected block (A) in the telencephalic wall of the 80-day monkey fetus. The cerebrum already contains well established frontal (F), occipital (O), and temporal (T) lobes. After the block is embedded in Maraglas and the orientation further adjusted (see MATERIALS AND METHODS), a series of smaller blocks in a vertical row from the ventricular zone (Z) to the cortical plate (CP) was taken and remounted for sectioning either parallel (a) or transverse (b) to the axis of cell migration.

series of thick (1–2 μ) with series of thin sections. Thick sections were stained with toluidine blue in 1% sodium borate for light microscopic observation. Thin sections were mounted on large mesh grids stained with lead citrate, and examined with a Zeiss 9S electron microscope at direct magnifications from 1,900 to 40,000 diameters. Rapid Golgi-impregnated material from the other cerebral hemisphere in each case was prepared and analyzed as described previously (Rakic, '71a). Selected sections were stained with cresyl violet, toluidine blue, or the periodic acid-Schiff method.

RESULTS

The monkey telencephalon at midgestation is already a complex assembly of cell bodies and processes. During the limited fetal period examined in this study the lateral cerebral wall at the parieto-occipital junction more than doubles in thickness (from less than 2 mm at 75 days to 5 mm at 97 days). By 75 days the cerebral wall consists of ventricular, subventricular and intermediate zones, cortical plate and lamina zonalis (fig. 2A). The ventricular zone is already less than 60 μ thick and continues to decrease in thickness until it has almost disappeared in the 97-day specimen. The subventricular zone, however, maintains a relatively uniform thickness of more than 300 μ; it first begins to decrease in the oldest specimens of this series. At midgestation both zones appear to contain cells and cell processes of several different classes and numerous cells in division (fig. 2B, C).

The intermediate zone at 75 days already contains numerous fiber components. Among them, the axons of the optic radiations form a particularly distinct layer of closely-packed, transversely cut fibers of small diameter immediately external to the subventricular zone, as seen in coronal sections at the parieto-occipital junction (figs. 2A, 3). Numerous other fiber constituents situated external to the optic radiation were not identified but most probably represent a mixture of afferent and efferent projections and immature cortico-cortical connections.

This report focuses on a population of bipolar cells most of which presumably originate in the subventricular zone and

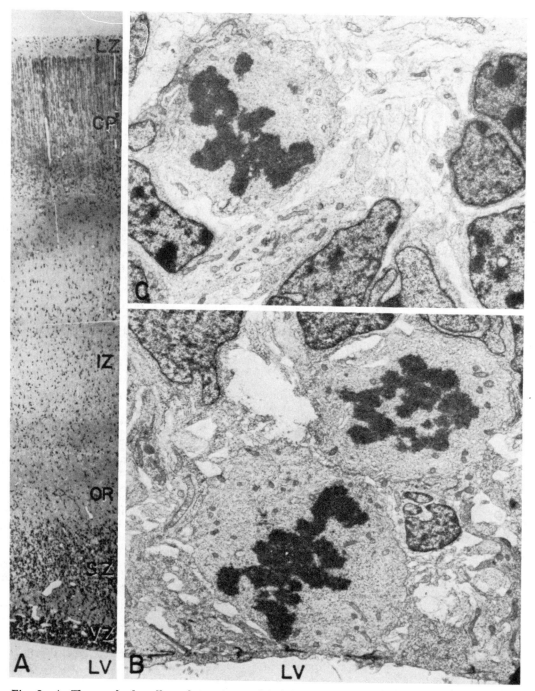

Fig. 2 A. The cerebral wall at the parieto-occipital junction in the brain of an 80-day monkey fetus. One micron section stained with toluidine blue. × 60. Abbreviations: CP, cortical plate; IZ, intermediate zone; LV, lateral ventricle; LZ, lamina zonalis; OR, optic radiation; SZ, subventricular zone; VZ, ventricular zone. B. Same specimen, electronmicrograph at the surface of the lateral ventricle (LV) to show mitotic figures. × 6,200. C. A mitotic figure in the middle of the subventricular zone of the same specimen. × 6,200.

migrate across the complex intermediate zone to the cortex (figs. 2A, 3), but before describing the cytology of the migrating cell, it is necessary to describe a prominent scaffolding of elongated fibers that penetrate radially across the telencephalic wall at these fetal ages.

A. *Fetal radial fibers*

A striking feature of the fetal macaque telencephalon at the migestational period is the presence of numerous radially oriented fibers which in most instances traverse the entire width of the cerebral wall (fig. 3). In younger fetuses (75-87 days of gestation) the radial arrangement is very regular. In slightly older specimens (95–97 days), the fibers systematically curve in areas where fissures are beginning to form, but even in such areas the basic radial alignment is preserved (figs. 3A, 5A). In the younger specimens the cell bodies from which radial fibers originate are situated predominantly in the ventricular and subventricular zones, whereas later, by 97 days, relatively large numbers of these cell somas have moved to the intermediate zone, and have lost their attachments to the ventricular surface.

In Golgi-stained specimens, the radial fibers are easily recognized by their elongated linear form extending from the parent cell body to the pial surface, where they terminate in a characteristic endfoot (figs. 3, 4). Frequently the radial fiber divides at the border of marginal zone and cortical plate into two or more terminal branches, each forming an endfoot at the pial surface (figs. 3, 4C). In electronmicrographs endfeet are displayed as pyramidal-shaped electronlucent cytoplasmic enlargements filled with characteristically dispersed smooth endoplasmic reticulum (fig. 4D). The hemispheric surface consists of palisades of these endfeet coated externally with basement membrane (BM in fig. 4D). The appearance is that of an immature glia limitans similar to that formed by the endfeet of Bergmann glial fibers in the developing cerebellar cortex. The periodic acid-Schiff stain, applied to light microscopic sections, gives a strong positive reaction for glycogen in the endfeet. The apparent absence of glycogen particles in the electronmicrographs may result from extraction during *en bloc* staining with uranyl acetate. A comparable result was obtained with Bergmann glia fibers (Rakic, '71a).

In the intermediate zone, the radial fiber shafts appear as rather coarse cylinders 0.8–1.2 μ thick, whereas most other processes are less than 0.5 μ thick. In younger specimens they display relatively small numbers of lamellate expansions, which radiate at a right angle from the main shaft. The number and size of these expansions increase in older specimens and become a characteristic feature of this specific cell process (LE in figs. 5C,D). The frequency and size of the expansions along the length of a given cell gradually decrease from cell body towards the cortical plate. At the point where the fibers penetrate vertically between the densely-packed cell bodies of the cortical plate, thy become difficult to trace because they intermingle with numerous ascending vertical processes of cortical neurons (figs. 3, 5A). Only in selected areas of Golgi preparations where cortical neurons are not impregnated, was it possible to demonstrate the entire course of the radial fibers. In such cases they terminate in endfeet at the pial surface (figs. 4A,B,C,E).

In spite of their characteristic silhouette in Golgi specimens, the electronmicroscopic identification of radial fibers and particularly of their parent somas posed a problem. Key criteria for their identification in the already complex neuropil of the intermediate zone were their straight radial orientation, the relatively large caliber of the shaft, and the lamellate expansions. Other helpful but less critical characteristics included the moderately electronlucent cytoplasmic matrix in which numerous longitudinally oriented microtubules and occasional elongated mitochondria were seen (RF in figs. 6A-D, 7D, 9, 10). The microtubules were straight 180 Å cylinders of indefinite length; they were never observed within the lamellate expansions. In several instances a membrane bounded electron-dense body filled with dense core vesicles was encountered in the main shaft (fig. 7D,E).

Although the radial fibers are linear throughout most of their course (figs. 5B,C,D, 6D) they become somewhat vari-

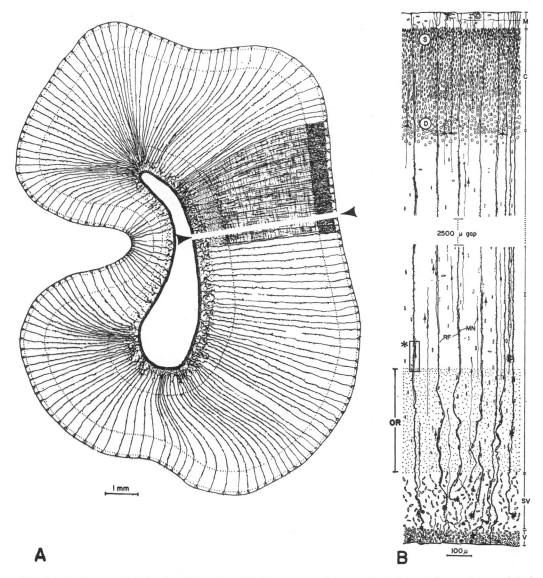

A

B

Fig. 3   A. Camera lucida drawing of a Golgi-impregnated coronal section at the parieto-occipital level of the brain of a 97-day monkey fetus.   The radial fibers are inscribed in slightly thicker lines than in the actual specimen in order to illustrate their arrangement at such a low magnification. (Scale equals 1 mm.)   The area delineated by the white strip between the arrowheads is drawn in B at higher magnification.   B. Composite camera lucida drawing of the cerebral wall in the area indicated by the white strip in A, combined from a Golgi section (black profiles) and an adjacent section stained with toluidine blue (outlined profiles).   The middle 2500 μ of the intermediate zone, similar in structure to the sectors drawn, is omitted.   The rectangle marked with an asterisk shows the approximate position of the three-dimensional reconstruction in figure 14.   100 μ scale indicates the magnification.   For further details, see text.   Abbreviations: C, cortical plate; D, deep cortical cells; I, intermediate zone; M, marginal layer; MN, migrating cell; OR, optic radiation; RF, radial fiber; S, superficial cortical cells; SV, subventricular layer; V, ventricular zone.

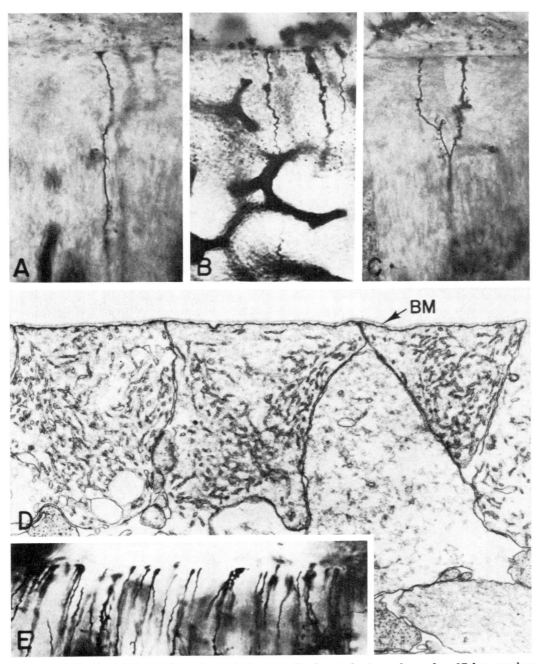

Fig. 4 A, B, C, and E. Endfeet of radial fibers at the hemispheric surface of a 97-day monkey fetus, impregnated by the Golgi method. × 400. D. Electronmicrograph of the external cerebral surface of the same specimen. Conical contiguous endfeet filled with smooth endoplasmic reticulum are coated externally with basement membrane (BM). × 16,200.

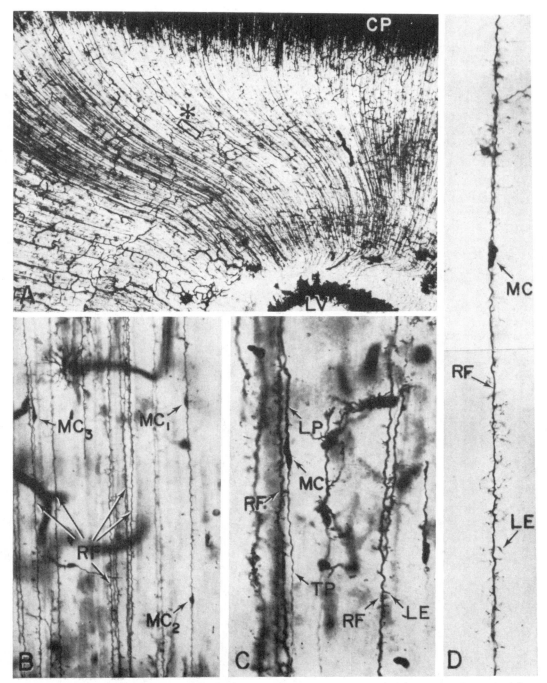

Fig. 5 Photomicrographs of the Golgi impregnated telencephalon of 97 day monkey fetus. A. A low power view of cerebral wall extending from the surface of the lateral ventricle (LV) to the cortical plate (CP) which displays a characteristic distribution of the radial fibers. The rectangle indicated by the asterisk is represented at higher magnification in D. × 32. B. A section cut parallel to the direction of radial fibers (RF) and migrating cells (MC₃). The cells MC₁ and MC₂ are discussed in the text. × 250. C. This micrograph displays at higher magnification the parallel orientation of the migrating cell soma (MC) its leading processes (LP) and trailing process (TP) with the radial fiber (RF). × 400. D. The portion of radial fiber (RF) at the level of the intermediate zone indicated by the rectangle marked with the asterisk in A. Note numerous lamellate expansions (LE) and the close apposition of the migrating cell (MC) whose leading process spirals around the radial fiber. For details see text. × 400.

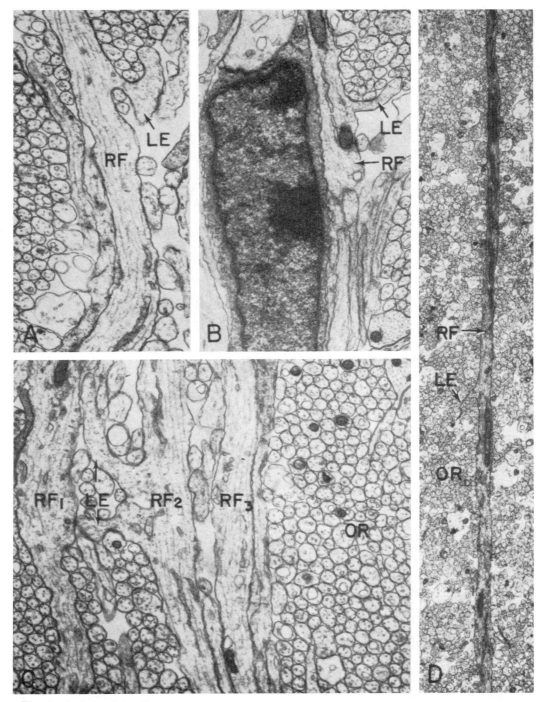

Fig. 6 A, B, and C. Electron micrographs of sections cut parallel to the radial fibers (RF) in an 80-day fetus. Note a presence of lamellate expansions (LE). At B the migratory cell lies apposed to a radial fiber (RF). All figures × 16,500. D. Lower power electron micrograph of a 97-day fetal brain at the level of the densely packed fibers of the optic radiation (OR). Note straight course of radial fiber (RF), oriented at a right angle to the transversely cut axons of the optic radiation (OR); its relatively large diameter contains many longitudinally oriented microtubules, elongated mitochondria and characteristic lamellate expansions (LE). × 6,200.

cose and curve as they emerge from the subventricular zone (figs. 3, 5A, 12). The plane of section in a few fortuitous instances, or the analysis of semiserial sections in other instances, allowed fibers to be followed in a retrograde direction from the intermediate zone to their origin in large and oval-shaped cell bodies in the superficial portion of the subventricular zone. The nucleus is variably lobulated, with homogeneously dispersed chromatin (fig. 7A,B). The cytoplasm contains, among the usual organelles, an elongated rough endoplasmic reticulum with parallel membranes arranged in a relatively unusual pattern (fig. 7A). Thin processes emerging from the cell body have been visualized in both Golgi micrographs (fig. 7C) and electronmicrographs (fig. 7A,B). In the limited number of positively identified cell bodies, no cytoplasmic process was found oriented towards the ventricle. The Golgi images indicate that it may no longer be present in cells with perikarya located some distance from the ventricular surface.

It was not possible on electronmicrographs to trace individual radial fibers inward through the subventricular zone. Therefore, in an attempt to identify more deeply situated cell bodies, the search was pursued outward from the ventricular surface. The shapes of cells in the Golgi preparations served for identification (compare fig. 8A,B). In cells thus identified, the process oriented towards the ventricle is a thick varicose stem with a dense cytoplasmic matrix and a very high concentration of microtubules and microfilaments (fig. 8). At the ages studied, the ventricular surfaces of these processes contain a variable number of microvilli and occasional cilia which protrude into the lumen of the lateral ventricle. Adjacent cells are connected by gap junctions (fig. 8B).

B. *Migrating cells in the intermediate zone*

The migrating cell in the intermediate zone can be recognized by its distinct bipolar, elongated form in Golgi preparations (figs. 3B, 5C, 9A). The leading cytoplasmic process, oriented toward the cortical plate, is an irregular voluminous cylinder with an average diameter of 1.5 to 2.5 μ. In most instances it does not exceed 70 μ in length. The trailing process oriented toward the ventricle is several times thinner (average 0.3 to 0.5 μ). Although the trailing process often could be followed for several hundred microns (figs. 5C, 9A), its mode of termination could not be established with certainty. Whether this was because it loses affinity for silver or leaves the plane of section was not resolved.

As a rule the longitudinal axis of the cell strictly parallels the orientation of a nearby radial fiber (fig. 5B, C), and this rigid cell orientation further simplified its identification in electronmicrographs. Its nucleus in spindle- or pear-shaped, occasionally lobulated with dispersed chromatin of moderate electron density. The leading process contains the usual organelles: mitochondria, Golgi apparatus, smooth endoplasmic reticulus, some rough endoplasmic reticulum, microtubules and numerous polyribosomes (figs. 9C, 10A). In some instances one or two centrioles were seen (CN in figs. 9C, 10A,B). The leading process usually terminates in thin (0.2–0.5 μ) pseudopodia of various lengths (figs. 9B, 12), some of them measuring almost 50 μ. It would require analysis of serial sections to establish their absolute length. The cytoplasm of the trailing process is very scanty close to the nucleus and abruptly attenuates into a thin elongated process almost devoid of organelles except for longitudinally-oriented microtubules (figs. 9E, 10C). In fortuitous planes of sections, such processes were followed for long distances in electronmicrographic montages (see, for example, fig. 1A in Rakic, '71b). The appearance of the migrating cells closely resembles the description of the immature migrating granule cell in the cerebellum (Mugnaini and Forstrønen, '66; Rakic, '71a).

C. *Migrating cell-radial fiber relationship*

The Golgi method rarely impregnates two adjacent cells (Ramón-Moliner, '70). Therefore it cannot be used with confidence to study interrelationships between contiguous elements such as radial fibers and migrating cells. Only in a few instances in our Golgi material is a migrating cell depicted in intimate apposition to a radial fiber. In some of these cases, close

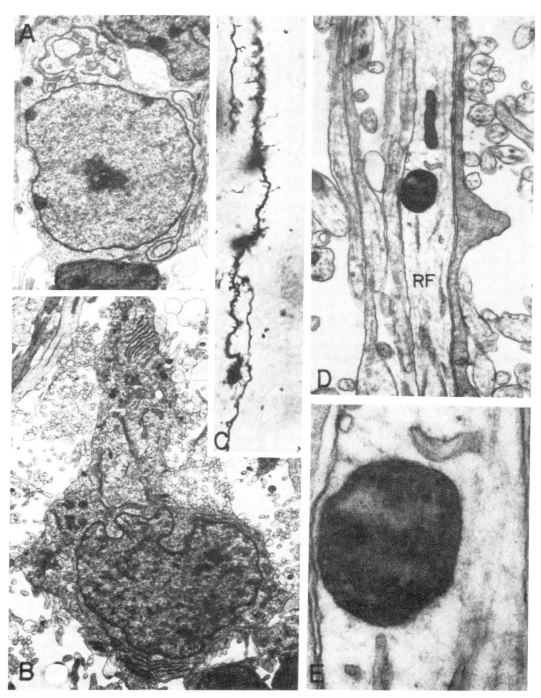

Fig. 7 A and B. Cell somas of radial glial cells situated in the external portion of the subventricular zone close to the border of the intermediate zone. Ninety seven day fetus. × 6,200. C. Similar cell in the same position as the cells in A and B, impregnated by the Golgi method. × 400. D. A longitudinal section through a radial fiber. Note the numerous microtubules, the mitochondrion and the dense body. × 22,000. E. Dense body at higher magnification. × 83,000.

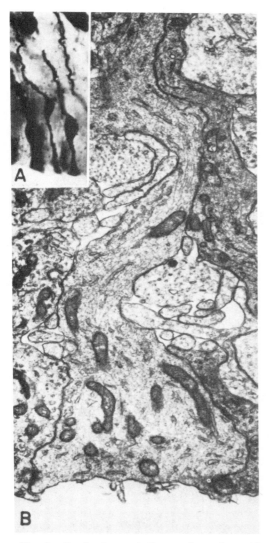

Fig. 8 Cerebral ventricular surface of an 80-day monkey fetus. Insert A represents Golgi images of the cell somas and their processes directed toward the ventricle. × 500. At B is the electronmicrograph of the similar process attached with gap junctions to the other cells at the ventricular surface. × 6,200.

examination through a range of focal planes suggests that the leading process of the migrating cell actually spirals around the radial fiber, though this point is difficult to demonstrate in the single plane of a photograph (fig. 5D). In other cases the migrating cell and radial fiber

are so closely apposed that it is virtually impossible to distinguish one from the other. Thus, for example, it is impossible to resolve whether the enlargements MC_1 and MC_2 in figure 5B represent two nuclei in the same fiber or two separate migrating cells aligned and closely apposed to a single radial fiber. The size and shape of the "lumps" (compare the migrating cell MC_3 to MC_1 and MC_2 in fig. 5B) support the possibility that two cells migrate across the same radial fiber, but adequate resolution of this relationship was possible only with the electron microscope.

Electronmicroscopic examination of the intermediate zone in a plane parallel to the main axis of the migrating bipolar cells reveals that they are directly apposed to radial fibers consistently along their entire course (figs. 6B, 9B-E, 10A-F). Even in ultrathin sections in which such an apposition is not observed, further serial sections almost always demonstrate the relationship. In the area of mutual contact the cells display smooth surfaces with a distance of about 200 Å between outermost dense lines of the apposed surface membranes. Occasionally the site of apposition is filled with an electrondense material (fig. 11F, arrows) representing either a fixation artifact, a membrane specialization, or a substance in the intercellular gap; this issue could not be resolved because membranes in this fetal material appeared not to be fixed satisfactorily enough for reliable study at high magnifications.

The constancy of the relationship between migrating cell and radial fiber was verified in sections cut transverse to the major axis of the cells. The soma of the migrating cell in such sections appears round or slightly oval, and is always in contact with several transversely cut fibers, which collectively form a distinct fascicle (fig. 11A-F). The fibers in such a fascicle vary in diameter and differ slightly in electron density, but have no distinguishing ultrastructural features at the fetal ages studied. Some of the thinner profiles are probably trailing processes of cells whose somas have crossed the level of the intermediate zone under examination and lie closer to the cortical plate. Other processes may be afferent axons originating in the thalamus or possible efferent axons of cor-

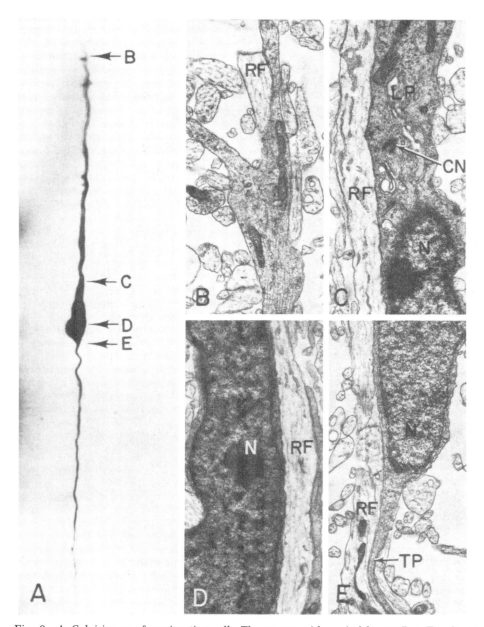

Fig. 9 A. Golgi image of a migrating cell. The arrows with capital letters B to E indicate approximate levels of electron photomicrographs of similar cells. × 1,000. B. Leading tip with ventrical expansion aligned with radial fiber (RF). C. Cytoplasm of leading process (LP) in front of the nucleus (N) containing Golgi apparatus, mitochondria, ribosomes and a centriole (CN). D. The midportion of the cell soma and nucleus (N). E. The inner pole of the nucleus (N) and the beginning of the trailing process (TP). Note a constant approximately 200 Å wide space between the apposed migrating cell and radial fibers (RF), in spite of the large extracellular spaces in the tissue. All electronmicrographs. × 15,000.

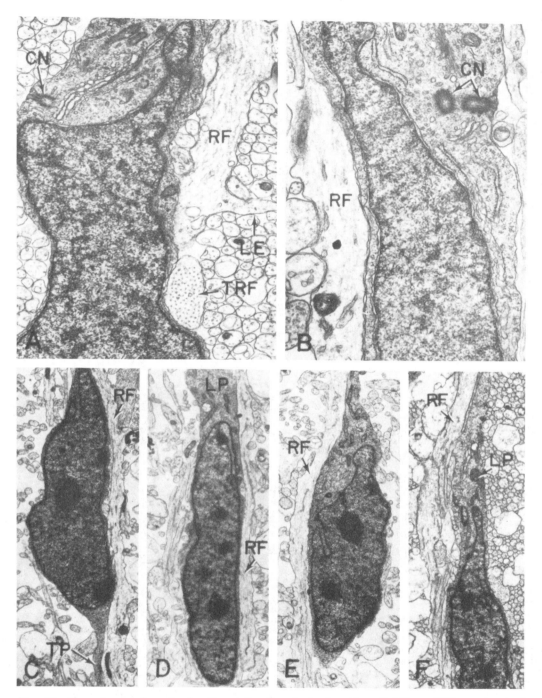

Fig. 10   Several examples of migrating cells aligned closely with radial fibers (RF) as seen in the plane parallel to the main cell axis. A. 80-day fetus, × 22,000; B. 97-day fetus, × 22,000; C. 97-day fetus, × 6,200; D. 97-day fetus, × 6,200; E. 97-day fetus, × 6,200; F. 75-day fetus, × 6,200. For further details see text. Abbreviations: CN, centriole; LE, lamellate expansion; LP, leading process; RF, radial fibers; TP, trailing process; TRF, transversely cut radial fibers.

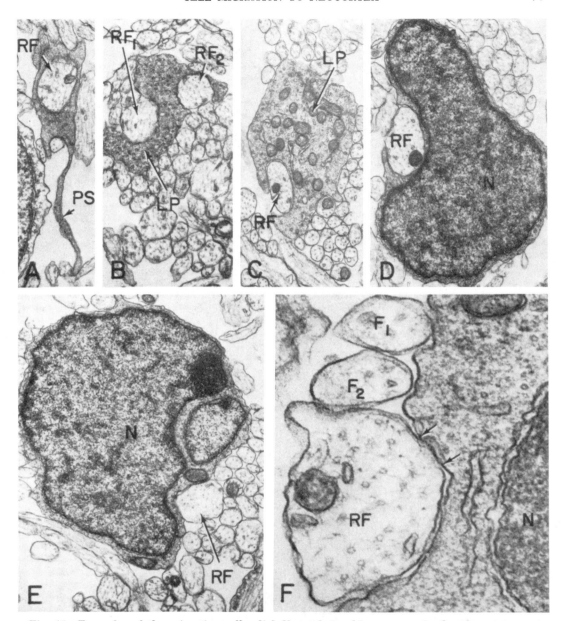

Fig. 11 Examples of the migrating cell-radial fiber relationships as seen in the plane transverse to the main cell axis at different levels of the intermediate zone. 80-day monkey fetus. A to E, × 16,200. F, × 83,000. Abbreviations: F_1, F_2, nerve fibers; LP, leading process; PS, pseudopodia; N, nucleus of migrating cell; RF, radial fibers. Arrows in F indicate surface appositions which represent possible specialized contact points, as discussed further in text.

tical neurons. One or more fibers in most fascicles were at least one order of magnitude thicker than the rest (RF in fig. 11). The caliber (0.8 to 1.2 μ), the density, and the disposition of microtubules indicate that these profiles are probably the radial fibers, especially since they are as a rule in direct contact with the migrating cells. Occasionally the leading cytoplasmic process of the migrating cell partially envelops the radial fiber (fig. 11B,C,D) and in some instances, actually encircle it (fig. 11A). Such an "embrace," is however, not a constant finding; it has been demonstrated only intermittently along the leading process and soma of the migrating cell. The thin trailing process was not seen to enter such a relationship (fig. 14).

The apposition of migrating cell and radial fiber is apparently established, at least in some instances, in the subventricular zone. Cells entering the deep portion of the intermediate zone follow closely the radial fibers as they penetrate between the densely packed axons of the optic radiations and other fiber systems (figs. 2A,B, 14). In a particularly fortuitous section through the junction of subventricular zone and optic radiation four pseudopodial expansions are seen emanating from one leading process (fig. 12A). The expansion of the right side of the electronmicrograph (PS$_4$ in fig. 12A) is closely apposed to the curved radial fiber for a distance of several microns. Presumably the cell becomes committed in some way to follow one probing pseudopodium (fig. 12B), so that as the cell moves along that pathway, the other pseudopodia are withdrawn. Although at certain points the migrating cell may be detached from the radial fiber for a short distance, perhaps by the intercession of other thin fibers, as schematically illustrated at the level of the asterisk in figure 14, it in general adheres to the fiber throughout its curving radial trajectory to the cortical plate (fig. 12B).

The migrating cell penetrates the cortical plate and passes outward between differentiating neurons which had arrived earlier. In contrast to the relatively immature migrating cells which stain darkly (C3, C5, C6, C7 and C8 in fig. 13), the neurons that already reside in the cortex have relatively lucent cytoplasm and more oval or round nuclei with lighter chromatin (C1, C4, and C10 in fig. 13). Neuron somas in the more superficial cortical levels are generally smaller, spindle shaped, and darker, i.e., appear less mature. This gradient in cell differentiation is consistent with the "inside out" sequence

of cell birthdays shown by autoradiography (see INTRODUCTION).

A vertical columnar arrangement of cells in the cortical plate is a prominent feature of this developmental stage (C1 to C5 in fig. 13). The gradient of cell differentiation suggests that a given vertical column may be composed of successive generations of cells all of which followed the same migratory path. The darker, less differentiated cell (C5 in fig. 13) presumably moved to its position along the same radial fiber that guided its more differentiated and more deeply located predecessor (C4 in fig. 13), both cells sharing a vertical axis determined by a common radial fiber. However, the relationship between migrating cell and radial fiber has not been analyzed in detail at the level of the cortical plate because the radial fibers become thinner, lose their lamellate expansion and are indistinguishable from other immature process of similar caliber, character, and orientation (VF in fig. 13).

DISCUSSION

The telencephalon is already very complex in the monkey fetus at the midgestational stages analyzed in this report. The cortical plate alone is several hundred microns thick. It is composed of 30 to 50 rows of cell somas and will gain still more cells as .development continues. In order for these new cells generated in the ventricular and subventricular zones to attain positions in the cortical plate, they must cross the intermediate zone, which by this stage has become more than 1500 μ wide and is packed with numerous fiber systems in various orientations. The main contribution of the present report is the demonstration that these late-arising cells find their way to the cortex by assuming a bipolar form and moving outward in direct and constant apposition to radial glial processes that span almost the entire width of the telencephalic wall (see also Rakic, '71b,c).

Three general questions will be considered concerning this intercellular relationship.

1. *Do the young neurons actually migrate?*

The assumption made in classical studies and in more recent autoradio-

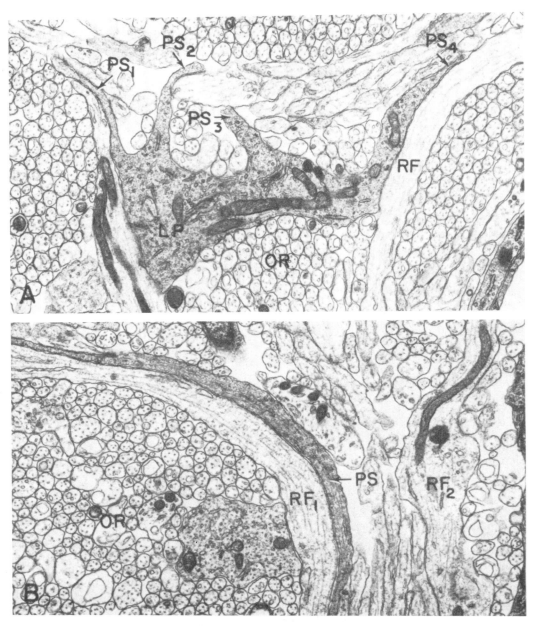

Fig. 12 Electronmicrographs of the portion of the intermediate zone slightly above the subventricular zone, filled with transversely cut fibers of the optic radiation (OR). A. Four pseudopodia (PS₁₋₄) radiate from the leading process (LP). The pseudopodium at the right (PS₄) has the longest area of apposition to the radial fiber (RF). B. Another field of the same section in which an elongated pseudopodium (PS) remains aligned with the radial fiber (RF) for even a longer distance. Both electronmicrographs, × 16,200.

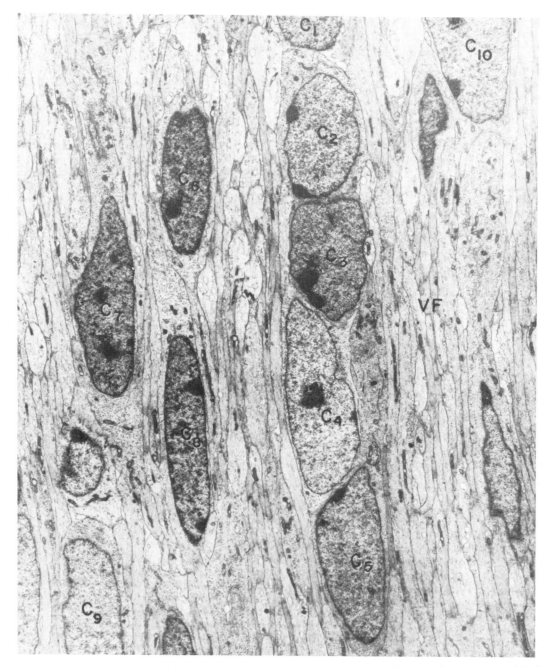

Fig. 13   Electronmicrograph of the medial portion of the cortical plate at the parieto-occipital junction of a 97-day fetus. Cells C_1- to C_5 are clearly aligned in the straight vertical column parallel to the numerous vertical fibers (VF). For explanation, see text. $\times$ 5,000.

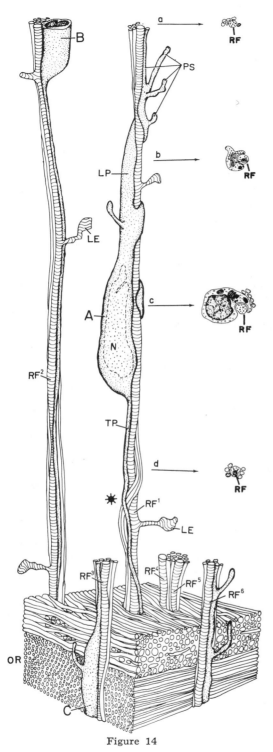

Figure 14

graphic work that young neurons migrate (see INTRODUCTION) has been questioned on the basis of Golgi data on the developing brains of small mammals (Berry and Rogers, '65; Morest, '69, '70). The autoradiographic evidence, previously cited, is not conclusive, for only the position of the nucleus is charted in standard autoradiograms. The issue of migration must be delineated in terms of the variations in shape of the whole cell as it changes its position with time (Morest, '69). In opossum pouch young, some postmitotic young neurons early in the course of cortical histogenesis develop processes which span the entire cerebral wall. The interpretation was offered that the nucleus then becomes translocated outward, even though the overall position of the cell remains fixed (Morest, '70). However, little account was taken of the probability that many of the cells with radial processes are still premitotic. Such a cell becomes round when it divides near the ventricular surface (Stensaas and Stensaas, '68; Hinds and Ruffett, '71), and a key unresolved problem is how its subsequently-generated external process will come to attain a radial orientation. In recognition of this issue,

Fig. 14 Three dimensional semi-diagrammatic reconstruction of the relationships between migrating cells and radial fibers in the intermediate zone at approximately the level indicated by the rectangle and asterisk in figure 3B. The subventricular zone lies some distance below the area selected for reconstruction, whereas the cortex is more than 1,000 μ above it. The lower portion of the diagram contains uniform, parallel fibers of the optic radiation (OR) and the remainder is occupied by more variable and irregularly disposed fiber systems; the border between the two systems is easily recognized. Except at the lower portion of the figure, most of these fibers are deleted from the diagram in order to expose the radial fibers (striped vertical shafts RF$_{1-6}$) and their relationships to the migrating cells (A, B, and C) and to other vertical processes. The soma of migrating cell A, with its nucleus (N) and voluminous leading process (LP) is within the reconstructed space, except for the terminal part of the attenuated trailing process and the tip of the vertical ascending pseudopodium. Cross sections of cell A in relation to the several vertical fibers in the fascicle are drawn at levels "a" to "d" at the right side of the figure and should be compared to figure 11. The perikaryon of cell B is cut off at the top of the reconstructed space, whereas the leading process of cell C is shown just penetrating between fibers of the optic radiation (OR) on its way across the intermediate zone. Further explanation in text.

Berry and Rogers ('65) suggested that only the nucleus divides at the ventricular surface and that the two daughter cells become separated later, after one nucleus has moved to the cortex within the elongated cylinder of undivided cytoplasm. They occasionally observed two separate somatic enlargements along one fiber traversing the cerebral wall by light microscopic examination of Golgi-stained sections or by dark field examination of teased fresh brain tissue. The greater resolving power of the electron microscope now allows clear recognition that the image of apparent binucleate cells probably represents two cells in close apposition to a single radial fiber, as described in the present report. The important qualification must be added that the cell types and the details of their relationship remain to be examined by electron microscopy at early stages of development. Several earlier observers did describe bipolar migrating cells with their outer process, inner process, or both failing to reach a cerebral surface (Ramón y Cajal, '11; Godina, '51; Åström, '67; Stansaas, '67b; Stensaas and Stensaas, '68).

In the fetal monkey cerebrum at the relatively late stages studied in the present report, the postmitotic neurons appear in both Golgi and electronmicroscopic preparations to assume bipolar shapes. The leading process is usually not more than 50 to 70 μ long. Attenuated expansions of pseudopodia sprout from the tip of each leading process, and while their exact length could not be established, few or none of them were noted to reach the pial surface, even in sections cut transverse to the direction of cell movement. Thus, migration appears to constitute a real event, though in some instances, the young neuron may transiently anchor its extended processes at the inner or outer surfaces of the cerebral wall and translocate its nuclear region within a fixed cytoplasmic cylinder.

2. What is the source of the radial fibers?

The presence of elongated, radially disposed glial fibers which traverse the fetal cerebral wall as described in many species soon after the introduction of the Golgi method (Golgi, 1883; Magini, 1888; Retzius, 1893; Sala y Pons, 1894; Thomas, 1894) and later was confirmed repeatedly (Castro, '20; Lorente de Nó, '33; Penfield, '39; Godina, '51; Stensaas, '67a; Åström et al., '67). Nevertheless, difficulties in classification of embryonic neuroglia, and misconceptions about their time and place of genesis, have led to confusion concerning the nature of this class of cells (e.g., His, 1889; Hardesty, '04; Streeter, '12) and at times even to a denial of their existence.

At all ages examined by the Golgi method in the present study, the radial fibers were recognized as belonging to a distinct, though probably transient, class of glial cells. The radial orientation, straight course, relatively large caliber, and the lamellate expansions collectively define the radial fibers in Golgi preparations, and serve further for their identification in low magnification electronmicroscopic montages and thence in more highly magnified images.

Such cells as these with radially-disposed processes were classified by Ramón y Cajal ('11) as primitive or modified astrocytes. Consistent with his interpretation are the new observations in the monkey fetus that these cells show relatively electronlucent cytoplasm, lamellate expansions at a right angle to the main shaft of the fiber, and glycogen granules in their expanded distal terminals. The abundance of microtubules, though not a diagnostic feature, was seen also in immature cells of astrocytic lineage in other regions of the central nervous system in the rat (Peters and Vaughn, '67; Vaughn, '69) and in the fetal monkey cerebellum (Rakic, '71a). Finally, even within the short developmental period examined in the present study, there were transitional forms between these cells and cells of more typical astrocytic morphology. This was evident as a function both of increasing age and of increasing distance from the ventricular surface.

3. Is the relationship between migrating cell and radial fiber merely fortuitous?

A three-dimensional reconstruction summarizing present and earlier observations

(Rakic, '71b,c), obtained by combining data from Golgi images, electronmicroscopic montages, and semiserial thin sections in carefully selected planes, is illustrated in figure 14. Although the migrating cell encounters myriad processes in various orientations, it remains constantly apposed to radially-oriented fibers. A strong affinity between them is suggested also by images showing the precision of apposition even where the processes follow a curving course between subventricular and intermediate zones. The same close contact is found in areas of the intermediate zone where large extracellular spaces separate other cell processes from each other but do not interrupt the migrating cell-radial fiber relationship. In transverse sections the processes of the migrating cell are seen to "embrace" the radial fiber intermittently, thereby increasing the area of contact.

Speculation might be entertained that the radial fiber provides some graded signal along its length so as to provide directionality for the migrating neuron. However, it is pertinent to note that the somatic region of the immature granule cell neuron of the cerebellar cortex crosses the molecular layer from outside inward by moving along a radially-oriented Bergmann glial fiber in chick (Mugnaini, and Frostrønen, '66), monkey (Rakic, '71a), and mouse (Landis, '71). In the cerebellum the direction of migration is toward the glial cell soma, whereas in the cerebral cortex the direction is away from the glial cell soma. Gradients of opposite sign would have to be hypothesized in the two cases.

The consistency of the relationship between migrating neuron and glial fiber suggests a stronger affinity between these two cell types than between most other cell pairings, but the observations do not contribute to the issue of specificity of contact. Possibly the migrating cell would follow any fiber that maintains a radial orientation. It should be noted that radially-oriented processes typically occur in fascicles (fig. 14). Some afferent axons might be incorporated into these fascicles in addition to the one or two glial processes and the several neuronal bipolar processes. Also, the several migrating cells that follow successively along the same

pathway might guide one another, rather than depending on the glial fiber. Such a neuron-to-neuron guidance might be particularly appropriate to consider at earlier stages of cortical genesis, when identification of cell types is very difficult and almost all cells maintain a radial orientation and elongated shape. Conversely, young glial cells as well as neurons might move to the intermediate zone and cortical plate along guiding radial fibers.

The evidence for passage of several neurons in succession along a common radial path comes from electronmicroscopic analysis. The significance of the sequential migration probably relates to the columnar organization of cerebral neocortex (Lorente de Nó, '49; Mountcastle, '57; Hubel and Wiesel, '62, '69; Bonin and Mehler, '71). The cells that follow a given radial fiber appear to stack in a common vertical row within the cortical plate, the more mature-appearing cells generally lying deep to the less mature ones. This vertical columnar organization of cell somas is very pronounced at early and middle developmental stages, though later it will become obscured by the growth of lateral dendrites and other horizontally and obliquely oriented processes.

ACKNOWLEDGMENTS

I am pleased to express my appreciation to Dr. T. C. Jones and Dr. F. Garcia of the New England Regional Primate Research Cetner, Southboro, Mass. for making timed pregnancies available for this study. Expert Caesarean section by Dr. F. Garcia are greatfully acknowledged.

LITERATURE CITED

Angevine, J. B., Jr., and R. L. Sidman 1961 Autoradiographic study of cell migration during histogenesis of cerebral cortex in the mouse. Nature, 192: 766–768.

Aström, K. E. 1967 On the early development of the isocortex in fetal sheep. In: Progress in Brain Research, Developmental Neurology. C. B. Bernhard and J. P. Schadé, eds. Elsevier, Amsterdam, 26: 1–59.

Berry, M., and A. W. Rogers 1965 The migration of neuroblasts in the developing cerebral cortex. J. Anat., 99: 691–709.

Bonin, G. von, and W. R. Mehler 1971 On columnar arrangement of nerve cells in cerebral cortex. Brain Research, 27: 1–9.

Boulder Committee 1970 Embryonic vertebrate central nervous system: Revised terminology. Anat. Rec., 166: 257–262.

Castro, F. de 1920 Algunas observaciones sobre la histogénesis de la neuroglia en el bulbo olfactivo. Trabajos, Lab. Invest., *18:* 83–109.

Godina, G, 1951 Istogenesis e differenziazione del neuroni e degli element gliali della corteccia cerebrale. Z. Zellforsch., *36:* 401–435.

Golgi, C. 1883 Sulla fina anatomia degli organi centrali del sistema nervoso. Republished in: Opera Omnia, Hoepli, Milan, 1903 pp. 397–536.

Hardesty, I. 1904 On the development and nature of the neuroglia. Am. J. Anat., *3:* 230–268.

Hicks, S. P., and G. J. D'Amato 1968 Cell migrations to the isocortex in the rat. Anat. Rec., *160:* 619–634.

Hinds, J. W., and T. L. Ruffett 1971 Cell proliferation in the neural tube: An electron microscopic and Golgi analysis in the mouse cerebral vesicle. Z. Zellforsch., *115:* 226–264.

Hines, M. 1934 Cyto-architecture of the cerebral cortex in man. In: Localization of Function in the Cerebral Cortex. Res. Publ. Assn. Res. Nerv. Ment. Dis. Proc., *8:* 26–28.

His, W. 1889 Die Neuroblasten und der Entstehung im embrionalen Mark. Arch. Anat. Psychol., Anat. Abth., pp. 249–300.

———— 1904 Die Entwickelung des menschlichen Gehirns wahrend der ersten Monte. Hirzel, Leipzig, 176 pages.

Hubel, D. H., and T. N. Wiesel 1962 Receptive fields, binocular interaction and functional architecture in cat's visual cortex. J. Physiol., *160:* 106–154.

———— 1969 Anatomical demonstration of columns in the monkey striate cortex. Nature, *221:* 747–750.

Karnovsky, M. J. 1965 A formaldehyde-glutaraldehyde fixative of high osmolarity for use in electronmicroscopy. J. Cell Biol., *27:* 137A–138A.

Kölliker, A 1896 Handbuch der Gewebelehre des Menschen. Vol. 2. Nervensystem des Menschen under die Thiere. Engelman, Leipzig, 409 pages.

Landis, R. M. 1971 Development of the cerebellar cortex in the normal and staggerer mouse. Thesis, Harvard Medical School, 59 pages.

Lorente de Nó, R. 1933 Studies on the structure of the cerebral cortex. J. Psychol. Neurol., Lepizig, *45:* 381–438.

———— 1949 Architectonics and structure of the cerebral cortex. In: Physiology of the Nervous System. Fourth ed. J. F. Fulton, ed. Oxford University Press, New York, pp. 288–330.

Magini, G. 1888 Sur la néuroglie et les cellules nerveuses cérébrales chez les foetus. Arch. ital. Biol., *9:* 59–60.

Morest, D. K. 1969 The differentiation of cerebral dendrites: a study of post-migratory neuroblast in the medial nucleus of the trapezoid body. Z. Anat. Entwickl.-Gesch., *128:* 271–289.

———— 1970 A study of neurogenesis in the forebrain of oppossum pouch young. Z. Anat. Entwickl.-Gesch., *130:* 265–305.

Mountcastle, V. B. 1957 Modality and topographic properties of single neurons of cat's

somatic sensory cortex. J. Neurophysiol., *20:* 408–434.

Mugnaini, E., and P. F. Forstrønen 1967 Ultrastructural studies on the cerebellar histogenesis. I. Differentiation of granule cells and development of glomeruli in the chick embryo. Z. Zellforsch., *77:* 115–143.

Penfield, W. 1939 Neuroglia, normal and pathological. In: Cytology and Cellular Pathology of the Nervous System. Vol. 2. W. Penfield, ed. Hafner, New York, pp. 423–479.

Peters, A., and J. E. Vaughn 1967 Microtubules and filaments in the axons and astrocytes of early postnatal rat optic nerves. J. Cell Biol., *32:* 113–119.

Poliakov, G. I. 1966 Embryonal and postnatal development of neurons of the human cerebral cortex. In: Evolution of the Forebrain. R. Hassler, and H. Stephan, eds. G. Thieme, Stuttgart, pp. 249–258.

Rakic, P. 1971a Neuron-glia relationship during granule cell migration in developing cerebellar cortex. A Golgi and electronmicroscopic study in macacus rhesus. J. Comp. Neur., *141:* 283–312.

———— 1971b Guidance of neurons migrating to the fetal monkey neocortex. Brain Research, *33:* 471–476.

———— 1971c Radial glial fibers as guides for cell migrating to the superficial layers of fetal monkey neocortex. Abst. Am. Soc. Cell Biol., *11:* 238.

Ramón-Moliner, E. 1970 The Golgi-Cox technique. In: Contemporary Research Methods in Neuroanatomy. W. J. H. Nauta and S. O. E. Ebbesson, eds. Springer, New York, Heidelberg, Berlin, pp. 32–55.

Ramón y Cajal S. 1891 Sur la structure de l'écorce ⁼éérébrale de quelques mammifères. La Cellule, *7:* 125–178.

———— 1911 Histologie de Système Nerveux de l'Homme et des Vertébrés. Vol. 2. Paris, Maloine. Reprinted by Consejo Superior de Investigaciones Cientificas, Madrid, 1955, pp. 847–861.

Retzius, G. 1893 Studien über Ependym und Neuroglia. Biologische Untersuchungen (Stockholm), *5:* 9–26.

Sala y Pons, C. 1894 La Neuroglia de los Vertebrados. Casa Provinial de Caridad, Barcelona, 44 pages.

Shimada, M., and J. Langman 1970 Cell proliferation, migration and differentiation in the cerebral cortex of the golden hamster. J. Comp. Neur., *139:* 227–244.

Stensaas, L. J. 1967a The development of hippocampal and dorsolateral pallial regions of the cerebral hemisphere in fetal rabbits. I. Fifteen millimeter stage, spongioblast morphology. J. Comp. Neur., *129:* 59–70.

———— 1967b The development of hippocampal and dorsolateral pallial regions of the cerebral hemisphere in fetal rabbits. II. Twenty millimeter stage, neuroblast morphology. J. Comp. Neur., *129:* 71–84.

Stensaas, L. J., and S. S. Stensaas 1968 An electron microscope study of cells in the matrix and intermediate laminae of the cerebral hemisphere of the 45 mm rabbit embryo. Z. Zellforsch., *91:* 341–365.

Streeter, G. L. 1912 The development of the nervous system. In: Manual of Human Embryology. Vol. 2. F. Keibel and F. P. Mall, eds Lippincott, Philadelphia and London, pp. 1–116.

Thomas, M. A. 1894 Contribution a l'étude du dévelopment des cellules d'écorce cérébrale par méthode de Golgi. Compt. Rend. Soc Biol., *46:* 66–68.

Vaughn, J. E. 1969 An electron microscopic analysis of gliogenesis in rat optic nerves. Z. Zellforsch., *94:* 293–324.

Vignal, W. 1888 Recherches sur le développment des éléments des couches corticales du cerveau et du cervelet chez l'homme et les mammiféres. Arch. Physiol. norm. path, (Paris), *2:* 228–254.

DEVELOPMENTAL BIOLOGY 42, 106–130 (1975)

An Analysis of the Migratory Behavior
of Avian Cephalic Neural Crest Cells[1]

DREW M. NODEN[2]

Department of Biology, Washington University, St. Louis Missouri 63130

Accepted September 17, 1974

The neural crest cells migrate from their origin into many regions of the vertebrate embryo. Upon reaching their terminal destinations, members of this population undergo cytodifferentiation into a wide range of diverse cell types. To follow the early migratory behavior of avian cephalic neural crest cells, neural fold tissue was transplanted orthotopically from a ^{3}H-thymidine-labeled donor into an unlabeled host. The hosts were sacrificed at subsequent stages and the positions of all labeled neural crest-derived cells ascertained radioautographically. Crest cells emigrating from each of three different preotic regions of the brain displayed unique patterns of migration, which are described in detail.

Having established these normal patterns of neural crest cell migration, the following question was posed: Are the unique migratory patterns of the developing neural crest cell population determined within the individual cells prior to their exodus, or are they imposed upon the crest cells by the environment through which the cells move?

To resolve this problem neural folds were removed from one of the three cranial regions described above and replaced with a segment of ^{3}H-thymidine-labeled neural fold from either a different cephalic region or the brachial spinal cord level. In nearly every case the heterotopically transplanted cells mimicked the normal patterns of migration, and the embryos were indistinguishable from those which had received orthotopic transplants.

This proves that the precise patterns of migration of chick neural crest cells are not irreversibly determined within the cells prior to their emigration. Rather, their complex yet highly organized migratory behavior is largely directed by environmental influences.

INTRODUCTION

From a band of cells originating along the dorsomedial aspect of the closing neural folds the neural crest cells migrate into many regions of the vertebrate embryo and subsequently differentiate into numerous, often unrelated cell types. The migratory behavior of neural crest cells is not random, but rather is spatially and temporally patterned (Weston, 1963, 1971; Johnston, 1966; Chibon, 1966; Noden, 1972, 1973). The derivatives of this embryonic population include sensory and autonomic neurons, cephalic chondroblasts and osteoblasts, odontoblasts, chromaffin cells and several other types of secretory cells, and chromatophores (see reviews by Hörstadius, 1950, and Weston, 1970). More recent experiments suggest that the full repertoire of neural crest derivatives has yet to be discovered (Pearse, 1969; Pearse *et al.*, 1973).

In the acquisition and expression of these characteristics the neural crest cells touch upon a central problem in development: determination. At what stages and under the influence of what factors are the migratory behavior and subsequent cytodifferentiation of neural crest cells determined? While some evidence indicates that amphibian crest cells are initially delineated from adjacent neuroepithelial tissue as a result of primary induction by a particular region of the archenteron roof (Raven and

[1] Investigation performed in partial fulfillment of the requirements for the degree of Ph.D., and supported by N.I.H. training Grant no. HD00012 and Grant no. NS-05721 from the N.I.N.D.S. to Dr. V. Hamburger.

[2] Author's current address: Department of Zoology, University of Massachusetts, Amherst, Massachusetts, 01002.

106

Kloos, 1945; Seno and Nieuwkoop, 1958), the degree of determination of crest cells at the time of their emigration has not been well defined in any organism.

Similarly, certain inductive interactions have been shown to be a necessary prerequisite for the cytodifferentiation of some neural crest derivatives, including amphibian visceral arch chondroblasts (Hörstadius and Sellman, 1946; Okada, 1955; Holtfreter, 1968), avian sympathoblasts (Cohen, 1972; Norr, 1973), scleral chondroblasts (Newsome, 1972), and odontoblasts (Slavkin, 1971). However, these investigations do not reveal the degree of commitment of neural crest cells previous to such interactions. Nor do they clearly define the role of environmental influences in directing their highly patterned migrations and spatial distribution.

This investigation focuses on the migratory behavior which normally precedes cytodifferentiation of neural crest cells. Included in this migratory phase are all the movements by which individual members of the population approach and become localized at specific regions of the embryo, and all their associations with other cells, of either crest or noncrest derivation.

The first problem was to investigate in detail the normal migratory behavior of crest cells in the preotic regions of the chick embryo. Previous accounts of avian cephalic neural crest development either failed to satisfactorily identify crest cells after their association with placodal and mesodermal cells (van Campenhout, 1946), or emphasized the terminal locations of these cells more than their distribution en route (Johnston, 1966). By performing orthotopic transplantations of ^{3}H-thymidine-labeled neural fold tissue, I was able to follow radioautographically the patterns of distribution of the preotic crest population. Based on the results three unique, region-specific patterns of neural crest migratory behavior were defined.

Next, in order to investigate both the degree of determination of these crest cells

at the time of their emigration and the influences of the environment on their migratory patterns, labeled neural fold tissue was transplanted heterotopically, either between different regions of the head, or from the trunk into the head. In nearly all cases the patterns of migration of heterotopic crest cells were identical to those normally found in the recipient site, and were indistinguishable from the patterns observed following orthotopic transplantation.

These results warrant two conclusions. First, the patterns of neural crest cell migration, condensation, and distribution in the preotic regions of the head of the chick embryo are under the directing influences of factors within the environment into which these cells actively migrate. Furthermore, neural crest cells are not irreversibly determined with respect to their migratory behavior at the time of their emigration.

MATERIALS AND METHODS

Experimental Design

Three series of neural fold transplantations have been performed on chick embryos: one orthotopic and two heterotopic sets of operations. Each involves the replacement of a unilaterally excised piece of cephalic neural fold tissue with a similar-sized length of neural fold from a ^{3}H-thymidine-labeled donor. Figure 1 illustrates the design of two of the three series and also outlines the delineation of the preotic cephalic region of a Hamburger–Hamilton (1951) stage 9$^+$ embryo into five areas, which will be described separately in the Results section.

In the orthotopic series neural fold tissue was transplanted from the donor into an identical region in the host. The cephalic heterotopic series involved the replacement of the neural fold from one area with ^{3}H-thymidine-labeled neural fold tissue from a different, nonadjacent area. In the brachiocephalic heterotopic transplants a

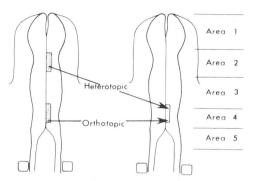

FIG. 1. Schematic illustration showing the design of the transplantations and the approximate morphological regions corresponding to Areas 1–5 in the head of a stage 9⁺ chick embryo.

segment of neural fold from the future brachial level was grafted in the place of cephalic neural fold tissue.

Operations

White Leghorn chick eggs were incubated in a forced-draft incubator at 38°C and 60–70% relative humidity. At approximately 26 hr of incubation, by which time the embryos had developed to stage 8, prospective donor embryos were exposed by grinding windows in the shell (Narayanan, 1970). Donor eggs for the brachiocephalic series were not opened until stage 11. ^{3}H-Methyl–thymidine in 0.02 ml warmed Tyrode's solution was pipetted directly onto the vitelline membrane. Dosage ranged from 1 to 5 µCi with a specific activity of 3–55 Ci/mmole. These embryos were then sealed with tape and incubated again for a minimum of 5 hr before being used as donors.

Prospective hosts were opened in a similar manner at approximately 32 hr of incubation. Using an ocular micrometer the distance from the anterior end of the prosencephalon to the first somite and also the length of apposed neural folds were measured. This provided a precise indication of the stage of development of the head of each embryo, as well as a record of the size of the organism.

Immediately prior to the operation both donor and host embryos were lightly stained with neutral red. A small hole was then made in the vitelline membrane of each directly over the appropriate region of the body (Hamburger, 1960). Short lengths of neural fold tissue were excised from the host and donor with glass needles. The graft was then transferred to the host in a Spemann pipette and carefully positioned in the prepared gap. Correct anteroposterior orientation was maintained, but it was often difficult to insure proper mediolateral orientation since the grafted tissue was nearly cylindrical in shape.

Following transplantation the windows were sealed with a flamed cover slip placed upon a paraffin ring which had been applied on the shell around the window, and returned to an incubator. Relative humidity was maintained above 90% for several hours after the operation, during which time the eggs were gently rocked at frequent intervals to prevent the extraembryonic surface from adhering to the vitelline membrane (Silver, 1960). After approximately 6 hr, the embryos were exposed and moistened with warm chick Ringer's solution, resealed, and returned to an incubator at 60–70% relative humidity.

Radioautography and Reconstructions

Embryos were fixed in Carnoy's at stages from 4 hr to 3 days following the operation, then dehydrated and embedded in paraffin. Specimens were sectioned at 8 µm, mounted on albumin-coated slides, and dipped in liquid NTB-2 emulsion (Eastman Kodak, Co.) according to the method of Kopriwa and Leblond (1962). The slides were exposed at 4°C in the presence of Drierite for 2–45 weeks, 4–6 weeks being the average length of time, and developed in Kodak D-19. Following fixation most slides were stained with 0.05% toluidine blue in 0.02 M sodium benzoate–benzoic acid buffer at pH 4.4 (Sidman, 1970).

Since the neural crest cells migrate into and arrange themselves throughout a three-dimensional field, it was necessary to reconstruct representative cases. By this method the position of neural crest cells relative to all other structures could be appreciated. Reconstructions were made from camera lucida sketches. Every second or third section was drawn and the position of all labeled cells in that section indicated.

The results are based upon analyses of 64 cases which showed no postoperative malformations that could have interfered with the normal course of neural crest cell migration.

RESULTS

Normal Migratory Patterns

Area 4, the metencephalon, and Area 5, the anterior myelencephalon. The pattern of neural crest cell migration is similar in both Area 4, which includes crest cells destined to contribute to the trigeminal ganglion and mandibular arch mesenchyme, and Area 5, from which the crest cells will form the geniculate ganglion and hyoid arch cartilages. Although the transplantation procedure may cause a slight delay in the onset of neural crest cell emigration or a diminution in the number of crest cells formed, these departures from normal do not usually interfere with the migratory behavior of cells from the graft.

By stage 12 the labeled crest cells have migrated laterally and ventrally, and are found distributed throughout the entire space between the metencephalon, the superficial epidermis, and the lateral extension of the pharynx (Fig. 2). An approximately equal number of labeled cells is usually found on both sides of the midline (Fig. 3), demonstrating the extent of mixing of crest cells across the midline prior to migration. Even at this early stage of development a few Area 4 neural crest cells exhibit behavior strikingly different from the others. These cells cease their ventrally directed migration near the dorsolateral surface of the anterior cardinal vein, adjacent to the middle of the metencephalon (arrows, Fig. 3). Stage-by-stage analysis indicates that this characteristic condensa-

tion of Area 4 crest cells represents the initial formation of the presumptive mandibulomaxillary portion of the trigeminal ganglion, and marks the site at which trigeminal efferent nerve fibers will later emerge.

At stage 13 labeled cells are found distributed from the trigeminal primordium to the mesodermal mesenchyme beneath the pharynx (Figs. 4 and 5). The earliest crest cells ventral to the pharynx are usually found adjacent to the pharyngeal endoderm. Those which enter later contribute to the mesenchyme which fills the enlarged area between the foregut and the epidermis, forming the mandibular visceral arch. In addition there is a caudally oriented movement of crest cells beside and beneath the pharynx.

Figures 5 and 6 reveal the presence of labeled neural crest cells throughout the trigeminal primordium. The absence of labeled cells adjacent to this primordium and the presence of labeled mitotic figures within the condensed tissue suggest that growth is the result of both cell division and aggregation of nearby crest cells. This enlargment is augmented at stage 14 by the influx of cells from the ophthalmic and mandibulo–maxillary placodes (Ham-

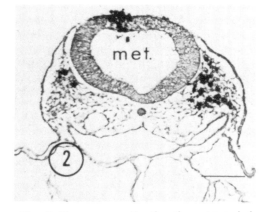

FIG. 2. Transverse section thru the metencephalon (met.) of a stage 12⁺ embryo (14 hr postoperative) following orthotopic transplantation into Area 4. Note the distribution of labeled cells throughout the region ventrolateral to the metencephalon. Bar = 0.1 mm.

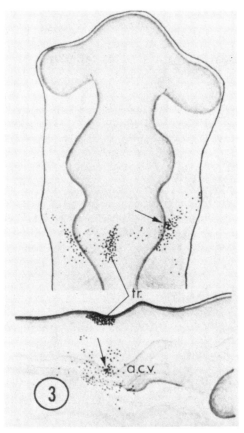

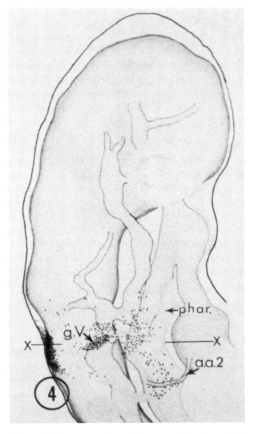

FIG. 3. Dorsal and lateral reconstructions of a stage 12+ embryo following orthotopic transplantation. Crest cells have migrated bilaterally from the site of neural fold implantation (tr.); some are clustered (arrows) dorsal to the anterior cardinal vein (a.c.v.) beside the metencephalon.

FIG. 4. Reconstruction of a stage 13 embryo (18 hr postoperative) which had received an orthotopic Area 4 transplant. Labeled cells are found in the trigeminal ganglion (g. V) and the presumptive mandibular arch. A few have migrated caudally beneath the pharynx (phar.) into the hyoid arch. (a.a. 2, second aortic arch). X--X indicates the level of sectioning of Fig. 5.

burger, 1961; Johnston, 1966). These two foci of cell proliferation begin to produce migratory presumptive neuroblasts at stages 12 and 14, respectively. As shown in Fig. 8 a trail of labeled cells extends from the ganglion into the mandibular arch; however, this connection is less densely populated by crest cells than either the ganglion or the visceral arch.

Within the mandibular arch labeled cells are most numerous lateral to the ventral aortae, although some are located more medially, either along the endothelial wall of these vessels or beneath the ventral surface of the pharynx. Many subpharyngeal crest cells continue to migrate caudally at later stages.

The pattern of early migration of Area 5 neural crest cells is similar to that found in Area 4, as shown in Fig. 8. Labeled cells are scattered through the future geniculate ganglion and extend into the hyoid arch. At 2 days of incubation the hyoid arch has not yet expanded ventrally beyond the level of the pharynx. However, the region posterior to the first pharyngeal pouch, between the lateral margin of the pharynx and the

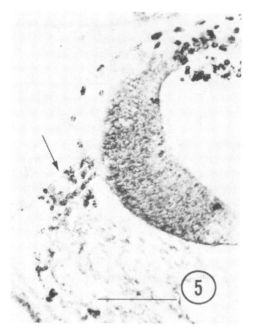

Fig. 5. Transverse section through the stage 13 embryo pictured in Fig. 4. Labeled cells are seen dispersed ventral to and condensed within the trigeminal ganglion (arrow), in the roof of the metencephalon and overlying superficial epidermis. Bar = 0.1 mm.

epidermis, is densely packed with labeled cells (Fig. 7). These cells surround the second aortic arch, and also move medially along both the floor and the roof of the pharynx. The cellular bridge between the VIIth ganglion and the hyoid visceral arch is very pronounced, due in part to a massive influx of cells from the hyoid epibranchial placode.

Neural crest cells in Areas 4 and 5 do not enter the parachordal mesenchyme, nor do they migrate medial to the dorsal aortae during the first three days of incubation. While they are found in apposition to the pharyngeal endoderm and the aortic endothelium, they do not appear to enter either epithelium.

With the onset of degeneration of the ventral aorta and ventral aspects of the first aortic arches beginning at stage 15, labeled Area 4 crest cells invade the medial

part of the future lower jaw. Thus, except for the mesodermal condensation representing principally muscle primordia, the mesenchyme of the mandibular arch is derived from the neural crest, as described by Johnston (1966).

Area 3, the posterior mesencephalon. The migratory behavior of neural crest cells emigrating from Area 3 is strikingly different from that found in Area 4. These cells migrate en masse away from the neural tube between the epidermis and the underlying mesoderm (Figs. 9 and 10). No crest cells remain adjacent to the mesencephalon, nor are there any condensations of crest cells in this region as was observed in Areas 4 and 5.

By stage 14 the Area 3 neural crest population has increased greatly throughout both the region ventrolateral to the mesencephalon and the future maxillary process (Figs. 11 and 12). In addition there is a caudally directed movement of cells in the visceral arch tissue around the ventral aorta; this migration extends nearly to the level where the second aortic arch leaves the unpaired ventral aorta.

During the third day of development axons of the oculomotor and ophthalmic nerves grow towards the eye and become infiltrated with labeled Area 3 crest cells, which are probably presumptive Schwann sheath cells. As shown in Fig. 13 these crest cells can travel along the oculomotor nerve proximally to its root. By stage 18 a condensation of labeled cells can be found medial and caudal to the optic cup along the oculomotor nerve tract. This represents the primordium of the parasympathetic ciliary ganglion. These crest cells apparently migrate to this position along the outgrowing nerve fibers, since all other neural crest cells in this region are of Area 2 origin. A few labeled cells are observed in the trigeminal ganglion. However, it could not be determined whether these represented presumptive neurons, glia, or Schwann sheath cells.

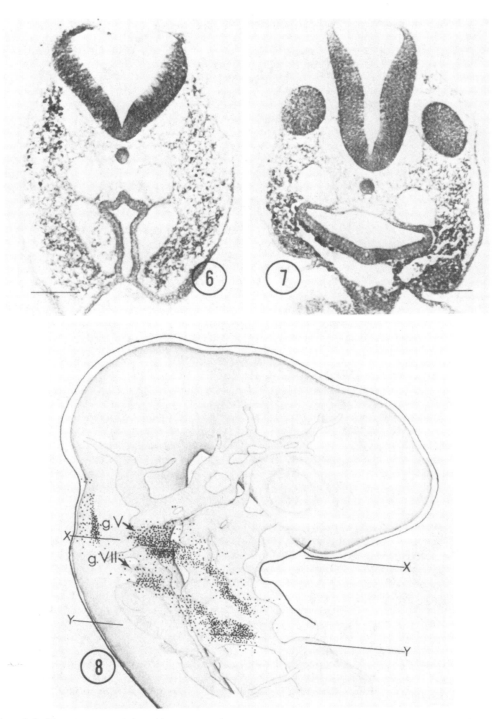

FIGS. 6–8. Transverse sections and reconstruction of a stage 14⁺ embryo (22 hr postoperative) which had received an orthotopic transplant occupying Areas 4 and 5. Figures 6 and 7, which correspond to levels X and Y indicated in Fig. 8, reveal the distribution of labeled crest cells in the trigeminal ganglion and hyoid arch, respectively. Bar = 0.1 mm. Note in Fig. 8 the columns of labeled cells between the Vth and VII ganglia (g. V; g. VII) and the corresponding visceral arches, with a crest cell-free area between the columns.

112

73

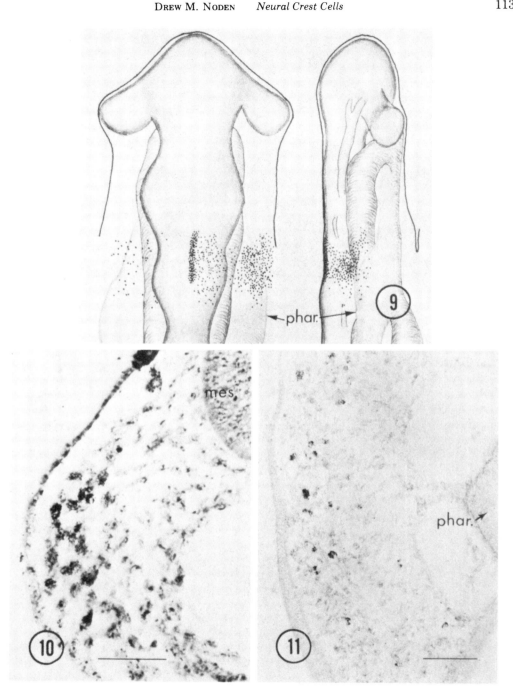

FIGS. 9 and 10. Reconstruction and transverse section showing the positions of crest cells at stage 12, 15 hr following an orthotopic transplantation into Area 3. A few cells have migrated below the lateral limit of the pharynx (phar.). Figure 10 illustrates the location of labeled cells migrating away from the mesencephalon (mes.) between the superficial epidermis and underlying mesoderm. Bar = 0.05 mm.

FIG. 11. This transverse section, which is from level Y indicated on Fig. 12, shows the distribution at stage 14 of labeled neural crest cells derived from an orthotopic Area 3 transplantation. Bar = 0.05 mm.

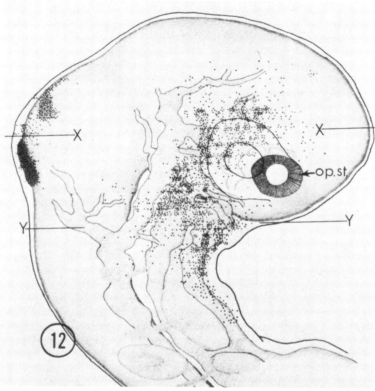

FIG. 12. In this case, a reconstruction of an embryo at stage 14 (22 hr postoperative), the graft separated into two portions which healed into Areas 3 and 2. Note the dispersal of labeled cells around and deep to eye (shown in outline; op. st., optic stalk), throughout the rostral portion of the first visceral arch, and caudally below the pharynx. X and Y indicate the levels of the transverse sections shown in Figs. 16 and 11.

Labeled cells are found throughout the maxillary and to a lesser extent the mandibular portions of the first visceral arch. Many are closely applied to the remnants of the ventral aortae; the fate of these cells following the degeneration of this vascular network is unknown. Some crest cells have moved medially into the region between the anterior cardinal vein and first aortic arch. However, crest cells are not found in the parachordal mesenchyme.

Area 2, the anterior mesencephalon and posterior diencephalon. The early migration of cells from neural folds transplanted into Area 2 is unique in that the majority of these crest cells initially move rostrally rather than laterally. Thus, by stage 10 the Area 2 crest cells are localized dorsal to the future optic stalk regions.

Between stages 11 and 12 the crest cells move ventrally around the posterior surface of the constricting optic stalks (Figs. 14 and 15). By stage 12 labeled cells are found dorsal, posterior, and ventral to the optic stalks and medial portion of the optic vesicles. Prior to this invasion the region immediately posterior to the future eye is sparsely populated with mesodermal mesenchyme. At later stages these crest cells overlap with those derived from Area 3, contributing to the formation of the maxillary process. In addition the Area 2 neural crest cells contribute to the mesenchyme found around the base of Rathke's pocket and the future oral region. Most of the mesenchyme lateral to the diencephalon, and later the telencephalon, is composed of crest cells (Figs. 12 and 16).

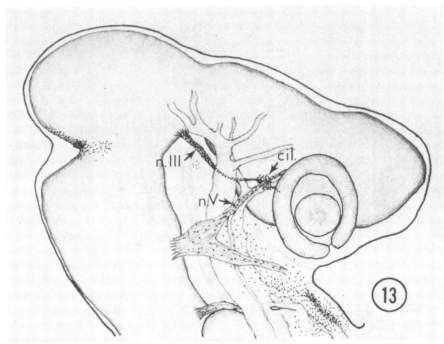

FIG. 13. A reconstructed stage 18⁻ embryo which had received a small Area 3 orthotopic transplant 40 hr prior to fixation. Note the presence of labeled cells along the oculomotor (n. III) and ophthalmic (n. V) nerves, in the presumptive ciliary ganglion (cil.), and around the ventral aorta.

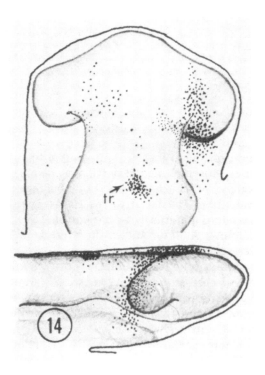

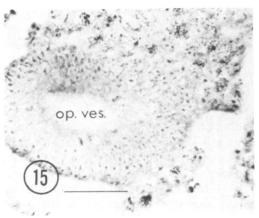

FIG. 15. A transverse section from immediately behind the right optic stalk of the embryo illustrated in Fig. 14. Labeled cells are seen dorsal, ventral, and medial to this posterior part of the optic vesicle (op. ves.). Bar = 0.05 mm.

FIG. 14. Reconstruction of a stage 12 embryo illustrating the rostral and subsequent ventral movement of neural crest cells during 13 hr following an orthotopic Area 2 transplantation. Part of the transplant (tr.) healed into the roof of the mesencephalon.

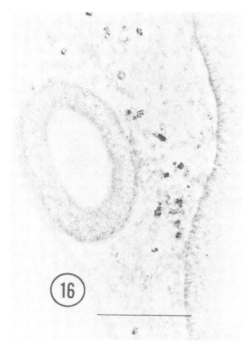

FIG. 16. Transverse section showing the presence at stage 14 of labeled crest cells between the eye and the diencephalon following an orthotopic, Area 2 transplantation. Bar = 0.1 mm.

On the third day of incubation some Area 2 neural crest cells condense along the outer wall of the neural epithelium; these probably represent presumptive leptomeningeal cells (Raven, 1936; Triplett, 1958; Johnston, 1966). Neural crest cells are also found associated with the endothelium of vascular tissue. The condensation of crest cells around the optic cup to form the sclera and choroid layers (Ris, 1941; Johnston, 1966) and the movement of these cells into the corneal stroma (Hay and Revel, 1969; Trelstad and Coulombre, 1971) do not occur until later stages.

Area 1, the mid- and rostral prosencephalon. As has been shown in urodeles (Hörstadius and Sellman, 1946) and chicks (Johnston, 1966), no appreciable number of crest cells arise from the neural folds in the presumptive telencephalic regions. All crest cells found in this region originate in Area 2.

Migratory Behavior of Heterotopically Transplanted Crest Cells

In each of the cases described in this section the area in the donor from which the graft was taken was nonoverlapping and nonadjacent to the area of implantation in the host. There were no appreciable differences between this and the previous series of transplants in the ability of the grafts to heal into the neural epithelium, although there was a slightly higher incidence of abnormal fusion with the contralateral neural fold.

Area 4 grafted into Area 2. The picture which emerges following heterotopic transplantation is clear and unequivocal: The pattern of migration in all cases was essentially identical to that seen in the analogous series of orthotopic Area 2 grafts. Labeled crest cells migrated rostrally to the furrows overlying the optic stalks (Fig. 17) and then moved ventrally as the stalks constricted. The later spatial distribution of these crest cells lateral to the diencephalon and beneath the optic vesicle in the future maxillary process (Fig. 19) is completely normal, as is the juxtaposition of labeled cells to the base of Rathke's pocket (Fig. 18), the outer layer of the optic cup, and the endothelium of the anterior vascular network.

The only departure from a normal pattern of Area 2 neural crest migration was one case in which labeled cells were found clustered around the proximal root of the oculomotor nerve. Possibly the precursor(s) of this cluster migrated along the lateral wall of the mesencephalon from the site of implantation to the ventrolateral margin of the midbrain. If true, this migratory behavior would be similar to that seen in the interaction between Area 4 crest cells and the metencephalon, and quite unlike that normally seen in Area 2. In no cases did the heterotopically transplanted Area 4 crest cells form a condensation.

Following neural crest cell emigration, the alar region of the neural tube in Areas 4

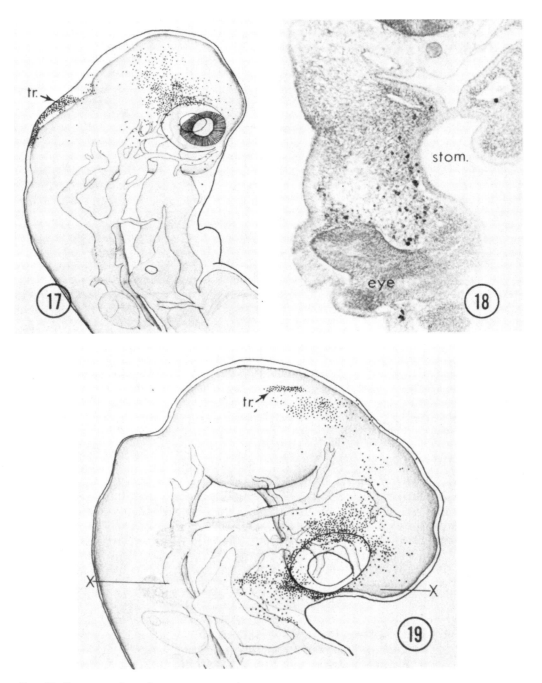

Fig. 17. Reconstruction of a stage 14⁻ embryo which had received a heterotopic Area 4-into-Area 2 transplant (tr.) 22 hours prior to fixation. The crest cells migrated rostrally in a manner characteristic of Area 2, although they have not yet moved ventrally around the optic primordium.

Figs. 18 and 19. These illustrate the distribution of labeled crest cells in a stage 15 embryo 25 hr following a heterotopic Area 4-into-Area 2 transplantation. Figure 18 is a transverse section corresponding to level X indicated on Fig. 19. Bar = 0.1 mm. The distribution of these neural crest cells around the eye and throughout the maxillary mesenchyme, lateral to the stomodeum (stom.) is indistinguishable from that normally seen in this area. This is clearly evident when comparing Fig. 19 with Fig. 12.

117

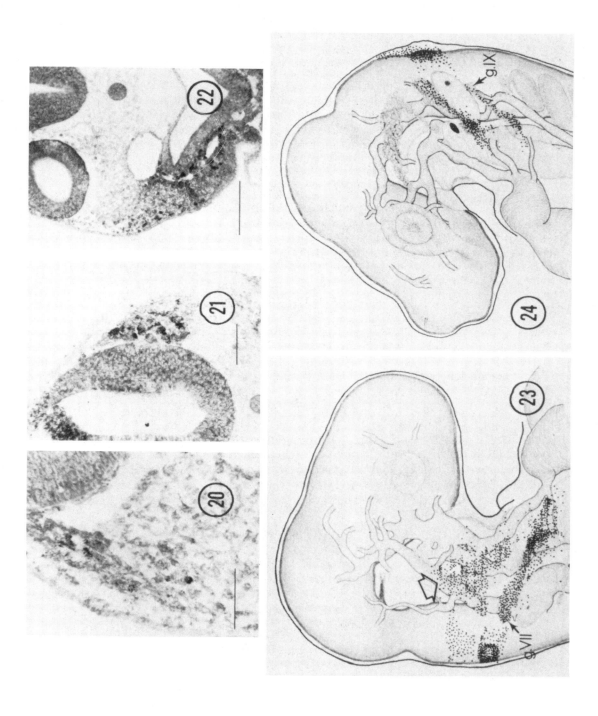

and 5 normally becomes drastically reduced, in contrast to Areas 2 and 3 in which the dorsal neuroepithelium remains thickened. However, no such reduction occurs when Area 4 neural fold is grafted into Area 2. It would be of interest to know what fate befalls those heterotopic neuroepithelial cells which remain in the roof in the grafted region; for example, would they be capable of differentiating into sensory cells of the mesencephalic trigeminal nucleus?

Areas 2 grafted into Area 4 or 5. The capacity of heterotopically transplanted Area 2 crest cells to migrate into the Area 4 environment is illustrated in Fig. 20, a transverse section through a stage 13.5 embryo. The presence of these labeled cells in the condensed primordium of a cranial sensory ganglion is in marked contrast to the behavior normally exhibited in Area 2 neural crest cells. The migration of these cells into a visceral arch is documented in Fig. 22.

Two reconstructed stage 15 embryos which received grafts of Area 2 neural fold into Area 4 (Fig. 23) and Area 5 (Fig. 24) dramatically confirm the above results. The latter clearly demonstrates the presence of labeled cells in the proximal and distal condensations of cranial ganglia VII and IX, and in the second and third visceral arches. Representative transverse sections illustrate the capacity of these heterotopic crest cells to condense into the geniculate ganglion primordium (Fig. 21) and invade the hyoid arch region (Fig. 22). In one embryo of this series labeled cells were found distributed through three cranial sensory ganglia (Fig. 25).

Only one case showed a significant departure from the normal pattern of Area 4 and 5 migration. In this embryo (Fig. 23) neural crest cells from the rostral part of a graft implanted into Area 4 entered the region medial to the anterior cardinal vein and condensed interspersed with the mesodermal primordia of the external rectus muscle (Adelmann, 1927), which is derived from the most caudal of three transient preotic somites. Since it is extremely unlikely that any mesodermal cells could have been accidently included in the transplanted tissue, the basis for this anomalous localization of neural crest cells is unknown.

Some embryos in this series were allowed to develop for 3 days postoperatively. The distribution of labeled cells in the mandibular and hyoid arches was normal. In addition a prominent stream of labeled crest cells was found running from the junction of the first and second visceral arches medially to the thyroid diverticulum, which is similar to the movement of Area 4 crest cells seen on the fourth day of incubation following orthotopic transplantation (Johnston, personal communication). Labeled cells were also found in the trigeminal ganglion, along the mandibulo–maxillary and abducens nerves, and in the posterior portion of the ciliary ganglion.

Thus the overall normal pattern of migration into the visceral arches and condensation to form the primordia of the sensory cranial ganglia is faithfully reproduced by Area 2 neural crest cells. This is in striking contrast to the behavior of these cells in their own region where they never condense as sensory ganglia.

Brachial neural fold grafted into Area 4.

Figs. 20–22. These transverse sections illustrate the migratory behavior of labeled neural crest cells following heterotopic Area 2-into-Area 4 and Area 5 transplantations. Figure 20 shows the presence of these cells in the trigeminal ganglion at stage 13.5. Bar = 0.05 mm. Figure 21 is a transverse section through the geniculate ganglion of the stage 15 embryo reconstructed in Fig. 24. Bar = 0.05 mm. The movement of these heterotopic crest cells into the hyoid visceral arch of a stage 15 embryo is pictured in Fig. 22 (bar = 0.1 mm), which is comparable to the normal movement of Area 5 crest cells seen in Fig. 7.

Figs. 23 and 24. These two reconstructed stage 15 embryos (24 hr postoperative) clearly demonstrate that Area 2 neural crest cells are capable of mimicking the migratory behavior of rhombencephalic, Area 4 and 5 crest cells (compare these with Fig. 8). The arrow, Fig. 23, indicates the position of some neural crest cells which migrated to an abnormal location (see text).

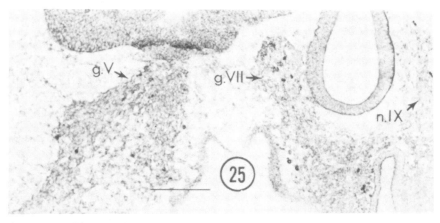

FIG. 25. A parasagittal section through a stage 17 embryo fixed 33 hr postoperatively. In this case a large segment from Area 2 had been implanted overlapping Areas 4 and 5. Labeled cells are found in the trigeminal (g. V) and geniculate (g. VII) ganglia, along the glossopharyngeal nerve (n. IX), and in the mandibular and hyoid arches. Bar = 0.1 mm.

The results of these transplants can be divided into two groups. Nearly half of the survivors had labeled heterotopic neural crest cells in their trigeminal ganglia but not in their visceral arches. The morphology of these hosts, including the size of their visceral arches, was normal.

The remaining cases reveal strikingly different situations. In each of these the patterns of neural crest cell behavior are indistinguishable from the normal patterns seen following orthotopic transplantation. Figure 26 shows the reconstruction of a stage 18.5 experimental embryo in which many of the cells in the trigeminal ganglion are heavily labeled. More importantly, the majority of the neural crest-derived cells are in the proximomedial parts of the ganglion (Fig. 27). This means that the trunk neural crest cells not only condensed to form the apparent primordium of a cranial sensory ganglion, but they also interacted in a perfectly normal manner with cells from the trigeminal placodes. In their normal environment these brachial crest cells would never encounter placode-derived neuroblasts. Labeled cells are found both in and around the distal stalk of the mandibulo–maxillary nerve, and a few are seen along the distal oculomotor nerve. The distribution of crest cells in the mandibular arch is also normal (Fig. 28).

These labeled cells are found most abundantly in the lateral parts of the arch, with some around the mandibular muscle condensation. A few labeled cells are observed within this mesodermal condensation, a normal condition described by Johnston (1966). Transplanted cells are found apposed to the pharyngeal endoderm, but very few are associated with the vascular endothelium. Comparing Fig. 26 with Fig. 8 leaves no doubt as to the remarkable capacity of the brachial neural crest cells to reproduce the behavioral patterns of the Area 4 crest cells.

DISCUSSION

Migratory Behavior

The orthotopic series of transplantations provides a detailed account of the early migratory patterns of avian preotic neural crest cells. These data corroborate earlier investigations on the regional distribution of crest cells derived from different cephalic areas of the neural tube in urodeles (Hörstadius and Sellman, 1946; Chibon, 1966) and chicks (Johnston, 1966). More importantly, these results reveal that crest cells emigrating from different parts of the fusing cephalic neural folds display unique region-specific patterns of migration, as summarized in Fig. 29.

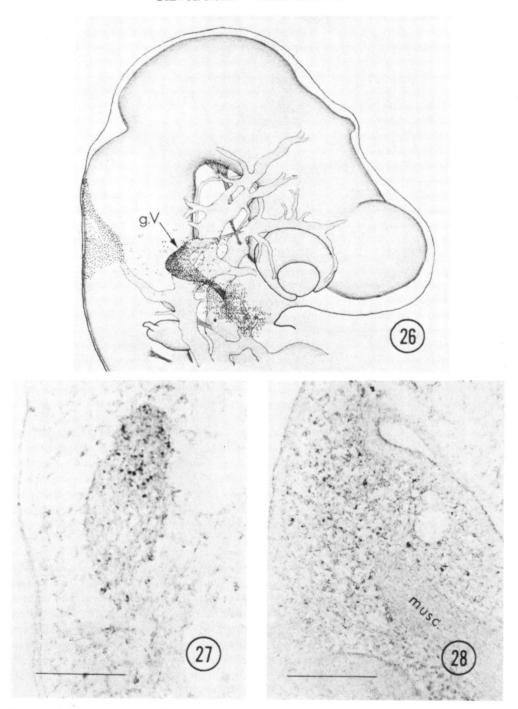

FIGS. 26–28. Reconstruction and transverse sections through a stage 18.5 embryo which had received a heterotopic brachial-into-Area 4 neural fold transplant 45 hr prior to fixation. Figure 27 shows the nonuniform distribution of labeled neural crest cells in the trigeminal ganglion. Figure 28 reveals the presence of these grafted cells in the mandibular arch surrounding the mandibular muscle anlagen (musc.). Bar = 0.1 mm.

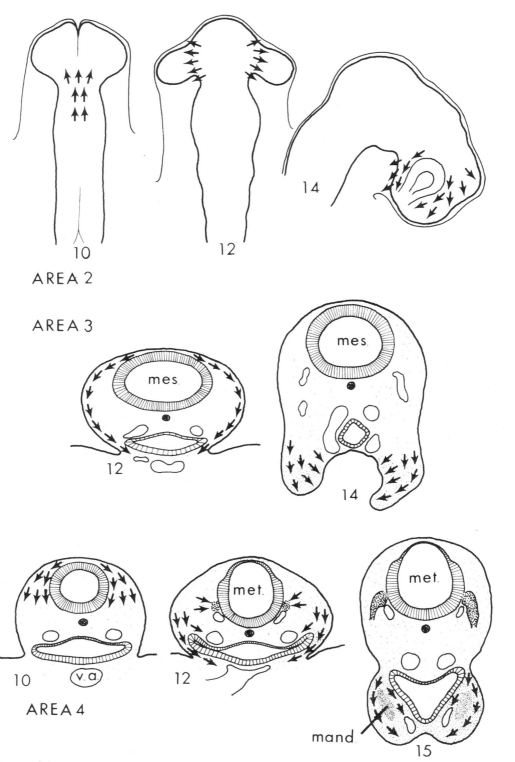

FIG. 29. Schematic summary of the early migratory behavior of neural crest cells in Areas 2–4. The numbers below each drawing indicate the stage of development. mes., mesencephalon; met., metencephalon; mand., mandibular muscle primordium.

122

83

In describing these patterns and attempting to elucidate some of the influences responsible for their establishment it is useful to consider separately homotypic and heterotypic neural crest cell associations and interactions. Homotypic associations are those which occur within the neural crest population, whereas heterotypic associations involve those between members of the neural crest population and the non-neural crest environment. Orthotopic grafts reveal that both types of associations occur; heterotopic transplantations suggest the relative roles each type plays in the determination of neural crest cell migratory behavior.

Homotypic associations. Neural fold apposition and fusion and the subsequent onset of crest cell migration begin in Area 2 then spread both rostrally and caudally. Unlike the neural crest cells in the avian trunk (Weston, 1963), the cephalic crest cells form a distinct, tightly packed mass prior to their emigration di Virgilio *et al.*, 1967; Hillman and Hillman, 1965). During the first 4–6 hr of migration all crest cells within each area become dispersed, reflecting an obvious alteration in their homotypic associations. Ectopic grafts of neural crest primordia to the flank region in urodeles (Twitty, 1945) and chicks (Weston, 1963) or beneath the pharynx in urodeles (Hörstadius and Sellman, 1946) have demonstrated that movement away from their zone of formation and initial dispersal are innate capacities. The *in vitro* analyses by Twitty (1949; Twitty and Niu, 1948, 1954) suggested that a mutual repulsion between neural crest cells occurs; however, other hypotheses have since been proposed (reviewed by Weston, 1972).

Between approximately 36 and 72 hr of incubation Area 2 crest cells disperse throughout the future orbital regions, moving also to surround the prosencephalon and contribute to the maxillary process. These cells invade a region which, except for the vascular elements, is relatively free of mesodermal mesenchyme. On the other hand, crest cells emanating from Areas 3–5 encounter both mesodermal tissue and, later, the lateral pharyngeal endoderm, forming heterotypic associations with each.

The pattern of homotypic associations in Areas 4 and 5 is identical and contrasts with that of the more rostral areas in several ways. First, the initial migratory behavior of crest cells emigrating from Areas 4 and 5 differs from Area 3 in that the latter population moves laterally and then ventrally as a compact mass between the mesoderm and the overlying epidermis, while rhombencephalic crest cells initially disperse, filling the region between the wall of the hindbrain and the lateral epidermis (see Fig. 29). Second, as these crest cells from the hindbrain continue their ventral migration they do not form a continuous sheet, but rather form delineated cords leading to the visceral arches. Observations presented by Hörstadius and Sellman (1946) suggest that in urodeles the formation of these cords is the result of outgrowth of the pharyngeal pouches. However, in the chick these discontinuities appear at a relatively earlier stage of neural crest migration; the pharyngeal pouches merely accentuate them.

The most striking deviations from the migratory patterns described for Areas 2 and 3 which some of the rhombencephalic crest cells exhibit are their cessation of ventral migration and reaggregation to form the primordia of cranial sensory ganglia. While similar events occur in the trunk region during spinal gangliogenesis, several differences exist between these two populations. The cephalic neural crest cells exhibit condensation much earlier than their counterparts in the trunk (Weston, 1963, 1970). Perhaps as in the other systems (Wessells, 1968; Deuchar, 1969; Drews *et al.*, 1972) a minimum population size or density must be attained before a developmental event, in this case condensation, can occur. Such a relationship would favor precocious condensation of presumptive cranial ganglion cells since greater numbers of crest cells are produced in each of the cephalic areas, and they emigrate en masse over a 4–6 hr period in contrast to the staggered emigration of trunk crest cells which requires approximately 15 hr (Weston, 1963).

A second major regional difference is the absence of definitive somites rostral to the otic vesicle. Experiments of Lehmann (1927), Detwiler (1934), and Weston (1963) indicate that heterotypic interactions between crest cells and the metameric somitic mesenchyme are a necessary prerequisite for the segmental distribution of trunk neural crest cells which condense to form the anlagen of spinal sensory ganglia. The transient preotic somites, whose principal derivatives are the extrinsic ocular muscles (Adelmann, 1927), are not morphologically detectable until after the Area 4 and 5 neural crest condensations have formed. Furthermore, these somites condense ventromedial to the anterior cardinal veins, while cranial gangliogenesis occurs dorsolateral to them. Hence, the cranial condensations are independent of these particular heterotypic interactions.

A third distinctive aspect of cranial ganglion formation is the contribution of cells derived from epidermal placodes. This has been demonstrated in amphibians (Landacre, 1910; Coghill, 1916; Stone, 1922, 1926) and chicks (van Campenhout, 1937; Hammond and Yntema, 1958; Hamburger, 1961; Johnston and Hazelton, 1972). The two populations do not mix randomly. Rather, neuroblasts derived from the neural crest preferentially contribute to the proximal, "root" ganglia while those of placodal origin settle in the distal, "trunk" portions of the ganglia (Yntema, 1937, 1943, 1944; Johnson, 1966). In the avian trigeminal ganglion neural crest-derived neuroblasts occupy the dorsomedial region, while the more lateral, distal neuroblasts are largely of placodal origin (Hamburger, 1961; Johnston and Hazelton, 1972).

The importance of homotypic interactions is further revealed by an examination of the surviving donor embryos. Following the removal of short lengths of neural fold tissue, embryos frequently showed no re-duction in the corresponding neural crest derivatives, and in later stages were often indistinguishable from normal embryos. Such restitution of a missing part of the neural crest population, noted also by Hörstadius and Sellman (1946) and Chibon (1966) in urodeles, is accomplished by immigration of crest cells from adjacent areas. A similar longitudinal movement of crest cells has been reported following extirpation of large segments of the avian trunk neural crest primordia (Yntema and Hammond, 1945; Hammond and Yntema, 1947; Nawar, 1956). These studies demonstrate that the migrating neural crest cells are not irreversibly determined with respect to their migratory behavior, and can assume different properties following reduction of the population, in a manner reminiscent of the morphogenetic field.

Corroboration of the idea that homotypic interactions play an essential role in the migratory behavior of the neural crest population comes from the investigations of Twitty and Bodenstein (1939, 1944), who performed both xenoplastic and heterochronic transplantations in urodeles. Their experiments were designed to allow the grafted crest cells to begin their migration earlier than the adjacent host crest cells. Melanoblasts emigrating from the transplant entered the epidermis but then spread anteriorly and posteriorly into adjacent crest-free regions, which is unlike their normal well-defined, ventrally directed migratory pathway. Later, when the crest cells of the host began their migration, they were prevented from entering the regions already occupied by crest cells from the graft.

These experiments suggest an explanation for the anomalous cases described in the Results in which crest cells implanted into Area 4 failed to migrate distally into the visceral arch regions. If, due to transplantation trauma, the onset of migration of these grafted cells was delayed, host crest cells from the adjacent areas might have already occupied the crest-free regions. The occurrence of this atypical pattern would be enhanced if the implanted cells had intrinsically a later onset of emigration than the cells which they replaced. In fact, this anomalous condition was found most frequently following implantation of brachial-level neural folds into Area 4, the former region producing emigrating crest cells somewhat later and over a longer period of time than the latter.

A similar situation was described by Weston and Butler (1966) in the chick embryo, but interpreted differently. They found that if a "young" segment of ³H-thymidine labeled spinal cord, from which neural crest migration was just beginning, was transplanted into a gap made by removing a segment of "older" spinal cord, from which most crest cells had already emigrated, few ³H-thymidine-labeled crest cells were found in the more distal regions of the host, such as the presumptive sympathetic ganglia. These workers discounted the idea that the failure of "young" crest cells to migrate further in an "older" environment could be "... caused only by previous filling of distal niches" (Weston and Butler, 1966, p. 258). Rather, they conclude, "...that the environment through which the crest cells migrate probably changes in its ability to support cell motility during embryogenesis" (Weston and Butler, 1966, p. 261). While I favor the former argument to explain the anomalous migratory behavior of certain cephalic crest cells, definitive resolution of this problem awaits further experimentation.

Heterotypic associations. The importance of heterotypic cell interactions in directing cell and tissue movements has been amply documented in many different systems (Holtfreter and Hamburger, 1955; Gustafson and Wolpert, 1967; Trinkhaus, 1969; Sidman, 1972). Within heterotypic reaggregates *in vitro* cells from different tissues show tissue-specific patterns of association (Townes and Holtfreter, 1955; Moscona, 1961; Curtis 1967; Steinberg, 1970).

During the course of their migration, cephalic neural crest cells form transient associations with many other tissues. Some of these associations are common to preotic crest cells from several areas, such as the apposition of neural crest cells to vascular endothelium and to nerve fibers, while the pattern of others is area-specific.

My data suggest that while en route towards the visceral arch regions cells from the neural crest do not penetrate appreciably into the mesodermal mesenchyme. The apparent absence of neural crest–mesodermal mixing is in contrast to the pattern described for the avian trunk crest cells by Weston (1963), in which neural crest cells migrate through the somitic mesenchyme. Weston (1970) suggests that an organized cellular environment such as somitic mesenchyme influences the migratory behavior of neural crest cells by facilitating migration. Possibly the epidermal–mesodermal interface which the pioneering cephalic crest cells pentrate serves an analogous role. However, since transplanted cells commingle with unlabeled crest cells from the contralateral neural fold prior to emigration, I am not able to exclude the possibility of some neural crest–mesodermal mixing.

As discussed earlier, Area 3 differs from the more caudal areas in that its crest population remains compact beneath the epidermis while moving tangentially away from the dorsal margin of the mesencephalon. In contrast, the neural crest population from Areas 4 and 5 spreads out between the body epidermis and the lateral wall of the hindbrain. Orthotopic grafts do not tell us whether this difference is due to the existence within these rhombencephalic crest populations of a distinct subgroup of cells whose members exhibit a modified migratory behavior, or is the result of environmental influences unique to Areas 4 and 5.

Following orthotopic transplantation cephalic neural crest cells are frequently found along nerve fibers, which they use as substrata for further migration. These cells, which are probably destined to become Schwann sheath cells, thus display a change in migratory behavior as a result of this heterotypic interaction. This example illustrates a sequence of events frequently seen during neural crest cell development: the formation of heterotypic associations, an alteration in migratory behavior and eventual specific cytodifferentiation. The basic question to be asked of such systems is whether there exists a causal relationship between these events.

Neural Crest Cell Determination

In undertaking a causal analysis of neural crest development one must distinguish between migratory behavior and acquisition of cell strain specificity. The analytical part of this investigation deals only with migratory behavior since, due to progressive dilution of the radioactive label, I did not raise embryos to stages at which terminal cytodifferentiation occurs. Thus, the inquiry has to focus on the stage(s) at which the migratory behavior becomes determined, and the specific factors that are involved.

These experiments clearly demonstrate that the migratory behavior of chick cephalic neural crest cells is the result of heterotypic interactions between the crest cells and their environment. When caused to migrate into Area 2, the neural crest population grafted from Area 4 disperses beside the prosencephalon and moves ventrally around the optic vesicles. These heterotopic cells never show any signs of condensation into ganglia, indicating the absence in Area 2 of the appropriate environmental influences. More convincingly, the Area 2 crest cells which normally never condense to form the anlagen of a cranial sensory ganglion will do so when transplanted heterotopically into Area 4 or 5. Furthermore, these cells move into the visceral arch regions in a manner indistinguishable from that normally seen in Area 4. Obviously the crest cells possess the capacities to recognize and respond to foreign environmental influences in a highly specific manner characteristic of

their new location, indicating that their migratory behavior is not irreversibly determined prior to the onset of emigration.

This demonstration of the essential role of the environment in directing neural crest migratory behavior is in contrast to the results obtained by Twitty (1936, 1945), who investigated the movements of urodele presumtive melanoblasts both following xenoplastic transplantation and *in vitro*. He found that the behavioral pattern of future pigment-producing cells is due in large part to properties inherent to the cells and independent of outside influences.

The ability of neural crest cells from the brachial spinal cord region to reproduce perfectly a cranial Area 4 behavioral pattern is equally remarkable. These cells, which normally condense as sensory ganglion primordia only after entering somitic mesenchyme, have the capacity to respond precociously to the local conditions responsible for the aggregation of cranial sensory ganglia. The striking manner in which brachial crest cells and trigeminal placode cells are able to interact and combine to form a morphologically normal presumptive Vth ganglion could not have been anticipated, since there is no placodal component in the trunk. The ability of these two populations to mimic the normal topographic distribution within the trigeminal ganglion, with neural crest cells forming the medial part and placodal cells the lateral part, clearly indicates both the essential role that heterotypic interactions play in directing patterns of migratory behavior and the apparent lack of region-specific neural crest cell surface properties. The movements of trunk-derived neural crest cells into the mandibular arch and the formation of a cellular bridge between the condensed ganglion and the arch are equally unparalled in their normal environment. In the foreign, Area 4 environment these cells are capable of forming visceral arch mesenchyme, surrounding the presumptive mandibular muscle condensation.

This ability of avian trunk crest cells to penetrate the visceral arch regions is at variance with the behavior of heterotopically grafted crest cells observed by Hörstadius and Sellman (1946) and Chibon (1966). They found significant depletions in the visceral arch cartilages following such transplantations in urodeles. Chibon was unable to find labeled cells in the arches following transplantation of ^{3}H-thymidine-labeled trunk neural fold tissue. This difference in the migratory behavior of heterotopically grafted urodele trunk crest cells might be due to unique taxonomic properties. On the other hand, it is possible that ventrally migrating heterotopic crest cells in Chibon's hosts might have gone undetected. This could occur if, being fewer in number than the normal population, they proliferated at an accelerated rate and thus prematurely diluted the label. Moreover, the presence of abnormalities following heterotopic trunk-into-head grafts in urodeles which are more severe than those found after unilateral ablation of neural folds (Hörstadius and Sellman, 1946; Chibon, 1966) strongly suggests that the heterotopic cells prevented adjacent crest cells from entering the operated region.

Since I did not follow the later fates of heterotopically transplanted neural crest cells, I do not know whether Area 2 crest cells will actually differentiate into sensory neurons after incorporation into morphologically normal presumptive trigeminal ganglia, or whether avian trunk crest cells are able to undergo chondrogenesis after incorporation into a visceral arch. Nor is it known whether the later morphogenesis of the avian visceral arch skeleton is largely the result of inherent, region- and species-specific properties of neural crest cells, as is the case in urodeles (Hörstadius and Sellman, 1946; Raven, 1931; Andres, 1949; Wagner, 1959), or rather is due to heterotypic interactions between neural crest cells and their environment.

To resolve this central problem experiments are currently in progress in which a replicating nuclear marker (LeDouarin, 1971, 1973) is being used for the purpose of analyzing the later cytodifferentiation and morphogenesis of heterotopic neural crest cells. Using this technique, LeDouarin and Teillet (1973) have shown that neural crest cells from vagal and thoracic regions are equipotential with respect to the migration and cytodifferentiation of catecholamine-containing derivatives of these regions.

The heterotopic transplantation of ^{3}H-thymidine-labeled neural fold tissue does prove that the migratory behavior of chick neural crest cells is strongly influenced by heterotypic interactions with their environment. All neural crest cells regardless of their region of origin, have the capacity to recognize and respond to highly specific local cues which direct their migration. If the cells at the time of their transplantation had any inherent disposition for a particular migratory pattern, such disposition is completely reversible. Few other developing systems, if any, require such a degree of "instruction" from their environment for the performance of their specific tasks.

The author wishes to express his gratitude to Professor Viktor Hamburger for his guidance, support, and constructive criticism during the course of this investigation and preparation of the manuscript.

REFERENCES

ADELMANN, H. B. (1927). The development of the eye muscles of the chick. *J. Morphol. Physiol.* **44,** 29–87.

ANDRES, G. (1949). Untersuchungen an Chimären von Triton und Bombinator. *Genetica* **24,** 387–534.

CHIBON, P. (1966). Analyse expérimentale de la régionalisation et des capacités morphogénetiques de la crête neurale chez l'Amphiben Urodèle *Pleurodeles waltlii* Michah. *Mem. Soc. Zool. France* **36,** 4–117.

COGHILL, G. E. (1916). Correlated anatomical and physiological studies of the growth of the nervous system of amphibia. II. The afferent system of the head of Amblystoma. *J. Comp. Neurol.* **26,** 247–340.

COHEN, A. M. (1972). Factors directing the expression of sympathetic nerve traits in cells of neural crest origin. *J. Exp. Zool.* **179,** 167–182.

CURTIS, A. S. G. (1967). "The Cell Surface: Its

Molecular Role in Morphogenesis." Logos Press, New York.

DETWILER, S. R. (1934). An experimental study of spinal nerve segmentation in Amblystoma with reference to the plurisegmental contribution to the brachial plexus. *J. Exp. Zool.* **67**, 395–441.

DEUCHAR, E. M. (1969). Effect of cell number on the type and stability of differentiation in amphibian ectoderm. *Exp. Cell Res.* **59**, 341–343.

DIVIRGILIO, G., LAVENDA, N., and WORDEN, J. L. (1967). Sequence of events in neural tube closure and the formation of neural crest in the chick embryo. *Acta Anat.* **68**, 127–146.

DREWS, U., KOCHER-BECKER, U., and DREWS, U. (1972). Die Induktion von Kiemenknorpel aus Kopfneuralleistenmaterial durch präsumptive Kiemendarm in der Gewebekultur und das Bewegungsverhalten der Zellen während ihrer Entwicklung zu Knorpel. *Wilhelm Roux' Arch. Entwicklungsmech. Organ.* **171**, 17–37.

GUSTAFSON, T., and WOLPERT, L. (1967). Cellular movement and contact in sea urchin morphogenesis. *Biol. Rev.* **42**, 422–498.

HAMBURGER, V. (1960). "A Manual of Experimental Embryology." University of Chicago Press, Chicago, IL.

HAMBURGER, V. (1961). Experimental analysis of the dual origin of the trigeminal ganglion in the chick embryo. *J. Exp. Zool.* **148**, 91–124.

HAMBURGER, V., and HAMILTON, H. L. (1951). A series of normal stages in the development of the chick embryo. *J. Morphol.* **88**, 49–92.

HAMMOND, W. S., and YNTEMA, C. L. (1947). Depletions of the thoraco–lumbar sympathetic system following removal of neural crest in the chick. *J. Comp. Neurol.* **86**, 237–266.

HAMMOND, W. S., and YNTEMA, C. L. (1958). Origin of the ciliary ganglion in the chick. *J. Comp. Neurol.* **110**, 367–390.

HAY, E. D., and REVEL, J. P. (1969). Fine structure of the developing avian cornea. *In* "Monographs in Developmental Biology" (A. Wolsky and P. S. Chen, eds.) Vol. 1, Karger, Basel.

HILLMAN, N. H., and HILLMAN, R. (1965). Chick cephalogenesis. The normal development of the cephalic region of stages 3 through 11 chick embryos. *J. Morphol.* **116**, 357–370.

HOLTFRETER, J. (1968). On mesenchyme and epithelia in inductive and morphogenetic processes. *In* "Epithelial-Mesenchymal Interactions" (R. Fleischmajer and R. E. Billingham, eds.), pp. 1–30. Williams and Wilkins, Baltimore, MD.

HOLTFRETER, J., and HAMBURGER, V. (1955). Amphibians. *In* "Analysis of Development" (B. H. Willier, P. A. Weiss, and V. Hamburger, eds.), pp. 230–296. Saunders, Philadephia, PA.

HÖRSTADIUS, S. (1950). "The Neural Crest." Oxford University Press, London.

HÖRSTADIUS, S., and SELLMAN, S. (1946). Experimentelle Untersuchungen über die Determination des Knorpeligen Kopfskelettes bei Urodelen. *Nova Acta Regiae Soc. Sci. Upsaliensis* (4) **14**, 1–170.

JOHNSTON, M. C. (1966). A radioautographic study of the migration and fate of cranial neural crest cells in the chick embryo. *Anat. Rec.* **156**, 143–156.

JOHNSTON, M. C., and HAZELTON, R. D. (1972). Embryonic origins of facial structures related to oral sensory and motor function. *In* "Third Symposium on Oral Sensation and Perception: The Mouth of the Infant" (J. Bosma, ed.), pp. 76–97. Thomas, Springfield, IL.

KOPRIWA, B. M., and LEBLOND, C. P. (1962). Improvements in the coating techniques of radioautography. *J. Histochem. Cytochem.* **10**, 269–284.

LANDACRE, F. L. (1910). The origin of cranial ganglia in Ameirerus. *J. Comp. Neurol.* **20**, 309–411.

LEDOUARIN, N. (1971). Charactéristiques ultrastructurales du noyau interphasique chez la caille et chez le poulet et utilisation de cellules de caille comme "marquers biologiques" en embroyologie experimentale. *Ann. Embryol. Morphol.* **4**, 125–135.

LEDOUARIN, N. (1973). A biological cell labeling technique and its use in experimental embryology. *Develop. Biol.* **30**, 217–222.

LEDOUARIN, N., and TEILLET, M. A. (1973). Recherches sur le déterminisme de le migration des cellules issues de la crête neurale. *C. R. Acad. Sci. Paris* **277**, 1929–1932.

LEHMANN, F. (1927). Further studies on the morphogenetic role of the somites in the development of the nervous system of amphibians. The arrangement and differentiation of spinal ganglia in *Pleurodeles waltlii*. *J. Exp. Zool.* **49**, 93–132.

MOSCONA, A. (1961). Rotation mediated histogenetic aggregation of dissociated cells. *Exp. Cell Res.* **22**, 455–475.

NARAYANAN, C. H. (1970). Apparatus and current techniques in the preparation of avian embryos for microsurgery and for observing embryonic behavior. *Bioscience* **20**, 869–871.

NAWAR, G. (1956). Experimental analysis of the origin of the autonomic ganglia in the chick embryo. *Amer. J. Anat.* **99**, 473–506.

NEWSOME, D. A. (1972). Cartilage induction by retinal epithelium of chick embryo. *Develop. Biol.* **27**, 575–579.

NODEN, D. M. (1972). The control of neural crest cell migration in the head region of the chick embryo. *Amer. Zool.* **12**, xxi (Abstract).

NODEN, D. M. (1973). The migratory behavior of neural crest cells. *In* "Fourth Symposium on Oral Sensation and Perception: Development in the Fetus and Infant" (J. Bosma, ed.), pp. 9–33. DHEW Pub. No. (NIH) 73–546.

NORR, S. C. (1973). *In vitro* analysis of sympathetic neuron differentiation from chick neural crest cells.

Develop. Biol. **34,** 16–38.

Okada, E. W. (1955). Isolationsversuche zur Analyse der Knorpelbildung aus Neuralleistenzellen bei Urodelenkeim. *Mem. Coll. Sci. Kyoto B* **22,** 23–28.

Pearse, A. G. E. (1969). The cytochemistry and ultrastructure of polypeptide hormone-producing cells of the APUD series and the embryologic, physiologic and pathological implication of the concept. *J. Histochem. Cytochem.* **17,** 303–313.

Pearse, A. G. E., Polak, J. M., Rost, F. W. D., Fontaine, J., LeLievre, C., and LeDouarin, N. (1973). Demonstration of the neural crest origin of type 1 (APUD) cells in the avian carotid body using a cytochemical marker system. *Histochemie* **34,** 191–203.

Raven, C. P. (1931). Zur Entwicklung der Ganglienleiste. I. Kinematic der ganglienleisten Entwicklung bei der Urodelem. *Wilhelm Roux' Arch. Entwicklungsmech. Organ.* **125,** 210–292.

Raven, C. P. (1936). Zur Entwicklung der Ganglienleiste. V. Uber die Differenzierung des Rumpfganglienleistenmaterials. *Wilhelm Roux' Arch. Entwicklungsmech. Organ.* **134,** 122–146.

Raven, C. P., and Kloos, J. (1945). Induction by medial and lateral pieces of the archenteron roof, with special reference to the determination of the neural crest. *Acta Neerland. Morphol.* **5,** 348–362.

Ris, H. (1941). An experimental study on the origin of melanophores in birds. *Physiol. Zool.* **14,** 48–66.

Seno, T., and Nieuwkoop, P. D. (1958). The autonomous and dependent differentiation of the neural crest in amphibians. *Koninkl. Ned. Akad. Wettenschap. Proc. C* **61,** 489–498.

Sidman, R. L. (1970). Autoradiographic methods and principles for study of the nervous system with thymidine-H³. *In* "Contemporary Research Methods in Neuroanatomy" (W. J. H. Nauta and S. O. E. Ebbesson, eds.), pp. 252–283. Springer-Verlag, New York.

Sidman, R. L. (1972). Cell interactions in the developing mammalian central nervous system. *In* "Cell Interactions" (L. G. Silvestri, ed.), pp. 1–13. American Elsevier, New York.

Silver, P. H. S. (1960). Special problems of experimenting *in ovo* on the early chick embryo, and a solution. *J. Embryol. Exp. Morphol.* **8,** 369–375.

Slavkin, H. C. (1971). The dynamics of extracellular and cell surface protein interactions. *In* "Cellular and Molecular Renewal in the Mammalian Body" (I. L. Cameron and J. D. Thrasher, eds.), pp. 221–276. Academic Press, New York.

Steinberg, M. S. (1970). Does differential adhesion govern self-assembly processes in histogenesis? Equilibrium configurations and the emergence of a hierarchy among populations of embryonic cells. *J. Exp. Zool.* **173,** 395–434.

Stone, L. S. (1922). Experiments on the development of the cranial ganglia and the lateral line sense organs in *Amblystoma punctatum. J. Exp. Zool.* **35,** 421–496.

Stone, L. S. (1926). Further experiments on the extirpation and transplantation of mesectoderm in *Amblystoma punctatum. J. Exp. Zool.* **44,** 95–131.

Townes, P. L., and Holtfreter, J. (1955). Directed movements and selected adhesion of embryonic amphibian cells. *J. Exp. Zool.* **128,** 53–120.

Trelstad, R. L., and Coulombre, A. J. (1971). Morphogenesis of the collagenous stroma in the chick cornea. *J. Cell Biol.* **50,** 840–858.

Trinkhaus, J. P. (1969). "Cells Into Organs." Prentiss-Hall, Englewood Cliffs, N.J.

Triplett, E. L. (1958). The development of the sympathetic ganglia, sheath cells, and meninges in amphibians. *J. Exp. Zool.* **138,** 283–311.

Twitty, V. C. (1936). Correlated genetic and embryological experiments on Triturus. I. Hybridization: Development of three species of Triturus and their hybrid combinations. II. Transplantation: The embryological basis of species differences in pigment pattern. *J. Exp. Zool.* **74,** 239–302.

Twitty, V. C. (1945). The developmental analysis of specific pigment patterns. *J. Exp. Zool.* **100,** 141–179.

Twitty, V. C. (1949). Developmental analysis of amphibian pigmentation. *Growth* **13,** Suppl. **9,** 133–161.

Twitty, V. C., and Bodenstein, D. (1939). Correlated genetic and embryological experiments on Triturus. III. Further transplantation experiments on pigment development. IV. The study of pigment cell behavior *in vitro. J. Exp. Zool.* **81,** 357–398.

Twitty, V. C., and Bodenstein, D. (1944). The effect of temporal and regional differentials on the development of grafted chromatophores. *J. Exp. Zool.* **95,** 213–231.

Twitty, V. C., and Niu, M. C. (1948). Causal analysis of chromatophore migration. *J. Exp. Zool.* **108,** 405–437.

Twitty, V. C., and Niu, M. C. (1954). The motivation of cell migration studied by isolation of embryonic pigment cells singly and in small groups *in vitro. J. Exp. Zool.* **125,** 541–574.

van Campenhout, E. (1937). Le rôle des placodes épiblastiques au cours du développement embryonnaire du porc et du poulet. *Bull. Acad. Roy. Med. Belg.* 169–184.

van Campenhout, E. (1946). The epithelioneural bodies. *Quart. Rev. Biol.* **21,** 327–347.

Wagner, G. (1959). Untersuchungen an Bombinator-Tritor Chimaeren. *Wilhelm Roux' Arch. Entwicklungsmech. Organ.* **151,** 136–158.

Wessells, N. K. (1968). Problems in the analysis of determination, mitosis, and differentiation. *In* "Epithelial-Mesenchymal Interactions" (R. Fleischmajer and R. E. Billingham, eds.), pp. 132–151. Williams and Wilkins, Baltimore, MD.

WESTON, J. A. (1963). A radioautographic analysis of the migration and localization of trunk neural crest cells in the chick. *Develop. Biol.* **6,** 279–310.

WESTON, J. A. (1970). The migration and differentiation of neural crest cells. *Advan. Morphog.* **8,** 41–114.

WESTON, J. A. (1971). Neural crest cell migration and differentiation. *In* "Cellular Aspects of Growth and Differentiation in Nervous Tissue" (D. Pease, ed); *UCLA Forum in Medical Sciences* **14,** 1–19.

WESTON, J. A. (1972). Cell interaction in neural crest development. *In* "Cell Interactions" (L. Silvestri, ed.), pp. 286–292. American Elsevier, New York.

WESTON, J. A., and BUTLER, S. L. (1966). Temporal factors affecting localization of neural crest cells in the chicken embryo. *Develop. Biol.* **14,** 246–266.

YNTEMA, C. L. (1937). An experimental study of the origin of the cells which constitute the VIIth and VIIIth cranial ganglia and nerves in the embryo of *Amblystoma punctatum. J. Exp. Zool.* **75,** 75–102.

YNTEMA, C. L. (1943). An experimental study of the origin of the sensory neurons and sheath cells of the IXth and Xth cranial nerves in *Amblystoma punctatum. J. Exp. Zool.* **92,** 93–120.

YNTEMA, C. L. (1944). Experiments on the origin of the sensory ganglia of the facial nerve in the chick. *J. Comp. Neurol.* **81,** 147–167.

YNTEMA, C. L., and HAMMOND, W. S. (1945). Depletions and abnormalities in the cervical sympathetic system of the chick following extirpation of neural crest. *J. Exp. Zool.* **100,** 237–263.

Reprinted from Science, Vol. 189, pp. 340–347. 1975

Compartments and Polyclones
in Insect Development

Clones made in early development keep within certain
fixed boundaries in the insect epithelium.

F. H. C. Crick and P. A. Lawrence

In this article our aim is to describe recent work on the development of intact epithelia and in particular the important results and ideas of Professor Antonio Garcia-Bellido (*1*) and his group in Madrid which are not yet widely known. We try to explain as clearly as possible what these ideas are and what sort of experiments have been done to support them. Some of the more obvious questions arising from the results and how the new concepts may relate to other ideas such as "gradients" are listed.

Development of *Drosophila*

The development of an adult *Drosophila* is a complex process. The nucleus of the fertilized egg divides a number of times to form a compact mass of about 250 nuclei, near the center of the egg, without cell walls. These nuclei then migrate outward to the inner surface of the egg where for the first time cell membranes are formed. The cells divide several more times to form a single layer of cells, about 4000 in all, lin-

Drs. Crick and Lawrence work in the Cell Biology Division of the Medical Research Council Laboratory of Molecular Biology, Cambridge, CB2 2QH, England.

ing the inside of the egg. This is called the blastoderm. Behaving as a sheet of cells, the blastoderm undergoes complex folding movements generating a multilayered germ band, which soon becomes visibly segmented. The egg hatches after 24 hours and the animal then goes through three larval stages each separated by a molt. After these larval stages, lasting in all about 96 hours, the animal then pupates and metamorphoses into the adult fly.

This adult is formed mainly from special groups of cells in the larva which themselves take little or no part in larval development or function. These are the histoblasts and the imaginal discs. There are 19 of the latter (nine pairs of discs plus the single genital disc). We shall concentrate mainly on one pair of these, the so-called wing disc. The left wing disc, within the left side of the larva, produces the left wing of the insect and that part of the dorsal left side of the thorax next to the wing.

The wing disc is seen in the first larval stage as a small patch of embryonic epidermal cells (*2*). These cells remain diploid, while the surrounding larval epidermal cells become polyploid (*3*). There are probably only about 15 to 30 cells forming the wing disc at this early stage (*4–6*). During the course of larval growth these disc cells

divide in all about 10 or 11 times (on average) to give a total of some 50,000 cells (*5*). Shortly after puparium formation cell division of the disc stops. The disc has now a characteristic size and shape, being somewhat like a flattened and heavily folded balloon (*7*).

At metamorphosis a complicated set of cell movements occurs, and these result in the disc being turned inside out so that it can form the adult structure. The wing itself, for example, is first formed as a bag. The bag is then collapsed to form the adult wing, which thus becomes a single sheet of epithelial cells folded and collapsed to form a double layer of epithelial cells.

Basic Ideas of Clonal Analysis

For the purposes of exposition we now temporarily leave the wing and describe a hypothetical sheet of "white" epithelial cells on the adult fly. We imagine that we have at our disposal a special technique that enables us to mark (say black), at random, a single cell in a developing disc. The mark is such that it does not interfere in any way with the normal development of the animal. Moreover, all the descendants of this marked cell retain the mark and can be recognized in the adult. The method of marking has the advantage that we can choose fairly precisely when, in development, we mark the cell; but it has the disadvantage that we cannot mark a particular cell at that time, but only one chosen at random, and in early stages we usually mark only one cell in any one individual. If we assume that the significant features of the process are effectively the same in all individuals, we can piece together what is happening in development by combining experiments on many different individuals.

What do we find? Naturally, we see a set of black cells in the adult, but how many of them are there, and how are they arranged?

The first observation is what might be

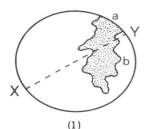
(1)

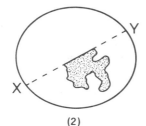
(2)

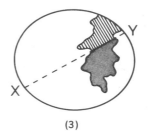
(3)

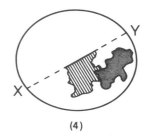
(4)

Fig. 1. A clone descending from a cell marked prior to the formation of the compartment border (XY). The clone is smooth at the edge of the structure (*a*) but rough elsewhere (*b*). Fig. 2. A clone descending from a cell marked after the formation of the compartment border. Fig. 3. The clones made by the two daughter cells of that cell generating the clone shown in Fig. 1. Fig. 4. The clone made by a cell marked prior to the formation of the compartment border, both of whose daughter cells give rise to clones within one subcompartment.

expected. In general, the earlier a cell is marked in development, the more black cells we find in the adult. A cell marked early leaves more descendants than a cell marked late.

The next obvious question is: What fraction of the total cells are marked? By the total cells we mean the number of cells in that portion of the adult epithelium which has come from the set of cells under consideration in the larva (for example, the 50,000 epithelial cells that come from a single wing disc).

The number of black cells produced by marking at a fixed time is not exactly constant, but the variation is such that we can usefully calculate its average value. If the average number of black cells in the adult is, say, a tenth of the total then making certain reasonable assumptions there were, on average, about ten cells in the larval set at the time they were marked (*8*). As the time of marking gets later and later in development this fraction gets smaller and smaller, and the frequency of marked clones produced increases.

From the arrangement of the black cells we can learn something about their movement during the interval between irradiation and observation. For instance, if there is a pepper and salt mixture, the cells must have been intermingling; while a coherent patch suggests that all the daughter cells have remained in contact during growth. The shape of the patch is also informative. For example, if it is long and thin this may result from the cell divisions being predominantly oriented in one direction. In the case of the wing disc, it is found that the patches are usually both coherent and elongated so that the long axes of the patches are parallel to the long axis of the wing (*4, 5, 9*).

We must next ask: Even though a patch is irregularly shaped, is the shape the same in different individuals? The experimental results show that it is not so. Consider a set of experiments in which the mark was made at more or less the same time in the development of a number of different indi-

viduals. Then it is found that the patches produced, when all drawn on the surface of a single idealized adult, do not neatly cover the entire epithelial surface, without either overlapping or leaving spaces (like a jigsaw puzzle). On the contrary, if two patches from separate individuals have ended up in roughly the same place, then it is always found that each partly overlaps the other and are usually of different size. This result shows that the cell lineage in *Drosophila* epithelium is not strictly determined in the same way in all individuals.

After all these preliminaries we can now approach the important result. Let us assume that our hypothetical piece of epithelium is smooth in outline, as shown in Fig. 1. Then perhaps it is not too surprising to learn that a black patch near the borders of this piece of epithelium has itself a rather smooth outline where it follows the boundary of the area but has a rough outline elsewhere. We assume that at the earliest stage of marking (that is, when the disc is first formed) a black patch can be produced anywhere within our area. In particular it may have the size and shape shown in Fig. 1. We now ask: Suppose the mark is made a little later, say, one cell generation later, what will the patch be like? Naturally, it will, on an average, be half the size, and we expect it to have an irregular outline except where it touches the area border. But now in some cases a new and totally surprising restriction appears. When all the results from many different patches are combined, it is found that a rather smooth line (marked XY) can be drawn, dividing our hypothetical area into two distinct parts, such that no black patch, made at this later time, will ever cross this line. Moreover, the outline of a patch touching this line is smooth where it runs along the line but rough elsewhere (Fig. 2). And this in spite of the fact that a patch marked one cell generation earlier can cross this special line.

The surprising nature of this result can be seen by going back and considering the entirely irregular patch illustrated in Fig.

1. We drew this particular patch (marked at the earlier stage) across the special boundary XY. We now ask: What would Fig. 1 look like if instead of just marking that particular cell we had been able to put a different mark on each of its two daughter cells, produced one generation later? We should now find two adjacent patches, each with an irregular outline except where the patches touched. Along the line of contact their outlines would be smooth and fairly straight (Fig. 3). This result is true only if the double patch crosses the special line XY. Otherwise the contact outline of the two daughter patches would be irregular (Fig. 4).

Garcia-Bellido, Ripoll, and Morata (*10*) have called an area bounded by these special demarcation lines a *compartment*. The progeny of a cell marked at about the time of the drawing of boundary lines never fills a compartment completely, but often occupies an appreciable proportion of it. A compartment is thus made by the descendants of a small group of cells. We propose to call the cells in the compartment a *polyclone*. Just as a clone is a group of cells which are all, without exception, the descendants of a single cell, so a polyclone is a group of cells that are descended from a certain (small) group of cells—the founder cells—which were present in the embryo at an earlier time. Moreover, in our terminology they are *all* the (surviving) descendants of that small group. This last point is vital since necessarily all the cells in a compartment are, for example, descendants of the fertilized egg. The distinction is that some of the descendants of the egg make up other parts of the body; that is, they end up in other compartments. The members of a polyclone, however, all fall within one compartment and account for all the cells in that compartment.

This point can be made more sharply. Consider the small group of cells, the founder members of the polyclone, and then consider their immediate ancestors. Then (except in rare cases) this earlier group will not form a polyclone for the compartment under consideration. That is, we will usually find that some of the descendants of these cells end up outside the compartment we are considering. The cells in the compartment are necessarily all descended from this smaller group, but they are not all the surviving descendants. Therefore, this earlier group are not the founder members of the polyclone for that compartment.

The other side of the idea must also be mentioned: a compartment is never a clone, except perhaps accidentally in rare cases. That is, for most cases, the cells in a compartment cannot be traced back to any single cell, all of whose descendants fall within the compartment. This idea, which implies that for these properties cells are switched not singly but in groups, is important (*11*).

We thus see that the idea of a compartment and the idea of a polyclone are, at the moment, intimately connected. As things stand at present we have no other reliable criterion for the sharply defined region we call a compartment except that a marked clone produced after a certain time in development will never cross over the compartmental boundary and include any part of any other compartment; whereas clones formed earlier may well do so. Reciprocally, we cannot say that a group of cells form a polyclone unless we first define the compartment to which the polyclone refers.

We must now consider the second major fact about certain compartments, namely that as time goes on they become subdivided. Let us call a certain compartment comp 1; at a later time it will be subdivided into two compartments which we may call comp 1A and comp 1B. These two subcompartments are not necessarily equal either in area or in number of cells but together they add up exactly to comp 1.

By definition all these compartments are polyclones. That is, the ancestors of all the cells contained in each compartment can be traced back to a founder group, early in the embryo, all of whose descendants end up in a compartment being considered. It is an experimental fact that one marked clone of cells, started from a single cell at a certain early stage, may stay entirely within comp 1 and yet go across the border between comp 1A and comp 1B. A marked clone made at a slightly later stage, however, will never cross this boundary. This implies that in any particular case the cells that are the founder members of the polyclone for comp 1 form three classes: those whose descendants will fall (i) wholly within comp 1A, (ii) wholly within comp 1B, and (iii) partly into comp 1A and partly into comp 1B.

It is this third class which explains why early clones can cross a subcompartment boundary whereas later ones cannot. However, at a slightly later stage in embryogenesis some further developmental step must take place, since at that time the descendants of the founder members of comp 1 will fall strictly into the first two classes listed above. No cell will then be found with the properties of class iii. Every cell in this enlarged group will be either a founder member for comp 1A or a founder member for comp 1B. In short, whereas before only one polyclone existed, that polyclone can now be considered as the sum of two distinct polyclones.

The work of Garcia-Bellido and his colleagues shows that this process of forming subcompartments within larger compartments can happen several times in succession. The data suggest, but do not prove, that the division takes place each time into just two parts.

The Methods

We shall now illustrate the methods used in clonal analysis by describing in outline the techniques employed by Garcia-Bellido *et al.* (*10*) in their detailed studies of the wing disc of *Drosophila melanogaster*. The wing disc is strictly called the dorsal mesothoracic disc. There are two of them in each larva, one for each side of the adult animal. Each disc produces the entire epithelium for a wing and that part of one side of the thorax near the wing. The dorsal part of the thorax is called the notum and the lateral part the pleura.

The method used to mark a clone is mitotic recombination produced by x-rays delivered at a chosen time in development, usually during the larval stages. The genetic makeup of the animal is designed so that certain mitotic recombinants will be phenotypically different. For example, if the animal is heterozygous for the recessive gene *yellow* ($y/+$) then mitotic recombination may produce two daughter cells. One of these ($+/+$), will be phenotypically wild-type and therefore indistinguishable from unaltered cells, but the other will be homozygous for *yellow* (y/y). All the descendants of this cell will also be (y/y). If such a descendant in the adult is colored at all then it will be yellow rather than the normal darker color.

An ideal genetic marker would be easily scored in all types of cell, have complete expression, and be cell-autonomous. That is, the phenotype would depend only on the genetic makeup of the cell in question and not at all on that of neighboring cells. Unfortunately few such markers are known. Markers often used are: *multiple wing*

hairs (*mwh*) which produces groups of two to five hairs (trichomes) on the wing instead of one per cell as in the wild type; and *forked* (*f*) and *singed* (*sn*), which produce deformed bristles and hairs. To assist recognition, the mutant allele with the most extreme phenotype among those available is usually used; and to minimize mistakes more than one marker is often employed. Double marking also allows the degree of expression and cell autonomy to be checked.

The markers used so far in this work do not allow a marked cell to be recognized when it is first produced in the imaginal disc, or even after a few divisions. The cell phenotypes employed can only be scored by the observer at the adult stage when the cells have differentiated. Moreover, only cells that form (or can be induced to form) hairs or bristles can be scored at all easily, so that if these are lacking or sparse in some particular area it is often difficult to find the exact edges of a marked clone in such regions. Fortunately most of the wing disc derivatives, being covered with hairs, are relatively easy to score.

If the growing disc in the larva is irradiated at the early stages of development, there will be few target cells and most individuals examined will not show any mutant patches. This cannot be overcome by increasing the x-ray dose (which is usually 1000 roentgens) as too big a dose will interfere with development. One simply has to examine a fairly large number of flies. If the x-rays are given later in development, more mutant clones are produced (since there are more target cells); but the average size of each clone will be smaller since a cell altered at a later stage produces few descendants. This small clone size means that it is more difficult to recognize compartment boundaries since most of the clones will be in the middle of a compartment rather than near its edge and even those at the boundary, being small, will not display the boundary so graphically. This is somewhat offset by the subdivisions making the compartments smaller as time goes on but in spite of this it becomes progressively more difficult to recognize compartment boundaries. It would in any case involve much more work if enough patches are to be scored to make an apparent boundary statistically significant.

However, Garcia-Bellido *et al.* devised a method of overcoming this difficulty. There exist a series of dominant *Minute* loci (*12*) which are lethal when homozygous. When heterozygous, the insects grow slowly and the bristles are small. They needed a mutant which (after mitotic recombination) would make the marked clone grow faster than the unaltered cells

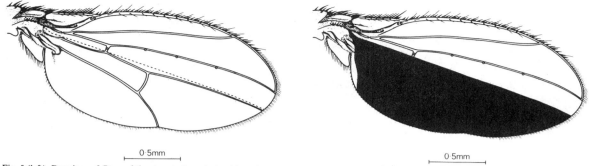

Fig. 5 (left). Drawings of *Drosophila* wing to show the position of the antero-posterior compartment border. Fig. 6 (right). Outline drawing of *Drosophila* wing to show the area covered by a typical M^+/M^+ clone in a M/M^+ background.

and thus produce a much bigger patch. Morata and Ripoll (*13*) showed that homozygous wild-type cells (M^+/M^+) produced by mitotic recombination divided more rapidly than the slow-growing heterozygous *Minute* (M/M^+) background, which was the effect they needed. In addition, for reasons which are obscure, the frequency of mitotic recombination for (M/M^+) larvae after irradiation is apparently increased (*14*). This is especially useful in the early stages of development when the normal rate is inconveniently low. A second somewhat unexpected result was that in spite of the (M^+/M^+) clones being much larger than normal, the overall size and shape of the wing was not altered (*13*). This implies that there are special mechanisms to regulate size and shape which can cope with differential cell division rates—an important result in its own right. These mechanisms can also regulate for the loss of cells both due to x-rays and the formation of M/M cells.

The Results

Having given an indication of the methods used in this type of clonal analysis we must now mention some of the earlier results. Becker (*15*) was the first to use x-rays to produce clones at particular stages of development, in his study of the *Drosophila* eye. Later Garcia-Bellido (*9*) noted that clones produced after the 1st instar larva never crossed from dorsal to ventral on the wing; and Bryant and Schneiderman (*8*) that they were confined to single leg segments when larvae older than early third-stage larva were irradiated. Bryant (*4*) made the important observation that clones in the wing disc could cross from dorsal to ventral if produced early enough, but not when produced late. Similarly, in *Oncopeltus* (*16–18*) up until the late blastoderm stage, clones may extend to two or more abdominal segments, but after that stage clones are strictly confined to a

single segment. These observations all show that within three different discs of *Drosophila* and in the *Oncopeltus* abdomen the "anlagen are represented by separate populations of proliferating cells" (*4*).

The most detailed results so far have been obtained by Garcia-Bellido and his colleagues studying the development of the wing disc. As might have been expected the earliest clones (irradiation of first-stage larvae) are contained exclusively within the fairly large area of the adult cuticle produced by the entire disc. This shows that effective separation of the wing disc from the other discs producing the adult epithelium must have occurred before the first larval stage. However, even at these early times a compartment boundary is apparent within the disc. This was first clearly demonstrated by the Madrid school using the *Minute* technique. The boundary, which separates anterior regions from posterior regions, runs along the middle of the wing between the third and fourth vein. The actual demarcation line is near the fourth vein but is distinct from it (Fig. 5). The line runs along both surfaces of the wing and continues on the body where it divides the notum into two distinct areas. Even a very large clone (Fig. 6) will observe this demarcation line although at this stage it may well cross the wing margins, thus appearing on both dorsal and ventral surfaces and extending onto the notum.

The edges of the clone are somewhat irregular except where they run along the demarcation line. It is not very likely that this line marks the frontier where two initially remote and separate groups of cells have moved together, since both anterior and posterior regions are within the same nascent imaginal disc and thus probably fairly close together (*6*). Since about twice as many clones appear in the anterior compartment as in the posterior one, it is surmised that at this early time there are about twice as many anterior as posterior cells. That is, the antero-

posterior division is not exactly into two equal parts but more like a 2 : 1 ratio (*10*).

Some time later, during larval development (the exact time is not quite clear), each of these two compartments is found to be divided into four parts, giving eight compartments in all. The demarcation lines divide dorsal from ventral areas and wing from thorax. The final size of these compartment areas varies somewhat (from 10^4 cells to 10^3 cells or less). The evidence that late clones really observe these demarcation lines is very strong. They are observed by very large clones, which in some cases make up as much as 90 percent of a compartment. Such clones may border a demarcation line for as many as a thousand cells. Nor is the effect solely due to the fact that clones are often elongated in a direction roughly parallel to a demarcation line. The main axis of these clones meets the demarcation line at various angles, sometimes even perpendicularly. Nor on any simple model can the demarcation lines be lines of fusion of quite separate groups of cells if only for the fact that marked clones made at a slightly earlier stage will go straight across these lines.

As development proceeds the recognition of new subcompartments again becomes somewhat more difficult because the effects of differential growth (due to M^+/M^+ cells in a M/M^+ background) have less time to produce larger clones. Garcia-Bellido, Ripoll, and Morata suggest that there may be two further demarcation lines formed about the same time. On the adult fly these separate two areas on the body, one dividing the notum into two parts and the other the pleura. These compartments were all discovered by the use of M/M^+ flies, but similar experiments on non-*Minute* flies (which have, of course, smaller clones), show that the demarcation lines are also observed in this more normal situation. The *Minute* flies thus serve to make the subcompartments more easy to observe: the phenomenon itself is not peculiar to them alone.

95

Further Problems

Having now described the results on compartments in outline we must ask how widely the idea is applicable and what are its limitations. One limitation is that the evidence obtained so far relates only to epidermal structures. This is mainly because in insects they are so easy to observe and so rich in detail. Internal structures, for example, the exact arrangement of the muscles, cannot be studied satisfactorily without the use of more difficult experimental methods.

However, the properties of internal tissues may be partly imposed by the pattern of the enclosing epithelium (19), and they may well also be compartmented.

With regard to compartments in imaginal discs, there are a series of outstanding questions that need answering. Are all subdivisions binary? We have seen how the first division of the wing disc, after the very early antero-posterior divisions, appears to yield four parts rather than two. It is natural to ask if this is really two separate binary steps in quick succession, and this question focuses attention on the exact timing of the subdivisions. Even for an obviously binary step one can ask whether the decision is an abrupt one or is spread over a period. Does it necessarily require cell division? Are compartment boundaries always smooth? The edge between the dorsal and ventral surface of the wing is very well defined, and clones that border it are smooth to the nearest cell (4, 5), but is this true for all boundaries?

The problem of how a compartment boundary is formed and how it gets so straight appears to be a difficult one. Factors that may have to be considered are strictly oriented mitoses near the boundary (17), straightening effects due to differential cell affinities, and possibly cell death for cells which get themselves into the wrong places, so that the compartment edges are trimmed. It is claimed (20) that extensive cell death is unlikely because otherwise clone size near the boundary would be smaller, which is apparently not the case.

Nor is it completely clear where the process of the subdivision of compartments stops. Even the technique for spotting compartment boundaries, using relatively fast-growing marked clones, has its limitations as, at later times, even these clonal patches are rather small. How can we be sure that these are not further subcompartments? Even the definition of a compartment becomes difficult at this point. Although formally, for example, the descendants of a single bristle mother cell [for example, the trichogen, the tormogen, the sense cell, and the neurilemma cell making up a bristle in *Oncopeltus* (21)] which are most certainly a clone and which stay together, could perhaps be regarded as a compartment, we feel that this is stretching the term too far. It would seem sensible to restrict the term "compartment" for the moment to fairly large groups of cells and to those groups which form a polyclone rather than a clone.

Other Possible Characteristics of Compartments

We have seen that, at the moment, a compartment is defined by its boundaries and these alone, since clones, made after a certain time in development, never cross them. Are there other properties that allow us to identify a compartment?

One such property may be the area affected by a homeotic mutant. There are mutants that shift an imaginal disc, or part of an imaginal disc, into another developmental pathway. For example, *aristapedia* (ss^a) transforms part of the antenna into leg segments (22).

It is rather rare for a mutant to turn one whole disc into another whole disc. Possibly such a drastic change would be lethal and thus escape observation. It is more common for a part of one disc to be turned into part of another one. Even in these cases the transformation is not always complete, because of partial and variable expressivity. We can, however, ask the general question: In such cases do the (maximum) boundaries of the transformation coincide with a compartment boundary found by the clonal method?

Morata and Garcia-Bellido (23) have shown by clonal analysis that the haltere disc (the metathoracic disc) has within it an antero-posterior boundary; but locating it precisely is difficult because of the absence of suitable landmarks on the haltere. It has been known for many years (24) that various mutants in the bithorax system turn various parts of haltere into wing (or vice versa) with different degrees of expressivity. A number of mutants appear to respect the antero-posterior boundary of wing with some precision and probably also of the haltere although here the precision is more difficult to judge. For example, an extreme allele of *bithorax* (bx^3) turns the anterior part of the haltere into anterior wing while leaving the posterior part of the haltere (which is much smaller) unaltered. The boundary of this transformed half-wing is very close or identical to the antero-posterior boundary found by clonal methods in the wild-type wing (Fig. 7). Another mutant in this complex locus (*postbithorax*) also delineates this boundary because its effect is restricted to the posterior part of the haltere.

The gene *engrailed* also delineates the boundary, and in an especially interesting way. In flies mutant for *engrailed* the posterior part of the wing is transformed and resembles a mirror image of the anterior part (25). The *Minute* technique has recently been used to show that the realm of action of the *engrailed* gene precisely coincides with the posterior compartment,

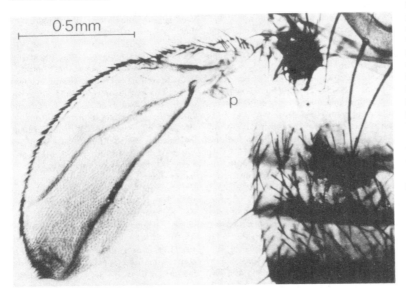

0·5mm

Fig. 7. A metathoracic appendage from a *Drosophila* carrying an extreme allele for *bithorax*. The posterior haltere develops normally (*p*) while the anterior haltere is transformed into an apparently normal and complete anterior wing compartment.

there being no effect on the anterior. If large *engrailed* (*en/en*) clones are made in a wide-type wing (*en/+*) they may fill the anterior compartment right up to the antero-posterior boundary but never cross it. They are completely without effect on the pattern. However, all *engrailed* clones in the posterior part express the phenotype (*26*) and, as discussed later, may cross the antero-posterior boundary.

Another possible correlation is between gradient discontinuities and compartment boundaries. These discontinuities can be of at least two kinds. The first has a discontinuity in the value of the gradient but not its slope, as shown in Fig. 8. The other has no discontinuity in the value but a change of slope, in particular a change of sign of the slope to give the mirror-image situation shown in Fig. 9.

The first of these is found between the segments of the insect cuticle in *Rhodnius* and *Oncopeltus*. Lawrence (*16, 18*) has shown in *Oncopeltus* that marked clones do not cross the intersegmental boundary, so here at least we have one clear case where a clonal boundary coincides at least approximately with a gradient discontinuity (*27*). Another possible case is suggested by the mutant *engrailed* mentioned above. Since this produces a rough mirror image across the antero-posterior compartment boundary of the wing, one might be tempted to think that the underlying gradient (or "prepattern") might have the mirror image form shown in Fig. 8 both in the mutant and the wild-type. Otherwise the experimental evidence for this possible correlation is either scanty or absent.

There are several other properties which we can speculate about. Experiments designed to show how mixtures of cells from imaginal discs appear to sort out show clearly that cells from different discs will segregate, suggesting rather strongly that they have different surface properties (*28*). Moreover, such segregation also occurs between marked cells from different parts of the same disc. For example, cells from the anterior part of the wing disc will segregate from those of the posterior part (*29*). This obviously suggests the generalization that each compartment has characteristic cell surface properties, different from every other compartment, which allow cells from any two compartments to segregate. Thus the normal development and maintenance of the antero-posterior boundary in the wing might depend on the confrontation of cells of a different type, that is "anterior" with "posterior" cells. If so, one might expect that boundary to be malformed or nonexistent in *engrailed* flies where the posterior cells are partially transformed into those of the anterior type. Clonal

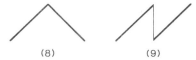

(8)   (9)

Fig. 8. The probable gradient situation in *Drosophila* wing; the slope, but not the altitude, changes near the antero-posterior compartment border. Fig. 9. The probable gradient situation in two adjacent abdominal segments of Hemiptera. The step probably coincides with the intersegmental compartment boundary.

analysis of *engrailed* flies has recently shown that clones do frequently cross the line where the border normally is (*26*). This never happens in flies wild-type for the *engrailed* locus, a result that strongly supports the idea that the role of the *en+* allele is both to control the development of the posterior pattern and to instruct the cells so that they do not intermingle with cells of the neighboring anterior type.

An additional possibility is that there is a gradient of cell surface properties within each compartment. This is certainly suggested by the observation (*30*) that in the epidermis of *Oncopeltus* a graft takes better if it is from the same level in the segmental gradient, even if from a different segment, than if moved to a different position in the gradient in the same segment. These speculations go far beyond the experimental data now available, but they do suggest that direct methods of characterizing cell surface properties, preferably in situ, would be very valuable. If such a method could be developed it would have the enormous advantage that it might work for the cells of the developing imaginal disc so that one could spot compartments and their boundaries at the moment, or soon after, they are formed.

It is also possible that, even though all the epithelial cells of a disc appear very similar, the compartments within them could differ by a particular enzyme or set of enzymes. For this reason there is a case for testing all the imaginal discs, both in their mature and their developing states, by as many histochemical tests as are available. A beginning has already been made in this approach by Janning (*31*) using a test for aldehyde oxidase.

Another histological feature that may correlate to some extent with compartments is the distribution of nerve axons. Hasenfuss (*32*), studying the epidermis of *Galleria* and *Rhyacophila*, noticed that the nerve axons of the sensillae in the abdominal epidermis were collected into groups each of which went to one segmental ganglion only. He suggested that this was because each group came only

from a single epidermal segment. This, however, was true only of the axons since the dendrites were observed to extend over considerable distances and thus could not be confined within one segment. A similar phenomenon has also been observed by Lawrence (*33*) in the abdomen of *Oncopeltus*. In this case, the intersegmental boundaries are clearly delineated by color and cell shape. No axons have been observed to cross these boundaries, although they do cross the midline. (It is known that the midline is formed in the embryo by the fusion of two separate groups of cells.)

One is thus led to the speculation that the fields outlined by well-defined groups of nerve axons may perhaps coincide in certain cases with compartments or subcompartments. This might be because compartmentalization may often occur before the separation of the neuroblasts from the presumptive epidermis, so that any cell surface differences or other labels associated with a compartment may be shared by both the epidermal cells and the neurons.

The hypothetical properties so far discussed would be possessed by all or most of the cells within a given compartment or subcompartment. They could be described as area properties. Another rather different property would be one which characterized boundaries between compartments, that is, an edge property. For example, the cells on one side of the intersegmental boundaries in *Oncopeltus* are markedly elongated in the direction of the boundary (*17*). Do all compartment boundaries have this property? For the antero-posterior wing boundary it seems that the adult cells have no unusual appearance; but nevertheless a detailed scrutiny of several such boundaries might be worthwhile. Another obvious hypothesis is that whereas there may be free diffusion of certain chemicals within compartments it may be greatly restricted across compartment boundaries. This suggests that compartments might not be electrically coupled to each other, but a direct test across the intersegmental boundary in *Rhodnius* (*34*) showed coupling to be normal. Moreover, a careful cytological study by electron microscopy has shown no observable difference in the various types of cell junctions (gap junctions, septate desmosomes, attachment desmosomes) for the corresponding intersegmental boundary in *Oncopeltus* (*35*). One is thus not exactly encouraged to look for these same differences at compartment boundaries in structures from imaginal discs. Nevertheless, it would be surprising if there were not some important cytological difference at compartment boundaries.

Possible Mechanisms for Compartment Formation

We must now consider the nature of the step which partitions the cells that are the ancestors of one compartment in such a way that some of them become the founder cells of one subcompartment while the others become the founders of the other subcompartment. As we have seen, this step is often a partition into two parts (rather than three, four, or more), and it is possible that this is always the case. For the moment we will only consider the case of binary partition.

At present, little can be said about any underlying biochemical mechanism, but we can usefully discuss the problem at the cellular level. Unfortunately, we have rather few facts to go on. In view of the existence of size and shape regulation (as shown by the experiments in which a relatively fast-growing clone within a compartment does not alter its dimensions), it is not obviously a requirement that the partition need be always exactly the same, since any variation, if it is not too big, can probably be corrected by subsequent growth. We consider three possible types of mechanism.

1) *The partition of daughters.* All the cells divide once, one daughter of each division being allocated to one subcompartment and one to the other.

2) *Random allocation.* The cells are allocated at random, with a fixed probability which we shall assume to be about one-half. Because of the number of cells involved, the chance of all the cells being accidentally allocated to one subcompartment is so small that it can be ignored (for example, for 20 cells this chance is 1 in 2^{19} or about 2 in 10^6). Even if all cells but one are allocated to one subcompartment, the single cell allocated to the other could, conceivably, compensate for this numerical handicap by an increased rate of multiplication.

3) *Geographical partition.* The patch of epithelial cells is divided, the dividing line separating the founder cells of one subcompartment from those of the other.

The difficulty with the first two mechanisms is that, in order to get the cells of each subcompartment together in one patch, a certain amount of relative cell movement would have to take place. Since the partitioning into subcompartments takes place several times in succession, one would not expect marked clones to stay in one piece, as they usually do. Thus these two mechanisms seem unlikely, except perhaps for the first of the several partitioning steps.

The mechanisms can be saved to some extent by an additional hypothesis; that any cell which is surrounded by cells of the other type commits suicide. It is difficult to make this model precise, but it would appear to lead to a fair amount of cell death. Moreover, the cells which migrated would still have to move to the correct place in the epithelium relative to other surrounding tissues.

The third proposed mechanism—geographical partition—seems to us to be by far the most likely one, especially as it does not need to be extremely precise. Consider, say, a patch of 20 cells. Let each cell divide once to give 40 cells. Each of these cells will be surrounded in the epithelium by several other cells (the average number is usually a little above five), one of which will be its sister cell. Now draw an arbitrary (but moderately straight) line partitioning the patch into two parts. This line will separate some cells which are sisters. The problem is to estimate the fraction (averaged over many cases) of the original 20 cells which will have daughters separated by the line. It is only these particular cells that can produce a clone of descendants which will go across the boundary between the subcompartments.

Several approximate estimates have been made by Ripley (*36*) using various simplifications. The fraction defined above can be written as equal to $C/N^{1/2}$ when N is the number of cells at the time the line is drawn (40 in the example above) and C is a parameter which is approximately constant. The values of C found were not far from 0.55. Thus for $N = 25$ the fraction is about 11 percent. This calculation shows rather clearly that on this simple mechanism the existence of clones which cross the subcompartment boundary will not be a rare event if they are marked one generation before the compartment is divided.

A more detailed mathematical study of this problem would be worthwhile since it is important to compare the detailed experimental data (what fraction of clones crosses a border, what fraction runs alongside one, and the like, as a function of exact time of irradiation) with what would be expected on the various theoretical models.

Conclusion

We have seen that the work of Garcia-Bellido and his colleagues has clearly brought out the formation of compartments and successive subcompartments in the epithelium produced by the wing disc of *Drosophila* and that there is evidence that a similar process occurs in the production of other regions of the insect epithelium. We have also seen that the phenomena, although clearly demonstrated in outline, need further detailed study, especially quantitative study. The mechanism that produces these subcompartments is obscure although a plausible model can be suggested for the general nature of the process.

It is therefore pertinent to ask what is the novelty of these ideas, viewed from the general perspective of development studies. To do this we must ask what the experiments show does not happen.

We are not talking about the determination of cell type in the usual sense—for example, a muscle cell as opposed to a fibroblast—but about cell position. In this system the determination and differentiation of cell types—for example, bristles as opposed to epithelial cells—probably comes later and may well also be dependent on the compartment to which the cells belong. What we are concerned with is geographical position in the organism and, moreover, not about exact geographical position but whether a cell is somewhere within one well-defined region or another one.

What has been demonstrated in this system is that once a major developmental step of this type has been taken by a cell it is not reversed in the progeny of that cell, at least in normal development. If reversal was possible, a cell which had been determined for the dorsal side of the wing and which found itself on the ventral side could be reprogrammed to be a ventral cell. What clonal analysis has shown is that this never happens. Either such a cell cannot get to the wrong side of the wing, or, if it does so, it must either move back to the right side or be killed. The exact mechanism is obscure. Whatever it is, it is clearly of interest, even though the basic concept, the irreversibility of major developmental steps, is not in itself especially novel.

But it would be both novel and exciting if it turns out that the compartments and subcompartments are used by the organism as units for the control of shape and size; if gradient systems meet at compartment boundaries, if cell surface properties changed abruptly there, if size regulation occurred partly independently within each of these domains, and so forth. It may be that the normal development of each imaginal disc can usefully be divided into a precise succession of major steps each of which produces a set of new compartments. If so, by studying compartment formation, one could both enumerate these steps and determine their times of action. On this picture each compartment would be specified by a unique combination of a small number of controlling genes [selector genes (*1*)] that are active in it. (The steps that follow—for example, the determination of a bristle in a particular position within a compartment—may be of a somewhat different and more complex character.) For the first time there is the real prospect of understanding the logic behind gene deployment in pattern formation. As we have seen, the speculative ideas about compartments in this section are not supported by hard evidence. The best we have so far is a series of hints. But it is exactly this possibility, that compartments may have a wider significance, which makes the study of them at the present time so important and so interesting.

References and Notes

1. A. Garcia-Bellido, in *Cell Patterning* (Associated Scientific Publishers, London, 1975), p. 161.
2. C. Auerbach, *Trans. R. Soc. Edinb.* **58**, 787 (1936).
3. M. J. Pearson, *J. Cell Sci.* **16**, 113 (1974).
4. P. J. Bryant, *Dev. Biol.* **22**, 389 (1970).
5. A. Garcia-Bellido and J. R. Merriam, *ibid.* **24**, 61 (1971).
6. P. Ripoll, *Wilhelm Roux' Arch. Entwicklungs-mech. Org.* **169**, 200 (1972).
7. C. A. Poodry and H. A. Schneiderman, *ibid.* **168**, 1 (1971).
8. P. J. Bryant and H. A. Schneiderman, *Dev. Biol.* **20**, 263 (1969).
9. A. Garcia-Bellido, *Genetics* **60**, 181 (1968).
10. ———, P. Ripoll, G. Morata, *Nat. New Biol.* **245**, 251 (1973); *Dev. Biol.*, in press.
11. W. Gehring, *Dev. Biol.* **16**, 438 (1967).
12. D. L. Lindsley and E. H. Grell, *Genetic Variations of* Drosophila melanogaster (Carnegie Institution of Washington, Washington, D.C., 1968).
13. G. Morata and P. Ripoll, *Dev. Biol.* **42**, 211 (1975).
14. A. Ferrus, *Genetics*, in press.
15. H. J. Becker, *Z. Indukt. Abstammungs-Vererbungsl.* **88**, 333 (1957).
16. P. Lawrence, *Symp. Soc. Exp. Biol.* **25**, 379 (1971).
17. ———, *Nat. New Biol.* **242**, 31 (1973).
18. ———, *J. Embryol. Exp. Morphol.* **30**, 681 (1973).
19. T. S. Sahota and W. E. Beckel, *Can. J. Zool.* **45**, 407 (1967).
20. P. Santamaria and A. Garcia-Bellido, in preparation.
21. P. A. Lawrence, *J. Cell Sci.* **1**, 475 (1966).
22. W. Gehring and R. Nöthiger, in *Developmental Systems: Insects*, S. Counce and C. H. Waddington, Eds. (Academic Press, New York, 1973), vol. 2, p. 211.
23. G. Morata and A. Garcia-Bellido, in preparation.
24. E. B. Lewis, *Am. Zool.* **3**, 33 (1963); in *Role of Chromosomes in Development*, M. Locke, Ed. (Academic Press, New York, 1964), p. 231; in *Heritage from Mendel*, P. A. Brink, Ed. (Univ. of Wisconsin Press, Madison, 1967), p. 17.
25. A. Garcia-Bellido and P. Santamaria, *Genetics* **72**, 87 (1972).
26. G. Morata and P. A. Lawrence, *Nature (Lond.)* **255**, 614 (1975).
27. P. A. Lawrence, F. H. C. Crick, M. Munro, *J. Cell Sci.* **11**, 815 (1972).
28. R. Nöthiger, *Wilhelm Roux' Arch. Entwicklungs-mech. Org.* **155**, 269 (1964).
29. A. Garcia-Bellido, *Dev. Biol.* **14**, 278 (1966).
30. P. A. Lawrence, unpublished data.
31. W. Janning, *Drosophila Inf. Serv.* **50**, 151 (1973).
32. I. Hasenfuss, *Verh. Dtsch. Zool. Ges.* **66**, 71 (1973); *Zool. Jahrb. Anat.* **90**, 1 (1973); *ibid.*, p. 175.
33. P. A. Lawrence, in *Cell Patterning* (Associated Scientific Publishers, London, 1975), p. 3.
34. A. E. Warner and P. A. Lawrence, *Nature (Lond.)* **245**, 47 (1973).
35. P. A. Lawrence and S. M. Green, *J. Cell Biol.* **65**, 373 (1975).
36. B. Ripley, personal communication.
37. We thank Professor A. Garcia-Bellido and Dr. G. Morata and our colleagues in the MRC Laboratory for many helpful comments and criticisms.

Zoon 6: 157–160, 1978

Proc. Symp. "Formshaping Movements in Neurogenesis," Uppsala, Sept. 12–15, 1977

Compartments and the Insect Nervous System

PETER A. LAWRENCE

MRC Laboratory of Molecular Biology, Cambridge, UK

ABSTRACT

Lawrence, P. A. (MRC Laboratory of Molecular Biology, Hills Road, Cambridge CB2 2QH, UK). *Compartments and the insect nervous system.*

Zoon 6 (Formshaping Movements in Neurogenesis): 157–160, 1978

A compartment is a precisely defined region of the adult insect which is made by all the progeny of a small group of cells. This group is set aside at a specific and early stage of development. The peripheral sensory neurons of insects develop from the epidermis: *a priori* one would expect them to share properties characteristic of the compartment to which they belong. In the abdominal epidermis of *Oncopeltus* (the milkweed bug) the behavior of the epidermal cells and the sensory axons is shown to be similar with respect to the segment borders, the lateral borders and the midline. One effect of these properties of the epidermal cells is that they become confined to specific regions, and the effect of the same properties on the axons is that all axons from one compartment will enter a single bundle.

We now know that insects are constructed piecemeal. Each piece of the adult epidermis (a *compartment;* García-Bellido et al., 1973) is precisely defined and is made by all the descendents of a small group of founder cells (a *polyclone;* Crick & Lawrence, 1975) which is set aside from other groups in early development. Sometimes the lines demarcating compartments fall in surprising places – as in the case of the wing (García-Bellido, 1973; García-Bellido et al., 1976) or the proboscis (Struhl, 1977) of *Drosophila* which are subdivided into two separate halves. Sometimes the lines fall more expectedly, as with the line between abdominal segments in *Oncopeltus* (Lawrence, 1973). We imagine that the development of polyclones is under the control of specific genes which are activated at the definition of a polyclone, and whose products are continually required by its constituent cells. The state of activity of these genes may, in combination, generate a binary code specifying the part

constructed (García-Bellido, 1975; Morata & Lawrence, 1977). Consequently the domain affected by mutation in these genes coincides with a compartment as defined by studies of cell lineage (García-Bellido et al., 1973; Morata & Lawrence, 1975). There is some evidence that compartments are the units of pattern formation; gradients specifying positional information may be set up in polyclones, and growth may be controlled from compartment borders (Crick & Lawrence, 1975).

So far these observations have been almost exclusively limited to the epidermal cells of insects, mainly because they can be easily labelled with genetic marker mutations. It is likely that other tissues are also subdivided into compartments, and here I discuss the possible significance of compartments to the organisation of the developing nervous system. The *peripheral* sensory organs of insects develop directly from epidermal cells and so must belong to particular compartments as defined by cell lineage. Further, it is possible that the neuroblasts which generate the *central* nervous system might separate from a defined polyclone and thus would have the determined state characteristic of that polyclone.

Peripheral nervous system

When an epidermal cell makes a sensillum, such as a bristle, it divides to generate cells which produce both the cuticular structures and the nerve cell (Wigglesworth, 1953). The outgrowing axon appears to grow at random until it meets another axon which it then follows to the central nervous system (Wigglesworth, 1953). In Hemiptera, where bristles are added every moult cycle, nerves from new bristles follow the pathway laid down previously. Hasenfuss (1973 *a, b*) was struck by the reliability with which particular sensilla send their central axons to the correct segmental ganglion. If growth of the axons were completely random one would

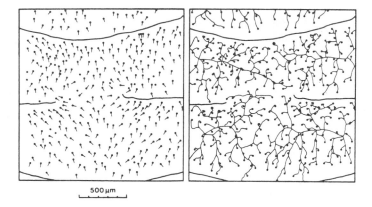

500 μm

Fig. 1. 5th stage *Oncopeltus fasciatus* bearing an interruption in the segment borders between dorsal tergites II and III On the left the orientation of bristles i shown, note the effects near the gap in the intersegmental boundary (*thick line*). On the right; the sensory innervation of the same region is shown. Bristles, *apparently* belonging to the upper segment (II), are connected to the axons of the lower segment (III). From Wright (unpublished).

expect that sometimes the nerve would cross to the next segment and go to the wrong ganglion. Detailed examination of *Oncopeltus* abdominal innervation (Lawrence, 1975) shows that this never happens—apparently because the growing axon will not transgress the intersegmental boundary. But why not? There seems to be no general barrier, because fine dendrites will cross from one segment to another (Hasenfuss, 1973 *a, b*). Moreover, the structure appears to be a simple interface between cells of the two abutting segments (Lawrence & Greene, 1975). It does seem to be the border itself which is respected, because when the boundary is locally missing, allowing interaction between adjacent segment gradients and consequent changes in cell polarity (Fig. 1; Lawrence, 1966); the nerves cross the line where the boundary normally is (Fig. 1; Wright, unpublished). Further, when grafts are exchanged between segments the nerves from the graft can grow out and join the host axons of a different segment (Lawrence, 1975).

Apparently the axons are behaving just like normal epidermal cells, which will not intermingle across the intersegmental boundary and instead form a straight interface there (Lawrence, 1973). Likewise, when the cells are transplanted to the same level in another abdominal segment they will intermingle during subsequent growth (Wright, unpublished). The effect of these properties of the epidermal cells is that precise compartments are formed with straight sharp edges, and the effect of the same properties in the axons is that *all* the nerves from the same compartment find their way into one bundle as they grow towards the central nervous system. This parallel can be extended to the lateral compartment boundary which intervenes

where dorsal meets ventral in the *Oncopeltus* abdomen. These polyclones are defined about the same time as the different segmental ones are formed (Lawrence, 1973). The dorsoventral interface in the mature larva is also straight and precise and is respected by axons growing out from the sensory bristles (Wright, unpublished). A similar comparison can be made between the behavior of epidermal cells and axons at the midline, where the left and the right parts of the segments meet. Although marked clones are generally confined to the left or the right they do not meet at a straight interface (Lawrence, 1973). Similarly, the peripheral nerve axons do not respect any sharp boundary at the midline, bristles arising on the left sometimes send their axons to the right nerve and *vice versa* (Lawrence, 1975). In *Drosophila*, fast-growing clones of cells are able to cross a long way from one side to the other in several organs, e.g. 1st leg (Steiner, 1976) and genitalia (Dubendorfer, Thesis. Univ. of Zurich 1977); an observation which underlines the identical cell affinities which characterise left and right sides of the same part of the body.

In conclusion, the characteristic behaviour of the epidermis which results in the formation of sharp compartment borders between homologous segments and between dorsal and ventral parts is paralleled exactly in the behavior of the axons within those compartments. Thus the hypothesis that the epidermal cells may bear specific compartmental 'labels' (Morata & Lawrence, 1975; Lawrence & Morata, 1976) can be directly extended to the peripheral nerve cells that they generate. One consequence of this idea is that in *Drosophila*, where organs such as the wings, legs and proboscis are subdivided into two separate polyclones at a very early stage, one might expect two bundles of sensory axons, one coming from each compartment.

Central nervous system

The epidermal cells and the central nervous system are closely related by lineage, as they both develop from the ectoderm. It is possible (Crick & Lawrence, 1975) that the neuroblasts and the epidermis could arise from the same specifically determined polyclones and therefore share the same inherited 'labels'. In both *Oncopeltus* (Lawrence, 1973) and *Drosophila* (Wieschaus & Gehring, 1976) the segmental polyclones are established at, or soon after, blastoderm formation; that is possibly before the divisions which generate the neuroblasts. If this were true, and there is no direct evidence, then it could be the basis for subsequent neuronal specificity. Particular axons growing into the centre would seek out their distant cousins in the ganglion, those with the best matching 'labels'.

Connections between the central and peripheral nervous system

We know little of the rules governing connections between the periphery and the centre. Experiments where limbs are transplanted in the cockroach show that outgrowing motor neurons and ingrowing peripheral axons are able to make appropriate (homologous) connections even when the limb and the central ganglion belong to different segments (Young, 1973). This could depend on a reiteration of positional information in each segment both in the peripheral epidermis (Locke, 1959; Lawrence et al., 1972), in the nerve cells generated within the epidermis and in the neuroblasts forming the central nervous system (Crick & Lawrence, 1975).

Young's experiments (Young, 1973) were performed on the mesothoracic and metathoracic legs of the cockroach, which are rather similar structures. The wing and haltere of *Drosophila* are also derivatives of the meso- and metathorax but are unlike in structure and function. The routes followed by ingrowing sensory axons are quite different in the two organs (Palka & Lawrence, unpublished). In an attempt to learn about the rules governing the routes taken by such axons we have made use of homeotic mutations which transform haltere into wing or *vice versa*. Because the effect of the mutations on the central nervous system is

unknown it seemed wise to make large clones of mutant cells in a wildtype animal, thus transforming entire peripheral compartments while leaving the centre unchanged. Such experiments are underway (Palka & Lawrence, unpublished).

ACKNOWLEDGEMENTS

I thank David Wright for permission to quote unpublished results.

REFERENCES

Crick, F. H. C. & Lawrence, P. A. 1975. Compartments and polyclones in insect development. Science *189*, 340–347.

García-Bellido, A. 1975. Genetic control of wing disc development in *Drosophila*. *In* Cell Patterning, Ciba Foundation Symposium, *29* (n.s.), pp. 161–178. Associated Scientific Publishers, Amsterdam.

García-Bellido, A., Ripoll, P. & Morata, G. 1973. Developmental compartmentalization of the wing disk of *Drosophila*. Nature New Biol. *245*, 251–253.

— 1976. Developmental compartmentalization in the dorsal mesothoracic disc of *Drosophila*. Dev. Biol. *48*, 132–147.

Hasenfuss, I. 1973 *a*. Vergleichend-morphologische Untersuchung der sensorischen Innervierung der Rumpfwand der Larven von *Rhyacophila nubila* Zett. (Trichoptera) und *Galleria mellonella* L. (Lepidoptera). Zool. Jahrb. Abt. Anat. Ontog. *90*, 1–54, 175–253.

— 1973 *b*. Über die Beziehung zwischen sensorischer Innervierung und primären Segmentgrenzen bei Arthropoden. Verh. Deutsch. Zool. Ges. *66*, 71–75.

Lawrence, P. A. 1966. Gradients in the insect segment: the orientation of hairs in the milkweed bug *Oncopeltus fasciatus*. J. Exp. Biol. *44*, 607–620.

— 1973. A clonal analysis of segment development in *Oncopeltus* (Hemiptera). J. Embryol. Exp. Morphol. *30*, 681–699.

— 1975. The structure and properties of a compartment border: the intersegmental boundary in *Oncopeltus*. *In* Cell Patterning, Ciba Foundation Symposium, *29*, (n.s.), pp. 3–16. Associated Scientific Publishers, Amsterdam.

Lawrence, P. A. & Green, S. M. 1975. The anatomy of a compartment border: the intersegmental boundary in *Oncopeltus*. J. Cell Biol. *65*, 373–382.

Lawrence, P. A. & Morata, G. 1976. Compartments in the wing of *Drosophila*: a study of the *engrailed* gene. Dev. Biol. *50*, 321–337.

Lawrence, P. A., Crick, F. H. C. & Munro, M. 1972. A gradient of positional information in an insect, *Rhodnius*. J. Cell. Sci. *11*, 815–853.

Locke, M. 1959. The cuticular pattern in an insect, *Rhodnius prolixus* Stal. J. Exp. Biol. *36*, 459–477.

Morata, G. & Lawrence, P. A. 1975. Control of compartment development by the *engrailed* gene in *Drosophila*. Nature *255*, 614–617.

160   *P. A. Lawrence*

— 1977. Homoeotic genes, compartments and cell determination in *Drosophila*. Nature 265, 211–216.

Steiner, E. 1976. Establishment of compartments in the developing leg imaginal discs of *Drosophila melanogaster*. Wilhelm Roux' Arch. *180*, 9–30.

Struhl, G. 1977. Developmental compartments in the proboscis of *Drosophila*. Nature *270*, 723–725.

Wieschaus, E. & Gehring, W. 1976. Clonal analysis of primordial disc cells in the early embryo of *Drosophila melanogaster*. Dev. Biol. *50*, 249–263.

Wigglesworth, V. B 1953. The origin of sensory neurones in an insect (*Rhodnius prolixus, Hemiptera*). Quart. J. Microsc. Sci. *94*, 93–112.

Young, D. 1973. Specific re-innervation of limbs transplanted between segments in the cockroach *Periplaneta americana*. J. Exp. Biol. *57*, 305–316.

103

Section 3
Neuronal Lineage and Differentiation

Patterson, P.H. and L.L.Y Chun. 1977. The induction of acetylcholine synthesis in primary cultures of dissociated rat sympathetic neurons. I. Effects of conditioned medium. *Dev. Biol.* 56: 263–280.

Furshpan, E.J., P.R. MacLeish, P.H. O'Lague, and D.D. Potter. 1976. Chemical transmission between rat sympathetic neurons and cardiac myocytes developing in microcultures: Evidence for cholinergic, adrenergic, and dual-function neurons. *Proc. Natl. Acad. Sci.* 73: 4225–4229.

Le Douarin, N.M. 1980. The ontogeny of the neural crest in avian embryo chimaeras. *Nature* 286: 663–669.

Horvitz, H.R. 1981. Neuronal cell lineages in the nematode *Caenorhabditis elegans*. In *Development in the nervous system.* British Society for Developmental Biology, Symposium 5 (ed. D. Garrod and J. Feldman), pp. 331–346. Cambridge University Press, Cambridge.

Goodman, C.S. and N.C. Spitzer. 1979. Embryonic development of identified neurones: Differentiation from neuroblast to neurone. *Nature* 280: 208–214.

As a class of cells becomes progressively distinct from other classes, the cells are said to differentiate. Differentiation obviously depends on a number of complex interactions; nonetheless, the acquisition of many specialized characteristics must be based ultimately on the modulation of gene expression during development. The details of such modulation are just beginning to be understood at the molecular level in eukaryotic cells, including neurons (Brown 1981; Schmitt et al. 1982). A major question about differentiation, relevant to all cells, concerns the relative contribution of extrinsic and intrinsic influences to this process. To what extent does development unfold according to rules built into each cell, and to what extent is it a result of influences impinging on developing cells from without? In fact, a cell's acquisition of the characteristics it will ultimately express appears to depend both on its lineage, i.e., its developmental history, and on cues from its environment.

Evidence for the importance of the cellular environment in differentiation first came from classical work on induction in amphibian embryos. As Spemann (1938) showed in experiments carried out early in this century, if the optic vesicle is removed from an early frog embryo, the lens that normally arises from the overlying ectoderm does not develop. Even more dramatic was Spemann's finding that the introduction of a particular piece of the amphibian embryo (the dorsal lip of the blastopore) into a host embryo organized the development of an entire second embryo in the host at the site of transplantation (Spemann and Mangold 1924).

The importance of the cellular and hormonal environment for neuronal differentiation is also evident in studies of neural crest cells and their neuronal derivatives. Thus far, most of the work in this area has examined the factors that

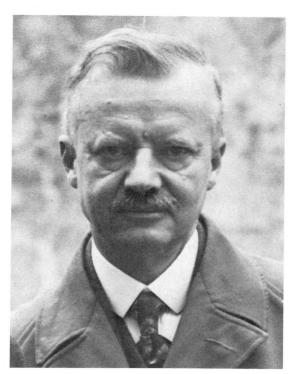

Hans Spemann, whose classical experiments on embryonic induction and regulation established the context for recent studies of cell differentiation.

cording electrophysiologically from individual neurons over a period of several weeks in culture (Potter et al. 1981). Since all of the neurons studied display noradrenergic properties at the beginning of the culture period and virtually all of them can be induced to display cholinergic properties, it was not surprising that some neurons expressed both properties simultaneously (Furshpan et al. 1976; Landis 1976; Reichardt and Patterson 1977; Higgins et al. 1981). This noradrenergic-to-cholinergic sequence may occur during the normal development of sympathetic cholinergic neurons in vivo (Landis and Keefe 1980), and perhaps in enteric neurons as well (Jonakait et al. 1979).

What is the nature of the environmental influence on transmitter choice? First, the embryonic milieu through which neural crest cells migrate and the site at which they come to rest are both thought to play a role (**Le Douarin 1980**; Bunge et al. 1978; Patterson 1978; Teillet et al. 1978). Second, certain nonneuronal cells, such as cardiac myocytes, can induce cholinergic properties through both diffusible and surface-bound factors (Patterson and Chun 1977; Hawrot 1980). Third, neuronal activity, at least in culture, appears to exert a stabilizing influence on the initial noradrenergic status, making the neurons less susceptible to the signal that influences cells to become cholinergic (Walicke et al. 1977). Finally, hormones such as glucocorticoids can also affect transmitter choice by inhibiting the synthesis and/or release of the cholinergic factor by heart cells (Fukada 1980; Jonakait et al. 1980; McLennan et al. 1980). The fact that neural crest cells and their derivatives can respond to cues in their environment does not rule out the possibility that crest cells have certain predetermined (but reversible) predilections about phenotype. Perhaps the best way to understand precursor cell predilections and the role of instructive signals is by means of cultures derived from single cells, as is being done for hematopoietic cells (Metcalf 1980; Sieber-Blum and Cohen 1980).

The relative roles of extrinsic and intrinsic influences in differentiation are also being studied in identified neurons in certain invertebrates. For example, in the tiny roundworm *Caenorhabditis elegans* it is possible to follow the lineage of each of its approximately 300 neurons with the light microscope as they divide, migrate, and differentiate in the living animal. A salient feature of the

regulate a developing neuron's choice of transmitter. That this choice is surprisingly malleable was first discovered by manipulating populations of neural crest cells and their neuronal derivatives, in particular, cholinergic and noradrenergic neurons in autonomic ganglia. Transplantation of crest cells to different positions in the embryo (Le Douarin and Teillet 1974), or addition of certain types of nonneuronal cells to postmitotic sympathetic neurons in cell culture (Patterson and Chun 1974), markedly affects the cholinergic-noradrenergic balance in these neuronal populations. That a given cell can alter its transmitter choice was first inferred from the observation that the cholinergic-noradrenergic balance can be shifted without a change in the number of nerve cells present (Johnson et al. 1976; **Patterson** and **Chun 1977**). This was demonstrated more directly by actually following this decision in single cells in culture (**Furshpan, MacLeish, O'Lague,** and **Potter 1976**; Reichardt and Patterson 1977). Transitions from noradrenergic function to dual function (i.e., secretion of both transmitters) and from dual function to cholinergic function, were observed by redevelopmental sequence in this organism is its invariance; the pattern of mitosis, the number of cells of each type, and their lineages are essentially identical from individual to individual (see Chitwood and Chitwood 1974; Sulston and Horvitz 1977; Deppe et al. 1978). This suggests a fairly rigid programming of cell fate. Support for this notion comes from ablation studies using a laser microbeam. In many cases, early development appears to be autonomous in that cells near a destroyed cell continue to develop normally, despite the fact that the undamaged cells sometimes differentiate in positions that normally would be occupied by cells with different fates (Sulston and Horvitz 1977).

Although the sequence of development for individual cells is highly predictable in C. elegans, even in these animals a cell's fate is not strictly determined by lineage. In certain groups of cells termed "equivalence groups" (see Kimble et al. 1979), ablation of one cell results in its replacement by an adjacent cell (Sulston and White 1980). This is presumably the cellular counterpart of the phenomenon called regulation, in which an embryonic structure is generated from alternative progenitors when its normal precursors are destroyed (see Spemann 1938). The cells in equivalence groups are unusual in that they have similar lineage histories and morphologies. They are therefore analogous to the polyclones that make up the compartments discussed in Section 2, since equivalence groups are nonclonally related collections of cells that generate specific regions (see Kimble et al. 1979). In a further example of regulation in C. elegans, it has recently been shown that the direction in which certain types of neurons extend axonal branches is also influenced by the local environment. That is, one neuron can adopt the morphology of another when it is placed in the other's location (see **Horvitz 1981**). In sum, despite the highly programmed fate of most cells in the nematode, environment can alter the course of events in some circumstances. Although induction and regulation are more obvious in the development of vertebrates, it seems unlikely that there is any fundamental phylogenetic difference in the ontogeny of vertebrates and invertebrates in this regard.

Lineage studies similar to those involving nematodes have been undertaken for the grasshopper (**Goodman** and **Spitzer 1979**) and the leech (Weisblat et al. 1980); in both of these cases the neurons and their precursors have the additional advantage of being large enough to impale with microelectrodes. This has enabled detailed study of electrical coupling, excitability, and chemosensitivity from the neuroblast stage to maturity (Spitzer 1979; Goodman et al. 1980). The acquisition or loss of some of these neuronal characteristics has been correlated with morphological changes and the onset of neurotransmitter production (Goodman et al. 1979; see also Sanes and Hildebrand 1976a,b,c). As in C. elegans, considerable functional diversity occurs among the descendants of a single precursor cell.

Although the relative contribution of extrinsic and intrinsic influences to the differentiation of identified neurons remains a matter of debate, increasingly well-defined systems both in vivo and in vitro have begun to show how the intrinsic programs of developing cells interact with the environment during the formation of the nervous system.

References

Brown, D.D. 1981. Gene expression in eukaryotes. *Science* 211: 667–674.

Bunge, R.B., M. Johnson, and C.D. Ross. 1978. Nature and nurture in development of the autonomic neuron. *Science 199:* 1409–1416.

Chitwood, B.G. and M.B. Chitwood. 1974. *Introduction to nematology.* University Park Press, Baltimore.

Deppe, U., E. Schierenberg, T. Cole, C. Krieg, D. Schmitt, B. Yoder, and G. Von Ehrenstein. 1978. Cell lineages of the embryo of the nematode *Caenorhabditis elegans. Proc. Natl. Acad. Sci.* 75: 376–380.

Fukada, K. 1980. Hormonal control of neurotransmitter choice in sympathetic neurone cultures. *Nature 287:* 553–555.

Furshpan, E.J., P.R. MacLeish, P.H. O'Lague, and D.D. Potter. 1976. Chemical transmission between rat sympathetic neurons and cardiac myocytes developing in microcultures: Evidence for cholinergic, adrenergic, and dual-function neurons. *Proc. Natl. Acad. Sci. 73:* 4225–4229.

Goodman, C.S. and N.C. Spitzer. 1979. Embryonic development of identified neurones: Differentiation from neuroblast to neurone. *Nature 280:* 208–214.

Goodman, C.S., K.G. Pearson, and N.C. Spitzer. 1980. Electrical excitability: A spectrum of properties in the progeny of a single embryonic neuroblast. *Proc. Natl. Acad. Sci. 77:* 1676–1680.

Goodman, C.S., M. O'Shea, R. McCaman, and N.C. Spitzer. 1979. Embryonic development of identified neurons: Temporal pattern of morphological and biochemical differentiation. *Science 204:* 1219–1222.

Hawrot, E. 1980. Cultured sympathetic neurons: Effects of cell-derived and synthetic substrata on survival and development. *Dev. Biol. 74:* 136–151.

Higgins, D., L. Iacovitti, T.H. Joh, and H. Burton. 1981. The immunocytochemical localization of tyrosine hydroxylase within rat sympathetic neurons that release acetylcholine in culture. *J. Neurosci. 1:* 126–131.

Horvitz, H.R. 1981. Neuronal cell lineages in the nematode *Caenorhabditis elegans.* In *Development in the nervous system.* British Society for Developmental Biology, Symposium 5 (ed. D. Garrod et al.), pp. 329–346. Cambridge University Press, Cambridge.

Johnson, M., D. Ross, M. Meyers, R. Rees, R. Bunge, E. Wakshull, and H. Burton. 1976. Synaptic vesicle cytochemistry changes when cultured sympathetic neurons develop cholinergic interactions. *Nature 262:* 308–310.

Jonakait, G.M., M.C. Bohn, and I.B. Black. 1980. Maternal glucocorticoid hormones influence neurotransmitter phenotypic expression in embryos. *Science 210:* 551–553.

Jonakait, G.M., J. Wolf, P. Cochard, M. Goldstein, and I.B. Black. 1979. Selective loss of noradrenergic phenotype characters in neuroblasts of the rat embryo. *Proc. Natl. Acad. Sci. 76:* 4683–4686.

Kimble, J., J. Sulston, and J. White. 1979. Regulative development in the post-embryonic lineages of *Caenorhabditis elegans. INSERM Symp. 10:* 59–68.

Landis, S.C. 1976. Rat sympathetic neurons and cardiac myocytes developing in microcultures: Correlation of the fine structure of endings with neurotransmitter function in single neurons. *Proc. Natl. Acad. Sci. 73:* 4220–4224.

Landis, S.C. and D. Keefe. 1980. Development of cholinergic sympathetic innervation of eccrine sweat glands in rat footpad. *Soc. Neurosci. 6:* 379. (Abstr.)

Le Douarin, N.M. 1980. The ontogeny of the neural crest in avian embryo chimaeras. *Nature 286:* 663–669.

Le Douarin, N.M. and M.-A.M. Teillet. 1974. Experimental analysis of the migration and differentiation of neuroblasts of the autonomic nervous system and of neuroectodermal mesenchymal derivatives, using a biological cell marking technique. *Dev. Biol. 41:* 162–184.

McLennan, I.S., C.E. Hill, and I.A. Hendry. 1980. Glucocorticoids modulate transmitter choice in developing superior cervical ganglion. *Nature 283:* 206–207.

Metcalf, D. 1980. Clonal analysis of proliferation and differentiation of paired daughter cells: Action of granulocyte-macrophage colony stimulating factor on granulocyte-macrophage precursors. *Proc. Natl. Acad. Sci. 77:* 5327–5330.

Patterson, P.H. 1978. Environmental determination of autonomic neurotransmitter functions. *Annu. Rev. Neurosci. 1:* 1–17.

Patterson, P.H. and L.L.Y. Chun. 1974. The influence of non-neuronal cells on catecholamine and acetylcholine synthesis and accumulation in cultures of dissociated sympathetic neurons. *Proc. Natl. Acad. Sci. 71:* 3607–3610.

———. 1977. The induction of acetylcholine synthesis in primary cultures of dissociated rat sympathetic neurons. I. Effects of conditioned medium. *Dev. Biol. 56:* 263–280.

Potter, D.D., S.C. Landis, and E.J. Furshpan. 1981. Adrenergic-cholinergic dual function in cultured sympathetic neurones of the rat. *CIBA Found. Symp. 83:* 123–138.

Reichardt, L.F. and P.H. Patterson. 1977. Neurotransmitter synthesis and uptake by isolated rat sympathetic neurones in microcultures. *Nature 270:* 147–151.

Sanes, J.R. and J.G. Hildebrand. 1976a. Structure and development of antennae in a moth, *Manduca sexta*. *Dev. Biol. 51:* 282–299.

————. 1976b. Origin and morphogenesis of sensory neurons in an insect antenna. *Dev. Biol. 51:* 300–319.

————. 1976c. Acetylcholine and its metabolic enzymes in developing antennae of the moth, *Manduca sexta. Dev. Biol. 52:* 105–120.

Schmitt, F.O., F.E. Bloom, and S.J. Bird. 1982. *Molecular genetics and neuroscience: A new hybrid.* Raven Press, New York. (In press.)

Sieber-Blum, M. and A.M. Cohen. 1980. Clonal analysis of quail neural crest cells. They are pluripotent and differentiate *in vitro* in the absence of noncrest cells. *Dev. Biol. 80:* 96–106.

Spemann, H. 1938. *Embryonic development and induction.* Yale University Press, New Haven, Connecticut.

Spemann, H. and H. Mangold. 1924. Über Unduktion von embryonalanlagen durch Implantation artfremder Organisatoren. *Wilhelm Roux' Arch. Entwicklungsmech Org. 100:* 599–638.

Spitzer, N.C. 1979. Ion channels in development. *Annu. Rev. Neurosci. 2:* 363–397.

Sulston, J.E. and H.R. Horvitz. 1977. Post-embryonic cell lineages of the nematode, *Caenorhabditis elegans. Dev. Biol. 56:* 110–156.

Sulston, J.E. and J.G. White. 1980. Regulation and cell autonomy during postembryonic development of *Caenorhabditis elegans. Dev. Biol. 78:* 577–597.

Teillet, M.A., P. Cochard, and N.M. Le Douarin. 1978. Relative roles of the mesenchymal tissues and of the complex neural tube-notochord on the expression of adrenergic metabolism in neural crest cells. *Zoon 6:* 115–122.

Walicke, P.A., R.B. Campenot, and P.H. Patterson. 1977. Determination of transmitter function by neuronal activity. *Proc. Natl. Acad. Sci. 74:* 5767–5771.

Weisblat, D.A., G. Harper, G.S. Stent, and R.T. Sawyer. 1980. Embryonic cell lineages in the nervous system of the glossiphoniid leech, *Helobdella triserialis. Dev. Biol. 76:* 58–78.

109

DEVELOPMENTAL BIOLOGY 56, 263–280 (1977)

The Induction of Acetylcholine Synthesis in Primary Cultures of Dissociated Rat Sympathetic Neurons

I. Effects of Conditioned Medium

PAUL H. PATTERSON AND LINDA L. Y. CHUN

Department of Neurobiology, Harvard Medical School, 25 Shattuck Street, Boston, Massachusetts 02115

Received September 27, 1976, and accepted in revised form November 27, 1976

Neurotransmitter metabolism in primary cultures of dissociated sympathetic neurons from the newborn rat has been examined. Previous studies have shown that neurons grown in the virtual absence of nonneuronal cells developed the ability to synthesize and accumulate radioactive norepinephrine (NE) from [³H]tyrosine, but synthesized little [³H]acetylcholine (ACh) from labeled choline. However, in the presence of certain types of nonneuronal cells, or in medium conditioned (CM) by them, the neurons produced considerable ACh from choline. Here we show that ACh production from choline depends on the concentration of CM in the growth medium. At 62% CM, the highest level of CM studied, ACh production is >40-fold higher than the control value. Furthermore, homogenates of mixed neuronal/nonneuronal cultures or CM-treated neuronal cultures contain 100- to 1000-fold more choline acetyltransferase activity than neuron-alone sister cultures. On the other hand, the ability to synthesize and accumulate NE is inversely related to the percentage CM in the growth medium; at high concentrations of CM, catecholamine production is depressed about 25-fold from the control. The effects of CM are rather specific, since CM does not affect the number of neurons surviving or their overall growth. These results suggest that CM acts by altering the differentiated fate of individual sympathetic neurons rather than by causing the selective survival or growth of a second population of neurons. CM from primary cultures of several tissues taken from the newborn rat induces neuronal ACh synthesis, as does CM from cultures of several, but not all types of rat cell lines. In contrast, CM from several non-rat cell lines as well as from primary cultures of mouse and chick heart is less effective in causing neuronal ACh production, suggesting some degree of species specificity in this phenomenon.

INTRODUCTION

A prominent characteristic of most differentiated neurons is the synthesis, storage, and release of neurotransmitters, and one of the most useful ways of classifying or identifying neurons is to determine which of the various transmitter candidates they utilize. Thus a critical decision made by developing neurons is which transmitter to produce. In the adult autonomic nervous system of mammals, the characteristic transmitters are acetylcholine (ACh)[1] and the catecholamines (CA), which are primarily utilized by parasympathetic and sympathetic neurons, respectively. The neuronal decision to become adrenergic or cholinergic has crucial functional consequences because these two transmitters have antagonistic effects on many autonomic target tissues such as the heart and blood vessels.

It has proved possible to influence experimentally the choice of transmitter produced in populations of developing autonomic neurons both *in vivo*, by transplantation of neural crest cells to abnormal sites (LeDouarin and Teillet, 1974; LeDouarin *et al.*, 1975), and *in vitro*, by manipulating the cellular (Patterson and

[1] Abbreviations used: acetylcholine, ACh; norepinephrine, NE; catecholamine, CA; (naphthylvinyl)pyridine, PVN; conditioned medium, CM; nerve growth factor, NGF; hemicholinium, HC-3; choline acetyltransferase, CAT.

263

Chun, 1974) or fluid (Patterson *et al.*, 1975) environment of sympathetic neurons. In the latter studies, cultures of developing sympathetic neurons synthesized and accumulated CA when grown in the virtual absence of nonneuronal cells, but produced substantial ACh when grown in the presence of certain types of nonneuronal cells or in medium conditioned by them. Since such manipulations may lead to improved understanding of the mechanisms involved in determining which type of neuron a cell will become, we have studied further the development of dissociated rat sympathetic neurons in cell culture and the influence of medium conditioned by a variety of types of nonneuronal cells on neuronal survival, growth and transmitter metabolism. A preliminary report of some of these findings has appeared (Patterson *et al.*, 1976).

MATERIALS AND METHODS

Sympathetic neurons were grown under four conditions: (i) in L-15 CO_2 medium using treatment with cytosine arabinoside to suppress proliferation of the ganglionic nonneuronal cells which are present in the original cell suspension along with the neurons; (ii) by themselves as in (i) but also treated with various concentrations of conditioned medium (CM) obtained from flasks containing nonneuronal cells; (iii) in mixed culture with the ganglionic nonneuronal cells which proliferate in permissive media, achieving a monolayer after several weeks; (iv) in mixed cultures on preplated heart cells which had been irradiated with ^{60}Co to block further division. These procedures are described in detail below.

Neuron Preparation

Dissociated sympathetic neurons were prepared by the mechanical procedure previously described (Mains and Patterson, 1973a). Briefly, 1- to 3-day-old rats (CD strain, Charles River Breeding Lab.) were killed by a blow to the head and the supe-

rior cervical ganglia were removed, cleaned, and teased apart with forceps. The resulting cells and chunks were vibrated in a test tube on a vortex mixer to produce standing waves but no swirling vortex (the latter being detrimental to cell survival). The resulting suspension was filtered through Nitex (10-μm pore size; Tobler, Ernst and Traber, Inc.) and the filtrate centrifuged. The cells were then resuspended and plated inside glass rings on modified culture dishes (Mains and Patterson, 1973a). The cultures were allowed to stand for 2 days before the glass rings were removed, and the first change of medium was made. Subsequently, the medium was changed either every 2 days (conditioned medium experiments) or every 4 days (control cultures) with 2 ml of growth medium. Forty to fifty dishes of about 5000 viable neurons each (after 3 weeks *in vitro*) were prepared from 40 pups.

Nonneuronal Cell Preparation

Primary cell cultures of nonneuronal cells from neonatal rats, mice, or 10-day chick embryos were prepared by mincing the particular tissue and then incubating it for 20 min in 1 mg/ml of collagenase (Worthington Biochem. Corp.) in phosphate buffered saline with frequent agitation. After allowing chunks to settle out, the cells were collected by centrifugation, washed several times and counted in a hemocytometer. Usually 5–10 $\times$ 10^6 cells were plated per 75-mm^2 flask in L-15 CO_2 medium (see below) with 10% fetal calf serum (Microbiological Associates).

The heart cell cultures consisted of synchronously beating muscle cells, fibroblasts, and a few endothelial-like cells. The blood vessel (common carotids) cultures contained primarily fibroblast-like cells (flat, noncontracting) and spindle-shaped cells which were probably smooth muscle cells. The brain (whole brain) cultures contained a background of flat cells with small cells of neuronal appearance on top, as in published pictures (Schrier, 1973). The liver cultures consisted primarily of fibroblast-like cells and some flat cells with highly refractile inclusions. Skeletal muscle (pectoral muscle) cultures contained spontaneously contracting myotubes on layers of fibroblast-like cells. For primary rat embryo fibroblasts, 16-day embryos were eviscerated and the body wall prepared as above.

In the cases where neurons were plated directly on to a preexisting monolayer of heart cells, the dissociated cells (atria or ventricles) were plated into the wells of the culture dishes (see below), and allowed to form a monolayer. Further proliferation was suppressed by irradiation (5000 rad) from a ^{60}Co-source. In addition, the cultures were sometimes irradiated again several days after the neurons were plated to inhibit proliferation of the accompanying ganglionic nonneuronal cells. We saw no evidence that the neuronal functions under study were affected by the irradiation (see also O'Lague *et al.*, 1975; Nurse and O'Lague, 1975). All cell lines were obtained from American Type Culture Collection except the RN22 Schwannoma line (gift of Dr. J. R. Sheppard), the L8 skeletal muscle line (gift of Dr. V. Ingram) and the Rat Embryo Fibroblast line (Microbiol. Assoc.) and were carried in L-15 CO_2 medium with 10% fetal calf serum.

Conditioned Medium

Flasks of nonneuronal cells to be used for conditioning medium, which had been grown in fetal calf serum were washed with medium containing rat serum and incubated 2–12 hr with the rat serum medium before the medium to be conditioned was placed in the flask. Only flasks with a dense layer of cells over a week old were used. In most cases 20–30 ml of complete L-15 CO_2 medium with methocel, rat serum, etc. was used for conditioning and it was left in the flask for 2 days and then removed and usually frozen at $-20°C$. In some cases medium without methocel was

used so that it could be passed thru a 0.22-μm filter to remove any nonneuronal cells before freezing and this alternative procedure made no apparent difference to the results. The conditioned media were thawed before use, mixed with fresh medium to yield the desired concentrations and used to feed the neuronal cultures. If the conditioned media contained methocel, the added fresh medium contained the usual concentration of methocel (0.6 g/100 ml). However, if conditioned media lacking methocel were used, the fresh media had a higher methocel concentration such that the final methocel concentration was 0.6 g/100 ml.

Isotopic Incubations and Assays

Synthesis and accumulation of neurotransmitters was determined by incorporation of radioactive precursors. Living cultures were incubated for 4 hr with [2,3-^{3}H]tyrosine (Amersham Searle) and [*methyl*-^{3}H]choline (Amersham Searle) in L-15 CO_2 as previously described (Mains and Patterson, 1973a) except that eserine was omitted and the glucose concentration was doubled. The final specific activities of the isotopes were 1–13.4 Ci/mmol of tyrosine and 2–10.1 Ci/mmol of choline. The radioactivity in NE, dopamine, tyrosine, choline, ACh, and acetylcarnitine was determined after electrophoresis of the culture extracts. Aliquots of the extracts were taken for measurement of total incorporation as described (Mains and Patterson, 1973a). The values for apparent moles of product were derived from the specific activities of the added isotopes, using 25% as the counting efficiency, and assuming full and rapid equilibration of the intracellular pool with the medium, subject to the qualifications outlined previously (Mains and Patterson, 1973a,b) and in the Discussion.

Choline acetyltransferase (CAT) activity was assayed in homogenates by measuring the conversion of [acetyl-^{3}H]coenzyme A to [acetyl-^{3}H]choline using electrophoresis at pH 1.9 (Mains and Patterson, 1973a) to separate the precursor and product. The final volume of the incubation was 30 μl and consisted of: 50 mM NaPO$_4$, pH 6.8, 200 mM NaCl, 0.5% Triton X-100, 0.1 mM eserine SO$_4$, 2 mM choline iodide or DL-carnitine, 0.11 mM [acetyl-^{3}H]coenzyme A (3.07 Ci/mmol, New England Nuclear), and 0.17 mg/ml of bovine serum albumin (Sigma). To inhibit the CAT activity, 0.5 mM (naphthylvinyl)pyridine (PVN, Sigma) was added. Culture extracts were made by scraping a thoroughly washed culture into 75 μl of a solution containing 50 mM NaPO$_4$, pH 6.8, 200 mM NaCl, 0.5% Triton X-100, and 20 mg/ml bovine serum albumin. The culture was then extensively homogenized in a microhomogenizer (Misco) at 0°C. Of this extract, 1–20 μl was used per assay tube. Reactions were run at 37°C for 20 min, and after addition of unlabeled ACh the tubes were frozen. In order to keep the boiled enzyme blanks at 100–200 cpm it was necessary to purify the isotope before use. One millicurie was applied to a Dowex 50-W-X8 column (100–200 mesh, Na$^+$ form, 6 cm in a Pasteur pipet) in H$_2$O and the eluate was lyophilized overnight. Yields from this purification were 80–90%. Product formation in extracts was linear for at least 30 min and for 0.5–20 μl of extract added.

Noncollagen protein was measured by the technique of Bonting and Jones (1957). Cultures were extensively washed and incubated with phosphate-buffered saline, drained well, and incubated in 40 μl of 1 M NaOH at 37°C for 60 min. Twenty microliters of this solution was removed to a 1-ml conical test tube (Misco). Fifty microliters of the bromo-sulfalein reagent solution was added and the tube was vortexed and centrifuged. Twenty-five microliters of the supernatant was removed and added to 350 μl of 0.1 M NaOH. After vortexing, the optical density was read at 580 nm. Collagen-coated dishes containing no cells served as blanks (1–2 μg of blanks vs 10–15 μg of protein per culture).

Lipid PO$_4$ was determined by PO$_4$ assays on chloroform-extracted and Folch-washed (Patterson and Lennarz, 1971) cultures. Cultures (2 per determination) were extensively washed and incubated in 0.9% NaCl, thoroughly drained, and scraped into 6 ml of chloroform–methanol (2:1). After vortexing, 0.35 ml of 0.9% NaCl was added and the tube was vortexed again. NaCl (0.9%, 2.5 ml) was then added and the tube was vortexed again. After chilling on ice, the tube was centrifuged and the CHCl$_3$ layer was transferred to a tube and taken to dryness. Total PO$_4$ was then assayed by the method of Ames and Dubin (1960).

RESULTS

Kinetics of ACh and CA Synthesis and Accumulation

In order to measure rates of transmitter synthesis and accumulation in cultured neurons, it is necessary to establish conditions under which precursor levels in the medium are saturating and rates of incorporation of label into the transmitters are linear with time. Although these conditions have been previously determined for neuronal cultures (Mains and Patterson, 1973b), mixed neuronal/nonneuronal cultures have greater cell mass and thus may require somewhat different conditions.

The kinetics of labeling of various pools with [^{3}H]choline and [^{3}H]tyrosine were analyzed in 2-week-old L-15 CO$_2$ cultures. These cultures consisted of neurons and the ganglionic nonneuronal cells which proliferate in this permissive medium and induce ACh production by the neurons (Patterson and Chun, 1974). The intracellular precursor pools labeled quickly and rapidly achieved a steady state equilibration with the medium as seen previously with neuron-alone cultures (Mains and Patterson, 1973b). Figure 1 shows that under these incubation conditions total incorporation of the precursors into protein and lipid (Fig. 1A) was linear for at least 4 hr. Similarly, incorporation of tyrosine into the catecholamines, norepinephrine and

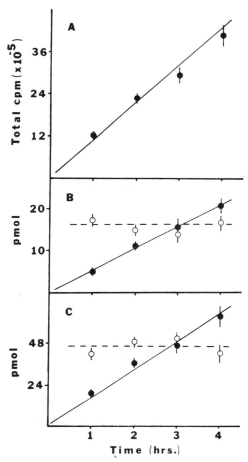

FIG. 1. The dependence of tyrosine and choline metabolism on the time of incubation was determined by incubating 2-week-old L-15 CO_2 cultures (neurons plus ganglionic nonneuronal cells) for varying times with 220 μM [³H]tyrosine and 100 μM [³H]choline. The radioactivity as (A) total incorporation (●), (B) free tyrosine (○) and CA (●), and (C) free choline (○) and ACh (●) was determined as described in Materials and Methods and expressed on a per culture basis. The bars in all figures represent the SEM of determinations on four cultures.

the other hand, the free choline pool expanded linearly with increased extracellular choline to at least 200 μM external choline, where other factors besides choline uptake were limiting ACh synthesis.

Similar data was obtained for tyrosine uptake and utilization by mixed cultures (Fig. 3). Higher tyrosine concentrations were necessary to saturate total uptake and catecholamine production with mixed cultures than with neuron-alone cultures (Mains and Patterson, 1973b). Accordingly, 125–250 μM tyrosine was used for the mixed cultures in the rest of these studies.

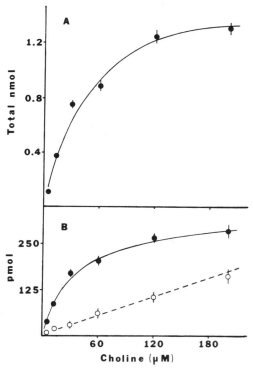

FIG. 2. The dependence of choline incorporation on the choline concentration in the medium was determined by plating neurons on rat heart cells and irradiation of the cultures at Day 2 after the neuron plating, as described in Materials and Methods. After 23 days, the cultures were incubated for 2 hr with varying concentrations of [³H]choline and assayed for (A) total incorporation (●) and (B) free choline (○) and ACh (●) as described in Materials and Methods. The values are expressed on a per culture basis.

dopamine (Fig. 1B), and of choline into ACh (Fig. 1C) were linear throughout the incubation period. Therefore measurements of ACh and CA at these times represent rates of synthesis and accumulation. As shown in Fig. 2, a choline concentration of 100 μM was necessary for saturation of total incorporation and ACh synthesis in mixed neuron–heart cultures. On

114

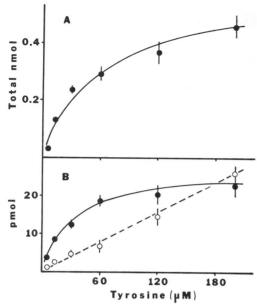

FIG. 3. The dependence of tyrosine incorporation on the tyrosine concentration in the medium was determined by the same methods as given for Fig. 2, except that the isotope was [³H]tyrosine rather than [³H]choline. The results for (A) total incorporation (●) and (B) free tyrosine (○) and CA (●) are expressed on a per culture basis.

Effects of Conditioned Medium

Cultured sympathetic neurons produce little or no labeled ACh from [³H]choline when grown in the virtual absence of nonneuronal cells, but mixed cultures of neurons plus certain types of nonneuronal cells produced 100- to 1000-fold higher ACh (Patterson and Chun, 1974). To determine whether the neurons were being stimulated to produce ACh by the nonneuronal cells or vice versa, medium from cultures containing only nonneuronal cells was transferred to neuronal cultures and the rate of ACh synthesis by the neurons determined. These experiments showed that medium conditioned (CM) by the appropriate nonneuronal cells can induce increases of 300- to 1000-fold in neuronal ACh production, and suggested that the nonneuronal cells exert their effect via the bulk medium (Patterson et al., 1975).

Because the presence of nonneuronal cells can increase ACh synthesis (Patterson and Chun, 1974), it was important to determine if the effect of CM was to increase the number of nonneuronal cells in the neuronal cultures (Fig. 4). Although the neurons, both controls and CM-tested, were grown in L-15 Air medium which does not normally permit nonneuronal proliferation, further precautions were taken. Some cultures were irradiated with ⁶⁰Co on Day 2, thus blocking cell division by the nonneuronal cells that might be caused by the CM treatment. Other cultures were treated with 10^{-5} M cytosine arabinoside in order to kill any dividing nonneuronal cells. To monitor the effectiveness of these treatments some cultures were fixed and stained with toluidine blue and the nonneuronal cells counted (Patterson et al., 1975). As seen in Fig. 4 these treatments reduced the number of nonneuronal cells 3- to 10-fold with little effect on the ACh production per neuron. With approximately the same number of nonneuronal cells present, the CM-treated neurons synthesized and accumulated about 150-fold more ACh than control neurons. Although the number of neurons per culture was largely unaffected by treatment with cytosine arabinoside, irradiation in the absence of background nonneuronal cells caused a 30–50% drop in neuronal number. However, the surviving neurons performed nearly as well as the untreated neurons as judged by total incorporation of choline and tyrosine per neuron and CA production per neuron (data not shown). The ratio of neuronal somas to nonneuronal cells varied in the experiment shown from 7.3 to 40.5 and in other experiments from 10 to >50. It is worth pointing out that the total mass of the cultures was overwhelmingly neuronal both because of the small numbers of nonneuronal cells and because the neuronal somas make up a small proportion of the overall neuronal mass. We conclude from this and similar experiments that CM treatment can stimulate neuronal ACh production without

115

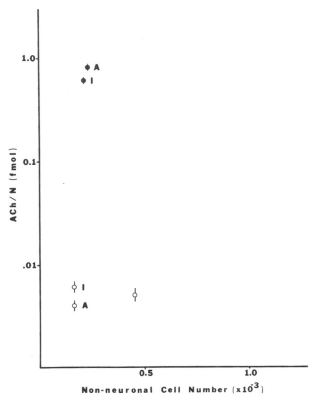

Fig. 4. The relationship of nonneuronal cell number to the ACh induction caused by CM treatment was determined on 16-day-old cultures grown in L-15 Air medium. The CM-treated cultures (●) were fed every 2 days with L-15 Air medium taken off confluent rat heart cultures and mixed 1:1 with fresh medium. Control cultures (○) were fed every 2 days with 100% fresh L-15 Air medium. Some cultures were irradiated with ^{60}Co on Day 2 (I) or treated with 10^{-5} M cytosine arabinoside (A) on Days 2 and 6 as described in Materials and Methods. On Day 16 neuronal somas were counted with the phase microscope and some cultures were fixed and stained with toluidine blue to count nonneuronal cells. Other cultures were incubated with [^{3}H]choline and labeled ACh was determined as described in Materials and Methods. The ACh data are expressed on a per neuron basis.

causing an increase in the number of nonneuronal cells.

Since CM causes such large changes in ACh synthesis and accumulation it was natural to ask what other effects it has on the neurons. Thus far, we have assayed its effect on neuronal survival, neuronal growth, CA production, and choline acetyltransferase (CAT) activity. The data in Table 1 show that the neuronal number after 20 days in culture was not appreciably affected by CM treatment. Similarly, cultures treated with 0 and 62% CM showed no significant differences in total neuronal protein or total neuronal lipid

PO_4, even though there was >150-fold difference in the ACh/CA ratio. Therefore, the signal in the CM appears to be a specific differentiation cue not directly related to neuronal survival or growth. The conditioned medium dose–response curves for neuronal survival and ACh and CA production are shown in Fig. 5. Again, neuronal number was not detectably altered by CM up to 62%. However, ACh production was dependent on CM concentration, rising about 40-fold over this concentration range. This was expected since previous experiments with mixed neuron/nonneuronal cell cultures demonstrated that in-

TABLE 1

EFFECT OF CM TREATMENT ON NEURONAL GROWTH[a]

	Neurons/culture ($\times 10^3$)	Total protein (ng/neuron)	Lipid PO₄ (pmol/neuron)	ACh/CA
−CM	1.32 ± 0.06	10.3 ± 0.5	17.5 ± 0.3	0.12 ± .01
+CM	1.38 ± 0.07	9.1 ± 0.8	17.4 ± 0.2	16.36 ± 1.07

[a] Cultures were grown for 29 days with or without 62% CM taken from flasks of rat heart cells. The assays employed are described in Materials and Methods and the data are means of four cultures, ± SEM.

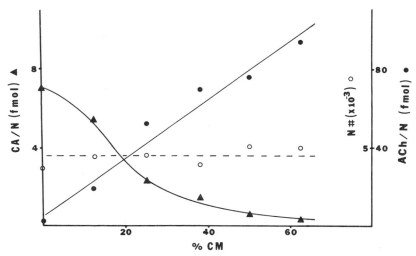

FIG. 5. The dependence of ACh and CA production and neuronal survival on CM concentration was determined on 20-day-old L-15 CO₂ cultures which had been treated with 10^{-5} M cytosine arabinoside on Days 2 and 8 to virtually eliminate all nonneuronal cells. CM from confluent rat heart flasks was mixed with fresh medium at the concentrations shown and added every 2 days, beginning at Day 2. On Day 20 neuronal somas were counted (○) and the cultures incubated with [³H]choline and [³H]tyrosine. Radioactive ACh (●) and CA (▲) were determined as described in Materials and Methods and the values are expressed on a per neuron basis.

creased nonneuronal cell number caused higher ACh production (Patterson and Chun, 1974). On the other hand, as the magnitude of the ACh effect was increased, CA production was significantly decreased. Over the CM concentration range 0–62% there was about a 25-fold decrease in CA production (Fig. 5). Thus the ratio of ACh to CA produced by the 62%-treated cultures was almost 1000-fold higher than that of the 0% controls.

While overall neuronal growth is unchanged by CM treatment, there must be enzymatic changes to account for the gross changes in transmitter metabolism. One obvious possibility is an induction of CAT activity, the enzyme responsible for the synthesis of ACh. It seemed unlikely that the differences in ACh accumulation observed in the whole cells could result simply from decreased ACh breakdown since, in previous work, incubations with [³H]choline were carried out in the presence of eserine, an acetylcholinesterase inhibitor (Patterson and Chun, 1974). Evidence is presented in Table 2 that CAT activity is induced in the sympathetic neurons by nonneuronal cells or medium conditioned by them. A complication in the analysis of CAT activity is that both neurons and nonneuronal cells have a mitochondrial enzyme, carnitine acetyltransferase, which prefers carnitine as a substrate, but can utilize choline with a low

TABLE 2

Nonneuronal Induction of Neuronal Choline Acetyltransferase[a]

Culture extract	Cho-line	Car-nitine	PVN	cpm		% PVN	ACh cpm	ACh/CA*
				ACh	AcCarn	inhi-bition	N #	
Expt. 1.								
(A) Heart alone	−	−		0	210			−
	+	−		0	260			
	−	+		0	75,560			
	+	−	+	0	240			
	−	+	+	0	75,370	0		
(B) Neurons alone	−	−		40	240			
	+	−		260	60	<.05		<0.1
	−	+		100	43,920			
	+	−	+	60	200			
	−	+	+	200	44,820	0		
(C) Neurons and heart	−	−		740	610			
	+	−		43,340	550			17.2 ± 0.8
	−	+		800	116,280	27.30		
	+	−	+	4,130	660	90		
	−	+	+	770	105,400	9		
(D) Neurons and heart −NGF	−	−		0	240			
	+	−		660	200		20.60	12.1 ± 1.3
	−	+		0	61,270			
	+	−	+	120	870	82		
	−	+	+	0	60,740	1		
(E) B + C	+	−		42,560	500			
Expt. 2.								
− CM neurons	+			2,130				0.1 ± 0.1
	+		+	1,720		19		
+ CM neurons	+			127,200				26.7 ± 0.6
	+		+	19,100		85		

[a] In Expt. 1, 24-day-old cultures grown in L-15 CO_2 either on preplated heart with and without added NGF, or on collagenized dishes and treated with 10^{-5} M cytosine arabinoside, were homogenized and assayed for production of labeled acetylcholine (ACh) or acetylcarnitine (AcCarn) from [³H]Acetyl CoA as described in Materials and Methods. One microliter of each extract was assayed under each condition. In E 1 μl of extracts from B and C were assayed in the same tube. In Expt. 2, 43-day-old cultures treated with 0 or 62% rat heart CM as described for Table 1, were homogenized and 5 μl of the extracts assayed as previously described. A 100 cpm blank has been subtracted from all values. * Sister cultures were incubated with labeled tyrosine (200 μM) and choline (100 μM) as described in the Materials and Methods to determine the rates of ACh and CA production under each condition.

affinity to produce ACh (White and Wu, 1973). That such an enzyme activity is present in cultured heart cells and sympathetic neurons is shown in Table 2, Expt 1A and 1B, respectively. In the experiments reported here, CAT activity was distinguished from the carnitine-utilizing enzyme by the different substrate preferences of the enzymes (Expt 1A vs 1C) and the differential inhibition of CAT by the inhibitor (naphthylvinyl)pyridine (PVN; Expt 1A and 1C). Most of the CAT activity was localized to the induced neurons by (i) the loss of the PVN-sensitive, choline-preferring enzyme activity when most of the neurons die as a result of NGF omission from the mixed cultures (Expt 1D vs 1C), and (ii) the presence of such an activity in neuronal cultures virtually free of nonneuronal cells which were treated with CM (Expt 2). In a series of five experiments, CAT activity, identified by these methods, was found to be 50- to 1000-fold higher in CM-treated or mixed cultures than in neuron-alone cultures without CM. These findings on crude extracts correlate qualitatively with those on ACh synthesis and accumulation from choline by living cells (Patterson and Chun, 1974; Patterson et al., 1975). Mixed extract experiments (Expt 1E vs 1C) gave no evidence of an enzyme inhibitor in the neuron-alone cultures nor an activator in the mixed cultures. This suggests that neuronal synthesis of new CAT molecules may be induced by the nonneuronal cells. The data in Expt 2 indicate the presence of low levels of CAT in very old (43 days) neuron-alone cultures. This corroborates the previous finding of low levels of ACh synthesis and accumulation from choline in older control cultures (Mains and Patterson, 1973a). A few neurons survive on heart in the absence of added NGF, presumably because NGF is produced by the fibroblasts (Young et al., 1975), and these appear to possess some CAT activity (Expt 1D). This correlates with the low ACh production seen in living neurons grown on heart in the absence of added NGF (see Discussion). Finally, the specific activity of CAT (PVN-inhibitable and choline-requiring) in the induced sympathetic neuron cultures ranged from 1 to 4.5 nmol min^{-1} mg protein^{-1} for nerve–heart cultures and from 0.15 to 3.5 for the CM-treated neuron-alone cultures.

What Types of Nonneuronal Cells Can Induce ACh Production?

Sympathetic neurons were grown in CM from a variety of nonneuronal cells and transmitter production assayed. Representative data from such experiments are shown in Table 3. The control neuronal cultures treated with medium conditioned in an empty flask exhibited a low ACh/CA value as expected. Primary cells from a number of tissues of the neonatal rat were able to induce ACh production in the sympathetic neurons via the CM, although

TABLE 3

Effects of Conditioned Medium from Various Nonneuronal Cells[a]

Source of conditioned medium	CA/N (fmol)	ACh/N (fmol)	ACh/CA
Empty flask	27.8	1.5	<0.1
Rat primary cells			
Blood vessel	8.5	131.5	15.5
Heart	11.9	130.6	10.0
Brain	20.0	34.1	1.7
Liver	24.2	20.3	0.8
Skeletal muscle	10.3	160.2	15.5
Embryo fibroblasts	8.1	180.6	21.0
Rat cell lines			
Embryo fibroblasts	9.3	169.8	18.2
L8 skeletal muscle	7.8	190.7	24.4
C6 glioma	10.0	61.0	6.1
RN22 Schwannoma	15.0	10.5	0.7
R$_2$C Leydig tumor	33.1	1.5	<0.1
Mouse cell lines			
3T3 fibroblasts	30.1	8.5	0.3
L929 fibroblasts	27.8	1.1	<0.1
Hamster cell line			
BHK fibroblasts	28.2	6.1	0.2

[a] Flasks of confluent nonneuronal cells were used to produce CM as described in Materials and Methods. The CM was mixed with fresh medium at a concentration of 25% and added every 2 days to L-15 CO_2 neuronal cultures which were treated with cytosine arabinoside. After 22 days the neuronal cultures were assayed for radioactive ACh and CA production as previously described. The numbers shown all have standard errors of the mean of less than 10%.

some types were more effective than others. The absolute numbers varied somewhat from experiment to experiment, presumably due to differences in numbers of nonneuronal cells per flask, in types of cells that grew up, etc. Since primary rat embryo fibroblasts were effective inducers, it is possible that the fibroblasts of each dissociated tissue were the cells responsible for the conditioning effect.

The rat skeletal muscle line L8 was effective at ACh induction, as were several other rat cell lines. However, not all rat cells were positive in this regard; the R$_2$C testicular tumor line which secretes steroids (Shin et al., 1968) did not display any detectable conditioning capacity. Of course, the R_2C cells may not be totally ineffective; they may simply exert too weak an effect to be detected here. The reciprocity between ACh and CA production is well shown by comparing the R_2C and control results with those from other rat cells, such as blood vessel, heart, and skeletal muscle (Table 3).

In contrast to the rat fibroblast line, mouse and hamster fibroblast cell lines were weak in promoting neuronal ACh production. A more stringent test of species specificity was made by comparing cultures of heart cells derived from neonatal rat and mouse and from 10-day chick embryos. These cultures were grown to confluency in fetal calf serum, then washed extensively, and incubated with standard L-15 CO_2 medium containing adult rat serum. These experiments (Table 4) clearly showed a species specificity in the ACh inductive capacity. It seems unlikely that these results are due to a deleterious effect of the rat serum on the mouse and chick cells because (i) all the heart cells had a normal appearance in the phase microscope and the muscle cells were beating, and (ii) CM obtained from the mouse heart flasks, but containing mouse serum instead of rat serum was also ineffective in inducing ACh in the rat sympathetic neurons (data not shown).

TABLE 4

SPECIES SPECIFICITY OF THE EFFECTS OF CONDITIONED MEDIUM[a]

Source of CM	CA/N (fmol)	ACh/N (fmol)	ACh/ CA
Empty flask	14.33	0.07	<0.01
Rat heart	7.93	18.74	2.37
Mouse heart	16.58	0.55	0.04
Chicken heart	14.43	0.18	0.01

[a] Dissociated neonatal rat and mouse and 10-day chick embryo hearts were grown to confluency in flasks. CM from these flasks was added at 25% to L-15 CO_2 neuronal cultures (treated with cytosine arabinoside) every 2 days until Day 20 when the neurons were counted and assayed for ACh and CA production as previously described. The SEM of these data were all less than 5% of the values shown.

DISCUSSION

Kinetics

One of the primary techniques employed in this study to assay the differentiation of transmitter function was the precursor conversion method. This method measures a net sum of all the parameters involved in transmitter synthesis, storage, and breakdown. An important point about the precursor conversion method is ensuring that the data represent ongoing metabolic activity. This involves employing saturating precursor concentrations and ensuring linear incorporation with time. Under the conditions used in the present study it was found that tyrosine and choline concentrations above 100 μM ensured that availability of these precursors would not be limiting for transmitter synthesis. This information may have relevance for normal growth conditions as well, especially for monolayer cultures with proliferating cells covering the entire dish instead of a small well (1 cm diameter), as is the case here. This may be even more important in studies employing media with much lower amino acid concentrations than L-15 and without choline supplementation. Obviously, it may be of interest to study synaptic interaction or development under conditions where transmitter precursors are limiting, but this should be done intentionally, (cf. Lloyd and Breakefield, 1974; Yavin, 1976; Cohen and Wurtman, 1976; Fernstrom and Wurtman, 1971; Birks and MacIntosh, 1961) rather than by depleting the medium. In the context of the role of precursor uptake in transmitter function, it will be of interest to examine in more detail the choline and tyrosine uptake properties of sympathetic neuron cultures, virtually free of nonneuronal cells, which are almost exclusively adrenergic (0% CM) or highly cholinergic (62% CM).

Effects of Conditioned Medium

The use of CM for induction of ACh production enables better experimental control of the phenomenon. It is possible to carry out detailed dose–response studies and the experiments reported here yielded the expected increase in ACh production with increasing CM and an unexpected corresponding drop in CA production. We have previously reported that certain non-neuronal cells can induce ACh production without appreciably affecting CA synthesis and accumulation in the same cultures (Patterson and Chun, 1974; Patterson et al., 1975). However, this appears to be true only for low levels of ACh production (0–10% CM, Fig. 5). It is possible to increase the ACh/CA ratio not only by increasing the CM concentration but also by employing L-15 CO_2 as the medium to be conditioned. This medium is better for nonneuronal growth and proliferation than is the L-15 Air medium previously used. Furthermore, analysis of older cultures (20–30 days rather than 10–15 days) in which the adrenergic or cholinergic character is more completely expressed (Patterson and Chun, in preparation) also enhances the ACh/CA ratio. These differences are seen when comparing the 50% CM data obtained with 16-day-old L-15 Air cultures (Fig. 4; ACh/N = 0.8 fmol) with the 50% CM data obtained with 20-day-old L-15 CO_2 cultures (Fig. 5; ACh/N = 75 fmol). Interestingly, the control ACh values were also higher in L-15 CO_2 cultures than in those in L-15 Air. Furthermore, cholinergic synapses between the neurons are occasionally observed in control L-15 CO_2 cultures but are very rare in L-15 Air cultures (Furshpan, Potter, and O'Lague, unpublished). Although it was not directly tested here, it is possible that bicarbonate has a direct effect on the neurons as well as on the nonneuronal cells; bicarbonate has been found to increase ACh turnover in some preparations (Birks and Mac-Intosh, 1961; McLennan and Elliott, 1950; but see Browning and Schulman, 1968). The fact that CA production tended to be depressed as ACh production was induced to high levels is consistent with the hypothesis that both transmitters could be produced by the same individual neurons. Recent electrophysiological (Furshpan et al, 1976) and morphological (Landis, 1976) studies on individual sympathetic neurons developing in isolation indicate that single neurons can in fact secrete both transmitters.

The data in Fig. 5 and Table 3 show that highly induced "cholinergic" cultures were capable of synthesizing and accumulating ACh at rates much higher than those of CA production by "adrenergic" cultures. The mechanism whereby this is accomplished is not yet clear. However, changes in neuronal number or growth are not the explanation. While increasing the CM concentration from 0 to 62% raised the ACh/CA ratio almost 1000-fold, no significant changes in neuronal number were observed. This was a consistent finding and has important implications for evaluating the ACh induction effect (see below). However, when the cultures displayed signs of ill health, such as very poor overall survival or low transmitter production, which can be due, for instance, to a low NGF concentration, CM can have the effect of increasing neuronal survival. Since this does not occur with healthier cultures, we interpret it as a nonspecific conditioning effect seen with other types of cultured cells and unrelated to the ACh induction phenomenon (e.g., Eagle and Piez, 1962). In addition, in the virtual absence of nonneuronal cells, the cholinergic induction was accompanied by no change in overall neuronal growth as measured by total protein and total lipid PO_4; any significant changes in number or size of neuronal processes, etc. would be reflected in these measurements. The results reported here do not support the possibility that the small population of sympathetic cholinergic neurons thought to be normally present in some sympathetic ganglia (cf. Sjöqvist, 1963; Aiken and Reit, 1969; Yamauchi et al., 1973) survive in the cultures in the presence of CM, but die or grow poorly in the control medium. Thus the CM effect involves an induction rather than a selection.

In addition to high ACh/CA ratios, the proportion of electrophysiologically identified cholinergic neurons in the 62% CM cultures is quite high. In contrast, 0% CM sister cultures display 1000-fold lower ACh/CA ratios, very few cholinergic synapses, and frequent morphologically identified adrenergic synapses (Landis *et al.*, 1976). Since the same number of neurons are present under both conditions, these results might suggest that the sympathetic neurons were not yet committed to one path of transmitter differentiation at the time of explantation and may be able to express either adrenergic or cholinergic properties depending on the environment in which they develop. It is possible, however, that the majority of the neurons in culture are in fact, already determined to become cholinergic and under the 0% CM "adrenergic" condition do not express this differentiated fate, remaining silent as far as neurotransmitters are concerned. This would also imply that adrenergic neurons are a minority population and are largely silent in the 62% CM condition. These possibilities are being tested by analysis of single neuron cultures under both "adrenergic" and "cholinergic" conditions (Reichardt *et al.*, 1976).

The efficacy of CM in the cholinergic induction has aided in the interpretation of the phenomenon. Since the nonneuronal cells and neurons produced little ACh when cultured separately, but considerable ACh when cocultured (Patterson and Chun, 1974) either type of cell could have been stimulating the other to produce ACh. A precedent for the possibility that nonneuronal cells can be induced to produce ACh is the evidence for induction of cholinergic properties in Schwann cells at the denervated neuromuscular junction (Dennis and Miledi, 1974; Bevan *et al.*, 1973). In this vein it is possible to contend that the CM taken from nonneuronal cultures makes the few nonneuronal cells cocultured with the sympathetic neurons more receptive to a neuronal influence to produce ACh. However, there was strong evidence that at least some of the ACh was localized in the cultured neurons because they formed functional cholinergic synapses with themselves and with skeletal muscle (O'Lague *et al.*, 1974, 1975; Nurse and O'Lague, 1975). This argument is further strengthened by the observation that neuronal cultures containing only a small fraction of the usual number of nonneuronal cells could be induced through addition of CM to produce large quantities of ACh. Furthermore, the CM did not act by causing proliferation of the few nonneuronal cells cocultured with the neurons. In light of these observations, we prefer the simpler interpretation that the nonneuronal cells induced ACh production in the neurons.

If the induced neurons are indeed cholinergic, how do they compare with other cultured neurons in their capacity for ACh formation? Specific activities were obtained for CAT in the mixed and neuron-alone sympathetically derived cultures. The values obtained for choline-dependent, PVN-inhibitable activity per non-collagen protein ($0.15–4.50$ nmol min^{-1} mg protein^{-1}) compare favorably with values obtained for other neuronal culture systems ($0.01–1.00$; Schubert *et al.*, 1974; Amano *et al.*, 1972; McMorris and Ruddle, 1974; Amano *et al.*, 1974; Ebel *et al.*, 1974; Schrier and Shapiro, 1974; Schrier, 1973; Wilson *et al.*, 1972; Peterson *et al.*, 1973; Godfrey *et al.*, 1975; Giller *et al.*, 1973; Kim *et al.*, 1974; Seeds, 1971). Given the presence of proliferating nonneuronal cells and the heterogeneous neuronal populations in most of these systems, the only cases which can be quantitatively compared are the neuroblastoma clones and the sympathetic neuron-alone cultures. In the future it may be possible to make direct comparisons of ACh production by single cells in these various systems because it is now possible to grow isolated sympathetic neurons and assay them for ACh and CA production (Reichardt *et al.*, 1976; Furshpan *et al.*, 1976). In any case, it is clear that the ACh production by the synpathetic neurons is not a metabolic by-product, for it enables them to form functional cholinergic synapses.

Nonneuronal Cell Specificity

The question of which types of nonneuronal cells can induce ACh production in the sympathetic neurons is of interest because the answer could shed light on the role of this inductive phenomenon in normal autonomic development. Initially we found that when neurons were grown with homologous ganglionic nonneuronal cells or C6 rat glioma cells, increased ACh production resulted, while addition of 3T3 mouse fibroblasts did not cause a significant increase (Patterson and Chun, 1974). An ambiguity in this type of experiment is that the particular nonneuronal cell type added (i.e., C6 cells) could act by causing a proliferation of ganglionic nonneuronal cells and thereby cause an increase in ACh production without itself directly affecting the neurons. With the use of CM, however, it is possible to grow and assay the neurons in the presence of only a very few ganglionic nonneuronal cells, making the interpretation clearer. Several significant observations emerged from the data in Table 3: rat fibroblasts, both primary and continuous cell lines, and rat glioma (C6), Schwannoma (RN22), and skeletal muscle (L8) lines were all able, with various degrees of effectiveness, to induce neuronal ACh production by conditioning the medium. However, one rat cell line (R_2C) and all non-rat lines (BHK, 3T3, L929) as well as the non-rat primary cells tested, were relatively weak at conditioning the medium. Since rat fibroblasts were positive it will be possible to attribute the results from all the rat primary tissues to mesenchymal fibroblast-like cells until tests

have been made of primary cells free of fibroblasts.

That fibroblasts can induce the ACh effect is of interest because they are known to produce several molecules important in development such as collagen, glycosaminoglycans (Hay, 1973), and NGF (Young *et al.*, 1975). Are any of these molecules responsible for the ACh induction? Raising the NGF concentration 50-fold above the dose normally employed (1 μg/ml; 7S) did not induce ACh production in the absence of CM. Furthermore, the effectiveness of CM was not impaired if it was produced in the absence of exogenously added NGF (Chun and Patterson, in preparation). Thus mouse submaxillary gland NGF alone could not induce ACh, nor was the exogenously added NGF modified in some manner by the nonneuronal cells to carry out a different mission. Regarding collagen, it is of interest that the RN2 (Schwann cell line cloned from the same neurinoma as RN22 by S. E. Pfeiffer), L6 (cloned from the same muscle line as L8 by D. Yaffe), and C6 cell lines as well as primary fibroblasts have all been shown to secrete proteins with some of the properties of collagen (Church *et al.*, 1973; Schubert *et al.*, 1973; Schubert, 1973). Therefore these cell types may have more in common than might be first suspected. However, collagen itself does not appear to be the key factor in the ACh induction because (i) collagen is present on the surface of control cultures, and (ii) 3T3 cells also secrete collagen (Schubert *et al.*, 1973). There may, of course, be different types or physical forms of collagen involved. The glycosaminoglycans remain to be tested for involvement in the ACh induction.

The species specificity of the ACh effect may provide important clues for understanding the phenomenon. This specificity is in contrast with the relative nonspecies specific nature of many hormones and growth factors. NGF, the molecule about which we have the most developmental information, is effective across species lines, in mammals, birds, reptiles and amphibians. On the other hand, Varon *et al.* (1974) reported a species specificity for an NGF-like effect by ganglionic nonneuronal cells on sympathetic and sensory neurons. Furthermore, Gospodarowicz *et al.* (1976) found that bovine fibroblast growth factor displayed some species specificity. The role of species specificity in such a basic phenomenon as control of cholinergic differentiation is unknown. Perhaps the species differences described here reflect quantitative differences in postganglionic cholinergic neurons in these three species *in vivo*.

Comparisons with Other Systems

Of interest are reports that nonneuronal cells may influence CAT activity in central nervous system neurons in culture. There is evidence consistent with CAT induction by nonneuronal cells in surface cultures from rat brain (Schrier and Shapiro, 1974). Most importantly, Giller *et al.* (1973) found that addition of skeletal muscle cells to spinal cord cultures caused an increased CAT activity compared to spinal cord and muscle cells cultured alone. This effect can also be transmitted via CM from skeletal muscle cultures (Nelson, 1975), indicating that neuromuscular junction formation is not necessary for the stimulation. The cell specificity of the effect was not absolute as fibroblasts also stimulated CAT activity in combined cultures with spinal cord. Without the ability to identify and assay cholinergic neurons in the control and untreated cultures, it is difficult to assess whether the stimulation was due to an increase in plating efficiency, growth, or differentiation in the affected neurons. It is also possible that the CM acts via the monolayer of nonneuronal cells in the spinal cord-alone cultures. It will be of great interest to see if there is any similarity between the phenomenon in spinal cord and that described here for sympathetic neurons. Characterization of some of the properties of the active factor(s) in the medium, nonneuronal cell specificity (skeletal muscle CM is posi-

tive for both), and species specificity would be good starting points for comparison.

Transplantation of neural crest cells to abnormal sites has demonstrated the importance of the environment in controlling development of transmitter metabolism *in vivo* and in explant culture (Cohen, 1972; Norr, 1973; LeDouarin and Teillet, 1974; LeDouarin *et al.*, 1974, 1975). Cells from the presumptive adrenergic crest (giving rise normally to sympathetic neurons or adrenal medulla) can be made to differentiate into parasympathetic cholinergic neurons by transplantation to the presumptive cholinergic region of the crest (LeDouarin *et al.*, 1975). Although the decision made by the neurons in the present culture experiments may be to become either sympathetic adrenergic or sympathetic cholinergic rather than sympathetic adrenergic or parasympathetic cholinergic, it will be of interest to determine if the cholinergic induction by the nonneuronal cells in culture is related to the influences brought to bear on presumptive parasympathetic neurons during their migration from the neural crest and/or at their final sites in ganglia. Concerning potential influences exerted within autonomic ganglia, the question arises why the neurons *in situ* remain primarily adrenergic if sympathetic ganglionic nonneuronal cells can induce ACh synthesis in sympathetically derived cultured neurons? Of course, the answer to this puzzle will not become clear until the nature of the inductive effect is understood, but several hypotheses can be offered at this point. (i) Principal neurons are normally ensheathed by a special cell type (satellite cells) *in vivo* and it could be that they are "protected" from the nonneuronal cholinergic influence (and the minority of cholinergic sympathetic neurons are not?). Recent observation of cholinergic innervation of the iris by explants of sympathetic ganglia (Hill *et al.*, 1976) may not support this idea if the neurons in the explants remain ensheathed and if that innervation involved a large proportion of the neurons. The latter point is difficult to establish with explant cultures. A similar observation was made by Crain and Peterson (1974) using sympathetic explants and skeletal muscle. (ii) A second possibility is that the ganglionic cell type which flourishes in culture (fibroblasts?) and thereby greatly outnumbers the other cell types, is not so numerous within the ganglion *in vivo*. (iii) It may also be that the cholinergic induction involves the serum in the culture medium, and the neurons *in vivo* are not directly in contact with the serum. (iv) Finally, the cholinergic influence could be present normally *in vivo* but counterbalanced by an adrenergic influence not yet added to the cell cultures, such as the spinal cord innervation of the ganglion. Hypothesizing such a finely balanced situation has the advantage of easily explaining adrenergic/cholinergic differences among the various ganglia in the sympathetic chain (Buckley *et al.*, 1967; Yamauchi *et al.*, 1973), between developing and adult ganglia (Boatman *et al.*, 1965; Burn, 1968), and between ganglia of different species (Burn and Rand, 1962).

In this context, certain developmental questions become especially relevant. Over what developmental time course do the cultured neurons differentiate adrenergically and cholinergically, at what age are they susceptible to the cholinergic signal, and are either the cholinergic or adrenergic decisions reversible? These are the points considered in another paper (Patterson and Chun, in preparation).

It is a pleasure to acknowledge the conscientious assistance of Doreen McDowell and Karen Fischer with the culturing. We also thank Eleanor P. Livingston, Shirley E. Wilson, Joe Gagliardi, and Zach Hall for excellent help with the manuscript, Ed Kravitz for the use of his equipment, Darwin Berg for help with the choline acetyltransferase assays, and Dick Mains for assistance with the initial experiments.

This research was supported by a grant-in-aid (93-877) from the American and Massachusetts Heart Associations and a USPHS Grant (1 R01 NS 11027) from the National Institute of Neurological and Communicable Diseases and Stroke. P.H.P. is a Research Career Development Awardee of the NINCDS (1 K04 NS 70806) and L.L.Y.C. is a PHS Trainee (T01 NS 05731).

REFERENCES

AIKEN, J., and REIT, E. (1969). A comparison of the sensitivity to chemical stimuli of adrenergic and cholinergic neurons in the cat stellate ganglia. *J. Pharmacol. Exp. Ther.* **169**, 211–223.

AMANO, T., RICHELSON, E., and NIRENBERG, M. (1972). Neurotransmitter synthesis by neuroblastoma clones. *Proc. Nat. Acad. Sci. USA* **69**, 258–263.

AMES, B. N., and DUBIN, D. T. (1960). The role of polyamines in the neutralization of bacteriophage deoxyribonucleic acid. *J. Biol. Chem.* **235**, 769–775.

BEVAN, S., MILEDI, R., and GRAMPP, W. (1973). Induced transmitter release from Schwann cells and its suppression by actinomycin D. *Nature New Biol.* **241**, 85–86.

BIRKS, R. I., and MACINTOSH, F. C. (1961). Acetylcholine metabolism of a sympathetic ganglion. *Canad. J. Biochem. Physiol.* **39**, 787–827.

BOATMAN, D. L., SHAFFER, R. A., DIXON, R. L., and BRODY, M. J. (1965). Function of vascular smooth muscle and its sympathetic innervation in the newborn dog. *J. Clin. Invest.* **44**, 241–246.

BONTING, S. L., and JONES, M. (1957). Determination of microgram quantities of deoxynucleic acid and protein in tissues grown *in vitro*. *Arch. Biochem. Biophys.* **66**, 340–353.

BROWNING, E. T., and SCHULMAN, M. P. (1968). [^{14}C]Acetylcholine synthesis by cortex slices of rat brain. *J. Neurochem.* **15**, 1391–1405.

BUCKLEY, G., CONSOLO, S., GIACOBINI, E., and SJÖQVIST, F. (1967). Cholinacetylase in innervated and denervated sympathetic ganglia and ganglion cells of the cat. *Acta Physiol. Scand.* **71**, 348–356.

BURN, J. H. (1968). The development of the adrenergic fibre. *Brit. J. Pharmacol.* **32**, 575–582.

BURN, J. H., and RAND, M. J. (1962). A new interpretation of the adrenergic nerve fiber. *Adv. Pharmacol.* **1**, 1–30.

CHURCH, R., TANZER, M. L., and PFEIFFER, S. E. (1973). Collagen and procollagen production by a clonal line of Schwann cells. *Proc. Nat. Acad. Sci. USA* **70**, 1943–1946.

COHEN, A. (1972). Factors directing the expression of sympathetic nerve traits in cells of neural crest origin. *J. Exp. Zool.* **179**, 167–182.

COHEN, E. L., and WURTMAN, R. J. (1976). Brain acetylcholine: control by dietary choline. *Science* **191**, 561–562.

CRAIN, S. M., and PETERSON, E. R. (1974). Development of neural connections in culture. *Ann. N.Y. Acad. Sci.* **228**, 6–33.

DENNIS, M., and MILEDI, R. (1974). Electrically induced release of acetylcholine from denervated Schwann cells. *J. Physiol.* 237, 431–452.

EAGLE, H., and PIEZ, K. (1962). The population-dependent requirement by cultured mammalian cells for metabolites which they can synthesize. *J. Exp. Med.* 116, 29–43.

EBEL, A., MASSARELLI, R., SENSENBRENNER, M., and MANDEL, P. (1974). Choline acetyltransferase and acetylcholinesterase activities in chicken brain hemispheres *in vivo* and in cell culture. *Brain Res.* 76, 461–472.

FERNSTROM, J. D., and WURTMAN, R. J. (1971). Brain serotonin content: increase following ingestion of carbohydrate diet. *Science* 174, 1023–1025.

FURSHPAN, E. J., MacLEISH, P. R., O'LAGUE, P. H., and POTTER, D. D. (1976). Chemical transmission between rat sympathetic neurons and cardiac myocytes developing in microcultures: evidence for cholinergic, adrenergic and dual-function neurons. *Proc. Nat. Acad. Sci. USA*, 73, 4225–4229.

GILLER, E. L., SCHRIER, B. K., SHAINBERG, A., FISK, H. R., and NELSON, P. G. (1973). Choline acetyltransferase activity is increased in combined cultures of spinal cord and muscle cells from mice. *Science* 182, 588–589.

GODFREY, E. W., NELSON, P. G., SCHRIER, B. K., BREUER, A. C., and RANSOM, B. R. (1975). Neurons from fetal rat brain in a new cell culture system: a multidisciplinary analysis. *Brain Res.* 90, 1–21.

GOSPODAROWICZ, D., WESEMAN, J., MORAN, J. S., and LINDSTROM, J. (1976). Effect of fibroblast growth factor on the division and fusion of bovine myoblasts. *J. Cell Biol.* 70, 395–405.

HAY, E. (1973). Origin and role of collagen in the embryo. *Amer. Zool.* 13, 1085–1107.

HILL, C. E., PURVES, R. D., WATANABE, H., and BURNSTOCK, G. (1976). Specificity of innervation of iris musculature by sympathetic nerve fibres in tissue culture. *Pflügers Arch.* 361, 127–134.

KIM, S. U., OH, T. H., and WENGER, E. L. (1974). Biochemical and cytochemical studies of the development of choline acetyltransferase and acetylcholinesterase in organotypic cultures of chick neural tube. *J. Neurobiol.* 5, 305–315.

LANDIS, S. C. (1976). Rat sympathetic neurons and cardiac myotubes developing in microcultures: correlation of the fine structure of endings with neurotransmitter function in single neurons. *Proc. Nat. Acad. Sci. USA*, 73, 4220–4224.

LANDIS, S. C., MacLEISH, P. R., POTTER, D. D., FURSHPAN, E. J., and PATTERSON, P. H. (1976). Synapses formed between dissociated sympathetic neurons: the influence of conditioned medium. *Sixth Ann. Soc. Neurosci.*, Abstract 280.

LEDOUARIN, N. M., and TEILLET, M. M. (1974). Experimental analysis of the migration and differentiation of neuroblasts of the autonomic nervous system and of neuroectodermal mesenchymal de-

rivatives using a biological cell marking technique. *Develop. Biol.* 41, 162–184.

LEDOUARIN, N., RENAUD, D., TEILLET, M., and LE-DOUARIN, G. (1975). Cholinergic differentiation of presumptive adrenergic neuroblasts in interspecific chimeras after heterotopic transplantations. *Proc. Nat. Acad. Sci. USA* 72, 728–732.

LLOYD, T., and BREAKEFIELD, X. O. (1974). Tyrosine-dependent increase of tyrosine hydroxylase in neuroblastoma cells. *Nature (London)* 252, 719–720.

MAINS, R. E., and PATTERSON, P. H. (1973a). Primary cultures of dissociated sympathetic neurons. I. Establishment of long-term growth in culture and studies of differentiated properties. *J. Cell Biol.* 59, 329–345.

MAINS, R. E., and PATTERSON, P. H. (1973b). II. Initial studies on catecholamine metabolism. *J. Cell Biol.* 59, 346–360.

McLENNAN, H., and ELLIOTT, K. A. C. (1950). Factors affecting the synthesis of acetylcholine by brain slices. *Amer. J. Physiol.* 163, 605–613.

McMORRIS, F. A., and RUDDLE, F. H. (1974). Expression of neuronal phenotypes in neuroblastoma cell hybrids. *Develop. Biol.* 39, 226–246.

NELSON, P. G. (1975). Central nervous system synapses in cell culture. *Cold Spring Harbor Symp. Quant. Biol.* 40, 359–371.

NORR, S. (1973). *In Vitro* analysis of sympathetic neuron differentiation from chick neural crest cells. *Develop. Biol.* 34, 16–38.

NURSE, C. A., and O'LAGUE, P. H. (1975). Formation of cholinergic synapses between dissociated sympathetic neurons and skeletal myotubes of the rat in cell culture. *Proc. Nat. Acad. Sci. USA* 72, 1955–1959.

O'LAGUE, P. H., MacLEISH, P. R., NURSE, C. A., CLAUDE, P., FURSHPAN, E. J., and POTTER, D. D. (1975). Physiological and morphological studies on developing sympathetic neurons in dissociated cell culture. *Cold Spring Harbor Symp. Quant. Biol.* 40, 399–407.

O'LAGUE, P. H., OBATA, K., CLAUDE, P., FURSHPAN, E. J., and POTTER, D. D. (1974). Evidence for cholinergic synapses between dissociated rat sympathetic neurons in cell culture. *Proc. Nat. Acad. Sci. USA* 71, 3602–3606.

PATTERSON, P. H., and CHUN, L. L. Y. (1974). The influence of nonneuronal cells on catecholamine and acetylcholine synthesis and accumulation in cultures of dissociated sympathetic neurons. *Proc. Nat. Acad. Sci. USA* 71, 3607–3610.

PATTERSON, P. H., CHUN, L. L. Y., and REICHARDT, L. F. (1976). The role of nonneuronal cells in the development of sympathetically derived neurons. Proc. ICN-UCLA Conf. on Neurobiol (C. F. Fox, ed.). *J. Supramolec. Struc.* in press.

PATTERSON, P. H., and LENNARZ, W. J. (1971). Studies on the membranes of bacilli. I. Phospholipid biosynthesis. *J. Biol. Chem.* **246**, 1062–1072.

PATTERSON, P. H., REICHARDT, L. F., and CHUN, L. L. Y. (1975). Biochemical studies on the development of primary sympathetic neurons in cell culture. *Cold Spring Harbor Symp. Quant. Biol.* **40**, 389–397.

PETERSON, G. R., WEBSTER, G. W., and SHUSTER, L. (1973). Characteristics of choline acetyltransferase and cholinesterases in two types of cultured cells from embryonic chick brain. *Develop. Biol.* **34**, 119–134.

REICHARDT, L. F., PATTERSON, P. H., and CHUN, L. L. Y. (1976). Norepinephrine and acetylcholine synthesis by individual sympathetic neurons under various culture conditions. *Sixth Ann. Soc. Neurosci.*, Abstract 327.

SCHRIER, B. K. (1973). Surface culture of fetal mammalian brain cells: effect of subculture on morphology and choline acetyltransferase activity. *J. Neurobiol.* **4**, 117–124.

SCHRIER, B. K., and SHAPIRO, D. (1974). Effects of fluorodeoxyuridine on growth and choline acetyltransferase activity in fetal rat brain cells in surface culture. *J. Neurobiol.* **5**, 151–159.

SCHUBERT, D. (1973). Protein secretion by clonal glial and neuronal cell lines. *Brain Res.* **56**, 387–391.

SCHUBERT, D., HEINEMANN, S., CARLISLE, W., TARIKAS, H., KIMES, B., PATRICK, J., STEINBACH, J. H., CULP, W., and BRANDT, B. L. (1974). Clonal cell lines from the rat central nervous system. *Nature (London)* **249**, 224–227.

SCHUBERT, D., TARIKAS, H., HUMPHREYS, S., HEINEMANN, S., and PATRICK, J. (1973). Protein synthesis and secretion by a myogenic cell line. *Develop. Biol.* **33**, 18–37.

SEEDS, N. (1971). Biochemical differentiation in reaggregating brain cell culture. *Proc. Nat. Acad. Sci. USA* **68**, 1858–1861.

SHIN, S., YASUMURA, Y., and SATO, G. H. (1968). Studies on interstitial cells in tissue culture. II: Steroid biosynthesis by a clonal line of rat testicular interstitial cells. *Endocrinology* **82**, 614–616.

SJÖQVIST, F. (1963). The correlation between the occurrence and localization of acetylcholinesterase-rich cell bodies in the stellate ganglion and the outflow of cholinergic sweat secretory fibers to the forepaw of the cat. *Acta Physiol. Scand.* **57**, 339–351.

VARON, S., RAIBORN, C., and BURNHAM, P. A. (1974). Selective potency of homologous ganglionic nonneuronal cells for the support of dissociated ganglionic neurons in culture. *Neurobiology* **4**, 231–252.

WHITE, H. L., and WU, J. C. (1973). Choline and carnitine acetyltransferases of heart. *Biochemistry* **12**, 841–846.

WILSON, S. H., SCHRIER, B. K., FARBER, J. L., THOMPSON, E. J., ROSENBERG, R., BLUME, A., and NIRENBERG, M. (1972). Markers for gene expression in cultured cells from the nervous system. *J. Biol. Chem.* **247**, 3159–3169.

YAMAUCHI, A., LEVER, J., and KEMP, J. (1973). Catecholamine loading and depletion in the rat superior cervical ganglion. *J. Anat.* **114**, 271–282.

YAVIN, E. (1976). Regulation of phospholipid metabolism in differentiating cells from rat brain cerebral hemispheres in culture. *J. Biol. Chem.* **251**, 1392–1397.

YOUNG, M., OGER, J., BLANCHARD, M., ASDOURIAN, H., AMOS, H., and ARNASON, B. (1975). Secretion of a nerve growth factor by primary chick fibroblast cultures. *Science* **187**, 361–362.

Reprinted from
Proc. Natl. Acad. Sci. USA
Vol. 73, No. 11, pp. 4225–4229, November 1976
Neurobiology

Chemical transmission between rat sympathetic neurons and cardiac myocytes developing in microcultures: Evidence for cholinergic, adrenergic, and dual-function neurons

(autonomic transmitters/autapses/culture methods/ neuron-heart cell interaction)

E. J. FURSHPAN*, P. R. MACLEISH*, P. H. O'LAGUE†, AND D. D. POTTER*

* Department of Neurobiology, Harvard Medical School, Boston, Massachusetts 02115; and † Department of Biology, University of California, Los Angeles, Calif. 90024

Communicated by David H. Hubel, September 7, 1976

ABSTRACT   Electrophysiological studies were made on microcultures (300–500 μm in diameter) in which solitary sympathetic principal neurons from newborn rats grew on previously dissociated rat heart cells. Some neurons inhibited, some excited, and others first inhibited and then excited the cardiac myocytes. Application of drugs provided evidence for secretion of acetylcholine by the first group, catecholamines by the second, and both acetylcholine and catecholamines by the third. Solitary neurons which inhibited the myocytes usually excited themselves at nicotinic synapses (autapses).

The transmitter functions of rat sympathetic principal neurons developing in culture can be influenced in a striking way by a variety of nonneuronal cells. Neurons cultured in the near absence of nonneuronal cells develop adrenergic functions including synthesis, storage, release, and uptake of norepinephrine (NE); these neurons form synapses of adrenergic appearance (i.e., containing small granular vesicles) on each other (1–4). Adrenergic transmission has not yet been detected at such synapses, apparently because of the insensitivity of the neurons to NE (unpublished; see ref. 5). Moreover, acetylcholine (AcCh) synthesis is usually negligible, and cholinergic transmission is rarely seen (1, 6, 7, 8). In contrast, when the neurons are cultured in the presence of nonneuronal cells (e.g., from ganglia or heart), or in medium conditioned by such cells, the neuronal population synthesizes both AcCh and NE (2, 9), and many neurons form nicotinic cholinergic synapses on each other (6–8, 10, 11). These effects are graded. A higher proportion of conditioned medium or a greater number of nonneuronal cells gives a higher ratio of AcCh synthesis to catecholamine synthesis (12), a higher incidence of cholinergic transmission, and a higher proportion of synapses which lack small granular vesicles (13). This shift to cholinergic functions occurs without appreciable change in the number of neurons per culture (2, 12). This and other evidence indicates that at least a majority of the neurons isolated from ganglia of newborn rats are plastic with respect to transmitter functions; many apparently remain so for at least two weeks in culture (12).

It is unclear whether in cultures with both adrenergic and cholinergic functions individual neurons are exclusively adrenergic or cholinergic, or whether they can display, at least temporarily, both functions simultaneously. To investigate this question with biochemical methods, Reichardt, Patterson, and Chun (14) developed techniques for growing single neurons and assayed AcCh and catecholamine synthesis. To investigate this question with electrophysiological methods, MacLeish grew neurons in mass cultures with atrial myocytes (thousands of dissociated neurons and cardiac cells per dish), because each

myocyte is sensitive to both AcCh and NE (MacLeish, unpublished). He found that the incidence of detectable neuron-myocyte interaction was too low to be useful, perhaps in part because the endings of each neuron were sparsely distributed in the large field of myocytes; the few cases found all appeared to be cholinergic.

It was plausible that the incidence of detectable interaction would increase if the innervation field of a given neuron was concentrated on a few cardiac myocytes. Thus, we made microcultures containing a single neuron and a small number of myocytes in an area only a fraction of a millimeter in diameter. In this paper, we report physiological observations on such microcultures; in the accompanying paper, Landis (15) reports electron microscopic observations on the same microcultures.

In two previous studies (16, 17), explants of sympathetic ganglia were found to make functional contacts with explants of heart.

METHODS

Several methods for making microcultures suitable for electrophysiology and microscopy were successful, but none routinely so. The simplest method was, in brief, to apply 25 to 50 equally spaced droplets of dissolved collagen to a nonwetting polystyrene surface. When dried, these produced a grid (*ca* 50 mm²) of collagen islands, each island 300–500 μm in diameter. Cardiac cells (myocytes and fibroblasts) were dissociated from hearts of newborn rats by use of collagenase (EC 3.4.24.3) (Worthington Type I; 1 mg/ml), and allowed to settle on the grid for about 2 hr. Almost all cells not adhering to the collagen islands could then be washed away with medium. Proliferation of the cardiac cells was suppressed after 1–2 days by γ-irradiation (^{60}Co; 5000 rads in 25–30 sec, where one rad equals 1 $\times$ 10^{-2} J/kg). One to 5 days later, principal neurons were dissociated from superior cervical ganglia of newborn rats (Charles River CD) as previously described (1, 18), and plated at a density such that many islands received only one or a few neurons. The cultures were grown in L-15 CO$_2$ medium (1) containing 5% adult rat serum or 10% fetal calf serum (Microbiological Associates, 14-414), but lacking bovine serum albumin and Methocel. Six platings (about 30 dishes per plating) were used in experiments reported here.

For electrophysiological recording, cultures were placed on a microscope stage and perfused continuously with fluid similar to that used previously (6) but containing 6 mM NaHCO$_3$, 0.14 mM ascorbate and fetal calf serum (1% vol/vol). A change to fluid containing drugs could be made while maintaining impalement of the cells. The culture was kept at 34–36°. Microelectrodes filled with 3 M KCl (60–150 Mohm) were used

Abbreviations: AcCh, acetylcholine; NE, norepinephrine; e.p.s.p.'s, excitatory postsynaptic potentials.

to pass current and record membrane potential in neurons and myocytes. In some experiments, an optical method was used to record the beating of myocytes (cf. ref. 19). At the end of many experiments, the microculture was fixed for electron microscopic examination as described by Landis (15).

RESULTS

In microcultures, the neurites grew rapidly, as in mass cultures of dissociated neurons on heart cells (7); two islands containing single neurons (called "solitary neurons" below) are shown in two figures below. A typical island had several clusters of myocytes which usually beat spontaneously and synchronously. The neurites crisscrossed the island and sometimes grew around the perimeter. Occasionally the neurites were seen to extend for short distances from the island to nonneuronal cells or even from island to island. In the cases reported below, no inter-island cellular connections were present.

The resting and action potentials recorded from solitary neurons were similar to those of dissociated neurons in mass cultures (6, 7, 10). Stable impalements of neurons for many hours were routine; repeated impalements of myocytes were often necessary. Action potentials recorded in the myocytes were up to 120 mV in size and were preceded by pacemaker potentials.

Cholinergic synapses formed by solitary neurons on themselves

In mass cultures of dissociated neurons grown on heart cells, the neurons frequently form cholinergic synapses on each other (ref. 7; see also refs. 6, 8, 10, and 11). One question was whether a solitary neuron would form such synapses on itself; many did so. Examples are shown in Fig. 1a$_{1-3}$. A single action potential in the neuron often evoked a barrage of excitatory postsynaptic potentials (e.p.s.p.'s) (Fig. 1a$_1$). The initial e.p.s.p. had such short latency that it began during the action potential. The longer-latency e.p.s.p.'s suggested the presence of long conduction pathways. Hexamethonium chloride (150–1000 μM), or d-tubocurarine chloride (350 μM) greatly reduced or abolished the e.p.s.p.'s (Fig. 3a–c), but atropine sulfate had little effect in concentrations which blocked the cholinergic inhibition of the myocytes by these neurons (see below). This leaves little doubt that the e.p.s.p.'s were produced by secretion of AcCh at nicotinic synapses. The useful name *autapse* was proposed by Van Der Loos and Glaser (20) for a synapse made by a neuron on itself. In the microcultures, almost all neurons that made nicotinic autapses also produced atropine-sensitive inhibition of myocytes (next section).

The action of the neurons on the myocytes

To test for effects on the myocytes, we stimulated neurons repetitively with one microelectrode while recording myocyte activity with a second electrode.

Evidence for Cholinergic Action. Many solitary neurons hyperpolarized the myocytes (Fig. 1b$_1$, and c$_1$) and stopped their spontaneous activity (e.g., Fig. 1b$_1$). The hyperpolarization of the myocytes always had a longer latency and a much slower time course than did the e.p.s.p.'s on the same neuron. In two cases, hyperpolarization was evoked by a single neuronal impulse; the latency was about 50 msec (cf. ref. 21). An increase in myocyte membrane conductance during the hyperpolarization was demonstrated either with small test current pulses (three cases) or by reversal of the hyperpolarization (one case; Fig. 1c$_1$–c$_3$).

In the mammalian heart, hyperpolarization and an increase in K$^+$ permeability are caused by AcCh acting on atropine-

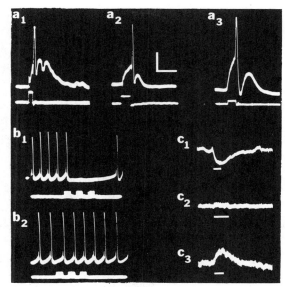

FIG. 1. Cholinergic transmission at autapses and at neuron-myocyte contacts. (a$_1$–a$_3$) autaptic e.p.s.p.'s after evoked spikes in three neurons (stimulating current pulses on lower traces). Culture ages in days: (a$_1$) 17; (a$_2$) 14; (a$_3$) 30. (b$_1$) inhibition of spontaneous impulses in a myocyte (upper trace) evoked by three trains of neuronal stimuli (35 per sec; lower trace). Culture age is 13 days. (b$_2$) perfusion with atropine sulfate (0.1 μM) blocked the inhibition. (c$_1$–c$_3$) reversal of neurally-evoked hyperpolarization of a myocyte when the myocyte resting potential (c$_1$) was shifted to inside-more-negative values (c$_2$, c$_3$) with applied currents. White bar under each trace is the duration of neuronal stimulation. Culture age is 30 days. Scales (y and x axis, respectively) are for (a$_1$–a$_3$) 20 mV and 20 msec; (b$_1$) or (b$_2$) 40 mV and 2 sec; (c$_1$–c$_3$) 10 mV and 10 sec.

sensitive muscarinic receptors (for references, see 22 and 23). Fig. 1b$_2$ shows that atropine (0.1 μM) blocked the inhibitory action of a solitary neuron on the myocytes. This effect of atropine (0.02–0.1 μM) was present in all cases tested and was readily reversible (not shown). Similar concentrations block vagal and AcCh effects on mammalian hearts (22, 24, 25). AcCh (0.6 μM) in the presence of eserine (1 μM) hyperpolarized the myocytes and stopped their beating (not illustrated; cf. ref. 5).

The inhibition of the myocytes, its time course, and its sensitivity to atropine, taken with the evidence that these solitary neurons simultaneously secreted AcCh at autapses, leave little doubt that the neurons secreted AcCh onto the myocytes. Moreover, there is biochemical evidence that these neurons synthesize substantial amounts of AcCh in mass cultures containing cardiac cells (12), as do single neurons grown in isolation (14).

Evidence for Adrenergic Action. Many solitary neurons which did not form cholinergic autapses had an excitatory effect on myocytes. The action potentials of two such neurons are shown in Fig. 2 (inset of phase micrograph and Fig. 2a); no autaptic effect was observed even after an impulse train (not illustrated). Trains of neuronal impulses did, however, produce a depolarization of slow onset and time course in the myocytes and gave rise to a train of cardiac impulses lasting about 20 sec (Fig. 2b). In mammalian heart, these effects are produced by sympathetic stimulation or application of catecholamines and are blocked by propranolol, a β-blocker, at a concentration of

Neurobiology: Furshpan *et al.*

Proc. Natl. Acad. Sci. USA 73 (1976)   4227

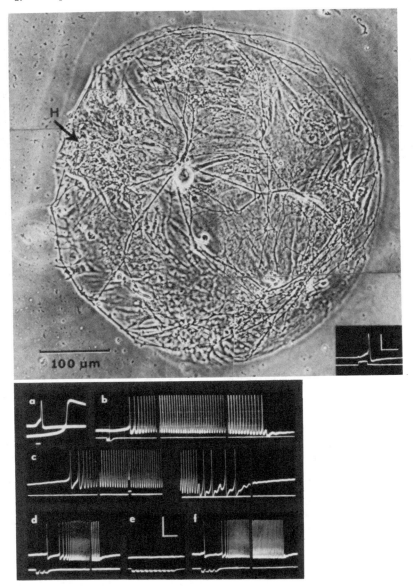

FIG. 2.   A microculture containing a solitary neuron; arrow at H indicates a cluster of myocytes. Neuron at 19 days in culture. Inset shows impulse in this neuron (scales are 50 mV, 20 msec for y and x axis, respectively); (d–f) were also from this neuron. (a) impulse in a similar neuron (upper trace), and a slower impulse in a myocyte; duration of stimulus in neuron shown by bar. (b) depolarization and impulses in the myocytes (upper trace) evoked by a train of neuronal impulses (22 per sec at deflection of lower trace). Brief gaps in both traces in this and other records mark start of new sweeps. (c) response of same myocytes to 0.1 μM NE. Pulse on lower trace marked return to normal fluid. Large gap in record is about 40 sec. Tops of impulses are not shown. (d) three trains of neuronal impulses (33 per sec) excited the myocytes. (e) ten trains had no effect in propranolol (1 μM). (f) subsequent recovery in normal fluid. Scales for y and x axis, respectively are (a) 50 mV and 20 msec; (b) 50 mV and 2 sec; (c) 25 mV and 2 sec; (d–f) 50 mV, 5 sec.

1 μM or less (see ref. 22 for references). Fig. 2d–f show that propranolol (1 μM) reversibly blocked the depolarization and initiation of beating; it consistently had this effect in the concentration range 0.3–1 μM. Fig. 2c shows that 0.1 μM NE mimicked the depolarization and initiation of beating produced by the solitary neuron; compare Fig. 2b and c.

The excitatory neuronal effect on the myocytes, its time course, its sensitivity to block by propranolol, and its similarity to the effect of applied NE all suggest that these solitary neurons secreted catecholamines, presumably including NE, onto the myocytes. Further evidence is provided by Landis' observations on these solitary neurons; varicosities near the myocytes con-

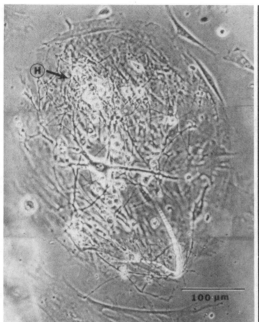

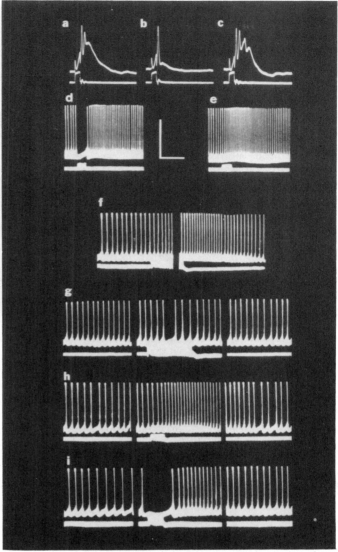

FIG. 3.   A microculture containing a dual-function solitary neuron after 13 days in culture. Arrow at H shows cluster of myocytes. All records were from this neuron. (a–c) neuronal impulse and autaptic e.p.s.p.'s before (a), during (b), and after (c) perfusing with hexamethonium (0.5 mM). (d) a train of neuronal impulses (deflection of lower trace) produced inhibition, and then excitation of spontaneous myocyte activity (upper trace). (e) inhibition was blocked by atropine (0.1 μM). In (d) and (e) hexamethonium (0.5 mM) was present. (f) the effect of atropine (0.1 μM; no hexamethonium in (f–i)) at higher sweep speed. (g) block of excitation by propranolol (0.6 μM; atropine still present). (h) about 45 min after removal of propranolol (atropine still present) with excitation restored. (i) the dual effect restored by perfusion with drug-free fluid. Scales are (for y and x axis, respectively) (a–c) 50 mV and 30 msec; (d) and (e) 100 mV and 12.5 sec (f–i) 100 mV and 5 sec.

tained many small granular vesicles (15). Moreover, when grown on cardiac cells either in mass cultures or in isolation some of the neurons synthesize NE (12, 14), and when grown in the absence (2) or presence (3) of ganglionic nonneuronal cells they release NE by a Ca^{++}-dependent mechanism.

Evidence for Dual-Function. In seven microcultures, stimulation of solitary neurons first inhibited and then accelerated the beating of the myocytes, as if both adrenergic and cholinergic transmission were present. One of these cases is illustrated in Fig. 3. Fig. 3d shows the initial hyperpolarization, a pause of about 5 sec in the beating, and the subsequent accelerated beating which lasted about 25 sec. In the presence of atropine (0.1 μM), the hyperpolarization and pause was eliminated, and the excitation enhanced (Fig. 3e). The inhibition was promptly restored after removal of atropine (not shown). This left little doubt that the neuron secreted AcCh onto the myocytes. To see whether the excitation which persisted in the presence of atropine (Fig. 3f; note change in time scale) was sensitive to propranolol, we added this drug at a concentration of 0.6 μM. The excitation was eliminated (Fig. 3g). It was gradually restored by perfusion with normal solution for about 45 min (Fig. 3h). In other experiments, propranolol alone (0.6 μM) abolished the excitation of the myocytes but left intact the secretion of AcCh at autapses and onto the myocytes; this is consistent with its conventional effect of blocking β-receptors, and rules out a general interference with secretion at nerve endings. In the experiment of Fig. 3 and others, hexamethonium alone had little influence on the action of the neuron on the myocytes, at concentrations which nearly eliminated transmission at cholinergic autapses. The presence of only one neuron in the microculture of Fig. 3 was confirmed by electron microscopic examination (15). Occasional small granular vesicles were present in the synaptic endings and varicosities of this neuron; see Landis (15) for discussion. Thus, a single neuron appeared to secrete two transmitters which activated three receptors: nicotinic-cholinergic and β-adrenergic (excitatory); muscarinic-cholinergic (inhibitory).

Burn and Rand (e.g., ref. 26) proposed that adult sympathetic neurons secrete both AcCh and NE, and that the acetylcholine acts on nicotinic receptors to stimulate NE secretion; it should be noted that the apparent secretion of NE by solitary neurons onto myocytes persisted in concentrations of hexamethonium which nearly eliminated cholinergic transmission at nicotinic autapses. There is evidence that certain molluscan neurons synthesize (27, 28) and use (29) more than one transmitter.

Multi-Neuron Microcultures. Many islands containing two to six neurons were examined. Further examples of block of neuron-myocyte interactions by atropine and propranolol were obtained. By these criteria, both adrenergic and cholinergic neurons were often present in the same island. In several cases, the cell bodies of two neurons, one apparently adrenergic, the other cholinergic, were in direct contact; we do not yet know whether this difference in transmitter functions arises because of heterogeneity among the neurons at the time of plating or because of environmental differences within a microculture. As they do in mass cultures (6–8, 10, 11), the neurons in these islands often activated each other by cholinergic synapses, and in one case by electrical transmission. Although hexamethonium or curare blocked the cholinergic interaction, the determination of the effects of individual neurons on myocytes remained uncertain because of the possibility of electrical interaction.

DISCUSSION

We began this work by asking whether individual sympathetic neurons developing in culture express, at any moment, only one set of transmitter functions, adrenergic or cholinergic, or both sets simultaneously. Three lines of evidence (ref. 14, this paper, and ref. 15) demonstrate that some of the developing neurons are at least predominantly adrenergic, and others at least predominantly cholinergic. In preliminary biochemical assays, dual-function neurons were not detected (14); physiological and morphological assays, which may be more sensitive than existing biochemical ones, have now provided preliminary evidence that, at least at shorter times in culture, some neurons use both transmitters (this paper, 15). If further work confirms the existence of such neurons, several questions of interest will be: (*i*) whether such neurons are capable of *synthesizing* both transmitters, since it is conceivable that the neurons take up and secrete catecholamines synthesized by adrenergic neurons in nearby islands; (*ii*) whether two transmitter systems in a single

neuron can be expressed in any proportion; and (*iii*) whether a particular proportion is stable. The microcultures have several advantages over mass cultures for investigating these questions. One advantage, which may have wide application, is that confinement of the growing neurites to a small number of target cells increases the probability of synapse formation on these cells and therefore the intensity of synaptic action.

This work was done in continuous collaboration with S. Landis (see ref. 15). We thank L. Chun for nerve growth factor, and our colleagues for helpful discussion. Essential help was provided by Delores Cox, William Dragun, Karen Fischer, Joseph Gagliardi, James LaFratta, Michael LaFratta, and Doreen McDowell. We thank Dr. John Little, Harvard School of Public Health for use of the ^{60}Co-source. Support was received from National Institutes of Health Research Grants NS02253, NS03273, NS11576, RR-7009, and Training Grant MH14275.

1. Mains, R. E. & Patterson, P. H. (1973) *J. Cell. Biol.* **59,** 329–345.
2. Patterson, P. H., Reichardt, L. F. & Chun, L. L. Y. (1975) *Cold Spring Harbor Symp. Quant. Biol.* **40,** 389–397.
3. Burton, H. & Bunge, R. P. (1975) *Brain Res.* **97,** 157–162.
4. Rees, R. & Bunge, R. P. (1974) *J. Comp. Neurol.* **157,** 1–12.
5. Obata, K. (1974) *Brain Res.* **73,** 71–88.
6. O'Lague, P. H., Obata, K., Claude, P., Furshpan, E. J. & Potter, D. D. (1974) *Proc. Natl. Acad. Sci. USA* **71,** 3602–3606.
7. O'Lague, P. H., MacLeish, P. R., Nurse, C. A., Claude, P., Furshpan, E. J. & Potter, D. D. (1975) *Cold Spring Harbor Symp. Quant. Biol.* **40,** 399–407.
8. Johnson, M., Ross, D., Meyers, M., Rees, R., Bunge, R., Wakshull, E. & Burton, H. (1976) *Nature* **262,** 308–310.
9. Patterson, P. H. & Chun, L. L. Y. (1974) *Proc. Natl. Acad. Sci. USA* **71,** 3607–3610.
10. Nurse, C. A. & O'Lague, P. H. (1975) *Proc. Natl. Acad. Sci. USA* **72,** 1955–1959.
11. Burton, H., Ko, C. P. & Bunge, R. (1975) *Fifth Annual Meeting, Society for Neuroscience* Abstr. 1251.
12. Patterson, P. H., Chun, L. L. Y. & Reichardt, L. F. (1976) Proceedings of the ICN-UCLA Conference on Neurobiology, ed. Fox, C. F., *J. Supramol. Struct.* **50,** in press.
13. Landis, S. C., MacLeish, P. R., Potter, D. D., Furshpan, E. J. & Patterson, P. H. (1976) *Sixth Annual Meeting, Society for Neuroscience,* in press.
14. Reichardt, L. F., Patterson, P. H. & Chun, L. L. Y. (1976) *Sixth Annual Meeting, Society for Neuroscience,* in press.
15. Landis, S. (1976) *Proc. Natl. Acad. Sci. USA* **73,** 4220–4224.
16. Crain, S. M. (1968) *Anat. Rec.* **160,** 466.
17. Purves, R. D., Hill, C. E., Chamley, J. H., Mark, G. E., Fry, D. M. & Burnstock, G. (1974) *Pflügers Arch.* **350.** 1–7.
18. Bray, D. (1970) *Proc. Natl. Acad. Sci. USA* **65,** 905–910.
19. Okarma, T. B. & Kalman, S. M. (1971) *Exp. Cell Res.* **69,** 128–134.
20. Van Der Loos, H. & Glaser, E. M. (1972) *Brain Res.* **48,** 355–360.
21. Purves, R. D. (1976) *Nature* **261,** 149–151.
22. Trautwein, W. (1963) *Pharmacol. Rev.* **15,** 277–322.
23. Ten Eick, R., Nawrath, H., McDonald, T. F. & Trautwein, W. (1976) *Pflügers Arch.* **361,** 207–213.
24. Amory, D. W. & West, T. C. (1962) *J. Pharmacol. Exp. Ther.* **137,** 14–23.
25. Leaders, F. E. (1963) *J. Pharmacol. Exp. Ther.* **42,** 31–38.
26. Burn, J. H. & Rand, M. J. (1965) *Annu. Rev. Pharmacol.* **5,** 163–182.
27. Brownstein, M. J., Saavedra, J. M., Axelrod, J., Zeman, G. H. & Carpenter, D. O. (1974) *Proc. Natl. Acad. Sci. USA* **71,** 4662–4665.
28. Hanley, M. R., Cottrell, G. A., Emson, P. C. & Fonnum, F. (1974) *Nature* **251,** 631–633.
29. Cottrell, G. A. (1976) *J. Physiol.* (*London*) **259,** 44–45P.

Reprinted from Nature, Vol. 286, pp. 663–669. 1980
© 1980 Macmillan Journals Ltd.

The ontogeny of the neural crest in avian embryo chimaeras

Nicole M. Le Douarin

Institut d'Embryologie du CNRS et du Collège de France, 49bis, avenue de la Belle-Gabrielle, 94130 Nogent-sur-Marne, France

The migration and subsequent development of autonomic ganglion cell precursors can be followed in suitably constructed chimaeric quail–chick embryos, thanks to the distinctive structures of quail and chick interphase nuclei. The decisive role of environmental factors arising from non-neuronal tissues on the chemical differentiation of neurones was demonstrated together with the lability of their phenotype during ontogeny.

EMBRYONIC development involves extensive movements of cells to achieve histogenesis and modelling of the body. With a few exceptions, such movements are extremely difficult to follow precisely by classical embryological methods. In fixed tissues, migrating cells, if they can be identified at all, can usually only be recognized in favourable situations, as for example when they are just leaving their site of origin. Since the expression of a particular differentiated phenotype generally occurs only after cell migration has taken place, the cells rapidly become indistinguishable from the equally undifferentiated surrounding tissues. The construction of embryonic 'fate maps' thus involves marking presumptive migrating cells so that their movements can be followed during ontogeny. This type of study, from which fundamental data on the formation and the fate of the germ layers have been obtained[1,2], entails differential labelling of relatively large tissue areas with rather crude methods, such as the application of vital dyes or small marking particles to specified embryonic regions. To investigate the migratory behaviour of individual cells, more precise means had to be found. One important way of achieving such refinement has been the use of techniques for combining early embryonic cells of different genotype. Such chimaeras develop normally and can be used to trace cell lineages through characteristic genetic markers.

In recent years, cell migration, cell derivation and cell–cell interactions during ontogeny of the avian embryo have become better understood, through the development of such a marking technique based on differences of the nuclear structure in two species of birds—the chick (*Gallus gallus*) and the quail (*Coturnix coturnix japonica*).

The quail–chick marking technique

The presence in all embryonic and adult cell types of the quail of a large amount of heterochromatin associated with the nucleolus was first described in 1969, and this characteristic was proposed as a cell-marking technique in combinations of embryonic cells from the quail and the chick[3]. Taxonomically, the two birds are closely related, but they differ significantly in the duration of their incubation period (16 days for the quail, 21 days for the chick) and their size at birth: the newly hatched chick weighs about three times as much as the quail. However, as shown by the tables of development of the two species[4,5], the chronology of development and also the size of the embryo differ only slightly during the first half of the incubation period, when the most decisive events of embryogenesis occur. Quail and chick cells can readily be recognized in sectioned material with the Feulgen–Rossenbeck stain or in the electron microscope after the routine uranyl acetate-lead citrate staining procedure. In undifferentiated cells, characterized by a high proliferation rate, the nucleolus is enlarged and made up of intimately associated

DNA- and RNA-containing structures[6]. In most differentiated cell types, the nucleolus is formed of a compact mass (sometimes 2 or 3) of heterochromatin, distinct from the nucleolar RNP, which occur as 'satellites' in contact with the heterochromatin. The structure of the nucleolus thus varies somewhat according to the cell type considered and the degree of differentiation reached. Nevertheless, the differences in their structures in quail and chicken cells are always conspicuous enough to make them easy to identify[6].

Quail–chick chimaeras can be constructed either *in vivo* or in culture. In the latter case, interactions between cell types from each species can be analysed in the course of a definite histogenetic process. Organotypic culture *in vitro* or grafting of the combined tissues on the avian chorioallantoic membrane (CAM) provides suitable conditions for these kinds of experiment[7,8]. The quail–chick system has also been applied to cell culture for recognition of nuclei in heterokaryons after acridine-orange staining[9]. However the domain in which it has so far been the most profitable is in the analysis of chimaeric embryos constructed *in ovo* by implanting quail cells into chick, or vice versa.

This method has been applied in my laboratory to study the ontogeny of two systems that involve extensive cell migrations in the embryo, the neural crest and the haemopoietic organs.

Migration pattern and fate of neural crest cells

The neural crest is a transitory structure of the vertebrate embryo arising from the lateral ridges of the nervous primordium and giving rise, among other cell types, to the neurones and supporting cells of the peripheral nervous system (sensory ganglia of the head and the rachis and autonomic sympathetic and parasympathetic ganglia), to the melanocytes and to mesenchymal derivatives in the head. As the elements derived from the neural crest are dispersed in various locations, the neural crest cells have to migrate throughout the developing body before reaching the embryonic rudiment in which they differentiate. This structure is, in many ways, an attractive model for the study of certain developmental problems and the fate of its cells has been widely investigated. Although they yielded much important information, the experimental techniques used by earlier workers for investigating differentiating capabilities of crest cells (excision and electrocauterization of the neural anlage, and various cell labelling techniques: see refs 6, 10, 11) did not provide a complete and detailed picture of the migration pattern and the developmental fate of the whole population derived from the crest. The application of the quail–chick marker to this problem brought additional information on the role of the neural crest in the construction of the head in higher

Nature Vol. 286 14 August 1980

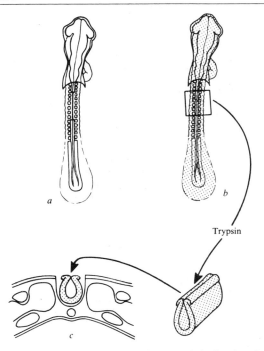

Fig. 1 Schematic representation of the isotopic-isochronic grafting technique of neural primordium between quail and chick embryos. *a*, Chick host embryo following the removal of the neural anlage from somite 4 to somite 10. *b*, Quail donor embryo from which the corresponding fragment of the neural tube + neural fold is isolated by enzymatic digestion. *c*, Graft of the quail neural primordium into the chick embryo.

vertebrates[12-16] and allowed new crest derivatives to be identified[17-19]. The method used, derived from that described by Weston[20], involved (1) surgical removal of a defined region of the neural primordium in a host embryo before the onset of crest cell migration at this level; and (2) its replacement by the strictly equivalent neural area originating from a donor embryo of the alternative species, at the same developmental stage (that is, isotopic and isochronic grafts) (Fig. 1). Since the graft is correctly positioned in the host, it develops normally in the chimaera (Fig. 2). Furthermore, the regulation processes that often follow extirpation of embryonic territories do not take place in the chimaera since the empty space is occupied by an equivalent structure originating from the donor embryo. Immunological mechanisms do not function during embryonic life and tissues of the two species are thus tolerated by each other. In the cephalic region, where the neural fold is larger than in the trunk, selective substitution of pieces of the neural crest alone can be carried out[12,13]. Migration of crest cells is followed on serial sections of the host embryos at various developmental stages. Recognition of the phenotype displayed by the grafted cells requires identification of both nuclear characteristics and an appropriate differentiation marker in the same cell. Electron microscopy can sometimes do this but, more often, the successive application of a cytochemical method (for example Falck's technique to evidence catecholamines[21]) and the Feulgen–Rossenbeck stain on the same section, have to be used.

Differentiation of the peripheral nervous system

Cells originating from the neural crest differentiate into constituents of two major neuronal systems: the sensory and the autonomic. Considerable interest has been focused in recent

years on the development of autonomic nerve cells and particularly on their chemical differentiation in terms of neurotransmitter synthesis. In complementary approaches the migratory behaviour and capabilities for differentiation of the presumptive autonomic neuroblasts have been studied by means of transplantation experiments *in vivo*, and the stability of neurotransmitter synthesis in developing autonomic neurones has been examined *in vitro*.

Although the ganglia of the autonomic nervous system and the adrenomedullary cells have long been recognized to be of neural crest origin, the migration pathways followed by their precursor cells were controversial (see ref. 22). By using the quail–chick chimaera system, we investigated their origin in normal development in the avian embryo. Isotopic and isochronic grafts of small fragments (corresponding to a length of 4–6 somites) of quail neural primordium into chick embryos (and vice versa) were systematically carried out along the whole length of the neural axis. The migrating neural crest cells were thereafter observed on serial sections of the host trunk (in the sympathetic chain and the adrenal medulla) and digestive tract (in the enteric and intravisceral ganglia). A correspondence could be established between the level of the graft and the definitive location of ganglion cells. In this way, the fate map of the autonomic cell precursors could be established (Fig. 3).

One of the striking observations made during these experiments was the finding that in the cervico-dorsal region (between somites 7 and 28) neural crest cell migration was strictly confined to the dorsal mesenchyme derived from the somites and the intermediate cell mass. Except for the melanocytes and for the Schwann cells that followed the nerve bundles to the periphery, neural crest derivatives were restricted to the sensory and sympathetic chain ganglia, the aortic and adrenal plexuses and the adrenomedullary paraganglia. No ganglion cell precursors penetrated the dorsal mesentery to contribute to either the ganglion of Remak or the enteric plexuses. In contrast, isotopic grafts carried out at the vagal (from somites 1 to 7) and lumbosacral (behind the 28th somite pair) levels of the neural primordium resulted in colonization of both the dorsal mesenchyme and the splanchnopleure. The myenteric plexuses are derived mainly from the crest at the level of somites 1–7; the contribution of the lumbosacral crest is restricted to the ganglion of Remak and to some ganglion cells of the post-umbilical gut. Crest cells continue to migrate ventrally from the vagal region between the 7- and 14-somite stages (approximately) and become incorporated into the mesodermal wall of the fore-gut, where they subsequently undergo a long cranio-caudal migration. Penetration of the hind-gut by either vagal or lumbo-sacral crest cells does not occur before days 7 to 8 of incubation[22,23].

The neural crest can therefore be divided into several different axial regions with respect to the development of the autonomic nervous system. One (level of somites 1–7) gives rise

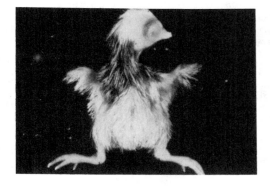

Fig. 2 Transverse pigmented stripe resulting when a fragment of a quail neural tube was grafted into a White Leghorn chick embryo.

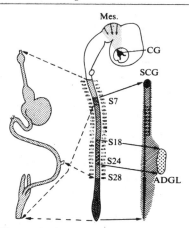

Fig. 3 Diagram showing the origin of adrenomedullary cells and autonomic ganglion cells. The spinal neural crest caudal to the level of the fifth somite gives rise to the ganglia of the orthosympathetic chain. The adrenomedullary cells originate from the spinal neural crest between the level of somites 18–24. The vagal neural crest (somites 1–7) gives rise to the parasympathetic enteric ganglia of the pre-umbilical region, the ganglia of the post-umbilical gut originating from both the vagal and lumbosacral neural crest. The ganglion of Remak is derived from the lumbosacral neural crest (posterior to the 28th somite level). Ciliary ganglion (CG) is derived from the mesencephalic neural crest. ADGL, adrenal gland; Mes., mesencephalon; SCG, superior cervical ganglion.

to the enteric ganglia of the gut. Another (somites 7–28) is the precursor of sympathoblasts of the trunk (within this area, the 'adrenomedullary' level of the crest contributes to the adrenal glands) and, finally, there are two regions from which both enteric and sympathetic ganglion cells arise (somites 5–7 and behind the 28th pair of somites). Next, neural primordia were transplanted heterotopically between quail and chick embryos, as shown in Fig. 4. This was to find out whether the migratory behaviour and phenotypic expression of crest cells from these regions were irreversibly fixed before migration and if experimental rearrangement of the axial levels of the neural crest would lead to developmental disturbances in the distribution and development of crest cell derivatives. Analysis of the resulting chimaeras showed that the neural crest cells of the adrenomedullary region, grafted at the vagal level, were able to colonize the gut (which they never do in normal development) and give rise to functional cholinergic enteric ganglia; second, neural crest cells from the quail mesencephalon or rhombencephalon, grafted at the chick adrenomedullary level, produced adrenergic sympathetic ganglia, populated the adrenal gland and differentiated into adrenomedullary-like cells[24,25]. This indicated that the migratory behaviour of the crest cells depends on the pathways available when they leave the neural primordium rather than on some specificity related to their origin in the neural axis. The vagal and the adrenomedullary regions of the embryo provide preferential pathways leading crest cells to the gut and to the suprarenal gland, respectively. In addition, the phenotypic expression of the crest cell population is regulated by environmental factors which elicit either cholinergic or adrenergic cell differentiation, irrespective of their fate in normal development. Furthermore, the potentialities for giving rise to cholinergic parasympathetic cells, adrenergic sympathetic ganglia and adrenomedullary paraganglia are not restricted to the areas identified in the isotopic-isochronic experiments, but are present in the entire crest.

Two questions thus arise. First, do the environmental signals for differentiation act on neural crest cells during their migration or after they have reached their definitive location? And second, when do the developing autonomic neurones become irreversibly differentiated into adrenergic or cholinergic cells?

When is the chemical differentiation of the autonomic neurone precursor determined?

To determine if chemical differentiation occurs before migration, we investigated the kind of transmitter synthesized by neurones when their extraintestinal migratory phase was eliminated. Since neural crest cells reach the hind gut only at 7 to 8 days of incubation, the colorectum remains totally aneural if it is removed from the embryo before this stage and grown on the CAM. When such an aneural rectum was associated with trunk neural crest for 10 to 12 days on the CAM, the crest cells migrated into it and differentiated into Auerbach's and Meissner's plexuses, in which catecholamine (CA)-containing cells were never observed. In contrast, significant levels of choline acetyltransferase (CAT) and acetylcholinesterase (AchE) activities were present in the explants[7,26]. Thus the induction of cholinergic metabolism does not depend on environmental signals received by autonomic neurone precursor cells during migration.

In contrast, the expression of the adrenergic phenotype in sympathoblasts does seem to be influenced by developmental cues during the dorso-ventral migration of the neural crest cells. By associating the neural crest with various trunk structures, Cohen[27] and Norr[28] reached the conclusion that the crest cells receive differentiating signals on their route and that the notochord, ventral neural tube and somitic mesenchyme are of decisive importance in promoting CA-synthesis in crest neuroblasts.

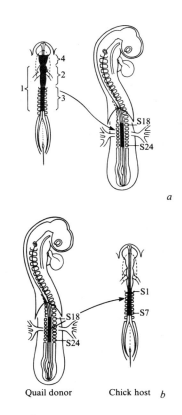

Fig. 4 Heterotopic grafts of quail neural primordium into the chick embryo. *a*, The quail primordium is removed from the mesencephalon; the anterior rhombencephalon or at the vagal level and grafted into the adrenomedullary region. *b*, The neural tissue is taken at the adrenomedullary level and grafted at the vagal level.

Nature Vol. 286 14 August 1980

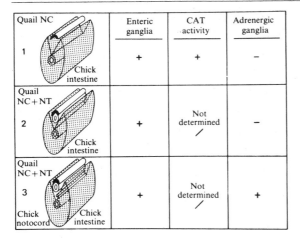

Fig. 5 Association of the aneural colorectum of a 5-day chick embryo with various dorsal trunk structures of 2-day embryos: (1) chick intestine + quail neural crest (NC). (2) chick intestine + quail neural crest and neural tube (NT). (3) chick intestine + quail neural crest/neural tube and chick notocord. CAT, choline acetyltransferase. Cholinergic ganglia develop in all cases. Adrenergic ganglia differentiate only in explants containing the notocord.

It is striking that the first CA-containing neuroblasts appear in the somitic mesenchyme (in fact in the sclerotomal part of the somite) in the immediate vicinity of the notochord and of the dorsal aorta. We therefore decided to reinvestigate the respective roles of each of these dorsal trunk structures (neural tube, notochord and somitic mesenchyme) in sympathoblast differentiation. When trunk neural primordium was isolated and inserted in aneural gut wall mesenchyme (Fig. 5), the neural crest gave rise to enteric plexuses; but in spite of the presence of the neural tube in the explants, no CA-containing cells could be detected in the ganglia. The result was therefore similar to the differentiation observed when the neural crest alone was associated with the gut[26]. In contrast, the inclusion of the notochord in the tissue associations resulted in the development of cholinergic myenteric plexuses and also in the formation of a series of adrenergic ganglia, located in the wall of the gut and characterized by the greenish fluorescence of CA. It is therefore clear that among the dorsal trunk structures, the notochord is of decisive importance in eliciting adrenergic differentiation in sympathoblasts, since, in its presence, adrenergic cells develop in the splanchnopleural gut mesenchyme, which normally supports only cholinergic differentiation. Moreover, this finding is in contradiction with the conclusions previously reached by Cohen[27] that the somite was the only structure of the embryo able to provide a convenient mesenchymal environment for adrenergic differentiation of crest-derived neuroblasts. In fact, culture experiments (unpublished) show that both the notochord and the sclerotomal part of the somitic mesenchyme are equally able to induce CA metabolism in the crest neuroblasts. This accounts perfectly for the distribution of the adrenergic cells in the trunk structures of the early embryo.

A recent observation made by Cochard *et al.*[29] in the rat embryo supports the notion that notochord induces the adrenergic phenotype. Both tyrosine hydroxylase and CA first appear at 11.5 days of gestation in the sympathetic ganglia of the trunk. But, in addition, cells with an adrenergic phenotype are transiently detectable in the gut wall from day 11.5 to about day 14.5. Thus CA differentiation in these cells may have been induced by interactions with the somite-notochord-neural tube environment during their dorso-ventral migration towards the gut. The resulting adrenergic phenotype is expressed for a time after cells have left the dorsal trunk structures and while they are

pursuing their migration in the gut, but it cannot be maintained in the gut, either because of the lack of appropriate stimulation, or because other factors intervene.

Lability of transmitter phenotype in developing autonomic neurones

If the neurotransmitter phenotype of neural crest cells is selected by the tissue environment during early development what is the stability of the chemical differentiation in the developing autonomic neurones? We have investigated this by attempting to change the fate of already differentiating ganglion cells.

Cholinergic ciliary ganglion from 4.5–6 day quail embryos were incubated and implanted into the dorsal trunk environment of a 2-day chick host at the level of somites 18 to 24, the idea being to subject the maturing cholinergic cells to the adrenergic signals normally operating from day 3 to 4 on the precursors of sympathoblasts and adrenomedullary cells (Fig. 6). The ciliary ganglion, which normally never contains adrenergic cells at any stage, exhibited cholinergic activity at the time of grafting[30–33]. Examination of the host embryos at 8 to 10 days showed that, irrespective of its age when grafted, the ciliary ganglion never remained intact at the site of implantation. Quail cells were found dispersed in the host trunk structures, but not randomly: they were always localized exclusively in normal sites of neural crest cell arrest and participated in the formation of various host crest derivatives, that is sympathetic ganglia, aortic and adrenal plexuses, adrenomedullary cords, ganglion of Remak and enteric plexuses. However, quail cells were virtually never found in the host sensory ganglia; in contrast, the Schwann cells of the rachidian nerve were mostly of the quail type at the site of the graft.

The ability of cells of a differentiating ganglion to migrate anew when grafted into the microenvironment which normally sustains crest cell migration is remarkable enough. However, the result obtained by treating the sections with the combined FIF–Feulgen–Rossenbeck techniques was even more striking: the quail cells which had homed to the sympathetic ganglia, the aortic and adrenal plexuses and the suprarenal gland exhibited the bright greenish fluorescence of CA (Fig. 7). In electron microscopy, most of the quail cells of the suprarenal gland, recognizable by their large DNA-rich nucleolus, were also seen to contain the electron-dense secretory granules characteristic of adrenomedullary cells.

Although in some cases sympathetic chain ganglia in the host were found to be totally (or mainly) made up of quail cells, grafted and host cells were usually intermingled. The possibility that the fluorescence observed in the quail cells resulted merely from an uptake of CA released by host sympathoblasts was ruled out by experiments in which the host neural crest was removed before the graft of the quail parasympathetic ganglion. In this case, adrenergic nervous structures entirely made up of quail cells developed at the site of the operation and showed the same CA fluorescence as in the previous series[33].

The cells of the ciliary ganglion which colonized the splanchnopleure and became localized in the host Remak and enteric ganglia were not CA-positive after FIF treatment, and presumably developed as cholinergic cells.

In recent (unpublished) experiments, pieces of ciliary ganglia taken from quail embryos as old as 9 days of incubation were similarly grafted into 2-day chick embryos. Quail cells were found in the same locations in the host structures as in the previously described experiments except that their migration was practically restricted to the dorsal trunk and generally did not penetrate the dorsal mesentery. Many quail cells were found with CA fluorescence in the sympathetic host ganglia in the adrenal gland and in the aortic plexuses.

We are currently examining in detail the ability of the grafted cells to proliferate in a young host. Merely from the extent of quail cell distribution in the 8-day host following the graft of a 4.5-to 6-day-old ciliary ganglion, it is clear that their number is higher than the total number of neurones of the mature ciliary ganglion. Detailed counts of the number of quail cells labelled one hour after ^{3}H-thymidine injection at various intervals after grafting, show that many mitoses occur both during the migration of ciliary ganglion cells and after their stabilization in host structures. Numerous quail neurones and adrenomedullary cells are labelled with ^{3}H-thymidine at all stages up to 9 days of incubation of the host. These observations are in agreement with the recent findings[34] that developing sympathoblasts, actually synthesizing CA, divide until late in development.

Such proliferative potential is not maintained as long in the cholinergic ciliary ganglion since, according to the work of Landmesser and Pilar[31], mitotic activity has virtually stopped in chick neuroblasts at stage 25 (4.5 to 5 days of incubation), while the definitive number of neurones, after physiological cell death has occurred, is reached around day 12. Therefore, transplantation of a cholinergic ganglion into a younger host changes its developmental program profoundly enough to modify not only its chemical differentiation but also the number of cell cycles that the neuroblasts undergo before reaching maturity.

In summary, our results demonstrate that CA synthetic ability exists in cells of developing cholinergic ganglia; although not expressed in normal development, it can be elicited by the dorsal trunk structures and the adrenal gland environment.

Since all our experiments deal with the transplantation, not of single cells but of a population, our results do not allow us to state that the appearance of CA-producing cells results from the conversion of initially cholinergic cells. It may well be that the ciliary ganglion, even as late as 9 days of incubation, contains a pool of still undifferentiated neuroblasts which may be destined to disappear later on in normal development. It should nevertheless be emphasized that the capacity for a developing

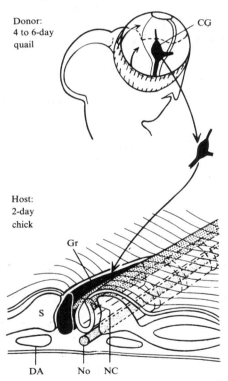

Fig. 6 Experimental design for back-transplantation of differentiating cholinergic ganglia from 4- to 6-day quail donor embryos into 2-day chick hosts. The ciliary ganglion (CG) is dissected and inserted either whole or in pieces into a slit made between the neural primordium and the somites (S). DA, dorsal aorta; Gr, graft; NC, neural crest; No, notochord.

autonomic neurone to change its transmitter metabolism in response to environmental influences has been indisputably demonstrated by experiments *in vitro*[35-38].

Manipulation of the fluid environment in which dissociated post-mitotic neurones from the newborn rat superior cervical ganglion are growing has been shown to influence the choice of transmitters and the type of synapse they make. These elegant experiments (reviewed by Patterson[39]) have revealed the existence of a soluble factor mediating the conversion of an adrenergic to a cholinergic phenotype. Moreover, during the switch in transmitter metabolism in culture, neurones with both adrenergic and cholinergic functions have been identified in single-cell cultures[40,41].

Although cell physiology may be profoundly altered by culture conditions, the results obtained *in vitro* are important in defining the mechanisms regulating autonomic nervous system development *in vivo*, particularly in two respects. First, the discovery that a change in transmitter synthesis can occur in post-mitotic nerve cells and the demonstration of dual-function neurones in culture strengthen the view that in the transplantation experiments *in vivo*, the environment imposes the choice of phenotypic expression on bipotential neuroblasts. The alternative hypothesis, that the microenvironment merely selects from a mixed population of committed adrenergic and cholinergic neuroblasts, becomes more unlikely. If the dual-function neurones detected in culture represent a transitional state between the adrenergic and the cholinergic condition, it seems probable that a similar process takes place in reverse when the cholinergic ciliary ganglion cells become adrenergic after back-transplantation into a younger host. Second, the demonstration that cholinergic differentiation can be triggered *in vitro* by a factor of non-neuronal cell origin suggests that an analogous mechanism might operate *in vivo*. In particular our experiments suggest that adrenergic differentiation is regulated by 'factors' produced by cells of the notochord or by the sclerotomal part of the somite and released into the extracellular matrix. Alternatively, an integral membrane component of the somitic mesenchyme might influence crest cell differentiation through intimate cell–cell contacts. The developmental relationships between sclerotomal and neural crest cells during ontogenesis support such a hypothesis but, experiments involving cultures of neural crest *in vitro*, to be described below, show that such cell–cell contacts are not necessary for eliciting CA metabolism in the developing sympathoblasts.

Developmental capabilities of neural crest cells *in vitro*

From their study of the *in vitro* differentiation of crest cells in the absence of any other tissue of the embryo, Greenberg and Schrier[42] reported CAT activity in mesencephalic neural crest cells after 7 days in culture and Cohen[43] described the appearance of adrenergic cells in trunk crest cultures. In both cases, the total neural anlage was explanted for 48 hours and, after the migration of crest cells had taken place, the neural tube was mechanically removed. This technique cannot avoid possible contamination of the crest cultures by central neurones or possible influence of the neural tube itself on peripheral neuroblast differentiation[44]. Therefore our approach has been to excise neural crest from quail embryos, at both mesencephalic and truncal levels, by a microsurgical procedure that leaves the neural tube in place. Cultures of pure crest explants from each region underwent morphological differentiation and were able to synthesize both ACh and CA. Although the amount of neurotransmitter synthesized could be increased by co-culturing with a variety of embryonic tissues, the ratio of ACh to CA formed in a given culture was markedly dependent on the composition of the liquid medium. In particular, horse serum was found to favour ACh synthesis, whilst fetal calf serum preferentially enhanced CA production. These studies, together with those of other workers[42,43], strongly suggest that direct intercellular contact with non-neural tissue is not essential for inducing neurotransmitter synthesis.

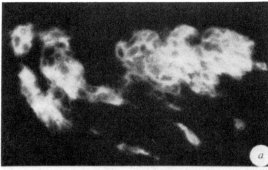

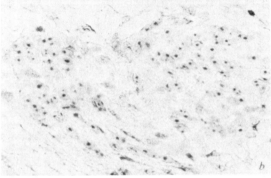

Fig. 7 Result of the experiment of back-transplantation of a quail autonomic ganglion into a 2-day chick embryo (as represented in Fig. 6). Transverse section of the host at 7 days of incubation at the level of the sympathetic ganglia. *a*, CA-containing cells shown after application of Falck's technique. *b*, Post-staining of the same section with the Feulgen reaction shows that the fluorescent cells originate from the grafted ciliary ganglion since they have the nuclear marker. ×460.

The choice between the cholinergic and the adrenergic pathways made *in vivo* by future neuroblasts could thus be the result of selective induction by soluble factors encountered at the opportune moment. If such an interpretation is correct, one has to assume that differentiating factors for both ACh and CA synthesis are present in the culture medium. They might be provided by the serum and/or by the embryo extract. Another possibility is that neuroblast precursors have the ability to synthesize neurotransmitters while still in the neural primordium; the role of environmental cues would then be limited to stabilizing and enhancing the appropriate phenotype.

As far as the adrenergic system is concerned, a number of histochemical studies have shown that the earliest detectable appearance of tyrosine hydroxylase and of CA synthesis in presumptive sympathoblasts coincides with their aggregation into the primary sympathetic chain[29,45,46]. This suggests that the first of the above mentioned alternatives is correct and that an inductive event occurs during the crest cells' dorso-ventral migration which gives them a bias towards the adrenergic pathway. On the other hand, recent results from our laboratory cast serious doubt on the applicability of this hypothesis to cholinergic differentiation[47]. We were, in fact, able to show that mesencephalic crest, excised from quail embryos of 8–12 somites (when the crest appears as an actively migrating sheet of cells under the ectoderm[44]) is able to convert ³H-choline to ³H-ACh and that this transformation is due to CAT. Furthermore, this activity can also be detected at an even earlier stage (5–7 somites), when migration is just beginning. In other words, mesencephalic crest cells already contain a cholinergic system

when they start to migrate. We cannot yet say whether all or only some of the crest cells are involved. However, if we assume that the early cholinergic differentiation concerns the presumptive parasympathetic neuroblast (the ciliary ganglion is derived from the mesencephalic crest[13,48]), the obvious implication is that no inductive stimulus is necessary once the latter have reached their definitive site, and cholinergic maturation involves consolidation and augmentation of already acquired properties. There is one clear case in which external cues have been shown to stabilize synthesis of a particular kind of transmitter and decrease the lability of neuronal chemical differentiation: Walicke *et al.*[49] have shown that the chemical differentiation of sympathetic neurones is stabilized by neuronal activity itself.

Conclusions

In our laboratory and elsewhere quail–chick chimaeras have proved most useful in the investigation of the early stages of the differentiation of the nervous system[48,50,51]. We have already identified some new derivatives of the neural crest and analysed certain aspects of the development of the autonomic nervous system; comparison of the *in vivo* transplantation and *in vitro* culture experiments has been particularly fruitful.

Future experiments will explore the developmental relationships which may exist between the neuroblasts that give rise to the sensory neurones of the dorsal root ganglia and those which become autonomic cells. It would be of great interest to know when the commitment of these different cell types occurs and whether the choice in this case also, remains labile for a while. The relationships between the glial satellite cells of the ganglia and the neural cell lines will also be examined. Furthermore the chemical differentiation of the peripheral neurones needs to be reconsidered in terms of neurotransmitters other than just ACh and CA and including neuropeptides.

Note that the chimaeric cell labelling technique has also been of great value in analysing many other aspects of embryonic development such as the ontogeny of the haemopoietic system[52–59], the development of the kidney[60,61] and limb[62–67] and the early movements of cells in gastrulation[68,69].

This work was supported by the CNRS, the Délégation Générale à la Recherche Scientifique et Technique and by a Research Grant from the US National Institutes of Health (5 R01 DE04257-03).

1. Vogt, W. *Arch. Entw. Mech.* **106**, 542–610 (1925).
2. Pasteels, J. *Archs Biol.* **48**, 381–488 (1937).
3. Le Douarin, N. *Bull. Biol. Fr. Belg.* **103**, 435–452 (1969).
4. Hamburger, V. & Hamilton, H. L. *J. Morph.* **88**, 49–92 (1951).
5. Zacchei, A. M. *Archs Anat.* **66**, 36–62 (1961).
6. Le Douarin, N. *Expl Cell Res.* **77**, 459–468 (1973); *Devl Biol.* **30**, 217–222 (1973); *Med. Biol.* **52**, 281–319 (1974); *Ciba Fdn Symp.* **40**, 71–101 (1976).
7. Smith, J., Cochard, P. & Le Douarin, N. M. *Cell Different.* **6**, 199–216 (1977).
8. Jotereau, F. V. & Le Douarin, N. M. *Devl. Biol.* **63**, 253–265 (1978).
9. Le Douarin, N. M. & Rival, J. M. *Devl. Biol.* **47**, 215–221 (1975).
10. Hörstadius, S. in *The Neural Crest: Its Properties and Derivatives in the Light of Experimental Research*, 111 (Oxford University Press, London, 1950).
11. Weston, J. A. *Adv. Morphogenesis* **8**, 41–114 (1970).
12. Johnston, M. C., Bhakdinaronk, A. & Reid, Y. C. in *Oral Sensation and Perception: Development in the Fetus and Infant* (ed. Bosma, J. F.) (U.S. Govt. Printing Office, Washington, 1974).
13. Noden, D. M. *Devl. Biol.* **67**, 296–312 (1978); **67**, 313–329 (1978); in *The Specificity of Embryological Interactions* (ed. Garrod, D.), 4–49 (Chapman and Hall, London, 1978).
14. Le Lièvre, C. *J. Embryol. exp. Morph.* **31**, 453–477 (1974); **47**, 17–37 (1978).
15. Le Lièvre, C. & Le Douarin, N. *J. Embryol. exp. Morph.* **34**, 124–154 (1975).
16. Le Douarin, N. & Le Lièvre, C. in *Birth Defects* (Excerpta Medica Intern. Congr. Ser. no. 432), (eds Littlefield, J. W. & de Grouchy, J.) 141–153 (1978).
17. Le Douarin, N. & Le Lièvre, C. *C.r. hebd. Séanc. Acad. Sci., Paris* **270**, 2857–2860 (1970).
18. Le Douarin, N., Le Lièvre, C. & Fontaine, J. *C.r. hebd. Séanc. Acad. Sci., Paris* **275**, 583–586 (1972).
19. Le Douarin, N. M. in *Gut Hormones* (ed. Bloom, S. R.) 49–56 (Churchill Livingstone, Edinburgh, 1978).
20. Weston, J. A. *Devl. Biol.* **6**, 279–310 (1963).
21. Falck, B. *Acta physiol. scand.* **56**, Suppl. 197, 1–25 (1962).
22. Le Douarin, N. & Teillet, M. A. *J. Embryol. exp. Morph.* **30**, 31–48 (1973).
23. Teillet, M. A. *W. Roux'Arch. dev. Biol.* **184**, 251–268 (1978).
24. Le Douarin, N. & Teillet, M. A. *Devl. Biol.* **41**, 162–184 (1974).
25. Le Douarin, N., Renaud, D., Teillet, M. A. & Le Douarin, G. H. *Proc. natn. Acad. Sci. U.S.A.* **72**, 728–732 (1975).
26. Teillet, M. A., Cochard, P. & Le Douarin, N. M. *Zoon* **6**, 115–122 (1978).
27. Cohen, A. M. *J. exp. Zool.* **179**, 167–182 (1972).
28. Norr, S. C. *Devl. Biol.* **34**, 16–38 (1973).
29. Cochard, P., Goldstein, M. & Black, I. *Proc. natn. Acad. Sci. U.S.A.* **75**, 2986–2990 (1978).
30. Landmesser, L. & Pilar, G. *J. Physiol., Lond.* **222**, 691–713 (1972).
31. Landmesser, L. & Pilar, G. *Fedn Proc.* **37**, 2016–2022 (1978).

32. Chiappinelli, V., Giacobini, E., Pilar, G. & Uchimura, H. *J. Physiol., Lond.* **257**, 749–767 (1976).
33. Le Douarin, N. M., Teillet, M. A., Ziller, C. & Smith, J. *Proc. natn. Acad. Sci. U.S.A.* **75**, 2030–2034 (1978).
34. Rothman, T. P., Gershon, M. D. & Holtzer, H. *Devl. Biol.* **65**, 322–341 (1978).
35. Patterson, P. H. & Chun, L. L. Y. *Proc. natn. Acad. Sci. U.S.A.* **71**, 3607–3610 (1974).
36. Patterson, P. H. & Chun, L. L. Y. *Devl. Biol.* **56**, 263–280 (1977).
37. Burton, H. & Bunge, R. P. *Brain Res.* **97**, 157–162 (1975).
38. Johnson, M. *et al. Nature* **262**, 308–310 (1976).
39. Patterson, P. H. A. *Rev. Neurosci.* **1**, 1–17 (1978).
40. Furshpan, E. J., MacLeish, P. R., O'Lague, P. H. & Potter, D. D. *Proc. natn. Acad. Sci. U.S.A.* **73**, 4225–4229 (1976).
41. Landis, S. C. *Proc. natn. Acad. Sci. U.S.A.* **73**, 4220–4224 (1976).
42. Greenberg, J. H. & Schrier, B. K. *Devl. Biol.* **61**, 86–93 (1977).
43. Cohen, A. M. *Proc. natn. Acad. Sci. U.S.A.* **74**, 2899–2903 (1977).
44. Ziller, C., Smith, J., Fauquet, M. & Le Douarin, N. M. *Prog. Brain Res.* **51**, 59–74 (1979).
45. Enemar, A., Falck, B. & Håkanson, R. *Devl. Biol.* **11**, 268–283 (1965).
46. Teitelman, G., Baker, H., Joh, T. H. & Reis, D. J. *Proc. natn. Acad. Sci. U.S.A.* **76**, 509–513 (1979).
47. Smith, J., Fauquet, M., Ziller, C. & Le Douarin, N. *Nature* **282**, 853–855 (1979).
48. Narayanan, C. H. & Narayanan, Y. *J. Embryol. exp. Morph.* **47**, 137–148.
49. Walicke, P. A., Campenot, R. B. & Patterson, P. H. *Proc. natn. Acad. Sci. U.S.A.* **74**, 5767–5771 (1977).
50. Saxod, R. *Devl. Biol.* **32**, 167–178 (1973).
51. Narayanan, C. H. & Narayanan, Y. *J. Embryol. exp. Morph.* **43**, 85–105 (1978).
52. Jotereau, F. V. & Le Douarin, N. M. *Devl. Biol.* **63**, 253–265 (1978).
53. Houssaint, E., Belo, M. & Le Douarin, N. *Devl. Biol.* **53**, 250–264 (1976).
54. Le Douarin, N. in *Differentiation of Normal and Neoplastic Hematopoietic Cells* 5–31 (Cold Spring Harbor Laboratory, New York, 1978); in *Mechanisms of Cell Change* (eds Ebert, J. E. & Okada, T. S.) 293–326 (Wiley, New York, 1979).
55. Le Douarin, N. & Jotereau, F. *Nature new Biol.* **246**, 25 (1973); *J. exp. Med.* **142**, 17–40 (1975).
56. Dieterlen-Lièvre, F. *J. Embryol. exp. Morph.* **33**, 607–619 (1975).
57. Martin, C., Beaupain, D. & Dieterlen-Lièvre, F. *Cell Differentiation* **7**, 115–130 (1978).
58. Beaupain, D., Martin, C. & Dieterlen-Lièvre, F. *Blood* **53**, 212–225 (1979).
59. Kahn, A. J. & Simmons, D. J. *Nature* **258**, 325–327 (1975).
60. Gumpel-Pinot, M., Martin, C. & Croisille, Y. *C.r. hebd. Séanc. Acad. Sci., Paris* **272**, 737–739 (1971).
61. Martin, C. J. *Embryol. exp. Morph.* **35**, 485–498 (1976).
62. Gumpel-Pinot, M. *C.r. hebd. Séanc. Acad. Sci., Paris* **279**, 1305–1308 (1974).
63. Christ, B., Jacob, H. J. & Jacob, M. *Experientia* **30**, 1446–1449 (1974); 1449–1451 (1974); **34**, 241–242; 514–516 (1978).
64. Chevallier, A. J. *Embryol. exp. Morph.* **42**, 275–292 (1977); *W. Roux's Archiv.* **184**, 57–73 (1978); *J. Embryol. exp. Morph.* **49**, 73–88 (1979).
65. Chevallier, A. J., Kieny, M., Mauger, A. & Sengel, P. in *Vertebrate Limb and Somite Morphogenesis* (eds Ede, D. A., Hinchliffe, J. R. & Balls, M.) 421–432 (Cambridge University Press, 1977).
66. Dhouailly, D. & Kieny, M. *Devl. Biol.* **28**, 162–175 (1972).
67. Kieny, M. in *Vertebrate Limb and Somite Morphogenesis* (eds Ede, D. A., Hinchliffe, J. R. & Balls, M.) 87–103 (Cambridge University Press, 1977).
68. Kieny, M. & Pautou, M. P. *W. Roux's Archiv.* **179**, 327–338 (1976); **183**, 177–191 (1977).
69. Saunders, J. W., Gasseling, M. T. & Errick, J. E. *Devl. Biol.* **50**, 16–25 (1976).
70. Vakaet, L. *C.r. hebd. Séanc. Acad. Sci., Paris* **167**, 781–783 (1973); 1053–1055 (1973); *Année. Biol.* **13**, 35–41 (1974).
71. Hornbruch, A., Summerbell, D. & Wolpert, L. *J. Embryol. exp. Morph.* **51**, 51–62 (1979).

Reprinted from Development in the Nervous System. British Society for Developmental Biology. Symposium 5 (ed. Garrod and Feldman), pp. 331–346. 1981

Neuronal cell lineages in the nematode *Caenorhabditis elegans*

H. ROBERT HORVITZ

Dept of Biology, Massachusetts Institute of Technology, 77 Massachusetts Avenue, Cambridge, Massachusetts 02139, USA

A neuron can be characterized by its morphology, transmitter(s?), receptor(s) and the nature of its synaptic contacts (chemical or electrical; excitatory or inhibitory; number and distribution of synapses; identity of the cells to which it is presynaptic or postsynaptic). It is clear that according to such criteria nervous systems consist of neurons of many distinct types. The origin of neuronal diversity is unknown. Both how such diversity is generated during development and how the relevant developmental programme is encoded in the genome remain to be elucidated.

One approach to these problems is to examine the development of a simple nervous system in an organism appropriate for detailed anatomical, developmental and genetical studies. The small free-living soil nematode *Caenorhabditis elegans* is such an organism. *C. elegans* consists of relatively few cells; for example, the adult hermaphrodite contains only 811 non-gonadal nuclei (Sulston & Horvitz, 1977). *C. elegans* is essentially invariant in cellular anatomy, which allows identified cells to be examined in different individuals and at different developmental stages. Because *C. elegans* is only about 1 mm in length, it has been possible to obtain serial electron micrographs through the entire animal. From such micrographs, essentially the complete neuroanatomy of *C. elegans* has been elucidated; the morphologies and synaptic connections of almost all of its 300 neurons are known (Ward *et al.*, 1975; Ware *et al.*, 1975; White *et al.*, 1976; Albertson and Thomson, 1976; J. White, N. Thomson & S. Brenner, personal communication).

C. elegans is well suited for genetical research (Brenner, 1974; Herman & Horvitz, 1980). Its attractive features include: ease of culture, maintenance and handling (10^5 animals can be grown on a

140

single petri dish); small genome size (haploid DNA content of only about 20 times that of the bacterium *Escherichia coli* and only about 2000 essential genes); rapid generation time (3 days); and reasonably large numbers of progeny per parent (about 300). *C. elegans* reproduces either as a self-fertilizing hermaphrodite or as a result of hermaphrodite–male matings. Hermaphroditic reproduction provides additional advantages: for example, continued subculturing rapidly drives strains to homozygosity, ensuring the isogenicity of all individuals within a population and thereby eliminating any variability in anatomy and development introduced by genetic differences; also, because mating is not necessary for reproduction, even severely abnormal behavioural mutants can be isolated and maintained. To date, nearly 300 genes have been mapped onto the six *C. elegans* linkage groups; more than 100 of these genes affect behaviour.

Cell lineage and cell fate in the ventral nervous system

One basic problem concerning the origin of neuronal diversity is the relationship between developmental history and neuronal type. For example, it is conceivable that all neurons of a given class are formed at the same time and/or in the same area; alternatively, all could be derived from a single precursor cell. Studies of neuronal cell lineages in *C. elegans* (Sulston & Horvitz, 1977; Sulston, Albertson & Thomson, 1980) have revealed a different and, to us, unexpected relationship between cell history and cell fate: neurons of a particular type are generated as lineally equivalent progeny derived from similar cell lineages. For example, the 12 'dorsal AS' neurons of the ventral nervous system, which are uniquely identified by their morphologies and synaptic connections (White *et al.*, 1976), are the anterior daughters of the posterior daughters of 12 morphologically indistinguishable neuroblasts. A more detailed consideration of the development of the ventral nervous system will further illustrate this point.

The ventral nervous system of *C. elegans* consists of a longitudinal fibre bundle extending along most of the length of the animal and a series of neuronal cell bodies arranged linearly along this nerve cord (Fig. 1 indicates aspects of the nervous system of *C. elegans* that are discussed here). Most of the axons of the ventral cord synapse onto the somatic musculature and control locomotion. In the young first stage (or L1) larva, there are 15 neuron cell bodies located along the ventral cord; these neurons are of three distinct classes. Substantial development occurs in the ventral cord during the period of postembryonic growth. The developmental changes have been studied by directly observing the divisions, migrations and deaths of identified cells in living nematodes. When appropriately mounted on a microscope slide and provided with *E. coli* for

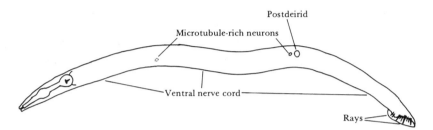

Fig. 1. Adult *C. elegans* male, left lateral view. Aspects of the nervous system discussed in the text are indicated. The ventral nerve cord runs longitudinally slightly right of the ventral midline. There are nine sensory rays, which are used in copulation, on each side of the male tail. A sensory postdeirid is located laterally on both the right and left sides. For simplicity, only the left rays and postdeirid are shown in this figure. The microtubule-rich neurons are asymmetrically located; the anterior cell (Q1. paa) is on the right side, and the posterior cell (Q2. paa) is on the left side. The microtubule-rich neurons and the two neurons of each postdeirid have their major processes in the ventral nerve cord. These anatomical features are similar in the hermaphrodite, except that the hermaphrodite tail is not specialized for copulation (e.g. no rays are present).

food, a young nematode develops normally. Observation of such an animal with Nomarski differential interference contrast optics allows every nucleus to be resolved. Individual nuclei can be followed in an animal as it develops. In this way, the complete postembryonic cell lineages of *C. elegans* have been elucidated (Sulston & Horvitz, 1977; Kimble & Hirsh, 1979). The fates of all of the cells produced have been determined using a combination of light and electron microscopy.

Ventral cord development begins about the middle of the L1 stage, when 12 precursor cells (P1–P12) migrate from ventro-lateral positions to the region of the ventral cord. All 12 of these cells then undergo the same asymmetric pattern of cell divisions (Fig. 2), generating one large epithelial-like daughter (a 'hypodermal' cell) and five progeny with neuron-like nuclei. Certain of the neuron-like progeny die within an hour of their formation. Electron microscopic studies have revealed that progeny that are equivalent in lineage history generally differentiate into neurons of a particular class. Thus, the five neuronal descendants of each P cell become neurons of five distinct types; the lineally equivalent progeny of different P cells differentiate into neurons of the same type.

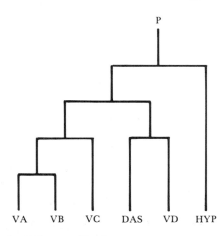

Fig. 2. Ventral cord cell lineage. Twelve precursor cells, P1–P12, all undergo the pattern of cell divisions shown. Each P cell divides to produce an anterior neuroblast (Pn.a) and a posterior hypodermal cell ('Hyp') (Pn.p). In this and the other figures, anterior ('a') daughters are represented by left branches and posterior ('p') daughters are represented by right branches. All divisions discussed in this article are along an anterior–posterior axis. 'Pn' refers to any of the 12 P cells. Each daughter cell is named by adding an additional character to the name of its mother cell; anterior daughters are named with an 'a', and posterior daughters are named with a 'p'. Pn.a divides to produce two neuroblasts, Pn.aa and Pn.ap. Pn.ap divides to generate Pn.apa and Pn.app, and Pn.aa divides to generate Pn.aap and another neuroblast, Pn.aaa. Finally, Pn.aaa divides to produce Pn.aaaa and Pn.aaap. All five progeny derived from Pn.a have neuron-like nuclei and, in general, differentiate to become neurons of five distinct classes that have been described by White *et al.* (1976). Lineage history and neuron fate are correlated as follows: Pn.aaaa is a ventral A ('VA') motoneuron; Pn.aaap is a ventral B ('VB') motoneuron; Pn.aap is a ventral C ('VC') neuron, which innervates vulval muscles; Pn.apa is a dorsal AS ('DAS') motoneuron; Pn.app is a ventral D ('VD') motoneuron. In a few instances, alternative fates are assumed. Thus, P1.aaaa becomes an AVF interneuron. Eight cells (P1.aap, P2.aap, P9.aap, P10.aap, P11.aap, P12.aap, P11.aaap and P12.aaap) undergo programmed cell death. This and all other lineages are adapted from Sulston & Horvitz (1977).

Other neuronal cell lineages

A similar correlation between lineage history and cell fate has been observed in many cell lineages in *C. elegans*. For example, there are 18 'rays' embedded in the non-cellular cuticular webbing of the male tail; these rays most likely function as sensory elements during copulation. Each ray consists of two distinct types of neurons and one structural cell (Sulston *et al.*, 1980). The three cells of each ray are derived from a single precursor (Fig. 3), and all 18 rays are

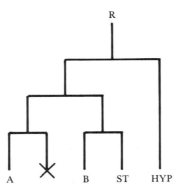

Fig. 3. Ray cell lineages. Each of 18 ray precursor cells, R, generates neurons of two distinct types ('A', Rn.aaa; and 'B', Rn.apa), one ray structural cell ('ST', Rn.app) and one hypodermal cell that is not associated with the ray ('HYP', Rn.p). The Rn.aap progeny cell undergoes programmed cell death ('X'). There are nine bilaterally symmetrical pairs of rays, which are denoted R1–R9. The fates of the R cell progeny have been determined by Sulston, Albertson & Thomson (1980).

generated after the same pattern of cell divisions from 18 morphologically similar precursors. As in the ventral cord, all neurons of a particular class have experienced similar series of divisions.

Additional examples are provided by the two lateral microtubule-rich mechanosensory neurons (Chalfie & Thomson, 1979; Chalfie & Sulston, 1981) derived from neuroblasts Q1 and Q2 (Fig. 4) and by the dopaminergic neurons of the postdeirids (Sulston, Dew & Brenner, 1975; Sulston & Horvitz, 1977) (Fig. 5). Each postdeirid is a small sensory organ consisting of two neurons (only one of which is dopaminergic) and two distinct structural cells. All four cells of each postdeirid are derived from a single precursor. The close ancestral relationship between neuronal and non-neuronal cells of a simple functional unit, as seen in the development of the rays and postdeirids, has been observed directly in other sensilla in *C. elegans* (Sulston *et al.*, 1980) and has been suggested for a variety of innervated structures found in insects (e.g. Lawrence, 1966).

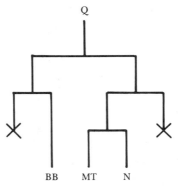

Fig. 4. Lateral neuroblast cell lineage. Each of two lateral neuroblasts, Q1 and Q2, generates three neurons. Progeny cell Qn.ap has a characteristic basal body ('BB'); cell Qn.paa contains a characteristic array of microtubules ('MT'); and cell Qn.pap is another type of neuron ('N'). Cells Qn.aa and Qn.pp undergo programmed cell death ('X'). The fates of the Q cell progeny are described by Chalfie, Horvitz & Sulston (1981).

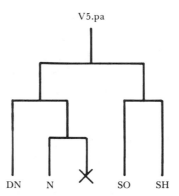

Fig. 5. Postdeirid cell lineage. A posterior lateral ectoblast, V5.pa, located on each side of the animal generates one dopaminergic neuron ('DN', V5.paaa), one neuron with a large, flattened nucleus ('N', V5.paapa) and two accessory structural cells known as socket ('SO', V5.papa) and sheath ('SH', V5.papp) cells. The V5.paapp daughter undergoes programmed cell death ('X'). The fates of these cells are from Sulston & Horvitz (1977).

Cases in which lineage and fate are not strictly correlated

Although neurons of equivalent lineage histories are generally of a given neuronal class, there are a number of exceptions to this rule. The two microtubule cells Q1.paa and Q2.paa, although similar in many of their morphological and synaptic characteristics, differ essentially in one way: only the more anteriorly located Q2.paa grows an axonal branch into the circumpharyngeal nerve ring, where synapses with interneurons form that allow Q2.paa to function autonomously in mediating a response to tactile stimulation. M. Chalfie (personal communication) has demonstrated that this difference appears to result from factors extrinsic to the microtubule cells. Specifically, if Q1.paa is generated in the region where Q2.paa is normally (as occurs in the mutant *mab-5*, which is altered in the cell migrations of the Q1 progeny), Q1.paa acquires the characteristics of Q2.paa; if Q2.paa is generated in the region where Q1.paa is normally (using a laser microbeam to prevent the migration of its progenitor Q2), Q2.paa appears to acquire the characteristics of Q1.paa. Thus, it is likely that Q1.paa and Q2.paa, which are equivalent in lineage history, are also équivalent in developmental potential; their precise differentiation depends upon their location in the animal.

Other exceptions may be similarly explained. For example, the AVF interneurons located near the anterior region of the ventral cord (P0.aaaa and P1.aaaa) are lineally equivalent to the VA motoneurons (P2.aaaa–P12.aaaa). Laser ablation experiments in which P1.aaaa has been eliminated have revealed that P2.aaaa has the potential to develop into an AVF neuron (Sulston & White, 1980).

The 18 rays of the male tail are similar but not identical. The two R6.apa neurons are morphologically distinct from the other Rn.apa neurons (Sulston *et al.*, 1980). Also, 6 of the 18 Rn.aaa neurons are dopaminergic (Sulston & Horvitz, 1977). It is possible that, as in the cases above, these differences are also defined by factors extrinsic to the neurons themselves. For example, it has been demonstrated that individual sympathetic neurons isolated from the rat superior cervical ganglion can be either adrenergic or cholinergic, depending upon their environment (Patterson, 1978).

In most of these exceptional cases, the differences between neurons

146

of a particular lineage history are relatively minor. Furthermore, at least for those cases tested, such neurons appear to be competent to acquire any of a limited number of possible fates. Thus, even in these examples, neurons of a particular lineage history appear to be of a single class, as defined by their developmental potential.

Programmed cell death

The strong correlation between lineage history and cell fate indicates that a particular series of cell divisions may be necessary for the generation of a particular cell type. If so, there may be instances when some but not all of the progeny of a given lineage are needed; it may then be necessary to generate all such progeny and eliminate those cells that are not required. This hypothesis provides one possible explanation for the programmed cell death that occurs during neuronal development in *C. elegans* (Sulston & Horvitz, 1977) and in other organisms (e.g. Lewis, 1980).

There are a number of cell deaths associated with the development of the *C. elegans* ventral nervous system (Sulston & Horvitz, 1977). In these cases cells die very soon after they are formed, before any overt signs of neuronal differentiation can be detected. For example, of the Pn.aap progeny, six (P3.aap–P8.aap) differentiate into ventral C neurons and six (P1.aap, P2.aap, P9.aap – P12.aap) die. The ventral C neurons modulate egg-laying and innervate the vulval muscles (White *et al.*, 1976), which are located about mid-way along the anterior–posterior axis of the animal. The ventral C neurons appear to be needed only in the region of the vulva and not near the head (where P1.aap and P2.aap are generated) nor near the tail (where P9.aap – P12.aap are generated). However, the other daughters of the ventral cord lineage are motoneurons (Fig. 2) and are needed throughout the length of the cord. In particular, there may be no way to generate ventral A (Pn.aaaa) and ventral B (Pn.aaap) neurons without necessarily generating presumptive ventral C progeny.

The deaths of P11.aaap and P12.aaap, the presumptive ventral B neurons generated in the posterior-most region of the ventral cord, may similarly reflect the elimination of unwanted cells formed because their sister cells (ventral A neurons P11.aaaa and P12.aaaa) are required. Ventral B neurons, which have axonal branches that project posteriorly and synapse onto body muscles (White *et al.*, 1976), may not be needed near the posterior end of the animal.

Characteristics of undivided neuroblasts

Given the relationship between lineage history and cell fate, it would be of interest to learn how determination varies during the course of a cell lineage. For example, if a particular cell division failed during the development of the ventral nervous system, what would be the characteristics of the undivided cell? Would it differentiate at all? If so, would it acquire neuronal features? Would these characteristics be those of one of its normal progeny or those of another class of neuron?

Such undivided cells have been studied in a number of ventral cord cell lineage mutants isolated on the basis of their abnormal behaviour and cellular anatomy (Horvitz & Sulston, 1980; Sulston & Horvitz, 1981). These mutants generate undivided Pn.aaa cells (the precursors to ventral A and ventral B neurons), Pn.ap cells (the precursors to dorsal AS and ventral D neurons) and P cells (the precursors to all six postembryonically derived ventral cord progeny). The morphologies and synaptic connections of these cells have been determined by electron microscopy. Each of these undivided precursors acquires characteristics of progeny cells it normally would generate. For example, mutants in *unc-59* or *unc-85* generate undivided Pn.aaa and Pn.ap cells. Undivided Pn.ap cells assume the characteristics of ventral D neurons, and undivided Pn.aaa cells assume the characteristics of either ventral A or ventral B neurons (J.White, personal communication). In a *lin-5* animal, undivided P cells are generally neuronal in character and appear to be hybrids, combining properties of normal ventral A, ventral B, ventral D and/or AVF neurons (Albertson, Sulston & White, 1978).

Two conclusions can be drawn from these studies. First, the characteristics of different neuron types can be expressed within a common cytoplasm, i.e. the expression of one neuronal state does not preclude the expression of another. Second, features associated with particular progeny cells can appear in a progenitor cell in the absence of cell division. That undivided precursors can specifically express the differentiated characteristics of progeny cells they would normally generate has also been observed in studies of non-neuronal cells in both *C. elegans* (Laufer, Bazzicalupo & Wood, 1980) and other organisms (e.g. Whittaker, 1973).

Thus, lineage history and cell fate are correlated, but cell division is not required for the expression of the differentiated state. Perhaps another cell cycle event is related to the series of changes in cell fate that appear to occur during a cell lineage. DNA replication is a reasonable candidate. In all of the experiments described above, DNA replication continues and, in those cases examined, the ploidy of the undivided precursors is essentially equivalent to that expected if a normal number of rounds of DNA synthesis had occurred. Thus, it is possible that in both neuronal and non-neuronal development an event coupled to DNA replication (perhaps affecting either the DNA itself or associated proteins) is responsible for activating the differentiative programme normally associated with the progeny cells produced.

Other neuronal cell lineage mutants

The developmental mutants described above (*mab-5, unc-59, unc-85, lin-5*) generate neuronal cells abnormal in position and/or lineage and have been used to indicate aspects of the relative influences of these two factors on neuronal cell fate. Similar mutants might be utilized in two additional ways. (1) Mutants lacking specific neurons might reveal the functions of those neurons. For example, all mutants defective in ventral cord cell lineages (*lin-5, lin-6, unc-59, unc-83, unc-84, unc-85*) can move forward but not backward, indicating that at least some post-embryonically derived ventral cord neurons control backward locomotion; furthermore, these mutants also undergo displacement and/or loss of the two 'hsn' neurons, suggesting that interactions with some ventral cord neurons may be necessary for hsn survival and/or development (Sulston & Horvitz, 1981). Similarly, in *lin-6* mutants, which fail in essentially all postembryonic cell divisions, the 'rewiring' of the dorsal D neurons that occurs during the L2 stage proceeds normally (White, Albertson & Anness, 1978); thus, no postembryonically-derived cell is required for this neuronal reorganization. (2) Certain mutants may directly affect genetic elements that control neuronal development and so reveal the nature of these elements.

Neuronal cell lineage mutants have been isolated on the basis of either their behavioural or their cellular defects (Horvitz & Sulston, 1980; W. Fixsen & R. Horvitz, unpublished). Many locomotory mutants are abnormal in the cell lineages of the ventral nerve cord. A variety of mutants isolated because they are defective in egg-laying have proved to have neuronal cell lineage lesions. All of these mutants are pleiotropic and affect other cells in addition to those needed for egg-laying; current evidence suggests that no post-embryonically generated neurons are essential for egg-laying (R. Horvitz & J. Sulston, unpublished). Mutants with abnormal numbers of neurons have been identified by screening populations of mutagenized animals in two ways. First, the number and locations of neuronal cell bodies have been examined in animals exposed to stains for DNA; in some experiments abnormalities in the pattern of neuronal cell deaths have been identified using the mutant *nuc-1*, which lacks an endodeoxyribonuclease and allows visualization of the DNA in the pycnotic nuclei of dying cells (Sulston, 1976). Second, the presence of the single dopaminergic neuron of each postdeirid has been checked in animals stained by the technique of formaldehyde-induced fluorescence.

The neuronal cell lineage mutants that have been obtained vary considerably in their phenotypes and specificities. Some appear behaviourally normal, whereas others are grossly uncoordinated and/or defective in other behaviours, such as egg-laying and response to tactile stimulation. In many mutants, cell lineage lesions alter non-neuronal as well as neuronal cells; in some cases ectoblasts that normally generate both hypodermal and neuronal cells are affected, whereas in other cases multiple (and sometimes all) postembryonic lineages are abnormal. All of the mutants studied so far are of variable expressivity, i.e. not all individuals of a given genotype display the same set of cell lineage alterations. It seems plausible that this variable expressivity could result from having isolated alleles of essential genes for which some residual gene activity remains. However, genetic studies (Horvitz & Sulston, 1980) have indicated that this variability occurs even in mutants completely lacking gene activity. One possible interpretation of this observation is that there exists significant genetic redundancy for functions that control neuronal (and non-neuronal) cell divisions.

150

P cell migration mutants

The postembryonic development of the ventral cord begins when cytoplasmic protrusions from the ventro-lateral P cells enlarge and the P cell nuclei migrate along these protrusions into the ventral cord. Twenty mutants have been isolated that fail in the migrations and subsequent divisions of the P cell nuclei (Sulston & Horvitz, 1981; W. Fixsen, E. J. Hess & R. Horvitz, unpublished); these mutants define two loci, *unc-83* and *unc-84*. Mutants in *unc-83* and *unc-84* are missing most of the neurons of the ventral nervous system and for this reason display uncoordinated locomotory behaviour. Because three of the hypodermal daughters of the P cells (P5.p – P7.p) normally generate the vulva (the structure through which eggs are laid), these mutants are egg-laying defective. The *unc-83* and *unc-84* mutants also fail in the embryonic migrations of a set of hypodermal nuclei, and for this reason are abnormal in hypodermal anatomy. That incorrectly positioned P cell nuclei do not divide suggests that P cells must be located in the ventral cord for divisions to occur. Alternatively, a single defect intrinsic to the P cells might prevent both migration and division.

Mutants that generate supernumerary neurons

The *unc-86* mutants contain extra copies of certain neuronal cell types and lack other neuronal cell types (Horvitz & Sulston, 1980; Sulston & Horvitz, 1981; Chalfie, Horvitz & Sulston, 1981; H. Ellis & R. Horvitz, unpublished). For example, each of the two postdeirids contains between two and four dopaminergic neurons, instead of the usual one; these supernumerary dopaminergic neurons appear to be normal in morphology. Also, *unc-86* animals lack the microtubule cells that mediate response to tactile stimulation. A variety of behavioural abnormalities result from these and other aberrations in neuroanatomy.

Most, and possibly all, of the anatomical lesions of *unc-86* mutants result from alterations in cell lineage (Chalfie *et al.*, 1981). During postembryonic development three neuroblasts on each side of the animal generate abnormal cell lineages. In each case a neuroblast divides to produce a normal anterior daughter and a posterior daughter apparently like itself in morphology and developmental potential. The posterior daughter then divides to produce an anterior daughter like that already formed and a posterior daughter once again like itself. Such division patterns, which are repeated from two to four times, result in the generation of supernumerary cells equivalent to the original anterior daughter and the absence of cells normally derived from the original posterior daughter.

One cell affected in *unc-86* mutants is the posterior lateral neuroblast V5.paa, which generates the neurons of the postdeirid (see Fig. 5). Normally, the anterior daughter of V5.paa is a dopaminergic neuron; the posterior daughter divides to produce an anterior daughter (V5.paapa) that becomes a neuron with a characteristic large and flattened nucleus and a posterior daughter that dies. In *unc-86* animals multiple dopaminergic neurons are formed and no cells like V5.paapa are found. The lineages of the lateral neuroblasts Q1 and Q2 (see Fig.4) are similarly altered. For example, Q1 normally divides to produce an anterior daughter (Q1.a) that divides to produce an anterior daughter (Q1.aa) that dies and a posterior daughter (Q1.ap) that becomes a neuron with a characteristic basal body. In *unc-86* mutants Q1.a behaves normally but the posterior daughter (Q1.p) of Q1 behaves like Q1; thus, its anterior daughter (Q1.pa) divides to produce an anterior daughter (Q1.paa) that dies and a posterior daughter (Q1.pap) that becomes a neuron with a basal body. One of the posterior descendants of Q1 normally is a microtubule neuron; this neuron is missing in *unc-86* animals. The third neuroblast altered in *unc-86* is T.pp. The effects on the T.pp lineage are more difficult to define, because the neurons produced by this lineage are not well characterized; nonetheless, the patterns seen for V5.paa and the Q cells seem to apply.

Several cells produced embryonically are either absent or over-produced in *unc-86* animals, and it seems likely that embryonic lineages, which are currently being elucidated for the wild-type (Deppe *et al.*, 1978; J. Sulston & E. Schierenberg, personal communication), are similarly affected. For example, the juvenile microtubule cells are missing and the juvenile deirids (which are morphologically similar to the postdeirids) contain multiple dopaminergic neurons. It seems likely that lineages responsible for generating these embryonic cells are similar to those that generate their postembryonic homologues, and that *unc-86* mutants affect these embryonic and postembryonic lineages in equivalent ways.

Another cell lineage mutant that affects postdeirid development is *lin(n372)* (W. Fixsen & R. Horvitz, unpublished). Whereas *unc-86* animals develop two postdeirids each of abnormal neuronal composition, the *lin(n372)* mutant appears to develop eight postdeirids each of normal composition. In the wild-type animal V5.pa generates the postdeird (Fig. 5), and a set of five cells that are similar in lineage history (V1.pa–V4.pa, V6.pa) divide to form non-neuronal ectodermal cells. In *lin(n372)*, V2.pa – V4.pa appear to acquire the fate of V5.pa, with respect to both their pattern of cell divisions and the differentiated states of the cells they generate, and produce three ectopic supernumerary postdeirids on each side of the animal.

Genetic control of neuronal cell lineages

Mutants in *unc-86* and *lin(n372)* are altered so that specific cells assume fates normally associated with certain other cells. Thus, in *lin(n372)*, ectoblasts V2.pa – V4.pa appear to behave like neuroblast V5.pa. In *unc-86*, a number of cells acquire the characteristics of the parental cells that produced them. Such alterations appear to reflect changes in specific determinative events, suggesting that the *lin(n372)* and *unc-86* genes may play primary roles in cell determination.

Since *unc-86* mutants are recessive, their effects are likely to reflect a reduction or loss of gene activity. Thus, the wild-type product of the *unc-86* gene (assuming such a product exists) is probably necessary for the generation of normal lineages. If so, *unc-86* mutations may not induce *de novo* cell lineages. Instead, *unc-86* mutations may reveal underlying aspects of the normal developmental programme. This hypothesis has led to the suggestion (Chalfie *et al.*, 1981) that at least two levels of programming instructions control neuronal cell lineages in *C. elegans*. At one level, a cell is instructed to divide either symmetrically, to produce two daughters like itself, or asymmetrically, to produce one daughter like itself and one new cell type; such asymmetric divisions, sometimes referred to as stem cell divisions, appear to occur in many developing neuronal (Poulson, 1950; Nordlander & Edwards, 1969; Goodman & Spitzer, 1979) and non-neuronal systems (e.g. Sulston & Horvitz, 1977; Le Douarin, 1979). At the second level of programming, the 'parental-like' daughter is instructed to assume a novel, non-parental fate. The existence of *unc-86* mutants, which presumably fail in executing this second set of instructions, suggests that these (and perhaps additional) levels of programming may be separately encoded in the genome.

I thank Marty Chalfie, Bill Fixsen, John Sulston and John White for sharing their unpublished data and thoughts. The work described that was done at MIT was supported by US Public Health Service grants GM24663 and GM24943.

References

Albertson, D., Sulston, J. & White, J. (1978). Cell cycling and DNA replication in a mutant blocked in cell division in the nematode *Caenorhabditis elegans*. *Developmental Biology,* **63,** 165–78.

Albertson, D. & Thomson, N. (1976). The pharnyx of *Caenorhabditis elegans*. *Philosophical Transactions of the Royal Society of London, Series B,* **275,** 299–325.

Brenner, S. (1974). The genetics of *Caenorhabditis elegans*. *Genetics,* **77,** 71–94.

Chalfie, M., Horvitz, R. & Sulston, J. (1981). Mutations that lead to reiterations in the cell lineages of *Caenorhabditis elegans*. *Cell,* **24,** in press.

Chalfie, M. & Sulston, J. (1981). Developmental genetics of the mechanosensory neurons of *Caenorhabditis elegans*. *Developmental Biology,* in press.

Chalfie, M. & Thomson, N. (1979). Organization of neuronal microtubules in the nematode *Caenorhabditis elegans*. *Journal of Cell Biology* **82,** 278–89.

Deppe, U., Schierenberg, E., Cole, T., Krieg, C., Schmitt, D., Yoder, B. & Von Ehrenstein, G. (1978). Cell lineages of the embryo of the nematode *Caenorhabditis elegans*. *Proceedings of the National Academy of Sciences, USA,* **75,** 376–80.

Goodman, C. & Spitzer, N. (1979). Embryonic development of identified neurones: differentiation from neuroblast to neurone. *Nature (London),* **280,** 208–14.

Herman, R. & Horvitz, R. (1980). Genetic analysis of *Caenorhabditis elegans*. In *Nematodes as Biological Models*, ed. B. Zuckerman, vol. 1, pp. 227–61. New York & London: Academic Press.

Horvitz, R. & Sulston, J. (1980). Isolation and genetic characterization of cell lineage mutants of the nematode *Caenorhabditis elegans*. *Genetics,* **96,** in press.

Kimble, J. & Hirsh, D. (1979). The postembryonic cell lineages of the hermaphrodite and male gonads in *Caenorhabditis elegans*. *Developmental Biology,* **70,** 396–417.

Laufer, J., Bazzicalupo, P. & Wood, W. (1980). Segregation of developmental potential in early embryos of *Caenorhabditis elegans*. *Cell,* **19,** 569–77.

Lawrence, P. (1966). Development and determination of hairs and bristles in the milkweed bug, *Oncopeltus fasciatus* (Lygacidae, Hemiptera). *Journal of Cell Science,* **1,** 475–98.

Le Douarin, N. (1979). *Stem Cells, Cell Lineages and Cell Determination*. Amsterdam: Elsevier/North-Holland.

Lewis, J. (1980). Death and the neurone. *Nature (London)*, **284**, 305–6.

Nordlander, R. & Edwards, J. (1969). Postembryonic brain development in the monarch butterfly, *Danaus plexippus plexippus*, L. I. Cellular events during brain morphogenesis. *Wilhelm Roux' Archiv für Entwicklungsmechanik der Organismen*, **162**, 197–217.

Patterson, P. (1978). Environmental determination of autonomic neurotransmitter functions. *Annual Review of Neuroscience*, **1**, 1–17.

Poulson, D. (1950). Histogenesis, organogenesis and differentiation in the embryo of *Drosophila melanogaster* Meigen. In *Biology of Drosophila*, ed. M. Demerec, pp. 168–274. New York: Hafner.

Sulston, J. (1976). Post-embryonic development in the ventral cord of *Caenorhabditis elegans*. *Philosophical Transactions of the Royal Society of London, Series B*, **275**, 287–97.

Sulston, J., Albertson, D. & Thomson, N. (1980). The *Caenorhabditis elegans* male: postembryonic development of nongonadal structures. *Developmental Biology*, **78**, 542–76.

Sulston, J., Dew, M. & Brenner, S. (1975). Dopaminergic neurons in the nematode *Caenorhabditis elegans*. *Journal of Comparative Neurology*, **163**, 215–26.

Sulston, J. & Horvitz, R. (1977). Postembryonic cell lineages of the nematode *Caenorhabditis elegans*. *Developmental Biology* **56**, 110–56.

Sulston, J. & Horvitz, R. (1981). Abnormal cell lineages in mutants of the nematode *Caenorhabditis elegans*. *Developmental Biology*, **82**, in press.

Sulston, J. & White, J. (1980). Regulation and cell autonomy during postembryonic development of *Caenorhabditis elegans*. *Developmental Biology*, **78**, 577–97.

Ward, S., Thomson, N., White, J. & Brenner, S. (1975). Electron microscopical reconstruction of the anterior sensory anatomy of the nematode *Caenorhabditis elegans*. *Journal of Comparative Neurology*, **160**, 313–38.

Ware, R., Clark, C., Crossland, K. & Russell, R. (1975). The nerve ring of the nematode *Caenorhabditis elegans*. *Journal of Comparative Neurology*, **162**, 71–110.

White, J., Albertson, D. & Anness, M. (1978). Connectivity changes in a class of motor neurones during the development of a nematode. *Nature (London)*, **271**, 764–6.

White, J., Southgate, E., Thomson, N. & Brenner, S. (1976). The structure of the ventral nerve cord of *Caenorhabditis elegans*. *Philosophical Transactions of the Royal Society of London, Series B*, **275**, 327–48.

Whittaker, J. (1973). Segregation during ascidian embryogenesis of egg cytoplasmic information for tissue-specific enzyme development. *Proceedings of the National Academy of Sciences, USA*, **70**, 2096–100.

(Reprinted from Nature, Vol. 280, No. 5719, pp. 208–214, July 19 1979) © *Macmillan Journals Ltd., 1979*

Embryonic development of identified neurones: differentiation from neuroblast to neurone

Corey S. Goodman* & Nicholas C. Spitzer

Department of Biology B-022, University of California at San Diego, La Jolla, California 92093

Individually identified neurones are sufficiently large and accessible in grasshopper embryos to permit visualisation and impalement with intracellular microelectrodes from the time of their birth to their maturation. In this article part of the temporal pattern of differentiation from an identified neuroblast (precursor cell) to a group of identified neurones is described.

THE development of nerve cells involves the acquisition of specific neuronal phenotypes. Precursor cells proliferate and give rise to progeny which differentiate into neurones. During neuronal differentiation, processes grow out, arborise and reach their targets where synaptic connections are formed. The neurones acquire a responsiveness to neurotransmitters, an ability to make action potentials and a capacity for their own neurotransmitter synthesis, storage and release. The temporal sequence in which these and other phenotypes appear has not yet been determined for any group of nerve cells *in vivo*. A knowledge of the timing in any one instance would be a useful step in understanding the rules and mechanisms of neuronal development. For example, must the appearance of one specific phenotype precede the appearance of another?

It is possible to identify single unique neurones in the nervous systems of both invertebrates[1-3] and vertebrates[4]; they are usually identified on the basis of their characteristic location, morphology, physiology and biochemistry. Identified neurones are attractive for the study of neuronal development, as it is possible to follow the timetable of single cells from their birth to their maturation, thus avoiding the problems involved in examining the developmental average of a heterogeneous and asynchronous population.

We have been studying the embryonic central nervous system (CNS) of the grasshopper and have focused our attention on the development of the dorsal unpaired median (DUM) neurones because they represent a population of relatively large, identifiable and accessible embryonic cells. The adult CNS of the grasshopper consists of the brain and a chain of segmental ganglia running along the ventral surface of the thorax and abdomen. The DUM cells are a group of identified neurones (80–100) situated on the dorsal surface of the thoracic and abdominal ganglia, near the midline. The properties of the mature DUM neurones are well known from studies of adults[5-11]. The embryonic DUM neurones can be visualised and impaled with intracellular microelectrodes at the earliest stages of their development. Furthermore, the lineage of these neurones can be determined by serial examination of dissected preparations of increasing age, with interference contrast optics, as has been demonstrated for some neurones in the nematode[12,13]. We are now able to write down part of the developmental timetable of some of the identified DUM neurones of the thoracic ganglia in the embryo of the grasshopper. Preliminary accounts of this work have appeared[14,15].

The present study begins with the day 5 embryo, a stage at which the precursor cells (neuroblasts) for the segmental ganglia have already differentiated from the epidermis. The embryonic

nervous system of the day 8 embryo is shown in Fig. 1A. At the centre of each body segment are the left and right plates of ventral neuroblasts (Fig. 1Aiii) which give rise to the chain of segmental ganglia[16-20].

Each ventral neuroblast is ~30 μm in diameter (Fig. 1Aiv). There are about 31 ventral neuroblasts in each left or right plate. Bate[20] found that the pattern and number of neuroblasts at early embryonic stages was at least as constant as that of the identified neurones of the adult segmental ganglia. Each neuroblast (NB) is a stem cell which will not in itself become a neurone. Rather, each NB maintains its large size while budding off a chain of smaller cells (Fig. 1Av). Each of these progeny divides into two cells which are postmitotic and differentiate into neurones. The neuroblasts eventually degenerate at precise times during embryogenesis[20].

Each segmental array of neuroblasts also contains a single unpaired neuroblast, called the median or dorsal unpaired median (DUM) neuroblast, at the posterior end of the segment and dorsal to the paired plates of ventral neuroblasts[16,18,20] (Fig. 1Aiii, iv, v). As Wheeler[16] first described, the progeny of the single DUM neuroblast extend anteriorly across the dorsal surface of the developing ganglion, quite separate from the neuronal progeny of the ventral neuroblasts. Thus, neuronal differentiation in this lineage can be viewed by removing the embryo from the egg, removing the chain of segmental ganglia from the embryo, desheathing the dorsal surface of the ganglion, and viewing the dorsal surface under a ×40 water immersion lens of a compound microscope with Nomarski interference contrast optics.

The dorsal unpaired median neurones

In the adult grasshopper the somata (cell bodies) of most of the 3,000 neurones in each thoracic ganglion (pro-, meso- and metathoracic) lie on the ventral surface or lateral edge of the ganglion and the neuropil lies dorsal to them. These cells are paired, that is, each cell has a contralateral homologue that is its mirror image. The left and right plates of ventral neuroblasts give rise to these ventral paired neurones[16,18,20]. However, there is a group of 80–100 somata clustered along the midline on the dorsal surface of the ganglion. These neurones, called dorsal unpaired median neurones[7], have the following distinctive characteristics. The cells thus far examined in the adult are unpaired and have medium neurites which bifurcate into bilaterally symmetrical processes. The DUM neurones are the only neurones in the segmental ganglia whose somata generate overshooting action potentials. The soma spikes of the DUM neurones depend on both Na+ and Ca2+ while the axon spikes are predominantly Na+ dependent[11].

Whereas DUM neurones have certain characteristics in common, many if not all of them can be uniquely identified by their morphology. The largest DUM neurone in the grasshopper metathoracic ganglion (diameter ~40–60 μm) is a unique identified neurone with axons emerging bilaterally in nerve 5 and innervating the extensor tibiae (ETi) muscle in the femur of the leg (this neurone is called DUMETi (ref. 7)).

Only 6–8 of the DUM neurones have large-diameter somata (40–60 μm); most are somewhat smaller (15–30 μm in diameter). The somata of the DUM neurones stain with neutral red[8,9], a dye which selectively stains monoamine-containing neurones in the leech[21] and lobster[22,23]. Both the soma and axons of DUMETi have been shown to contain octopamine[9]. In

*Present address: Department of Biological Sciences, Stanford University, Stanford, California 94305.

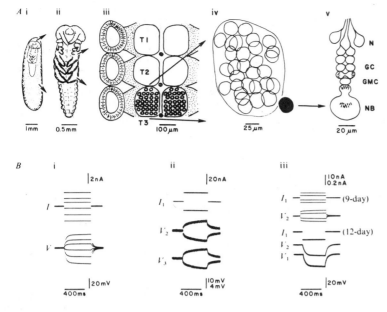

Fig. 1 *A*, Grasshopper embryo (*Schistocerca nitens*) at day 8; diagrams and camera lucida drawings of living specimens. Location of neuroblasts (precursor cells) and formation of neurones are shown (hatching occurs on day 20 at 35 °C[45]). (i) Embryo at day 8 viewed within the egg case. The embryo metabolises yolk, shown stippled. (ii) The day 8 embryo viewed from the ventral surface, showing the three prominent thoracic limb buds and the equivalent segmental appendages forming the mouth parts. (iii) Removal of the thoracic limb buds exposes the paired plates of ventral neuroblasts (enlarged ectodermal cells, open circles), and the single dorsal unpaired median (DUM) neuroblast (filled circles), also called the median (MNB) neuroblast, at the posterior margin of each segmental array of ventral neuroblasts. The contiguous chain of paired plates of neuroblasts gives rise to the chain of segmental ganglia (T1, pro; T2, meso-; T3, metathorax). (iv) Camera lucida drawing of the left hemiganglionic plate of neuroblasts in the metathoracic segment, also showing the dorsal unpaired median neuroblast, viewed with a ×40 water immersion lens and interference contrast optics. (v) A schematic drawing showing a neuroblast (in this case, the DUM neuroblast) as a stem cell; it maintains its large size while budding off a chain of ganglion mother cells (GMC) which each divide into two ganglion cells (GC) and then differentiate into neurones (N). *B*, Input resistance (R_{in}) and extent of electrical coupling of cells at different stages of development of the grasshopper embryo. (i) R_{in} for a ventral neuroblast at day 8 of development (~10 MΩ). Current (*I*) and voltage (*V*) electrodes in the same cell. (ii) Electrical coupling of one ventral neuroblast (I_1) to a second ventral neuroblast (V_2) and to an epithelial cell of the limb bud (V_3), in a day 8 embryo. (iii) Electrical coupling of DUM neuroblast (I_1) to nearby progeny cell (V_2) at day 9 (note large current); DUM neuroblast is still coupled to the rest of the embryo at this stage. Coupling of DUM neuroblast (I_1) to nearby progeny cell (V_2) at day 12 (note small current); DUM neuroblast becomes uncoupled from most of the rest of the embryo at day 10. R_{in} for the DUM neuroblast (V_1) and for the coupled network is ~200 MΩ.

fact, most if not all of the DUM neurones (particularly the large ones) contain octopamine[24].

Electrical and dye coupling

All cell types examined at early embryonic stages of the grasshopper are electrically coupled to each other; development involves a process of selective uncoupling. Dissected embryos were perfused with a simple saline (NaCl 125 mM; KCl 3 mM; $CaCl_2$ 10 mM; HEPES buffer 5 mM; adjusted to *p*H 7.4). Cells were impaled with intracellular microelectrodes, each with recording and current passing capability. Neuroblasts (~30 μm diameter) had resting potentials of −60 to −80 mV; non-neuronal cells (~10 μm diameter) often had recorded resting potentials of −40 to −60 mV, that may have been the result of damage during impalement. Records made by inserting two microelectrodes into the same ventral or dorsal neuroblast at easly stages (Fig. 1*B*i) show that the input resistance (R_{in}) is quite low (~10 MΩ), probably as a result of the extensive electrical coupling. The input resistance of a single ventral neuroblast was found to be about 150 MΩ after mechanically removing it from the network of neighbouring cells to which it was coupled, and impaling it with two electrodes. This is likely to be less than the true value because of possible damage during the isolation.

Ventral neuroblasts are electrically coupled to one another within a hemiganglion (Fig. 1*B*ii). Coupling also exists between left and right hemiganglia, between the DUM neuroblast and ventral neuroblasts, and between neuroblasts of a given segment and those of a segment either anterior or posterior to it. Furthermore, the neuroblasts are coupled to the smaller and morphologically distinct epithelial cells (termed cap cells) which lie just over them, and even to the more distant epithelial cells of the developing limb bud (Fig. 1*B*ii). Confirmation of the positions of the electrode tips and the identities of the coupled cells was achieved by injecting cells with the dyes Fast Green or Procion Rubine (2% dye in 0.25 M KCl). No evidence for rectification of electrical coupling was seen. In all such experiments, the coupling recorded between any two cells disappeared when either intracellular electrode was withdrawn from the cell. Ventral neuroblasts become electrically uncoupled from the limb buds at day 10, but remain electrically coupled to each other until they stop dividing and degenerate by day 15.

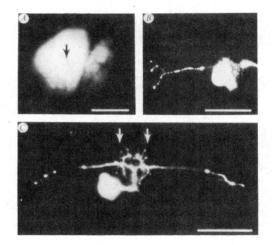

Fig. 2 Lucifer Yellow (450 MW) injections of a neuroblast and two identified neurones of grasshopper embryos. Fluorescence viewed with UV illumination. Scale bar, 100 μm. *A*, Injection of a ventral neuroblast (arrow) in the left hemiganglionic plate of neuroblasts of the metathoracic segment of an 8-day embryo. Dye spreads rapidly through other ventral neuroblasts and some of their progeny in the left plate, and within a few minutes through cells in the right plate. Note absence of spread to adjacent limb buds. *B*, *C*, Injection of identified neurones in the metathoracic ganglion of a 13-day embryo. Cell bodies appear unusually large because of intense fluorescence. The dye does not spread to other cells. Axons are truncated at points of exit from the ganglion. *B*, DUM 3, 4, 5: median neurite bifurcates, and left axon sends branches out nerves 3, 4 and 5 (top to bottom). *C*, DUMETi (DUM 5): axons extend out nerve 5 only. Arrows indicate beginnings of relatively symmetrical central arborisations.

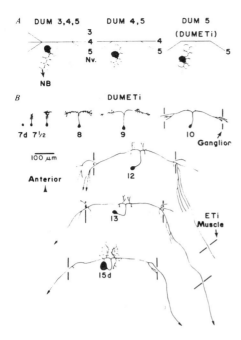

Fig. 3 *A*, DUM neuroblast gives rise to identified DUM neurones. The DUM neoroblast (NB), not shown here, gives rise to chains of progeny; some of the oldest of these progeny become identified DUM neurones. At days 12–13, we find two chains of progeny, generally two cells in width. We have examined the identities of the first three cells on the outside of the oldest chain of progeny (*n* = 10). The morphology of the DUM neurones is revealed by intracellular injection of Lucifer Yellow. In this schematic diagram, the most anterior cell on the outside bifurcates and bilaterally extends out peripheral nerves 3, 4, and 5; the second cell bilaterally extends out nerves 4 and 5; and the third cell extends out bilaterally only nerve 5 (this cell is DUMETi). *B*, Morphological development of the single identified DUM neurone, DUMETi (*n* ≥ 3 for each time point). The DUM neuroblast begins dividing at about day 6. Many extra branches and growth cones are produced at the distal end, whether it be in the central nervous system or periphery, and these extra neurites later disappear as the correct branch for DUMETi continues to grow. 'Ganglion' marks the border of the metathoracic ganglion, and 'ETi muscle' marks the proximal boundary of the extensor tibiae muscle in the femur of the limb bud. Arrows mark points of axonal extension beyond the margins of the figure.

We examined the movement of low molecular weight tracers from the interior of one cell to the interior of another by injecting the dye Lucifer Yellow (450 MW), which has a high fluorescent quantum efficiency and rapid rate of diffusion. When iontophoresed into single cells (from electrodes filled with 5% dye in distilled H_2O), it will often spread to other cells to which the injected cell is electrically coupled[25]. When a single ventral neuroblast is filled with Lucifer Yellow in a day 8 embryo, the dye spreads to other ventral neuroblasts and some of their progeny in the hemiganglion within a few minutes (Fig. 2*A*). The fluorescence can be detected in the contralateral hemiganglion shortly thereafter, but spreads to anterior and posterior ganglia much more slowly. However, dye was not seen to spread to limb-bud epithelium, even though the neuroblasts are electrically coupled to the limb-bud cells. In control experiments, dye was not taken up by the cells when simply applied in the bath.

We next examined the electrical and dye coupling of the DUM neuroblast and its progeny. The DUM neuroblast begins dividing at day 6. At first, all of its progeny are electrically coupled to the DUM neuroblast (Fig. 1*B*iii). Until day 9, large currents injected into the DUM neuroblast produce small voltage changes in progeny cells (Fig. 1*B*iii, top), consistent with the extensive electrical coupling of the DUM neuroblast to the rest of the embryo. As early as day 10 (Fig. 1*B*iii, bottom, similar

records from day 12) much smaller currents produce large voltage changes in progeny cells. Day 10 is the time at which the DUM neuroblast becomes electrically uncoupled from most embryonic cells other than its own progeny. Input resistance (R_{in}) for the coupled network of neuroblast and progeny (as well as the R_{in} of the DUM neuroblast) increases from < 10 MΩ at day 9 to ~200 MΩ by day 12 (Fig. 1*B*iii). All progeny remain electrically coupled to the neuroblast until day 11, when the oldest progeny (identified DUM neurones described below) are first becoming electrically uncoupled. (Mature DUM neurones are not electrically coupled to one another.)

Lucifer Yellow injected into the DUM neuroblast at day 7 spreads throughout all of its progeny. However, at day 8, its oldest progeny are dye-uncoupled. Dye does not spread into or out of these identified DUM neurones, although they are still electrically coupled to other cells (Fig. 2*B*, *C*).

DUM neuroblast gives rise to identified DUM neurones

The evidence that the DUM neuroblast gives rise to identified DUM neurones is described by considering day 12–13 embryos, although these cells can be followed from day 6 by serial examination of dissected preparations of increasing age. Viewing the desheathed dorsal surface of the metathoracic ganglion reveals chains of progeny extending anteriorly from the DUM neuroblast. Cells close to the neuroblast are young progeny which are the result of recent divisions (the neuroblast continues dividing until it degenerates on day 16), whereas those at the anterior (distal) end of the elongating chains are the oldest progeny. The DUM neuroblast is ~30 μm in diameter, the progeny at first are ~10 μm and quickly enlarge to ~15 μm in diameter. Several of the somata increase to a diameter of over 40 μm during embryogenesis. Some of the oldest progeny of the DUM neuroblast become identified as DUM neurones because within a few days they assume the characteristic location (dorsal midline), the characteristic morphology (median neurites which bifurcate and extend bilaterally, Figs 2, 3), the characteristic physiology (spiking somata, Fig. 5) and the characteristic histochemistry (somata which stain with Neutral Red[24]).

At days 12–13, we see two chains of progeny, each being generally two cells in width, with one chain extending anteriorly on the left side and the other chain on the right side of the midline. Initially the older chain is dorsal to the younger (day 7). Between days 7 and 11, the plane in which the two chains lie changes in orientation, from dorso-ventral to horizontal. When the orientation changes, there is a 50% probability (*n* = 24) that the dorsal (older) chain will assume either the left or right position in the horizontal plane. It can easily be distinguished, however, by the morphology of its cells throughout this period (C. M. Bate, C.S.G. and N.C.S., in preparation).

We have examined the identities of the first three cells on the outside of the oldest chain of progeny, and find the same identified neurone in the same position along the chain (*n* = 10) (Fig. 3*A*). The morphology of the DUM neurones is revealed by intracellular injection of Lucifer Yellow, and later visualisation in either living or fixed tissue, with UV illumination (Fig. 2*B*, *C*). (Tissue is fixed in 4% formaldehyde, dehydrated in an ethanol series, cleared in methyl benzoate and mounted in fluoromount.) The most anterior cell on the outside bifurcates and extends bilaterally out as peripheral nerves 3, 4 and 5; the second cell on the outside bifurcates and extends bilaterally out as peripheral nerves 4 and 5; and the third cell on the outside bifurcates and extends bilaterally out only peripheral nerve 5. The axons of this third cell run out nerve 5 to the extensor tibiae (ETi) muscle; this cell is DUMETi. In the mesothoracic ganglion, the first cell also bifurcates and extends bilaterally out as peripheral nerves 3, 4 and 5. Thus, from animal to animal, the cell in the same position along the chain, presumably having the same mitotic ancestry, develops into the same identified neurone.

Morphological development of identified DUM neurones

The outgrowth of processes by the single identified DUM neurone, DUMETi, was followed as a function of developmental age ($n \geq 3$ for each time point). Axonal outgrowth of DUMETi begins on about day 7 with the extension of a median neurite (Fig. 3B). At this time, the framework for the neuropil, nerve connectives and peripheral nerves already exists in the form of two longitudinal fibre tracts, two commissures in each segment, and lateral fibre tracts to the periphery. The distal end of the growing axon produces multiple branches with growth cones extending in different directions, often for over 20 μm in the wrong direction. As the correct branch continues to extend and send out branches at its distal tip, the extra incorrect neurites disappear, leaving a relatively naked proximal axon.

By day 8, the axon of DUMETi has bifurcated and both lateral axons appear fuzzy because of the presence of many fine branches. During day 9, the distal end of the axon grows out to the edge of the ganglion, and many of the proximal branches disappear. By day 10, the neurone sends axons out many of the available peripheral nerves and branches of those nerves, even though ultimately these extra branches will disappear and the axon of DUMETi will extend out only nerve 5 (and branch 5b1d) to the ETi muscle. By day 12, the distal axon reaches the ETi muscle. Three prominent features at this age are the occurrence of extra peripheral branches, the start of the central bilateral arborisations and the relatively naked central axon. By day 13, the axon has extended over the entire ETi muscle, but the cell body and arborisations are still relatively small.

After the axon of DUMETi reaches its target, there are three clear morphological changes: the extra peripheral neurites disappear, leaving behind only one axon in nerve 5; the central arborisations greatly increase in the extent and number of their fine branches; and the cell body greatly enlarges. A similar initial overproduction of distal branches and eventual disappearance of these extra branches was found also for DUM 3, 4, 5 and DUM 4, 5.

Onset of chemosensitivity

At day 7, neither the DUM neuroblast nor its progeny show responses to bath application of acetylcholine (ACh) or γ-aminobutyric acid (GABA) at 10^{-3} M. In contrast, by 13 days the oldest identified DUM neurones (described above) are sensitive to bath application and iontophoresis of both of these agents. This latter result is illustrated in Fig. 4B, which shows the intracellularly recorded responses of a developing DUM neurone to iontophoretic application of ACh and GABA from a double-barrelled electrode. These responses involve a membrane conductance increase (not illustrated). The observed reversal potential for GABA is -70 mV, while the extrapolated reversal potential for ACh lies above $+20$ mV. The ACh response is abolished by removal of Na^+ (replacement with choline); the GABA response is abolished by removal of Cl^- (replacement with isethionate). The ACh response is reduced by the nicotinic antagonists curare (10^{-4} M), hexamethonium (10^{-3} M) and decamethonium (10^{-3} M); nicotine is an agonist. However, α-bungarotoxin does not significantly reduce the response at 10^{-6} M. The ACh response is unaffected by the muscarinic antagonists atropine (10^{-6} M) and quinuclidinyl benzilate (QNB, 10^{-7} M); pilocarpine has no effect (10^{-3} M). The GABA response is rapidly blocked by picrotoxin (10^{-4} M); muscimol is an agonist.

The oldest DUM neurones first become sensitive to ACh and GABA at day 8 of development, and seem to become sensitive to both neurotransmitters at the same time. Young progeny in close proximity to the DUM neuroblast show no response to iontophoretic application of ACh. In contrast, the oldest progeny at the distal end of the chain, which are still electrically coupled (Fig. 1Biii) and already possess neurites (Fig. 3B), are depolarised by iontophoretic application of ACh onto their

somata. (No desensitisation is seen in response to prolonged application of these agents.)

The processes of the oldest DUM neurone are also depolarised by iontophoretic application of ACh on day 8. Processes seem to be sensitive over their entire length. It seems that chemosensitivity is distributed over the whole surface of the cell, at or soon after the time that it first appears. Identified DUM neurones thus develop chemosensitivity to ACh and GABA while still electrically coupled, and may be sensitive to other neurotransmitters as well. The reversal potential and ionic dependence of the response to ACh and GABA appear similar at days 8, 13 and 18 of development.

Onset of electrical excitability

We have examined the onset of electrical excitability in the oldest DUM progeny by observing the responses of cells to depolarising current pulses injected through an intracellular

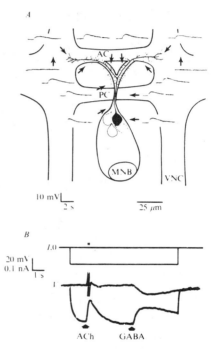

Fig. 4 Chemosensitivity of identified DUM neurones in the grasshopper embryo (the three oldest progeny as described above). A, Response to iontophoretic application of ACh in a day 8 embryo. The diagram shows the embryonic neuropil of a single segmental ganglion (T3), as viewed from the dorsal surface (anterior at top). The DUM neuroblast (NB) is shown with its packet of progeny; those most anterior (oldest) send their axons anteriorly in a median bundle of processes which cross the posterior commissure (PC) and bifurcate near the anterior commissure (AC). The extent of branching of an individual neurone was determined by intracellular injection of Lucifer Yellow. The longitudinal connectives extend into the ventral nerve cords (VNC) and are seen on either side. The lateral neuropil extends (beyond the margin of the figure) into three fibre tracts which become peripheral nerves 3, 4 and 5. The response to application of ACh at the points indicated by the arrows were recorded by an intracellular electrode in the cell body. Processes are sensitive to ACh over their whole length. Small vertical or lateral displacements of the iontophoretic electrode abolished the response. B, Responses to sequential iontophoretic application of ACh and GABA from a double-barrelled micropipette, recorded with an intracellular electrode in a day 13 embryo. At a resting potential of -55 mV, ACh depolarises the cell to threshold, eliciting overshooting action potentials, while GABA hyperpolarises the cell. When the cell is hyperpolarised by injected current, the response to ACh is larger, but remains subthreshold; the cell is then depolarised by GABA.

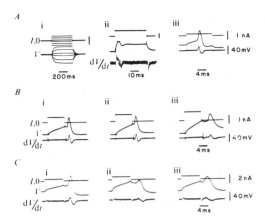

Fig. 5 Electrical excitability of the oldest DUM neurones in the grasshopper embryo. *A*, Responses in the oldest DUM progeny between days 11 and 12. (i) The DUM neuroblast is impaled with one microelectrode to inject current, and an electrically coupled progeny is impaled with a second microelectrode to record voltage. These cells have resting potentials of −50 to −70 mV and appear electrically coupled. Depolarisation and hyperpolarisation of the neuroblast and its progeny by 50 mV reveals a constant membrane resistance. (ii) As the cells become uncoupled they develop neurite action potentials in which the inward current is carried predominantly by Na⁺ (data not shown). The early embryonic neurites bifurcate at a T-junction, and in many cases the first embryonic axon spikes have the adult characteristic of appearing double-peaked; each peak in the adult and presumably in the embryo corresponds to a separate site of initiation along one of the two lateral axons. (iii) Current injected into a DUM neurone at a later time yields an overshooting action potential that appears to arise in the cell body. *B*, Ionic dependence of the somatic action potential in a day 12 embryo. The overshoot of the spike seen in normal saline (i) is not greatly affected by replacement of Na⁺ with Tris (ii) or addition of 30 mM Co²⁺ (iii). *C*, Ionic dependence of the action potential of a DUM neurone in a day 18 embryo. The overshoot (i) is reduced by either removal of Na⁺ (ii) or addition of Co²⁺ (iii). In both day 12 and day 18 action potentials, simultaneous removal of Na⁺ and addition of Co²⁺ (not shown here) abolishes the action potential.

recording electrode. They are generally incapable of producing action potentials at day 11. They become electrically excitable between days 11 and 12 (Fig. 5*A*), while they are becoming electrically uncoupled. It seemed possible that voltage-dependent channels were not revealed while the cells were electrically coupled because of the long time constant of the coupled network of cells, preventing depolarisation to threshold before channel inactivation occurred. This possibility was tested by exposing the cells to veratridine 10^{-5} g ml^{-1}, which specifically depolarises cells possessing voltage-dependent Na⁺ channels[26]. The treatment has no effect on the resting potentials of any of the ventral neuroblasts, the DUM neuroblast, or its progeny up to day 11. In contrast, the oldest DUM progeny are depolarised by the treatment by day 12 (we thank A. Willard for suggesting this approach).

Between days 11 and 12, the oldest DUM neurones first produce small action potentials which fail to overshoot the zero potential and often have a characteristic double-peaked appearance (Fig. 5*A*). These action potentials are likely to be produced in the neurites, because this response has been shown in adult DUM neurones to be the sum of action potentials arising from two symmetrical neurites distal to the point of bifurcation[10]. These action potentials depend largely on an inward Na⁺ current, because they are rapidly blocked by removal of Na⁺ or addition of 10^{-9} g ml^{-1} tetrodotoxin (TTX). These cells and those in older embryos are depolarised by 25 mV or more when exposed to veratridine. This depolarisation is blocked by prior removal of Na⁺ or addition of TTX.

Within a day, the oldest DUM neurones are capable of producing overshooting action potentials, 2–4 ms in duration, that appear to arise in the cell body ($R_{in} \cong 300$ MΩ). These action potentials depend on Na⁺ and Ca²⁺ for their inward current. Removal of Na⁺ or addition of 30 mM Co²⁺ (to block Ca²⁺ channels) has little effect on the overshoot (Fig. 5*B*), although simultaneous application of both treatments abolishes the action potential. However, by 18 days, blockage of either inward current reduces the overshoot in these same neurones (Fig. 5*C*). It is known that in at least one adult DUM neurone, DUMETi, the blockage of either inward current alone is sufficient to abolish the action potential[11]. The basis for these developmental changes is not yet known.

Development of later phenotypes

The transmitter of the DUM neurones, octopamine, begins to appear in the thoracic ganglion on day 13, after the axons of the oldest DUM neurones reach their peripheral target[24]. Shortly thereafter, the somata of the oldest DUM neurones begin to stain with Neutral Red.

The first spontaneous synaptic activity, from unidentified synaptic input, is recorded in DUM neurones at 15 days, 1 week after the appearance of chemosensitivity. The source of these synaptic inputs is not yet known.

Temporal sequence of development

There is a distinct order in the acquisition of particular phenotypes by the identified DUM neurones that are the oldest progeny of the DUM neuroblast (Fig. 6). This developmental sequence occurs first in the oldest progeny; younger progeny may be as much as several days behind in their differentiation.

Some of the phenotypes initially express change during the course of further embryonic development whereas others do not. There are changes in the morphology of identified neurones: the initial fine branches and the extra peripheral neurites all eventually disappear. Similarly an initial overproduction and later disappearance of many central branches around the site of the main arborisation has been observed in an identified neurone in the brain of the grasshopper (D. Bentley and A. Raymond, personal communication). In other systems, gap junctions[27] and profiles of chemical synapses[28] appear transiently on cell bodies shortly before the outgrowth of their processes. In the embryonic DUM cells, there appears to be no change in the ionic basis of the responses to ACh and GABA, as indicated by the ion substitution experiments and the reversal potential determinations. In contrast, there is a change in the ionic requirements for electrical excitability of the cell body, consistent with, although not qualitatively as great as, the changes reported for the development of excitability in other neurones[29-33].

The initially extensive electrical coupling and eventual uncoupling are consistent with observations in other embryos[34-36]. The outgrowth of processes and the appearance of chemosensitivity of the identified DUM neurones begin after their terminal mitoses but while they are still extensively electrically coupled. The observation that cells become dye uncoupled before they become electrically uncoupled suggests that there may be some progressive restriction on the molecular size of substances that can pass freely between cell interiors. Further work will be needed to determine the mechanisms involved in these changes and the role of uncoupling in further differentiation.

How general is the sequence of appearance of neuronal phenotypes observed in the DUM neurones? Studies of the development of amphibian spinal cord have shown that Rohon-Beard neurones become electrically excitable a substantial time after their final DNA synthesis[30,37]. They are already depolarised by GABA at this time, but it is not known how early chemosensitivity first appears[38]. The development of electrical excitability of the neurites of embryonic amphibian neurones seems to precede the cell body by a small time interval[33]. The identity of the neurotransmitter of Rohon-Beard cells is not known. The known portion of the developmental sequence for these cells is compatible with the sequence for DUM neurones.

Neurotransmitter synthesis is a relatively early phenotype for

Fig. 6 The developmental timetable for the oldest DUM neurones of the grasshopper embryo *in vivo* [DUM 3, 4, 5; DUM 4, 5; and DUM 5 (DUMETi)]. The egg is laid at day zero, and at 35 °C hatching occurs at day 20. The time of onset or first appearance of a phenotype in these neurones is indicated by a vertical bar. The morphology of the embryo, viewed from the ventral surface in the egg case, is illustrated below as traced from camera lucida projections. Note that the embryo makes a major rotation (blastokinesis) at day 10, and thus from day 10 onward the embryo is viewed from the opposite side of the egg case.

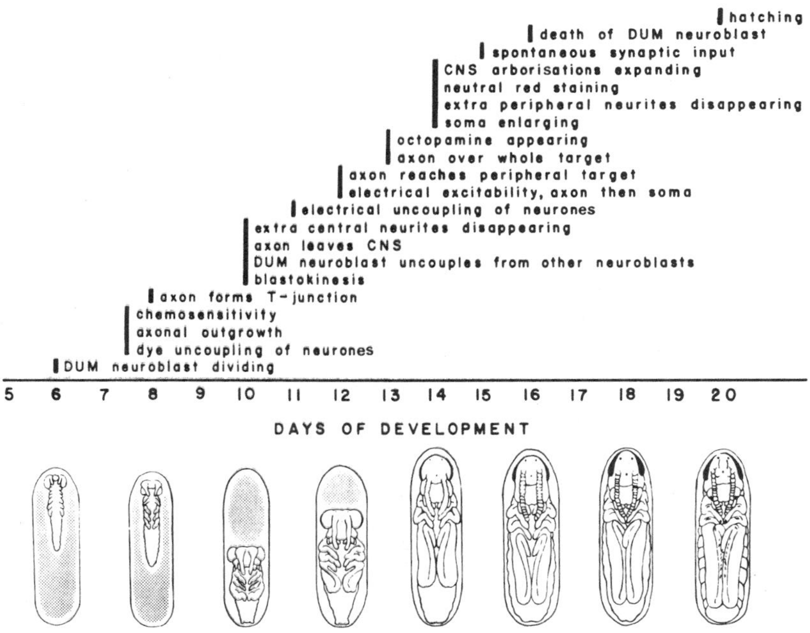
hatching
death of DUM neuroblast
spontaneous synaptic input
CNS arborisations expanding
neutral red staining
extra peripheral neurites disappearing
soma enlarging
octopamine appearing
axon over whole target
axon reaches peripheral target
electrical excitability, axon then soma
electrical uncoupling of neurones
extra central neurites disappearing
axon leaves CNS
DUM neuroblast uncouples from other neuroblasts
blastokinesis
axon forms T-junction
chemosensitivity
axonal outgrowth
dye uncoupling of neurones
DUM neuroblast dividing
5 6 7 8 9 10 11 12 13 14 15 16 17 18 19 20
DAYS OF DEVELOPMENT

vertebrate superior cervical ganglion cells[39,40], whereas it is a relatively late phenotype for invertebrate DUM neurones. However, vertebrate ciliary ganglion neurones show a late large increase in neurotransmitter synthetic enzyme activity after their axons have reached and synapsed on their targets[41]. Neurotransmitter synthesis may differentiate earlier in other neurones in grasshopper embryos, since high levels of ACh are already present by day 5, before differentiation of central neurones[24]. Sanes and Hildebrand[42] found that antennal sensory cells in the pupae of the moth *Manduca* were capable of synthesising and storing ACh before the axons arrived at their targets in the central nervous system. If the onset of neurotransmitter synthesis requires particular environmental cues[43,44], then these cues may exert their influence at different points in the lives of these different types of cells. Alternatively, different types of neurones may simply be reading out different intrinsic programmes.

Further work will be needed before any causal relationship in the sequence of phenotypes of the embryonic DUM neurones can be established or ruled out. However, it is worth noting that several events are closely linked temporally. The outgrowth of processes and the onset of chemosensitivity occur at about the same time. Cells become electrically uncoupled and electrically excitable at about the same time. Neurotransmitter storage is detected just after cell processes have reached their targets. Cell body enlargement, Neutral Red staining, the disappearance of extra peripheral neurites, and the expansion of central arborisations occur at this time. It may now be possible to manipulate one phenotype and examine the consequences for the later expression of others.

We thank Michael Bate and Michael O'Shea for stimulating discussions, Janet Lamborghini and Darwin Berg for critical reading of the manuscript, William Kristan and Allen Selverston for providing facilities, James Coulombe for technical assistance, and Nino Cooley for preparation of the figures. Bungarotoxin was supplied by P. Ravdin and D. Berg, Lucifer Yellow by Walter Stewart, and QNB by M. Nirenberg and Hoffman-LaRoche. This work was supported by NIH and NSF grants to N.C.S. and a Helen Hay Whitney Fellowship to C.S.G.

Received 27 December 1978; accepted 4 June 1979.

1. Kuffler, S. W. & Nicholls, J. G. *From Neuron to Brain* (Sinauer, Boston, 1976).
2. Kandel, E. R. *Cellular Basis of Behavior* (Freeman, San Francisco, 1976).
3. Hoyle, G. (ed.) *Identified Neurons and Behavior of Arthropods* (Plenum, New York, 1977).
4. Faber, D. S. & Korn, H. (eds) *Neurobiology of the Mauthner Cell* (Raven, New York, 1978).
4. Plotnikova, S. I. *J. evolut. biochem. Physiol.* **5**, 339–341 (1969).
6. Crossman, A. R., Kerkut, G. A., Pitman, R. M. & Walker, R. *J. comp. Biochem. Physiol.* **40A**, 579–596 (1971).
7. Hoyle, G., Dagan, D., Moberly, B. & Colquhoun, W. *J. exp. Zool.* **187**, 159–165 (1974).
8. O'Shea, M. & Evans, P. *Soc. Neurosci.* **3**, 187 (1977).
9. Evans, P. & O'Shea, M. *Nature* **270**, 275–279 (1977); *J. exp. Biol.* **73**, 235–260 (1978).
10. Heitler, W. J. & Goodman, C. S. *J. exp. Biol.* **76**, 63–84 (1978).
11. Goodman, C. S. & Heitler, W. J. *Soc. Neurosci.* **3**, 426 (1977); *J. exp. Biol.* (in the press).
12. Sulston, J. E. *Phil. Trans. R. Soc.* B **275**, 287–297 (1976).
13. Sulston, J. E. & Horvitz, H. R. *Devl Biol.* **56**, 110–156 (1977).
14. Goodman, C. S. & Spitzer, N. C. *Soc. Neurosci.* **4**, 113 (1978).
15. Spitzer, N. C. & Goodman, C. S. *Soc. Neurosci.* **4**, 127 (1978).
16. Wheeler, W. M. *J. Morph.* **4**, 337–343 (1891); **8**, 1–160 (1893).
17. Baden, V. *J. Morph.* **60**, 159–190 (1936).
18. Roonwal, M. L. *Phil. Trans. R. Soc.* B**227**, 175–244 (1937).
19. Anderson, D. T. in *Developmental Systems: Insects* (eds Counce, S. J. & Waddington, C. H.) (Academic, New York, 1972).
20. Bate, C. M. *J. Embryol. exp. Morph.* **35**, 107–123 (1976).
21. Stuart, A. E., Hudspeth, A. J. & Hall, Z. W. *Cell Tissue Res.* **153**, 55–61 (1974).
22. Wallace, B. G., Talamo, B. R., Evans, P. D. & Kravitz, E. A. *Brain Res.* **74**, 349–355 (1974).
23. Evans, P. D., Kravitz, E. A., Talamo, B. R. & Wallace, B. G. *J. Physiol., Lond.* **262**, 51–70 (1976).
24. Goodman, C. S., O'Shea, M., McCaman, R. E. & Spitzer, N. C. *Science* **204**, 1219–1222 (1979).
25. Stewart, W. W *Cell* **14**, 741–759 (1978).
26. Narahashi, T. *Physiol. Rev.* **54**, 813–889 (1974).
27. Lopresti, V., Macagno, E. R. & Levinthal, C. *Proc. natn. Acad. Sci. U.S.A.* **70**, 433–473 (1974).
28. Schacher, S. & Kandel, E. R. *Soc. Neurosci.* **4**, 126 (1978).
29. Spitzer, N. C. & Baccaglini, P. I. *Brain Res.* **107**, 610–616 (1976).
30. Baccaglini, P. I. & Spitzer, N. C. *J. Physiol., Lond.* **271**, 93–117 (1977).
31. Baccaglini, P. I. *J. Physiol., Lond.* **283**, 585–604 (1978).
32. Spitzer, N. C. & Lamborghini, J. E. *Proc. natn. Acad. Sci. U.S.A.* **73**, 1641–1645 (1976).
33. Willard, A. L. *Soc. Neurosci.* **3**, 123 (1977); and in preparation.
34. Potter, D. D., Furshpan, E. J. & Lennox, E. S. *Proc. natn. Acad. Sci. U.S.A.* **55**, 328–336 (1966).
35. Warner, A. E. in *Simple Nervous Systems* (eds Newth, D. R. & Usherwood, P. N. R.) (Arnold, London, 1975).
36. Blackshaw, S. E. & Warner, A. E. *J. Physiol., Lond.* **255**, 209–230 (1976).
37. Spitzer, N. C. & Spitzer, J. L. *Am. Zool.* **15**, 781 (1975).
38. Spitzer, N. C. *Soc. Neurosci.* **2**, 204 (1976).
39. Cochard, P., Goldstein, M. & Black, I. B. *Soc. Neurosci.* **4**, 109 (1978); *Proc. natn. Acad. Sci. U.S.A.* **75**, 2986–2990 (1978).
40. Rothman, T. P., Gershon, M. D. & Holtzer, H. *Devl Biol.* **65**, 322–341 (1978).
41. Chiappinelli, V., Giacobini, E., Pilar, G. & Uchimura, H.K Physiol., Lond. **257**, 749–766 (1976).
42. Sanes, J. R. & Hildebrand, J. G. *Devl Biol.* **52**, 105–120 (1976).
43. LeDouarin, N. M., Renaud, D., Teillet, M. A. & LeDouarin, G. H. *Proc. natn. Acad. Sci. U.S.A.* **72**, 728–732 (1975).
44. LeDouarin, N. M., Teillet, M. A., Ziller, C. & Smith, J. *Proc. natn. Acad. Sci. U.S.A.* **75**, 2030–2034 (1978).
45. Bentley, D., Keshishian, H., Shankland, M. & Raymond, A. *J. Embryol. exp. Morph.* (in the press).

Section 4
Axon Guidance

Lance-Jones, C. and L. Landmesser. 1980. Motoneurone projection patterns in the chick hind limb following early partial reversals of the spinal cord. *J. Physiol. 302:* 581–602.

LoPresti, V., E.R. Macagno, and C. Levinthal. 1973. Structure and development of neuronal connections in isogenic organisms: Cellular interactions in the development of the optic lamina of *Daphnia. Proc. Natl. Acad. Sci. 70:* 433–437.

Edwards, J.S., S.-W. Chen, and M.W. Berns. 1981. Cercal sensory development following laser microlesions of embryonic apical cells in *Acheta domesticus. J. Neurosci. 1:* 250–258.

Letourneau, P.C. 1975. Cell-to-substratum adhesion and guidance of axonal elongation. *Dev. Biol. 44:* 92–101.

How do the axonal processes of developing neurons find their targets? This basic question in developmental neurobiology has proved difficult to answer because axon outgrowth occurs early in embryonic life, when observation and manipulation are difficult. Unfortunately, regenerating axons in adult animals, for the reasons outlined below, do not provide a completely satisfactory substitute for outgrowth in embryos.

Although there were many studies of axon growth earlier in the century (see, for example, Weiss 1934; Harrison 1935; Speidel 1941; Ramón y Cajal 1960, 1968), the phenomenology of this process is perhaps best exemplified in recent studies of the development of limb innervation in chick embryos (Landmesser 1980). For many years neurobiologists debated the degree to which initial innervation might be random (see, for example, Weiss 1936; Sperry 1959). Extracellular recordings from embryonic nerves to the chick hindlimb show that the distribution of peripheral axons is, in fact, similar to the adult pattern from the earliest times at which such recordings can be made (about 8 days of incubation) (Landmesser and Morris 1975). Injection of small amounts of the enzyme horseradish peroxidase (HRP) into muscle masses at even earlier stages (4–5 days of incubation) confirmed this view. HRP is transported along axons either anterogradely or retrogradely and can be demonstrated histochemically; it thus provides an excellent means of tracing neural pathways. Even though these injections were made before individual muscle masses had fully cleaved, the motor neurons that took up the enzyme occupied the same positions in the embryonic spinal cord as the adult motor neuron pools (Landmesser 1978; Hollyday 1980; Oppenheim 1981; see, however, Pettigrew et al. 1979; Lamb 1976; Dennis and Harris 1979). Furthermore, the axons

163

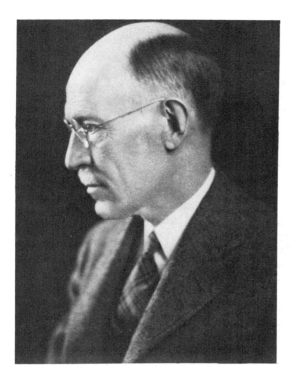

Ross G. Harrison, who made many early contributions to the study of axons and the mechanism of their outgrowth.

of motor neurons could still find their way to appropriate muscles after deletion or reversal of short (but not long) segments of lumbar spinal cord (**Lance-Jones** and **Landmesser 1980**a,b; Hollyday et al. 1977). Thus, chick motor axons appear to make very few errors finding their targets. There are some apparent counterexamples in the development of invertebrates, however, and how widely this conclusion can be generalized is still uncertain (see Goodman et al. 1981).

Another important phenomenon described in work on the chick limb is that growing axons segregate while still far from their destinations. When Lance-Jones and Landmesser (1981) traced the course of anterogradely labeled axons after HRP injection into the embryonic cord, they found that motor axons sorted themselves into the correct nerve branches of the relevant plexus in the proximal limb bud. Thus, these axons appear to follow directional cues from the very beginning of their growth to the periphery. Studies of Mauthner cells in lower vertebrates (see Kimmel and Model 1978) and of abnormally positioned cells in mammalian cortex (Van der

Loos 1965; Caviness and Rakic 1978) also provide evidence that some aspect of the local environment influences the direction in which axons grow. The idea that axons are locally guided in this way can be traced back to Harrison (1935; see also Hamburger 1980, reprinted in Section 1).

Several possible mechanisms that might account for axon guidance have been considered. A possibility favored in some older literature (see Weiss 1934) is that of preexisting mechanical guides. A recent expression of this general concept is the "blueprint hypothesis," which states that specific pathways—in the form of holes or spaces in the neuroepithelial matrix—are generated before axon outgrowth (Singer et al. 1979). Evidence for this idea comes from the observation that axons in the embryonic newt spinal cord grow into open spaces which appear to guide them to appropriate destinations. Additional evidence for preexisting channels for axon outgrowth has come from studies of mouse and chick retinas, where ganglion-cell axons normally grow into preexisting spaces in the optic cup (Silver and Robb 1979; Silver and Sidman 1980; Krayanek and Goldberg 1981). In a mutant mouse in which these spaces are partially obliterated, axon outgrowth is impeded (Silver and Robb 1979), indicating that such spaces are necessary for axon outgrowth from the eye. In most situations, however, such axon channels are not evident.

A different observation related to the concept of preexisting pathways is that in some invertebrates a small number of "lead" or "pioneer" fibers reach the target first and apparently serve to guide axons that develop later (**LoPresti, Macagno,** and **Levinthal 1973;** Sanes and Hildebrand 1975; Bate 1976; Edwards 1977). In the embryonic locust, for example, two solitary pairs of processes grow out from sensory neurons in the antennae to the central nervous system (Bate 1976). Axons from sensory receptors that differentiate somewhat later in development accumulate around the original axons, thus forming the adult nerve bundle. A similar sequence occurs in the ingrowth of sensory axons from the locust limb and moth antenna (Sanes and Hildebrand 1975). In another insect, the cricket, **Edwards, Chen,** and **Berns (1981)** have provided experimental evidence for the importance of pioneer fiber guides for axon outgrowth. When pioneer fibers are destroyed by a laser-beam microlesion, the outgrowth of subsequent axons forms multiple bundles instead of a single nerve. Of course, one still has to explain how the pioneers find their way. One possibility is that the pioneer fibers grow out when the distance to the target is very small. Some other important aspects of initial contact by a "lead" axon are discussed by LoPresti et al. (1973).

Another possible mechanism of axon guidance is a gradient of a diffusible agent emanating from the axon's target. The experimental basis for this proposal is that the axons of cells sensitive to nerve growth factor (NGF—see Section 6) are capable of changing the direction of their growth in response to an NGF concentration gradient (Campenot 1977; Letourneau 1978; Menesini-Chen et al. 1978; Gundersen and Barrett 1980). There are, however, some problems with the idea that tropic agents released from targets provide a primary guide to axons. First, normal concentrations of NGF are much lower than the concentrations necessary to demonstrate axonal tropism in vitro. Second, the targets of neurons sensitive to NGF are ubiquitous; therefore it is hard to imagine how NGF gradients could be established that, by themselves, could cause the stereotyped branching patterns one sees in nerves carrying NGF-sensitive axons. Finally, the same nerves that carry NGF sensitive axons also carry NGF-insensitive axons to other targets. It may well be that the *tropic* influence of peripherally secreted agents is a local one, acting on sensitive axons once they have reached the general vicinity of an appropriate target. It is interesting in this regard that the growth of some cortical projections appears to occur in two stages, as if axons were required to wait for the emergence of a local signal once they reached the right vicinity (see, for example, Wise and Jones 1976, 1978).

A third possible mechanism axon guidance is that the growing ends of axons (the growth cones) recognize molecular cues on the surfaces they contact (see Hamburger 1980, reprinted in Section 1, for the early history of this idea). The potential importance of surface qualities in axon guidance was apparent from the outset of tissue-culture experiments and has been demonstrated dramatically by **Letourneau (1975)**. If neurons are seeded onto a culture plate whose surface consists of geometrical patterns of artificial materials to which neurites adhere differentially, axons follow the pattern described by the substance they adhere to best. Although the materials used presumably play no role in vivo, similar responses to cell surfaces of different adhesivity may be important not only in axon guidance, but in cell migration and morphogenesis generally (see Section 2). A detailed knowledge of the properties of growth cones (and of the surfaces of the cells contacted along the path of outgrowth) will be critical in resolving the nature of such surface interactions. In fact, considerable progress has been made recently in determining the fine structure of growth cones and some of the factors involved in their navigation (Bray and Bunge 1973; Pfenninger and Rees 1976; Shaw and Bray 1977; Bray 1979; Letourneau 1981).

The apparent loss of guidance mechanisms in adult mammals (but not some lower vertebrates) provides some additional insight into the way this feat is normally accomplished in development. Most classes of peripheral axons readily regenerate after they are severed and often reinnervate their normal targets (e.g., muscles or sensory receptors in the skin). In fact, regenerating axons have a strong predilection for original sites of termination within a target. Thus, motor axons reoccupy the original end-plate zones of muscle fibers (Bennett et al. 1973; Letinsky et al. 1976; Sanes et al. 1980), and at least some sensory axons return quite precisely to specialized sensory receptors in the skin (Burgess and Horch 1973; Burgess et al. 1974) or to muscle spindles (Thulin 1960; Bessou et al. 1965; Brown and Butler 1976). Although regenerating axons often are able to find appropriate postsynaptic elements within a target, in most higher vertebrates (mammals in particular) they have little luck finding their original targets within the larger context of a limb or some other part of the body (Bernstein and Guth 1961; Brushart and Mesulam 1980). Thus, when motor axons regenerate, they appear to innervate deprived muscles on a first-come, first-served basis. Furthermore, as shown by Sperry (1941, 1959), there is no mechanism of central rewiring that can compensate for these peripheral mistakes. In short, regenerating mammalian axons are no longer guided to the proper position within the body. Whether this reflects axonal incompetence or a disappearance of the cues present during development is not known.

It is therefore surprising that such topographic

guidance does operate during peripheral nerve regeneration in some lower vertebrates. Sperry and Arora (1965) showed that regenerating axons of the third cranial nerve in fish partition themselves correctly between the several extraocular muscles that the nerve normally supplies. This sorting out has been demonstrated more directly in nerve-regeneration experiments carried out using salamander limbs. These animals, unlike mammals, are fully capable of coordinated function after injury or even transplantation of adult limbs (Weiss 1936; see also Section 9). In lower vertebrates like the salamander, it is as if the tissues of the mature limb continue to provide cues that regenerating axons are able to interpret. The basis of this difference between higher and lower vertebrates remains a mystery.

Given the evidence briefly reviewed here, a reasonable conclusion is that axon outgrowth is directed by a number of influences including mechanical factors, diffusible agents, and surface cues. A central question at present concerns the relative importance of each of these influences at various stages of development and the relationship of these mechanisms of axon guidance to other phenomena that appear to involve interpretation of position. An interesting question is whether the molecular cues that axons respond to during outgrowth are similar to the molecular cues that guide migration, morphogenesis, and perhaps some aspects of selective synapse formation.

References

Bate, C.M. 1976. Pioneer neurones in an insect embryo. *Nature 260:* 54–55.

Bennett, M.R., E. McLachlan, and R.S. Taylor. 1973. The formation of synapses in reinnervated mammalian striated muscle. *J. Physiol. 233:* 481–500.

Bessou, P., Y. Laporte, and B. Pages. 1965. Observations sur la reinnervation de fuseaux neuro-musculaires de chat. *C.R. Soc. Biol. 160:* 408–411.

Bernstein, J.J. and L. Guth. 1961. Nonselectivity in establishment of neuromuscular connections following nerve regeneration in the rat. *Exp. Neurol. 4:* 262–275.

Bray, D. 1979. Mechanical tension produced by nerve cells in tissue culture. *J. Cell Sci. 37:* 391–410.

Bray, D. and M.B. Bunge. 1973. The growth cone in neurite extension. *CIBA Found. Symp. 14:* 195–209.

Brown, M.C. and R. Butler. 1976. Regeneration of afferent and efferent fibres to muscle spindles after nerve injury in adult cats. *J. Physiol. 260:* 253–266.

Brushart, T.M. and M.-M. Mesulam. 1980. Alteration in connections between muscle and anterior horn motoneurons after peripheral nerve repair. *Science 208:* 603–605.

Burgess, P.R. and K.W. Horch. 1973. Specific regeneration of cutaneous fibers in the cat. *J. Neurophysiol. 36:* 101–114.

Burgess, P.R., K.B. English, K.W. Horch, and L.J. Stensaas. 1974. Patterning in the regeneration of type I cutaneous receptors. *J. Physiol. 236:* 57–82.

Campenot, R.B. 1977. Local control of neurite development by nerve growth factor. *Proc. Natl. Acad. Sci. 74:* 4516–4519.

Caviness, V. and P. Rakic. 1978. Mechanisms of cortical development: A view from mutations in mice. *Annu. Rev. Neurosci. 1:* 297–326.

Dennis, M.J. and A.J. Harris. 1979. Elimination of inappropriate nerve muscle connections during development of rat embryos. *Prog. Brain Res. 49:* 359–364.

Edwards, J.S. 1977. Pathfinding by arthropod sensory nerves. In *Identified neurons and behavior of arthropods* (ed. G. Hoyle), pp. 484–493. Plenum Press, New York.

Edwards, J.S., S.-W. Chen, and M.W. Berns. 1981. Cercal sensory development following laser microlesions of embryonic apical cells in *Acheta domesticus. J. Neurosci. 1:* 250–258.

Goodman, C.S., M. Bate, and N.C. Spitzer. 1981. Embryonic development of identified neurons: Origin and transformation of the H cell. *J. Neurosci. 1:* 94–102.

Gundersen, R.W. and J.N. Barrett. 1980. Characterization of the turning response of dorsal root neurites toward nerve growth factor. *J. Cell Biol. 87:* 546–554.

Hamburger, V. 1980. S. Ramón y Cajal, R.G. Harrison and the beginnings of neuroembryology. *Perspect. Biol. Med. 23:* 600–616.

Harrison, R.G. 1935. On the origin and development of the nervous system studied by the methods of experimental embryology. The Croonian Lecture. *Proc. R. Soc. Lond. B 118:* 155–196.

Hollyday, M. 1980. Organization of motor pools in the chick lumbar lateral motor column. *J. Comp. Neurol. 194:* 143–170.

Hollyday, M., V. Hamburger, and J.H.G. Farris. 1977. Localization of motor neuron pools supplying identified muscles in normal and supernumerary legs of chick embryo. *Proc. Natl. Acad. Sci. 74:* 3582–3586.

Kimmel, C.B. and P.G. Model. 1978. Developmental studies of the Mauthner cell. In *Neurobiology of the Mauthner cell* (ed. D. Faber and H. Korn), pp. 183–220. Raven Press, New York.

Krayanek, S. and S. Goldberg. 1981. Oriented extracellular channels and axonal guidance in the embryonic chick retina. *Dev. Biol. 84:* 41–50.

Lamb, A.H. 1976. The projection patterns of the ventral horn to the hind limb during development. *Dev. Biol. 54:* 82–99.

Lance-Jones, C. and L. Landmesser. 1980a. Motoneurone projection patterns in embryonic chick limbs following partial deletions of the spinal cord. *J. Physiol. 302:* 559–580.

———. 1980b. Motoneurone projection patterns in the chick hind limb following early partial reversals of the spinal cord. *J. Physiol. 302:* 581–602.

———. 1981. Pathway selection by embryonic chick motoneurons in an experimentally altered environment. *Proc. R. Soc. Lond. B 214:* 19–52.

Landmesser, L. 1978. The development of motor projection patterns in the chick hind limb. *J. Physiol. 284:* 391–414.

———. 1980. The generation of neuromuscular specificity. *Annu. Rev. Neurosci. 3:* 279–302.

Landmesser, L. and D.G. Morris. 1975. The development of functional innervation in the hind limb of the chick embryo. *J. Physiol. 249:* 301–326.

Letinsky, M.S., K.H. Fishbeck, and U.J. McMahan. 1976. Precision of reinnervation of original postsynaptic sites in frog muscle after a nerve crush. *J. Neurocytol. 5:* 691–718.

Letourneau, P.C. 1975. Cell-to-substratum adhesion and guidance of axonal elongation. *Dev. Biol. 44:* 92–101.

———. 1978. Chemotactic response of nerve fiber elongation to nerve growth factor. *Dev. Biol. 66:* 183–196.

———. 1981. Immunocytochemical evidence for colocalization in neurite growth cones of actin and myosin and their relationship to cell-substratum adhesions. *Dev. Biol. 85:* 113–122.

LoPresti, V., E.R. Macagno, and C. Levinthal. 1973.

Structure and development of neuronal connections in isogenic organisms: Cellular interactions in the development of the optic lamina of *Daphnia*. *Proc. Natl. Acad. Sci.* 70: 433–437.

Menesini-Chen, G.M., J.S. Chen, and R. Levi-Montalcini. 1978. Sympathetic nerve fibers ingrowth in the central nervous system of neonatal rodents upon intracerebral NGF injections. *Arch. Ital. Biol.* 116: 53–84.

Oppenheim, R.W. 1981. Cell death of motoneurons in the chick embryo spinal cord. V. Evidence on the role of cell death and neuromuscular function in the formation of specific peripheral connections. *J. Neurosci.* 1: 141–151.

Pettigrew, A.G., B. Lindemann, and M.R. Bennett. 1979. Development of the segmental innervation of the chick forelimb. *J. Embryol. Exp. Morphol.* 49: 115–137.

Pfenninger, K.H. and R.P. Rees. 1976. From growth cone to synapse: Properties of membranes involved in synapse formation. In *Neuronal recognition* (ed. S.H. Barondes), pp. 131–178. Plenum Press, New York.

Ramón y Cajal, S. 1960. *Studies on vertebrate neurogenesis.* (Translation of the 1929 edition by L. Guth.) C.C. Thomas, Springfield, Illinois.

———. 1968. *Degeneration and regeneration of the nervous system.* Facsimile of 1928 edition in two volumes. Hafner, New York.

Sanes, J.R. and J.G. Hildebrand. 1975. Nerves in the antennae of pupal *Manducca sexta Johanssen (Lepidoptera: Sphingidae). Wilhehm Roux's Arch.* 178: 71–78.

Sanes, J.R., L.M. Marshall, and U.J. McMahan. 1980. Reinnervation of skeletal muscle: Restoration of the normal synaptic pattern. In *Nerve repair and regeneration: Its clinical and experimental basis* (ed. D.L. Jewett and H.R. McCarroll), pp. 130–138. Mosby, St. Louis, Missouri.

Shaw, G. and D. Bray. 1977. Movement and extension of isolated growth cones. *Exp. Cell Res.* 104: 55–65.

Silver, J. and R.M. Robb. 1979. Studies on the development of the eye cup and optic nerve in normal mice and in mutants with congenital optic nerve aplasia. *Dev. Biol.* 68: 175–190.

Silver, J. and R.S. Sidman. 1980. A mechanism for the guidance and topographic patterning of retinal ganglion cell axons. *J. Comp. Neurol.* 189: 101–111.

Singer, M., R.H. Nordlander, and M. Egar. 1979. Axonal guidance during embryogenesis and regeneration in the spinal cord of the newt: The blueprint hypothesis of neuronal pathway patterning. *J. Comp. Neurol.* 185: 1–22.

Speidel, C.C. 1941. Adjustments of nerve endings. *Harvey Lect.* 36: 126–158.

Sperry, R.W. 1941. The effect of crossing nerves to antagonistic muscles in the hind limb of the rat. *J. Comp. Neurol.* 75: 1–19.

———. 1959. The growth of nerve circuits. *Sci. Am.* 201: 68–75.

Sperry, R.W. and H.L. Arora. 1965. Selectivity in regeneration of the oculomotor nerve in the cichlid fish, *Astronatus ocellatus. J. Embryol. Exp. Morphol.* 14: 307–317.

Thulin, C.A. 1960. Electrophysiological studies of peripheral nerve regeneration with special reference to small diameter (γ) fibres. *Exp. Neurol.* 2: 598–612.

Van der Loos, H. 1965. The "improperly" oriented pyramidal cell in the cerebral cortex and its possible bearing on problems of neuronal growth and cell orientation. *Bull. Johns Hopkins Hosp.* 117: 228–250.

Weiss, P. 1934. *In vitro* experiments on the factors determining the course of the outgrowing nerve fiber. *J. Exp. Zool.* 68: 393–448.

———. 1936. Selectivity controlling the central-peripheral relations in the nervous system. *Biol. Rev.* 11: 494–531.

Wise, S.P. and E.G. Jones. 1976. The organization and postnatal development of the commissural projection of the rat somatic sensory cortex. *J. Comp. Neurol.* 168: 313–343.

Wise, S.P. and E.G. Jones. 1978. Developmental studies of thalamocortical and commissural connections in the rat somatic sensory cortex. *J. Comp. Neurol.* 178: 187–208.

J. Physiol. (1980), **302**, pp. 581–602
With 1 *plate and* 8 *text-figures*
Printed in Great Britain

581

MOTONEURONE PROJECTION PATTERNS IN THE CHICK HIND LIMB FOLLOWING EARLY PARTIAL REVERSALS OF THE SPINAL CORD

By CYNTHIA LANCE-JONES AND LYNN LANDMESSER

*From the Biology Department, Yale University,
New Haven, Connecticut 06520, U.S.A.*

(*Received* 11 *July* 1979)

SUMMARY

1. The development of motoneurone projection patterns in the chick hind limb from reversed spinal cord segments was studied from the onset of axonal outgrowth (St. 24) to the establishment of mature connectivity patterns (St. 36). Approximately the first three lumbosacral cord segments were reversed along the anterior–posterior axis at St. 15–16.

2. Projection patterns from reversed cord segments were assessed electrophysiologically by direct spinal cord and spinal nerve stimulation and anatomically by retrograde horseradish peroxidase (HRP) labelling of motoneurones in St. 30–36 embryos. In younger embryos, paths taken by reversed axons were characterized by orthograde HRP labelling of motoneurones in specific reversed cord segments.

3. Lumbosacral motoneurones formed appropriate functional connexions with individual limb muscles in spite of anterior-posterior shifts in their spinal cord position and consequent shifts in their spinal nerve entry point into the limb bud. Reversed motoneurones supplying individual hind limb muscles formed discrete nuclei in the transverse plane of the cord. Each nucleus and the lateral motor column as a whole showed reversed topographical characteristics when compared to control embryos. These observations were made both before (St. 30) and after (St. 35–36) the major period of motoneurone cell death.

4. Correct connectivity resulted from specific alterations in axonal pathways within the plexus or major nerve trunks proximal to the branching of individual muscle nerves. Further such directed outgrowth was present from the earliest times that axons could be traced into the limb which is before the onset of motoneurone cell death and muscle cleavage.

5. It is concluded that motoneurones are specified to project to individual muscles or to follow particular pathways prior to motoneurone birthdays and limb bud formation. The establishment of specific motoneurone connectivity can not be accounted for by passive or mechanical guidance models alone. Rather, motoneurones must also actively respond to cues within the limb or interact among themselves on the basis of an early central specification.

INTRODUCTION

Anatomical and electrophysiological studies have shown that the motoneurones which innervate individual limb muscles are located in discrete pools within the spinal cord (Romanes, 1964; Cruce, 1974; Landmesser, 1978*a*), exit the cord in specific spinal nerves (Landmesser & Morris, 1975) and seem to form compact bundles within a specific region of the plexus and major nerve trunks (Ueyama, 1978; Stirling & Summerbell, 1979). Further, a general correlation exists between a neurone's anterior–posterior position in the cord and its target muscle's position in a normal limb (Landmesser, 1978b). These discrete spatial relationships may reflect an orderly axonal outgrowth pattern during development. Motoneurones may be passively guided to a particular target determined by their cord or plexus position (Horder, 1978). Motoneurones might also grow out in an orderly temporal sequence and form connexions with the nearest uninnervated muscle (Jacobson, 1978). Experimental evidence suggests that a spatio-temporal model for axonal outgrowth and synapse formation can account for the formation of specific optic fibre connexions in vertebrates (Bunt & Horder, 1978; Gaze, 1978) and invertebrates (Anderson, 1978; Macagno, 1978). While these models are economical in not requiring that each motoneurone and muscle have a specific identity, other characteristics of limb motoneurone projection patterns in the chick are not as compatible with a strictly passive contact guidance model for the establishment of specific connexions.

Motoneurone pools overlap extensively along the anterior–posterior axis of the cord and as a result their axons must cross one another in the periphery. It has been suggested that these discontinuities result from secondary events during development such as competition for targets or limb morphogenetic movements (Horder, 1978). However, the experimental evidence presented in the previous paper (Lance-Jones & Landmesser, 1980) excludes competition as necessary for the establishment of normal motoneurone projection patterns. In these deletion experiments, motoneurones appeared to recognize appropriate targets and did not innervate foreign but uninnervated tissue. Further, in the chick limb motoneurone projection patterns are correct and specific at early developmental stages prior to limb muscle morphogenesis (Landmesser & Morris, 1975; Landmesser, 1978b). These results are compatible with a hypothesis that motoneurones are specified to innervate a particular target or recognize correct pathways upon outgrowth. Such specificity might be imparted by the limb or develop independently. In either case, axonal outgrowth might be actively guided by cues within the limb (Morris, 1978). Studies *in vitro* (Letourneau, 1975, 1978; Ebendal, 1977) and *in vivo* (Hibbard, 1965) in other systems clearly demonstrate that axonal growth cones are active structures capable of responding differentially to environmental cues.

In order to address the question of whether motoneurones are specified prior to outgrowth an experiment was designed to provide lumbosacral motoneurones with a choice of pathways and targets within an unaltered and localized limb region. Specific lumbosacral cord segments were reversed prior to limb bud formation and lumbosacral motoneurone differentiation. Thus, axons from reversed segments were offered a choice between originally appropriate and spatially appropriate targets. Motoneurone projection patterns from the reversed cord segments were characterized from the time of initial axonal outgrowth to the establishment of the mature pattern using electrophysiological and anatomical horseradish peroxidase labelling techniques. A preliminary report of the results has been presented elsewhere (Lance-Jones & Landmesser, 1978).

METHODS

Surgical procedure

White Leghorn chick embryos were incubated until Stage (St.) 15–16 ($2\frac{1}{2}$–3 days) of Hamburger & Hamilton (1951). A window was made in the egg above the embryonic area with a dental drill and the embryo stained over the lumbosacral region with a small drop of a 1–2 % neutral red saline solution. After opening the vitelline membrane, the part of the spinal cord to be transposed was identified by reference to adjacent somites.

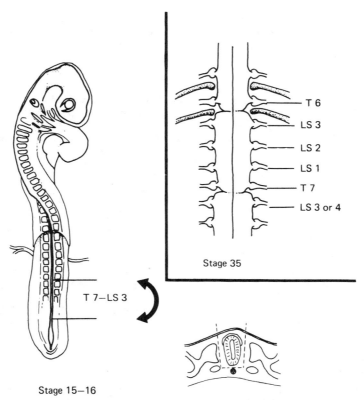

Fig. 1. Diagrams of the position and morphology of the cord segments reversed at the time of the operation (left) and at a representative time of examination (top right). The structures removed and reversed in the operation are shown in cross-section at the bottom right (within dashed lines). Not drawn to scale.

The anterior part of the lumbosacral enlargement, including cord segments 1 and 2 or 1–3 (segments 23–25 of Hamburger, 1975) were chosen for manipulation. In order to reverse these segments it was necessary to isolate that part of the cord opposite somites 26–29 (see Fig. 1). Variability in the actual extent of the reversal resulted from (1) slight changes in the developmental relationship between somite and cord segment number (see Wenger, 1951), (2) the necessity of estimating the position of the more posterior somites which have not formed at St. 15–16 and (3) the observation that between a quarter and one segment was often lost or damaged during the operation.

The spinal cord segments were freed laterally from the somitic tissue with tungsten needles. Transverse cuts were then made and the piece of cord separated from the underlying tissue. It was then rotated 180° along the anterior–posterior axis and placed back in line with the rest of the cord. In most cases the notochord was rotated with the spinal cord in order to minimize damage. Controls in which the notochord was not rotated gave similar results. Following the operation the embryo and vitelline membrane were moistened with Tyrode solution. The window was covered with a glass coverslip and sealed with paraffin, and the egg returned to the incubator.

Dissection

Experimental embryos were incubated until stages ranging from 24 to 36. The embryos were removed from the egg, placed into oxygenated Tyrode solution at 20–22 °C, staged, and dissected as described in a previous study by Landmesser (1978a). Following a ventral laminectomy of the thoracic and lumbosacral spinal cord, the extent of the reversal could be characterized visually (see Fig. 1). Small indentations on the ventrolateral edges of the cord were visible at the cranial and caudal ends of the transposed region. The lateral outline of the spinal cord usually expanded abruptly at the cranial end of the reversal, tapered down gradually, and expanded again just beyond the end of the reversal.

Electrophysiology

Techniques used to assess the innervation pattern of the embryonic limb have been described in earlier studies of normal projection patterns (Landmesser & Morris, 1975; Landmesser, 1978b). In St. 30 and 35–36 embryos muscle contraction was elicited by direct cord stimulation and/or by spinal nerve stimulation which were found to give equivalent results. Direct cord stimulation involved the use of suction electrodes at selected sites along the ventrolateral margin of the cord or just over ventral root exit regions. Stimulation points were mapped on a drawing of the cord. In order to examine spinal nerve patterns, the cord was removed and individual nerves isolated and stimulated with suction electrodes. Muscle contraction was scored for each cord point or nerve either visually or by recording electromyograms. Suction or bipolar silver electrodes were used to record electrical activity from the medial surface of individual muscles.

Retrograde labelling with horseradish peroxidase

Three muscles, the sartorius, femorotibialis and adductor have motoneurone pools which are located in specific regions of the first three segments of the lumbosacral lateral motor column (Landmesser, 1978a). In order to examine the topography of these pools muscles were injected with horseradish peroxidase (HRP) in St. 30 or St. 35–36 experimental embryos, after ascertaining the extent of the reversal by direct cord stimulation. The procedures for HRP injection, histological processing, and the counting and mapping of labelled motoneurones were described by Landmesser (1978a). Limbs were also histologically processed for visualization of the injection site.

Orthograde labelling with HRP

In order to characterize the pathways of limb innervating motor axons during the outgrowth period, an orthograde HRP labelling technique was designed (see Lance-Jones & Landmesser, 1980). The segment at the anterior end of the reversal region was filled directly with HRP on one side of an experimental embryo, the segment at the posterior end on the other. These segments corresponded in most cases to the 3rd and 1st lumbosacral segments, respectively. Camera lucida drawings and graphic reconstructions were made of the nerve patterns within the limbs of embryos ranging in age from St. 24 to 30. Control injections were also made into normal embryonic cords at an equivalent stage of development.

RESULTS

Anatomy of the reversed segments and spinal nerves

At St. 30 and St. 35–36 individual lumbosacral segments can be identified on the basis of the size and concomitant lateral expansion of the lateral motor column. The number of lateral motoneurones increases as one progresses caudally through the lumbosacral enlargement, reaching a maximum number per segment around LS 6 and then declining through LS 8 (see Hamburger, 1975). In LS 1 and LS 8 the lateral motor column projects very little beyond the external contours of the ventrolateral grey matter. Between these segments the lateral motor column is large and extends well beyond the rest of the grey matter. Within this area, the glycogen body aids further in segment identification as it usually is found in segments 4–7.

In embryos in which the first three segments have been reversed, the characteristic morphology of the individual cord segment is maintained despite 180° rotation. A series of representative sections taken from progressively more posterior segments through the posterior thoracic and lumbosacral spinal cord of a control and experimental St. 36 embryo is shown in Pl. 1. The reversed LS 3 has a large and laterally expanded motor column even though it is now in a more anterior position adjacent to thoracic segments. The reversed LS 1, now posterior to LS 3, nevertheless has a very small lateral motor column like its counterpart in the control. Sections taken from segments beyond the reversal region appeared anatomically normal. These morphological characteristics account for the abrupt expansion and then tapering of the reversed cord seen after the ventral laminectomy (see Fig. 1). The development of normal segmental morphology despite an altered anterior–posterior orientation suggests that the form of the lateral motor column is determined prior to St. 15–16. It should be noted that a disordered or abnormal cord region equivalent to about a quarter to half a segment was usually found at each end of the reversed cord. These regions were frequently characterized by whorls of commonly oriented cells projecting beyond the normal contours of the grey matter, a displaced central canal and poor development of the dorsal white matter. As a result, in small reversals (less than two segments) a morphological reversal was not as evident.

Spinal nerves emanating from the region of a reversal appeared anatomically discrete and could be identified as specific spinal nerves corresponding in number to the number of segments reversed. In a few cases, small extra spinal nerves or fibre groups projected from the junctional regions but usually these could be identified as parts of the major spinal nerves. Further, spinal nerve patterns within the limb and plexus formation appeared normal despite the fact that these nerves were projecting from transposed segments. Thus, spinal nerves appeared to be taking routes anatomically appropriate to their new position.

Segmental and spinal nerve projection patterns from the reversed cord region to individual muscles in the St. 35–36 embryonic limb.

The normal motoneurone and spinal nerve projection patterns from the first three segments of the lumbosacral cord to the limb of a St. 36 embryo are schematically shown in Fig. 2. This diagram represents a summary of data from the studies of Landmesser & Morris (1975) and Landmesser (1978a). Four muscles, the sartorius, femorotibialis, adductor and ischio-flexorius receive all or most of their motor innervation from these segments. Of these muscles, the sartorius and femorotibialis were chosen for close electrophysiological examination. These two muscles have motoneurone pools which overlap only slightly in the anterior half of segment two. The sartorius, one of the most anterior muscles of the thigh normally contracts in response to stimulation of spinal nerves 1 and 2. The femorotibialis, a slightly more posterior muscle, contracts in response to stimulation of spinal nerves 2 and 3.

E.m.g.s recorded from these muscles following spinal nerve stimulation in a normal and an experimental St. 36 embryo are shown in Fig. 3. When the first three spinal segments were reversed, the spinal nerve projection pattern was reversed. The sartorius was innervated by the last two spinal nerves of the reversal. These nerves projected from the reversed first and second segments indicating that they had established appropriate muscle connexions. Similarly, the femorotibialis contracted in response to stimulation of anterior spinal nerves which projected from the displaced posterior segments.

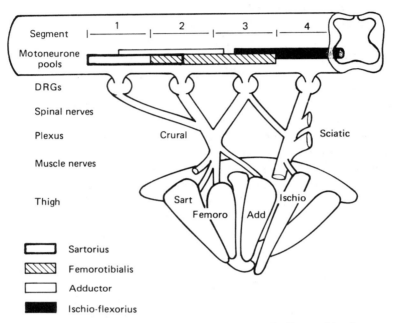

Fig. 2. Schematic diagram of the spinal cord and hind limb illustrating the motoneurone projection patterns from the first four lumbosacral segments to the sartorius, femorotibialis, adductor and ischio-flexorius muscles. The cranio-caudal extents of motoneurone pools innervating each muscle are graphically represented. While pools overlap on this axis, they are discrete in the transverse plane. DRG, dorsal root ganglion.

In twenty-five experimental St. 35 or 36 embryos, projection patterns were mapped by direct cord stimulation and/or spinal nerve stimulation. Visual observation of muscle contraction in all cases revealed that appropriate connexions were established in spite of the altered anterior-posterior position of cord segments. In twenty-two of these embryonic limbs, e.m.g.s monitored in the femorotibialis and sartorius muscles confirmed visual observations. A schematic tabulation of muscle responses is presented in Fig. 4. In individual embryos, stimulation of a given spinal nerve or the cord adjacent to it produced the same response. Therefore, axons did not take aberrant courses of exit from the cord; rather, they projected from individual cord segments via the corresponding spinal nerve.

The length of cord which was reversed without damage varied from 1 to $2\frac{1}{2}$ segments, the largest reversal encompassing LS 1, LS 2 and the anterior part of LS 3. The sequence of muscle contractions in response to sequential stimulations is a mirror image of the normal innervation pattern. In all reversals contraction of the femorotibialis was always elicited by stimulation at the anterior end of the transposed region. In large reversals, a mid-reversal stimulation elicited both sartorius and femorotibialis responses and more posterior stimulation elicited only sartorius contraction. In some embryos only small sections of the reversed cord gave rise to muscle contractions presumably as a result of damage to the ends of the reversed segments. The projection patterns from these small areas matched discrete and identifiable parts of the control in mirror image. As can be seen in Fig. 4, these areas usually corresponded to a reversed LS 2. The undamaged sections of the cord thus seemed to behave as a mosaic showing no indication of compression of the whole projection pattern.

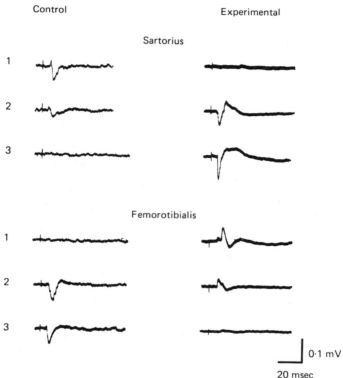

Fig. 3. E.m.g. recordings from the sartorius and femorotibialis muscles at St. 36 in a control embryo (left) and in an experimental embryo in which the first three cord segments had been reversed (right). Stimulation of spinal nerves 1 and 2 elicited responses from the sartorius in the control embryo. In the experimental embryo, spinal nerves 2 and 3 (numbered according to their order of projection from the cord after the reversal, not according to their origin prior to reversal) caused sartorius contraction. The femorotibialis contracted in response to stimulation of LS 2 and 3 in the control but LS 1 and 2 in the reversal embryo.

In some cases, electrophysiological evidence indicated that motoneurone pools to individual muscles had been split and parts of the pools reversed, giving rise to separation along the anterior–posterior axis of the cord. Two examples of spatially separated projections to the femorotibialis are illustrated in Fig. 4. Stimulation at the anterior end of the reversed cord and at the beginning of the normal cord posterior to the operated area elicited femorotibialis contraction. The femorotibialis was thus appropriately innervated by the reversed second segment and by segment 3 which was not included in the reversal. The segmental projection to the sartorius muscle was also split in the first example. Here a part of segment 1 had not been reversed. Stimulation just anterior to the reversal region and at its posterior end gave rise to sartorius contraction. Thus the topography of individual projection patterns as well as the relationship between them are altered by a reversal.

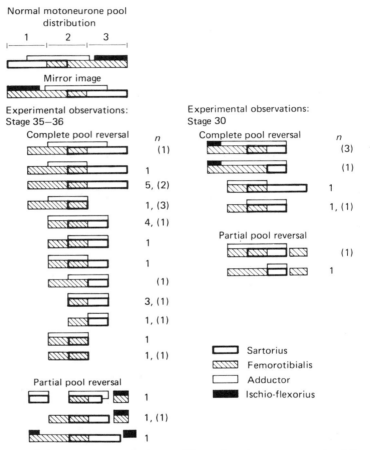

Fig. 4. Summary of the anterior–posterior position of motoneurone pools, following partial spinal cord reversals in St. 35–36 (left) and St. 30 (right) embryos as determined electrophysiologically. The normal motoneurone pool distribution and the mirror image appearance expected following complete reversal are shown at the top. Each change in muscle response along the horizontal axes marks a shift to a new recording site on the cord or to the next spinal nerve. In the partial pool reversals, gaps along the horizontal axis represent transitions between non-reversed and reversed cord regions. The complete pool reversal diagrams are vertically organized according to the size of the reversal discounting disorganized cord regions. In a few cases only sartorius and femorotibialis contractions were scored. Reversed motoneurone pools generally are similar to all or part of the mirror image control. n = number of limbs in which e.m.g.s were recorded. (n) = additional limbs in which muscle contraction was scored visually.

Projection patterns from reversed cord segments to the adductor and ischio-flexorius muscles were less easily interpreted than those to the sartorius or femoro-tibialis. In only one St. 35–36 embryo was there a clear indication of a reversal of a part of the ischio-flexorius motoneurone pool, which normally lies in LS 3 and 4. As shown in Fig. 4, stimulation at the anterior end of the reversed cord segments and just posterior to them, gave rise to contraction of the ischio-flexorius. While the low frequency of this occurrence might suggest that motoneurones are only capable of establishing appropriate connexions, if displaced only limited distances, it appears more likely that the motoneurones to the ischio-flexorius were often damaged as a result of the reversal. In most cases where part or all of segment 3 had been reversed, no contraction of the ischio-flexorius could be elicited from any part of the cord at all. The extent of cord contributing to the innervation of the femorotibialis also appeared shorter than normal in these operations (see Fig. 4). Further, segment 4 which also innervates the ischio-flexorius, was frequently damaged. Projection of cord segments posterior to the reversal region normally corresponded to those of normal segments 5–8. It thus appears that the disorganized cord areas usually included the moto-neurone pool of the ischio-flexorius. Identification of segments on the basis of cord morphology supported this. However, even larger cord reversals are necessary before this can be definitely determined.

The adductor muscle of a normal embryo is primarily innervated by spinal nerves 1 and 2. However, most of the motoneurones which project to the adductor are located in segment 2 (see Landmesser, 1978a). Thus, a reversal of LS 1, 2 and part of 3 alters the position of the pool, as a whole, only slightly, and little information about the appropriateness of projection patterns to the adductor can be gained from the type of analysis presented in Fig. 4. However, in some muscles including the adductor, segmental and spinal nerve projection patterns vary depending on the region of the muscle from which one is recording. In a normal embryo, stimulation at the cranial end of segment 1 consistently elicits contraction at the posterior border of the adductor and little or no contraction at the anterior border. Further posteriorly in segments 1 and 2 stimulation gives rise to contraction at both borders of the adductor. Following the reversal of segments 1 and 2, this innervation pattern was observed to be reversed as well.

Topography of motoneurone pools in a St. 35–36 embryo

The electrophysiological data indicate that motoneurones within a particular segment establish appropriate limb muscle connexions in spite of the alterations in their position along the anterior–posterior axis of the cord. However, these data provide little information about the topographical relationships of motoneurone pools in the transverse plane of the cord or about the normality of the spatial distri-bution of motoneurones to an individual muscle. In order to localize motoneurones in the reversed and adjacent segments of the lumbosacral cord which project to an individual muscle, the retrograde transport of HRP was utilized. HRP was injected into either the sartorius, femorotibialis or adductor in each limb of ten St. 35–36 experimental embryos after the extent of the reversal had been characterized electro-physiologically.

In all cases, reversed motoneurones which were labelled by injection of a single muscle were found in a discrete nucleus positioned normally in the transverse plane. In segments where two or more affected motoneurone pools overlapped along the anterior–posterior axis, the individual pools were separated in the dorso-ventral and medio-lateral axes. Individual motoneurone pools could thus be identified by their location in transverse cord sections, as in the normal condition (see Landmesser, 1978*a*).

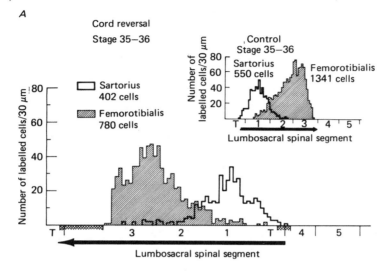

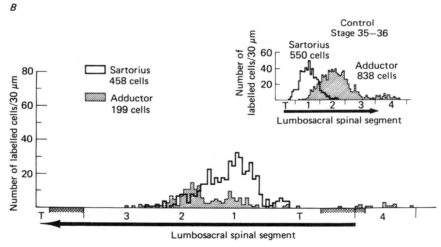

Fig. 5. Anterior–posterior positions of motoneurones projecting from reversed cord segments to individual limb muscles determined anatomically. *A*, histogram of labelled motoneurones in a St. 35–36 experimental embryo in which the femorotibialis had been injected on one side, the sartorius on the other. Inset at top shows a similar injection in a control embryo. *B*, histogram of St. 35–36 experimental and control (inset) embryos in which the adductor and sartorius had been similarly injected. Note that the adductor motoneurone pool has been split into two parts as a result of the operation in the experimental embryo. The arrows indicate cord segments reversed and the corresponding region in a control. Cross-hatched areas represent damaged cord sections.

In order to characterize the distribution of motoneurones within a nucleus, histograms of the number of labelled motoneurones per 30 μm increment of lumbosacral cord were constructed and compared to histograms of normal motoneurone pools compiled from the original data of Landmesser (1978a). It should be noted that while motoneurone distribution could be compared in the control and experimental embryos, the actual number of motoneurones could not be readily compared due to segmental damage following a reversal and variability in the number of motoneurones normally projecting to individual muscles.

As is clearly evident in Figs. 5 and 6, the spatial distribution of the reversed motoneurones to an individual muscle confirms the electrophysiological data. In the case illustrated in Fig. 5A, the sartorius and femorotibialis motoneurone pools were totally reversed by the reversal of segments LS 1–3. Both nuclei have peaks in reversed normal positions; the sartorius in LS 1, the femorotibialis in LS 3. Injections into both muscles gave rise to at least a small number of labelled cells in all segments. While this is often the case following femorotibialis injections in normal embryos (see Fig. 6), labelled cells are not normally found in segment 3 as a result of HRP injection into the sartorius. Although these might represent a few aberrant connexions, some leakage of HRP into the adjacent femorotibialis is a more likely possibility. In normal and most experimental St. 35–36 embryos, the sartorius motoneurone nucleus is distinctly more lateral than that of the femorotibialis. In the experimental embryo illustrated in Fig. 5A, the bulk of labelled cells in the reversed segments 1 and 2 were positioned quite laterally in the cord and formed a nucleus of cells unseparated by unlabelled cells. The few labelled cells in segment 3 were isolated from one another and in a position in the transverse plane characteristic of femorotibialis motoneurones.

Fig. 5B shows a cord reversal in which the adductor muscle had been injected on one side and the sartorius on the other. Again the spatial pattern of each motoneurone pool has been conserved. A small portion of the adductor motoneurone pool in segment 4 was not reversed in the operation and formed a separate small nucleus of labelled cells which projected to the adductor. Although the number of motoneurones was lower than normal (603 ± 43) in this embryo, injections into other embryonic adductor muscles following a reversal have given normal sized pools.

A more striking case of a split motoneurone pool is presented in Fig. 6. In the example illustrated, only one of the segments which normally projects to the femorotibialis, LS 2, was reversed. Following HRP injection into this muscle, labelled motoneurones were found in two separate pools along the cranio-caudal axis of the lateral motor column, whereas in the normal embryo a similar number of motoneurones are found in one pool in segments LS 2 and 3. Direct cord stimulation at four points confirmed that the femorotibialis muscle was mainly innervated by the reversed second segment and by segment 3 which was not included in the reversal.

Motoneurone projection patterns prior to the peak of cell death

It has been suggested that the large amount of cell death which occurs in the lateral motor column in the chick between St. 30 and 35 might be the result of the loss of cells which have formed inappropriate or an insufficient number of appropriate connexions in the limb (Hamburger, 1975). If such an event occurred one might postulate that although inappropriate connexions are not seen in St. 35 or 36 embryos following a partial lumbosacral cord reversal, such connexions may have been present earlier in development. In order to examine this possibility, motoneurone projection patterns were characterized in experimental embryos at St. 30, preceding the peak of cell death in the lateral motor column. In nine embryos in which part or all of LS 1–3 had been reversed, electrophysiological and anatomical observations yielded results comparable to those obtained at St. 35–36. No evidence of incorrect connexions or connexions in accord with a new cord position was found.

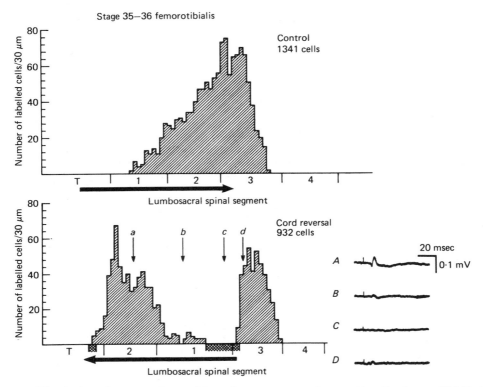

Fig. 6. Anterior–posterior position of motoneurones innervating the femorotibialis following a reversal that split the motoneurone pool. A control femorotibialis motor nucleus (top) extends from the end of segment 1–3. In a St. 35–36 experimental embryo (bottom) femorotibialis motoneurones are found in two nuclei, one in reversed segment 2, the other posterior to the reversal in segment 3. Inset shows e.m.g.s recorded from the femorotibialis in response to stimulation at four points (a–d) along the cord whose spatial distribution is indicated above the histogram.

Axonal pathways

The electrophysiological evidence presented above demonstrates that motoneurones in reversed cord segments projected via adjacent spinal nerves into the limb. Alterations in their pathways must have been made distal to this point in order to account for the establishment of appropriate connexions. One possibility is that motoneurones projected initially to targets in accord with their new anterior-posterior position, 'recognized' the incorrectness of the muscle, and then altered

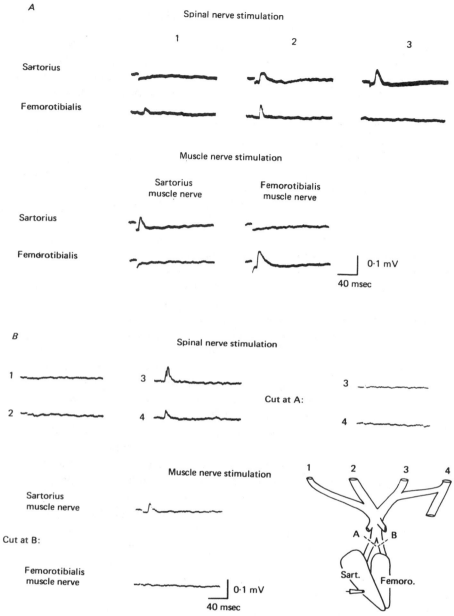

Fig. 7. Pathways taken by reversed sartorius and femorotibialis motoneurones determined electrophysiologically. *A*, e.m.g. recordings from both muscles in a St. 34 embryo in which the first three segments were reversed. Spinal nerve projection patterns are reversed (compare to Fig. 3, control), but muscle nerve pathways are normal, each muscle contracting only in response to stimulation of the appropriate muscle nerve. *B*, e.m.g. recordings from the sartorius muscle in a St. 34 embryo. Sartorius contraction was elicited by stimulation of the 3rd and 4th spinal nerves projecting from the reversed cord. These responses disappeared after transecting the sartorius muscle nerve (level *A* in the diagram). Stimulation of the cut distal stumps of the sartorius and femorotibialis muscle nerves (A and B) indicates that axons innervating the sartorius course through the sartorius muscle nerve only.

their course to establish connexions with the correct muscle. While the anatomical pattern of muscle nerves appeared to be normal, small branches might go undetected if they projected between muscles. In order to examine this possibility individual muscle nerves of St. 34–36 embryos were isolated and stimulated with suction electrodes and e.m.g.s recorded from muscles innervated by reversed motoneurones. The sartorius and femorotibialis were chosen for examination as they are directly apposed to one another in the limb. In a normal embryo, each muscle is innervated by discrete branches off the femoral trunk (Landmesser & Morris, 1975). Anatomically similar muscle nerves could be identified in experimental embryos.

These muscle nerves were cut and stimulated after an electrophysiological identification of spinal nerve projection patterns to the femorotibialis and sartorius. Two examples of the results obtained are shown in Fig. 7. In the first experimental embryo (Fig. 7*A*) sequential stimulation of spinal nerves projecting from the reversal region indicated that the sartorius and femorotibialis motoneurones exited the cord in a reversed order. However, muscle nerve stimulation showed that motoneurone axons coursed through appropriate muscle nerves. Thus, reversed motoneurone axons corrected their pathways between the level of the spinal nerves and the muscle nerves. In the second example (Fig. 7*B*), stimulation of spinal nerves 3 and 4 elicited responses in the sartorius which disappeared after transection of the sartorius muscle nerve. We did not detect any connexions which might have been made by axons taking aberrant pathways to the sartorius. Since the sartorius muscle was activated by stimulation of the sartorius muscle nerve, but not the femorotibialis muscle nerve, we can conclude that displaced sartorius motoneurones did not first grow down the femorotibialis muscle nerve and then cross over to innervate the sartorius muscle. These results suggest that axons can recognize or are directed to their target at some distance from its actual location.

However, it is possible that a period of pathway modification might occur between the time of initial axonal outgrowth and St. 35–36. Experimental evidence in the amphibian limb (Lamb, 1976; 1977; McGrath & Bennett, 1979) and the chick wing (Pettigrew, Lindeman & Bennett, 1979) suggests that some incorrect projections are made and subsequently removed during normal embryogenesis. Further, these events occur just prior to and at the onset of motoneurone cell death periods in the cord. Orthograde labelling of motoneurones with HRP (see Methods) lends itself particularly well to this question as it allows the visualization of regionally identified motoneurones and their axons from the time of initial axonal outgrowth into the chick hind limb (St. 23–24) to the time at which correct connectivity patterns are seen and muscle cleavage has occurred (St. $28\frac{1}{2}$–30). Twenty-two cord reversal embryos ranging from St. 24–30 were examined utilizing this technique.

At all stages labelled axons projected into the limb in discrete bundles as they do in normal embryos (C. Lance-Jones & L. Landmesser, unpublished observations). No indications of random or diffuse outgrowth were found even in the youngest material. Axonal pathway differences between control and experimental embryos, were visible as early as St. 24 (Fig. 8). In a normal St. 23–24 embryo labelled axons from lumbosacral segment 1 maintain an anterior topographical position as they project via spinal nerve 1 to the base of the limb. Axons destined for axial musculature branch off the anterior proximal border of the spinal nerve. In an experimental embryo in which T7–LS 3 had been reversed, labelled axons from T7 and LS 1 mainly project straight into the limb as normal LS 3 motoneurones do. However, a few labelled axons clearly cross in the plexus region and appear to be growing towards the anterior axial musculature. No such crossing is visible following the labelling of LS 3 motoneurones in a normal embryo.

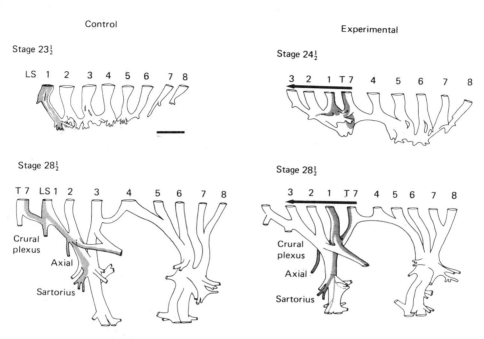

Fig. 8. Pathways taken by motoneurones projecting from segments T 7 and LS 1. Paths of axons labelled by direct HRP injection into the cord are stippled. Left: control embryos injected at stages before (top) and after (bottom) the onset of motoneurone cell death and muscle cleavage. Right: experimental embryos in which four segments had been reversed (T7–LS3) injected at similar stages. Calibration bar = 255 μm.

At later stages, labelled axons can be followed to individual muscle primordia (see Fig. 8). Labelled motoneurones projecting from reversed segments exited the cord in adjacent spinal nerves as they do in a normal embryo. Distally, however, they alter their course either within the plexus or proximal nerve trunks to project to correct targets. In the control St. 28½ embryo labelled T7 and LS 1 motoneurone axons projecting to the sartorius and the axial musculature maintain an anterior position within spinal nerves, the plexus, and nerve trunks. In the experimental embryo the labelled axons course from a posterior to anterior position just prior to the branching of the discrete muscle nerves. Thus, motor axons appeared to pass over inappropriate muscles or muscle regions directly in their path. A few labelled axons project to other muscles. While not seen in the control illustrated, such projections from segment 1 were found in other normal embryos. Similar results were obtained following injections of a reversed LS 3. Labelled motoneurones crossed from the anterior to the posterior side of the femoral trunk and projected to the femorotibialis muscle via the femorotibialis muscle nerves. Such pathway alterations were visible as early as sartorius and femorotibialis muscle nerves could be identified (St. 25½–26) and before muscle cleavage. Thus, motoneurone axons do not seem to follow inappropriate pathways even transiently.

DISCUSSION

Morphological polarity

Previous investigations have shown that, in general, regional determination along the anterior-posterior axis of the neural tube occurs between the neural plate stage and the time of neural fold closure. Anterior-posterior reversals or displacements of prospective brain tissue in the amphibian neural plate or tube indicate that individual regions behave as mosaics in spite of inappropriate surrounding tissue (Jacobson, 1964; Chung & Cooke, 1978). Similarly, chick brachial, thoracic and lumbosacral cord regions differentiate in accordance with their origin in spite of early alterations of their position along the anterior–posterior axis of the cord (Bueker, 1945; Wenger, 1951). Experiments involving limb ablations or additions confirm these observations and suggest that the initial pattern of motoneurone proliferation and differentiation is independent of the periphery (Hamburger, 1939, 1958; Hollyday, Hamburger & Farris, 1977).

Our study demonstrates that the morphology of the lateral motor column in individual segments of the lumbosacral cord is also determined prior to limb bud formation and axonal outgrowth. The size of the lateral motor column in reversed cord segments is characteristic of its origin before the reversal. That this is not a result of differential motoneurone survival following the establishment of appropriate peripheral connexions is demonstrated by segmental morphological differences at St. 30 prior to the major motoneurone cell death peak.

Active vs. passive mechanisms

The present study demonstrates that motoneurones from reversed cord segments establish functional connexions in accord with their original cord position. The size, form and topographical positions of individual motoneurone pools within the reversed segments are conserved in a mirror image of the normal condition. Reversed motoneurones exit the cord via adjacent spinal nerves and therefore are confronted with a foreign environment. Motoneurones then demonstrate a specific pathway or target preference by altering their course and establishing correct connexions. These pathway alterations are apparent from the onset of axonal penetration into specific limb regions. At no time in their development did reversed motoneurones project to incorrect muscle primordia.

These observations provide the first clear evidence that the establishment of specific motor connexions is an active process. Limb motoneurones do not form a homogeneous or unspecified pool prior to outgrowth. Rather, by St. 15 intrinsic differences between motoneurones exist such that upon outgrowth axons are capable of 'choosing' appropriate pathways or targets. The acquisition of these differences or target specificities is independent of direct limb interactions. Cord segments were reversed before limb bud formation and the birth of lumbosacral motoneurones (see Hollyday & Hamburger, 1977). If the limb normally determines motoneurone identity, one would have expected the specification of reversed motoneurones in accord with their new cord position.

Two major hypotheses implicating passive contact guidance mechanisms alone in the establishment of specific connectivity in the limb are thus ruled out by our results. Horder (1978) has argued that at the time of initial fibre outgrowth parallel arrays of neurones and muscles exist and that motoneurone distribution to particular muscles is dictated solely by fibre arrangement and by morphogenetic events within the limb. Although there is an early general correspondence between motoneurone position along the anterior–posterior axis of the cord and muscle position in the limb (Landmesser, 1978b), the present experiments clearly refute Horder's hypothesis. In the cord reversed embryos, axons exit the cord in a disrupted topographical order and course through foreign tissue yet are able to find appropriate pathways to their respective targets.

The second hypothesis invokes a temporal as well as spatial gradient of axonal outgrowth into the limb (Jacobson, 1978). Motoneurones that grew as a result of general spatial constraints to a particular limb region would bypass muscles innervated by axons which had grown out earlier and would innervate the neighbouring uninnervated target. In our experimental embryos, axons from reversed cord segments clearly bypassed muscles which would have been innervated by motoneurones exiting from that cord level in a normal embryo. In order to account for these results in terms of this model, one would have to suggest that muscles are innervated in a disrupted temporal order in the cord reversal embryos. It is possible that motoneurones are prespecified only with respect to time of outgrowth. The observed correct patterns after a reversal might then be due to an unaltered time of axonal outgrowth. However, the temporal sequence of limb innervation in both the normal and cord reversed chick embryos does not show sufficient variability along the anterior–posterior axis to account for selective connectivity. As early as St. 24, all but the eighth spinal nerve contribute to the formation of the plexus and are at parallel levels along the proximo–distal limb axis. Thus observations of correct and specific motoneurone projection patterns in partial cord reversal and also deletion experiments (Lance-Jones & Landmesser, 1980) refute this hypothesis.

Limb directed processes

We do not mean to suggest that passive or mechanical factors are not involved in the establishment of connectivity. Although motoneurone axons clearly alter their pathways to reach appropriate targets in our experiments, the anatomical pattern of the plexus and major trunks is similar to that in a normal embryo. Further, the major muscle nerves affected, those to the sartorius and femorotibialis muscles, branch from the femoral trunk in a normal sequence and spatial pattern. These observations are compatible with results following other experimental manipulations of the cord or limb. Nerves projecting from foreign cord segments into a normal or supernumerary limb form a grossly normal pattern in chicks (Hamburger, 1939; Wenger, 1951; Straznicky, 1967; Hollyday, Hamburger & Farris, 1977; Morris,

1978) and amphibians (Detwiler, 1920, 1936; Piatt, 1956; Szekely, 1963). Following anterior–posterior and anterior–posterior, dorsal–ventral reversals of the chick limb (Narayanan, 1964; Morris, 1978; Stirling & Summerbell, 1979; Ferguson, unpublished observations) or complete brachial cord reversals in amphibians (Detwiler, 1923), the form of the plexus mirrors the orientation of the limb rather than that of the cord. Further, the pathways taken by nerves in chick wings following proximo-distal deletions, truncations (Stirling & Summerbell, 1977) and duplications (Lewis, 1978) appear to be appropriate for the limb region approached by the outgrowing axons. All of these experiments, including ours, suggest that limb directed processes can affect anatomical nerve branching patterns.

What then is the relationship between passive and active processes in the development of specific connectivity in the limb? When a disparity is experimentally created between the anterior–posterior position of the cord and limb, two conflicting results are obtained. In the cord reversal experiments, motoneurones appear to actively recognize the disparity and establish correct connexions. However, following other experimental manipulations, the polarity of the limb appears totally to govern axonal outgrowth and incorrect connexions are formed (Hollyday et al. 1977; Morris, 1978; Stirling & Summerbell, 1979). Several hypothesis may account for these differences and define conditions necessary for the formation of correct connexions.

The conditions for the establishment of specific connectivity patterns

Although our results indicate that motoneurones differ at St. 15, we know little of the nature of these differences. One possibility is that each motoneurone bears a specific label corresponding to a particular muscle and that correct connexions are established as a result of differential chemo-affinities between axons and specific targets or pathways (see Sperry, 1963). An active target or pathway recognition could then account for the formation of correct connexions in the cord reversal experiments and also in deletion experiments (see Lance-Jones & Landmesser, 1980). The apparent absence of such recognition following other experimental manipulations might result because motoneurones have been radically displaced. Following an anterior–posterior limb reversal or the addition of a supernumerary limb, axons which would normally course through the anterior half of the limb in the crural plexus are confronted with posterior limb tissue and ischiadic plexus pathways. In a three or four segment cord reversal correct pathway alterations need only be made within the crural plexus. It might be hypothesized that motoneurones are only capable of responding to local cytochemical cues. Normally, passive or general limb-directed processes may ensure that axons get to muscle regions in which they can respond to such cues. Further displacements may give rise to connectivity determined by passive mechanisms which only generally approximates a normal spatially ordered pattern. Alternatively, a hierarchy of neuronal specificities may exist such that motoneurones chose the most appropriate muscle in a particular region (see Hollyday et al. 1977). It is not possible to distinguish between these possibilities with the data presently available. Although it is known that patterned connexions are formed in anterior–posterior reversed or supernumerary limbs and that their polarity corresponds to that of the limb (Hollyday et al. 1977; Morris, 1978), topographical relationships between motoneurone pools in the cord have not been sufficiently characterized. Thus, the degree of selectivity shown by motoneurones in a foreign environment has yet to be determined.

One need not suggest that each muscle and neurone bears a specific biochemical label. Rather, motoneurones might be specified to respond differentially to a gradient of some sort distributed along the anterior–posterior axis in the periphery. An axial gradient might guide axons to a particular limb region where separate mechanisms would operate to define innervational boundaries and specific synaptic connectivity. Such secondary processes might include limits on the number of synapses a moto-neurone can form, physical boundaries created by dividing muscles, or competition for a trophic factor in the periphery (see Feldman, 1977; Lance-Jones & Landmesser, 1980). A likely site for the axial gradient is within the tissue between the cord and limb proper. Preliminary evidence based on tracings of retrograde HRP labelled axons suggests that axons sort out into discrete bundles destined for a particular muscle within a short distance from the cord (Landmesser, 1978*b* and unpublished observations). Further, reconstructions of axonal pathways following the ortho-grade labelling of individual reversed cord segments demonstrate that the displaced axons alter their course by crossing through the plexus or femoral nerve trunk before entering specific muscle regions. Thus, motoneurones may be actively choosing pathways on the basis of cues emanating from tissue immediately adjacent to the cord, such as somitic or lateral mesenchyme. Such a proximal sorting out process might account for the differing results in anterior–posterior limb reversal and cord reversal experiments. In the former, motoneurones grow into an immediate periphery which is not reversed. Consequently, motoneurone axons would take spatially normal pathways which would lead them to incorrect muscles in the reversed limb. However, following a cord reversal, the outgrowing axons would immediately encounter tissue of reversed polarity and thus alter their course appropriately.

Alternatively or in addition to active interactions between neurones and peripheral structures, interactions between neurones may determine the pathways taken by limb motoneurones. Models implicating fibre sorting mechanisms based on a neurone's original position (Cook & Horder, 1977; Hope, Hammond & Gaze, 1976) and the maintenance of neighbour relationships between two structural arrays (von der Malsberg & Willshaw, 1977) have been proposed to account for the formation of retino-tectal connexions. It is possible that motoneurones acquire topological speci-ficity on the basis of their position in the cord which is manifested in a subsequent sorting out process within the limb. For example, motoneurones regardless of their relative level in the cord (i.e. brachial, thoracic or lumbosacral) may distribute to particular peripheral paths or targets by interacting among themselves according to their relative early cranio-caudal axial position and that of their neighbours. This hypothesis is compatible with anterior–posterior limb and cord reversal results if one assumes that cues within the immediate periphery provide the polarity information necessary to orient the sorting out process. In addition, it can account for the orderly innervation of supernumerary and adjacent ipsilateral limbs by a less than normal complement of spinal nerves. It is possible that differences between motoneurones are quantitative or graded rather than qualitative. Thus, axons within four spinal nerves would sort out spatially in a manner similar to those in the normal eight spinal nerves innervating the limb on the basis of relative differences. However, a neuronal interaction model cannot account for the results of our cord deletion experiments in which remaining motoneurones innervate only their normal targets, leaving some limb regions entirely devoid of innervation. If a fibre sorting mechanism does operate during normal development, one must suggest that additional factors determine the area over which neurones can interact.

It is not possible to fully explain the establishment of chick limb connectivity without invoking the operation of active as well as passive mechanisms. Our results clearly demonstrate that motoneurones possess specific identities prior to axonal outgrowth and direct limb interactions. However, several conditions may be necessary before specific and correct connexions can be established. If such conditions are not met, motoneurones may obey other laws governed by their origin within the cord, by cues emanating from the limb, or by a hierarchy of target or pathway preferences. Alternatively, only passive mechanisms may be operative. In order to examine these possibilities, precise characterizations of motoneurone projection patterns to individual muscles are necessary under various experimental conditions.

We would like to thank Miss Betty Ferguson and Miss Marcia Honig for critically evaluating the manuscript, Mr Matthew Winer for his technical help and Mrs Frances Hunihan for her expert secretarial assistance. Supported by NIH grant NS 10666 and postdoctoral fellowship NS 05990.

REFERENCES

ANDERSON, H. (1978). Postembryonic development of the visual system of the locust, *Schistocera gregaria*. II. An experimental investigation of the formation of the retina-lamina projection. *J. Embryol. exp. Morph.* **46**, 147–170.

BUEKER, E. D. (1945). The influence of a growing limb on the differentiation of somatic motor neurones in transplanted avian spinal cord segments. *J. comp. Neurol.* **82**, 335–361.

BUNT, S. M. & HORDER, T. J. (1978). Evidence for an orderly arrangement of optic axons in the central pathways of vertebrates and its implications for the formation and regeneration of optic projections. *Neurosci. Abstr.* **4**, 468.

CHUNG, S-H. & COOKE, J. (1978). Observations on the formation of the brain and of nerve connections following embryonic manipulation of the amphibian neural tube. *Proc. R. Soc.* B **201**, 335–373.

COOK, J. E. & HORDER, T. J. (1977). The multiple factors determining retinotopic order in the growth of optic fibres into the optic tectum. *Phil. Trans. R. Soc.* B **278**, 261–276.

CRUCE, W. L. R. (1974). The anatomical organisation of hind limb motor neurones in the lumbar spinal cord of the frog, *Rana catesbeiana*. *J. comp. Neurol.* **153**, 59–76.

DETWILER, S. R. (1920). Experiments on transplantation of limbs in *Amblystoma*. The formation of nerve plexuses and the function of the limbs. *J. exp. Zool.* **31**, 117–169.

DETWILER, S. R. (1923). Experiments on the reversal of the spinal cord in *Amblystoma* embryos at the level of the anterior limb. *J. exp. Zool.* **38**, 293–321.

DETWILER, S. R. (1936). *Neuroembryology: An Experimental Study.* New York: Macmillan.

EBENDAL, T. (1977). Extracellular matrix fibrils and cell contacts in the chick embryo. *Cell & Tissue Res.* **175**, 439–458.

FELDMAN, J. (1977). Specific junction formation between neurones and their target cells. In *Intercellular Junctions and Synapses*, eds. Feldman, J, Gilula, N. B. & Pitts, J. D., pp. 183–214. London: Chapman and Hall.

GAZE, R. M. (1978). The problem of specificity in the formation of nerve connections. In *Specificity of Embryological Interactions.* ed. Garrod, D. R., pp. 53–93. London: Chapman and Hall.

HAMBURGER, V. (1939). The development and innervation of transplanted limb primordia of chick embryos. *J. exp. Zool.* **80**, 347–389.

HAMBURGER, V. (1958). Regression versus peripheral control of differentiation in motor hypoplasia. *Am. J. Anat.* **102**, 365–410.

HAMBURGER, V. (1975). Cell death in the development of the lateral motor column of the chick embryo. *J. comp. Neurol.* **160**, 535–545.

HAMBURGER, V. & HAMILTON, H. L. (1951). A series of normal stages in the development of the chick embryo. *J. Morph.* **88**, 49–92.

HIBBARD, E. (1965). Orientation and directed growth of Mauther's cell axons from duplicated vestibular nerve roots. *Expl Neurol.* **13**, 289–301.

HOLLYDAY, M. & HAMBURGER, V. (1977). An autoradiographic study of the formation of the lateral motor column in the chick embryo. *Brain Res.* **132**, 197–208.

HOLLYDAY, M., HAMBURGER, V. & FARRIS, J. M. G. (1977). Localization of motor neuron pools supplying identified muscles in normal and supernumerary legs of chick embryo. *Proc. natn. Acad. Sci. U.S.A.* **74**, 3582–3586.

HOPE, R. A., HAMMOND, B. J. & GAZE, R. M. (1976). The arrow model: retinotectal specificity and map formation in the goldfish visual system. *Proc. R. Soc.* B **194**, 447–466.

HORDER, T. J. (1978). Functional adaptability and morphogenetic opportunism, the only rules for limb development? *Zoon* **6**, 181–192.

JACOBSON, C. -O. (1964). Motor nuclei, cranial nerve roots, and fibre pattern in the medulla oblongata after reversal experiments on the neural plate of axolotl larvae. I. Bilateral operations. *Zool. Bidr. Upps.* **36**, 73–160.

JACOBSON, M. (1978). *Developmental Neurobiology*, 2nd edn., p. 310. New York: Plenum

LAMB, A. (1976). The projection patterns of the ventral horn to the hindlimb during development. *Devl Biol.* **54**, 82–99.

LAMB, A. H. (1977). Neuronal death in the development of the somatotopic projections of the ventral horn in *Xenopus*. *Brain Res.* **134**, 145–150.

LANCE-JONES, C. & LANDMESSER, L. T. (1978). Effect of spinal cord deletions and reversals on motoneuron projection patterns in the embryonic chick hindlimb. *Neurosci. Abstr.* **4**, 118.

LANCE-JONES, C. & LANDMESSER, L. T. (1980). Motoneurone projection patterns in embryonic chick limbs following partial spinal cord deletions. *J. Physiol.* **302**, 559–580

LANDMESSER, L. (1978*a*). The distribution of motoneurones supplying chick hind limb muscles. *J. Physiol.* **284**, 371–389.

LANDMESSER, L. (1978*b*). The development of motor projection patterns in the chick hind limb. *J. Physiol.* **284**, 391–414.

LANDMESSER, L. & MORRIS, D. G. (1975). The development of functional innervation in the hindlimb of the chick embryo. *J. Physiol.* **249**, 301–326.

LETOURNEAU, P. (1975). Cell-to-substratum adhesion and guidance of axonal elongation. *Devl Biol.* **44**, 92–101.

LETOURNEAU, P. (1978). Chemotactic response of nerve fibre elongation to nerve growth factor. *Devl Biol.* **66**, 183–196.

LEWIS, J. (1978). Pathways of axons in the developing chick wing: evidence against chemospecific guidance. *Zoon* **6**, 175–179.

MACAGNO, E. R. (1978). Mechanism for the formation of synaptic projections in the arthropod visual system. *Nature, Lond.* **275**, 318–320.

MALSBERG, VON DER CH. & WILLSHAW, D. J. (1977). How to label nerve cells so that they interconnect in an ordered fashion. *Proc. natn. Acad. Sci. U.S.A.* **74**, 5176–5178.

McGRATH, P. A. & BENNETT, M. R. (1979) The development of synaptic connections between different segmental motoneurones and striated muscles in an axolotl limb. *Devl Biol.* **69**, 133–145.

MORRIS, D. G. (1978). Development of functional motor innervation in supernumerary hindlimbs of the chick embryo. *J. Neurophysiol.* **41**, 1450–1465.

NARAYANAN, C. H. (1964). An experimental analysis of peripheral nerve pattern development in the chick. *J. exp. Zool.* **156**, 49–60.

PETTIGREW, A. G., LINDEMAN, R. & BENNETT, M. R. (1979). Development of the segmental innervation of the chick forelimb. *J. Embryol. exp. Morph.* **49**, 155–137.

PIATT, J. (1956). Studies on the problem of nerve pattern. I. Transplantation of the fore-limb primordium to ectopic sites in *Amblystoma*. *J. exp. Zool.* **131**, 173–202.

ROMANES, G. (1964). The motor pools of the spinal cord. *Prog. Brain Res.* **11**, 93–119.

SPERRY, R. W. (1963). Chemoaffinity in the orderly growth of nerve fibre patterns and connections. *Proc. natn. Acad. Sci. U.S.A.* **50**, 703–710.

STIRLING, R. V. & SUMMERBELL, D. (1977). The development of functional innervation in the chick wing-bud following truncations and deletions of the proximal–distal axis. *J. Embryol. erp. Morph.* **41**, 189–207.

STIRLING, R. V. & SUMMERBELL, D. (1979). The segmentation of axons from the segmental nerve roots to the chick wing. *Nature, Lond.* **278**, 640–642.

STRAZNICKY, K. (1967). The development of the innervation and the musculature of wings innervated by thoracic nerves. *Acta biol. hung.* **18**, 437–448.

SZEKELY, G. (1963). Functional specificity of spinal cord segments in the control of limb movements. *J. Embryol. erp. Morph.* **11**, 431–444.

UEYAMA, T. (1978). The topography of root fibres within the sciatic nerve trunk of the dog. *J. Anat.* **127**, 277–290.

WENGER, B. S. (1951). Determination of structural patterns in the spinal cord of the chick embryo studied by transplantation between brachial and adjacent levels. *J. erp. Zool.* **116**, 123–146.

EXPLANATION OF PLATE

Transverse sections through the spinal cord in St. 36 control and experimental embryos. LS 1–3 were reversed at St. 16 in the latter. Section *A* in the control embryo was made through T7, the last thoracic segment. A slightly more anterior thoracic segment is illustrated in *A* of the reversal as T7 was lost in the operation. The size discrepancy is normal. Sections *B* and *C* were taken from LS 1 and LS 3 in the control and from similarly positioned segments within the reversal region of the experimental embryo. The segments in the reversal, which correspond to the reversed LS 1 and LS 3, show a morphology characteristic of their position prior to the operation. The lateral motor column (outlined in black) expands abruptly at the anterior end of the reversal (section *B*) in a manner similar to LS 3 (section *C*) in the control. Cord segments posterior to the reversed ones appear anatomically normal when compared to segments at an equivalent level in the control (sections *D*). Calibration bar = 250 μm.

Reversal

Control

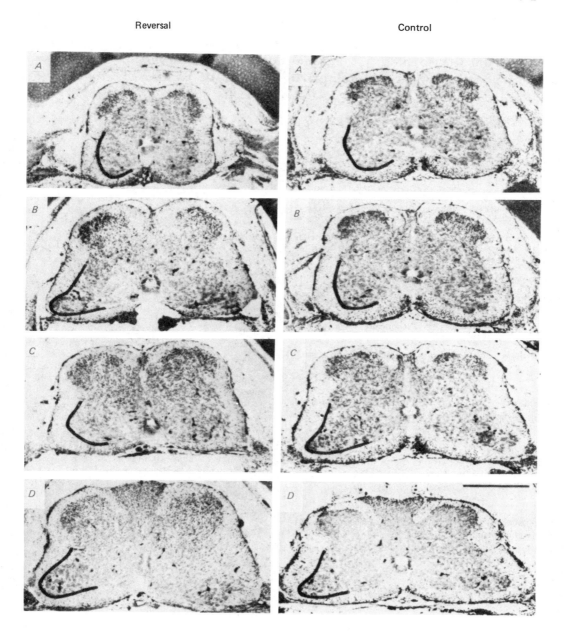

C. LANCE-JONES AND L. LANDMESSER

(*Facing p.* 602)

Reprinted from
Proc. Nat. Acad. Sci. USA
Vol. 70, No. 2, pp. 433–437, February 1973

Structure and Development of Neuronal Connections in Isogenic Organisms: Cellular Interactions in the Development of the Optic Lamina of *Daphnia**

(neuronal specificity/serial section reconstruction/crustacea)

V. LOPRESTI, E. R. MACAGNO, AND C. LEVINTHAL

Department of Biological Sciences, Columbia University, New York, N.Y. 10027

Contributed by C. Levinthal, December 4, 1972

ABSTRACT Some details of the growth and initial cellular interactions of optic nerve axons were examined in a parthenogenetic clone of *Daphnia magna*. Results are summarized as follows: (*i*) the final structure of the optic lamina is dependent upon interactions between growing optic nerve fibers and optic lamina neuroblasts closest to the midplane of the animal, which trigger the morphological differentiation of the neuroblasts; the specificity of connections is achieved by well-defined sequences of cell migration in the ganglion; (*ii*) only one of the eight optic nerve axons growing back from each ommatidium in the eye possesses a structure similar to the growth cones seen on termini of nerve fibers growing *in vitro*; and (*iii*) undifferentiated neuroblasts in the ganglion react to surface contact by this "lead axon" by enveloping the axon in a glial-like relationship.

The formation of specific neuronal connections has been studied by various methods in several different biological systems (1, 2). Very little is known, however, about either the morphological or biochemical phenomena that take place at the cellular level and are responsible for the resulting adult neuronal patterns. A straightforward procedure for studying the anatomy of embryological events is to examine serial electron micrographs of identified growing nerve fibers at various well-defined stages, especially at the time when the target cells are contacted and functional interactions established. Studies of this type have been made with the computer method of three-dimensional reconstruction from serial sections (3, 4). We have examined embryos of the small crustacean, *Daphnia magna*, grown under conditions in which the organisms reproduce as a parthenogenetic clone. It is possible to obtain embryos that are accurately staged with respect to time of development and to identify individual optic nerve axons as they grow from the eye to the optic ganglion where primary synaptic contacts take place in the adult organism. The comparison of three-dimensional reconstructions at various stages allows a determination of the sequence of events from which overall patterns of development can be deduced.

In several instances, the nature of the phenomena only became apparent after the three-dimensional reconstructions were done on the computer. But in virtually every case it was then possible to confirm the findings by examination of the electron micrographs themselves. For example, one of the early interactions between an undifferentiated target cell and the first optic nerve axon that touches its surface involved a wrapping of the target cell around the optic axon. Once this process was recognized, it was possible to examine the details in a high-magnification electron micrograph.

There are three general aspects of the interactions between optic axons and ganglion cells that have been clarified in the initial studies. *First*, a well-defined temporal sequence of growth and migration can account for most, if not all, of the spatial specificity of the nerves that are establishing their connections between the eye and the optic ganglion. *Second*, only a small fraction of the fibers that grow from the eye to the ganglion have the flattened expansions with filopodial-like projections at their termini that have been called growth cones for fibers growing *in vitro* (5). *Third*, neuroblasts in the ganglion with which the growing axons first make contact respond with rather elaborate and characteristic changes, which are associated with the onset of morphological differentiation and seemingly with establishment of functional contacts. These results raise a series of questions concerning the nature of the information transfer between optic fibers and ganglion neuroblasts that can, at least in principle, be answered by further experiments.

MATERIALS AND METHODS

Embryos are staged by isolation of large females with dark ovaries and observation of the time at which the eggs are passed from the ovaries into the dorsal brood pouch. This time is taken as time zero of development; the total gestation time *in vivo* is about 55 hr. In almost all animals, no more than 5 min elapse between entrance of the first and last eggs into the brood pouch, the brood size ranging between 10 and 30 for these large adults. Broods that did not enter the brood pouch within a 5-min interval were not used in these studies. The embryos are allowed to develop *in vivo* at 24° until the desired stage is reached (between 26 and 38 hr for these studies), at which time they are removed and placed into fixative. Alternatively, only part of the brood is immediately fixed; the remainder are allowed to develop further *in vitro* at 24° and subsequently fixed. We have found that in order for development *in vitro* to occur, embryos must remain in the mother for the initial 7 hr of gestation. They may then be transferred to plastic trays containing standard medium at 24°; development then proceeds with a gestation time equivalent to that *in vivo*.

All other techniques are identical to those described in the first paper of this series (3) with the following exceptions: the fixative and buffer contain 0.40% NaCl rather than 0.85% (this reduction in osmolarity is necessary to prevent cell shrinkage in embryos); the fixation time is 45 min rather than 1 hr, any longer times resulting in extensive leaching of membranes; finally, the uranyl acetate staining solution used was 3% in 50% ethanol rather than 0.5%.

---

* This is paper no. II in a series. The previous paper is ref. 3.

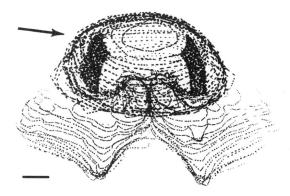

Fig. 1. Computer reconstruction of the outline of the embryonic eye (*arrow*) at 35 hr of gestation, with the two lobes of the optic ganglion displayed in their proper position relative to the eye. The approximate areas of eye pigmentation at this stage have been added to the reconstruction. *Bar* = 20 μm.

RESULTS

The following results were obtained from studies of five embryonic stages, namely 29, 32, 34, 35, and 37.5 hr of gestation. The uniqueness and reproducibility of each stage have been checked by looking at various embryos of a single brood, fixed at the same time. We find that the relevant features are the same for all specimens at any one stage.

In adult *Daphnia*, each bundle of eight optic nerve axons from the receptor cells of one ommatidium is surrounded, as the bundle enters the ganglion, by the cell bodies of five optic lamina neurons, forming a structure similar to an optic cartridge, as seen in other crustaceans and insects (6, 7). The axons† of these five lamina cells receive primary afferent input from the optic axons (3). There are 22 such structures, 11 in each lobe of the optic lamina. In discussing their formation, the term "proximal" refers to locations close to the eye, and hence anterior.

Early in the development of a cartridge, all five lamina cell bodies are located at different anteroposterior levels; progression toward adult morphology involves proximal migration of the cells as one of its aspects until all five cell bodies come to be located in about the same plane. The five lamina cells of any cartridge can be numbered sequentially 1 through 5, a lower number indicating both an earlier association with optic axons and a more proximal initial location.

At these embryonic stages, the ganglion consists of two symmetric and separate lobes, which develop simultaneously (Fig. 1). In each lobe the 11 sets of optic nerve axons grow into the lamina over a period of about 10 hr, from gestation times of 28 hr to about 38 hr. Table 1 shows the numbers and relative positions of developing optic cartridges present at the five stages examined within this period (see Fig. 2). Two features of the system are evident in this table. First, the number of cartridges formed increases with time in a regular fashion; and second, the older cartridges have migrated laterally away from the midplane, at any stage the youngest cartridges being closest to the midplane. This observation is illustrated in Figs. 2a and 2b. At 35 hr (Fig. 2a), optic axons IIIa, b, and c occupy the midplane position and interact with the neuroblasts present there. At 37.5 hr (Fig. 2b), cartridges IIIa, b, and c have moved laterally with the arrival of new neuroblasts in the midplane; these neuroblasts are contacted by optic axons IVa, b, and c, which come from the last ommatidia to differentiate.

As a consequence of the sequential growth of optic axons into the midplane of the lamina, one finds cartridges at different stages of development within one embryo. The most lateral cartridges are always closest to the adult morphology, the most medial are the youngest. We can, therefore, follow the time course of cartridge development both by examining the same cartridge at different developmental stages and by comparing the morphology of cartridges at different mediolateral levels in one embryo.

In 35-hr embryos, three general stages of cartridge development can be found. In cartridge IIIb, located adjacent to

TABLE 1. *Numbers and relative positions of developing optic cartridges present in both lobes of the optic lamina at five different embryonic stages*

Hr of gestation				V				
29				2	2			
32			1 2	3 4 5	3 4 5	1 2		
34		1 2	3 4 5	6 7	6 7	3 4 5	1 2	
35		1 2	3 4 5	6 7 8	6 7 8	3 4 5	1 2	
37.5	1 2	3 4 5	6 7 8	9 10 11	9 10 11	6 7 8	3 4 5	1 2

D

For reference to Fig. 2: *1* and *2* in this table correspond to *Ia* and *Ib*, respectively; *3, 4,* and *5* to *IIa, IIb,* and *IIc; 6, 7,* and *8* to *IIIa, IIIb,* and *IIIc;* and *9, 10,* and *11* to *IVa, IVb,* and *IVc*. *D* = dorsal; *V* = ventral; *L* = lateral. The *double line* represents the midplane of the animal.

---

† The term "axon" refers to a process containing the normally observed ultrastructural aspects of axonal processes. For monopolar invertebrate neurons the term is used independently of whether the process is pre- or post-synaptic. "Neurite," on the other hand, refers to a process extending from the cell body whose cytoplasmic morphology resembles that of the cell body and that does not yet show characteristic axonal elements such as organized microtubular arrays.

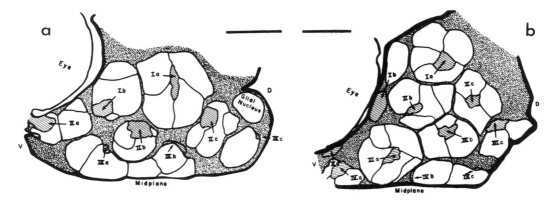

FIG. 2.   Tracings made from electron micrographs of sections at equivalent anteroposterior levels of the optic lamina in 35-hr (*a*) and 37.5-hr (*b*) embryos. *Clear areas* represent lamina cell cytoplasm; *stippled area*, glial cell cytoplasm; and *slanting parallel-lined areas*, the bundles of optic axons. Note that the relative positions of the cartridges are the same in each embryo (e.g., *Ia* with respect to *IIb* and *IIc*), but that lateral movement of those present at 35 hr has occurred at 37.5 hr with the arrival of new undifferentiated cells and lead optic axons (*IVa, b, c*) in the midplane. In (*b*) there is seemingly a shift in the positions of *Ib* and *IIa* with respect to their positions relative to the other cartridges in (*a*). This is solely a function of a difference in sectioning plane between the two animals; the three-dimensional reconstructions confirm that these two cartridges do maintain the same position relative to the others at 37.5 hr. *D* = dorsal; *V* = ventral. *Bar* = 10 μm.

the midplane at this stage, the central of the eight optic axons has grown much further than the rest, and is the only one to possess a terminal dilation which resembles the growth cones described *in vitro*. Filopodia are short and few in number, a feature consistently observed for all growth cones in these studies. The seven "follower fibers" in this cartridge grow along, and in contact with, the "lead fiber," but do not possess any terminal dilations (Fig. 3*a* and *b*). The lead axon in this cartridge has contacted only three midplane neuroblasts out of the final number of five; the growth cone makes surface contact with the two more distal cells (cells 2 and 3). None of the three cells shows any signs of axon proliferation. In cartridge IIb, located more laterally at the 35-hr stage, the lead and follower relationship is evident, although the fol-

lowers are further advanced in growth with respect to the lead than in IIIb. Of the five associated lamina cells, cells 1 and 2 have short neurites along the surface of the optic bundle and, like the follower optic fibers, do not show terminal growth cones; cells 3, 4, and 5 are devoid of distal processes. In a most lateral optic cartridge, Ia, in the same embryos, all eight optic axons have grown to more or less the same level and all possess terminal dilations. Lamina cells 1 and 2 have well-defined axons without growth cones, cells 3 and 4 have short neurites, and cell 5 is morphologically undifferentiated (devoid of processes). The lamina cell axons lie along the bundle of eight optic axons and are in contact with its surface, thus forming what is finally a fascicle of thirteen nerve fibers. In addition, the five lamina cell bodies in the cartridge are

TABLE 2.   *General structure of cartridge Ia at five different stages*

	\multicolumn{5}{c}{Hr of gestation}				
	29	32	34	35	37.5
Optic axons					
+GC	1	1	6	8	2
−GC	7	7	2	0	0
+S	0	0	0	0	6
Lamina neurons					
1	U*	N	A	A	A_b
2	U	U	N	A	A_b
3	U	U	N	N	A
4		U	U	N	A
5		U	U	U	A

For the eight optic axons, +GC indicates the number of axons with growth cones, −GC the number without growth cones, and +S the number with nascent synapses. For lamina neurons, U = morphologically undifferentiated; N = distally directed neurite; A = axon; A_b = branched axon. U* for cell 1 at 29 hr indicates that the cell is wrapping around the lead axon as shown in Fig. 5.

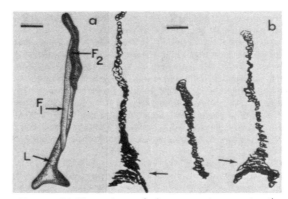

FIG. 3.   (*a*) Illustration made from computer reconstruction of a lead axon (*L*) with two of its follower axons (*F*₁, *F*₂). (*b*) Computer reconstruction of two different lead axons showing their growth cones (*arrows*) and one follower axon displayed separately. The receptor cell bodies would be at the top of the figure. The follower is not shown in its correct relative position with respect to either lead. *Bar* = 2 μm.

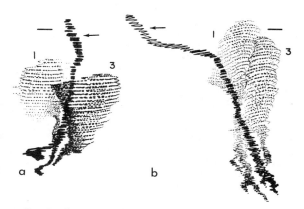

FIG. 4. Computer reconstruction of cells 1 and 3 of cartridge Ia displayed with only one of the eight optic axons (*arrow*) at 35 hr (*a*) and 37.5 hr (*b*). Note that at 35 hr, cell 1 has a well-defined axon, cell 3 has a short neurite in the eventual direction of the axon, and the terminal dilation of the optic axon appears to be a growth cone. At 37.5 hr, the axon of cell 1 is longer with significant branching, while cell 3 now has a well-defined axon. The terminus of the optic axon at this stage contains forming synapses. *Bar* = 2 μm.

significantly closer to their adult coplanar positioning than are the five lamina cells of cartridge IIb at this stage.

The same and additional stages in cartridge development have been investigated by tracing cartridge Ia at various times. These results are summarized in Table 2. Computer reconstructions of part of this cartridge at 35 and 37.5 hr are shown in Figs. 4a and 4b. In Fig. 4b, the terminal portion of the optic axon shown contains forming synapses. It follows from the data in this table and from data obtained for other cartridges that axon proliferation by lamina cells in a cartridge occurs in the order 1 to 5, which corresponds to the order in which the cells are contacted by the lead axon in the midplane.

The results for the 35-hr embryo show that the optic nerve axons from the eight receptor cells in an individual ommatidium are not proliferated at the same time. It was consistently found in all newly differentiated ommatidia that there is a lead axon and that it is the only one to possess a growth cone. It was also found that it is always the lead axon from each ommatidium that makes the initial cellular contacts in the midplane. Although they are clearly growing, the followers lag behind without growth cones, until the stage when the lamina cells of the cartridge have begun to proliferate axons. The followers then catch up to the lead, and the optic fibers form synaptic expansions onto the lamina cell axons.

In both cartridge Ia at 29 hr and cartridges IIIa and b at 35 hr, the lead axon has contacted only three midplane cells of the final five, the growth cone touching the cell surface of the two distal neuroblasts (cells 2 and 3). The most proximal and, therefore, the first contacted neuroblast wraps itself around the axon in a glial-like relationship (Figs. 5a and 5b). The relationship is clearly transient, as at 37.5 hr the cell body is adjacent to the entire bundle of eight optic axons (Fig. 5c), rather than surrounding any one of the eight. Three-dimensional reconstructions not shown here demon-

strate that at 34 hr, IIIb is in a configuration where the growth cone of the lead axon is touching the surface of two midplane neuroblasts, confirming, by comparison with 35 hr, that the lead axon first contacts a cell with its growth cone and the cell then wraps around the axon as the growth cone moves distally to contact additional midplane cells. In IVa and b, midplane cartridges at 37.5 hr, the lead axon has contacted four neuroblasts, the growth cone touching the surface of the distal two cells (cells 3 and 4). Cell 2 is wrapped around the lead in the same fashion as above, while cell 1 is only partially wrapped around the bundle of eight optic axons, the followers having grown to this level.

DISCUSSION

Three-dimensional reconstructions of growing optic nerve axons and of the neurons they contact in the optic lamina make it possible to identify and visualize various stages in the development of these structures. From a comparison of these stages and the variations in morphology of the cells involved, several generalizations appear to be justified:

(*i*) Growth of new axons from receptor cells toward the optic lamina occurs along the midplane. When the lead axon in the group of eight from one ommatidium has contacted five

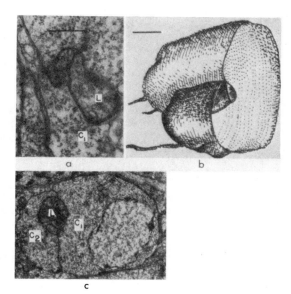

FIG. 5. (*a*) Electron micrograph showing the glial-like relationship between a lead axon (*L*) and one of its recently contacted midplane neuroblasts (C_1) *Bar* = 0.5 μm. (*b*) Illustration made from computer reconstruction of the anterior half of the cell shown in (*a*). *Bar* = 1 μm. (*c*) Electron micrograph of the same cell (C_1) shown in (*a*), but 2.5 hr later in development. Seven followers now surround the lead axon (*L*) and C_1 is only partially surrounding the whole bundle of eight. The second cell originally touched by the lead fiber in the midplane (C_2) now lies almost on the same anteroposterior level as C_1. *Bar* = 1 μm. The lead axon in this figure was traced from its receptor cell body in the eye to its cellular contacts in the lamina in a low magnification series of electron micrographs. It was the examination of the three-dimensional reconstruction that then led to the higher-magnification electron micrograph shown in (*a*).

undifferentiated neuroblasts in one lobe and formed an optic cartridge, the whole structure migrates laterally, even while many of its fibers are still growing and making connections. The process is then repeated by the next arriving group of axons and by the neuroblasts that have moved into the midplane position. Previous results on adults (3) have shown that the arrangement of cartridges and the ommatidia that map on to them is the same in all genetically identical animals studied, reflecting the constancy of the developmental sequence just described.

Within any one cartridge, axon proliferation by the five neuroblasts occurs in the same temporal order as the order in which the cells were originally contacted by the lead axon from the eye. When surface contact is first made, the neuroblasts are spread out in the anteroposterior direction, and, therefore, the first one contacted is closest to the eye and the last one is furthest away. As the cartridge develops, the lamina cell axons grow distally along the surface of the bundle of eight optic nerve axons to form a bundle of 13 fibers. Concomitant with axon formation is the proximal migration of the lamina cell bodies in order to achieve their final adult positioning within a cartridge.

(*ii*) The overall pattern of cell and fiber migration summarized above allowed us to study in detail the structure of the end of the growing axons. In all cases, the initial cellular contacts are made solely by one axon among the eight from one ommatidium. This lead axon is the only one to possess a growth cone; the seven follower axons clearly grow along the surface of the lead, but end in a rounded tip with no terminal enlargements. Except for the close proximity between the lead and its followers, we have not yet observed any specialized interactions between them.

(*iii*) At least for the first two lamina cells to be touched by lead fibers, there is a characteristic response of the neuroblasts that results in their being wrapped around the lead axon in a glial-like relationship. This reaction has not yet been observed for cells 3, 4, or 5 in any of the cartridges studied, but this may well be because our methods give us only brief glimpses of the ongoing developmental processes. In any case, the wrapping around lasts for only a short time, and the type of close interaction shown in Fig. 5*a* has not been observed except for the lead fiber. By the time the followers have grown beyond the positions of neuroblasts 1 and 2, these cells have loosened their grasp on the lead axon and have taken a position adjacent to the bundle of eight nerve fibers without the individual wrapping that is evident earlier.

There are several interpretations that seem to us to be suggested by the above results. First, although the adult *Daphnia* optic system is connected with a well-defined three-dimensional geometry, it is possible to design a model for the events that occur during establishment of neural connections that only requires cells or fibers to receive very limited signals to determine their positions or appropriate targets for connections. Wolpert (8) discussed the need for developing systems to establish "positional information" to which individual cells could respond, depending on their genes and their physiological states. In the present case, the only "positional information" that the growing axons seem to require is an indication as to whether or not they are near the midplane, and which positions are anterior and posterior. If we assume

that only morphologically undifferentiated neuroblasts are able to act as targets for growing axons, then the relatively complex three-dimensional relationships could be determined if cell behavior were simply controlled by (*i*) contact with a landmark, such as the midplane column of glial cells of the embryonic eye, and (*ii*) a more or less stereotypic response of a neuroblast when it is touched by the growth cone of a lead axon. A model of this type would imply that the connections between eye cells and optic ganglion cells are made with whatever undifferentiated neuroblast happens to be touched by the growing lead axon. After a cartridge has been completed and moved laterally, the next optic axons that grow back from the eye are limited in their available contact to those cells that are now undifferentiated midplane cells. All lateral cells facing the base of the eye are already occupied and in the process of further differentiation.

The type of model outlined here suggests that the particular cell that is contacted by a lead axon is not necessarily identified before being touched. The wrapping around process could be thought of as the equivalent of the neuroblasts responding to a particular lead fiber in the manner, "You touched me, I am yours." A different type of model, more similar to the one proposed by Sperry (9), would imply that the appropriate phrase for the neuroblasts to express before contact is made would be, "I am yours, come and get me."

The first type of model discussed above is functionally equivalent to that proposed by Jacobson (1), in which neuroblasts in the optic system are assumed to be "labeled" by the first optic nerve fiber to grow back from the eye and make contact with them. The transient wrapping around reaction of the neuroblasts could then be thought of as a morphological representation of Jacobson's proposed labeling.

Finally, it should be emphasized that only one of the eight members of a bundle of axons from a single ommatidium has a growth cone at its terminus. This terminal flattened enlargement resembles those described *in vitro*, except that where filopodia are present they are rather short. The other seven optic axons grow without such a terminal specialization, as do the five axons from the lamina neuroblasts. It is clear that growth *per se* does not require the so-called "growth cone." It seems, therefore, likely that the growth cone is in fact functionally associated with the process of "recognizing" cell surfaces or otherwise detecting position in space, and that this information can be then shared with other growing processes in order to create a spatial arrangement.

We thank Yu-Chih Jao for technical assistance and Dorothea Goldys for illustrations. This work was supported by NIH Grants RR00442(04) and 5R01-A1-08902(04), and a gift from the RGK Foundation.

1. Jacobson, M. (1970) in *Developmental Neurobiology* (Holt, Rinehart and Winston, Inc.), pp. 252–260 and 305–330.
2. Gaze, R. M. (1970) in *The Formation of Nerve Connections* (Academic Press, London), pp. 178–215.
3. Macagno, E. R., LoPresti, V. & Levinthal, C. (1973) *Proc. Nat. Acad. Sci. USA* **70**, 57–61.
4. Levinthal, C. & Ware, R. (1972) *Nature* **236**, 207–210.
5. Yamada, K. M., Spooner, B. S. & Wessells, N. K. (1970) *Proc. Nat. Acad. Sci. USA* **66**, 1206–1212.
6. Hamori, J. & Horridge, G. A. (1966) *J. Cell Sci.* **I**, 257–270.
7. Trujillo–Cenóz, O. (1963) *J. Ultrastruc. Res.* **13**, 1–33.
8. Wolpert, L. (1969) *J. Theor. Biol.* **25**, 1–47.
9. Sperry, R. W. (1963) *Proc. Nat. Acad. Sci. USA* **50**, 703–709.

The Journal of Neuroscience
Vol. 1, No. 3, pp. 250–258
March 1981

CERCAL SENSORY DEVELOPMENT FOLLOWING LASER MICROLESIONS OF EMBRYONIC APICAL CELLS IN *ACHETA DOMESTICUS*[1]

JOHN S. EDWARDS,* SU-WAN CHEN,* AND MICHAEL W. BERNS‡

* Department of Zoology, University of Washington, Seattle, Washington 98195 and ‡ Department of Developmental and Cell Biology, University of California, Irvine, California 92717

Abstract

The hypothesis that pioneer fibers, which develop relatively early in the differentiation of insect appendages, serve to organize the peripheral sensory nerves was tested by ablating apical regions of the cercal rudiments in embryos of *Acheta domesticus*. Multiple nerve bundles rather than the normal mid-dorsal and midventral pair of nerves were formed within the cercus following ablation of the cercal tip before pioneer fiber differentiation, but the cercal nerve was normal when lesions were made after formation of the pioneer fiber tracts and associated glia. These results indicate a necessary morphogenetic role for the pioneer fibers.

A guidance function has been proposed for sets of neuron-like cells, the so-called pioneer fibers, that appear in insect appendages during early embryonic development in advance of sensory neuron differentiation (Bate, 1976; Edwards, 1977; Keshishian, 1980). The basis for this inference is the relative timing of their differentiation, the pioneer fibers appearing before the elongation of appendage primordia and forming central projections when the distances separating periphery and center are smallest. It is proposed that, by following these pioneer fibers, later differentiating sensory axons reach their central targets along pathways that, in the course of organogenesis, become considerably longer and more tortuous than that required of the pioneers, but it remains to be shown that pioneer fibers are necessary for the organization of the definitive sensory nerve. Proof of their necessity requires demonstration that the sensory axons arising from functional sensilla late in embryogenesis do not become organized into a normal nerve in the absence of the pioneer fiber pathway.

In this study, we have used the abdominal cerci of the house cricket, *Acheta domesticus*. These posteriorly placed sensory appendages contain purely sensory nerves formed by aggregation of different axons that arise from cell bodies situated in the epidermis, as is typical of insects. Since the cerci lack intrinsic muscles, they provide appropriate material for the study of guidance of sensory nerves alone. The normal embryonic development of the cercal sensory system has been described elsewhere (Edwards and Chen, 1979).

The initial attempts to produce localized lesions in embryonic cercal rudiments were made with tungsten microneedles. Eggs were penetrated under saline and the tip of the cercal rudiment was pricked so that apical cells or the entire structure was ablated. In most embryos so treated, the damaged embryonic epithelium became attached to the egg membranes at the site of puncture and further development was grossly distorted as a result of the adhesion. The few embryos that completed development after puncture and hatched with reduced or no cerci had also suffered damage to the anal and adjacent areas during the egg penetration and were not able to develop beyond the midpoint of the first instar. Since mechanical damage could not be localized to the cercal tip, an alternative approach using an ultraviolet laser microbeam was used for the work described below.

We report here that ablation of the apical region of embryonic abdominal cerci, at a time before the centripetal processes of pioneer fibers develop, yields cerci in which sensory nerves are not organized to form normal bundles within the cercus. A brief report of the principal finding has been published earlier (Edwards et al., 1979).

Materials and Methods

Eggs of *Acheta domesticus* were obtained and cultured essentially as described by Edwards and Chen (1979).

[1] Dedicated in memory of Professor William T. Keeton of Cornell University who was an inspiration as both a teacher and researcher in neurobiology.

This work was supported by National Institutes of Health Grants NB 07778 (J. S. E.) and GM 23445 (M. W. B.). Irradiation was conducted in the Laser Microbeam Facility under Biotechnology Resource Grant RRO 1192-1. We thank Drs. J. Palka and M. Meyer for their critiques of the manuscript.

197

Embryos selected for electron microscopy were fixed for a minimum of 2 hr in a mixture of 2% paraformaldehyde and 0.5% glutaraldehyde in Millonig's phosphate buffer, followed by postfixation in 2% osmium tetroxide in Millonig's buffer. Tissues were embedded in Epon 812. Sections for light microscopy were stained with Richardson's stain (Richardson et al., 1960). Thin sections were stained with saturated uranyl acetate and lead citrate (Reynolds, 1963) and examined with a Philips 300 electron microscope.

For microlaser lesions, selected eggs at appropriate stages were transferred to a drop of saline on a microslide and covered with a quartz coverslip. The laser microbeam system employed a neodymium Yag laser as described elsewhere (Berns et al., 1979). The 265-nm beam of a frequency-quadrupled Yag laser was reflected into a Zeiss photomicroscope equipped with quartz optics. The output of the laser at 265 nm was 400 W and the phase duration of each laser shot was 80 nsec. Various neutral density filters were used to attenuate the beam so that the beam intensity was sufficient to kill the target cells without destroying neighboring tissue. The energy density of the 1- to 2-μm focused laser spot was between 10 and 50 μJ. A quartz $\times$ 32 Ultrafluar glycerin immersion objective was positioned with the cercal rudiment in focus and aligned for irradiation while under observation on a television monitor. A cross-hair on the monitor screen denoted the point of laser focus in the cercus. During irradiation, the embryo was moved and the focus was altered to ensure that the beam traversed appropriate epithelial cells. Where damage of the chorion and serosa were avoided, little damage was observed outside the target tissue, but damage to egg membranes, which occurred frequently when the cercal rudiment was in contact with them at the time of irradiation, caused rapid blackening and subsequent adhesion of embryonic tissue to the serosa. The resulting embryos were deformed and were not used for studies of nerve distribution. After lesioning, eggs were placed singly in the wells of an LKB electron microscope grid holder in a drop of saline and maintained in a moist chamber at 28°C. They were examined periodically under a dissecting microscope, and the saline was changed every 1 or 2 days. Transfer of eggs to the surface of moist filter paper late in development allowed for normal eclosion.

Results

Laser lesions were made on cercal rudiments of embryos at stages 19 through 22 (Edwards and Chen, 1979) with the objective of ablating pioneer fiber cell bodies or their precursors before, or shortly after, the formation of their centripetal processes. Since the exact time of axon formation cannot be determined precisely in the intact embryo, a range of embryos was irradiated, some of which preceded the time at which first pioneer fibers are detectable at stage 20. Several embryos were irradiated during the rapid phase of cercal elongation (stages 21 to 23). The general effects of laser irradiation on the cercal rudiments are described below as a context for the analysis of effects on the developing sensory system.

Effects of focal laser irradiation on cercal tissue

The distance between the cercal rudiment and enclosing egg membranes changes during development and varies among individual embryos. In embryos where the cercal tissue lay close to the egg membranes at the time of irradiation, adhesions developed at the lesion site and the subsequent development of the abdomen was arrested. Blackening, presumably due to polyphenol synthesis, developed at the wound site and became distributed throughout the embryonic fluid only if the serosal membrane was damaged by irradiation.

Localized lesions in the region of the cercal tip reduced the length of the cercus (Fig. 1*a*), while more basal lesions eliminated or severely reduced cercal development (Fig. 1*c*). Where massive lesions were sustained, the cercus failed to develop; regeneration of damaged cerci did not occur during embryogenesis. Occasional duplication of the normally single sub-basal clavate mechanoreceptor hair (Fig. 1*c*) was the only morphogenetic effect observed in the integumental structure.

The effects of apical lesions designed to eliminate presumptive pioneer fiber cell bodies included retardation of elongation on that side so that the normal cercus tended to grow across the midline, curving over its lesioned partner. This did not affect cuticular development (Fig. 1*d*) or the differentiation of sensilla, although the numbers of sensilla were reduced in proportion to the loss of tissue. The cerci selected for ultrastructural studies, in most cases, were modified only in general form at the apex, with minimal modification of the basal shaft of the cercus where thin sections were taken for nerve mapping.

Visible effects on the tissue at the time of irradiation, notably a localized increased opacity in the zone of the lesion, made it possible to monitor the lateral extent of the lesion (Fig. 1*e*). Since the depth of the zone of cell disruption was about 5 μm, a single traverse could be made which affected cells on one side of the cercus only.

At the ultrastructural level, the immediate effect of the lesion is manifested in a disruption of most intracellular membranes, although the nuclear envelope frequently survives (Fig. 2*a*). Within 24 hr, collapse of the affected cells is accompanied by condensation of chromatins within the nuclei, swelling of the remaining mitochondria, and clumping of the remaining cytoplasmic contents (Fig. 2*b*). Hemocyte-like cells appear in the region of the wound within 24 hr and become filled with lysosomes. Such cells characteristically have elaborately folded profiles, with multiple invaginations (Fig. 2*c*). Cellular debris is largely removed from the wound site within 2 to 3 days, and intact neighboring cells join to restore a continuous epithelium. Lysosomes persist in hemocytes throughout development and postembryonic stages and in trichogen cells (Fig. 3*a*). The embryonic hemocytes appear to be mobile, for lysosome-laden cells appeared in the untreated cercus within 24 hr of irradiation. Where laser lesions damaged established pioneer fiber bundles, the distal segments degenerated rapidly (Fig. 3*b*), but the surrounding glial cells showed no marked short term reaction. The destruction of pioneer fibers in the cercus was followed within 24 hr by the

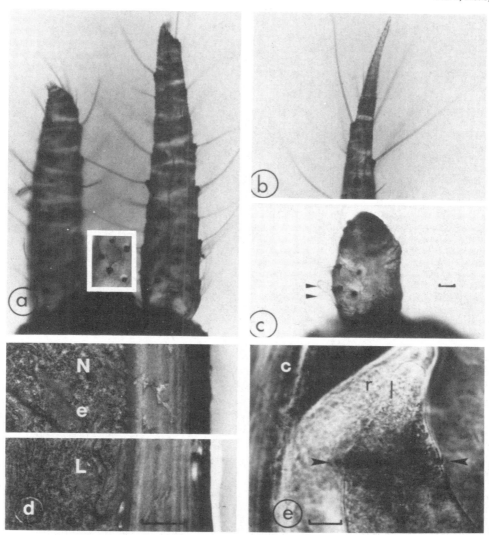

Figure 1. a, Cerci of newly hatched first instar *Acheta* larva. The *left* cercal rudiment was irradiated before differentiation of pioneer fibers (stage 20). Apical development was suppressed in both cerci as compared with normal cerci (*b*). *Inset*, single clavate hair situated on medial surface at base of first instar cercus. *Scale* for *a, b*, and *c*: 50 μm. *b*, Apical segment of normal first instar cercus. *c*, Strongly suppressed cercus lesioned at stage 20. Development of the entire distal region is suppressed. The normally single clavate hair near the medial base is duplicated (*arrows*). *d*, Comparison of cuticular structure from integument of normal (*N*) and lasered (*L*) areas from an embryo near hatching. The number and thickness of the cuticular laminae are closely comparable. *e*, epidermal cell. *Scale*: 0.5 μm. *e*, Right (*r*) and left (*l*) cercal rudiments immediately after irradiation. The lesion site on the *left* cercus lies between the *arrows*. Chorion (*c*) is at *left* margin. Cercal tips are at *upper right* margin. *Scale*: 10 μm.

Figure 2. a, Subapical transverse section of embryonic cercus (about stage 20) fixed 5 min after irradiation. Lumen (*lu*) is at the *left*. The path of the focal point passed through cells on the *upper right*, disrupting most intracellular structures but leaving nuclear membranes intact. The investing lamina (*la*), the so-called first embryonic cuticle, remains intact. *Scale* for *a* and *b*: 1 μm. *b*, Detail of cercal epithelium 24 hr after irradiation. Below the investing lamina (*la*), chromatin of nuclei is clumped (*c*). Surviving mitochondria (*m*) are swollen. The surface of intact cells has become highly folded. *c*, Detail of hemocytic-like cell packed with lysosomes (*ly*). This cell type, which may also be the source of glia that surround pioneer fibers, assemble in the region of irradiation within 24 hr and subsequently are found in the state shown here in other regions of the embryo. *Scale*: 0.5 μm.

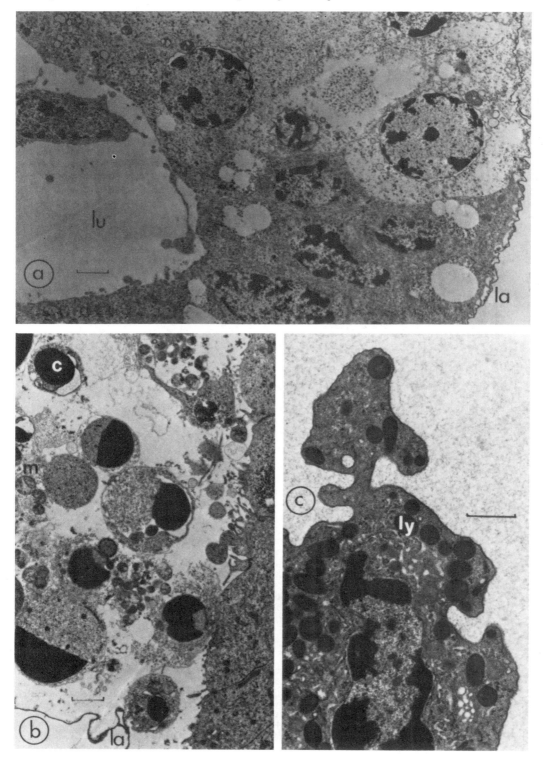

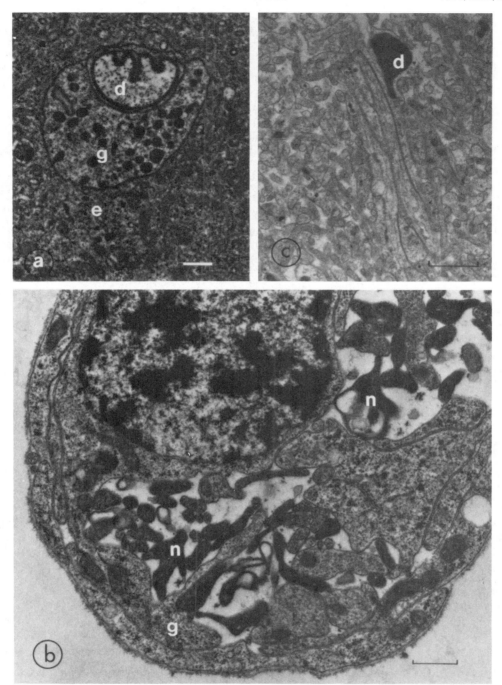

Figure 3. a, Dendrite (*d*) of mechanoreceptor (filiform hair) in irradiated cercus surrounded by trichogen cell (*g*) containing lysosomes comparable to those in Figure 2*c*. The surrounding epidermal cell (*e*) contains no comparable lysosomes. *Scale* for *a* and *c*: 1 μm. *b*, Degenerating pioneer fibers in cercal tract 12 hr after lesion. While the hitherto electron-lucent cells become densely osmiophilic (*n*), the surrounding glia (*g*) show no significant change. *Scale*: 0.5 μm. *c*, Subterminal degeneration (*d*) of pioneer fiber within neuropile of embryonic terminal abdominal ganglion.

appearance of dense osmiophilic figures in the ventral neuropile of the terminal ganglion (Fig. 3c). The similarity to degeneration figures described for crickets (Edwards and Palka, 1974) and elsewhere (e.g., Stocker et al., 1976) suggests that these are the terminal or subterminal segments of pioneer fibers.

Effects of irradiation on the organization of pioneer fibers and cercal sensory nerves

The assessment of effects of apical lesions on nerve growth was made on embryos that were allowed to approach complete embryonic development when they were fixed for electron microscopy. The distribution of sensory nerve axons in the irradiated cercus was compared with the normal member of the pair. The conformation of the sensory nerves within the cercus has been described elsewhere (Edwards and Chen, 1979). In essence, a mid-dorsal and midventral nerve in each cercus lie in contact with the basal lamina of the cercal epithelium. Axons from sensilla distributed over the cercus reach the dorsal and ventral nerves by the shortest path where they join more distal axons. Shortly before embryonic development is completed, the dorsal and ventral nerves detach from the basal lamina and come to lie in the hemocoel. They remain as separate nerves within the cercal lumen but coalesce as they leave the cercus to form the single cercal sensory nerve. The following description of treated cerci is based on a comparison of their nerve distribution.

Effects of earliest lesions. Of nine embryos irradiated before termination of katatrepsis movements and before pioneer fiber formation, one was fixed for electron microscopy 1 day after treatment. No differentiation of pioneer fiber tracts was evident nor had glial cells aggregated in mid-dorsal and midventral position of the presumptive pioneer tracts.

Of the eight fixed later in embryogenesis, four had multiple axon bundles in the treated cercus (Fig. 4, a and b), while the untreated member of the pair showed the normal mid-dorsal and midventral configuration (Fig. 4c) that is identical to that of a normal cercus (Fig. 4d). In the absence of dorsal and ventral pioneer tracts, subsequently differentiating sensory axons appear to have wandered within the cercus and aggregated with other sensory axons encountered during their growth. In two cases where the early irradiation was restricted to the dorsal side of the cercal rudiment, no cercal sensory nerve developed on that surface, and the axon number was increased in the remaining nerve within that cercus (Fig. 5b). Most of the multiple bundles had glial envelopes (Figs. 4, a and b and 5a), but several smaller groups did not.

Lesions at stage 21+. Eight embryos lesioned at the time of, or shortly after, pioneer fiber differentiation were fixed for electron microscopy. Of these, three were fixed immediately after lesioning in order to assess the immediate effects and extent of the irradiation and are described above. One embryo, fixed 3 days after irradiation, showed no evidence of pioneer fiber formation. The remaining four embryos, fixed at or near completion of embryogenesis, all showed the normal configuration of dorsal and ventral bundles within the cercus (Fig. 5, c and d).

Lesions during cercus elongation (stages 22 and 23)

Four embryos were fixed at hatching after receiving cercal lesions during the latter half of cercal elongation. Of these, three had normal cercal nerves. The fourth, which received a severe lesion resulting in distortion of the cercus, had multiple nerve bundles within the cercus comparable to those seen in embryos irradiated at stages 19 to 21.

Three embryos were fixed 1 day after lesioning. In all cases, the axons were degenerating within the cercal nerve bundle on the lesioned side, but the glial sheath showed no significant change in ultrastructural appearance (Fig. 3b).

In a comparison of all cases described above, three general categories can be recognized. The nerve distribution was either normal, asymmetric, or multiple in embryos lesioned before the termination of katatrepsis movements. Multiple bundles were found in only one other embryo which was irradiated late in elongation and in which the cercus was distorted during development. Asymmetric patterns of nerve fiber distribution appear to have been due to the elimination of pioneer fiber on one side of the cercus only. A lesion track that did not pass through the entire target area on both sides of the apex of the cercus would produce this result.

Later lesions generally did not affect the conformation

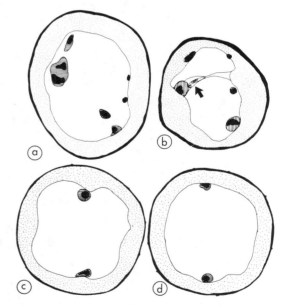

Figure 4. Tracings of cerci based on electron micrograph montages. *a* and *b*, Multiple sensory nerves in cerci that were irradiated before formation of pioneer tracts. *c* shows the position of the chordotonal organ shown in Figure 5a. The area of axon bundles is shown in *black*. Epidermal cells are *stippled* and the surrounding cuticle is shown *black*. *c*, Normal configuration of cercal nerves in cercus irradiated after the formation of the pioneer fiber pathways. *d*, Normal distribution of cercal sensory nerves at mid-dorsal and midventral positions shortly before they detach.

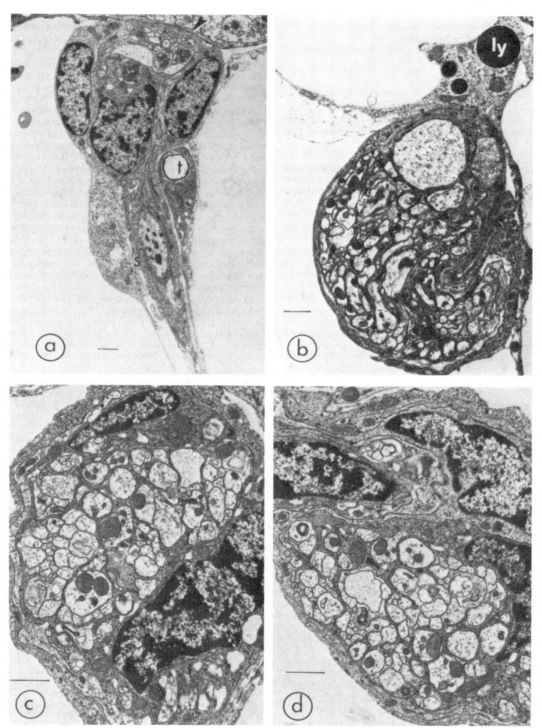

TABLE I
Summary of cercal sensory nerve configuration within embryonic cerci subjected to laser lesions at successive stages of development

Stages	Nerves Normal	Multiple Nerves	Nerves Absent
19–21	2	4	2
21–22	4	0	0
22–23	3	1	0

of the cercal nerves within the cercus. The results are summarized in Table I.

Discussion

The paths taken by growing axons during embryogenesis in insects are laid down early. In the first axons in appendages of grasshoppers (Bate, 1976; Keshishian, 1980) and crickets (Edwards, 1977; Edwards and Chen, 1979), the pioneer fibers occupy constant positions and establish pathways along which subsequently differentiating sensory axons travel to reach their central destinations. Similar functions are served by temporary processes of central neurons (Goodman et al., 1979). Our objective in this study was to determine whether this proposed guidance role is essential to the organization of the functional peripheral nerves during their development in the last 15% of embryogenesis. The use of microlaser lesions provided the potential for localizing damage to the site of pioneer fiber cell bodies, thus reducing the possibility that more extensive tissue damage alone might cause disruption of sensory axon development. Ultrastructural examination of cercal rudiments immediately after lesion indicated that the lesions were indeed local, except for the appearance of lysosomes in hemocyte-like cells which subsequently were found to be distributed through the affected and the neighboring normal cercus. Later lesions did not affect the normal development of cercal sensory nerves except for a reduction in the number of sensilla related to reduced total area of the smaller cercus, and we conclude that a localized lesion per se had no effect in sensory differentiation. Epidermal function appeared normal as judged by comparison of the sequences of cuticular layers formed in lesioned and normal cerci and neighboring abdominal integument.

The largest proportion of modified cercal sensory nerves were found in cerci where lesions were produced at or before the formation of the pioneer fibers. The presence of multiple bundles of sensory axons that showed no particular orientation within the cercus and the absence of bundles in the normal position indicate that normal organization of the cercal sensory nerves does not proceed if the pioneer fiber tract is not laid down.

The pioneer fibers become enveloped by companion cells that occupy the position of glia in the final nerve and which may be considered pioneer glia without necessarily implying that they take up their positions before the axons grow. The precise temporal relationship between the differentiation of the pioneer fibers and their glia is not known yet and it may be that the glial cells are in the vicinity of the dorsal and ventral midlines of the cercal lumen before the formation of the pioneer fibers. If so, they seem to be unable to function alone as organizers of the sensory bundles. The outcomes of later lesions to the pioneer fiber tracts, in which the axons degenerate but glia persist, show that the glial conduit once formed during the early association of pioneer fiber processes and glia can function as an organizing focus for the functional sensory fibers.

We have noted earlier (Edwards and Chen, 1979) that the mid-dorsal and midventral lines of the basal lamina underlying the cercal epithelium invariably serve as the surface on which the pioneer fibers make their transit to the base of the cercus. The pioneer fibers remain in contact with this surface until late in embryogenesis when the functional nerves of sensory axons have traversed the length of the cercus *en route* to the center. The glia retain their association with this surface after distal lesions kill the pioneer fibers and they can persist to form the aggregation site for the functional nerves.

Some uncertainty persists concerning the capacity of the pioneer cells to regenerate processes in cases where the axon was severed by the lesion but the cell body persisted. This possibility cannot be eliminated yet, but the more extreme case of regulation following loss of the cell bodies of pioneer fibers appears most unlikely for two reasons: first, because pioneer tracts did not appear in expected positions where the terminal lesion had clearly damaged the site of pioneer fibers and second, because the capacity for regeneration or regulation of the embryonic cercus appears to be restricted. Wound healing occurs in early massive lesions, but conpensatory growth does not occur and a normal cercus is never formed even though 50 to 60% of developmental period is available.

The persistence of the pathway between the base of the cercus and the ganglion was not investigated in this phase of the study in which attention was restricted to events within the cercus. We note, however, that degenerating axon profiles were observed in ventral positions within the embryonic ganglia after lesions of the cercal apex in stage 20, that is shortly after differentiation of the pioneer fibers, a finding in accord with Shankland's (1979) observation on the central projection of cercal pioneer fibers in the grasshopper *Schistocerca nitens*. Connections between cerci and the center were estab-

---

Figure 5. a, One of several axon bundles (*arrow top right*) from lesioned cercus shown in Figure 4*b*. The scolopale (*s*) of a chordotonal organ within the cercus lies adjacent to the nerve. A trachea (*t*) lies in contact with the chordotonal organ. *Scale* for *a* to *d*: 1 μm. *b,* Cercal sensory nerve within cercus in which the pioneer fiber pathway of one side was eliminated by laser lesion. In this case, all sensory axons have aggregated with the remaining tract. Lysosomes (*ly*) are in neighboring hemocyte. *c,* Normal cercal sensory nerve from normal cercus fixed shortly before hatching. *d,* Normal cercal nerve formed in cercus after irradiation at stage 21 after the differentiation of the pioneer fiber tract.

lished in animals lesioned after formation of the pioneer fibers but before differentiation of sensilla, suggesting, but not proving, that the pathway to the ganglion is preserved under these conditions.

References

Bate, C. M. (1976) Pioneer neurons in an insect embryo. Nature *260:* 54–56.

Berns, M. W., L. K. Chong, M. Hammer-Wilson, K. Miller, and A. Siemens (1979) Genetic surgery by laser: Establishment of a clonal population of rat kangaroo cells (PTK$_2$) with indirected deficiency in a chromosomal nucleolar organiser. Chromosoma *73:* 1–8.

Edwards, J. S. (1977) Pathfinding by arthropod sensory nerves. In *Identified Neurons and Behavior of Arthropods,* G. Hoyle, ed., pp. 484–493, Plenum Press, New York.

Edwards, J. S., and S.- W. Chen (1979) Embryonic development of an insect sensory system, the abdominal cerci of *Acheta domesticus.* Wilhelm Roux's Arch. Dev. Biol. *186:* 151–178.

Edwards, J. S., and J. Palka (1974) The cerci in abdominal giant fibers of the house cricket *Acheta domestica.* I. Anatomy and physiology of normal adults. Proc. R. Soc. Lond.

(Biol.) *185:* 83–103.

Edwards, J. S., M. W. Berns, and S.- W. Chen (1979) Laser lesions of embryonic cricket cerci disrupt guidepath role of pioneer fibres. Soc. Neurosci. Abstr. *5:* 158.

Goodman, C. S., M. Bate, and N. C. Spitzer (1979) Origin transformation and death of neurons from an identified precursor during grasshopper embryogenesis. Soc. Neurosci. Abstr. *5:* 161.

Keshishian, H. (1980) The origin and morphogenesis of pioneer neurons in the grasshopper metathoracic leg. Dev. Biol., in press.

Reynolds, E. S. (1963) The use of lead nitrate at high pH as an electron-opaque stain in electron microscopy. J. Cell Biol. *17:* 208–212.

Richardson, K. C., L. Jarrett, and E. H. Finke (1960) Embedding in epoxy resins for ultrathin sectioning in electron microscopy. Stain Technol. *35:* 313–323.

Shankland, M. (1979) Development of pioneer and sensory afferent projections in the grasshopper embryo. Soc. Neurosci. Abstr. *5:* 178.

Stocker, R. F., J. S. Edwards, J. Palka, and G. Schubiger (1976) Projection of sensory neurons from a homestic mutant appendage, *antennapedia* in *Drosophila melanogaster.* Dev. Biol. *52:* 210–220.

DEVELOPMENTAL BIOLOGY 44, 92–101 (1975)

Cell-to-Substratum Adhesion and Guidance of Axonal Elongation

PAUL C. LETOURNEAU[1]

Department of Biological Sciences, Stanford University, Stanford, California 94305

Accepted January 8, 1975

The behavior of axonal growth cones on surfaces with patterned variations in substratum was observed. Cells from sensory ganglia of 8-day-old chicken embryos were cultured on plastic petri dishes, plastic tissue culture dishes, and polyornithine-coated tissue culture dishes, all of which contained gridlike patterns of palladium (Pd) deposition.

The results indicated that growth cones elongated on the Pd-shadowed areas vs areas lacking Pd deposits depending on the relative adhesivity of the growth cones to the substrata. In petri dishes, growth cones stay on the Pd; in tissue culture dishes, they cross from one surface to the other; and in polyornithine-coated dishes, they elongate for great distances on the Pd-free areas. Analyses of time-lapse movies showed that, on Pd-shadowed polyornithine dishes, growth cones often approach the Pd-coated areas and microspikes touch the Pd surface. Yet, the axon tip continues to elongate on the Pd-free polyornithine surface.

The conclusion is offered that interactions between microspikes and the substratum adjacent to the growth cone are important determinants of the directions and pathways of axonal elongation.

INTRODUCTION

The assumption is often made that the complexity and specificity which exist in the nervous system result at least partially from an ordered or directed growth of nerve fibers during embryogenesis. The constancy of architecture observed in the nervous systems of some invertebrates also suggests that the embryonic growth of axons is not random (Burrows, 1973; Macagno *et al.*, 1973). However, the basic mechanisms that operate to produce such ordered growth have not yet been elucidated (Jacobson, 1970; Harrison, 1910).

One directive force in axonal growth may be contact guidance (Harrison, 1910). Elongating axons seem to be oriented by extracellular topographic features (Goldberg, 1974; Nornes and Das, 1972; Speidel, 1933), cell surfaces (Das *et al.*, 1974; Lopresti *et al.*, 1973, 1974; Rakic, 1971; Rakic and Sidman, 1973), and other axons and axonal growth cones (Dunn, 1971; Nornes

and Das, 1972; Lopresti *et al.*, 1973, 1974; Weiss, 1941). Such contact-mediated interactions may restrict axon elongation to certain pathways, but might not specify the particular direction taken. Growing axons that have been experimentally or naturally disoriented from their normal pathways can reverse their incorrect vector of growth and make appropriate connections (Hibbard, 1965; Sperry and Hibbard, 1968). This suggests that other forces may operate in addition to mere contact guidance.

Chemotaxis is another guiding force in cell movements (Adler, 1973; Bonner, 1947). Attempts to demonstrate chemotaxis of growing axons have produced both positive and negative results (Chamley *et al.*, 1973; Coughlin, 1975; Weiss and Taylor, 1944). Hence, chemotaxis should not be excluded as a possible guiding force of axon elongation (Ramon y Cajal, 1928).

Adhesion to the substratum may influence cell movements. Fibroblastic cells move up a gradient of metal deposition on a surface (Carter, 1965). Harris (1973)

[1] Present address: Department of Pediatrics, Stanford University School of Medicine, Stanford, CA 94305.

92

showed that cells will actively accumulate on portions of a patterned substratum to which they adhere most strongly. In these studies elongating axons of embryonic sensory neurons were presented with such patterned substrata. The results show that growth cones prefer to elongate on surfaces to which they adhere most firmly. This suggests a role for cell-to-substratum adhesion in determining the pathways of nerve fiber growth.

MATERIALS AND METHODS

Preparation of substrata. Four types of culture dishes were used: plastic petri dishes (Falcon Plastics, Oxnard, CA), plastic tissue culture dishes (Falcon Plastics), collagen-coated tissue culture dishes, and polyornithine-coated tissue culture dishes. The last two types were prepared as described in Letourneau (1975).

The patterned substrata were made as follows: Several size #2200 Effa, general electron microscope grids (Ernest F. Fullman, Inc., Schenectady, NY) were put into an open dish. Palladium (Pd) wire was shadowed onto the dishes using a vacuum evaporator. The dishes were inverted to remove the copper grids, and a clear pattern of Pd deposition was seen. The patterns consisted of 80-μm squares of Pd deposition with 27-μm-wide lanes of unshadowed Pd-free surface between the squares (see Figs. 1–7). Each shadowed dish was washed overnight with sterile water before use.

Cell culture. Dorsal root ganglia from 8-day-old chicken embryos were dissected and dissociated into single cells as described in Letourneau (1975). To a culture dish cells were added (8–12 $\times$ 10^4) in 2.5–3.0 ml of modified F12 (Spooner, 1970) with 10% fetal calf serum (Pacific Biological Supplies) and nerve growth factor (prepared as in Letourneau, 1975). Cultures were incubated overnight in a 37°C, humidified, 5% CO_2 incubator before being filmed, photographed, or otherwise manipulated.

Cell–substratum adhesion. The Gail and Boone air-blaster method of assaying cell-to-substratum adhesion was used to compare the adhesion of growth cones to a Pd-shadowed surface and to tissue culture plastic (Gail and Boone, 1972; Letourneau and Wessells, 1974; Letourneau, 1975).

Time-lapse cinematography. Time-lapse movies were made on a Zeiss inverted microscope, using a Bolex 16 mm movie camera, controlled by a Sage cinematographic apparatus. The culture medium was changed to L-15 (Pacific Biological Supplies) supplemented with 10% fetal calf serum and nerve growth factor just before filming was begun. L-15 maintained the medium at pH 7.4 in the absence of 5% CO_2 concentrations. During filming, the dish was kept at 37°C with a Sage Aircurtain Incubator.

RESULTS

The adhesion of growth cones to Pd-shadowed tissue culture dishes and to Pd-free tissue culture dishes was compared with the air-blaster method. As seen in Table 1, there is no significant difference in the adhesion of growth cones to Pd or to tissue culture plastic. This equality is further indicated by the fact (Table 1) that the percentage of neurons which form axons and the average length of axon per neuron at 24 hr *in vitro* on Pd-coated polyornithine or tissue culture plastic is not different from data for neurons on Pd-free tissue culture plastic (Letourneau, 1975). Growth cones are more adhesive to collagen, polyornithine, and the upper surfaces of glial cells than to tissue culture plastic (Table 1; Letourneau, 1975).

Growth cone–substratum adhesion was not assayed in plastic petri dishes because too few neurons form axons in petri dishes to do an adhesion assay (except in serum-free medium; Ludueña, 1973). Many cell types do not adhere well to Falcon petri-dish plastic (Harris, 1973; Martin and Rubin, 1974). We, therefore, assume that

TABLE 1

GROWTH CONE ADHESION, AXON INITIATION, AND MEAN AXON LENGTH AT 24   HR[a]

Dish	% Initiation	Axon/neuron (μm)	% Distracted
Pd-coated tissue culture	27 (n = 137)	158 (n = 20)	48 (n = 54)
Pd-coated polyornithine	29 (n = 86)	148 (n = 20)	—
Tissue culture	25 (n = 642)[b]	154 (n = 60)[b]	53 (n = 95)

[a] Growth cone–substratum adhesion was assayed at a blasting distance of 2.4 cm and an air flow-rate of 3.0 l/min. Duration of blast was 0.085 sec. The difference in percentage of growth cones distracted on these substrata is not significant. Methods of determining percent of axon initiation and average μm of axon/neuron are described in Letourneau (1975). n, number of neurons counted.

[b] Data taken from Letourneau (1975).

growth cone–petri-plastic adhesion is relatively weak.

From these data a hierarchy of substrata for growth cones can be postulated, based on the relative strengths of growth cone–substratum adhesion; Glia ≈ polyornithine > collagen > tissue culture plastic ≈ Pd > petri plastic. Hence, the patterned substrata used in these studies consisted of Pd squares surrounded by lanes of substrata to which growth cones are less, equally, or more adhesive (i.e., petri plastic; tissue culture plastic; collagen or polyornithine, respectively).

Cultures were observed after approximately 16 hr *in vitro*. On the Pd-shadowed petri and tissue culture dishes axons were seen which extended from Pd onto the unshadowed plastic and vice versa (Figs. 1–5). Growth cones also were seen on both the Pd squares and on the unshadowed lanes.

In marked contrast to these results, in collagen or polyornithine-coated dishes with Pd patterns, axons extended for long distances along the unshadowed lanes between the Pd squares (Figs. 6–11). After 48 hr, axons longer than 1000 μm extended down the collagen or polyornithine lanes. Frequently, axons bent around 90° corners

---

FIG. 1. A neuron cultured in a Pd-shadowed plastic petri dish. The nerve cell body (N) and the axons (A) are on a Pd square (Pd) surrounded by unshadowed petri plastic. One axon extends to the edge of the Pd surface. × 180. All of these photographs were taken after 16–24 hr of culture.

FIG. 2. Neurons cultured in a Pd-shadowed petri dish. One axon tip (GC) is at the edge of the Pd, and another (a) is on the unshadowed side of the boundary. × 180.

FIG. 3. These growth cones have crossed the unshadowed petri plastic from one Pd square to another. Note that the glial cells (G) tend to be on the Pd squares (see Table 3). Axon (A); nerve cell body (N). × 180.

FIG. 4. A neuron cultured in a Pd-shadowed tissue culture dish. The axons (A) have elongated from the Pd surface (Pd) across the unshadowed lanes. Nerve cell body (N); glial cell (G). × 170.

FIG. 5. Neurons cultured in a Pd-shadowed tissue culture dish. Nerve cell bodies (N); glial cells (G). × 180.

FIG. 6. Neurons cultured in a Pd-shadowed, polyornithine-coated tissue culture dish. Note how the axons extend only along the unshadowed lanes of the dish. Nerve cell body (N); polyornithine surface (porn). × 170.

FIG. 7. Neurons cultured in a Pd-shadowed, polyornithine-coated tissue culture dish. One axon (a) has elongated on the Pd surface, but most axons (A) stay on the unshadowed lanes. Several axons appear to have made 90° turns (arrows). Polyornithine surface (porn). × 145.

FIG. 8–11. Four frames from a time lapse movie of a neuron cultured on Pd-shadowed collagen. (8) The axon (A) has several terminal growth cones (arrows). Nerve cell body (N); collagen (col.). × 215. (9) Taken 36 min after Fig. 8. Two growth cones (GC) have elongated along the unshadowed lane. Collagen (col.). × 215. (10) Taken 53 min after Fig. 9. Note how the growth cones do not stay in the middle of the unshadowed lane (arrows) but wander from one side of the lane to the other (compare to Fig. 9). One growth cone has contacted a glial cell (G). Collagen (col.). × 215. (11) Taken 35 min after Fig. 10. The axons have elongated further along the unshadowed lane. Collagen (col.). × 215.

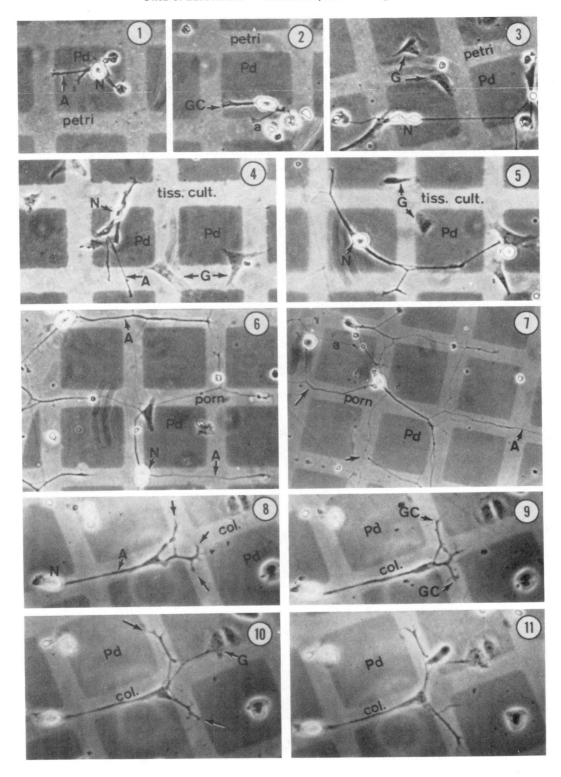

or had branches going down several lanes at an intersection (Figs. 6, 7). Some nerve cell bodies were located on Pd squares with axons which had crossed onto and continued along the Pd-free lane.

Although axons did extend along the unshadowed lanes in petri and tissue culture dishes, the frequency of such observations and the lengths of axons were much less than in collagen or polyornithine dishes.

In order to estimate the preference of growth cones for various substrata, the percentage of growth cones that were on (a) Pd, (b) unshadowed lanes, and (c) upper surfaces of flattened glial cells were determined in the petri dishes, tissue culture dishes, and polyornithine-coated dishes. The data are presented in Table 2. If the percentage of growth cones on a surface is a measure of relative preference for that surface, then on petri dishes, growth cones prefer (1) glia, (2) Pd, and (3) petri plastic; in tissue culture dishes the order is (1) glia, (2) Pd, and (3) plastic, but the differences

are small; and on polyornithine dishes growth cones prefer (1) polyornithine, (2) glia, and (3) Pd.

These numbers are not absolute indications of the preference of growth cones for a surface because of the geometry of the patterns. The Pd squares comprise about 67% of the surface area, but they are islands surrounded by continuous lanes of unshadowed substratum. Obviously, growth cones can elongate for long distances on the lanes but not for more than 115 μm on the Pd squares. Glia cover little (less than 5%) of the surface, at the cell densities plated here. However, glia do migrate, and opportunities for encounter with an axon or growth cone are greater than suggested by the 5% figure.

From photographs of the cultures, the numbers of glia on the Pd or on the unshadowed lanes were counted. As seen in Table 3, the distribution of glia is similar to that for growth cones. In addition, it conforms with Harris' (1973) results with several cell types, except that he reported that cells strongly prefer tissue culture plastic to Pd.

The 35 mm photographs and the proportions of growth cones situated on various substrata suggested that growth cones tend to remain on substrata to which they are more adhesive. Time-lapse cinematography was used to observe the behavior of growth cones on these dishes.

TABLE 2

PERCENT OF GROWTH CONES ON SUBSTRATA[a]

Dish	Substratum		
	Pd	Un-shad-owed lane	Glia
Petri plastic	35	18	47 (n = 98)
Tissue culture plastic	32	31	36 (n = 207)
Polyornithine-coated	4	74	22 (n = 274)
	Substratum		
	Pd	Unshadowed lane	
Petri plastic	65	35 (n = 52)	
Tissue culture plastic	51	49 (n = 132)	
Polyornithine-coated	5	95 (n = 214)	

[a] The distribution of growth cones on Pd, unshadowed lanes, and glia, respectively, was determined by counting the number of growth cones on these substrata in several randomly selected microscope fields. The data for growth cones on glial cells was omitted in calculating the percentages shown in the lower panels. n, number of neurons counted.

TABLE 3

PERCENT OF GLIA ON SUBSTRATA[a]

Dish	Substratum	
	Pd	Unshadowed lane
Petri plastic	86	14 (n = 50)
Tissue culture plastic	59	41 (n = 66)
Polyornithine-coated	29	71 (n = 55)

[a] The distribution of glia on Pd and on the unshadowed lanes, respectively, was determined from photographs of cell cultures. Only those glial cells that were wholly on one substratum type or almost wholly, except for marginal areas, were counted. n, number of glia counted.

On Pd-shadowed petri dishes growth cones would move across the Pd to the edge of a square. Several behaviors followed. Often, they would remain active (i.e., intensive microspike activity; Ludueña and Wessells, 1973) but not advance onto the plastic. This was occasionally followed by retraction of the growth cone and axon. Another observation was that the growth cone would move laterally along the border, staying on the Pd. There were cases of the growth cone crossing from Pd onto petri plastic. When this happened, the growth cone usually would not elongate far, although it did continue microspike activity. It seemed as though the growth cones were "slipping back" after accomplishing a short advance.

On Pd-shadowed tissue culture dishes, growth cones frequently crossed from Pd to plastic and from plastic to Pd. One filming sequence of 5.5 hr was a particularly good example. An axon started on Pd and moved onto the plastic, where it elongated about 80 μm in 2 hr. Then, it crossed onto a Pd square and grew 100 μm or more to the other side and moved onto plastic again. Another axon from the same cell body elongated on the plastic for over 4 hr and then crossed onto the Pd.

On Pd-shadowed collagen and polyornithine dishes, growth cones of axons elongating along an unshadowed, Pd-free lane did not stay in the middle of a lane; instead, they meandered from one edge of the lane to the other (Figs. 8–11). Microspikes waved about in close proximity to the Pd surface (Figs. 12–17). It seemed that microspikes protruded from various edges of the growth cone and were contacting the Pd and the unshadowed substrata simultaneously. Yet, the growth cone continued to elongate on the unshadowed surface. In addition to microspikes many thin veillike expansions of microspikes formed on collagen and polyornithine. These veils are reminiscent of the distinctive flattening of growth cones observed in cultures with elevated Ca^{2+} levels (Letourneau, 1975).

Such flattened veils may result from a strong adhesion to the substratum. Related to this is the impression that microspikes adhere to the collagen or polyornithine surface for longer time periods than to the Pd.

Growth cones were observed extending around a corner at the intersection of two unshadowed lanes. The growth cone stayed on the collagen or polyornithine as it moved from one lane to the other. In such cases, if the axon was not adherent to the substratum, it straightened out across the corner, thereby extending over the Pd surface. This arrangement could give the impression that the axon had elongated directly across the Pd from one lane to the next. However, the film shows clearly that the growth cone grew *around* the corner and the axon slipped sideways in a passive fashion (as predicted by Ludueña (1973) and above).

Another interesting series of observations with time-lapse cinematography was the movement of growth cones onto the upper surfaces of glia. The actual adhesion of the growth cone to a glial surface was often not observed, but the result was (Figs. 18–21), the axon rapidly straightened as if pulled tight. The cause of this is unknown, but a possible explanation is that the adhesion of the growth cone, followed by an advance, created tension to pull the axon toward the glial cell.

DISCUSSION

The basic results of these experiments are: (1) A hierarchy of growth cone–substratum adhesion can be postulated; glia $\approx$ polyornithine $>$ collagen $>$ tissue culture plastic $\approx$ Pd $>$ petri plastic. (2) On Pd-shadowed petri dishes, growth cones do not move well on petri plastic and often do not cross from Pd to petri plastic. (3) On Pd-shadowed tissue culture dishes, growth cones cross from plastic to Pd and vice versa frequently. (4) On Pd-shadowed collagen or polyornithine dishes, growth cones elongate for hundreds of μm's on the un-

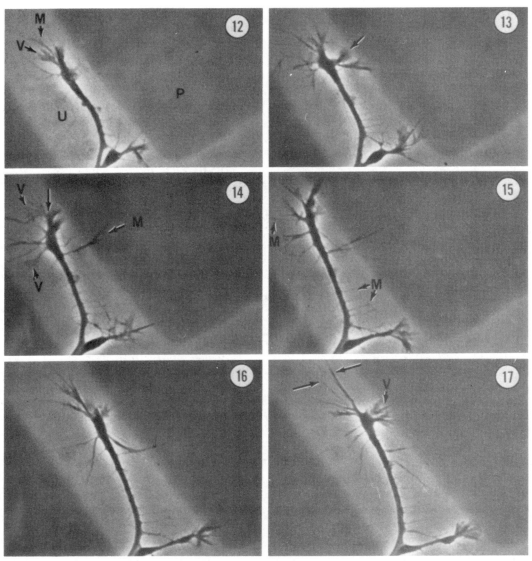

Fig. 12–17. Frames from a time-lapse movie of a growth cone elongating along the unshadowed lane between two Pd-shadowed squares in a polyornithine-coated tissue culture dish. (12) Note the microspikes (M) and veillike expansions of cell surface. The microspikes are distributed over the substratum adjacent to the growth cone. Pd surface (P); unshadowed lane (U). × 880. (13) Taken 200 sec after Fig. 12. Note how the morphology of the growth cone has changed due to microspike formation and movement. Some microspikes (arrow) are out of the plane of focus, meaning they are moving in the fluid medium. × 880. (14) Taken 200 sec after Fig. 13. The growth cone has elongated in the area indicated by the arrow. A microspike (M) has extended onto the Pd surface. Veil (V). × 880. (15) Taken 200 sec after Fig. 14. Note the microspikes (M) that extend from the growth cone and the sides of the axon. × 880. (16) Taken 200 sec after Fig. 15. × 880. (17) Taken 200 sec after Fig. 16. Note the forward extending microspikes (arrows) and the veillike expansion (V) that is close to the Pd surface. × 880.

shadowed lanes, even though the growth cones approach the Pd surface very closely.

These results may have important implications for neuronal axon formation.

One can understand why growth cones will not cross from Pd to petri plastic if they adhere only weakly to petri plastic (adhesion may occur in the absence of serum;

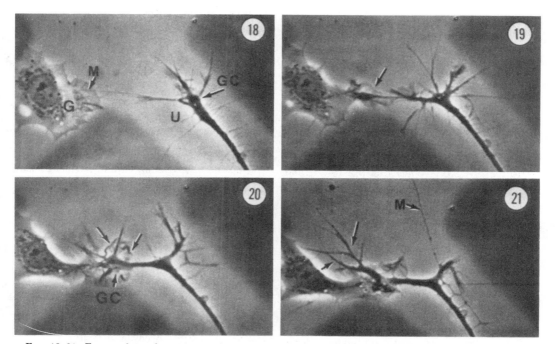

FIG. 18–21. Frames from the same movie of a growth cone as shown in Figs. 12–17. (18) The growth cone (GC) is near the middle of an unshadowed lane (U). A microspike (arrow) has just contacted the upper surface of a glial cell (G). × 880. (19) Taken 296 sec later. The growth cone is beginning to extend towards the glial cell. Also, note the movement of the glial cell's leading edge towards the growth cone (arrow). × 880. (20) Taken 312 sec after Fig. 19. The growth cone has moved onto the upper glial cell surface. Note the increased ruffling (arrows) of the glial cell margin where it contacts the growth cone. × 880. (21) Taken 288 sec after Fig. 20. The growth cone has elongated across the glial cell surface and microspikes (arrows) are extending over the dish substratum on the far side of the glial cell. Note the extremely long microspike (M), which is touching the dish substratum. × 880.

Ludeña, 1973). Harris (1973) reports that 3T3 cells undergo vigorous ruffling activity on petri dishes, giving the impression of "a frantic, but unsuccessful struggle to spread, which is continually frustrated by repeated de-adhesions at the margin."

However, what can be offered to explain the response of growth cones to the same substratum, Pd, in different ways? Growth cones do not often cross from collagen or polyornithine surfaces onto Pd. Yet, Pd is a perfectly acceptable substratum for axon elongation, when petri or tissue culture plastic is the alternative substratum! Do growth cones prefer to stay on collagen or polyornithine because they adhere more tightly? Or are they unable to move onto the Pd-coated surface? The fact that neurons do initiate and extend axons on Pd-shadowed, polyornithine-coated dishes

which lack patterned deposits eliminates the possibility that Pd-coated polyornithine is an unacceptable surface for growth cone function.

These results suggest a mechanism for regulating the directions in which axons elongate. Microspikes and their veillike expansions often contact the substratum ahead of the growth cone (Wessells *et al.*, 1973). Bray (1973) has postulated that microspikes and other filopodia grow via addition of intracellular vesicles to the surface of the microspike tip. It could be that addition of vesicles and microspike enlargement are enhanced by adhesion of the microspike to a surface (Letourneau, 1975; Rovensky and Slavnaya, 1974; Vasiliev and Gelfand, 1973, p. 326). This may lead to expansion of the microspike and advancement of the growth cone in that direction. In this manner the growth cone will advance on that substratum adjacent to the growth cone to which microspikes adhere more often or more strongly.

A criticism of these experiments is the artificial nature of the patterned substrata, which are not likely to represent accurately the subtle differences of the microenvironment in an embryo. Nevertheless, the results, however crude, do suggest a way of guiding an axon to its destination. Pathways of relatively high adhesion or adhesion gradients may be crucial elements for both gross axonal routing and for aspects of neuronal connection specificity.

This model does not rule out chemotaxis as a possible directive force. If a chemical concentration gradient could make microspike interactions with the substratum more effective in a particular direction, elongation would be similarly guided. The diffusing molecule could act either on the growth cone surface or on the substratum. Jacobson (1970) has stated well the error of making a hard distinction between chemical and mechanical guidance of nerve fiber growth because "at short range they boil down to the same thing; the physicochemical interaction between the nerve fiber and its environment."

I thank Dr. Norman K. Wessells for advice and support in conducting these experiments and preparing the manuscript. I am also grateful to Dr. Frank E. Stockdale and Dr. Merton R. Bernfield for reading and criticizing the manuscript.

This work was supported by an NIH predoctoral traineeship provided to the author and by NIH Grant No. HD-04708 to Dr. Wessells.

REFERENCES

ADLER, J. (1973). A method for measuring chemotaxis and use of the method to determine optimum conditions for chemotaxis by Escherichia coli. J. Gen. Microbiol. 74, 77–91.

BONNER, J. T. (1947). Evidence for formation of cell aggregates by chemotaxis in the development of the slime mold Dictyostelium discoideum. J. Exp. Zool. 106, 1–26.

BRAY, D. (1973). Model for membrane movements in the neural growth cone. Nature (London) 244, 93–96.

BURROWS, M. (1973). The morphology of an elevator and depressor motor neuron of the hind wing of a locust. J. Comp. Physiol. 83, 165–178.

CARTER, S. B. (1965). Principles of cell motility. The directionality of cell movement and cancer invasion. Nature (London) 208, 1183–1187.

CHAMLEY, J. H., GOLDER, I., and BURNSTOCK, G. (1973). Selective growth of sympathetic nerve fibers to explants of normally densely innervated autonomic effector organs in tissue culture. Develop. Biol. 31, 362–379.

COUGHLIN, M. D. Target organ stimulation of parasympathetic nerve growth in the developing mouse submandibular gland. Develop. Biol. 43, 140–158.

DAS, G. D., LAMMERT, G. L., and MCALLISTER, J. P. (1974). Contact guidance and migratory cells in the developing cerebellum. Brain Res. 69, 13–29.

DUNN, G. (1971). Mutual contact inhibition of extension of chick sensory nerve fibers in vitro. J. Comp. Neurol. 143, 491–508.

GAIL, M. H., and BOONE, C. W. (1972). Cell-substrate adhesivity. Exp. Cell Res. 70, 33–40.

GOLDBERG, S. (1974). Studies on the mechanisms of development of the visual pathways in the chick embryo. Develop. Biol. 36, 24–43.

HARRIS, A. (1973). Behavior of cultured cells on substrata of variable adhesiveness. Exp. Cell Res. 77, 285–297.

HARRISON, R. G. (1910). The outgrowth of the nerve fiber as a mode of protoplasmic movement. J. Exp. Zool. 9, 787–848.

HIBBARD, E. (1965). Orientation and directed growth of Mauthner's cell axons from duplicated vestibular nerve roots. Exp. Neurol. 13, 289–301.

LETOURNEAU, P. C. (1975). Possible roles for cell-to-substratum adhesion in neuronal morphogenesis. Develop. Biol. 44, 77–91.

LOPRESTI, V., MACAGNO, E. R., and LEVINTHAL, C. (1973). Structure and development of neuronal connections in isogenic organisms: Cellular interactions in the development of the optic lamina of Daphnia. Proc. Nat. Acad. Sci. USA 70, 433–437.

LOPRESTI, V., MACAGNO, E. R., and LEVINTHAL, C. (1974). Structure and development of neuronal connections in isogenic organisms: Transient gap junctions between growing optic axons and lamina neuroblasts. Proc. Nat. Acad. Sci. USA 71, 1098–1102.

LUDUEÑA, M. A. (1973). The growth of spinal ganglion neurons in serum-free medium. Develop. Biol. 33, 470–476.

MACAGNO, E. R., LOPRESTI, V., and LEVINTHAL, C. (1973). Structure and development of neuronal connections in isogenic organisms: Variations and similarities in the optic system of Daphnia magna. Proc. Nat. Acad. Sci. USA 70, 57–61.

MARTIN, G. R., and RUBIN, H. (1974). Effects of cell adhesion to the substratum on the growth of chick embryo fibroblasts. *Exp. Cell Res.* **85,** 319–333.

NORNES, H. O., and DAS, G. D. (1972). Temporal pattern of neurogenesis in spinal cord: cytoarchitecture and directed growth of axons. *Proc. Nat. Acad. Sci. USA* **69,** 1962–1966.

RAKIC, P. (1971). Neuron-glia relationship during granule cell migration in developing cerebellar cortex. A Golgi and electron microscopic study in *Macacus rhesus, J. Comp. Neurol.* **141,** 282–312.

RAKIC, P., and SIDMAN, R. L. (1973). Weaver mutant mouse cerebellum: Defective neuronal migration secondary to abnormality of Bergmann glia. *Proc. Nat. Acad. Sci. USA* **70,** 240–244.

RAMON Y CAJAL, S. (1928). *In* "Degeneration and Regeneration of the Nervous System" (R. M. May, ed.). Oxford Univ. Press. London and New York. 1959.

ROVENSKY, YU. A. and SLAVENAYA, I. L. (1974). Spreading of fibroblast-like cells on grooved surfaces. *Exp. Cell Res.* **84,** 199–206.

SPEIDEL, C. C. (1933). Studies of living nerves. II. Activities of amoeboid growth cones, sheath cells, and myelin segments, as revealed by prolonged observation of individual nerve fibers in frog tadpoles. *Amer. J. Anat.* **52,** 1–79.

SPERRY, R. W., and HIBBARD, E. (1968). Regulative factors in the orderly growth of retino-tectal connexions. *In* "Growth of the Nervous System" (Ciba Symposium) (G. E. Wolstenholme, and M. O'Conner, eds.), pp. 41–52. J. and A. Churchill, London.

SPOONER, B. S. (1970). The expression of differentiation by chick embryo thyroid in cell culture. I. Functional and fine structural stability in mass and clonal culture. *J. Cell. Physiol.* **75,** 33–48.

VAN DER LOOS, H. (1965). The "improperly" oriented pyramidal cell in the cerebral cortex and its possible bearing on problems of growth and cell orientation. *Bull. Johns Hopkins Hosp.* **117,** 228–250.

VASILIEV, JU. M., and GELFAND, I. M. (1973). Interactions of normal and neoplastic fibroblasts with substratum. *In* "Locomotion of Tissue Cells" (Ciba Foundation Symposium 14), pp. 311–329. Assoc. Scientific Publishers, Amsterdam.

WEISS, P. (1941). Nerve patterns: The mechanics of nerve growth. *Growth (Third Growth Symposium; suppl.)* **5,** 163–203.

WEISS, P., and TAYLOR, A. C. (1944). Further experimental evidence against "neurotropism" in nerve regeneration. *J. Exp. Zool.* **95,** 233–257.

WESSELLS, N. K., SPOONER, B. S., and LUDUEÑA, M. A. (1973). Surface movements, microfilaments, and cell locomotion. *In* "Locomotion of Tissue Cells" (Ciba Foundation Symposium 14), pp. 53–82. Assoc. Scientific Publishers, Amsterdam.

Section 5
Neuronal Death
in Normal Development

Hamburger, V. 1975. Cell death in the development of the lateral motor column of the chick embryo. *J. Comp. Neurol. 160:* 535–546.

Pilar, G., L. Landmesser, and L. Burstein. 1980. Competition for survival among developing ciliary ganglion cells. *J. Neurophysiol. 43:* 233–254.

Pittman, R. and R.W. Oppenheim. 1979. Cell death of motoneurons in the chick embryo spinal cord. IV. Evidence that a functional neuromuscular interaction is involved in the regulation of naturally occurring cell death and the stabilization of synapses. *J. Comp. Neurol. 187:* 425–446.

In addition to migration, differentiation, and axonal outgrowth, many neurons undergo a further striking change during normal development: They degenerate and die. Neuronal death occurs in both central and peripheral structures, and the magnitude of the loss is impressive; it is not unusual for half of all neurons initially present in a given nucleus or ganglion to die over a relatively short period (see Oppenheim 1981a).

Early on, it was recognized that cell death in many instances is not preprogrammed but is related to events occurring in the targets innervated by neurons (see Detwiler 1920, 1936; Piatt 1948; Cowan 1973; Oppenheim 1981a). Perhaps the most compelling evidence in this regard is that early ablation of the target causes severe depletion of the final population of innervating neurons. The nature of this phenomenon was debated for several decades but was generally interpreted in terms of a peripheral influence on the recruitment of neuronal precursors (see Oppenheim 1981a). This idea was brought into question by the experiments of Hamburger and Levi-Montalcini (1949) which showed that neuronal death in sensory ganglia is a normal phenomenon and that target ablation accentuates this process. Neuronal death and its accentuation by early target removal was subsequently described in a variety of systems, including spinal motor neurons, autonomic ganglia, brain-stem nuclei, and cells projecting entirely within the central nervous system (see, for example, **Hamburger** 1958, **1975;** Cowan and Wenger 1967; Landmesser and Pilar 1974a; Clarke and Cowan 1976; Hendry and Campbell 1976). Moreover, some of the normal neuronal loss can be diminished if the amount of target available to an innervating population is increased (Hollyday and Hamburger 1976; **Pilar, Landmesser,** and **Burstein 1980**). For example, if a motor neuron pool is supplied with an extra limb at an early embryonic stage, the number of neurons surviving is appreciably increased (Hollyday and Hamburger 1976). Finally, cell death is not simply a result of axonal misdirection or axons failing to reach the target (Prestige and Wilson 1972; Clarke and Cowan 1976; Landmesser and Pilar 1976). This has been demonstrated most convincingly by retrograde labeling of the innervating cells after injection of the target with horseradish peroxidase (Clarke and Cowan 1976; Chu-Wang and Oppenheim 1978; Pilar et al. 1980).

Taken together, this evidence has given rise to the prevailing view that there is competition among axons innervating a target and that the losers die. This idea is supported by the finding that removing two thirds of the neurons that normally innervate the iris of the chick results in the rescue of approximately 40% of the neurons that would have died (Pilar et al. 1980), presumably because the altered ratio of neurons to target makes the competition less stringent. Further support for the idea of competition at the level of the target comes from the observation that the neurons that eventually die appear to differentiate normally until the time their axons reach the periphery (Landmesser and Pilar 1974b; Oppenheim et al. 1978). It should be pointed out, however, that not all results are consistent with competition as the sole cause of neuronal death, even in vertebrates (see Lamb 1980). Cell death in invertebrates can be much more programmatic (see, for example, Sulston and Horvitz 1977; see also the introduction to Section 3), and some invertebrate neurons can survive in the absence of their targets (Sanes et al. 1976).

A more particular explanation of neuron death during normal development is that nerve cells compete for a survival or maintenance factor produced in limited quantities by their targets. Acquisition of the factor may be related to synapse formation, although this issue is by no means decided. There is, for example, some evidence that the formation of synapses per se does not protect a neuron against eventual death (Pilar and Landmesser 1976), although death or survival might depend on the number of synapses formed and the quality of their function. That synaptic function is an important aspect of neuronal survival in some systems, however, is suggested by the finding that blockade of neuromuscular transmission prevents the normal death

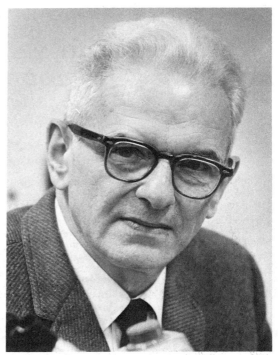

Viktor Hamburger, whose studies of neuronal death in chick embryos form much of the basis for present thinking about this phenomenon.

of some motor neurons (**Pittman** and **Oppenheim 1979**; Oppenheim 1981a,b; Hamburger et al. 1981). When the concentration of the blocking agent falls to the point where movement can begin, the surplus motor neurons belatedly die. According to the maintenance-factor hypothesis, the explanation of this result would be that as the muscle is innervated and becomes active, its production of the factor is lowered to a level that can support only some of the neurons originally projecting to it. Blockade of synaptic transmission might therefore keep innervated muscle in a state resembling its condition prior to nerve contact, in which the production and/or secretion of factor is high. Support for this idea comes from the observation that the production of nerve growth factor by the iris increases markedly after denervation, as discussed in the next section. An alternative to the idea of competition for a diffusible survival factor is that neurons compete for a limited number of postsynaptic sites. This concept is not consistent (at least in its simplest form) with what is presently known about synapse formation (see Sections 8, 9, and 11).

An unanswered question about neuronal death

is whether or not it is ubiquitous in normal development. For technical reasons, most of the neuronal populations that have been examined for cell death are those whose axons project to relatively distant targets. What about local interneurons which, after all, make up the bulk of the neurons in the nervous system? Another question is whether the number of neurons present at the end of embryonic development remains constant in maturity. Certainly there are some systems that continue to add neurons throughout life (see, for example, Birse et al. 1980; Johns 1981). Furthermore, in one particular mammalian system, the olfactory epithelium, neurons that degenerate are apparently replaced (Graziadei and Monti Graziadei 1977).

In summary, the death of many developing neurons is a widespread occurrence and in many instances depends on an interaction with neuronal targets. The maintenance factor hypothesis proposes that a majority of the neuronal deaths in vertebrates are caused by neither murder nor suicide, but by something akin to a starvation that arises from failure to compete successfully with other neurons for an agent produced by the target cells. Whatever the merits of this particular explanation, the degeneration of many nerve cells in normal vertebrate development appears to be based on feedback and consequent adjustment rather than on preordination. At least one result of this phenomenon (and thus a presumptive purpose) is to match the size of innervating populations to the capacity of their targets. In invertebrates, where single cells rather than populations are often charged with carrying out particular functions, this matching may be carried out by a more programmed (as opposed to competitive) degeneration of neurons. A similar programmed demise of neuronal precursors may also occur at earlier stages of vertebrate development, which has not been much studied in this context.

References

Birse, S.C., R.B. Leonard, and R.E. Coggeshall. 1980. Neuronal increase in various areas of the nervous system of the guppy, *Lebistes. J. Comp. Neurol.* 194: 291–301.

Chu-Wang, I.-W. and R.W. Oppenheim. 1978. Cell death of motorneurons in the chick embryo spinal cord. II. A quantitative and qualitative analysis of degeneration in the ventral root, including evidence for axon outgrowth and limb innervation prior to cell death. *J. Comp. Neurol.* 177: 59–86.

Clarke, P.G.H. and W.M. Cowan. 1976. The development of the isthmo-optic tract in the chick, with special reference to the occurrence and correction of developmental errors in the location and connections of isthmo-optic neurons. *J. Comp. Neurol.* 167: 143–164.

Cowan, W.M. 1973. Neuronal death as a regulative mechanism in the control of cell number in the nervous system. In *Development and aging in the nervous system* (ed. D.M. Rockstein and M.L. Sussman), pp. 19–41. Academic Press, New York.

Cowan, W.M. and E. Wenger. 1967. Cell loss in the trochlear nucleus of the chick during normal development or after radical extirpation of the optic vesicle. *J. Exp. Zool.* 164: 267–280.

Detwiler, S.R. 1920. On the hyperplasia of nerve centers resulting from excessive peripheral loading. *Proc. Natl. Acad. Sci.* 6: 96–101.

———. 1936. *Neuroembryology. An experimental study.* MacMillan, New York.

Graziadei, P.P.C. and G.A. Monti Graziadei. 1977. Continuous nerve cell renewal in the olfactory system. *Handbook of sensory physiology* (ed. M. Jacobson), vol. 9, pp. 55–83. Springer-Verlag, Berlin.

Hamburger, V. 1958. Regression versus peripheral control of differentiation in motor hypoplasia. *Am. J. Anat.* 102: 365–407.

———. 1975. Cell death in the development of the lateral motor column of the chick embryo. *J. Comp. Neurol.* 160: 535–546.

Hamburger, V. and R. Levi-Montalcini. 1949. Proliferation, differentiation and degeneration in the spinal ganglia of the chick embryo under normal and experimental conditions. *J. Exp. Zool.* 111: 457–501.

Hamburger, V., J.K. Brunso-Bechtold, and J.W. Yip. 1981. Neuronal death in the spinal ganglia of the chick embryo and its reduction by nerve growth factor. *J. Neurosci.* 1: 60–71.

Hendry, I.A. and J. Campbell. 1976. Morphometric analysis of rat superior cervical ganglion after axotomy and nerve growth factor treatment. *J. Neurocytol.* 5: 351–360.

Hollyday, M. and V. Hamburger. 1976. Reduction of the naturally occurring motor neuron loss by enlargement of the periphery. *J. Comp. Neurol.* 170: 311–320.

Johns, P.R. 1981. Growth of fish retinas. *Am. Zool.* 21: 441–453.

Lamb, A.H. 1980. Motoneuron counts in *Xenopus* frogs reared with one bilaterally-innervated hindlimb. *Nature* 284: 347–350.

Landmesser, L. and G. Pilar. 1974a. Synapse formation during embryogenesis on ganglion cells lacking a periphery. *J. Physiol.* 241: 715–736.

———. 1974b. Synaptic transmission and cell death during normal ganglionic development. *J. Physiol.* 241: 737–749.

———. 1976. Fate of ganglionic synapses and ganglion cell axons during normal and induced cell death. *J. Cell Biol.* 68: 357–374.

Oppenheim, R.W. 1981a. Neuronal cell death and some related regressive phenomena during neurogenesis: A selective historical review and a progress report. In *Studies in developmental neurobiology; essays in honor of Viktor Hamburger* (ed. W.M. Cowan), pp. 74–133. Oxford University Press, New York.

———. 1981b. Cell death of motoneurons in the chick embryo spinal cord. V. Evidence on the role of cell death and neuromuscular function in the formation of specific peripheral connections. *J. Neurosci.* 1: 141–151.

Oppenheim, R.W., I.-W. Chu-Wang, and J.L. Maderdrut. 1978. Cell death of motoneurons in the chick embryo spinal cord. III. The differentiation of motoneurons prior to their induced degeneration following limb-bud removal. *J. Comp. Neurol.* 177: 87–111.

Piatt, J. 1948. Form and causality in neurogenesis. *Biol. Rev.* 23: 1–45.

Pilar, G. and L. Landmesser. 1976. Ultrastructural differences during embryonic cell death in normal and peripherally deprived ciliary ganglia. *J. Cell Biol.* 68: 339–356.

Pilar, G., L. Landmesser, and L. Burstein. 1980. Competition for survival among developing ciliary ganglion cells. *J. Neurophysiol.* 43: 233–254.

Pittman, R. and R.W. Oppenheim. 1979. Cell death of motoneurons in the chick embryo spinal cord. IV. Evidence that a functional neuromuscular interaction is involved in the regulation of naturally occurring cell death and the stabilization of synapses. *J. Comp. Neurol.* 187: 425–446.

Prestige, M.C. and M.A. Wilson. 1974. A quantitative study of the growth and development of the ventral root in normal and experimental conditions. *J. Embryol. Exp. Morphol.* 32: 819–833.

Sanes, J.R., J.G. Hildebrand, and D.J. Prescott. 1976.

Differentiation of insect sensory neurons in the absence of their normal synaptic targets. *Dev. Biol.* 52: 121–127.

Sulston, J.E. and H.R. Horvitz. 1977. Post-embryonic cell lineages of the nematode *Caenorhabditis elegans*. *Dev. Biol.* 56: 110–156.

Reprinted from J. Comp. Neurol., Vol. 160, pp. 535–546. 1975

Cell Death in the Development of the Lateral Motor Column of the Chick Embryo

VIKTOR HAMBURGER

Department of Biology, Washington University, St. Louis, Missouri

ABSTRACT   Cell counts were made in the lumbar lateral motor column (l.m.c.) of chick embryos of 5.5, 6, 7, 8, 9, 12, 18 days of incubation and five days post-hatching (n = 68). Only nuclei with nucleoli were counted and corrections were made for double counting (Abercrombie, '46). The population attains a peak value of over 20,000 cells (corrected figure: over 17,000) at 5.5–6.5 days = stages 28 and 29 (Hamburger and Hamilton, '51). The l.m.c. loses between 7,000 and 8,000 cells between days 6.5 and 9.5, (between stages 29 and 36). In other words, 60% of the population survive. A plateau of approximately 12,300 cells (corrected figure: 10,300) is maintained through five days posthatching. Massive cell degeneration was observed in 7- and 8-day embryos. Counts of distinctly pyknotic cells indicate that at least 5–6% of the total population is in the process of degeneration at any particular time. This figure is probably an underestimation; hence it is virtually certain that the depletion of the l.m.c. is due entirely to cell death. Arguments are presented in support of the hypothesis that the naturally occurring cell death in the l.m.c. is due to the failure of their axons to survive in a competition process at the periphery. Observations of the time pattern of muscle differentiation and their neurotization in the leg further endorse this hypothesis. However, it is not clear whether the axons compete for contact sites on muscle fibers or for a "trophic" agent.

Cell loss seems to be a widespread phenomenon in neurogenesis. In a number of nerve centers small enough to permit cell counts of the entire population, such as brain stem nuclei and motor columns, precise data of cell loss during normal development have been obtained. In extreme cases, such as the mesencephalic V nucleus in the chick embryo (Rogers and Cowan, '73) and the lateral motor column of anurans (Hughes, '68; Prestige, '70), only one out of four neuroblasts survive. A recent review of naturally occurring neuron death by Cowan ('73) which deals also with theoretical aspects makes a further general discussion of this topic unnecessary.

It may seem redundant to investigate cell loss in yet another neuron population. The justification for undertaking such a study on the lateral motor column (l.m.c.) of the chick embryo lies in the hope that special features of this system may make it a particularly suitable object for further analysis of this interesting phenomenon. The early events in the development of the l.m.c. in the chick embryo are neatly programmed in a sequential order, without

overlap of the different phases. The production of prospective l.m.c. cells by proliferation in the ventral part of the spinal cord is nearly completed at four days, (Hamburger, '48; Corliss and Robertson, '63), hence cell production and cell loss do not overlap as they do, for instance, in spinal ganglia, making numerical analysis very difficult. Neuroblast migration and the formation of the l.m.c. is completed at five and one-half days. This date had been suggested previously (Hamburger, '58) and is confirmed in the present investigation. In the previous publication, massive cell degeneration was observed between six and eight days, following unilateral extirpation of an early limb bud. On that occasion degenerating cells had also been observed on the normal (control) side, and particularly high counts of degenerating cells had been found in 6.5- and 8-day embryos, suggesting a naturally occurring cell loss during a relatively short period. The present investigation gives a precise time table of the depletion process, based on cell counts of surviving as well as degenerating cells, in a large sample.

The clear-cut situation involving no overlap of the three major events: proliferation, l.m.c. assembly; and cell loss, and the compression of the latter phenomenon within a few days seems to be favorable for further analysis. Of particular interest is the observation that naturally occurring depletion occurs at approximately the same period (between 6.5 and 9 days) as the massive cell degeneration leading to a total destruction of the l.m.c. following early limb bud extirpation. The findings suggest that there might be a common cause for both events, an idea which had occurred to us many years ago in a study of the development of spinal ganglia. We had found a naturally occurring cell degeneration in thoracic and cervical ganglia, but not in brachial or lumbar ganglia. However, a massive cell degeneration occurred in the latter, following limb bud extirpations. Both events happen at approximately the same developmental stages (Hamburger and Levi-Montalcini, '49). We proposed the hypothesis that in general axons which fail to establish contacts of some sort at the periphery undergo retrograde degeneration which eventually results in the breakdown of their perikarya. This would explain selective survival in the normal situation and total loss in the case of complete absence of the periphery. This hypothesis, though widely accepted, has never been subjected to a critical test suggested at that time, namely, peripheral overloading; a supernumerary limb might accommodate additional fibers and thus spare some cells that would normally degenerate. We thought that it would be "very difficult to obtain quantitatively valid data to show that peripheral overloading can block degeneration." (Hamburger and Levi-Montalcini, '49, p. 496). This difficulty still holds true for spinal ganglia, but the more favorable situation in the l.m.c. may permit the execution of crucial experiments.

The hypothesis implies a certain sequential order of events. Cell degeneration should not begin until after the motor axons have reached the muscle primordia and entered into competition with each other for terminal sites or for specific "trophic" requirements, whatever their nature. Again, this aspect can be studied more easily in the neuro-muscular system than in the sensory or other systems. We shall report on the relations of motor nerve distribution and muscle differentiation in the hindlimb during the critical stages; they seem to support the hypothesis.

MATERIALS AND METHODS

Chick embryos (White Leghorn, obtained from Ken-Roy Hatchery, Berger, Mo.) were incubated in a forced-draft incubator at 99°F.

For motor cell counts, embryos were fixed at 5.5, 6, 7, 8, 9, 12 and 18 days of incubation and five days post-hatching (p.h.), and staged according to the Hamburger-Hamilton stage series ('51). Fixation was in Carnoy's fluid and staining with thionin. Some 6- to 8-day embryos were impregnated with silver, using the Cajal-de Castro method. In addition, isolated legs, sectioned in different planes and stained in phosphotungstic acid hematoxylin or impregnated with silver were used for the study of muscular differentiation and nerve distribution. Sections were 8 μ up to nine days, and 12 μ thereafter.

Motor cell counts. Motor neuroblasts were counted along the entire length of the lumbar lateral motor column (l.m.c.). The l.m.c. is clearly demarcated, and the motor neuroblasts clearly identifiable by their size and dark stain, from stage 28 (5.5 days) on. Reconstruction of the spinal ganglia and dorsal and ventral roots aided in the mapping. The only difficulty was encountered in determining the rostral and caudal ends of the column in stages 28 and 29 (5.5–6 days). At the rostral end, the thoracic median motor column and the l.m.c. are not clearly demarcated. Only those cells were counted which projected beyond the smooth contour of the ventrolateral grey matter. The same criterion was applied for the caudal border. L.m.c. neuroblasts have two nucleoli; only nuclei in which at least one nucleolus was identifiable were counted. Outlines of the nuclei to be counted were made, using a drawing tube, and the actual counts were made on the drawings. Magnification was 600 × for the early stages and 500 × or 400 × for older stages. Every sixth section was counted in the stage-28 embryos, every eighth section in 6- to 8-day embryos, and every tenth section in embryos nine days or older. This meant the counting of 41–49 sections in embryos up to 12 days, 56–68 sections in 18-day embryos and over 70 sections in 5-day p.h. chicks. Left or right sides were selected at random; in a few cases, both sides were counted (brackets in table 1). All counts were made by the author.

RESULTS

The cell counts are summarized in table 1. The figures are the actually counted cells multiplied by 6, 8 or 10, respectively (METHODS). At the earliest stage used, i.e., 28 (5.5 days), the l.m.c. is clearly demarcated and protrudes from the grey matter. The motor neuroblasts are distinguished from the adjacent interneurons by their larger size, deeper stain and more dense packing. The perikaryon is sparse; Nissl substance can be observed. The nuclei contain two nucleoli. Most cells are arranged in irregular rows extending from dorso-lateral to medio-ventral. The long axes of the oval nuclei are oriented in this direction. Silver-impregnated material shows a further distinct organization of the l.m.c. Three parallel longitudinal cell groups and a ventral horizontal group can be identified by their differential affinity for silver (Hamburger, '58, figs. 11, 24). No glia cells

were found at stage 28, but a few are present at stage 29, and they are numerous at stage 31 (7 days). In subsequent stages, growth and differentiation of neurons is accompanied by an increasingly wider spacing and increase in glia.

The cell counts indicate that in stages 28 and 29 (5.5–6 days) a peak in population size is attained, amounting to almost 20,200 motor neuroblasts per l.m.c. The correction for inclusion of nuclear fragments, using the equation of Abercrombie ('46) reduces the number to 17,140.

Depletion of the l.m.c.

During days 7 and 8 a substantial reduction occurs, resulting in the loss of 36% at day 9 (40% after Abercrombie correction). Between 9 and 12 days, a plateau is reached which remains constant at the 12,300 level until at least five days post-hatching (corrected figure: 10,300). The end of the depletion phase is probably near nine and one-half days, because the decline from day 9 to 12 is much less than during the preceding days, and the number of degenerating cells is already low at day 9. Figure 1 gives a graphic presentation of depletion. Extrapolation from the steep phase of de-

TABLE 1

Cell counts of lateral motor column

Stage	28	29	31	34	35	38	43	
Days	5.5	6	7	8	9	12	18	5 d.p.h.
	19.638	21.592	17.870	16.510	13.370	12.670	12.320	12.770
	20.748	18.936	18.320	18.550	12.740	⌈12.160	11.100	12.710
		20.488	18.970	17.584	12.820	⌊11.990	11.660	11.820
		19.504	18.360	17.752	12.820	⌈11.410	12.300	12.470
		20.576		[1] ⌈16.200		⌊11.510	12.350	12.600
		19.952		⌊16.100		11.680	⌈12.750	12.010
		20.304		⌈17.184		⌈12.340	⌊12.580	
		19.832		⌊17.320		⌊12.600	12.410	
		20.272		16.368		12.950	12.630	
				15.328		12.890	⌈12.210	
				⌈15.590		11.690	⌊11.910	
				⌊16.000		12.290	12.220	
				16.340		12.530	12.950	
						12.570	12.750	
						12.610		
						12.380		
Mean	20.193	20.161	18.380	16.615	12.937	12.267	12.295	12.396
Percent survival					64%	61%	61%	61%
Corrected mean [2]		17.137			10.350	10.304		10.041
Percent survival					60%	60%		59%

[1] Brackets indicate left and right side of the same embryo.
[2] Correction after Abercrombie ('46).

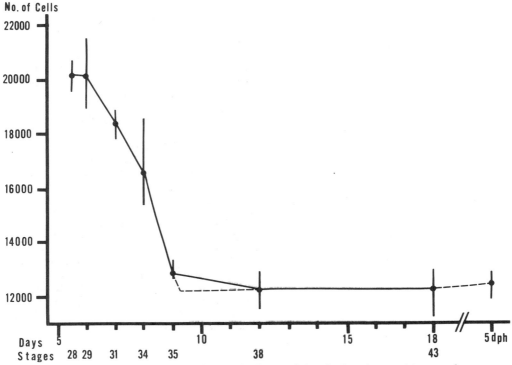

Fig. 1   Normally occurring cell loss in the l.m.c. of the chick embryo; with range between the maximum and minimum counts for each stage (uncorrected counts).

cline indicates that the end of depletion is around nine and one-half days (the corrected figure confirms this). The total loss amounts to 39% (40% after the Abercrombie correction). In other words, two out of every five cells degenerate and die. The rapidity of the depletion process is remarkable: 7,000 to 8,000 cells disappear within three days. As was to be expected, large numbers of degenerating cells in different stages of pyknosis were observed in 7- and 8-day embryos. Counts of the clearly pyknotic cells were made for a few embryos (table 2). The rate of degeneration on day 8 (5.4%) seems to be slightly higher than on day 7 (4.8%). After day 9, cell death seems to be a very rare event.

The distribution of pyknotic cells along the main axis is of some interest. Data were obtained by calculating the percentage of degenerating cells in successive groups of ten sections, along the craniocaudal extent of the l.m.c. This was done for several individual 7-day and 8-day em-

bryos. Two features were noticed. At the rostral and caudal ends of the column the relative number of degenerating cells was higher than in the main body of the column, amounting up to 10%. Perhaps the axons of these cells have a reduced chance to get into a ventral root. Furthermore, in the 7-day embryos, the percentage figures in the rostral half are much higher than in the caudal half. In fact, part of the posterior third is still fairly intact, except for the terminal sector of the l.m.c. In 8-day embryos, degeneration is equally high in the first and last third and lower in the middle third, indicating a gradient of progression of the degeneration process in rostro-caudal direction.

The distribution of the definitive cell loss along the main axis of the l.m.c. can be established by calculating the percentage loss in successive comparable sections of the 6-day and 12-day embryos. The 12-day column is longer and the packing of motor neurons is less dense compared to the 6-day column. But since in both age groups approximately the same number of sections per individual was counted, matching sections along the main axis (with adjustments for slight differences in length in each age group) could be compared. Calculations of average cell numbers for 43 equidistant levels along the axis were made, using a total of nine 6-day embryos and thirteen 12-day embryos. The percentage survival rate per level was then calculated (fig. 2). In general, the configuration of the two curves is very similar, including some details in local peaks and valleys. However, the curve for percentage survival reveals differentials in cell depletion along the axis. Remembering that the average neuron loss is approximately 40%, one observes that the survival rate in the rostral half is above the 60% line, and in the caudal half it is below this line, reaching a low of 40%, in the caudal quarter. An explanation may be necessary for the omission of percentage points at the rostral and caudal ends, and the rise near the two ends. As was mentioned under METHODS (p. 536), the beginning and end of the column were identified by the presence of a few cells (usually 5–20) that were slightly larger and positioned beyond the contour of

TABLE 2

Counts of degenerating cells

Embryo	Total, l.m. cells	Number, degener. cells	Percent degenerating cells of total pop.
6d 17 (stage 29)	19,504	81	0.4
6d 18 (stage 29)	20,576	41	0.2
6d 19 (stage 29)	19,952	88	0.4
7d 2 (stage 31)	17,870	848	4.7
7d 5 (stage 31)	18,320	872	4.8
7d 10 (stage 31)	18,360	888	4.8
8d 10 (stage 34)	17,752	952	5.4
8d 20 (stage 34)	16,340	880	5.4
8d 18 (stage 34)	15,328	915	5.9
9d 1 (stage 35)	13,370	72	0.5
9d 2 (stage 35)	12,740	95	0.7
12d 8 (stage 38)	12,890	3	
12d 20 (stage 38)	12,380	5	

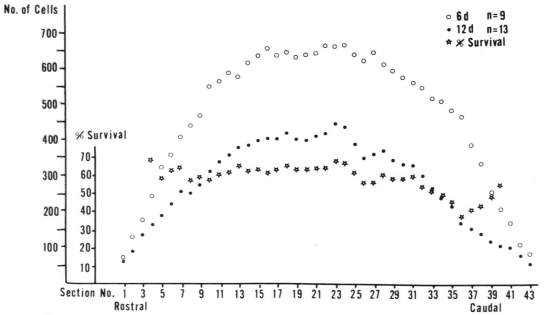

Fig. 2   Upper two curves: average (uncorrected) cell numbers in the l.m.c. of a group of 6-day embryos (n = 9), before onset of the degeneration process, and a group of 12-day embryos (n = 13) after termination of the degeneration process. Abscissa: equidistant points along the rostro-caudal axis; rostral end to the left. Notice the similarity in the general trend of the two curves and the presence of the same peaks and valleys (near the middle of the column) before and after cell loss. The lower curve represents percentage of surviving cells (see text).

226

thoracic or sacral columns, respectively. Hence, the first three counted sections showed in both age groups similar average totals, which would give unrealistically high survival rates. Furthermore, it was mentioned above (p. 538) that a particularly high rate of degenerating cells was found at the rostral and caudal ends of the 7-day and 8-day embryos; hence it is likely that the extreme ends of the 6-day column disappear altogether and therefore the actual ends in the two age groups are perhaps not strictly homologous. However, the validity of the percentage curve for the major extent of the column is not in doubt.

The cytological picture. No detailed study was made of the cytological aspect of motor neuroblast degeneration, (for an EM study of degenerating neurons see O'Connor and Wyttenbach, '74). One finds a great variety of pictures representing different phases of pyknosis and cytoplasm disappearance, but no effort was made to arrange them in a series of progressive deterioration. Pyknosis is by no means uniform; rather, it assumes a variety of forms characterized by very deep stain of the basophilic nuclear material. One finds for instance one or several dark spheres, considerably larger than the nucleoli, in an otherwise empty nucleus. The spheres are usually surrounded by a less dark homogeneous material, floating in the otherwise transparent nucleus. In some instances, numerous small spheres are embedded in the lighter homogeneous material. The irregular chromatin mass characteristic of normal nuclei is usually not identifiable; it is apparently incorporated in the dark globules. Pyknotic nuclei were often greatly swollen. The stain was not favorable for distinction of the contour of the cytoplasm. Some pyknotic nuclei were surrounded by a small amount of cytoplasm. In some instances, large irregular masses of the size of several normal cells, were found in the l.m.c. These were probably macrophages or gliocytes filled with debris.

Nerve and muscle differentiation in the leg. We have indicated in the introduction that a favored explanation of naturally occurring death of nerve cells links this process with the failure of their axons to establish connections at the periphery. This hypothesis presupposes that cell death in the motor column is approximately synchro-nous with the penetration of nerves into muscles and the formation of provisional neuro-muscular contacts. In the following, a brief account is given of nerve and muscle differentiation in the leg, based on older studies of Tello ('23), Romer ('27), Wortham ('49) and Hamburger ('58) and supplemented by new observations on hematoxylin-stained and silver-impregnated embryos. The emphasis is on the time sequence of events and not on details of histogenesis or nerve distribution.

At *stage 23* (4 days), the elongated leg bud is composed of undifferentiated cells. Loose bundles of nerve fibers have reached its base but not yet entered it. Half a day later, at *stage 24*, the leg bud terminates in a rounded toe plate with no indication of individual toes. The segregation of a dense core of precartilage in the femur and tibia-fibula region and less dense dorsal and ventral muscle masses flanking the precartilage is in progress. The contours of the three skeletal elements are barely outlined, the distal part of the bud is undifferentiated. Two fairly strong nerve fiber bundles emerging from the crural and ischiadic plexus, respectively, have grown along opposite sides of the interface between precartilage and muscle masses. They reach the level of the knee at *stage 25*. The remarkably stout nerves consist of intertwining strands of loosely arranged fibers; the nerves appear to end rather abruptly.

At *stage 26* (5 days) the limb is elongated and its three subdivisions are indicated; three toes are demarcated. The precartilaginous femur, tibia, and fibula are more distinct; condensations appear in the center of the toes. Dorsal and ventral muscle masses begin to subdivide, but individual muscles are not yet identifiable. In the thigh muscle mass one observes the beginning of columnar arrangement of nuclei in preparation for myotube formation. The two major strong nerve bundles are still loosely textured; they begin to form side branches. Fine nerves can be found down to the level of the base of the toe plate.

During the sixth day, that is, at *stage 27* and *stage 28*, all three systems; skeleton, muscles, peripheral nerve pattern, undergo a remarkably rapid differentiation. Individual muscles become segregated, except for the distal region; and they receive nerve branches. The three main parts of the leg are set apart and the upper and lower leg form a distinct angle. The toe plate becomes pointed due to the differential growth of the third toe. The individual precartilage primordia have distinct contours; phalanges become discernible. The subdivision of the dorsal and ventral muscle masses proceeds in several steps which have been followed in great detail for the thigh muscles by Romer ('27) and for lower leg and foot by Wortham ('48). Both authors agree that the major phase of individualization of muscles is during the sixth day, and that by day 8 the adult condition has been attained. Our preparations show that beginning with stage 27, myotube formation is in progress in most muscle groups in the thigh and shank. Myofibrils with cross striation were observed at *stages* 27 and 28 in muscles as far distal as the lower tibial region, but they are sparse with considerable spaces between them. The three major nerves, femoral, peroneal and tibial, (Romer, '27) are clearly discernible. Side branches taking off perpendicularly to the main longitudinal nerves were seen entering muscle tissue. Small groups of fibers or even individual fibers belonging to these side branches can be traced to myotubes, though the mode of their termination could not be established. In other words, formation of individual muscles and of myofibrils is synchronous with the formation of nerve branches to these muscles. This process begins early on day 5 and extends through days 6 and 7. Thigh and shank proceed rather synchronously; there is some delay in the foot. It will be remembered that at *stage* 28 the full numerical complement of lateral motor neuroblasts is present. To judge from the substantial size of the ventral roots and of the massive plexus nerves it appears that most of these neuroblasts have sent out axons to the periphery, by *stage* 28.

Hamburger and Balaban ('63) have found the first movements within the leg at *stage* 29 (6–6.5 days). I have observed distinct upward-downward movements of the foot in the tarsal region and slight movements in the knee at stage 28 +. These movements were performed in conjunction with trunk activity, though not during every activity phase. The coincidence of incipient muscle differentiation, nerve fiber penetration into muscle tissue and first visible movements can be taken as a further argument that we are dealing with neurogenic and not myogenic motility, from start (for other arguments see Hamburger, '63; Alconero, '65; Ripley and Provine, '72; Bekoff, '74).

Stages 30 (6.5–7 d.) and *31* (7–7.5 d.). Differentiation of skeletal elements, muscle formation and nerve patterns have advanced considerably. All skeletal elements are distinct and in the process of chondrification, except for the distal phalanges which are still in the precartilage condition. Joints are in the process of formation but actual clefts have not yet appeared. Most individual muscles are present, but separation of adjacent muscles is not yet completed in distal parts. Myofibrils with cross-striation in register are present in most muscles, down to the metatarsal flexors and extensors of toes. The muscle fibers are more densely packed in the proximal than in the distal musculature. Neurotization of muscles (and skin) has occurred at a rapid pace between *stages* 28 and 30. One finds substantial nerve bundles in every muscle unit and the splitting up of intramuscular nerves into finer and finer branches and fiber groups. The smaller branches often leave the nerve at right angles or obliquely, running across muscle fibers; and terminal individual fibers or very small bundles changing direction again, follow the muscle fibers lengthwise. Nerves could be traced as far distally as to the base of the phalanges where they enter differentiating muscle tissue. Individual nerves were not identified, but it seems that at seven days most features of the adult pattern are established and that individual nerve fibers attach themselves to muscle fibers while the latter complete their differentiation.

In summary, the main distribution of nerve fibers in the muscles of the leg occurs between five and one-half days (*stage* 28) and seven days (*stages* 30–31). Cell death in the l.m.c. begins between *stages* 29 and 31, that is, at the same time when motor nerves begin to establish provisional contacts with muscle fibers.

DISCUSSION

Naturally occurring cell death in the lumbo-sacral l.m.c. of the chick embryo presents a particularly clear picture of this widespread phenomenon. Since the number of degenerating cells in 6-day embryos, is low (table 2), we consider the population size of somewhat over 20,000 (that is, somewhat over 17,000 after the Abercrombie correction) as the peak value in the l.m.c. Depletion of the l.m.c. begins shortly after it has attained its full numerical complement. A loss of 7,000–8,000 cells, or approximately 40%, occurs within three days; only three out of five cells survive. Due to the rapid speed of the depletion process, substantial numbers of degenerating cells are present in every 7- and 8-day embryo. In this respect, the l.m.c. gives a clearer picture of what actually happens during depletion than other systems in which the process extends over longer periods and affects fewer cells, whereby the probability of detecting degenerating cells is reduced. As shown in table 2, 5–6% of all cells are in the process of degeneration at any instant, during the period of depletion. These figures are undoubtedly an underestimation, since only cells showing conspicuous pyknosis were counted. Incipient stages were missed and the terminal phases represented by cellular debris and macrophages or glia filled with debris, defy counting. Hence it is reasonably certain that the numerical cell loss in the l.m.c. is due entirely to cell degeneration. This point is stressed because in other systems it is not always easy to exclude other possibilities. Cells of the original population may simply fail to grow or to differentiate or migrate to other sites or become glia. None of these alternatives seem to be applicable to the l.m.c.

From the end of the depletion process around nine and one-half days, the number of l.m.c. neurons remains remarkably constant at least until five days post-hatching. Individual variations between embryos at 12, 18 days and five days p.h. are also very small; maximal differences amount to 12% in 12-day embryos, to 14% in 18-day embryos, and 7% for chickens five days p.h. Differences between left and right sides of the same embryo are even smaller, ranging between 0.6% and 2.6%. The figures give an impressive illustration of the precision with which the mechanisms controlling population size in neuronal units operate.

Other investigators have calculated the duration of the breakdown process in individual neuroblasts based on counts of degenerating cells. I have not done this, because, as indicated above, I consider the counts as crude estimates which cannot be expected to give reliable degeneration times. The published data should perhaps be considered with some scepticism for the same reason.

It was pointed out that degeneration progresses in rostro-caudal direction and furthermore, that the caudal half loses more cells than the rostral half (for details see p. 538). There is no obvious explanation for this difference.

Comparison with other motor systems

A considerable depletion was found in the l.m.c. of the *fetal mouse* (Harris Flanagan, '69). A comparison with the chick is difficult, because the author gives figures only for the entire motor column including cervical, brachial, lumbo-sacral and caudal regions. A population size figure of 100,000 cells is given for *both* columns of 11-day fetuses. The loss between fetal days 11 and 14 is given as 75,000; that is, only 25% of the cells are supposed to survive. A plateau seems to have been reached at day 14.

A scrutiny of the data and illustrations indicates that these figures ought to be corrected. Specifically, the assumed loss of 40,000 cells between 11 and 12 days is probably not real. Description and figures show that at 11 days the l.m.c. is not clearly demarcated; motor neuroblasts cannot be distinguished from other mantle cells; they are "all at the same early stage of differentiation" (Harris Flanagan, '69, p 283). Furthermore, no degenerating cells are present at day 11 and 12, whereas they are abundant at days 13 and 14. The author states: "It seems that the fall in number between 11.25 and 12.25 days is probably due to the fact that not all the cells in the motor columns differentiate further into motor neuroblasts" (Harris Flanagan, '69, p. 293). If the motor and non-motor cells cannot be clearly distinguished, then the figure of 100,000 for the 11-day fetus is arbitrary. The motor column becomes distinct at 12 days; the population size of 60,000 at that stage (for both sides) represents probably the peak value, comparable to the 6-day chick embryo. The legs are also in comparable stages of development.

During the following two days, a cell loss of 35,000 cells occurs; that is, 41% of the 12-day column survives. This figure is lower than that for the chick; and the depletion process is even more precipitous than in the chick (if my correction is accepted). The absolute figures cannot be compared, since those for the mouse include the brachial and lumbo-sacral part of the l.m.c. In the mouse, altogether 12,500 cells survive on each side; this means that the absolute figures for the lumbo-sacral column alone are considerably lower than in the chick.

Romanes ('46) has described a second postnatal depletion process in the mouse. He found a further loss of approximately 30% during the first postnatal week. If a similar event occurs in the chick, this would happen after five days posthatching.

Extensive investigations have been concerned with motor neuroblasts depletion in *Anurans* (Hughes, '61, '68; Prestige, '67, '70; Kollros, '68). In all instances it was found to be of greater magnitude than in the chick. For instance, in *Xenopus*, the cell number declines from approximately 6,000 to 1,500, that is, by 75%, and in the brachial l.m.c. of *Rana pipiens* the loss is 62% (Pollack, '69). Even higher figures were reported for other species. In *Xenopus*, large numbers of degenerating cells were observed during the stages of most precipitous decline of cell members, indicating that the depletion of the l.m.c. can be accounted for by cell death, as was assumed for the chick. The period of cell degeneration in *Xenopus* extends over several weeks (Hughes, '68, p. 64), in contrast to the situation in the chick.

One other motor center has been investigated thoroughly, namely the *trochlear nucleus* in the chick embryo (Cowan and Wenger, '67). It is numerically complete at five and one-half days and maintains its maximum population size of approximately 1,300–1,400 neurons until day 9. A conspicuous decline of over 50% occurs between days 9 and 15; cell loss continues on a much lower scale until after hatching. No degenerating cells were observed. This is probably due to the prolonged period of depletion and the relatively small number involved. In these respects, the situation is different from that of the l.m.c. But the most interesting difference is the long survival time of the neuroblasts that die eventually. While the lumbo-sacral l.m.c. cells break down shortly after the formation of the column, those of the trochlear nucleus survive for ten days or longer before they die.

Mechanism of depletion

Finally, mechanisms that might account for neuroblast depletion will be considered. Cell loss is related to overproduction in the sense that one necessitates the other, if an adjustment of neuron numbers to peripheral requirements is to be achieved. It is not obvious why the attainment of the definitive population size requires two steps. Yet, this is what happens in nearly all neuronal units which have been investigated so far; only the limb-innervating spinal ganglia in the chick show little, if any, depletion. We know very little concerning the programming of either the mitotic activity that leads to overproduction or the subsequent depletion process, but they are certainly controlled by different sets of factors. The overproduction cannot be ascribed to an unprecise programming of the number of mitotic cycles because the total number of cells produced in 5.5- and 6-day embryos is relatively constant (table 1). Perhaps a safety factor had to be built into the production process, since the quantitative requirements of the periphery cannot be anticipated precisely at the time when proliferation goes on. In fact, the periphery for the l.m.c. does not yet exist at the time when mitotic activity in the basal plate which produces the motor neurons is at its peak. Another explanation will be offered below (p. 545).

At any rate, there is no evidence that agencies outside the neural tube are involved in the control of proliferation or in the switch from mitotic cycling to differentiation; whereas powerful arguments can be marshalled in support of the peripheral control of the depletion process. The possibility that a certain percentage of l.m.c. cells is *preprogrammed* for cell death has not been ruled out rigorously but it is usually disregarded, because the assumption that conditions at the periphery decide the fate of a given neuroblast has strong support. Of course, the two alternatives are not mutually exclusive; some cells may show differential susceptibility to adverse conditions at the periphery. In fact, Prestige ('67) makes such a claim for the l.m.c. of *Xenopus*. The motor neuroblasts which migrate out first, that is, the oldest ones which are also the largest appear to be more resistant to the effects of limb extirpation than later arrivals in the l.m.c. (Prestige, '73).

Peripheral control of depletion implies that most or all motor axons have reached the periphery before cell degeneration begins; and furthermore, that cellular breakdown is paralled by axon degeneration. These suppositions have been affirmed for *Xenopus* by axon counts in electron micrographs of a ventral root (Prestige and Wilson, '72). A close correspondence was found in the number of neurons and of fibers in stages before, during and after the naturally occurring neuron death. For the chick embryo, only qualitative data are available. In *stages* 28 and 29, that is, before depletion begins, strong ventral roots are present and the limbs are abundantly neurotized. In leg bud extirpation experiments, the motor roots are at first fully formed and then gradually reduced in size and only traces are left at eight days (Hamburger, '58), corresponding to the cell loss.

There are other arguments supporting the involvement of the periphery. It was pointed out in the introduction that the investigation of spinal ganglion development (Hamburger and Levi-Montalcini, '49) had directed our attention to the simultaneity of naturally occurring cell death and the more severe neuron degeneration following early limb bud extirpation. The synchronism had suggested a similar peripheral influence in both instances. In the experimental situation, the periphery is unquestionably implicated, and by analogy this would apply to normally occurring cell death. The same argument holds with equal force for the l.m.c. Both the normally occurring depletion and the spectacular breakdown following limb extirpation take place between six and nine days. Furthermore, the light-microscope picture of pyknosis is cytologically very similar in both instances. In other words, the effects of limb extirpation appear to be an aggravated manifestation of a normally occurring process. Hence, of the total loss of the l.m.c. in experimental cases, only 60% would be attributed to the removal of the limb.

A final argument is based on the synchronism of limb neurotization and neuroblast degeneration. The latter would be expected to occur at the critical period when motor axons are in the process of innervating the limb muscles. The brief account of leg innervation on p. 540 demonstrates very clearly that this is indeed the case. The depletion process in the l.m.c. begins exactly at the time when the muscle fibers differentiate and are contacted by nerve fibers.

In short, we are satisfied that all premises of the hypothesis of peripheral control of neuroblast death in the l.m.c. are fulfilled. But even the best structural and temporal coincidences do not substitute for a rigorous proof. Efforts have been made to obtain direct evidence by experiments of peripheral overloading, whereby axons which would otherwise die could be accommodated in an enlarged peripheral area. Hyperplasia of spinal ganglia following the transplantation of supernumerary limbs has been obtained consistently in amphibian (e.g., Detwiler, '20; Hughes, '68) and chick embryos (Hamburger and Levi-Montalcini, '49). However, in ganglia it is impossible to relate the increase in cell number directly to the survival of sensory neurons that would have died otherwise. The reason is that normally occurring cell death in limb ganglia is minimal (at least in the chick), and in thoracic ganglia it overlaps with cell proliferation. In contrast, the situation in the l.m.c. seems to be particularly favorable for such a test. In an earlier limb transplantation experiment (Hamburger, '39) a slight motor hyperplasia had been detected in overloaded segments of the brachial or lumbar l.m.c., respectively, but the results were far from convincing. The detailed numerical and temporal data on population size that are now on hand should make it possible to detect even moderate survival rates of motor neurons. The experiments are now being repeated in this laboratory.

While the general notion that the l.m.c. sends out more fibers than the periphery can sustain and that a certain fraction of axons loses out in competition is well supported, the crucial question concerning the nature of the competition remains unanswered. In the minds of most neuro-embryologists competition is equated with competition for attachment sites of axons at the periphery. This could take any one of a number of forms: There might be a membrane reaction after the contact of the first fiber, excluding all latecomers, as in fertilization; or an initial hyperneurotization might be corrected later. If, as may well be, the permanent neuro-muscular contacts are based on a high degree of biochemical matching specificity, then the recognition process would require some degree of trial and error; and a surplus of nerve fibers near the muscle fibers would be necessary to guarantee adequate chances for successful matching. Thus, the overproduction of neurons would find a ready explanation. A careful investigation on the EM level of the formation of incipient neuro-muscular contacts, in situ is urgently needed. If this information were available, a more precise working hypothesis could be formulated.

While this model of competition is plausible, it is certainly not the only one. The NGF should alert us to the alternative possibility that peripheral tissues produce metabolites which become indispensable for neuronal survival. In other words, we should consider a *"trophic"* relationship in a broader physiological sense which would imply the centripetal transfer of a "trophic" agent to the perikaryon by retrograde axoplasmic flow (Prestige, '67; Lamb, '74). Prestige ('67; '70) has proposed a similar hypothesis. He has postulated a "maintenance factor" and suggested that a certain quantity of this agent is stored in each neuroblast assuring a certain survival time in the absence of the periphery. But eventually, the agent would have to be replenished by the periphery, or else the cell will die. The available data do not permit a decision between the different alternatives. Once the analysis has been carried to the molecular level, the difference between a competition for contact sites and a competition for "trophic" agents might disappear.

ACKNOWLEDGMENTS

This investigation was supported by U.S.P.H.S. grant N50 5721 from the National Institute of Neurological Diseases and Stroke. I wish to thank Juanita Farris for technical assistance and Ruth Cowan for the preparation of figures 1 and 2.

LITERATURE CITED

Abercrombie, M. 1946 Estimation of nuclear population from microtome sections. Anat. Rec., 94: 239–247.

Alconero, B. 1965 The nature of the earliest spontaneous activity of the chick embryo. J. Embryol. Exp. Morph., 13: 255–266.

Beckoff, A. 1974 Abstract. In: Society for Neuroscience. Fourth Annual Meeting, p. 136.

Corliss, C. E., and G. G. Robertson 1963 The pattern of mitotic density in the early chick neural epithelium. J. Exp. Zool., 153: 125–140.

Cowan, W. M. 1973 Neuronal death as a regulative mechanism in the control of cell number in the nervous system. In: Development and Aging in the Nervous System. Academic Press, New York, pp. 19–41.

Cowan, W. M., and E. Wenger 1967 Cell loss in the trochlear nucleus of the chick during normal development and after radical extirpation of the optic vesicle. J. Exp. Zool., 164: 267–280.

Detwiler, S. R. 1920 On the hyperplasia of nerve centers resulting from excessive peripheral loading. Proc. Natl. Acad. Sci., 6: 96–101.

Hamburger, V. 1939 Motor and sensory hyperplasia following limb bud transplantations in chick embryos. Physiol. Zool., 12: 268–284.

———— 1948 The mitotic patterns in the spinal cord of the chick embryo and their relation to histogenetic processes. J. Comp. Neur., 88: 221–284.

———— 1958 Regression versus peripheral control of differentiation in motor hypoplasia. Am. J. Anat., 102: 365–410.

———— 1963 Some aspects of the embryology of behavior. Quart. Rev. Biol., 38: 342–365.

Hamburger, V., and M. Balaban 1963 Observations and experiments on spontaneous rhythmical behavior in the chick embryo. Devel. Biol., 7: 533–545.

Hamburger, V., and H. Hamilton 1951 A series of normal stages in the development of the chick embryo. J. Morph., 88: 49–92.

Hamburger, V., and R. Levi-Montalcini 1949 Proliferation, differentiation and degeneration in the spinal ganglia of the chick embryo under normal and experimental conditions. J. Exp. Zool., 111: 457–502.

Harris Flanagan, A. E. 1969 Differentiation and degeneration in the motor horn of foetal mouse. J. Morph., 129: 281–305.

Hughes, A. 1961 Cell degeneration in the larval ventral horn of Xenopus laevis (Daudin). J. Embryol. Exp. Morph., 9: 269–284.

Hughes, A. 1968 Aspects of Neural Ontogeny. Acad. Press, New York.

Kollros, J. 1968 Order and control of neurogenesis (as exemplified by the lateral motor column). Devel. Biol. Suppl., 2: 274–305.

Lamb, A. H. 1974 The timing of the earliest motor innervation to the hind limb bud in the Xenopus tadpole. Brain Res., 67: 527–530.

O'Connor, T. M., and C. R. Wyttenbach 1974 Cell death in the embryonic chick spinal cord. J. Cell Biol., 60: 448–459.

Pollack, E. D. 1969 Normal development of the lateral motor column in Rana pipiens. Anat. Rec., 163: 111–120.

Prestige, M. C. 1967 The control of cell number in the lumbar ventral horns during the development of Xenopus laevis tadpoles. J. Embryol. Exp. Morph., 18: 359–387.

———— 1970 Differentiation, degeneration and the role of the periphery: Quantitative considerations. In: The Neuro-Sciences: Second Study Program. F. O. Schmitt, ed. pp. 73–82.

———— 1973 Gradients in time of origin of tadpole motoneurons. Brain Res., 59: 400–404.

Prestige, M. C., and M. A. Wilson 1972 Loss of axons from ventral roots during development. Brain Res., 41: 467–470.

Ripley, K. L., and R. R. Provine 1972 Neural correlates of embryonic motility in the chick. Brain Res., 45: 127–134.

Rogers, L. A., and W. M. Cowan 1973 The development of the mesencephalic nucleus of the trigeminal nerve in the chick. J. Comp. Neur., 147: 291–320.

Romanes, G. J. 1946 Motor localization and the effects of nerve injury on the ventral horn cells of the spinal cord. J. Anat., 80: 117–131.

Romer, A. 1927 The development of the thigh musculature of the chick. J. Morph., 43: 347–385.

Tello, J. F. 1922 Die Entstehung der motorischen und sensiblen Nervenendigungen I. In dem lokomotorischen System der hoeheren Wirbeltiere. Zeitschr. f. Anat. u. Entw. gesch., 64: 348–440.

Wortham, R. 1948 The development of the muscles and tendons in the lower leg and foot of chick embryos. J. Morph., 83: 105–148.

233

Reprinted from J. Neurophysiol., Vol. 43, pp. 233–254. 1980
© 1980 The American Physiological Society

Competition for Survival Among Developing Ciliary Ganglion Cells

GUILLERMO PILAR, LYNN LANDMESSER, AND LARRY BURSTEIN

Physiology Section, Biological Sciences Group, University of Connecticut, Storrs, 06268, and Department of Biology, Yale University, New Haven, Connecticut 06510

SUMMARY AND CONCLUSIONS

1. Functionally different subgroups, each innervating a different part of the peripheral target, were defined within the ciliary population of the avian ciliary ganglion by electrical stimulation of the various ciliary nerve branches.

2. Although neurons innervating defined parts of the peripheral target consistently sent their axons through certain nerves, the technique of retrograde horseradish peroxidase (HRP) transport showed that the ganglion cell bodies were not spatially grouped but distributed throughout the ganglion, both before and after the period of naturally occurring cell death. However, such neurons tended to be clustered into groups of two or greater.

3. Ciliary and choroid populations, however, were found to be for the most spatially separate and recognizable by location and soma size before the period of cell death. Choroid cells did not project out the ciliary nerves even prior to the cell death period, confirming previous observations of selective axon outgrowth in the two populations.

4. Competition for survival was demonstrated within the ciliary population by experimentally removing approximately two-thirds of the neurons by axotomy-induced cell death at stage 32–34 just prior to the normal cell death period. This reduction in the number of competing neurons resulted in rescue of approximately 40% of the neurons that would have died, as assessed both by the number of axon profiles in the remaining intact nerve branch, as well as the number of somata that could be retrogradely labeled from this nerve.

5. It was concluded that many of the neurons that are normally removed during the cell death period are not destined to die, but can be rescued by reducing the number of neurons competing for a limited supply of some aspect of the peripheral target. Further, the postulated interaction with the target was shown to occur relatively late, just prior to the onset of cell death.

6. At the time of the peripheral interaction, the target was found to consist primarily of myoepithelial cells, which had migrated into the target region following the arrival of the ciliary axons. The target per se, therefore, cannot be involved in the selective growth of ciliary axons to the appropriate region. Well-defined synapses were rare, although many axonal endings were observed in close contact with both myoepithelial cells and the sparser differentiated muscle fibers, which increased to account for 60% of the target by the end of the cell death period.

7. Competition was also found to retard the rate of neuronal maturation because intact axons in the partially axotomized ganglion developed more rapidly than control axons, as assessed by axon diameter, conduction velocity, and degree of glial ensheathment.

8. Finally, at least some of the neurons in the partially axotomized ganglion expanded to innervate the peripheral territory of the axotomized branches, suggesting that competition between neurons is involved in the establishment of the observed peripheral innervation pattern.

INTRODUCTION

The naturally occurring cell death, which has been observed in many parts of the developing nervous system (see Ref. 10 for review), can be greatly enhanced by prior removal of the peripheral target (7, 14, 15, 27, 29, 44). In some cases it has been found that cell death occurs at about the time the neurons form peripheral synapses (15, 25, 27, 29), and further that the neurons that die have at least sent axons to the peripheral target (8, 28, 29, 40). These observations have given rise to the idea that during normal development, neurons compete for some aspect of the peripheral target, such as synaptic sites or a trophic factor(s), which is in limited supply.

If it is true that most neurons are not destined to die and that they merely lose out in a competitive struggle for survival, it should be possible to prevent cell death by increasing the amount of postulated peripheral factor per neuron. This has usually been attempted by experimentally increasing the size of the peripheral target by embryonic surgical manipulations. The best-documented cases show that a portion of avian preganglionic autonomic (48) and spinal cord motoneurons (20) can be rescued by such a procedure, and similar results have recently been reported for the avian ciliary ganglion (34).

However, since experimental increases or decreases in size of the peripheral targets are usually carried out at early developmental stages, it has not been possible to determine at what time the postulated interaction required with the periphery actually takes place. In addition, the altered peripheral geometry (supernumerary limb, two eyes, etc.) with attendant complexity of innervation hinders determining to what extent the neurons innervate the extra peripheral target. This makes it difficult to relate quantitatively the number of cells rescued to the amount of increase in peripheral target.

We have therefore studied neuronal competition during embryonic development in the avian ciliary ganglion by reducing the number of competing ganglion cells rather than by increasing the peripheral target. This manipulation can be carried out late in development just prior to the cell death period and leaves the peripheral target unaltered. We have also determined the effect of this manipulation on the in-

nervation of the peripheral target to see whether competition between neurons is involved in the establishment of specific territories of innervation, as has been proposed (45). A brief report of these results has appeared elsewhere (6).

METHODS

Embryonic surgery

White leghorn chick embryos were incubated in a forced-draft incubator until stage (st) 30–34 of Hamburger and Hamilton (16). For a correlation between stages and days of incubation see Fig. 7. Eggs were candled, a square opening made in the shell with a dental drill, and the shell and underlying membrane removed. In a sterile glove box, a small hole was made in the chorion and amnion. A vibrating needle (51) was then used to pierce the sclera and to cut some or all of the ciliary nerves. The cuts were made at the level of the scleral papilla and the nerve branches could be clearly visualized through the sclera. No muscles or major blood vessels were cut. The hole was sealed and the eggs returned to the incubator until st 36–42. Most embryos survived 4–5 days following surgery, but subsequently the mortality rate increased sharply and was apparently associated with the necessity of cutting the various extraembryonic membranes. Only 10–15% survived until the desired st 39–42, but these appeared normal in all respects.

Determination of number and distribution of ganglion cells

To determine the number and distribution of ganglion cells that projected out specific ciliary nerves, a method using the retrograde transport of horseradish peroxidase (HRP) was used. The ciliary ganglion with intact preganglionic and postganglionic nerves was dissected free, together with a ring of sclera including the iris and ciliary muscles, in a petri dish containing oxygenated Tyrode at room temperature. The ring of sclera with iris and ciliary muscles was placed in a small square chamber in the bottom of the petri dish and the ciliary nerves were pulled through a V-shaped channel in the side so that the ganglion lay outside the chamber. The top of the small chamber together with the side channel was coated with vaseline; 5% HRP (Sigma type VI) in Tyrode was put into the chamber to cover the preparation and the top was sealed with a cover slip. The level of Tyrode was then raised to cover the chamber and the temperature was increased to 33°C. After 1.5 h, the preparation was removed from the chamber after rinsing out the HRP, and was allowed to remain in the oxygenated Tyrode for an additional 3.5 h at 33°C. This time was sufficient for the HRP to be taken up by the nerve terminals in the iris and ciliary muscle and to be transported back to the parent cell bodies in the ganglion approximately 1 cm away. When all ciliary nerves were left intact, the entire ciliary population could be labeled. However, for most of the experiments the ciliary branches lying lateral to the main blood vessel to the ciliary muscle were transected close to the ganglion (see Fig. 1). This left only one medial branch, hereafter called branch 3, entering the chamber, so that the cell bodies with axons projecting out this nerve could be labeled in both control and partially axotomized ganglia.

Preparations were then pinned to small pieces of cardboard, fixed in 2% phosphate-buffered glutaraldehyde (pH = 7.2) overnight, and treated subsequently as previously described (24). The ganglia were dehydrated and embedded in paraffin and sectioned at 8 μm, transverse to the proximodistal axis of the ganglion. Although differing somewhat from the actual orientation in vivo, the surface of the ganglion in contact with the optic nerve will be referred to as ventral and the opposite surface dorsal, with the mediolateral axis at right angles to this.

The slides were counterstained with cresyl violet to aid in visualization of unlabeled cells. Labeled cells contained a dark brown granular reaction product, and were easily counted using a Zeiss microscope at a magnification of 500× for st 38–42 ganglia and at 980× for earlier stages. Every labeled cell profile in each section was counted. Concurrent measurement of the diameter of the labeled cells allowed a correction to be made for double counting (1). When the cut distal ends of ciliary nerves were placed in the HRP chamber, backfilled cells always contained diffuse reaction product, easily distinguished from the granular type. Thus in these experiments, only granularly stained cells were counted.

The spatial distribution of labeled cells in control ganglia was determined for the entire ciliary population or for only those neurons projecting out branch 3, by use of a Zeiss universal microscope with camera lucida attachment. Usually every third section through the ganglion was drawn on graph paper and the location of all labeled (and in a few cases unlabeled cells) was marked. These drawings were later used to make a reconstruction of the ganglion showing the position of the labeled cells. Labeled cells immediately adjacent to each other (i.e., not separated by an unlabeled cell) were connected with lines for cluster analysis. The number of clusters of two, three,

or more labeled cells projecting out branch 3 could therefore be determined for the entire ganglion.

To determine whether the number and size of clusters would be expected from a random spatial distribution of branch 3 cells within the ganglion, the number of labeled and unlabeled ciliary cells was determined for several sections through a st 34 ganglion. The ciliary cell area was divided into 20 squares, and the expected number of squares containing 0, 1, 2, . . . stained cells was determined according to the Poisson distribution from the mean number of labeled cells per square. The observed distribution of labeled cells clearly differed from a Poisson distribution, so a nonrandom or clustered distribution of cells was assumed.

To determine whether one would have expected contiguous pairs, triplets, etc., of stained cells, if these had been randomly distributed among the unlabeled cells, the ciliary area in a single section was divided into 320 squares, which was the total number of labeled cells in that section. The squares were each assigned a number from 1 to 320, and the 26 stained cells observed in that section were distributed randomly among the 320 cells, using a table of random numbers. On this basis no clusters containing more than two contiguous stained cells would have been expected, whereas single clusters of three, four, and six cells, and two clusters of five cells were also observed. A statistical analysis was applied to determine if there was any tendency for cell survival to be associated with cluster size, and is detailed in the APPENDIX.

The completeness of ganglion cell death resulting from transection of the postganglionic nerves at st 30–32 was determined by performing total axotomies of the ciliary nerves. These axotomized ganglia were not subjected to the retrograde HRP method but were otherwise processed according to the procedures above. Counts of all remaining cells were made at st 39–40, and the proportion of ciliary cells was estimated by using cell diameter as a criterion to distinguish between ciliary and choroid cells.

Electron microscopy

Tissue was processed for electron microscopy according to previously described methods (41). Ultrathin transverse sections were made of branch 3 of the ciliary nerves at one-third the distance between its entry into the optic cup and its entry into ciliary muscles. Sections were mounted on carbon-coated slot grids and were photographed at a magnification of 3,000×. Montages of the entire nerve were made from prints so that the total magnification was 10,000×.

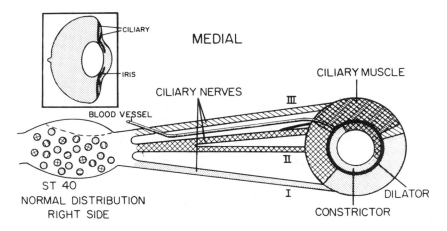

FIG. 1. Schematic diagram of peripheral innervation pattern of the ciliary population. Each of the main ciliary nerve branches emanating from the ganglion innervates different parts of the peripheral target: branch 1 (stippled) innervates the iris constrictor and the lateral portion of the ciliary muscle, branch 3 (hatched) innervates only the medial portion of the ciliary muscle, while branch 2 (crosshatched) innervates intermediate areas of the ciliary muscle as well as iris constrictor. A small branch (solid) emerging from branch 2 innervates the iris dilator. The cell bodies that project out of each of these nerves are not localized but distributed throughout the ciliary portion of the ganglion. Inset. Sagittal (bisecting the lens) section of the eye showing the position of the intrinsic eye muscles.

All the axons in the nerve were counted and their diameters measured. Iris and ciliary muscles were also observed at different stages to better define the peripheral target and the nature of axonal endings in both control and partially axotomized preparations.

Electrophysiology

The regions of the peripheral target innervated by neurons projecting out each of the three ciliary nerves was determined electrophysiologically at st 34–42. The ciliary nerves were dissected together with a ring of sclera containing the iris and ciliary muscles. The sclera was pinned to the bottom of a Sylgard-lined dish containing oxygenated Tyrode at 20–22°C.

Each ciliary nerve (see Fig. 1) was separately stimulated electrically with a suction electrode. The effect of this stimulation on the iris was determined by measuring the diameter of the iris with an eyepiece micrometer, at rest and after stimulation at 20 Hz for 10 s. To measure which regions of the ring of ciliary muscle was contracting (muscle fibers run radially), an eyepiece protractor was positioned over the ciliary muscle so that 0° coincided with the main blood vessel. Those parts of the ring contracting were expressed in degrees proceeding in a clockwise direction from the blood vessel, for control ganglia (left side), and a counterclockwise direction for axotomized ganglia (right side).

To confirm these visual observations the postsynaptic structures were also recorded from by gentle suction into the orifice of a suction electrode. The signals were passed through a Transidyne MPA-6 AC amplifier and photographed from an oscilloscope screen. To confirm that these responses were synaptic in nature, they were blocked with *d*-tubocurarine (*d*-TC), 10^{-5} M. At early stages, before synaptic potentials were elicited, responses could be recorded directly from the nerves. These could not be blocked by *d*-TC and were resistant to block with repetitive stimulation. The conduction velocity of the ciliary nerves was measured in a few cases as previously described (26).

Estimation of proportion of axons in ciliary nerve that are sensory

Sensory fibers, carried in a ramus of the ophthalmic nerve (33), enter the ciliary nerves just distal to the ganglion. Since axon counts were made from the ciliary nerves distal to the juncture with this ramus, it was necessary to obtain at least a rough estimate of the number of sensory axons in the ciliary nerves. First, the total number of axons in the ophthalmic ramus was determined with light microscopy, for 1- to 6-day-hatched chicks, from photographic montages of 1 μm Epon-embedded cross sections. The number was 650 ± 20 (mean ± SE) and the axon diameters were distributed unimodally. To determine what proportion of these fibers were distributed to each of the ciliary nerve branches, an electrophysiological technique was used. Electrical activity was recorded from the ramus with a suction electrode and each of the ciliary branches was sequentially stimulated. The area under each of these action potentials (see Ref. 26 for further details) was compared with the summed area of all three. This gave an estimate of the proportion of ophthalmic ramus axons in each ciliary branch. While the distribution of axons to the various branches varied considerably from animal to animal, the mean value for branch 3 in eight preparations, 30 ± 15% (mean ± SE), would represent approximately 200 axons. Since axon number in branch 3 does not vary greatly between st 39–40 and after hatching, we would estimate that sensory fibers make up about 15% of the axons in branch 3 at the stages in which we did most of the experiments. Since this number is small, it should not alter any of our conclusions, but it should be borne in mind that the graphs depicting axon counts have not been corrected and, therefore, include both ciliary postganglionic autonomic and sensory axons.

RESULTS

Distinct subpopulations within ciliary group of ganglion cells

Previous studies (26, 33) have defined two cell populations within the ciliary ganglion,

which have different peripheral targets; the ciliary cells projecting to the iris and ciliary muscles and the choroid cells to the vascular smooth muscle of the choroid coat. These populations also differ with respect to the conduction velocity of the pre- and post-ganglionic fibers and the mode of ganglionic transmission.

The present study, using retrograde transport of HRP, confirmed earlier observations that the ciliary population is composed primarily of large, ovoid cells, which are located dorsolaterally (see Fig. 2), while the choroid population consists of smaller more irregularly shaped cells, which are densely packed in the ventromedial part of the ganglion. In the st 40 preparation shown in Fig. 2, a count of stained cells showed that those projecting out the ciliary nerves numbered 1,391 cells while the unstained cells, presumably the choroid population, numbered 2,338 cells. The total number of ganglion cells, 3,729, was similar to previously published values at the same stage, which is after the main period of

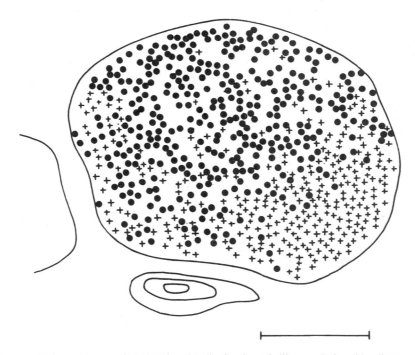

FIG. 2. Camera lucida reconstruction showing the distribution of ciliary and choroid cell somata in a st 40 ciliary ganglion. In this reconstruction of a transversely sectioned ciliary ganglion, the ciliary cells containing granular HRP reaction product transported by the intact ciliary nerves from the peripheral target, are shown as dots. The unlabeled choroid cells are shown as crosses. The ventral portion of this left ganglion is oriented down and overlies a major blood vessel, while medial is to the right. Calibration: 100 μm.

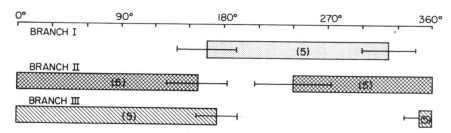

FIG. 3.   Regions of ciliary muscle innervated by each of the three main ciliary nerve branches. The extent of the innervation territory of each branch, determined in five electrophysiological experiments, is shown in degrees from the main blood vessel by bars representing mean ± SD.

naturally occurring cell death (27). In confirmation of previous indirect evidence (33) the stained, and therefore by definition, ciliary cells were larger (12.4 ± 2.9 μm; mean ± SD) than the choroid cells (7.3 ± 1.9 μm).

Although the ciliary cell population has been considered homogeneous in many aspects (26, 27, 33), electrical stimulation of individual ciliary nerves provided evidence of distinct subpopulations, each

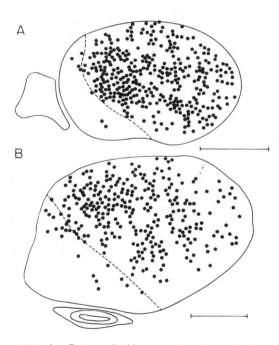

FIG. 4.   Camera lucida reconstruction showing the distribution of ciliary cell somata that project out branch 3 before (A) and after (B) the period of normal-occurring cell death. At st 34 (A) ciliary cell somata are distributed throughout the ganglion except for the ventromedial choroid region to the right of the dashed line. A similar distribution was found at st 40, following the cell-death period (B). Calibration: 100 μm.

innervating a different part of the peripheral target. In isolated preparations (st 40 to posthatching), each ciliary nerve was electrically stimulated and the area of ciliary muscle activated, determined by recording extracellularly from the muscle fibers at their midpoint. The extent of the innervation territories was determined for a number of preparations and was given in degrees around the circular ring of ciliary muscle, using the main blood vessel as 0° or the reference point (see Fig. 1).

In Fig. 3, the extent of the territories in degrees is displayed graphically in the form of bars. There is clearly overlap in the innervation territories, especially of branches 1 and 2 and branches 2 and 3. However, each branch can be seen to innervate a characteristic region of the target, and branch 3 was found never to innervate an extensive region of the ciliary muscles lying between approximately 200 and 340°. Further, the iris constrictor was always activated by branch 1, sometimes by branch 2, but never by branch 3.

Since the ciliary and choroid populations are spatially segregated, we wanted to determine if ciliary cells projecting to specific parts of the peripheral target were grouped in the ganglion. A camera lucida reconstruction of all cells sending their axons out branch 3 in one st 40 ganglion (Fig. 4B) shows that although the greatest density of branch 3 cells occurs in the medial part of the ganglion, labeled cells were found at all extremes of the ciliary region; medial, lateral, dorsal, and ventral (as well as along the proximodistal axis, which is not shown). Similar distributions of branch 3 cells were found for four other st 39–40 ganglia. In several other preparations branch 1, which innervates the iris con-

239

strictor as well as ciliary muscle, was labeled. While the peak density of labeled cells was located differently from branch 3 (more lateral), they were again distributed throughout the ciliary cell region. No size differences or other distinguishing characteristics were noted between the two.

The distribution of cells projecting out branch 3 at st 34 (Fig. 4A), which is prior to the cell death period when more than half of the ciliary cells are lost (27), was not noticeably different from st 40 (Fig. 4B). It can also be seen that the choroid region at st 34 is essentially free of labeled cells. Further, the characteristic size difference between ciliary and choroid cells is already apparent: unlabeled cells in the choroid region were 5.1 ± 1.0 μm (mean $\pm$ SD) in diameter versus 8.0 ± 1.2 μm for labeled branch 3 cells. Thus even prior to the cell death period, choroid cells do not appear to project out branch 3 to any great extent, supporting previous observations of selective outgrowth of ciliary and choroid axons (28, 29). Cell death also does not alter the distribution of branch 3 cells in a noticeable manner, although given the distributed location of branch 3 cells, it is not possible to rule out the occurrence of some projection errors within the ciliary population.

In all the preparations in which branch 3 cells were labeled, both before and after the cell death period, a clustering of labeled cells into groups of two, three, or more was noted. To better quantify this tendency, we analyzed the camera lucida drawings from one ganglion as described in the METHODS. The number of clusters of two, three, or more cells, as well as their percentage occurrence is shown in Table 1.

The clustering of branch 3 cells at st 34 was found (see Methods) to be too extensive to have resulted from a random distribution of labeled cells among the unlabeled cells of the ciliary population (excluding the choroid area, which rarely contains ciliary cells.) Therefore the probability that cells in a certain location will send their axons out branch 3 is not uniform throughout the ciliary region of the ganglion, but there is the tendency for small contiguous groups of cells to project to the same region of the target. A possible explanation of this phenomenon, although certainly not the

TABLE 1. *Clustering of branch 3 cells within ganglion*

No. of	St 34	St 40	% of Total Cells in Clusters of Each Number	
			St 34	St 40
Single cells	273	143	35	43
Clusters of 2	94	56	24	33
3	41	18	16	16
4	17	4	9	5
5	10	1	6	2
6	8	0	6	0
7	2	0	2	0
8	1	0	1	0
9	1	0	1	0

Total number of clusters occurring within a single ganglion cell are shown at st 34 and st 40.

only one, is that the clusters represent the progeny of single precursor cells, which are specified to send their axons out branch 3. Some cell proliferation continues as late as st 22, after the formation of the ganglion (L. Landmesser, unpublished observations). Clusters of cells destined for branch 3 might then occur if there was not extensive migration following terminal cell division. Similar clustering has been observed in other neural crest-derived ganglion (37; M. Honig, unpublished observations).

In order to see if there was any correlation between cluster size and cell survival, a statistical analysis was performed on the distribution of cluster sizes prior to and after the cell death period (Table 1). We initially hypothesized that cells in clusters might have less chance to survive since they might project to the same target region where competition would be more intense. Yet it was found that clustered cells actually survived better than single cells (see APPENDIX). However, since we are uncertain as to what such clustering represents, these results are not yet readily interpretable.

Characteristics of peripheral targets of different classes of ciliary cells

Not only do the ciliary cells project to different parts of the target, but the striated ciliary, iris constrictor, and iris dilator muscles, have distinguishing characteristics as well. These differences may partially explain the nonuniformity of innervation by branch 3 after axotomy (described later).

240

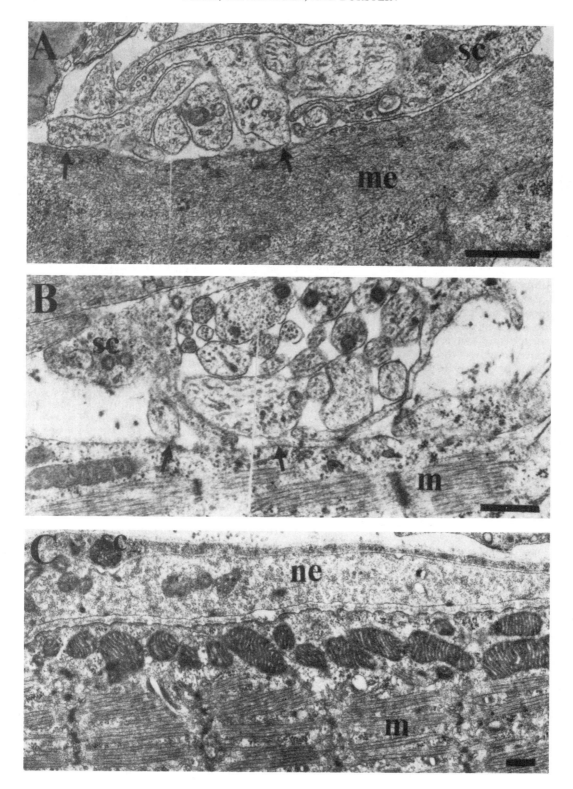

Anterior and posterior (Crampton and Brücke) ciliary muscles run radially from the periphery of the anterior chamber until their insertion near the level of the ora serrata; they are 12 μm in diameter (after hatching), and are singly innervated approximately midway along the fiber (53; and G. Pilar, unpublished observations). The iris fibers in contrast branch extensively, their diameter varies between 1 and 6 μm, and they are multiply innervated by two to three terminal endings (42, 53). Furthermore, there are differences in their embryological derivation; the ciliary muscle arising from the mesoderm, the iris from the ectoderm (11, p. 53–55). However, the ciliary cells form cholinergic nicotinic junctions in all muscles (42; G. Pilar, unpublished observations)

A brief description of the later embryological development of the iris muscle and its innervation will now be given. It will serve as a control, to compare with irises innervated by "foreign" branch 3 following partial axotomy (described in last section of paper).

The precursors of the striated muscle are myoepithelial cells, which originate from the inner retinal layer at st 34. These cells migrate to the iris primordium (31), and by st 40 have fused to form multinucleate cells whose cytoplasmic matrix is electron dense with a fibrillar appearance (Fig. 5A). They are found intermixed and running along with already differentiated striated muscle cells (Fig. 5B). From 40 to 60% of the iris musculature at st 40 is formed by these undifferentiated myoepithelial cells, which decrease with age of the embryo, some persisting after hatching (G. Pilar, unpublished observations).

It was known, from an earlier study (28) that by st 34½ some contractile cells have already been innervated. By st 36 nerves have projected to the entire extent of the peripheral target (Fig. 6), and by st 40, nerve stimulation causes as extensive iris constriction as found in the adult animal (28). In spite of this extensive functional innervation, few structurally defined endings could be identified in an exhaustive electron microscopic search (Figs. 5A , B). The paucity of ultrastructural synaptic specialization found here during early embryogenesis is characteristic of other types of neuromuscular junction development (9) and is in contrast to the ease with which synaptic endings as long as 10 μm can be found on iris muscle fibers after hatching, using similar electron microscope (EM) techniques (Fig. 5C). The innervation at st 36 for the most part is composed of bundles of unmyelinated axons, some with varicosities, running between muscle cells and occasionally coming into close apposition with muscle fiber membranes. Similar patterns of axon distribution were present with the precursor cells.

These observations allow several conclusions. First, since ciliary axons project to appropriate general target area (29) prior to the migration of the myoepithelial cells, the target itself cannot be involved in attracting or guiding the ciliary axons. Second, since myoepithelial cells make up the bulk of the target at st 34 or the onset of ganglion cell death, it is for some aspect of these cells that the ciliary neurons are presumably competing (see below).

Development of peripheral innervation territories

The development of the peripheral innervation territories was studied using electrophysiological techniques already described. The earliest responses in ciliary muscles were recorded from st 31–34. These responses apparently represented

FIG. 5.   Nerve-muscle contacts between ciliary axons and iris. Abbreviations: sc, Schwann cell; m, muscle cell; me, myoepithelial cell; ne, nerve terminal. Arrows indicate areas of close apposition between axons and postsynaptic elements. In all three illustrations the neural elements are wrapped by Schwann cells. A :   a st 39½ group of axons and nerve terminals in possible synaptic contact with a myoepithelial cell, which is characterized by a packed filamentous structure that confers to the cell and electron-dense appearance. B :   similar type of axonal endings abutting on a differentiated muscle also at st 39½. Note in A and B the scarcity of vesicles in the synaptic structures. C :   these endings can be compared with the well-developed neuromuscular junction shown here, from a 1-wk-old chick. A portion of a 15-μm nerve terminal full of vesicles, with presynaptic densities can be clearly recognized opposite to postsynaptic densities in the muscle. Calibration: 0.5 μm.

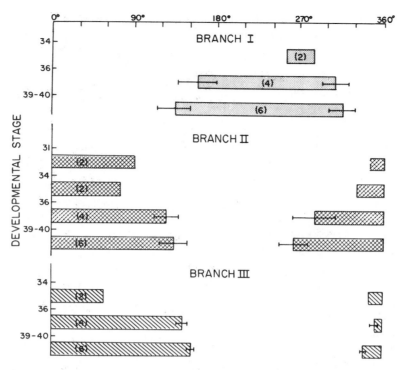

FIG. 6. Development of the peripheral innervation pattern in the ring of ciliary muscle. The area of ciliary muscle from which it was possible to record extracellularly either presynaptic (st 31–34) or postsynaptic (st 36–40) responses following stimulation of each of the ciliary nerve branches is shown by the position of the horizontal bars. 0° denotes the position of the main blood vessel and the error bars represent ±SD from the mean. Number of experiments in parentheses.

activity in the peripheral nerves and nerve endings as they were not blocked by d-TC (10^{-5} M) or lowered extracellular calcium. Later (st 36–40) responses were primarily postsynaptic in nature as they were blocked by these treatments. Figure 6 shows that the earliest responses are obtained from small areas of the target, which corresponded with the entry point of each nerve. Between st 34–40, there was a rapid expansion in the area activated by each branch until it conformed with the mature innervation pattern. There was no evidence for an initial diffuse innervation of the whole target by each branch. Rather, each branch appeared to ramify and form synapses only within appropriate regions of the territory. However, it is possible that small numbers of inappropriately projecting axons could have gone undetected. Also in accordance with the mature pattern, the iris was never activated by branch 3.

Reduction of ganglion cell population enhances survival of remaining neurons

Previous observations on the effect of axotomy at different developmental stages (G. Pilar and L. Landmesser, unpublished observations) indicated that postganglionic axotomy of the ciliary nerves at st 32, just prior to the normal cell death period, resulted in rapid death of many of the ciliary cells. Since we desired to use axotomy as an experimental tool to reduce the size of the ciliary cell population, the effectiveness of this procedure was assessed.

An attempt was made to cut all of the ciliary nerves (leaving the choroid nerves intact) at st 32 on the right side of a series of embryos. The contralateral, unoperated ganglia served as controls. Since the nerves were transected close to the ciliary muscles where some branching had already occurred, often one or more of the finer branches was not cut as intended, and

243

appeared intact and of normal appearance when the embryos were sacrificed at st 39–40. The branches that had been cut appeared only as faint traces of degenerating debris. Since all operated ganglia were grossly atrophic by st 39–40, it was clear that many cells had died in the intervening period, which included the normal cell death period (27). These results are similar to amphibian spinal cord (44) and rat sympathetic ganglia (19) where axotomized neurons also die during the period of normally occurring cell death.

The number of ciliary cells surviving axotomy was determined in several ganglia of this series by using cell diameter as well as soma shape, cell position, and location of the nucleus to distinguish ciliary from choroid cells. As seen in Table 2, the total number of ganglion cells was greatly reduced on the axotomized side. This reduction was restricted to the ciliary population whose mean number of 529 was only 35% of the control number. The number of choroid cells did not differ on the control and axotomized side.

Therefore, axotomy at st 32 is not completely effective in removing all ciliary cells, but does reduce their number considerably. Furthermore, it appears that most cells that are axotomized actually die and that the surviving cells can be accounted for by the branches that escaped transection since the proportion of ganglion cells that survives (35%) correlates with the proportion of the total ciliary nerve represented by the intact branches, 30 ± 11% (mean ± SD). This percentage of the total ciliary nerve represented by the intact branches was obtained from the ratio of the summed diameter of the intact branches over the summed diameter of all the ciliary branches on the contralateral side. Since sensory neurons contribute an equal proportion to all ciliary branches, they should not have affected this calculation.

In order to see whether reduction in the number of competing ganglion cells would reduce the amount of cell death in the remaining population, we axotomized at st 32–34 the two ciliary nerves that are lateral to the main blood vessel. The number of cell projecting out the remaining branch

TABLE 2. *Number of ciliary and choroid cells following total axotomy of ciliary nerves and of branch 3 ganglion cells following partial axotomy of ciliary nerves*

| | A. Total axotomy | | | |
| | Ciliary | | Choroid | |
	Control	Axotomized side	Control	Axotomized side
	1,894	396	2,242	2,498
	1,226	573	2,349	2,557
	1,451	618	3,206	2,551
Mean	1,523	529	2,599	2,535
SD	± 339	± 117	± 528	± 32

| | B. Partial axotomy | | |
| | Control Side | | Partial Axotomy Side |
	St 34	St 39–40	St 39–40
		270	546
		241†	716†
		328	479
		380	518
	1,067	230	484
	971	270	
	807	395	
Mean	948	302	549
SD	± 131	± 66	± 97

A, number of ciliary and choroid cells following total axotomy of ciliary nerves. *B*, number of branch 3 ganglion cells following partial axotomy of ciliary nerves. The surgical procedure actually transected on the average 70% of the ciliary axons (see text for explanation).   † Axotomized at st 34.

3 that survived the cell death period was determined at st 39–40 by using the technique of retrograde transport of HRP as detailed in the METHODS. This number was compared with the number of surviving cells projecting out branch 3 in control ganglia. Table 2 shows that in each of five cases, a large number of neurons, ranging from 138 to 475, were apparently rescued. The number of cells on the experimental side was significantly greater (P < 0.01, Wilcoxon test) than on the control side, resulting in a mean percentage increase of 98%. While four of these ganglia had been axotomized at st 32, one had been axotomized at st 34 (dagger) just one day before the onset of normal cell death. Even this

resulted in a substantial increase in cells (197%) on the experimental side. Two values from unoperated control animals (asterisks) are included, and can be seen to fall within the standard deviation of the contralateral control group.

This increase in cell number in experimental ganglia was not accompanied by an increase in the size of individual ganglion cells. The mean soma diameter values for the control group and the experimental group were not significantly different. However, it is possible that differences in size might become apparent later in development.

Reducing the size of the ciliary population at st 32–34 allowed a relatively large number of ciliary cells, which normally would have died, to survive. In order to see what proportion of the cell population had been rescued, it was necessary to determine the number of cells projecting out branch 3 before the cell death period. Table 2 shows that for controls the mean number of cells at st 34, before the cell death period, is 948 ± 131 and 302 ± 66 afterward; thus 69% of branch 3 cells normally die. This value is slightly larger than the previously published value of 54%, which included the total ciliary and choroid population (27). On the axotomized side only 42% of the cells die, so that 39% of the cells that would normally die (or 251 cells on the average) have been saved.

To make reasonable interpretations about the amount of cell death prevented, it is necessary to have some idea of the proportion of the ciliary population that has been removed by axotomy. A rough estimate can be obtained by measuring the diameter of branch 3 and the summed diameter of all the ciliary nerves. In 16 control ganglia from unoperated embryos at st 39–40, branch 3 was found to represent 22 ± 3% of the entire ciliary population, and in contralateral control ganglia from axotomized embryos, 22 ± 5% (n = 15). Thus ipsilateral axotomy of the ciliary nerves did not affect survival of contralateral branch 3 cells, a supposition that is supported by cell counts (Table 2). This means first that the contralateral ganglion can serve as an adequate control, and second that roughly 88% of the ciliary population would be

removed by total axotomy of nerves 1 and 2. The sensory component of the ciliary nerves (15%, see METHODS) should not affect these calculations, since the sensory fibers are distributed more or less equally to all ciliary branches.

However, as stated earlier, axotomy of nerves 1 and 2 generally was not complete. If one takes into account the nerves that were not cut for the five axotomized embryos shown in Table 2, the reduction in the ciliary population was only 63 ± 8% (mean ± SD). Therefore it can be concluded that reducing the ciliary population by an average of 63% resulted in saving 39% of the cells that would normally die.

Axon numbers in branch 3 in control and partially axotomized ganglia

It was previously shown for the entire ciliary population that normal-occurring ganglion cell loss was reflected in a proportionate loss of axons in the ciliary nerves (29). Furthermore, early in development, each ciliary cell had more axon collaterals than at later stages. To see if enhanced cell survival resulted in an increase of branch 3 axons and whether the number of axon collaterals per cell was altered, axon counts were made from EM montages of branch 3 at different developmental stages.

Figure 7 shows that the number of axons in control branch 3 (open bars) declines markedly between st 34 and 40, reflecting the ganglion cell death (27), and is similar to the axon loss previously described for the entire ciliary population (29). A secondary, smaller loss of axons occurs between st 40 and hatching. An enhanced survival of branch 3 axons was seen in partially axotomized ganglia at st 40, as shown by the cross-hatched area of the bar at st 39–40. This represents the rescue of approximately 700 axons per ganglion, a significant increase over the control side (P ≤ 0.01, Wilcoxon test).

The relative increase in both branch 3 axons and ganglion cells over control numbers is shown in Fig. 8. There was a greater increase in the number of ganglion cells (189% of control) than of axons (141% of control) at st 39–40. During normal development, the number of axons per cell is unaltered during the cell death period

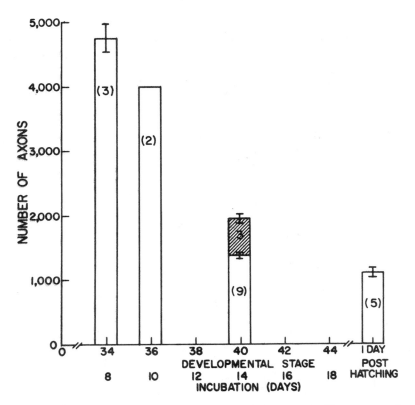

FIG. 7. Number of branch 3 axons during different stages of development. The mean number of axons in control branch 3 (open bars) declines markedly between st 34–40. The increase over the control value at st 40 in partially axotomized ganglia is shown by the hatched part of the bar. No experimental values were determined posthatching. The error bars represent SE and the number of individual samples contributing to each was three at st 34, nine for controls and three for experimentals at st 40, and three at 1 day posthatching.

(5.0 at st 34 versus 4.7 at st 40), but later declines to 3.7 by hatching. However, in partially axotomized ganglia, the number of axons per cell has already declined to 3.6 by st 39–40. This may merely reflect a speeding up of the maturational process in the experimental situation, as documented below. However, these calculations assume that the sensory component of the nerves is constant, and unproved supposition.

Competition between neurons retards rate of neuronal development

Competition between neurons not only causes a large proportion of neurons to die but actually delays the maturation of the cells that survive. This became apparent when comparing EM cross sections of branch 3 at st 38–39. Even the low-power EM micrograph of Fig. 9 shows that not only is the experimental branch 3 larger than

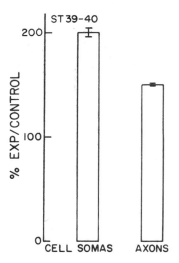

FIG. 8. Comparison of the increase in the number of branch 3 ganglion cells and axons in partially axotomized ganglia at st 39–40. Bars represent means ± SE.

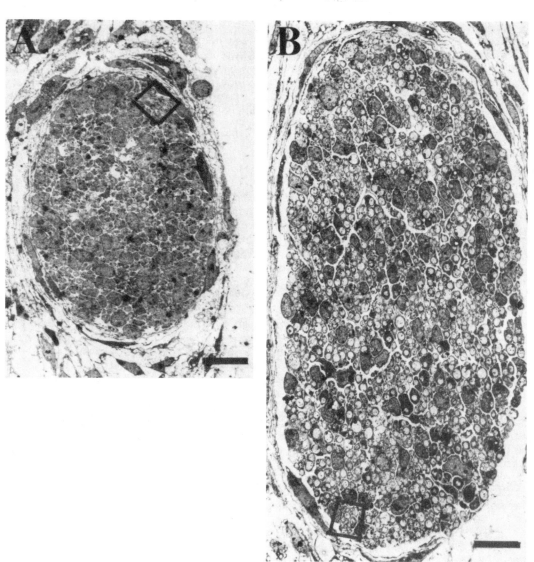

FIG. 9.   Cross sections of branch 3 nerves at st 39. *A* :   control; *B* :   experimental side. Micrographs were taken at same magnification. Area enclosed in square illustrated in Fig. 10 at higher magnification. Calibration: 1 μm.

its contralateral control, as would be expected from the larger number of axons, but the individual axons are considerably larger as well. The latter point can be better appreciated in Fig. 10, which compares the same nerves at higher magnification. The control axons are not only smaller in diameter but also less mature, bundles of naked axons being surrounded by single Schwann cells. In the experimental nerve, Schwann cell ensheathment of individual axons has

progressed further and few naked axons remain.

When diameters were measured the mean diameter of axons in the experimental branch 3 was 0.74 ± 0.01 μm, (mean ± SE), nearly double the diameter of the axons in control branch 3, 0.42 ± 0.01 μm. This increase in axon diameter should be reflected in an increase in conduction velocity. Indeed, when the conduction velocities of two additional pairs of experimental and control nerves were measured, conduction velocity was increased in both cases by approximately 150%; from 0.20 to 0.29 m/s and from 0.24 to 0.36 m/s.

Thus reduction of the ganglion cell population not only rescues a number of cells from death, but also allows the surviving cells to develop at a faster rate. This effect was most obvious at st 38–39, and by st 40–42 differences in axon diameter and degree of myelination were not marked. Therefore, nerves on the control side eventually catch up to those on the experimental side.

Expansion of branch 3 innervation territory in partially axotomized ganglia

As described earlier, each branch of the ciliary nerves innervates a discrete portion of the peripheral target; branch 3 innervates approximately 160° of the ring of ciliary muscle medial to the main blood vessel and does not innervate the iris constrictor. It was of interest of see if branch 3 would expand its peripheral field into the territory of the other branches when these were denervated by the partial axotomy procedure. Animals that had had branch 1 and 2 transected at st 32–34 were visually tested at st 39–40 for ciliary muscle contraction on electrical stimulation of branch 3, as described in the METHODS. In all 12 cases, branch 3 was found to have expanded into portions of the ciliary muscle not normally innervated by it. It caused a contraction of 284 ± 62° of the ring of ciliary muscle, compared with 157 ± 27° in control ganglia (Fig. 11A and B). In fact, in four of the cases, branch 3 caused the entire ring of ciliary muscle to contract. Furthermore, in 7 of 12 cases, nerve 3 also caused strong constriction of the iris.

While most of these preparations were only assessed visually, in some cases EMG recordings were made from different parts of the peripheral field as well. An example is shown in Fig. 11C and D where stimulation of branch 3 in a partially axotomized preparation activated muscle fibers situated at 60, 200, and 270° as well as in the iris. In the contralateral control, responses could only be evoked in the ciliary muscles up to 120° and were not obtained from the iris.

Expansion of the peripheral field is there-fore associated with saving a number of cells from death. However, since ganglion cell death begins at st 35 and we did not assess peripheral field expansion until st 39–40, it is not certain that field expansion actually occurred prior to cell death and was causally linked to preventing it.

Nonuniform innervation of available peripheral target

In all cases studied, branch 3 was found to expand its peripheral innervation territory. However, it did not, on the average, innervate the entire available target; for example, in only 7 of 12 cases did it innervate the iris and in only 4 of 12 cases the entire ciliary muscle.

We attempted to further assess the density and normalcy of nerve 3 endings in foreign target with an EM study. Our observations were restricted to the iris because it is never normally innervated by branch 3. Thin sections of 0.2–0.5 mm in length, cut parallel to the long axis of the constrictor fibers, were photographed with the electron microscope and montages of the whole section were constructed. Iris samples were obtained from the four different quadrants of each iris. Because of the difficulty in anatomically identifying iris neuromuscular junctions at the stages studied, the number and distribution of axons were used in assessing the density of innervation when nerve 3 innervated other regions of the target after partial axotomy.

In the control iris, bundles of seven to eight unmeylinated axons were seen running into the iris stroma between the pigmented layer and the muscle core, which is formed by four to six adjacent muscle cells. Other bundles of axons (four to six) were observed between the differentiated and precursor muscle cells.

Two irises of the seven innervated by branch 3 were studied. Bundles of unmyelinated axons were seen forming an outer ring under the pigmented layer, as in controls, but fewer than the control number of axonal bundles were observed to enter into the muscle core and they only contained two to three axons. Furthermore, there were decreases in the number of contractile cells, only three to four forming the muscle thickness, resulting in a 20% reduction of

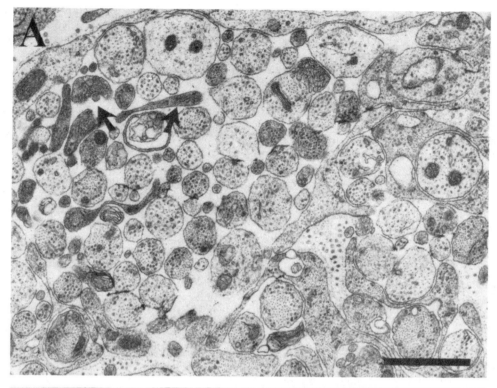

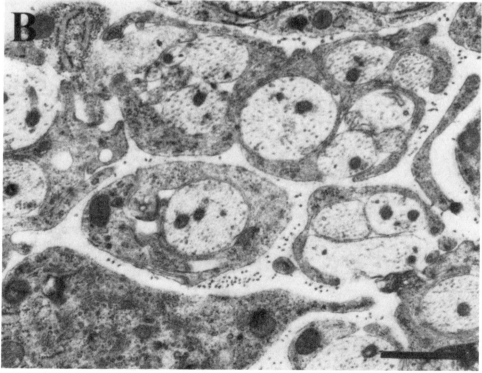

the muscle thickness. Finally the proportion of differentiated muscle to precursor cells was decreased to 20%.

To investigate the influence of the innervation on the final differentiation of muscle cells, two irises from partially axotomied embryos in which nerve 3 did not functionally innervate the iris, were studied with the electron microscope. First, the iris was substantially reduced in mass. Further, in extensive surveys of EM montages made from serial sections, only myoepithelial precursor cells were observed. This suggests that some influence from the nerve may be necessary to cause either the differentiation of muscle fibers from myoepithelial cells, or at least their continued maintenance.

DISCUSSION

A substantial portion of the ciliary cell population that would normally be eliminated during the cell death period can be rescued by reducing the number of competing cells. A similar result has recently been reported for *Xenopus* spinal cord (39). It is generally assumed that many neurons die during development because they fail to compete effectively for a limited supply of some aspect of their peripheral target, such as synaptic sites or a trophic substance. It would thus be interesting to calculate whether the number of neurons saved is what one would expect from the altered quantitative relationship between neuron population and peripheral target.

A total precell death ciliary population, of approximately 4,300 cells would be expected since branch 3, which represents $22 \pm 3\%$ of the ciliary population, contains roughly 950 cells. One can assume that there is sufficient peripheral factor for only 1,500 cells, which is the total number of ciliary cells that normally survive cell death. Since partial axotomy can be calculated to reduce the precell death ciliary population to 1,600,

one would expect almost all of the branch 3 cells to obtain sufficient peripheral factor and, therefore, survive, whereas 550 of them actually do.

Therefore, two-thirds of the cells that would be expected to survive (or 40% of those that normally die) can be saved by increasing the amount of peripheral target and presumably peripheral factor per neuron. This in turn suggests that these cells normally die because of competition. Clearly they are not preprogrammed to die nor are they grossly defective, a view borne out by tissue-culture studies where it appears that virtually all the cells can survive the cell death period (35, 50). Further, since branch 3 cells project to the correct region of the target prior to cell death, they presumably do not die in order to correct projection errors. In fact, since rescue of branch 3 cells is associated with expansion of branch 3 into foreign regions of the target, errors of this kind do not appear to be selected out by the cell death process. Cell death has, however, been observed to remove projection errors of a minor magnitude in several systems (8, 23).

While we cannot be certain why we were unable to rescue all the cells, total rescue would require the postulated peripheral factor to be distributed equally among the remaining neurons. Since we have in fact found nonuniform innervation of the peripheral target, neurons ending in the more densely innervated "original" region of the target would be under more severe competition for a postulated factor such as synaptic sites. Even, were a diffusible trophic factor responsible, the amount available per neuron could be reduced in densely innervated areas of the target. Therefore, given more appropriate conditions, all neurons might survive. The somewhat smaller proportion of neurons rescued in other studies where the periphery was doubled (approximately 29% for lumbosacral motoneurons following addition of a

FIG. 10. Cross section of branch 3 nerves at higher magnification. *A*: control; *B*: experimental. Notice the increase in axon diameter on the experimental side, in comparison with the control. Further, in the control, 6–10 axons are surrounded by a single Schwann cell, whereas there are only 1–3 axons per Schwann cell in the experimental nerve. Arrows point to degenerating axons, which were more prevalent on the experimental side. Calibration: 1 μm.

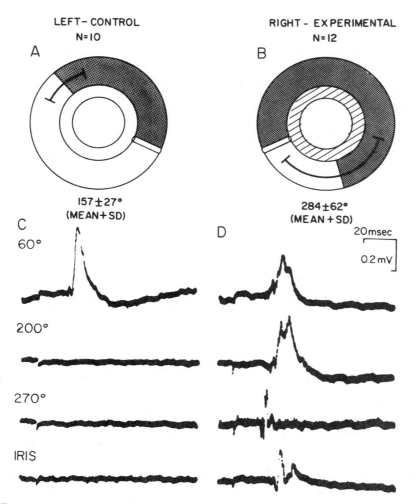

LEFT - CONTROL
N=10

RIGHT - EXPERIMENTAL
N=12

A

B

157±27°
(MEAN + SD)

284±62°
(MEAN + SD)

C

D

20 msec

0.2 mV

60°

200°

270°

IRIS

FIG. 11. Expansion of branch 3's innervation territory in partially axotomized preparations. The mean extent of the peripheral innervation territory of branch 3 is shown schematically for control (A) and partially axotomized (B) preparations by the stippling of the ciliary muscle extending from the main blood vessel dorsolaterally. Expansion of branch 3 to innervate the iris constrictor in 7/12 cases as indicated by crosshatching. Suction electrode recordings from the muscle fibers on stimulation of branch 3 is shown for a representative case on the control (C) and experimental (D) sides. The position of the recording site along the ring of ciliary muscle is in degrees dorsolaterally from the main blood vessel. Recordings from the iris constrictor are also shown.

supernumerary limb (20) or 23% for the ciliary ganglion after addition of a second eye (34) could be similarly explained. For example, while the periphery was apparently doubled in Hollyday and Hamburger's study (20), there was clearly nonuniform innervation of the peripheral targets, with only the first two of the eight lumbosacral segments innervating the supernumerary limb. Calculations, similar to those applied above to the ciliary ganglion, show that the maximum expected rescue of cells would be around 50%. The discrepancy

between this and the approximately 30% of the cells rescued is not great, whereas a truly effective doubling of the periphery should have rescued 100% of the cells. Additionally, in the Narayanan (34) study both eyes on the experimental side were considerably smaller than normal and there was no convincing evidence of innervation of the peripheral target.

The type of experiments reported here do not directly address whether the competition observed is for 1) synaptic sites, 2) a trophic factor, or 3) uptake of a trophic factor dependent on making a sufficient number of synapses. Considerable evidence shows that nerve growth factor is important in trophic interactions between sympathetic neurons and their peripheral targets (4, 18, 30, 36, 49) and may in fact be the factor competed for during normal development (18, 19). However, in the sympathetic as well as other systems, the importance of synapse formation has not been ruled out. Our experiments at least show that the interaction with the peripheral target during which neurons compete occurs relatively late in development at the time of peripheral synapse formation.

We cannot completely exclude another possibility. Neurons could be rescued not because of events in the periphery, but because reduction in cell number provides additional nutritive factors within the ganglion itself, coming from glial as well as other sources. We consider this possibility unlikely, however, because axotomy of all of the ciliary nerves greatly reduced this population yet the choroid cell number was not increased, being similar to control values.

A form of synaptic competition appears to be involved in the developmentally later elimination of polyneuronal innervation in skeletal muscle (5), although this is apparently achieved by collateral retraction rather than cell death (22, 52; but see Ref. 47). However, similar mechanisms might operate earlier during the cell death period as well. In fact Pittman and Oppenheim (43) have recently reported that blocking function with neuromuscular blocking agents (α-bungarotoxin and d-TC) can prevent cell death in about half of chick lumbosacral motoneurons that normally die (43). Presumed changes in function have also been shown to affect the postnatal elimination of polyneuronal innervation in mammals; tenotomy (3) and deafferentation (52) delaying the elimination while chronic nerve stimulation (38) and compensatory hypertrophy of muscle (52) speed it up. The process of competition might require synapses to function in order for one neuron to gain a competitive advantage, both during the cell death period and later during the process of synaptic elimination.

A novel finding of the present study was that competition between neurons normally retards their rate of development. In the face of competition it might take neurons longer to accumulate enough trophic factor or to make sufficient synapses, and the rate of neuronal maturation would then be influenced by the state of the axonal endings in the peripheral target. Zelena et al. (52) have recently observed a speeding up in the development of skeletal neuromuscular junctions following treatments that caused hypertrophy of the muscle, and a slowing of development following treatments that produced atrophy, which may be similar to the results reported here. However, the treatments used in that study were also considered to alter function. Changes in function per se might be directly associated with altering the rate of maturation, and we cannot at this time rule out changes in functional activity in the ciliary ganglion following partial axotomy.

Finally, competition between neurons has been suggested as a means of achieving specific connectivity both during reinnervation (12, 32) and initial development (17, 45). Various studies have shown that axons will sprout to invade foreign territory that has been previously denervated (2, 13, 46), suggesting that competition may be required to achieve specific connectivity during neuronal development. Our results are consistent with this idea and suggest that some form of competition normally restricts each ciliary nerve to the appropriate part of the target. However, in most studies of this sort, the expansion of neurons into foreign territory has been assessed in the adult or relatively late in development, so very little can be said about the actual mechanisms used in the initial development of the specific innervation territories. In our study branch 3 neurons were shown to have invaded foreign territory by st 39, only some 4 days after they establish their peripheral innervation territories. Thus if absolute constraints on nerve growth into foreign tissue operate in this system at all they must be very transient.

Leaving aside the question of mechanism, one may wonder why so many cells die when they have managed to project to the correct region of target. Earlier explanations of normal neuronal cell death primarily as a mechanism for quantitative matching of pre- and postsynaptic neuronal populations (10, 27–29) seem generally valid, although the apparent wastefulness of this process is more understandable in light of a recent proposal that considers evolutionary adaptability (21). Redundancy of neurons, with their final number determined by the size of the peripheral target, allows the balance to be maintained following evolutionary changes in the size of the target, without requiring concurrent changes in the neuronal cell population.

APPENDIX

Uwe Koehn and Samuel Zahl
Statistics Dept.,
University of Connecticut

We are given a number of clusters of cells of various sizes. After a time some of the cells die, and so the distribution of cluster sizes changes. We wish to determine whether the deaths occur at random among the cells or whether cluster size influences the deaths.

The original distribution of clusters is given, say there are n_j clusters of size j (with j cells). Some of the cells are survivors yielding L_i clusters of i living cells. If the distribution of living (and so dead) cells is random, we can liken the problem to having $N = \sum_{j=1}^{J} j n_j$ balls, J being the largest cluster size. Of the N balls, M are colored red

$$M = \sum_{i=1}^{J} i L_i$$

If a cluster has n_j balls, how many are red? This is just the probability distribution involved in choosing n_j balls from an urn with N balls, M of which are red, i.e., the hypergeometric distribution.

Let us define X_{ijk} to be associated with the kth cluster that has j balls. Let $X_{ijk} = 1$ if there are i red balls among the j, 0 if not; e.g., if $(X_{141}, X_{241}, X_{341}, X_{441}) = (0, 1, 0, 0)$, then the first ($k = 1$) cluster with 4 ($n_j = 4$) balls has 2 red ones. Using the hypergeometric

probability function, $h(x, N, M, n)$, $P(X_{ijk} = 1) = h(i, N, M, j) = E(X_{ijk})$.

A little thought reveals that the number of clusters with i red balls is

$$L_i = \sum_{j=i}^{J} \sum_{k=1}^{n_j} X_{ijk}$$

j beginning at i since if a cluster has i red balls, it has at least j balls.

Therefore, under the hypothesis of random deaths

$$E(L_i) = \sum_{j=i}^{J} \sum_{k=1}^{n_j} h(i, N, M, j) = \sum_{j=i}^{J} n_j h(i, N, M, j)$$

The covariance $(L_i, L_{i'})$ is elementary but tedious, being based on $E(X_{ijk}, X_{i'j'k'})$. The cases where $(j, k) = (j', k')$ are easy and only the cases where $(j, k) \neq (j', k')$ require a little thought.

In this case $E(X_{ijk}, X_{i'j'k'}) = P(\text{both } X_{ijk} \text{ and } X_{i'j'k'}$ are 1) $= P(i + i'$ red balls appear among the $j + j'$ chosen from the original N, of which M are red) $\times P(i$ red balls appear among the j chosen from $j + j'$ balls of which $i + i'$ are red).

Think of drawing first $j + j'$ balls and then splitting into two groups, the first with j and the second with j' balls. Thus

$E(X_{ijk}, X_{i'j'k'})$

$= h(i + i', N, M, j + j') h(i, j + j', i + i', j)$
if
$\qquad (j, k) \neq (j', k')$

$= h(i, N, M, j)$ if $(i, j, k) = (i', j', k')$

$= 0$ if $(j, k) = (j', k')$ and $i \neq i'$

Because the L_i satisfy the linear constraint

$$\sum_{i=1}^{J} i L_i = M$$

$\Sigma = (\text{covariance } (L_i, L_{i'}))$, the covariance matrix is singular of rank $J - 1$.

Thus, asymptotically, if the vector, $L^T = (L_1 - E(L_1), \ldots, L_{J-1} - E(L_{J-1}))$, $Q = L^T \Sigma^{-1} L$ has an X^2 distribution with $J - 1$ degrees of freedom.

If $Q > X^2_{J-1,\alpha}$ we would reject the hypothesis of random deaths throughout the clusters.

In our particular case, we have the following data:

Cluster size	1	2	3	4	5	6	7	8	9
Total observed no.	273	94	41	17	10	8	2	1	1
Expected no. living	188.16	42.17	11.98	3.66	1.02	0.23	0.04	0.01	0.00
Observed no. living	143	56	18	4	1	0	0	0	0

The table of covariances, Σ (writing only the lower triangular part) is

1	2	3	4	5	6	7	8	9
87,1073								
−25.4863	26.8770							
−7.2012	−5.5960	8.8345						
−2.4119	−1.8853	−1.3030	2.9840					
−0.8111	−0.5718	−0.4186	−0.2566	0.9074				
−0.2209	−0.1404	−0.1033	−0.0714	−0.0377	0.2194			
−0.0500	−0.0292	−0.0208	−0.0153	−0.0089	−0.0036	0.0427		
−0.0086	−0.0047	−0.0032	−0.0023	−0.0014	−0.0006	−0.0002	0.0060	
−0.0007	−0.0004	−0.0002	−0.0002	−0.0001	−0.0000	−0.0000	−0.0000	0.0004

The above values are calculated using a program written by one of the authors. Using the SAS package, we see that $Q = 24.93$ with 8 df, which is significant with $P < 0.002$, i.e., the observed numbers of the various size clusters is significantly different than the numbers expected under the hypothesis of random deaths.

ACKNOWLEDGMENTS

We thank Dr. Allen Wachtel for use of the Electron Microscope facility at the University of Connecticut, Ms. Amy Banford for her technical assistance, and Mrs. Frances Hunihan for typing the manuscript.

This study was supported by National Institutes of Health Grants NS10666 and NS10338, and the University of Connecticut Research Foundation.

Received 13 February 1979; accepted in final form 2 July 1979.

REFERENCES

1. ABERCROMBIE, M. Estimation of nuclear population from microtome sections. *Anat. Rec.* 94: 239–247, 1946.
2. BENNETT, M. R. AND RAFTOS, J. The formation and regression of synapses during the re-innervation of axolotl striated muscles. *J. Physiol. London* 265: 261–295, 1977.
3. BENOIT, P. AND CHANGEUX, J. P. Consequence of tenotomy on the evolution of multi-innervation in developing rat soleus muscle. *Brain Res.* 99: 354–358, 1975.
4. BLACK, I. B., HENDRY, I. A., AND IVERSON, L. Effects of surgical decentralization and nerve growth factor on the maturation of adrenergic neurons in a mouse sympathetic ganglion. *J. Neurochem.* 19: 1367–1377, 1972.
5. BROWN, M. C., JANSEN, J. K. S., AND VANESSEN, D. Polyneuronal innervation of skeletal muscle in new-born rats and its elimination during maturation. *J. Physiol. London* 261: 387–422, 1976.
6. BURSTEIN, L. G., LANDMESSER, L., AND PILAR, G. Competitive interactions between developing ciliary ganglion cells. *Soc. Neurosci. Abstr.* 3: 422, 1977.
7. CHU-WANG, I. W. AND OPPENHEIM, R. W. Cell death of motoneurons in the chick embryo spinal cord II. *J. Comp. Neurol.* 177: 59–86, 1978.
8. CLARKE, P. G. H. AND COWAN, W. M. The development of the isthmo-optic tract in the chick, with special reference to the occurrence and correction of developmental errors in the location and connection of isthmo-optic neurons. *J. Comp. Neurol.* 167: 143–164, 1976.
9. COHEN, M. W., LENTZ, T. L., AND KULLBERG, R. W. Development of the myotomal neuromuscular junction in *Xenopus laevis*: an electrophysiological and fine structural study. *Dev. Biol.* 60: 101–129, 1977.
10. COWAN, W. M. Neuronal death as a regulative mechanism in the control of cell number in the nervous system. In: *Development and Aging in the Nervous System*. New York: Academic, 1973, p. 19–41.
11. DAVSON, H. *The Eye.* New York: Academic, 1962, vol. 1.
12. DENNIS, M. J. AND YIP, J. W. Formation and elimination of foreign synapses on adult salamander muscle. *J. Physiol. London* 274: 299–310, 1978.
13. GUTH, L. AND BERNSTEIN, J. J. Selectivity in the re-establishment of synapses in the superior cervical sympathetic ganglion of the cat. *Exp. Neurol.* 4: 59–69, 1961.
14. HAMBURGER, V. Regression versus peripheral control of differentiation in motor hypoplasia. *Am. J. Anat.* 102: 365–410, 1958.
15. HAMBURGER, V. Cell death in the development of the lateral motor column of the chick embryo. *J. Comp. Neurol.* 160: 535–546, 1975.
16. HAMBURGER, V. AND HAMILTON, H. L. A series of normal stages in the development of the chick embryo. *J. Morphol.* 88: 49–92, 1951.
17. HARRIS, A. J. AND DENNIS, M. J. Deletion of "mistakes" in nerve-muscle connectivity during development of rat embryos. *Soc. Neurosci. Abstr.* 3: 316, 1977.
18. HENDRY, I. A. The response of adrenergic neurones to axotomy and nerve growth factor. *Brain Res.* 94: 87–97, 1975.
19. HENDRY, I. A. AND CAMPBELL, J. Morphometric analysis of rat superior cervical ganglion after axotomy and nerve growth factor treatment. *J. Neurocytol.* 5: 351–360, 1976.
20. HOLLYDAY, M. AND HAMBURGER, V. Reduction of the naturally occurring motor neuron loss by enlargement of the periphery. *J. Comp. Neurol.* 170: 311–320, 1976.
21. KATZ, M. J. AND LASEK, R. J. Evolution of the nervous system: role of ontogenetic mechanisms in the evolution of matching populations. *Proc. Natl. Acad. Sci. USA* 75: 1349–1352, 1978.
22. KORNELIUSSEN, H. AND JANSEN, J. K. S. Morphological aspects of the elimination of skeletal muscle fibres in newborn rats. *J. Neurocytol.* 5: 591–604, 1976.
23. LAMB, A. The projection patterns of the ventral horn to the hind limb during development. *Dev. Biol.* 54: 82–99, 1976.
24. LANDMESSER, L. The distribution of motoneurons supplying chick hindlimb muscles. *J. Physiol. London* 284: 371–389, 1978.
25. LANDMESSER, L. AND MORRIS, D. G. The development of functional innervation in the hindlimb of the chick embryo. *J. Physiol. London* 249: 301–326, 1975.
26. LANDMESSER, L. AND PILAR, G. The onset and development of transmission in the chick ciliary ganglion. *J. Physiol. London* 222: 691–713, 1972.
27. LANDMESSER, L. AND PILAR, G. Synapse formation during embryogenesis on ganglion cells lacking a periphery. *J. Physiol. London* 241: 715–736, 1974.
28. LANDMESSER, L. AND PILAR, G. Synaptic transmission and cell death during normal ganglionic development. *J. Physiol. London* 241: 737–749, 1974.
29. LANDMESSER, L. AND PILAR, G. Fate of ganglionic

synapses and ganglion cell axons during normal and induced cell death. *J. Cell Biol.* 68: 357–374, 1976.

30. LEVI-MONTALCINI, R. AND ANGELLETI, P. V. Nerve growth factor. *Physiol. Rev.* 48: 534–569, 1968.

31. LUCCHI, M. L., BORTOLAMI, R., AND CALLEGARI, E. Fine structure of intrinsic eye muscles of birds: development and postnatal changes. *J. Submicros. Cytol.* 6: 205–218, 1974.

32. MARK, R. F. Selective innervation of muscle. *Brit. Med. Bull.* 30: 122–126, 1974.

33. MARWITT, R., PILAR, G., AND WEAKLEY, J. N. Characterization of two cell populations in the avian ciliary ganglion. *Brain Res.* 25: 317–334, 1971.

34. NARAYANAN, C. H. AND NARAYANAN, Y. Neuronal adjustments in developing nuclear centers of the chick embryo following nuclear transplantation of an additional optic primordium. *J. Embryol. Exp. Morphol.* 44: 53–70, 1978.

35. NISHI, R. AND BERG, D. K. Dissociated ciliary neurons in vitro: survival and synapse formation. *Proc. Natl. Acad. Sci. USA* 74: 5171–5175, 1977.

36. NJA, A. AND PURVES, D. The effects of nerve growth factor and its antisera on synapses in the superior cervical ganglion of the guinea-pig. *J. Physiol. London* 277: 53–75, 1978.

37. NORCIO, R. AND DE SANTIS, M. The organization of neuronal somata in the first sacral spinal ganglion of the cat. *Exp. Neurol.* 50: 246–258, 1976.

38. O'BRIEN, R. A., PURVES, R. D., AND VRBOVÁ, G. Effect of activity on the elimination of multiple innervation in soleus muscles of rats. *J. Physiol. London* 271: 54–55P, 1977.

39. OLEK, A. J. AND EDWARDS, C. The effect of spinal nerve section on motor neuron loss during development in *Xenopus*. *Soc. Neurosci. Abstr.* 3: 115, 1977.

40. OPPENHEIM, R. S. AND CHU-WANG, I. W. Spontaneous cell death of spinal motoneurons following peripheral innervation in the chick embryo. *Brain Res.* 125: 154–160, 1977.

41. PILAR, G. AND LANDMESSER, L. Ultrastructural differences during embryonic cell death in normal and peripherally deprived ciliary ganglia. *J. Cell Biol.* 68: 339–356, 1976.

42. PILAR, G. AND VAUGHAN, P. C. Electrophysio-

logical investigations of the pigeon iris neuromuscular junctions. *Comp. Biochem. Physiol.* 29: 51–72, 1969.

43. PITTMAN, R. H. AND OPPENHEIM, R. W. Neuromuscular blockade increases motoneurone survival during normal cell death in the chick embryo. *Nature London* 271: 364–366, 1978.

44. PRESTIGE, M. C. The control of cell number in the lumbar ventral horns during the development of *Xenopus laevis* tadpoles. *J. Embryol. Exp. Morphol.* 18: 359–387, 1967.

45. PRESTIGE, M. C. AND WILLISHAW, D. J. On a role for competition in the formation of patterned neural connexions. *Proc. R. Soc. London Ser. B* 190: 77–98, 1975.

46. ROBSON, J. A., MASON, C. A., AND GUILLERY, R. W. Terminal arbors of axons that have formed abnormal connections. *Science* 201: 635–637, 1978.

47. ROSENTHAL, J. L. AND TARASKEVICH, P. S. Reduction of multiaxonal innervation at the neuromuscular junction of the rat during development. *J. Physiol. London* 270: 299–310, 1977.

48. SHIEH, P. The neoformation of cells of preganglionic type in the cervical spinal cord of the chick embryo following its transplantation to the thoracic level. *J. Exp. Zool.* 117: 359–396, 1951.

49. THOENEN, H., SANER, A., KETTLER, R., AND ANGELETTI, P. V. Nerve growth factor and preganglionic cholinergic nerves; their relative importance to the development of the terminal adrenergic neuron. *Brain Res.* 44: 593–602, 1972.

50. TUTTLE, J., SUSZKIW, J. B., AND ARD, M. Long-term survival and development of dissociated parasympathetic neurons in culture. *Brain Res.* In press.

51. WENGER, B. S. Construction and use of the vibrating needle for embryonic operations. *Bioscience* 18: 226–232, 1968.

52. ZELENA, J., VYSKOČIL, F., AND JIRANOVÁ, I. The elimination of polyneuronal innervation of endplates in developing rat muscles with altered function. In: *The Cholinergic Synapse*, edited by S. Tuček. Amsterdam: Elsevier, 1979, p. 365–372.

53. ZENKER, W. AND KRAMMER, E. Untersuchungen über Feinstruktur und Innervation der Augenmuskulatur des Hunnes. *Z. Zellforsch. Mikrosk. Anat.* 83: 147–168, 1967.

Reprinted from THE JOURNAL OF COMPARATIVE NEUROLOGY
Vol. 187, No. 2, September 15, 1979 © The Wistar Institute Press 1979

Cell Death of Motoneurons in the Chick Embryo Spinal Cord

IV. EVIDENCE THAT A FUNCTIONAL NEUROMUSCULAR INTERACTION IS INVOLVED IN THE REGULATION OF NATURALLY OCCURRING CELL DEATH AND THE STABILIZATION OF SYNAPSES

RANDALL PITTMAN [1] AND RONALD W. OPPENHEIM [2]
North Carolina Division of Mental Health and Mental Retardation Services,
Anderson Hall, Dorothea Dix Hospital, Raleigh, North Carolina 27611

ABSTRACT   Embryos immobilized with neuromuscular blocking agents for differing periods between 4.5 and 9 days of incubation had an increased number of motoneurons in the brachial and lumbar lateral motor columns. Treatment with α-cobratoxin (α-CTX) on days 4-9, for instance, was able to prevent virtually all natural cell death during this period; control embryos had an average of 22,500 lumbar motoneurons on day 5.5, and 13,500 on day 10, whereas treated embryos had approximately 21,000 cells on day 10. Curare, α-CTX, α-bungarotoxin (α-BTX) and botulinum toxin were all about equally effective in preventing cell death. Similar treatment *begun after* day 12, however, had no effect on cell number. If even a partial immobilization was continued after day 10 (in embryos totally immobilized earlier) most of the excess neurons were maintained, in some cases right up to hatching, at which time the embryos died due to respiratory failure. In contrast, when administration of the immobilizing agents was stopped, allowing the embryos' motility to return to control levels, the excess neurons underwent a delayed cell death and total cell number fell to below control levels by days 16-18.

Limb muscles from embryos with excess motoneurons exhibited relatively normal differentiation and had acetylcholinesterase (AChE) stained endplates which were innervated. Following curare treatment the two wing muscles, anterior and posterior latissimus dorsi, were found to have an increased number of AChE-stained endplates, whereas the only leg muscle examined quantitatively—the ischioflexorius (IFL)—did not; the IFL, did, however, have a markedly reduced variance in endplate distance, as well as other apparent differences suggesting an altered pattern of innervation.

Our findings imply that the number of motoneurons undergoing natural cell death is closely related to muscle activity. Thus, functional interactions at the developing neuromuscular junction seem to be critical in controlling cell death. If a retrograde trophic factor is involved its action is somehow related to muscle activity.

In a preliminary publication (Pittman and Oppenheim, '78) we reported that a neuromuscular blockade during the period of natural cell death of spinal motoneurons led to a substantial reduction in the number of such cells undergoing degeneration. Although we were not able to prevent all of the cells from dying, we did reduce natural cell death to a considerably greater extent than that following peripheral enlargement (e.g., Hollyday and

Hamburger, '76), the only previous manipulation known to prevent cell death; in some of our most favorable cases more than 60% of the neurons destined to die were maintained for more than a week after the cessation of natural cell death.

Our intention in pursuing this line of inves-

---

[1] Present address: Department of Pharmacology, University of Colorado, Denver, Colorado 80262.
[2] Address reprint requests to Ronald W. Oppenheim.

tigation was to gain a better understanding of the possible role of synaptic mechanisms in the regulation of neuronal cell death. In the system we have chosen to study—the motoneurons located in the lateral motor column (LMC) of the lumbar (and brachial) region—40-60% of the neurons that are produced and begin differentiation subsequently cease normal maturation and enter a phase of regression during which several thousand cells die and are phagocytosed over a period of only a few days (Hamburger, '75; Chu-Wang and Oppenheim, '78a; Oppenheim and Majors-Willard, '78). The period of maximal cell death coincides, in general, with the time of leg (and wing) innervation (Hamburger, '58; Oppenheim and Heaton, '75; Landmesser and Morris, '75; Atsumi, '77) and virtually all of the lumbar motoneurons which die send axons into the leg musculature prior to their death (Oppenheim and Chu-Wang, '77; Chu-Wang and Oppenheim, '78b). In fact, before the onset of frank degeneration we have been unable to detect any differences between the motoneurons that die and those that survive (Oppenheim et al., '78a). All of the evidence to date strongly indicates that the fate of the cells that die in this system are not in any sense preprogrammed. Instead, their future is decided by epigenetic events occurring at the target site following the initiation of differentiation; the prevention of cell death by neuromuscular blocking agents provides striking confirmation of this point.

The currently favored hypotheses of what events at the target control normal cell death involve the notion of either a competition between neurons for a limited number of synaptic sites and/or for a limited amount of trophic substance supplied by the target (Prestige, '70; Cowan, '73; Hamburger, '75). One of the critical unanswered questions concerning both of these putative mechanisms is the extent to which synaptic transmission may be involved (Changeux and Danchin, '76). It was the primary goal of the present experiments to elucidate this question with regard to spinal motoneurons and their normal targets in the limb musculature.

MATERIALS AND METHODS

Approximately 1,000 White Leghorn chick embryos ranging from 4.5 to 20 days of incubation were used. A large number of these died following treatment; thus motoneuron counts were obtained for only approximately 280. A few embryos had their right limb-bud removed on day 2.5 using the vibrating needle technique of Wenger ('68). Operations were carried out as described by Chu-Wang and Oppenheim ('78a).

1. *Drug administration*

For some experiments neurotoxins or saline were administered on day 6 (st. 28-29) by intramuscular injection into the ventral muscle mass of the right leg using a 33-gauge Hamilton microsyringe fitted with a 40 μ pipette. On day 12 injections were made into the region of the gastrocnemius of the right leg using a 33-gauge Hamilton microsyringe without the glass pipette. A few 12-day embryos were injected into the left gastrocnemius, and no difference in survival or motoneuron counts were seen when compared to those injected in the right leg. Injections were made using a dissecting microscope and by employing fine hair loops to manipulate and stabilize the legs (Oppenheim and Heaton, '75).

With one exception, in all groups of curare-treated animals, and in some groups of α-CTX and α-BTX animals, agents were administered by dropping solutions (0.1-0.25 ml) onto the highly vascularized chorioallantoic membrane (CAM) for four consecutive days beginning either on day 6 or 12. In one group, curare (1.5 mg) was administered daily on days 4-6 and the embryos sacrificed on day 8. One group of embryos received α-CTX on days 6-9 and curare on days 10-13 (α-CTX + curare), and one group received α-CTX on days 4-9. The CAM over the embryo was exposed by making a lateral window in the egg (Oppenheim et al., '73). Once the drug was administered, the opening was sealed with Parafilm and the egg returned to a temperature and humidity controlled incubator.

Drugs used in this study were: α-CTX (*Naja naja siamensis;* Miami Serpentarium, Miami, Florida); α-BTX (Miami Serpentarium); cobratoxin (CTX, *Naja naja atra;* Biological Unlimited, Baltimore, Maryland); d-tubocurarine (curare, Sigma Chemicals, St. Louis, Missouri); botulinum toxin (BoTX, gift from Dr. E. J. Shantz); and tetanus toxin (TeTX, gift from Dr. R. O. Thomson).

2. *Motility recordings and cell counts*

Prior to sacrifice, motility recordings were obtained for many of the embryos later examined histologically. Observations were carried out in a temperature and humidity controlled plexiglass box and embryonic motility was recorded for three to five minutes using a 10 × binocular dissecting scope and a simple hand counter (Oppenheim et al., '78b).

For motoneuron counts, embryos were sacrificed on days 5-10, 12-16, 18 or 20 and staged according to Hamburger and Hamilton ('51). The lumbar or brachial spinal column was removed and fixed in Carnoy's solution and the spinal cords were processed for paraffin histology, serially sectioned at either 8 μ (5-8 days) or 12 μ (9-20 days) and stained with thionin. The rostral and caudal ends of both the lumbar and brachial cord were identifiable at all ages (Hamburger, '75). Spinal ganglia were left attached to the cord for all embryos younger than 16 days; this aided in identifying the most rostral and caudal segments. The presence of the spinal ganglia was particularly useful in some treatment groups which had an apparent increase in the number of medial motoneurons with a resulting encroachment into the more lateral part of the cord thereby making the identification of segments difficult by other criteria.

Motoneurons in either one or both lateral motor columns were counted according to established criteria (Hamburger, '75; Chu-Wang and Oppenheim, '78a). Every tenth section was counted. No corrections were made for double counting of motoneurons since the section thickness at all stages was much greater than the entire nuclear diameter (Konigsmark, '70); moreover, a small sampling of nucleolar diameters comparing control and curare-treated embryos showed no appreciable difference between the two groups.

Cell counts for the 5- to 12-day-old embryos were carried out at a magnification of 500 ×, and at 312 × for those 13 to 20 days old. At least one animal in each group was counted on both sides to assure that no consistent discrepancies existed between the right and left LMC.

Either one or both legs were removed from some of the embryos. After blotting, wet weights were taken of the entire shank and the legs used for either biochemistry, histochemistry, or histological staining.

3. Histochemistry and biochemistry

Acetylcholinesterase (AChE) was demonstrated histochemically in wing and leg muscles using the El-Badawi and Schenk ('67) modification of the Koelle-Friedenwald technique. In the wing, the anterior and posterior latissimus dorsi (ALD, PLD) muscles were used for most experiments (some observations were also made on the brachially-innervated pectoral muscle). In the leg, most observations were on the ischioflexorius (IFL) a multiply-innervated thigh muscle innervated by spinal segments 25 and 26 (Landmesser, '78); some observations were also made on the sartorius muscle which is innervated by segments 23 and 24, and the gastrocnemius which is innervated by segments 26-29 (Landmesser and Morris, '75). Both the sartorius and the gastrocnemius contain a mixture of focally and multiply innervated fibers (Hess, '70; Ashmore et al., '78).

In most cases, either whole muscles or portions of whole muscles were dissected out and stained for AChE en bloc; a single layer of small fascicles of muscle fibers from the middle of the muscle was then dissected free using fine tungsten needles. These were placed on slides, covered with glycerine and cover-slipped. The sections were examined at 312 × and the distance between AChE-positive endplates was measured with an eyepiece micrometer. Although an attempt was made to make as many of these measurements as possible on single isolated fibers, this was not always possible. Instead it was often necessary to take measurements from small "fascicles" of fibers (i.e., 2-10) in which successive endplates were clearly demarcated. Although there is undoubtedly more room for error in measuring from such fascicles, comparisons of these values with those from single fibers were not significantly different. In some instances frozen sections (25-50 μ) from whole muscle were incubated for 60 to 90 minutes for AChE demonstration. Muscles were also examined for the simultaneous demonstration of endplates (AChE) and innervation (silver) by the technique recently described by Toop ('76). In some cases whole muscles were fixed in Carnoy's solution; serial sections were cut parallel to the long axis of the muscle and stained with hematoxylin and eosin.

AChE (EC 3.1.1.7) activity was determined radiometrically by the method of Potter ('67) using [acetyl-1^{14}C]-β-methylcholine (New England Nuclear, Boston, Massachusetts) as a selective substrate. Shank muscles were removed on day 16 and either stored at −30°C (BoTX and TeTX) along with control muscles, or were assayed immediately (curare and α-CTX). Protein was measured by the method

TABLE 1

Motility (movements/min) at various ages during and following curare, α-CTX, α-BTX or BoTX treatment

Treatment	N	Age (days)							
		7	8	9	10	13	16	18	20
Controls	18	7.0±0.7	11.1±2.3	13.9±2.7	15.0±1.1	16.8±1.9	14.5±1.5	7.2±2.6	3.6±1.3
Curare (CAM)									
1 mg d 6-9	3	5.3±1.2	8.6±2.8	11.8±1.8	9.0±2.1	—	14.4±7.1 [3]	—	—
1.5 mg d 4-6	3	2.7±1.1	2.3±1.6	—	—	—	—	—	—
2.5 mg d 6-9	16	2.5±0.5	2.1±1.7	1.0±0.4	2.5±1.4	4.9±2.2	5.6±2.3	5.0±2.5	2.6±1.2 [3]
4.0 mg d 6-9	3	2.2±0.8	2.0±0.3	0.2±0.4	0	—	0	—	—
5.5 mg d 6-9	3	0.6±0.5	1.0±0.7	0	0	—	0	—	—
α-CTX i.m.									
6 μg d 6	8	0	8.1±4.2	14.2±1.9 [3]	15.0±2.1 [3]	—	—	—	—
α-CTX (CAM) [1]	15	0	1.1±0.4	0	2.3±1.1	10.7±2.3	16.8±3.8 [3]	7.5±3.0 [3]	—
α-BTX (CAM) [1]	6	0	1.0±0.4	0.9±0.5	1.2±0.6	13.0±3.6	15.8±5.1 [3]	—	—
α-CTX + curare [2]	5	0	0	0	1.4±0.8	0.4±0.2	3.7±1.1	1.9±0.7	—
BoTX i.m.									
1200 LD₅₀ d 6	9	—	—	—	4.9±3.1	—	0	—	—

[1] Received 100 μg d 6; 85 μg d 7, 8; 50 μg d 9 of α-CTX or α-BTX.
[2] Received same levels of α-CTX as indicated in note-1 on days 6-9 and 2.5 mg curare on d 10-13.
[3] With these exceptions, all other treatments were significantly different from control at $p < 0.01$ or $p < 0.05$, Mann-Whitney Test. Mean ± S.D.

of Lowry et al. ('51) using bovine serum albumin as the standard.

RESULTS

1. *Motility and general morphological development*

Activity levels of saline and heat-inactivated BoTX-injected embryos, as well as uninjected control embryos, did not differ significantly, so their combined motility recordings are presented in table 1.

For those embryos receiving drugs daily, motility recordings were taken 22 to 23 hours after each treatment. Therefore, the activity levels presented in table 1 represent the maximum activity for the preceding 24-hour period. That these do represent the maximum activity levels is supported by previous observations that a single treatment with 2.5 mg of curare stopped all activity for a large portion of the 24-hour period, followed by a subsequent slow rise in motility (Oppenheim et al., '78b).

Solutions of curare are rapidly taken up into the embryonic circulation after placement onto the CAM, and although little or no degradation occurs, there is a redistribution within the egg (Oppenheim et al., '78b). Amounts of curare ranging from 1-5.5 mg were given daily from days 4-6, days 6-9 or days 12-15. All concentrations decreased activity levels below those of controls and the decreases were proportional to the concentration (table 1). Even on days 16-18, which is seven to nine days

after the last curare treatment in the 6- to 9-day groups, motility was still decreased in all animals except the group receiving 1 mg of curare daily.[3] This group maintained a motility deficit as long as curare was administered; however, once treatment was stopped, redistribution of the curare within the extra-embryonic system evidently decreased the amount of curare in the embryos below a level sufficient to maintain a motility decrease; by day 16 motility levels were comparable to controls.

A single i.m. injection of α-CTX (or either of the other irreversible snake toxins) on day 6 produced an almost total cessation of motility two hours after injection (0.1 ± 0.09 moves/min, n = 7, compared to 4.6 ± 1.3 moves/min, n = 10 for 6-day controls), and at 6 and 24 hours following injection no motility was observable. On day 8 (48 hours after injection), motility levels were beginning to approach control levels and by day 9 activity was comparable to controls. When α-CTX or α-BTX was given each day by dropping solutions onto the CAM, however, motility was essentially eliminated over the entire four days of treatment. As would be expected from the results of the i.m. injections, once the α-CTX treatment (CAM) was stopped, motility gradually re-

[3] It is important to point out that because most of the curare is not inactivated metabolically by the chick embryo (Oppenheim et al., '78b) it remains active long beyond the cessation of injections (e.g., on day 9). Thus, embryos receiving 2.5 mg of curare on days 6-9 have significant decrements in motility at least until day 18 of incubation.

TABLE 2

Leg weights (shank) in grams at various ages following curare or α-cobratoxin treatment

Age	Control	Curare (d 6-9)	α-CTX (d 6-9)	α-CTX + curare (d 6-9 + d 10-13)
10	0.065±0.002	0.055±0.002 [1]	0.049±0.003 [2,3]	—
13	0.340±0.04	0.280±0.07 [1]	0.240±0.06 [2,3]	0.22±0.08 [2,3]
16	1.100±0.2	0.780±0.1 [3]	0.600±0.08 [2,3]	0.50±0.06 [2,3]
18	1.300±0.1	0.950±0.3 [1]	0.850±0.07 [2]	0.70±0.05 [2,3]

Mann-Whitney Test. N = 4-5 per group. Mean ± S D. Curare = 2.5 mg; α-CTX and α-CTX + curare concentrations are the same as in table 1.
[1,2] p < 0.05 and p < 0.01, respectively, compared to control.
[3] p < 0.05 compared to curare.

turned to normal levels. In contrast, embryos receiving α-CTX + curare exhibited a continued motility decrement through day 18.

Following i.m. injection of BoTX on day 6, no obvious decrease in motility could be seen 18 hours later. Because BoTX produced a much higher mortality than other treatments and because mortality increased with repeated openings of the eggs, additional motility recordings were made only on days 10 and 16, prior to sacrificing the animals. On day 10, motility was about one-third that of controls and by day 16 no activity was present (table 1).

Decreasing or stopping motility for several days with curare causes a retardation in development (e.g., Oppenheim et al., '78b). In the present study, those embryos which had a substantial decrease in motility betweeen days 6 and 10 were consistently about one-half day "younger" than comparable controls. On day 16, embryos which had received either a single injection of BoTX on day 6, or curare or α-CTX on days 6-9 were retarded in development by approximately one day.

On day 16, some of the embryos in the 4-mg curare group showed an inordinate amount of muscle atrophy, had spinal cords that were reduced in size (fig. 8), and were retarded in overall development by two to three days. Others in the 4-mg curare group appeared similar to embryos receiving 2.5 mg of curare. It seems that 4 mg of curare may be a critical dosage in that embryos receiving lower dosages never showed gross muscular atrophy, whereas some receiving 4 mg or higher dosages (5.5 mg) did. Embryos showing extensive muscle atrophy are not included in the data on cell counts.

Consistent with the general morphological retardation in treated embryos was the observation that leg weight was reduced at 10, 13, 16 and 18 days of incubation (table 2). We have also found effects on muscle similar to those described by others (e.g., Drachman, '68; Giacobini et al., '73) — i.e., atrophy, degeneration, an increase in sarcolemmal nuclei and a tendency to retain a myotube appearance — however, differences between treated and control muscle did not appear as marked as those reported by Drachman ('68) or Giacobini et al. ('73) (figs. 1a,b). The shorter duration and less severe paralysis in our study is probably responsible for this difference.

Because many of the treated embryos which were sacrificed on day 10 were actually only 9 to 9.5 days old by staging criteria, cell counts for control 9-day embryos were made so that any increase in cell number due solely to age could be taken into account. No significant differences were found in the number of motoneurons between day 9 and 10 (Right LMC: day 9, st. 35+, 13,725 ± 420, n = 4; day 10, st. 36, 13,688 ± 491, n = 3).

2. *Cell counts*

(a) Curare treatment

No significant differences between right and left LMC's were found in any control or experimental embryos except those which had a limb-bud removed at stage 16. The cell counts for control animals presented in tables 3, 4 and 5 are from embryos which had saline solutions injected onto the CAM on days 6-9, as well as untreated embryos; [4] since there was no difference between the groups they were combined. Natural cell death in the lumbar

---

[4] The number of motoneurons in control embryos older than 12 days is about 20% less than previously reported by us (Oppenheim et al., '78b). The techniques for counting the cells were the same and White Leghorn eggs were used in both studies; however, different suppliers of eggs (i.e., different egg strains) were used in the two studies. A third strain of White Leghorns currently being used by us (but not included in the present report) appears to differ from both of the earlier strains in that cell numbers on day 16 are lower (e.g., 8,503 ± 750, n = 5 vs 11,407 ± 562, n = 13 for the strain used in the present study). Thus, significant strain differences in cell number appear to exist indicating that one must always be certain that experimental and control animals are from the same strain.

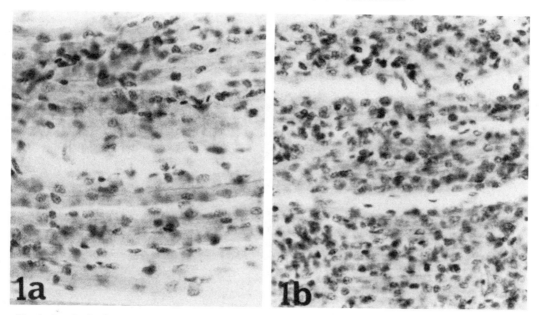

Fig. 1   Longitudinal sections of the ischioflexorius (IFL) muscle from an 18 day control (A) and curare-treated embryo (B) (st. 44). The muscle fibers are somewhat smaller in the curare-treated embryos and there is an apparent increase in sarcolemmal nuclei. A and B × 700.

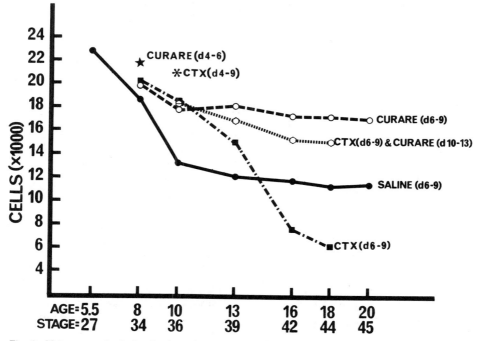

Fig. 2   Motoneurons in the lumbar lateral motor column (LMC) at different ages in controls and following various drug treatments. Each point is the average of two to ten embryos.

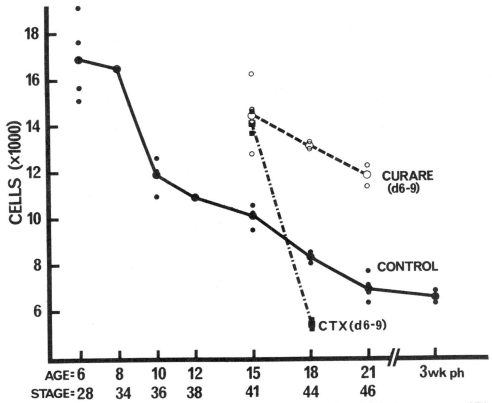

Fig. 3 Motoneurons in the brachial LMC at different ages in controls and following curare or α-CTX treatment. Large symbols are averages; small symbols are individual cases.

spinal cord of the chick occurs predominately between days 6 and 10 when 40-50% of the motoneurons present on day 6 degenerate and disappear (Hamburger, '75; Chu-Wang and Oppenheim, '78a,b; Oppenheim et al., '78a). Some cell death does occur prior to day 6, however, and the present study indicated that these early degenerating neurons can also be maintained if curare is administered between days 4-6 (table 3). It is also evident in table 3 and figure 2 that between days 10 and 16 an additional 1,500 to 2,000 cells degenerated in control embryos. The greatest part of this reduction occurred between days 10 and 13.

The control cell counts for the brachial spinal cord (fig. 3) are from Oppenheim and Majors-Willard ('78) in which cell death in this region was shown to begin later and extend for a longer duration than in the lumbar cord. Between embryonic days 8 and 21 there is a loss of about 11,000 brachial motoneurons

comprising almost 60% of the original population. Curare treatment between days 6 and 9 reduced this loss considerably such that by days 18-20 there were 60% more motoneurons in the curare-treated embryos. Treatment with α-CTX on days 6-9 resulted in 45% more brachial motoneurons than control on day 16; however, by day 18 these embryos had 34% fewer cells than controls.

Cell counts in the lumbar region for the groups receiving 1, 2.5, and 4 mg of curare on days 6-9 were comparable on day 10 and showed a consistent decrease in the extent of cell death (table 3; figs. 4, 5). Curare treatment *after* the period of cell death, however, had no effect on cell number.

Between days 10-16, the 1-mg curare group lost over 4,000 motoneurons and thus had only 13% more neurons than controls on day 16. This was the only curare group that had motility levels comparable to controls on day

TABLE 3

Cell counts (mean ± S.D.) of motoneurons following curare treatment [1]

Treatment		Age (days)						
		6	8	10	13	16	18	20
Control		22,635(7) ±1,337	18,608(3) ±952	13,330(15) ±408	12,109(3) ±891	11,407(13) ±562	11,175(3) ±784	11,400(3) ±587
Curare (CAM) 1.5 mg d 4-6		—	21,208(3) ±717	—	—	—	—	—
Curare (CAM) 1 mg d 6-9		—	—	17,035(4) ±571	—	12,793(3) ±1,516		
Curare (CAM) 2.5 mg d 6-9		—	19,830(3) ±797	17,750(7) ±666	18,121(3) ±878	17,600(3) ±527	17,230(4) ±598	17,050(3) ±813
Curare (CAM) 4.0 mg d 6-9		—	—	16,597(6) ±409	—	16,353(4) ±891	—	—
Curare (CAM) 2.5 mg d 12-15		—	—	—	—	11,351(6) ±797	—	—
Curare (CAM) 2.5 mg d 6-9	Exp.	—	—	2,675(5) [1] ±470	—	—	—	—
(Limb-bud removal)	Con.	—	—	17,331 (5) ±1,153	—	—	—	—

[1] Data are presented for both the right (exp.) and left (control) sides of the spinal cord. Numbers in parentheses are the number of animals examined in each treatment.

16 (table 1). Treatment with 2.5 mg of curare daily between days 6-9, on the other hand, resulted in a continued maintenance on day 16 of the excess motoneurons present on day 10 (table 3; figs. 6, 7). The increased percentage of motoneurons surviving on day 16 (50%), when compared to day 10 (35%), results from the additional normal cell death that occurs in control animals between days 10-13, and which has been prevented by the continued presence of unmetabolized curare.

In order to show that curare was not having a direct *central* effect on motoneurons and thereby causing a decrease in cell death, several embryos had their right hind limb-bud removed at stage 16 (day 2.5) and were then given 2.5 mg of curare daily on days 6-9. On day 10, the left LMC contained 31% more motoneurons than control, which is quite similar to that seen in the previous 2.5-mg curare group. The right LMC had an 87% decrease in motoneurons which is comparable to the previously reported decrease seen after limb-bud removal in embryos receiving no drug treatment (Hamburger, '58; Oppenheim et al., '78a).

The increase in cell number following curare treatment was still largely present as late as 19 to 20 days of incubation; cell counts after this time were not possible because virtually all embryos die after day 19 due to paralysis of respiratory muscles (prior to this time, oxygen requirements are met by the chorioallantoic vascular system).

(b) Irreversible snake toxins and botulinum toxin

Cell counts for CTX and α-CTX treated embryos (at similar concentrations) did not differ significantly and were combined for presentation in table 4; for clarity, the abbreviation α-CTX will be used in the text as being synonymous with both of these irreversible snake toxins.

No difference between the right and left LMC was seen in embryos that were injected i.m. on days 6 or 12; therefore, the injection procedure itself did not produce any differential effects on the number of motoneurons.

A single injection of α-CTX on day 6 had no effect on the number of motoneurons present on day 10, and a considerably larger injection on day 12 did not affect the number of neurons present on day 16. The single large injection of

Figs. 4, 5 Cross-sections of the lumbar spinal cord (Seg. 27) at ten days of incubation (st. 36) from a control (fig. 4) and curare-treated (2.5 mg) embryo (fig. 5). G, glycogen body. × 110. Inset: enlargement of the LMC. × 165.

Figs. 6, 7 Cross-sections of the lumbar spinal cord (Seg. 27) at 16 days of incubation (st. 42) from a control (fig. 6) and curare-treated (2.5 mg) embryo (fig. 7). × 35. Inset: enlargement of the LMC. × 80. Glycogen body inadvertently removed during dissection in figures 6 and 9.

Fig. 8 Cross-section of the lumbar spinal cord (Seg. 27) at 16 days of incubation (st. 42) from a 4.0-mg curare-treated embryo. × 35. Inset: enlargement of the LMC. Note general atrophy of spinal cord. G, Glycogen body. × 80.

Fig. 9 Cross-section of the lumbar spinal cord (Seg. 27) at 16 days (st. 42) from an α-CTX treated embryo (d 6-9). × 35. Inset: enlargement of the LMC. × 80.

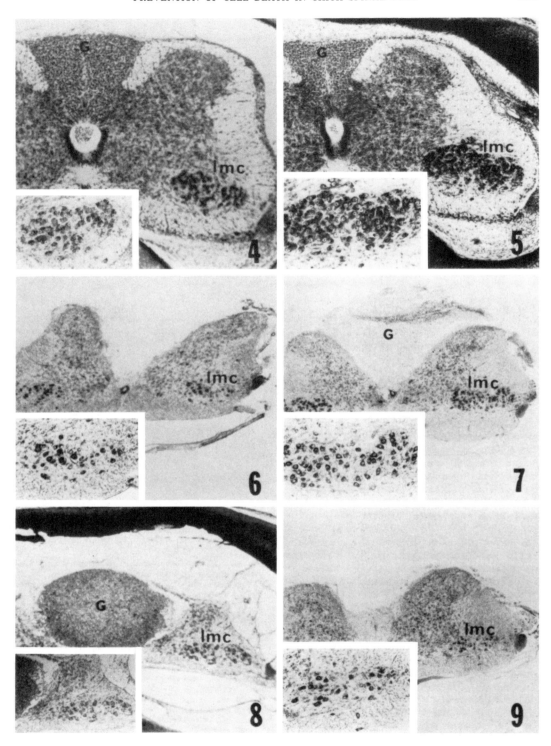

TABLE 4

Cell counts (mean ± S.D.) of motoneurons following α-cobratoxin or α-bungarotoxin treatment

Treatment	Age (days)					
	6	8	10	13	16	18
Control	22,635(7) ±1,337	18,608(3) ±952	13,330(15) ±408	12,109(3) ±891	11,407(13) ±562	11,175(3) ±784
α-CTX (9 μg i.m. d 6)	—	—	13,329(10) ±134	—	—	—
α-CTX (32 μg i.m. d 12)	—	—	—	—	11,097(9) ±394	—
α-CTX (d 4-9) [1]	—	—	21,000(4) ±773	—	—	—
α-CTX (CAM) (d 6-9) [2]	—	20,210(3) ±887	18,570(6) ±931	14,950(3) ±470	7,618(3) ±367	6,200(3) ±743
α-BTX (CAM) (d 6-9) [2]	—	—	18,780(3) ±1,075	12,800(3) ±711	8,735(3) ±466	—
α-CTX (CAM (d 6-9 + curare d 10-13) [3]	—	—	18,300(3) ±884	16,882(3) ±428	15,255(3) ±576	15,025(3) ±493

Note: Numbers in parentheses refer to the number of animals per treatment.
[1] Received 100 μg d 4; 90 μg d 5; 85 μg d 6-8; 60 μg d 9.
[2] Received 100 μg d 6; 85 μg d 7, 8; 50 μg d 9.
[3] Received 100 μg α-CTX d 6; 85 μg d 7, 8; 50 μg d 9 plus 2.5 mg curare d 10-13.

α-CTX on day 12 resulted in a 30% decrease in motility on day 16.

Whereas a single injection of α-CTX on day 6 had no effect on motoneuron survival on day 10, daily treatment with α-CTX or α-BTX on days 6-9 resulted in the maintenance of 40% more motoneurons than controls on day 10 (table 4; fig. 2). If, however, these animals were allowed to survive until day 16, a 25-30% *decrease* in cell number was observed and by day 18 the α-CTX group had a 45% decrease in cell number compared to controls. Motility levels were comparable to those of controls by days 14-16 (table 1). Beginning treatment with α-CTX on day 4, rather than day 6, and continuing through day 9 resulted in a 64% increase in cell number on day 10 (table 4; fig. 2).

The embryos treated with α-CTX were somewhat smaller than controls, and those injected on day 12 showed some ankylosis, but these embryos were in no way comparable to the developmentally retarded embryos receiving high concentrations (4 or 5.5 mg) of curare. Even though daily treatment (days 6-9) of α-CTX produced a decrease in cell number on days 16 and 18 the spinal cord looked quite healthy (fig. 9). Extensive muscular atrophy followed by secondary CNS degeneration seems a likely outcome of high concentrations of curare but is probably not the case for the α-CTX treatment.

Embryos given α-CTX on days 6-9 *plus*

curare on days 10-13 did not show this marked decrease of cell number below control levels. On days 16 and 18 these embryos had 36% more neurons than controls and almost 100% more than embryos receiving only α-CTX on days 6-9 (fig. 2).

Although the i.m. injection procedure itself did not produce any noticeable effect on motoneuron survival, as an added precaution the LMC contralateral to the injected leg was used for motoneuron counts in BoTX injected embryos.

A single injection of BoTX on day 6 resulted in 20-25% more motoneurons on day 10 and

TABLE 5

Cell counts (mean ± S.D.) of motoneurons following botulinum or tetanus toxin treatment

Treatment	Age	N	No. of cells
Heat-inactivated BoTX control (i.m. d 6)	10	6	13,816±531
BoTX (2,000 LD$_{50}$ [1] d 6 i.m.)	10	4	17,080±704
BoTX (750 LD$_{50}$ d 6 i.m.)	10	5	16,470±864
BoTX (750 LD$_{50}$ d 7 i.m.)	10	5	14,765±418
TeTX (6,000 LD$_{50}$ d 6 i.m.)	10	5	13,116±512
Control (uninjected)	16	13	11,407±562
BoTX (1,200 LD$_{50}$ d 6 i.m.)	16	5	16,402±438
TeTX (6,000 LD$_{50}$ d 6 i.m.)	16	3	8,520±490

[1] Doses expressed as LD$_{50}$ for 20-g mouse.

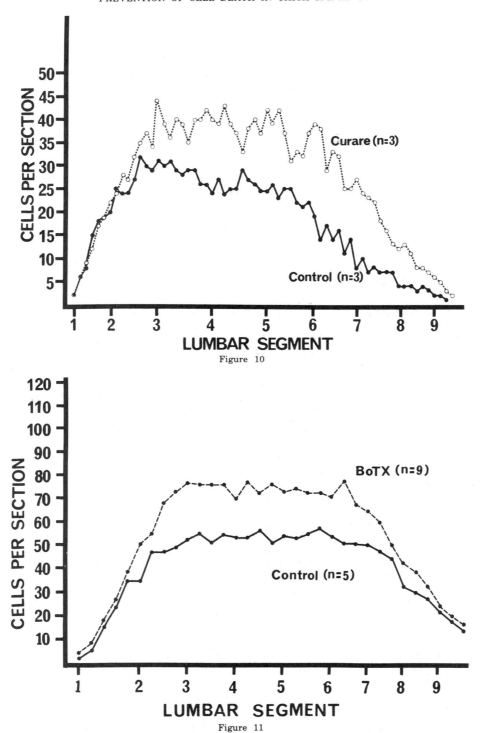

Figure 10

Figure 11

Figs. 10, 11   Rostral-caudal distribution of motoneurons in control and curare (d 6-9) treated embryos on day 16 (fig. 10) and control and BoTX (i.m. d 6) treated embryos on day 10 (fig. 11).

TABLE 6

Distance in microns between the endplates of curare-treated (2.5 mg, d 6-9) and control muscle at 17 and 19 days of incubation [1]

	ALD		PLD [2]		IFL	
	C	E	C	E	C	E
17-day						
N	100	100	50	100	150	150
Mean	158.3	130.1 [3]	471.2	123.5 [3]	273.9	283.9
SD	74.3	65.2	249.7	86.1	207.1	155.5
19-day						
N	100	100	50	150	100	100
Mean	162.8	130.4 [3]	577.7	220.7 [3]	146.0	176.1 [3]
SD	77.8	71.3	227.1	137.3	75.4	80.1

[1] See text for details of measurement.
[2] Many of the PLD muscle fibers were singly innervated; these measurements were only from fibers in which two or more endplates were clearly on the same fiber.
[3] $p < 0.005$, t-test. C, control; E, experimental. Each value is derived from muscles of 2-4 embryos.

44% more neurons than controls on day 16 (table 5). Injection of BoTX on day 7 was not as effective in preventing cell death as injection on day 6 and heat-inactivated BoTX had no effect on motoneuron number.

Treatment with TeTX (6,000 LD_{50}) on day 6 had little or no effect on the number of neurons present on day 10, but led to a 25% decrease in cell number on day 16 (table 5). Unfortunately the lack of readily available pure tetanus toxin prevented a repetition of this experiment; therefore, the results should be viewed as preliminary.

3. Distribution of excess motoneurons

The excess motoneurons present on days 10 or 16 following curare, α-CTX or BoTX treatment were not confined to a few segments but rather were distributed over a large portion of the lumbar cord (figs. 10, 11). The composite graphs have the same shape and distribution as data for individual embryos. The composite graphs for cell counts of BoTX, α-CTX, and curare-treated embryos were very similar on day 10, and graphs for BoTX, and curare-treated animals were essentially the same on day 16. On day 16, the 50% hypothanasia seen after curare treatment was found to extend from about the middle of the second lumbar segment (spinal segment 23) to the caudal end of the lumbar cord (fig. 10). A slightly different distribution was seen on day 10 (fig. 11), in that the last three caudal segments showed somewhat less hypothanasia than at 16 days. The difference in motoneuron number in the caudal lumbar region in control embryos between days 10 and 16 may be accounted for if the normal cell death which occurred between

days 10 and 13 is largely restricted to these segments.

4. Histochemistry and endplate distribution

With the exception of the embryos that received 4.0 mg curare on days 6-9 there was no difficulty in obtaining AChE-staining of endplates in either wing or leg muscles of 16- to 18-day-old treated embryos (figs. 12-17). Moreover, in embryos prepared by the Toop technique for simultaneous staining of endplates (AChE) and their innervation, it appeared that virtually all of the AChE-stained endplates were in fact innervated (figs. 18-21).

Preliminary observations of the PLD muscle from curare-treated embryos (Oppenheim and Majors-Willard, '78) suggested that this muscle, which in the adult is focally (i.e., singly) innervated (Ginsborg, '60; Hess, '61), had considerably more AChE-stained endplates than normal. Measurements of the distances between endplates on teased muscle fibers have now confirmed this suggestion. The average distance between endplates in the control

Figs. 12, 13 Small fascicles of teased fibers from the ALD of control (fig. 12) and curare (fig. 13) treated (2.5 mg) embryos on day 18 (st. 44) stained for AChE. Both at $\times$ 100. Inset: Two adjacent fibers exhibiting multiple sites of AChE-reaction (arrows). $\times$ 36.

Figs. 14, 15 Large fascicles of teased muscle fibers from the PLD of control (fig. 14), and curare (fig. 15) treated (2.5 mg) embryos on day 19 (st. 44) stained for AChE. Both at $\times$ 100.

Figs. 16, 17 Fascicles of teased muscle fibers from the IFL of control (fig. 16) and curare (fig. 17) treated (2.5 mg) embryos on day 18 (st. 44) stained for AChE. Both at $\times$ 45. Inset: An isolated, single muscle fiber exhibiting two sites of AChE-reaction (arrows). $\times$ 100.

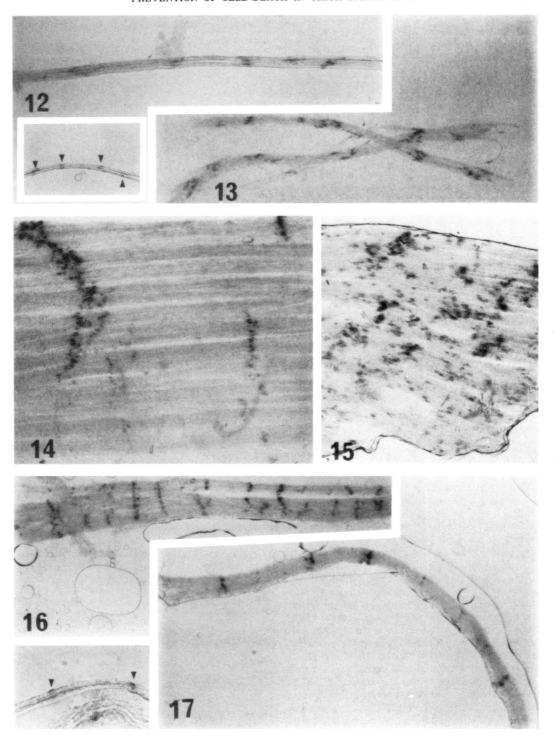

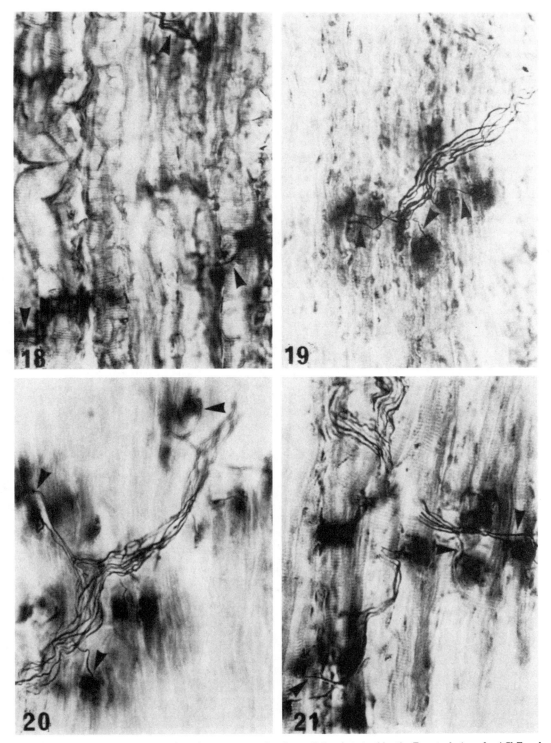

Figs. 18-21   Muscle from 18-day (st. 44) curare treated embryos (2.5 mg) stained by the Toop technique for AChE and innervation. Figure 18, ALD; figure 19, PLD; figure 20, IFL; figure 21, Gastroc. Note innervation of endplates (arrows). All at × 1,000.

PLD muscle was 471 μ at 17 days and 578 μ at 19 days, whereas the comparable values for the PLD of curare-treated animals were 123 μ and 220 μ, respectively (table 6).[5] Similar measurements on the normally multiply-innervated ALD muscle also showed a significant reduction in the distance between endplates of curare vs. control animals at both 17 and 19 days.[6] In contrast, the average distance between endplates in the ischioflexorius, a multiply-innervated thigh muscle, was unaltered in curare-treated embryos at 17 days and was slightly greater at 19 days. With one exception, in all treated muscles (ALD, PLD, IFL) the *variability* in the distances between endplates was reduced; no difference in variability was seen in the IFL at 19 days. Preliminary studies on the pectoralis, sartorius and gastrocnemius muscles suggest that the average distance between endplates is not altered following curare treatment. Despite the fact that the data for the IFL do not support the notion of increased multiple innervation of muscle in the curare-treated animals, this may be misleading. It was our impression that in many instances there were, in fact, additional endplates but that they were so closely spaced as to almost merge with one another, and for that reason defied accurate quantitation with our techniques. New histological techniques (Letinsky and DeCino, '78; Pestronk and Drachman, '78; Ashmore et al., '78) and ultrastructural studies may help resolve this problem.

5. *Biochemistry*

The overall size of embryos was decreased following the various drug treatments. It has also been shown that treatment with curare or BoTX leads to a considerable replacement of muscle with adipose tissue (Drachman, '68; Oppenheim et al., '78b). For these reasons, the most accurate and meaningful way of expressing AChE activity would be per milligram protein rather than per gram muscle or per muscle.

Concentrations of curare which maintained a decrease in motility from days 6-16 produced no significant change in the specific activity of AChE (table 7) although the *total* amount of AChE activity was decreased due to a decrease in muscle size.[7] Treatment with curare (1 mg) or α-CTX daily (days 6-9) resulted in a large decrease in the specific activity of AChE on day 16 (37% and 34%, respectively). Injections of BoTX or TeTX on day 6 also produced

TABLE 7

Muscle acetylcholinesterase activity for 16-day embryos

Treatment	N	AChE activity, (μmoles acetyl-β-methyl-choline hydrolyzed /mg protein/hr)	Percent change
Control (for curare and α-CTX)	3	2.01 ± 0.18	—
Curare (CAM d 6-9)			
1.1 mg	3	1.27 ± 0.17	-36.8
2.5 mg	3	2.07 ± 0.20	$+3.0$
4.0 mg	3	1.85 ± 0.35	-8.0
5.5 mg	2	2.12 ± 0.73	$+5.5$
α-CTX (CAM d 6-9) [1]	3	1.33 ± 0.27	-33.8
Control (for BoTX and TeTX)	3	1.52 ± 0.15	—
BoTX (1,200 LD$_{50}$ i.m. d 6)	3	1.06 ± 0.08	-30.3
TeTX (6,000 LD$_{50}$ i.m. d 6)	5	1.11 ± 0.27	-27.0

[1] 100 μg d 6; 85 μg d 7, 8; 50 μg d 9. Mean $\pm$ S.D.

a large decrease in the specific activity of AChE on day 16 (30% and 27%, respectively).

DISCUSSION

One of the primary goals of this study was to determine if altering normal physiological function at the neuromuscular junction would have any effect on motoneuron cell death. Motility in the chick embryo results from a direct nerve-muscle interaction (neurogenic) rather than from non-innervated muscle contractions (myogenic) (Hamburger, '63; Alconero, '65; Oppenheim, '74). Because of its neurogenic origin, an efficient means of interfering with embryonic activity would be to alter the nerve-muscle interaction.

Botulinum toxin blocks the release of acetylcholine (ACh) from motoneuron boutons (reviews by Drachman, '71; Simpson, '71),

[5] Although most fibers in the control PLD muscle at these stages were singly innervated there were also many that had two (or more) regions that stained intensely for AChE and it was these fibers that were used for measurements of endplate distance. More of these multiply innervated fibers were seen at 17 than at 19 days and unpublished observations on hatchlings indicate that they become increasingly rare (also see Hess, '70).

[6] It is important to make a distinction between multiple innervation which is spatially distributed over the muscle fiber vs. multiple innervation which is restricted to the endplate region. In the present paper, unless stated otherwise, we will always use *multiple innervation* (or hyperinnervation) to refer to the former and *polyneuronal innervation* for the latter.

[7] Choline acetyltransferase (ChAc) activity in the lumbar spinal cord is elevated by 60-70% in 11-day embryos receiving 2.5 mg curare on days 6-9 (Maderdrut and Oppenheim, in preparation), thereby mimicking the *cellular* hypothanasia produced by such treatment. Since ChAc activity per lumbar spinal cord increased approximately 6-fold between day 6 and day 11 these data also provide evidence that the excess neurons have differentiated normally.

whereas curare and the various snake toxins directly block the nicotinic receptors.[8] Therefore, all drugs used in this study decrease the amount of ACh interacting with receptors, resulting in a decrease of muscle contraction and motility. Motility levels are, therefore, a rough index of the drug's ability to interfere with normal neuromuscular function.

Innervation of the chick hindlimb begins on day 4.5 (Oppenheim and Heaton, '75; Hamburger, '75; Landmesser, '78) and innervation of the forelimb begins at least as early as day 8 (Atsumi, '77). Thus, initiating treatment with neuromuscular blocking agents on days 4-9 coincides with the onset of innervation as well as with the onset of cell death in the brachial (Oppenheim and Majors-Willard, '78) and lumbar (Hamburger, '75; Chu-Wang and Oppenheim, '78a) spinal cord of the chick.

The results of our study indicate that by decreasing normal function at the neuromuscular junction during the period of motoneuron cell death, a large number of neurons which would normally die are maintained. The decreased cell death occurs in both the brachial and lumbar spinal cord and the anterior and posterior latissimus dorsi muscles show an increased number of endplates. The additional motoneurons are viable as long as motility levels remain depressed; however, once activity returns to control levels, excess neurons are lost.

(1) Permanent hypothanasia

The term hypothanasia has been introduced by Hollyday and Hamburger ('76) as a more accurate and precise term than hyperplasia for the increase in motoneuron survival following peripheral enlargement. Hypothanasia is also more appropriate for describing the excess motoneurons we observe because they are the result of a decrease in cell death as opposed to increased neuronal production. Autoradiographic data have shown that motoneuron proliferation in the lumbar LMC occurs from stages 17-24 (Hollyday and Hamburger, '77), whereas the earliest stage at which embryos were treated in the present study was stage 25 (4.5 days of incubation).

Treatment with various neuromuscular blocking agents between days 6-9 decreased the extent of natural cell death and resulted in the survival of 4-5,000 excess motoneurons on day 10. By day 16, BoTX injected embryos as well as the 2.5- and 4-mg curare animals

still maintained the additional motoneurons, whereas the α-CTX and α-BTX treated embryos had considerably fewer cells than control 16-day embryos. At the present, it cannot be conclusively shown that the results with curare and BoTX represent a permanent hypothanasia because no embryos survive past day 20 as a result of paralysis of respiratory muscles. However, on days 18 and 20, 15-17,000 cells were still present in embryos in the α-CTX + curare and the 2.5-mg curare groups; so as long as the embryos survived they maintained most of the additional motoneurons. Motility levels were approaching control levels in the 2.5-mg curare groups between days 18-20, yet cell number remained constant. This suggests that perhaps by day 18 the cells had bypassed a critical period in which the hypothanasia is maintained by a decreased neuromuscular function.

Embryos in which treatment with neuromuscular blocking agents was begun on day 4 maintained considerably more neurons on days 8 and 10 than did those embryos in which treatment was begun on day 6; therefore, it would seem possible to prevent cell death to an even greater extent and to maintain more cells up until days 19 or 20 by beginning drug treatment on day 4. Laing and Prestige ('78) using the same preparations have recently reported that α-BTX treatment every other day from days 4 to 18 prevents substantial cell death (also see Creazzo and Sohal, '78; Olek and Edwards, '78).

Thus far, the easiest and most reproducible procedure for inducing and maintaining a high level of hypothanasia is the daily administration of 2.5 mg of curare onto the CAM from days 6-9 (or from days 4-9). This concentration is sufficient to maintain a motility deficit for most of the remainder of the incubation period but is not so large that muscular atrophy becomes the limiting factor in the maintenance of excess neurons.

In the case of the brachial motoneurons, in which cell death begins on day 8 and continues to hatching, we have also shown that curare

---

[8] It has recently been reported that curare depolarizes embryonic rat muscle (similar to the effects of depolarizing blocking agents in the adult), whereas by three to five days postnatally this effect disappears (Ziskind and Dennis, '78). It is not known whether curare also depolarizes chick muscle. Chronic treatment (days 6-9) with the depolarizing blocker decamethonium does, however, prevent cell death to the same extent as curare (Oppenheim and Maderdrut, in preparation). Since BoTX prevents cell death but does not depolarize muscle, however, it is unlikely that our results are due solely to the putative depolarizing effects of curare on embryonic muscle.

treatment on days 6-9, which induces a long-lasting motility deficit beyond day 9, prevents substantial cell death. And as might be expected in this system, an increased prevention of cell death occurs even beyond day 16; on days 18-20 there were about 60% more cells compared to controls, whereas on days 15-16 there were only 45% more cells than control.

An increase in motor and sensory neurons can be obtained by enlarging the peripheral area of innervation to which the neuronal population projects (Hamburger and Levi-Montalcini, '49; Jacobson, '78; Hollyday and Hamburger, '76); however, in no case had it been shown that the normal target area was capable of maintaining additional neurons (but see Burstein et al., '77). Hollyday and Hamburger ('76) found that transplantation of an additional limb onto the body wall of a chick embryo could produce as much as 27.5% hypothanasia in a few individual cases, although the average hypothanasia was only approximately 15%. Because the additional or supernumerary limb was rostral to the normal limb, it was less available to the motoneurons in the more caudal lumbar segments. This probably reduced the extent of hypothanasia below that which might have been expected by doubling the size of the periphery.

What was of great interest in our findings was that a single limb was capable of maintaining up to 50% more cells than controls and occasionally individual embryos showed an even greater increase in motoneurons. Therefore, it seems that virtually all of the motoneurons which normally degenerate are capable of surviving, and that most, if not all, motoneurons in the LMC which undergo normal cell death can be "spared" by altering conditions at the neuromuscular junction.

(2) Mechanisms

Although one possible mechanism that could decrease the extent of cell death would be an increase in the number of available targets (e.g., by increasing the number of muscle fibers) in fact we have found that the various drug and toxin treatments used here resulted in a *decreased* muscle mass as indicated by the weights of shank muscles on days 10, 13, 16 and 18. This would imply that if an increase in target number exists, then it may result from decreasing the area of the muscle membrane "controlled" by a single axon, or that additional axons can be maintained at the same endplate. An increase in the number of muscle fibers while maintaining a constant target size would seemingly have to result in an increase in muscle weight.

Another possible explanation of our findings is that the prevention of cell death results from the direct action of the various drugs on the motoneurons in the spinal cord rather than at the neuromuscular junction. The fact that the induced cell death following limb-bud removal was not prevented by curare treatment on days 6-9 makes this rather unlikely.

It is also conceivable that treatment with neuromuscular blocking agents causes an arrest in differentiation of motoneurons such that the cells are unable to advance to some hypothetical stage necessary for the manifestation of cell death. We are presently carrying out morphometric studies on several aspects of motoneuron differentiation in α-CTX and curare-treated embryos and have not seen any signs of arrested differentiation (also see footnote 7). Consequently we consider it unlikely that arrested neuronal differentiation, per se, can explain our findings.

The most important basic finding common to all embryos showing an increase in motoneuron survival on days 10 or 16 was that at the time hypothanasia was present, a decrease in activity had existed since day 6 (or in a few cases since day 4). That is, if motility was decreased during the period when a large portion of the motoneurons normally degenerate, then a large excess of neurons survived and were viable as long as muscular activity remained sufficiently depressed. Although a small continuous decrease in activity (20-40%) was not as effective in increasing motoneuron survival as a total cessation of activity, there was no clear graded increase in survival with decreasing activity; therefore, it seemed that muscle (or nerve) alterations resulted once muscle activity decreased below a certain level and was not altered with further decreases in activity. It is possible that some type of all-or-none phenomenon is triggered once the decrease in activity has fallen below a threshold.

Exactly what physiological modifications may account for this phenomenon are only speculative; however, a very interesting mechanism for determining the innervation pattern of muscle has recently been postulated (Gordon et al., '74, '75; Gordon and Vrbová, '75) and the findings partially confirmed (Oppenheim et al., '78b). These studies showed that by treating chick embryos with curare during the period of innervation of the PLD and ALD, the distribution (and density) of endplates as determined by cholinesterase staining was altered. Following curare treatment, the distance between successive endplates was less for muscles with multiple innervation, while focally innervated muscles showed areas of multiple innervation. From these results, Gordon and her colleagues have concluded that the distribution of endplates on a muscle fiber is dependent on the area of the muscle membrane which becomes "desensitized" by ACh at the time of initial innervation.

Our findings could be explained using this model. The decreased ACh interacting with receptors following curare, BoTX or α-CTX treatment would decrease the extent of membrane depolarization and allow muscles with multiple innervation to possibly accept additional synapses and/or it may allow muscles which under normal conditions are focally innervated to accept additional innervation. This would imply that the primary factor in determining whether a motoneuron survives or degenerates is its ability to form a synapse with a muscle fiber. Therefore, a competition for a limited number of targets would seem to be one of the critical determining factors in naturally occurring neuronal cell death. Our present findings that the density of neuromuscular endplates in the ALD and PLD muscles on days 17 and 19 is increased following curare treatment—and that these additional endplates are innervated—is consistent with such an interpretation. We have no explanation, however, for the fact that the IFL muscle does not exhibit additional multiple innervation since this muscle is innervated by spinal segments 25 and 26 both of which show a marked response (i.e., hypothanasia) to curare treatment on days 6-9. It is conceivable that the excess motoneurons in this case may "hyperinnervate" existing endplates (i.e., polyneuronal innervation) rather than forming additional synapses. It is also of interest, however, that the amount of variance in endplate distance was about 30% less in the 17-day curare-treated IFL muscle, indicating a greater regularity in endplate distribution compared to control. The same was seen in the PLD and to a lesser extent in the ALD of curare-treated animals. Although we assume that the hyperinnervation observed in the ALD and PLD of curare-treated embryos results from innerva-

tion by additional neurons, as opposed to axonal sprouting, we cannot decide between these alternatives on the basis of the available data.

Our present findings also do not allow us to determine whether during normal development muscle fibers are transiently hyperinnervated or whether the hyperinnervation observed here is wholly an outcome of the prevention of cell death. Kikuchi and Ashmore ('76) have reported that the M. complexus or hatching muscle of the chick, which is focally innervated in the adult, is multiply innervated at early embryonic stages.

The existence of high levels of extrajunctional ACh receptors is closely correlated with the ability of adult muscle to accept additional innervation (Jansen et al., '73; Brockes et al., '75). Thus, the presence of extrajunctional ACh receptors may "allow" innervation by more than one axon, or at least may be characteristic of a particular state of the muscle fiber (e.g., inactive) which allows multiple innervation. The normal decrease in extrajunctional ACh receptors of the chick PLD that follows innervation can be prevented by muscular paralysis with curare (Burden, '77a). Therefore, the neuro-muscular blockade in our study probably results in the maintenance of extrajunctional receptors, which in the adult muscle is highly characteristic of a state which can accept additional innervation. Adult muscles exposed to α-CTX are also capable of accepting additional "foreign" innervation (Duchen et al., '75). However, Robbins et al. ('77) have reported that neonatal rat muscle with high levels of extrajunctional ACh receptors does not accept additional innervation.

Direct stimulation of denervated muscle can prevent or reverse the development of increased extrajunctional sensitivity to ACh (Lømo and Rosenthal, '72; Drachman and Witzke, '72; Jones and Vrbová, '74; Purves and Sakmann, '74), and the ability of a foreign nerve to innervate a denervated muscle can also be blocked by direct electrical stimulation (Jansen et al., '73, '75). Neuromuscular activity is involved in the normal reduction of polyneuronal innervation in developing rat and chick muscle (Benoit and Changeux, '78; O'Brien et al., '78; Srihari and Vrbová, '78). Unlike cell death, however, the elimination of polyneuronal innervation does not involve the degeneration of motoneurons or axonal branches. The excess terminals are apparently resorbed or retracted into the parent axon (Korneliussen and Jansen, '76). Nevertheless, in both embryonic cell death and the elimination of polyneuronal innervation, the level of muscle activity seems of critical importance in determining the physiological state of the muscle with regard to the ability to accept and maintain additional innervation.

Recent findings by Kuffler et al. ('77) indicate that the elimination of synapses in rat muscle following experimental hyperinnervation is directly related to the distance between competing synapses. In cases where two synapses from different foreign nerves are both close to one another on a muscle fiber, one synapse is eliminated; similar synapses located farther apart, however, are retained. Although the synapses that are eliminated in this case also do not involve degeneration of the entire motor unit, the underlying competitive mechanism may nevertheless be similar to that observed during natural cell death and to the transient hypothanasia we observed. If our proposal regarding the role of activity in cell death and muscle innervation is correct, it would be expected that increased stimulation of the muscle should lead to increased cell death and to an enhanced rate of loss of polyneuronal innervation.

(3) Treatments failing to prevent cell death

There are two treatment groups in the present experiments which showed little or no hypothanasia following pharmacological immobilization. Since we have argued that inactivity is a critical factor in the prevention of cell death it is imperative that we examine these groups and attempt to explain the negative results.

A single injection of α-CTX on day 6 had no significant effect on the number of motoneurons present on day 10. The injection produced either a total or partial cessation of activity during the period between days 6 and 8, whereas from days 8.5 to 10 the motility was comparable to controls. This suggests that either the critical period for preventing cell death occurs after day 8, or once activity returns to normal levels on day 8.5, redundant synapses are lost, leading to a degeneration of excess neurons. In that α-CTX treatment on days 6 and 7, or curare treatment on days 4-6, leads to an increased number of motoneurons on day 8, the latter alternative seems correct.

BoTX injection on day 7 resulted in only a small decrease (8%) in cell death on day 10. Motility recordings from animals injected on day 6 indicated that it was at least 18 to 24 hours before BoTX began affecting motility levels. Therefore, in those embryos injected on day 7 only those neurons which were still viable and had axons in the periphery after day 8 would be capable of synapsing with any additional targets made available by BoTX treatment. It is known that a large number of neurons undergo degeneration between days 7 and 8 (Hamburger, '75; Chu-Wang and Oppenheim, '78a), so it would be expected that less hypothanasia would occur following BoTX injection on day 7.

(4) Transient hypothanasia

Treatments which produced an increase in motoneuron number on day 10 but failed to maintain these excess neurons also produced a decrease in activity up until day 10, after which levels subsequently returned to normal. The close association between the loss of excess neurons and the return to normal activity levels strongly suggests that once activity levels returned to a certain level, redundant synapses were lost and the additional neurons degenerated. The correlation between muscle activity and excess motoneuron survival is quite evident in the group of embryos receiving 1 mg of curare daily from days 6-9. On day 10, the LMCs of these embryos contained approximately 17,000 motoneurons and motility was 60% of control levels. On day 16 less than 13,000 motoneurons were present in each LMC (compared to 11,500 in controls) and motility levels were comparable to controls. Upon closer examination of cell counts versus motility on day 16, it was evident that the one embryo which had a decreased motility also contained more motoneurons than controls (14,500), whereas the other two embryos which had motility levels equal to or slightly greater than controls contained approximately the same number of neurons as controls (12,320 and 11,570) (also see section 2 of DISCUSSION).

α-CTX or α-BTX treatment daily from days 6-9 resulted in approximately 18,500 motoneurons present in each LMC on day 10, but only 6-8,000 of these survived until days 16-18. Essentially no motility was present in these embryos between days 6 and 10. Once α-CTX treatment was discontinued, it might be expected that motility would return to normal levels because of the reasonably fast receptor turnover in embryonic chick muscle ($t\frac{1}{2}$ = 30 hours; Burden, '77a,b). In fact, by day 13 motility levels were approaching that of controls and by day 16 there were no differences between controls and α-CTX and α-BTX treated embryos.

If our proposed hypothesis is correct, then it would be expected that once motility approached control levels, the excess motoneurons would degenerate, and by day 16 approximately 11,500 neurons would be present in each LMC. Not only was there a degeneration of the excess neurons, as expected, but an additional 3-4,000 motoneurons per LMC also degenerated. Although these embryos were somewhat smaller than controls, they did not show an inordinate amount of atrophy as did some of the embryos receiving high concentrations of curare. Hence, at the moment, it is not clear why cell number falls below control values. Our results from the combined α-CTX + curare group, however, do show that the loss of neurons to below control levels following α-CTX or α-BTX on days 6-9 can be largely prevented and the hypothanasia present on day 10 maintained by continued treatment with curare on days 10-13.

The return of motility to control levels seems to lead to a loss of excess neurons; however, we do not mean to imply that the activity levels must exactly reach control levels before redundant synapses begin to be lost. The level of activity at which excess neurons are lost is probably influenced by a number of factors, including the length and extent of the motility deficit as well as how quickly the increase in motility occurs. The pattern of muscle activity may also be an important factor (Lømo, '76).

In summary, a possible model for explaining both the permanent and transient hypothanasia seen following neuromuscular blockade would be that during early synapse formation an axon contacts a myotube and begins releasing small amounts of ACh which leads to a partial depolarization of the muscle membrane. Prior to and during this critical period of early membrane depolarization, more than one synapse could be maintained by each myotube. However, once the *frequency* and *extent* of membrane depolarization reached a certain level, the membrane properties would be altered such that only one synapse could be supported, and additional contacts would be lost. Following neuromuscular blockade, the amount of ACh interacting with receptors

would decrease considerably, thereby decreasing membrane depolarization. This would result in the critical period being maintained and an increase in motoneuron survival. For muscle fibers which are normally multiply-innervated, similar events could also occur. In the adult muscle, a similar membrane state would exist following denervation or neuromuscular blockade and the muscle fiber would be capable of accepting foreign innervation. In both the developing and adult muscle, neuromuscular blockade would decrease the size of a "target," and therefore increase the number of "targets."

If the neuromuscular blocking agents are removed from the system, then membrane depolarization would increase and excess synapses would be lost. If a postsynaptic supersensitivity develops, then a single neuromuscular synapse in a multiply-innervated muscle fiber may produce depolarization of the entire fiber with a resulting loss of synapses which under normal conditions would be maintained. This could account for the later drop in cell number below control levels in the embryos treated with α-CTX on days 6-9.

ACKNOWLEDGMENTS

This investigation was supported by NSF Grant BNS 77 20452 and by the North Carolina Division of Mental Health Research. We acknowledge the competent technical assistance of C. Willard and I-W. Chu-Wang and the careful clerical help of R. Daniels. J. L. Maderdrut suggested the limb-bud removal experiment and provided many other useful suggestions during the course of this study.

LITERATURE CITED

Alconero, B. B. 1965 The nature of the earliest spontaneous activity of the chick embryo. J. Embryol. Exp. Morph., *13:* 255-266.

Ashmore, C. R., T. Kikuchi and L. Doerr 1978 Some observations on the innervation patterns of different fiber types of chick muscle. Exp. Neurol., *58:* 272-284.

Atsumi, S. 1977 Development of neuromuscular junctions of fast and slow muscles in the chick embryo: a light and electron microscope study. J. Neurocytol., *6:* 691-709.

Benoit, P., and J.-P. Changeux 1978 Consequences of blocking the nerve with a local anesthetic on the evolution of multiinnervation of the regenerating neuromuscular junction of the rat. Brain Res., *149:* 89-96.

Brockes, J. P., D. K. Berg and Z. W. Hall 1975 The biochemical properties and regulation of acetylcholine receptors in normal and denervated muscle. In: Cold Spring Harbor Symposium on Quantitative Biology. The Synapse. Vol. *40:* 253-262.

Burden, S. 1977a Development of the neuromuscular junction in the chick embryo: the number, distribution, and stability of acetylcholine receptors. Dev. Biol., *57:* 317-329.

———— 1977b Acetylcholine receptors at the neuromuscular junction: Developmental change in receptor turnover. Dev. Biol., *61:* 79-85.

Burstein, L., G. Pilar and L. Landmesser 1977 Competitive interactions between developing ciliary ganglion cells. Neurosci. Abst., *3:* 422.

Changeux, J.-P., and A. Danchin 1976 Selective stabilization in developing synapses as a mechanism for the specification of neuronal networks. Nature, *264:* 705-712.

Chu-Wang, I-W., and R. W. Oppenheim 1978a Cell death of motoneurons in the chick embryo spinal cord. I. A light and electron microscopic study of naturally occurring and induced cell loss during development. J. Comp. Neur., *177:* 33-58.

———— 1978b Cell death of motoneurons in the chick embryo spinal cord. II. A quantitative and qualitative analysis of degeneration in the ventral root, including evidence for axon outgrowth and limb innervation prior to cell death. J. Comp. Neur., *177:* 59-86.

Cowan, W. M. 1973 Neuronal death as a regulative mechanism in the control of cell number in the nervous system. In: Development and Aging in the Nervous System. M. Rockstein, ed. Academic Press, New York, pp. 19-41.

Creazzo, T. L., and G. S. Sohal 1978 Effects of alpha and beta bungarotoxin on the development of trochlear nucleus and superior oblique muscle. Neurosci. Abst., *4:* 110.

Drachman, D. B. 1968 The role of acetylcholine as a trophic neuromuscular transmitter. In: Growth of the Nervous System. G. E. W. Wolstenholme and M. O'Connor, eds. Little, Brown, Boston, pp. 251-273.

———— 1971 Botulinum toxin as a tool for research in the nervous system. In: Neuropoisons: Their Pathophysiological Actions. L. L. Simpson, ed. Plenum Press, New York, pp. 325-347.

Drachman, D. B., and F. Witzke 1972 Trophic regulation of acetylcholine sensitivity of muscle: effect of electrical stimulation. Science, *176:* 514-516.

Duchen, L. W., W. Heilbron and D. A. Tonge 1975 Functional denervation of skeletal muscle in the mouse after the local injection of a postsynaptic blocking fraction of *Naja siamensis* venom. J. Physiol., *250:* 26-27P.

El-Badawi, A., and E. A. Schenk 1967 Histochemical methods for separate, consecutive and simultaneous demonstration of acetylcholinesterase and norepinephrine in cryostat sections. J. Histochem. Cytochem., *15:* 580-583.

Giacobini, G., G. Filogamo, M. Weber, P. Boquet and J. P. Changeux 1973 Effects of a snake α-neurotoxin on the development of innervated skeletal muscles in chick embryo. Proc. Nat. Acad. Sci. (U.S.A.), *70:* 1708-1712.

Ginsborg, B. 1960 Spontaneous activity in muscle fibres of the chick. J. Physiol., *150:* 707-717.

Gordon, T., and G. Vrbová 1975 Changes in chemosensitivity of developing chick muscle fibres in relation to endplate formation. Pflügers Arch., *360:* 349-364.

Gordon, T., R. Perry, A. R. Tuffery and G. Vrbová 1974 Possible mechanisms determining synapse formation in developing skeletal muscles of the chick. Cell Tiss. Res., *155:* 13-25.

Gordon, T., A. R. Tuffery and G. Vrbová 1975 A possible mechanism determining the pattern of innervation of skeletal muscle fibers. In: Recent Advances in Myology. W. G. Bradley, D. Gardner-Medwin and J. N. Walton, eds. Elsevier, New York, pp. 22-26.

Hamburger, V. 1958 Regression versus peripheral control of differentiation in motor hypoplasia. Am. J. Anat., *102:* 365-410.

———— 1963 Some aspects of the embryology of behavior. Quart. Rev. Biol., *38:* 243-365.

———— 1975 Cell death in the development of the lateral motor column of the chick embryo. J. Comp. Neur., *160:* 535-546.

Hamburger, V., and H. L. Hamilton 1951 A series of normal stages in the development of the chick embryo. J. Morph., *88:* 49-92.

Hamburger, V., and R. Levi-Montalcini 1949 Proliferation, differentiation and degeneration in the spinal ganglia of the chick embryo under normal and experimental conditions. J. Exp. Zool., *111:* 457-501.

Hess, A. 1961 Structural differences of fast and slow extrafusal muscle fibres and their nerve endings in chickens. J. Physiol., *157:* 221-231.

———— 1970 Vertebrate slow muscle fibers. Physiol. Rev., *50:* 40-62.

Hollyday, M., and V. Hamburger 1976 Reduction of the naturally occurring motoneuron loss by enlargement of the periphery. J. Comp. Neur., *170:* 311-320.

———— 1977 An autoradiographic study of the formation of the lateral motor column in the chick embryo. Brain Res., *132:* 197-208.

Jacobson, M. 1978 Developmental Neurobiology. Second ed. Plenum Press, New York.

Jansen, J. K. S., T. Lømo, K. Nicolaysen and R. H. Westgaard 1973 Hyperinnervation of skeletal muscle fibers: Dependence on muscle activity. Science, *181:* 559-561.

Jansen, J. K. S., D. C. van Essen and M. C. Brown 1975 Formation and elimination of synapses in skeletal muscles of rat. In: Cold Spring Harbor Symposium on Quantitative Biology. The Synapse. Vol. *40:* 425-434.

Jones, R., and G. Vrbová 1974 Two factors responsible for the development of denervation hypersensitivity. J. Physiol., *236:* 517-538.

Kikuchi, T., and C. R. Ashmore 1976 Developmental aspects of the innervation of skeletal muscle fibers in the chick embryo. Cell Tiss. Res., *171:* 233-251.

Konigsmark, B. W. 1970 Methods for the counting of neurons. In: Contemporary Research Methods in Neuroanatomy. W. J. H. Nauta and S. O. E. Ebbesson, eds. Springer-Verlag, New York, pp. 315-340.

Korneliussen, A., and J. K. S. Jansen 1976 Morphological aspects of the elimination of polyneuronal innervation of skeletal muscle fibres in newborn rats. J. Neurocytol., *5:* 591-604.

Kuffler, S., W. Thompson and J. K. S. Jansen 1977 The elimination of synapses in multiply-innervated skeletal muscle fibres of the rat: Dependence on distance between end-plates. Brain Res., *138:* 353-358.

Laing, N. G., and M. C. Prestige 1978 Prevention of spontaneous motoneurone death in chick embryos. J. Physiol., *282:* 33-34P.

Landmesser, L. 1978 The distribution of motoneurons supplying chick hind limb muscles. J. Physiol., *284:* 371-389.

Landmesser, L., and D. Morris 1975 The development of functional innervation in the hindlimb of the chick embryo. J. Physiol., *249:* 301-326.

Letinsky, M. S., and P. A. DeCino 1978 Structural organization of the developing amphibian neuromuscular junction. Neurosci. Abst., *4:* 371.

Lømo, T. 1976 The role of activity in the control of membrane and contractile properties of skeletal muscle. In: Motor Innervation of Muscle. S. Thesleff, ed. Academic Press, New York, pp. 289-321.

Lømo, T., and J. Rosenthal 1972 Control of ACh sensitivity by muscle activity in the rat. J. Physiol., *221:* 493-513.

Lowry, O. H., N. H. Rosenbrough, A. L. Farr and R. J. Randall 1951 Protein measurement with Folin phenol reagent. J. Biol. Chem., *193:* 265-275.

O'Brien, R. A. D., A. J. Ostberg and G. Vrbová 1978 Observations on the elimination of polyneuronal innervation in developing mammalian skeletal muscle. J. Physiol., *282:* 517-582.

Olek, A. J., and C. Edwards 1978 Effect of alpha and beta bungarotoxin on the naturally occurring motoneuron loss in *Xenopus* larvae. Neurosci. Abst., *4:* 122.

Oppenheim, R. W. 1974 The ontogeny of behavior in the chick embryo. In: Advances in the Study of Behavior. D. S. Lehrman, J. S. Rosenblatt, R. A. Hinde and E. Shaw, eds. Academic Press, New York, pp. 133-171.

Oppenheim, R. W., and I-W. Chu-Wang 1977 Spontaneous cell death of motoneurons following peripheral innervation in the chick embryo. Brain Res., *125:* 154-160.

Oppenheim, R. W., I-W. Chu-Wang and J. L. Maderdrut 1978a Cell death of motoneurons in the chick embryo spinal cord. III. The differentiation of motoneurons prior to their induced degeneration following limb-bud removal. J. Comp. Neur., *177:* 87-112.

Oppenheim, R. W., R. Pittman, M. Gray and J. L. Maderdrut 1978b Embryonic behavior, hatching and neuromuscular development in the chick following a transient reduction of spontaneous motility and sensory input by neuromuscular blocking agents. J. Comp. Neur., *179:* 619-640.

Oppenheim, R. W., and M. B. Heaton 1975 The retrograde transport of horseradish peroxidase from the developing limb of the chick embryo. Brain Res., *98:* 291-302.

Oppenheim, R. W., H. L. Levin and M. S. Harth 1973 An investigation of various egg-opening techniques for use in avian behavioral embryology. Dev. Psychobiol., *6:* 53-68.

Oppenheim, R. W., and C. Majors-Willard 1978 Neuronal cell death in the brachial spinal cord of the chick is unre-lated to the loss of polyneuronal innervation in wing muscle. Brain Res., *154:* 148-152.

Pestronk, A., and D. B. Drachman 1978 A new stain for quantitative measurement of sprouting at neuromuscular junctions. Muscle and Nerve, *1:* 70-74.

Pittman, R., and R. W. Oppenheim 1978 Neuromuscular blockade increases motoneurone survival during normal cell death in the chick embryo. Nature, *271:* 364-366.

Potter, L. T. 1967 A radiometric microassay for acetylcholinesterase. J. Pharm. exp. Ther., *156:* 500-506.

Prestige, M. C. 1970 Differentiation, degeneration, and the role of the periphery: quantitative considerations. In: The Neurosciences, Second Study Program. F. O. Schmitt, ed. Rockefeller University, New York, pp. 73-82.

Purves, D., and B. Sakmann 1974 The effect of contractile activity on fibrillation and extrajunctional acetylcholine sensitivity in rat muscle maintained in organ culture. J. Physiol., *237:* 57-82.

Robbins, N., J. Antosiak, R. Gerding and O. D. Uchitel 1977 Nonacceptance of innervation by innervated neonatal muscle. Dev. Biol., *61:* 166-176.

Simpson, L. L. 1971 The neuroparalytic and hemiagglutinating activities of botulinum toxin. In: Neuropoisons: Their Pathophysiological Actions. L. L. Simpson, ed. Plenum Press, New York, pp. 303-323.

Srihari, T., and G. Vrbová 1978 The role of muscle activity in the differentiation of neuromuscular junction in slow and fast chick muscles. J. Neurocytol., *7:* 529-540.

Toop, J. 1976 A rapid method for demonstrating skeletal muscle innervation in frozen sections. Stain Technol., *51:* 1-6.

Wenger, B. S. 1968 Construction and use of the vibrating needle for embryonic operations. Bioscience, *18:* 226-228.

Ziskind, L., and M. L. Dennis 1978 Depolarizing effect of curare on embryonic rat muscles. Nature, *276:* 622-623.

Section 6
Trophic Agents: Nerve Growth Factor

Levi-Montalcini, R. 1975. NGF: An uncharted route. In *The neurosciences, paths of discovery* (ed. F.G. Worden, J.P. Swazey, and G. Adelman), pp. 245–265. MIT Press, Cambridge, Massachusetts.

Gorin, P.D. and E.M. Johnson. 1979. Experimental autoimmune model of nerve growth factor deprivation: Effects on developing peripheral sympathetic and sensory neurons. *Proc. Natl. Acad. Sci.* 76: 5382–5386.

Gundersen, R.W. and J.N. Barrett. 1979. Neuronal chemotaxis: Chick dorsal-root axons turn toward high concentrations of nerve growth factor. *Science* 206: 1079–1080.

Johnson, E.M., Jr., R.Y. Andres, and R.A. Bradshaw. 1978. Characterization of the retrograde transport of nerve growth factor (NGF) using high specific activity [125I]NGF. *Brain Res.* 150: 319–331.

Ebendal, T., L. Olson, Å. Seiger, and K.-O. Hedlund. 1980. Nerve growth factors in the rat iris. *Nature* 286: 25–28.

The effects of early end-organ removal, discussed in Section 5, make plain that many types of neurons must contact suitable targets in order to survive. One way in which target organs could exert this influence is by secreting a survival or maintenance factor. There is now considerable evidence that the well-characterized protein called nerve growth factor (NGF) is such an agent. The discovery and early investigation of NGF was largely the work of Levi-Montalcini, Hamburger, and Cohen; the story makes fascinating reading and a first-hand account is reprinted here (**Levi-Montalcini 1975**).

In general, there are three important experimental results that indicate the biological function of NGF: (1) Injection of NGF into chick embryos results in a remarkable hypertrophy and hyperplasia of neurons in sympathetic and sensory ganglia (Levi-Montalcini and Hamburger 1951; Levi-Montalcini and Cohen 1956); (2) injection of an antiserum to NGF destroys most of the cells in sympathetic and sensory ganglia (Levi-Montalcini and Booker 1960; **Gorin** and **Johnson 1979**); and (3) NGF is essential for the survival and maintenance of sympathetic and some sensory neurons in dissociated cell culture (Levi-Montalcini and Angeletti 1963). Thus, NGF acts directly on particular classes of neurons that require it for survival during normal development.

In addition to being required for survival, NGF stimulates neuronal growth and differentiation; i.e., increasing the NGF concentration increases the amount of protein produced by each neuron and also the amount of neurotransmitter produced per unit of protein (see, for example, Chun and Patterson 1977). The ability of NGF to stimulate neuronal differentiation is also important in another context. There appears to be an interplay of NGF with corticosteroid hormones in controlling developmental decisions in the

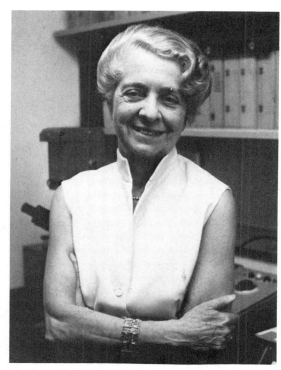

Rita Levi-Montalcini, who with Viktor Hamburger discovered nerve growth factor. Her studies of this agent for more than three decades, with many collaborators, established the nature of this molecule and its biological importance.

adrenal medulla and in sympathetic ganglia. Several studies have shown that the relative balance of neuronal and chromaffin cell features can be influenced by NGF and corticosteroids (Unsicker et al. 1978; Aloe and Levi-Montalcini 1979; Doupe and Patterson 1981).

If NGF is a survival factor for which neurons compete, it must be demonstrated that appropriate target tissues produce it and that it exerts effects on growing neurites. What is the evidence on these points? First, NGF can act locally on growing neurites both in vitro (Campenot 1977; Letourneau 1978; **Gundersen** and **Barrett 1979**, 1980); and in vivo (Menesini-Chen et al. 1978) (see also Section 4). Second, cutting the axons of immature sympathetic neurons results in neuronal death unless NGF is given exogenously (Hendry 1975; Hendry and Campbell 1976). This suggests that NGF is normally obtained peripherally. Third, NGF presented to axon terminals within the target tissue is retrogradely transported to the cell bodies (Stockel et al. 1975; **Johnson, Andres,** and **Bradshaw 1978**). Di-

rect evidence that NGF is normally produced by target organs has been difficult to obtain because it is present in extremely low concentration (see Harper and Thoenen 1980). A number of studies have shown that many tissues can produce an NGF-like molecule in vitro, but it was not clear that such production occurred in vivo. Therefore, the recent demonstration of NGF production by an intact sympathetic target (the iris) represents an important advance (**Ebendal, Olson, Seiger,** and **Hedlund 1980**).

Ordinarily, the isolation and characterization of NGF would have been very difficult, since in most targets it is present at vanishingly low concentrations. Thus, the chance discovery by Levi-Montalcini and Cohen that NGF is present in extraordinarily large quantities in snake venom and in the salivary glands of adult male mice has been of immense importance in identifying this molecule (Cohen and Levi-Montalcini 1956; Cohen 1960). NGF can be isolated as a multisubunit complex (7S) in which the biologically active subunit, β (Angeletti et al. 1973), is resistant to proteolysis (Moore et al. 1974). In the mouse salivary gland (which is probably not an important source of NGF for developing neurons), NGF is synthesized in a "pro" form and is subsequently cleaved to its final size (Berger and Shooter 1978). Although high-affinity receptors for β-NGF have been described (see, for example, Herrup and Shooter 1975), the mechanism of action of NGF is poorly understood and remains controversial (Greene et al. 1979; Halegoua and Patrick 1980). Many of these studies have used a clonal cell line (PC12) that responds to NGF with neurite outgrowth but does not require it for survival (see Greene and Trisler 1978). The advantage of such lines for biochemists is cellular homogeneity and the possibility of obtaining large amounts of material (e.g., NGF receptors) for molecular studies.

Since the survival of many types of neurons that are not influenced by NGF also depends on an interaction with their targets (see Section 5), it is natural to suspect that there are a variety of molecules that act selectively on other parts of the nervous system in a manner analogous to the action of NGF on sympathetic and dorsal-root ganglion cells. Indeed, pursuit of such molecules is a burgeoning area of contemporary research. Evidence has already been obtained for survival factors acting on ciliary ganglia (see, for example, Collins 1978; Nishi and Berg 1979, 1981; Adler et al. 1979; Hendry and Hill 1980), sensory ganglia (Barde et al. 1980), and spinal cord (Dribin and Barrett 1980). In these cases much work remains to be done. The putative trophic factors must be purified, their specificities assessed, and their in vivo roles tested. The importance of NGF in this context is that it stands as a model for these investigations, much as early knowledge of acetylcholine and noradrenaline facilitated the discovery of additional neurotransmitters. Just as neurotransmission has proved quite diverse in terms of the agents involved and their mechanisms of action, so NGF may eventually be regarded as a particular example of a variety of retrograde trophic agents that share certain functional characteristics.

References

Adler, R., K.B. Landa, M. Marthorpe, and S. Varon. 1979. Cholinergic neuronotrophic factors: Intraocular distribution of trophic activity for ciliary neurons. *Science 204:* 1434–1436.

Aloe, L. and R. Levi-Montalcini. 1979. Nerve growth factor-induced transformation of immature chromaffin cells *in vivo* into sympathetic neurons: Effects of antiserum to nerve growth factor. *Proc. Natl. Acad. Sci. 76:* 1246–1250.

Angeletti, R.H., M.A. Hermondson, and R.A. Bradshaw. 1973. Amino acid sequences of mouse 2.5S nerve growth factor. II. Isolation and characterization of the thermolytic and peptic peptides and the complete covalent structure. *Biochemistry 12:* 100–115.

Barde, Y.-A., D. Edgar, and H. Thoenen. 1980. Sensory neurons in culture: Changing requirements for survival factors during embryonic development. *Proc. Natl. Acad. Sci. 77:* 1199–1203.

Berger, E. and E. Shooter. 1978. Biosynthesis of β-nerve growth factor in mouse submaxillary glands. *J. Biol. Chem. 253:* 804–810.

Campenot, R.B. 1977. Local control of neurite development by nerve growth factor. *Proc. Natl. Acad. Sci. 74:* 4516–4519.

Chun, L.L.Y. and P.H. Patterson. 1977. Role of nerve growth factor in the development of rat sympathetic neurons *in vitro*. I. Survival, growth and differentiation of catecholamine production. *J. Cell Biol. 75:* 694–704.

Cohen, S. 1960. Purification of a nerve-growth promoting protein from the mouse salivary gland and its neurocytotoxic antiserum. *Proc. Natl. Acad. Sci. 46:* 302–311.

Cohen, S. and R. Levi-Montalcini. 1956. A nerve growth stimulating factor isolated from snake venom. *Proc. Natl. Acad. Sci. 42:* 571–574.

Collins, F. 1978. Induction of neurite outgrowth by a conditioned-medium factor bound to the culture substratum. *Proc. Natl. Acad. Sci. 75:* 5210–5213.

Doupe, A.J. and P.H. Patterson. 1982. Glucocorticoids and the developing nervous system. *Curr. Top. Neuroendocrinol.* (in press).

Dribin, L.B. and J.N. Barrett. 1980. Conditioned medium enhances neuritic outgrowth from rat spinal cord explants. *Dev. Biol. 74:* 184–195.

Ebendal, T., L. Olson, Å. Seiger, and K.-O. Hedlund. 1980. Nerve growth factors in the rat iris. *Nature 286:* 25–28.

Gorin, P.D. and E.M. Johnson. 1979. Experimental autoimmune model of nerve growth factor deprivation: Effects on developing peripheral sympathetic and sensory neurons. *Proc. Natl. Acad. Sci. 76:* 5382–5386.

Greene, L.A. and A.S. Trisler. 1976. Establishment of a noradrenergic clonal line of rat adrenal pheochromocytoma cells which respond to nerve growth factor. *Proc. Natl. Acad. Sci. 73:* 2424–2428.

Greene, L.A., D.E. Burstein, J.C. McGuire, and M.M. Black. 1979. Cell culture studies on the mechanism of action of nerve growth factor. *Soc. Neurosci. Symp. 4:* 153–171.

Gundersen, R.W. and J.N. Barrett. 1979. Neuronal chemotaxis: Chick dorsal-root axons turn toward high concentrations of nerve growth factor. *Science 206:* 1079–1080.

———. 1980. Characterization of the turning response of dorsal root neurites toward nerve growth factor. *J. Cell Biol. 87:* 546–554.

Halegoua, S. and J. Patrick. 1980. Nerve growth factor mediates phosphorylation of specific proteins. *Cell 22:* 571–581.

Harper, G.P. and H. Thoenen. 1980. Nerve growth factor: Biological significance, measurement, and distribution. *J. Neurochem. 34:* 5–16.

Hendry, I.A. 1975. The response of adrenergic neurons to axotomy and nerve growth factor. *Brain Res. 94:* 87–97.

Hendry, I.A. and J. Campbell. 1976. Morphometric analysis of rat superior cervical ganglion after axotomy and nerve growth factor treatment. *J. Neurocytol. 5:* 351–360.

Hendry, I.A. and C.E. Hill. 1980. Retrograde axonal transport of target tissue-derived macromolecules. *Nature 287:* 647–649.

Herrup, K. and E.M. Shooter. 1975. Properties of the β-nerve growth factor receptor in development. *J. Cell Biol. 67:* 118–125.

Johnson, E.M., R.Y. Andres, and R.A. Bradshaw. 1978. Characterization of the retrograde transport of nerve growth factor (NGF) using high specific activity [^{125}I] NGF. *Brain Res. 150:* 319–331.

Letourneau, P.C. 1978. Chemotactic response of nerve fiber elongation to nerve growth factor. *Dev. Biol. 66:* 183–196.

Levi-Montalcini, R. 1975. NGF: An uncharted route. In *The neurosciences, paths of discovery* (ed. F.G. Worden et al.), pp. 245–265. MIT Press, Cambridge, Massachusetts.

Levi-Montalcini, R. and P.U. Angeletti. 1963. Essential role of the nerve growth factor in the survival and maintenance of dissociated sensory and sympathetic embryonic nerve cells *in vitro*. *Dev. Biol. 7:* 653–659.

Levi-Montalcini, R. and B. Booker. 1960. Destruction of the sympathetic ganglia in mammals by an antiserum to a nerve growth protein. *Proc. Natl. Acad. Sci. 46:* 384–391.

Levi-Montalcini, R. and S. Cohen. 1956. In vitro and in vivo effects of a nerve growth-stimulating agent isolated from snake venom. *Proc. Natl. Acad. Sci. 42:* 695–699.

Levi-Montalcini, R. and V. Hamburger. 1951. Selective growth stimulating effects of mouse sarcoma on the sensory and sympathetic nervous system of the chick embryo. *J. Exp. Zool. 116:* 321–362.

Mensini-Chen, M.G., J.C. Chen, and R. Levi-Montalcini. 1978. Sympathetic nerve fibers ingrowth in the central nervous system of neonatal rodent upon intracerebral NGF injections. *Arch. Ital. Biol. 116:* 53–84.

Moore, J.B., W.C. Mobley, and E.M. Shooter. 1974. Proteolytic modification of the β-nerve growth factor protein. *Biochemistry 13:* 833–840.

Nishi, R. and D.K. Berg. 1979. Survival and development of ciliary ganglion neurones grown alone in cell culture. *Nature 277:* 232–234.

———. 1981. Two components from eye tissue that differentially stimulate the growth and development of ciliary ganglion neurons in cell culture. *J. Neurosci. 1:* 505–513.

Stockel, K., M. Schwab, and H. Thoenen. 1975. Specificity of retrograde transport of NGF in sensory neurons: A biochemical and morphological study. *Brain Res. 89:* 1–14.

Unsicker, K., B. Krisch, U. Otten, and H. Thoenen. 1978. Nerve growth factor-induced fiber outgrowth from isolated rat adrenal chromaffin cells: Impairment by glucocorticoids. *Proc. Natl. Acad. Sci. 75:* 3498–3502.

Reprinted from The Neurosciences: Paths of Discovery (ed. Worden et al.),
pp. 245–265. MIT Press, Cambridge. 1975

NGF : An Uncharted Route

Rita Levi-Montalcini

"A scientist should never attempt to judge his own contributions, whether significant or not, but especially when not." (Lwoff, 1966)

Introduction

A disclaimer of personal merit, such as phrased above by Lwoff, is not a disclaimer of the significance of a phenomenon that chance rather than calculated search has brought to one's attention, and for this reason I have accepted with pleasure the very flattering invitation to discuss the history of nerve growth factor (NGF). I am afraid, however, that the following account will not provide a unique glimpse into the paths of discovery that have shaped the course and content of neuroscience in recent decades. The NGF has in fact still not found its place in the broadening panorama of neuroscience, and, even worse, twenty years after its coming into existence this factor has disclosed only a few, perhaps the most trivial, of its traits. It keeps us wondering where it is heading, and whether its uncharted route has, indeed, any ending.

It is in the spirit of never-ending pursuit, which has characterized this search from its very beginning, that the present biography of the NGF is written by one who has watched with awe and wonder the birth of this "miracle" molecule from the sinister womb of malignant tissues.

Different moments of this experience were shared with three friends. Their names are Viktor, Stanley, and Piero. Their true identity, as well as their participation in this adventure, will emerge in the following pages.

Biographical Sketch of the Biographer

Starting a career

The start of what was supposed to be a medical career took place in Turin, in northern Italy, in the early 1930s. Eugenia Lustig, my cousin, Salvador Luria, and Renato Dulbecco were my schoolmates and became my lifelong friends. We had in common a tremendous respect and fear of our teacher, Giuseppe Levi (Figure 14.1), a towering figure in the biology of that period, and shared a lukewarm interest in histology, the subject that he taught with great enthusiasm and unique knowledge. To be honest, I should confess that I hated histology and that up to this day I have never mastered even the most common staining techniques. I suspect that my three schoolmates nursed the same feelings, but so high was our esteem for "the master" that this dislike never came out in the open, nor prevented us from becoming *allievi interni* in the Istituto di Anatomia which he di-

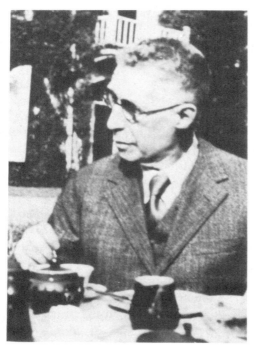

Figure 14.1   Professor Giuseppe Levi.

rected with enormous energy and iron rules. It was my good luck that the master, realizing my lack of histological talent, decided that I should learn instead to culture different cell types in vitro, a field which was at that time just beginning. My first study, on the formation of reticular fibers in vitro from connective and epithelial tissues, pleased Levi and signaled the beginning of a master–pupil association that was to last until his death 33 years later.

In 1936 graduated I from medical school and specialized in neurology and psychiatry, equally attracted by the clinical profession and by a pure academic career in the footsteps of Levi. My perplexity was not to last too long: in June 1938 Mussolini issued the "Manifesto per la difesa della razza," signed by ten Italian "scientists," which barred academic as well as professional careers to non-Aryan citizens. Intermarriage between Aryan and Semitic citizens was prohibited to protect the pure Italian Aryan blood from contamination with that of inferior non-Aryan races. In 1939 I received and accepted an invitation from a neurological institute in Brussels, and I moved there a few months before the declaration of war between Germany, France, and England. However, when the invasion of Belgium appeared imminent, I returned to Italy to join my family in Turin. In the meantime the situation had greatly worsened: the only two alternatives to total stagnation were either to abandon the country and emigrate to the United States (there were no more safe places in Europe), or to pursue some activity that would need neither support nor connection with the outside Aryan world in which we lived. My family did not want to consider the first alternative, and I then decided to build a small research unit at home. Though I had never performed neuroembryological experiments, I was familiar with the literature (non-Aryan citizens were no longer allowed to consult the university libraries), and I was thrilled at the idea of this experience à la Robinson Crusoe.

I built a laboratory in my bedroom with few indispensable pieces of equipment, such as an incubator, a light, a stereomicroscope, and a microtome. The object of choice was the chick embryo, and the instruments consisted of sewing needles transformed with the help of a sharpening stone into microinstruments. My Bible and inspiration was an article by Viktor Hamburger dated 1934, which I had happened to read some years earlier. The title of this excellent classic study was "The effects of wing bud extirpation on the development of the central nervous system in chick embryos." Through my training with Levi I had become an expert in silver techniques, and I decided to reinvestigate the problem of the effect of the periphery on the developing nerve centers by making use of the specific Cajal–De Castro technique. The project had barely started when Levi returned from Belgium, where he had also moved soon after being discharged from the university. Levi asked to join me in this investigation, and he became, to my great pride, my first and only assistant.

The trying years

Looking back to the period 1940–1943, I wonder how I could have found so much interest in and have devoted myself with such a burning enthusiasm to the study of a small neuroembryological problem when all the values I cherished were being crushed and the triumphant advance of the Germans all over Europe seemed to herald the end of Western civilization. The answer may be found in the well-known refusal of human beings to accept reality at its face value, whether it be the fate of an individual, of a country, or of the whole of human society. Without this built-in defense mechanism life would be unbearable, not only to those doomed to impending death by fatal illness, but also to those who approach the physiological end of their lives with all the misery and suffering that are the companions of old age.

I believe that I inherited from my father an unusually efficient defense mechanism that was to be of great help during those years. This was strengthened by the association with Levi, then in his seventies. The old master followed with unfailing enthusiasm (comparable to and tuned to an even higher pitch than my own) the development of our experiments. I still hear his thundering voice, used to frighten assistants and legions of students, which now resounded even more powerfully in the narrow precinct of my small bedroom laboratory. During the period 1940–1942 the anti-Semitic campaign reached its peak, and the daily press found great pleasure in spreading all the more hideous slogans borrowed from the Nazis; but Levi and I ignored the threats and abuses, so absorbed were we in our work. My bedroom became the meeting center for old pupils and friends of Giuseppe Levi, who worshiped in him not only the great scientist but also the valiant and undaunted anti-Fascist. It should, in fact, be remembered that the majority of Italians rebelled vigorously against the racial laws and were not afraid of expressing dissent even at the risk of being themselves persecuted. In July 1942, however, the heavy bombing of Turin and other industrial cities by the Allies forced my family and me to move to a small country house, where I rebuilt my laboratory under conditions far worse than in my previous bedroom, while Levi moved to a small mountain village. Shortages of eggs (the eggs were used first for experimentation and then, five days later, upon removal of the operated embryo, as scrambled eggs for food) and of electrical power, which was cut off every few days, made the work extremely difficult, not to say impossible. Yet, to my great satisfaction, I was able to complete an experimental study on the acousticovestibular centers of the chick embryo that was to come out in print many years later in the United States (Levi-Montalcini, 1949).

In July 1943, on the verge of military disaster and the total collapse of the country, Mussolini was disavowed by his (up to then) most loyal followers and was jailed by the king. One and a half months later Italy was invaded by hordes of Nazis, and the small Jewish-Italian population became the object of ferocious hunting, mass killing, and deportation to the extermination camps. My family and I escaped capture by flying to Florence, where we mingled with hundreds of other refugees living, as we did, with false identity cards. Of the long months spent there in seclusion, listening secretly to the news broadcasts from London, in continuous danger of being discovered, I shall mention only one episode, which is perhaps more amusing in retrospect than when it actually occurred. One day the bell rang, and I heard the familiar voice of Professor Levi asking the landlady in his usual authoritative way to call me immediately. He did not know my new family name, but, with a wisdom that I would never have expected from him, he gave my first name: Rita. To the question, whom should she announce, he answered: "Professor Giuseppe Levi, ah no, I keep forgetting, Professor Giuseppe Lovisato." The landlady, who was not aware of our true identity, became from that moment very suspicious of us and of our absent-minded friend; but, being a gentle soul and not at all curious, she kept her suspicions to herself.

With the end of the war in May 1945, I returned to Turin and became the assistant of Levi, who had resumed his position as professor of anatomy at the university. One year later, in the spring of 1946, I received a letter from Viktor Hamburger, who had come across the 1942 article by Levi and myself on the correlations between periphery and developing nerve centers. This manuscript, refused by Italian journals in view of the non-Aryan names of its authors, had been accepted by the Belgian *Archives de Biologie* (Levi-Montalcini and Levi, 1942). Hamburger was intrigued by the different mechanisms of action that had been postulated by us and by him for the interaction between nonnervous and nervous structures. He invited me to work for a one- or two-year period in his laboratory in Saint Louis to collaborate with him in reinvestigating this problem. However, it was not until the fall of 1947 that I left Turin for Saint Louis, where I was to spend the next 26 years, the happiest and most productive years of my life.

Viktor Hamburger, a Founding Father of Experimental Neuroembryology

If the beginning of my career was under the spell of Giuseppe Levi, the second period was under the influence of Viktor Hamburger, who had already played a key role in channeling my interests toward problems of growth and differentiation of nerve cells.

Viktor Hamburger was a former student and the "favorite son" of Hans Spemann, the great German embryologist who was awarded the Nobel Prize in 1934 for his discovery of the role played by induction in developmental embryonic processes. From his teacher Viktor had learned the trades and skills of the art, which requires both sharp thinking and sharp microinstruments. Spemann was a master in both fields; in fact he greatly enjoyed devising and forging his own microtools and, in the Renaissance tradition, passed on both skills to his pupil. In 1932, one year before Germany fell into the hands of Hitler, Viktor had come to the United States to spend one year in Chicago in the laboratory of Frank Lillie, a close friend of Spemann and himself a famous embryologist who had actually started experimental work on the chick embryo. The triumph of Hitler in 1933 persuaded Viktor to remain in the United States to pursue the analysis of the developing nervous system that he had started in Germany. In 1935 he moved from Chicago to Saint Louis where, in 1940, he succeeded F.O. Schmitt (who had moved to MIT) as chairman of the Department of Zoology of Washington University.

Viktor directed the department with rules that were quite different from those of Levi. Accustomed as I was to the thundering voice of Levi and to his explosive way of expressing dissent in political and scientific matters (a mild way of conveying his viewpoint to his interlocutor was: "I beg your pardon, but you are a perfect imbecile"), I was struck by the kindness and subtle dry humor of Viktor, who would never hurt other people's feelings nor show his disagreement with more than a few gentle remarks and a firm glance of disapproval. Working with him on the same problem that had absorbed so much of my time and thoughts in my secluded laboratory in Turin was a sheer pleasure. Instead of the sinister atmosphere of an Italian city during the fateful years 1940–1943, I was now surrounded by the cheerful environment of an American college. It was right after the war and the period of dissent was still far away; students strolled hand in hand on the university campus, which, to a European observer, seemed like the garden of Eden with no snake to tempt the naïve inhabitants of such a Paradise. (But, alas, the snake was there.) But even more than these novel surroundings, it was my association with Viktor that I enjoyed. While I dearly loved the "old master," it had often been difficult to adjust to his temperamental fits and dogmatic way of thinking. With Viktor, however, there was no problem of this sort. What I liked most was the clarity of his thinking and his superb control of the English language. Writing a scientific paper was a new experience for me, and I concentrated on the effort of learning how to do it. Up to this day, everytime I write one, my first thought is: Will Viktor like it?

In the fall of 1948, one year after my arrival in Saint Louis (the work had progressed so well that my return to Turin was postponed indefinitely), Viktor showed me a short article by one of his former students (Bueker, 1948) which was to change entirely the direction of my research. In this article Bueker reported on the results of a bold and ingenious experiment that he had performed to test the ability of developing nerve fibers to innervate fast-growing tissues, such as neoplastic tissues, and to adjust their growth rate to that of a rapidly expanding tumor. He selected for these studies a mouse tumor, sarcoma 180, and to his satisfaction he found that the results agreed with his expectation. Fragments of this particular tumor (other mouse tumors did not produce the same effect), implanted into the body wall of three-day chick embryos, became established and innervated by nerve fibers growing out from adjacent sensory ganglia of the host. Histological studies performed three to five days later showed that the ganglia providing fibers to the tumor were larger than contralateral ganglia innervating the leg.

These results were so much in line with current concepts of the interrelation between nerve centers and end organs that Bueker overlooked other, more perplexing aspects of the growth response. A reinvestigation of this effect by Viktor and myself showed that the growth response of sensory ganglia innervating the tumor was, in fact, much more pronounced than that of the same ganglia innervating a supernumerary limb. Furthermore, while the motor somatic nerve cells in the spinal segment facing the tumor transplant were not increased (they actually decreased in number), the sympathetic ganglia were tremendously enlarged and contributed to the innervation of the neoplastic tissues to a much larger extent than did sensory ganglia. Sensory and sympathetic nerve fibers branching into the tumor established no contact with the neoplastic cells but wandered aimlessly among the cells. And yet, even conceding that the effect was much more marked than that produced by implantation of a supernumerary limb bud, and differed in many respects from it, we were still not prepared in 1951 (Levi-Montalcini and Hamburger, 1951) to see in this response any flagrant deviation from normality, so difficult is it to refute generally accepted concepts and to evaluate novel results with an unprejudiced mind.

It was a spring day in 1951 when the block was suddenly removed, and it dawned on me that the tumor effect was *different* from that of normal embryonic tissues in that the tumor acted by *releasing* a growth factor of unknown nature rather than by making available to the nerve fibers a larger-than-usual field of innervation. This hypothesis, which became a certitude with me long before I obtained supporting evidence in its favor, was suggested by the observation that the viscera of embryos bearing transplants of mouse sarcomas 180 or 37 (the latter proved to produce the same effect as sarcoma 180) were invaded by sympathetic nerve fibers at a stage when there was still no innervation apparent in controls. Furthermore, and this was an even more remarkable infraction of normal rules, sympathetic nerve fibers forced their way inside blood vessels of the host where they formed large neuromas coated with red blood cells. How many times during the past two years had I seen but not perceived this most intriguing routing of nerve fibers into the blood vessels?

While I was lost in the contemplation of this, for me, stupendous phenomenon, I heard the familiar thundering voice of the "old master," who had just arrived from Italy and was paying me his first and only visit in the United States. In the excitement of the moment of discovery I showed him under the microscope the nerve bundles filling the viscera and entering into the blood vessels. Levi shook his powerful leonine head, still covered with a thick red mane in spite of his eighty-one years: "How can you say such nonsense? Don't you see that these are collagenous and not nerve fibers? Did it take you such a short time to forget all that you learned in Turin?" Soon after Levi left the room, I showed the slide to Viktor, who immediately grasped the far-reaching significance of these findings and was enthusiastic. I obtained decisive evidence for my hypothesis by grafting fragments of sarcomas 180 or 37 onto the chorioallantoic membrane of four- to six-day chick embryos, in such a position that the tumor and the embryo shared the circulation but no direct contact was established between neoplastic and embryonic tissues (Levi-Montalcini, 1952; Levi-Montalcini and Hamburger, 1953). The results were the same as in intraembryonic transplants.

The excitement of this discovery was tempered by the realization that it would be tremendously difficult to identify the tumor factor by using the ordinary exceedingly laborious and time-consuming embryological experiments. What was needed was a much simpler and faster bioassay. The tissue-culture method that I had learned in Turin with Levi seemed to offer a possible approach to this problem. A dear friend of mine, Herta Meyer, a former associate of Fisher in Berlin and then research assistant with Levi in Turin, was now in charge of the tissue-culture unit in the Biophysics Institute of the Medical School of Rio de Janeiro, directed by Professor Carlos Chagas. After an exchange of letters with Professor Chagas and Herta and with their consent, I submitted a travel-grant application to the Rockefeller Foundation, which would permit me to perform these experiments in Rio de Janeiro. The proposal was approved, and in October 1952 I boarded a plane for Brazil.

The NGF: Its Birth and Early Life History

The tumoral factor had given a first hint of its existence in Saint Louis; but it was in Rio de Janeiro that it revealed itself, and it did so in a theatrical and grand way, as if spurred by the bright atmosphere of that explosive and exuberant manifestation of life that is the Carnival in Rio.

I had come from Saint Louis with two mice bearing transplants of sarcomas 180 and 37 in my handbag. Immediately after arriving, I dissected small fragments of these tumors and cultured them in vitro in a hanging, semisolid drop of rooster plasma and embryonic extract; sensory or sympathetic ganglia from eight- to ten-day chick embryos were then transplanted in close proximity to neoplastic tissues. The first results were not only negative but worse: the ganglia cultured adjacent to the tumor produced less fibers than controls grown alone or in combination with embryonic chick tissues. It occurred to me that perhaps some other contaminants released from mouse tumors overshadowed or masked the tumor effect. I transplanted both tumors into chick embryos as intermediary hosts and then dissected out small fragments and cultured them in vitro, in proximity to sympathetic or sensory ganglia. Twenty years later I recall, as if it had just happened, the astonishment and wonder of that morning when, for the first time, I saw in the light microscope the outcome of these experiments. Figure 14.2 reproduces the drawing that I did with India ink (I did not have a camera and I could not wait long enough to search for one) and immediately sent in an express airmail letter to

Viktor, who returned it to me many years later. Nerve fibers had grown out in twelve hours from the entire periphery of sensory and sympathetic ganglia cultured in proximity to the neoplastic tissues and had spread out radially around the explants like the rays of the sun (Levi-Montalcini, Meyer, and Hamburger, 1954). The "NGF halo," as it soon became known, represents the most sensible and reliable index of the presence of this growth factor in any tissue or, as we shall see, in body fluids. Without this assay I very much doubt that we could ever have discovered and eventually identified this factor.

The news of the halo spread in no time throughout the Biophysics Institute and was celebrated at a party in the Chagases' most hospitable home. Three months later I returned to Saint Louis with my halo, a good dose of enthusiasm, and the naive belief that the identification and characterization of the tumoral factor would be only a matter of some months of solid work. How far we were from that goal we would learn in the subsequent twenty years; nor would we even today have solved the problem were it not for a most fortunate association with an outstanding biochemist and some fortuitous discoveries which, all of a sudden, made available far better sources of this factor than mouse sarcomas.

Enter Stanley Cohen

Stanley Cohen, or Stan as he became known to us from the very beginning, had never been interested in the nervous system. His first postdoctoral study was on the mechanism of urea excretion of the earthworm, and to this end he had spent long days collecting tons of them in the fertile ground around Denver, Colorado. Having solved this problem, he had then moved to Saint Louis, where he became associated with Martin Kamen.

I have wondered many times where we would stand now if Stan had not heard from Viktor about the halo effect and had not been tempted to work with us on this problem. Soon after joining the Department of Zoology as research associate, Stan fractionated the tumor homogenate and identified in the microsomal fraction the active tumoral principle. In 1954 this factor was christened "Nerve Growth Stimulating Factor" (Cohen, Levi-Montalcini, and Hamburger, 1954), a name shortened later to "Nerve Growth Factor" or, more simply, "NGF."

In a biological science, perhaps to a larger extent than in any other experimental

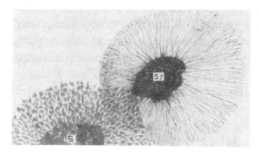

Figure 14.2   The "halo effect" at its first appearance in Rio de Janeiro in December 1952. This is an India ink drawing of a combined culture of sarcoma 180 (S) and a sympathetic ganglion (Sy) from an eight-day chick embryo after twelve hours of incubation.

science, chance and good luck play a notoriously great role. It is not only, as is so often stated, a matter of serendipity, or of the perception of a truth that is there all the time but goes unnoticed until the mind of the observer suddenly grasps it, but rather of a fortuitous stumbling into a cave of precious stones while hiking up a hill on a trail that is not expected to bring one anywhere but to the top of the hill.

When Stan, following the suggestion of Arthur Kornberg, made use of snake venom to purify further the tumoral factor, he did not, nor could he, anticipate the outcome of this routine experiment. The venom was used as a source of phosphodiesterase to degrade the nucleic acids present in the active fraction. If the nucleic acids were an essential component of the NGF, their enzymatic degradation would destroy the biological activity of this factor; if the activity remained, then the protein rather than the nucleic acids must be responsible for the growth effect.

It was again a spring morning (1956) when I inspected, as I used to do every morning, the cultures performed the day before and then, with no comment, asked Stan to do the same. Stan looked through the eyepiece of the microscope and mumbled: "Rita, I am afraid that with this we have used up all our good luck; we cannot count on it anymore." Fortunately he was wrong, but this will come out later.

The addition of the venom to the tumoral fraction endowed with NGF activity had so potentiated its effect as to transform the delicate fibrillar halo into one of tremendous density. Two alternatives were considered: either the venom had destroyed an inhibitor present in the tumoral fraction or it harbored the growth factor itself. Six hours later we knew the answer. The addition of minute amounts of snake venom to the culture medium evoked the same effect from sensory and sympathetic ganglia as when it was added in the presence of the tumoral fraction. Thus the venom was another most potent source of the NGF.

Between 1956 and 1958 Stan succeeded in purifying and characterizing the venom NGF (a feat that had not been possible with the tumoral NGF since in these tissues the factor is present in exceedingly small quantities) as a protein molecule of molecular weight 20,000. At the same time I studied the in vivo and in vitro effects of the venom NGF on sensory and sympathetic ganglia of the chick embryo. It soon became apparent that its biological activity was strikingly similar if not identical to that of the tumoral NGF, with only one important difference: the NGF factor was present in the venom at a concentration estimated as a thousand times higher than in the two mouse sarcomas (Cohen and Levi-Montalcini, 1956).

The finding of a protein molecule endowed with such a potent and selective biological activity in two unrelated sources, mouse tumors and snake venom, prompted a search for it in other tissues and body fluids. At the time of the discovery in Rio of the in vitro NGF effect of mouse sarcomas, other mouse tissues had been tested and I had found, to my dismay, that they also elicited a nerve growth effect similar to, but much milder than, that of the two sarcomas. This finding, reported in the 1954 article, seemed somewhat disturbing to the thesis that the production of this factor was the prerogative of some neoplastic tissues; but in the absence of clear-cut evidence against the hypothesis (other mouse tumors proved to elicit no growth effect), we did not pursue the study of normal mouse tissues any further.

The discovery of the venom NGF was a definite blow to the thesis and called for a reconsideration of the earlier findings. It was Stan who conceived the idea of testing the mouse salivary glands, a homologue of the venom gland, as another potential source of NGF. The results of in vitro experiments fully confirmed his guess: the mouse salivary glands proved to be a third and by far the most potent source of NGF (Figure 14.3). From 1958, when these experiments were first performed, to the present day, all our work and that of the other laboratories that have become interested in the NGF has centered on the purification and characterization of the salivary NGF. Stan identified the factor as a protein molecule of molecular weight 44,000, possibly a dimer of the venom NGF (Cohen, 1960). Extensive studies in newborn and adult mice and rats injected with the purified NGF gave evidence for the magnitude of the growth response elicited from sympathetic ganglia. While these ganglia remain receptive to the action of the NGF throughout their life, the sensory ganglia respond to it only during a restricted period of their embryonic development (Levi-Montalcini and Booker, 1960a).

In 1959 Stan made his last, but no less remarkable, contribution to the study of the NGF. He prepared an antiserum to the NGF and we tested its effects in vitro. When we found that it abolished the halo stimulated by the salivary factor around sensory and sympathetic ganglia, we injected the serum into newborn mice; treated and control animals of the same litter were sacrificed and inspected at the stereomicroscope twenty days later. On June 11, 1959, Stan and I saw for the first time in the stereomicroscope the outcome of this seemingly innocuous treatment. Control and injected mice were of the same size, and the vitality of the group injected daily with the antiserum to the NGF was in no way impaired; but the sympathetic chain ganglia, which in controls are easily detected at the two sides of the vertebral bodies, were no longer there. With considerable effort I succeeded in identifying them in two vanishingly thin translucent filaments. After dissection, fixation, and serial section, we saw in the light microscope what was left of each

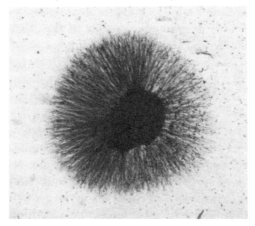

Figure 14.3   Fibrillar halo around a sensory ganglion from an eight-day chick embryo cultured in vitro in the presence of 0.01 μg/ml of the purified salivary factor. From Levi-Montalcini (1964).

ganglion: a population of glial cells with a few highly atrophic sympathetic neurons scattered among nonnervous cells. The entire para- and prevertebral population of sympathetic nerve cells was reduced to 3–5% of that of controls (Levi-Montalcini and Booker, 1960b).

These findings gave additional evidence for the key role played by the NGF in the life of the sympathetic adrenergic neuron, and at the same time provided a unique method of rearing mice and rats that are deprived of their sympathetic nervous system from birth. Subsequent studies showed that three to five injections of the antiserum to the NGF given in the first five days of life are sufficient to obtain the near-total destruction of sympathetic ganglia, and also showed that this effect is irreversible. This end result, which became known as "immunosympathectomy," has been utilized ever since 1959 in our laboratories and in several others to assess the role of the sympathetic nervous system in physiological and pathological conditions (Zaimis and Knight, 1972; Steiner and Schoenbaum, 1972).

Exit Stan; Enter Piero Angeletti

Shortly after this last discovery, Stan, to my great regret, abandoned our joint pursuit and moved to Nashville, to Vanderbilt University, where he started the study of another factor, also isolated from mouse salivary glands, that is endowed with an equally potent and selective growth-promoting effect on epithelial cells. With the same ingenuity and talent that he had displayed in the NGF chase, he now succeeded in uncovering the properties of this new growth factor, which he named the "Epithelial Growth Factor" or, more simply, the "EGF" (Cohen, 1962). His departure from his small and not too clean office on the first floor of Rebstock Hall, where he had labored for six years to unveil the mysterious nature of the NGF, signaled the end of the most romantic and picturesque phase of this adventure. Stan used to spend the entire day and most of his evenings there, meditating with eyes half-closed, smoking his pipe, and playing the flute (his main talents were, however, not in this direction), while Smog, his gentle, dirty, and all-bastard dog, looked fondly at his master or slept peacefully at his feet.

Shortly after the departure of Stan, Piero Angeletti joined our group and for twelve years became my partner in this exploration. Piero moved into Stan's office and brought to the problem his youth and imagination combined with a strong scientific drive and remarkable talent. The NGF pursuit now took a somewhat different direction.

By the time Piero made his entrance we no longer entertained the naive belief that the NGF phenomenon could be explained with a few more months of work. The rules of the game were clear by now, and while the problem was all the more challenging, especially for a newcomer, they warned against hasty conclusions and prepared us to accept defeat gracefully.

The strategy of Piero was markedly different from that of Stan and reflected their different backgrounds, personal inclinations, and, most of all, the natural history of the NGF. Now that it had revealed itself, the search demanded a new course and suggested a different tactic. Rather than concentrating all his efforts on elucidating the nature of this molecule, Piero, at the head of a small team (in 1961 we built a new study center in Rome, which remained in close connection with that in Saint Louis through the continuous commuting of members of the two groups), guided the attack in several directions, aiming at uncovering not only the nature of the NGF but also its origin, significance, and mechanism of action.

The extraction procedure of the salivary NGF was considerably improved, and, as a result, a highly purified NGF became the object of studies that paved the way to its complete characterization (Bocchini and Angeletti, 1969). It was, however, only in 1971 that this goal was reached (R. H. Angeletti and Bradshaw, 1971). This achievement climaxed twenty years of work and settled one of the most debated and crucial aspects of the whole phenomenon, namely, the nature of the NGF molecule, which had been conceived by some investigators in the mystic light of a Trinity, or as a triune entity whose biological activity would result from the cooperative action of three different subunits (Varon, Nomura, and Shooter, 1967). The NGF, as unveiled by Ruth Angeletti and Ralph Bradshaw, was instead identified as a rather small dimeric molecule consisting of two identical

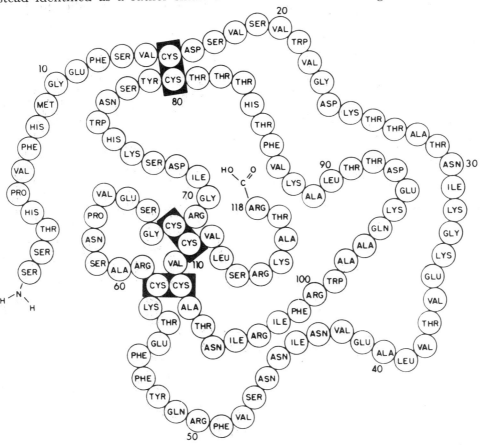

Figure 14.4 A portrait of the NGF: a schematic representation of the amino-acid sequence of the primary subunit of 2.5 S NGF from mouse submaxillary gland. From R. H. Angeletti and Bradshaw (1971).

subunits of molecular weight 13,259, each subunit consisting of 118 amino-acid chains held together by three disulfide bonds (Figure 14.4).

Among other advances that took place in the period 1960–1970 I shall mention here only the most significant ones. Biochemical and immunological studies gave evidence for the remarkable similarity of the venom and salivary NGF (Levi-Montalcini and Angeletti, 1968; Angeletti, Levi-Montalcini, and Zanini, 1971). The finding of such a potent growth factor in two exocrine glands such as the snake venom gland and mouse salivary gland raised the question of whether this factor is produced and released in a hormonal fashion from these glands, and should therefore be classified as a hormone, or whether growth factors such as the NGF and the EGF belong to a class of biologically active agents that is different from that of hormones. Extensive studies on the salivary NGF and its production and release mechanisms gave evidence for substantial differences between NGF and classical hormones (Levi-Montalcini, 1966; Levi-Montalcini and Angeletti, 1968); the question, however, is far from being settled, as indicated by the recent extensive reexamination of the problem by Hendry and Iversen (1973).

The mechanism of action of the NGF and the characterization of the growth response were studied at the metabolic and ultrastructural levels. Experiments in vitro showed that all anabolic processes are markedly stimulated in embryonic sensory and sympathetic cells; puromycin and cyclohexamide block the outgrowth of nerve fibers from the explanted ganglia, while actinomycin-D, at a concentration which inhibits RNA synthesis, does not entirely prevent the formation of the fibrillar halo, thus disproving the early hypothesis that this factor may act at the transcription level (Angeletti, Levi-Montalcini, and Calissano, 1968; Levi-Montalcini, 1964; Levi-Montalcini and Angeletti, 1971; Larrabee, 1972).

Electron-microscopic studies revealed that the most precocious and marked NGF effect is the production of neurofilaments and neurotubules, which fill the cell cytoplasm and from there are funneled into the axon (Levi-Montalcini et al., 1968). This effect, which is difficult to fit into the concept of a major role for neurotubules in intracellular transport processes (a role that would conceivably be called upon in the fully differentiated neuron rather than in nerve cells at their early inception), will be considered again in the last section.

While continuing these studies, our attention was focused on the sympathetic neuron, not only as the target cell of the NGF but also as a most convenient model of nerve-cell growth and differentiation. As is all-too-well known, we owe to this neuron the discovery of the chemical nature of nerve impulse transmission as well as the subsequent identification of the adrenergic neurotransmitter. These discoveries were soon followed by the elucidation of the metabolic pathways and of the enzymes involved in the synthesis and degradation of noradrenaline. The successful development of drugs that compete with noradrenaline for its storage sites or interfere with its release and uptake mechanisms opened a new field in neuropharmacology and was of immediate clinical significance. Among the drugs that were found to block the transmission of the nerve impulse from the sympathetic adrenergic neuron, a dopamine analogue, six-hydroxydopamine (6-OHDA), proved to be most effective. In 1968 Thoenen and Tranzer showed that, at variance with other adrenergic-neuron blocking agents, 6-OHDA suppresses the transmission of the nerve impulse by causing a selective destruction of the synaptic vesicles. The process is reversible, and four to eight weeks after discontinuation of the treatment both the integrity of these organelles and the sympathetic function are fully restored (Thoenen and Tranzer, 1968).

The extensive experience gained in our laboratory on the differential vulnerability of immature and mature sympathetic neurons (the former are destroyed by a specific antiserum to the NGF, while the latter are only temporarily impaired) suggested to Piero that we should assay 6-OHDA for its possible noxious effects in newborn animals. The dopamine analogue was injected daily in newborn mice and rats for a week, and the sympathetic chain ganglia were inspected by stereo and light microscopy weeks and months after discontinuation of the treatment. The results fully confirmed the hypothesis that immature sympathetic neurons are much more severely affected by this drug than are fully differentiated nerve cells. The 6-OHDA treatment resulted, in fact, in the destruction of 95–98% of neurons located in the sympathetic para- and prevertebral chain ganglia. The process is irreversible, as indicated by studies of treated animals one to two years later (Angeletti and Levi-Montalcini, 1970). Thus a new and most effective method to suppress the sympathetic system in newborn animals became available, known as "chemical sympathectomy."

Studies with the electron microscope showed that the lesions produced by 6-OHDA differ markedly from those caused by antibodies to the NGF. The latter are localized at first in the nuclear compartment and consist of disaggregation of the nucleolus and clumping of the chromatin (Levi-Montalcini, Caramia, and Angeletti, 1969), while the former consist of dilation and rupture of the cisternal lamellae and selective destruction of the synaptic vesicles in the nerve end terminals (Angeletti and Levi-Montalcini, 1972).

It seemed of interest to see whether NGF would prevent the lethal effects of 6-OHDA on the immature sympathetic neuron. Newborn mice and rats were injected daily for one- to four-week periods with NGF and 6-OHDA, and the ganglia were then dissected out, compared with those of controls or NGF-injected littermates, and examined at the optic and electron microscope. We expected that the ganglia would be equal in size to those of animals injected with only the NGF if the growth factor entirely obliterated the 6-OHDA effects, and of an intermediate size if the NGF and 6-OHDA effects added to and compensated for each other. Once again we were faced instead with a much more complex and, indeed, unpredictable result. The combined NGF and 6-OHDA treatment produced a dramatic enhancement of the NGF effects, as shown in Figure 14.5. Ganglia of rats injected with both agents undergo a further volume increase that amounts to three or four times that of NGF-injected littermates and about thirty times that of controls (Levi-Montalcini, 1974; Levi-Montalcini, Revoltella, and Calissano, 1974). Studies with light and electron microscopes showed that this effect is mainly due to an overproduction of axons by sympathetic neurons, which compare in size to those of NGF-treated rats. The mechanism and possible cause of this paradoxical effect are now under investigation.

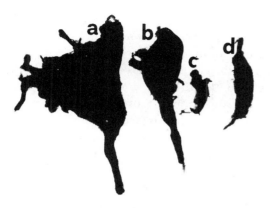

Figure 14.5 The paradoxical effect of NGF plus 6-OHDA. Whole mounts of the superior cervical ganglia of nineteen-day littermate rats injected since birth with: a, NGF plus 6-OHDA; b, NGF; c, 6-OHDA; d, saline. From Levi-Montalcini (1974).

The NGF and the Forgotten Organelle

"Although the ubiquity in living cells of these fibrous structures (microtubules) is now established, little is known concerning their role; they may be regarded as organelles vital to cell function. The status of our knowledge about these organelles is comparable with that about mitochondria a generation ago" (Schmitt, 1968b). Thus F.O. Schmitt, in his usual forceful way, called the attention of the neurobiologist to the function of these forgotten organelles in this as well as in several other articles that appeared between 1967 and 1970 (Schmitt, 1968a,b, 1970).

Interest in neuronal fibrous proteins, first identified in neurofibrils, goes back to the nineteenth century, when these filamentous structures were first detected, in the cell cytoplasm and in the axons of nerve cells, by their strong and selective affinity for metal salts. Their ubiquitous presence in nerve but not other cells was correlated with the unique function of nerve cells: the production and transmission of the nerve impulse. The hypothesis was abandoned at the beginning of this century when the membrane theory replaced the neurofibril theory. Interest in neuronal fibrous proteins in nerve cells was revived in the fifties, mainly because of Schmitt and his classic studies on the physicochemical properties of these organelles (Schmitt, 1950, 1957; Schmitt and Davison, 1961; Schmitt and Geren, 1950). More recently, various authors have presented evidence that neurotubules play an all-important role in axoplasmic flow (Weiss, 1967, Dahlström, 1969), as well as in several other intracellular transport processes (Tilney, 1971). At the same time a much clearer distinction has been made between three different fibrous proteins: the neurofilament (present only in nerve cells); the microfilament or actinlike filament; and the microtubule (Fine and Bray, 1971; Shelanski, Gaskin, and Cantor, 1973; Yamada, Spooner, and Wessells, 1970); both microfilaments and microtubules are regular constituents of most eukaryotic cells.

What is the significance, if any, of the NGF in relation to these fibrous proteins? We shall consider only one of them, the microtubule.

It will be remembered that the most outstanding feature of the NGF response is the massive production by its target cells of neurotubules and neurofilaments. This effect, which was noticed at the beginning of the investigation in 1951, came into sharper relief in 1969 when we studied at the electron microscope the earliest changes evoked by the NGF in vitro (Levi-Montalcini et al., 1968). It was, however, not until the spring of 1973 that the overproduction of neurotubules by NGF-treated sensory and sympathetic nerve cells in vitro suddenly became the object of intensive efforts to elucidate the role of microtubules in the NGF growth response. The credit for this new turn (for, as we shall see, this novel approach has already showns its validity as well as its potential for further development) must go to a neurochemist, Piero Calissano, and an immunologist, Roberto Revoltella, both of whom joined our group and explored the NGF phenomenon with an unprejudiced eye and with new tools. In the following section I shall summarize both lines of investigation, even if the overall picture that emerges is still hazy and is likely to undergo changes as it comes into sharper focus.

Calissano, who had had extensive experience in studies on the specific proteins of nervous tissue, conceived the idea of exploring a possible interaction of NGF with some brain proteins. This inspired guess was fully justified by preliminary experiments which showed that a solution of brain proteins undergoes an almost instantaneous and marked turbidity upon addition of the NGF. Electrophoretic analysis of the pellet revealed that NGF coprecipitates with one single protein band, which exhibits a molecular weight and amino-acid composition strikingly similar to those of tubulin (Calissano and Cozzari, 1974).

While these experiments were in progress, Roberto Revoltella and his coworkers explored the binding of the NGF to its target cells with immunological and biochemical techniques as a possible model system to analyze the mechanism of interaction between a ligand and its structural membrane receptor. In preference to the sympathetic nerve cells they selected murine neuroblastoma (NB) cells (C 1300), which share many properties in common with sympathetic neurons but have the advantage of being much larger and of growing in suspension as well as in monolayer; they can therefore be harvested in large quantity and used for immunological and biochemical tests. Studies with ^{125}I-NGF and with the rosette-forming technique showed that the NB cells bind NGF onto their surface with an avidity that is several orders of magnitude higher than that of a variety of other ligands. A binding capacity of the same order is exhibited by sympathetic but not by other normal or neoplastic cells (Levi-Montalcini, Revoltella, and Calissano, 1974).

Electron-microscopic studies of rosettes of NB- and NGF-coated sheep erythrocytes brought to light other features of the interaction between these two partners, strongly suggestive of a high specificity of the NGF binding for this "vicarious" cell target. At 37°C the NGF-coated erythrocytes are rapidly wrapped by folding of the NB-cell membrane and then phagocytized. At the contact point, immediately beneath the cell membrane, microtubules appear in large number. The tubulin polymerization, which is responsible for microtubule formation, is immediately followed by interiorization of NGF-coated erythrocytes into NB cells (Revoltella, Bertolini, and Pediconi, 1974; Revoltella et al., 1974). A protein extracted from

NB cells interacts and precipitates upon addition of the NGF. The amino-acid content, the electrophoretic pattern, and the molecular weight of this protein are remarkably similar to those of tubulin extracted from rat brain. These results suggest that, on the membrane of neuroblastoma and sympathetic cells (studies performed on the latter, although less extensive, are in agreement with those on NB cells), there is a protein that selectively interacts with NGF and exhibits physicochemical properties remarkably similar to those of tubulin.

These findings seem to indicate that microtubule proteins play a most prominent role in the chain of events triggered by NGF. Beside their generally acknowledged function in mediating intracellular transport processes, they would mediate the effects of agents such as the NGF at the membrane level. A similar role for neurotubule proteins has been suggested recently in many hormone-stimulated effects, in transduction processes, and in several immune reactions of lymphocytes or macrophages (Strom et al. 1973; Taylor et al., 1973; Taylor and Varela, 1971; Edelman, Yahara, and Wang, 1973; Inoué and Sato, 1967; Plaut, Lichtenstein, and Henney, 1973; Ukena and Berlin, 1972).

When compared with other similar or dissimilar systems, the one under investigation presents considerable advantages and recommends itself for this study. The target cell, the sympathetic neuron, has been the object of intense analysis, and its structural and functional properties are known to an extent unparalleled not only among nerve cells but even among other cells of simpler design than neurons. Hence, any deviation in growth and differentiation processes is easily noticed and tracked down. The microtubule proteins are unusually prominent in sympathetic nerve cells and lend themselves to exploration not only in this cell but also in its neoplastic counterpart, the neuroblastoma cell. Last, but not least, the NGF stands out today as one of the best known hormonal and growth factors, and its long-sought mechanism and site of action are slowly but steadily coming into focus.

Twenty Years Later

The long search for the identification of the NGF, which started under the sun of Rio de Janeiro in 1953, ended two years ago when the NGF with its small package of tightly coiled amino acids stood proudly in front of the photographer and of its admirers. But this achievement did not bring the exploration to an end.

In fact, the NGF, for all its feats, has still not found its place in the ever-changing game on the neuroscience chessboard, and this is, perhaps, the best sign of its vitality and of its potential rather than actual impact in a field that is itself in its most vigorous growth stage.

At the time of writing of this biography, the NGF, as has been its habit ever since it came to light, has driven its hunters into new surroundings. At variance with the past, however, and in line with prevailing trends, the new surroundings are not the open space of an unexplored world but, rather, the narrow precinct of a small field that has already been extensively explored but has still revealed only a few of its hidden treasures.

The chase is now taking place inside rather than outside the adrenergic neuron, a cell that many times in these last decades has generously rewarded its explorers. Thus, among other merits, the NGF deserves to be praised for once again bringing to the forefront this nerve cell that used to belong to the third world and is now asking for a long-overdue primary role on the widening stage of neurobiology.

Now that the NGF has come of age and the most picturesque and adventurous phase of its life is over, the biographer, who has had some part in the chase, entrusts it, with love, to younger and more skillful hands.

References

Angeletti, P.U., and Levi-Montalcini, R. (1970): Sympathetic nerve cell destruction in newborn mammals by 6-hydroxydopamine. *Proc. Natl. Acad. Sci. USA* 65:114–121.

Angeletti, P.U., and Levi-Montalcini, R. (1972): Growth inhibition of sympathetic cells by some adrenergic blocking agents. *Proc. Natl. Acad. Sci. USA* 69:86–88.

Angeletti, P.U., Levi-Montalcini, R., and Calissano, P. (1968): The nerve growth factor (NGF): Chemical properties and metabolic effects. *Adv. Enzymol.* 31:51–75.

Angeletti, P.U., Levi-Montalcini, R., and Zanini, A. (1971): Immunochemical properties of the nerve growth factor. *In: Hormones in Development.* Hamburgh, M., and Barrington, E.J.W., eds. New York: Appleton-Century-Crofts, pp. 731–738.

Angeletti, R.H., and Bradshaw, R.A. (1971): Nerve growth factor from mouse submaxillary gland: Amino acid sequence. *Proc. Natl. Acad. Sci. USA* 68:2417–2420.

Bocchini, V., and Angeletti, P.U. (1969): The nerve growth factor: Purification as a 30,000-molecular-weight protein. *Proc. Natl. Acad. Sci. USA* 64:787–794.

Bueker, E D. (1948): Implantation of tumors in the hind limb field of the embryonic chick and the developmental response of the lumbosacral nervous system. *Anat. Rec.* 102:369–389.

Calissano, P., and Cozzari, C. (1974): Interaction of NGF with the mouse brain neurotubule proteins. *Proc. Natl. Acad. Sci. USA* 71:2131–2135.

Cohen, S. (1960): Purification of a nerve-growth promoting protein from the mouse salivary gland and its neurocytotoxic antiserum. *Proc. Natl. Acad. Sci. USA* 46:302–311.

Cohen, S. (1962): Isolation of a mouse submaxillary gland protein accelerating incisor eruption and eyelid opening in the new-born animal. *J. Biol. Chem.* 237:1555–1562.

Cohen, S., and Levi-Montalcini, R. (1956): A nerve growth-stimulating factor isolated from snake venom. *Proc. Natl. Acad. Sci. USA* 42:571–574.

Cohen, S., Levi-Montalcini, R., and Hamburger, V. (1954): A nerve growth-stimulating factor isolated from sarcomas 37 and 180. *Proc. Natl. Acad. Sci. USA* 40:1014–1018.

Dahlström, A. (1969): Synthesis, transport, and life-span of amine storage granules in sympathetic adrenergic neurons. *In: Cellular Dynamics of the Neuron* (Symposia of the International Society for Cell Biology, vol. 8). Barondes, S.H., ed. New York: Academic Press, pp. 153–174.

Edelman, G.M., Yahara, I., and Wang, J.L. (1973): Receptor mobility and receptor-cytoplasmic interactions in lymphocytes. *Proc. Natl. Acad. Sci. USA* 70:1442–1446.

Fine, R.E., and Bray, D. (1971): Actin in growing nerve cells. *Nature [New Biol.]* 234:115–118.

Hamburger, V. (1934): The effects of wing bud extirpation on the development of the central nervous system in chick embryos. *J. Exp. Zool.* 68:449–494.

Hendry, I.A., and Iversen, L.L. (1973): Reduction in the concentration of Nerve Growth Factor in mice after sialectomy and castration. *Nature* 243:500–504.

Inoué, S., and Sato, H. (1967): Cell motility by labile association of molecules. The nature of mitotic spindle fibers and their role in chromosome movement. *J. Gen. Physiol.* 50 (Suppl.):259–288.

Larrabee, M.G. (1972): Metabolism during development in sympathetic ganglia of chickens: Effects of age, nerve growth factor and metabolic inhibitors. *In*: Zaimis and Knight (1972), pp. 71–88.

Levi-Montalcini, R. (1949): The development of the acoustico-vestibular centers in the chick embryo in the absence of the afferent root fibers and of descending fiber tracts. *J. Comp. Neurol.* 91:209–241.

Levi-Montalcini, R. (1952): Effects of mouse tumor transplantation on the nervous system. *Ann. NY Acad. Sci.* 55:330–343.

Levi-Montalcini, R. (1964): Growth control of nerve cells by a protein factor and its antiserum. *Science* 143:105–110.

Levi-Montalcini, R. (1966): The Nerve Growth Factor: its mode of action on sensory and sympathetic nerve cells. *Harvey Lect.* 60:217–259.

Levi-Montalcini, R. (1974): Control mechanisms of the adrenergic neuron. *In: Dynamics of Degeneration and Growth in Neurons* (Wenner-Gren Symposium Series, vol. 22). Fuxe, K., ed. New York: Pergamon Press, pp. 297–314.

Levi-Montalcini, R., Aloe, L., and Johnson, E.M., Jr. (1973): Interaction between the nerve growth factor (NGF), guanethidine and 6-hydroxydopamine in sympathetic neurons. *In: Frontiers in Catecholamine Research* (III International Catecholamine Symposium, Université de Strasbourg, 1973). Usdin, E., and Snyder, S.H., eds. New York: Pergamon Press, pp. 267–276.

Levi-Montalcini, R., and Angeletti, P.U. (1968): Nerve growth factor. *Physiol. Rev.* 48:534–569.

Levi-Montalcini, R., and Angeletti, P.U. (1971): Ultrastructure and metabolic studies on sensory and sympathetic nerve cells treated with the nerve growth factor and its antiserum. *In: Hormones in Development*. Hamburgh, M., and Barrington, E.J.W., eds. New York: Appleton-Century-Crofts, pp. 719–730.

Levi-Montalcini, R., and Booker, B. (1960a): Excessive growth of the sympathetic ganglia evoked by a protein isolated from mouse salivary glands. *Proc. Natl. Acad. Sci. USA* 46:373–384.

Levi-Montalcini, R., and Booker, B. (1960b): Destruction of the sympathetic ganglia in mammals by an antiserum to a nerve-growth protein. *Proc. Natl. Acad. Sci. USA* 46:384–391.

Levi-Montalcini, R., Caramia, F., and Angeletti, P.U. (1969): Alterations in the fine structure of nucleoli in sympathetic neurons following NGF-antiserum treatment. *Brain Res.* 12:54–73.

Levi-Montalcini, R., Caramia, F., Luse, S.A., and Angeletti, P.U. (1968): In vitro effects of the nerve growth factor on the fine structure of the sensory nerve cells. *Brain Res.* 8:347–362.

Levi-Montalcini, R., and Hamburger, V. (1951): Selective growth stimulating effects of mouse sarcoma on the sensory and sympathetic nervous system of the chick embryo. *J. Exp. Zool.* 116: 321–361.

Levi-Montalcini, R., and Hamburger, V. (1953): A diffusible agent of mouse sarcoma, producing hyperplasia of sympathetic ganglia and hyperneurotization of viscera in the chick embryo. *J. Exp. Zool.* 123:233–287.

Levi-Montalcini, R., and Levi, G. (1942): Les conséquences de la destruction d'un territoire d'innervation périphérique sur le développement des centres nerveux correspondants dans l'embryon de poulet. *Arch. Biol. (Liège)* 53:537–545.

Levi-Montalcini, R., Meyer, H., and Hamburger, V. (1954): In vitro experiments on the effects of mouse sarcomas 180 and 37 on the spinal and sympathetic ganglia of the chick embryo. *Cancer Res.* 14:49–57.

Levi-Montalcini, R., Revoltella, L., and Calissano, P. (1974): Microtubule proteins in the Nerve Growth Factor-mediated response (interaction between the Nerve Growth Factor and its target cells). *Recent Prog. Horm. Res.* 30:635–669.

Lwoff, A. (1966): The prophage and I. *In: Phage and the Origins of Molecular Biology.* Cairns, J., Stent, G.S., and Watson, J.D., eds. Long Island, N.Y.: Cold Spring Harbor Laboratory of Quantitative Biology, pp. 88–99.

Moran, D.T., and Varela, F.G. (1971): Microtubules and sensory transduction. *Proc. Natl. Acad. Sci. USA* 68:757–760.

Plaut, M., Lichtenstein, L.M., and Henney, C.S. (1973): Studies on the mechanism of lymphocyte-mediated cytolysis. III. The role of microfilaments and microtubules. *J. Immunol.* 110: 771–780.

Revoltella, L., Bertolini, L., and Pediconi, M. (1974): Unmasking of Nerve Growth Factor membrane-specific binding sites in synchronized murine C 1300 neuroblastoma cells. *Exp. Cell Res.* 85:89–94.

Revoltella, R., Bertolini, L., Pediconi, M., and Vigneti, E. (1974): Specific binding of Nerve Growth Factor (NGF) by murine C 1300 neuroblastoma cells. *J. Exp. Med.* 140:437–451

Schmitt, F.O. (1950): The structure of the axon filaments of the giant nerve fibers of *Loligo* and *Myxicola. J. Exp. Zool.* 113:499–515.

Schmitt, F.O. (1957): The fibrous protein of the nerve axon. *J. Cell. Comp. Physiol.* 49:165–174.

Schmitt, F.O. (1968a): The molecular biology of neuronal fibrous proteins. *Neurosci. Res. Program Bull.* 6:119–144. Also *In: Neurosciences Research Symposium Summaries.* Vol. 3. Cambridge, Mass.: The MIT Press (1969), pp. 307–332.

Schmitt, F.O. (1968b): Fibrous proteins, neuronal organelles. *Proc. Natl. Acad. Sci. USA* 60:1092–1101.

Schmitt, F.O. (1970): Molecular neurobiology: An interpretive survey. *In: The Neurosciences: Second Study Program*. Schmitt, F.O., editor-in-chief. New York: Rockefeller University Press, pp. 867–879.

Schmitt, F.O., and Davison. P.F. (1961): Biologie moléculaire des neurofilaments. *In: Actualités Neurophysiologiques*. 3ième série. Monnier, A.-M., ed. Paris: Masson et Cie., pp. 355–369.

Schmitt, F.O., and Geren, B.B. (1950): The fibrous structure of the nerve axon in relation to the localization of "neurotubules." *J. Exp. Med.* 91:499–504.

Shelanski M.L., Gaskin, F., and Cantor, C.R. (1973): Microtubule assembly in the absence of added nucleotides. *Proc. Natl. Acad. Sci. USA* 70:765–768.

Steiner, G., and Schoenbaum, E., eds. (1972): *Immunosympathectomy*. Amsterdam: Elsevier.

Strom, T.B., Garovoy, M.R., Carpenter, C.B., and Merrill, J.P. (1973): Microtubule function in immune and nonimmune lymphocyte-mediated cytotoxicity. *Science* 181:171–172.

Taylor, A., Mamelak, M., Reaven, E., and Maffly, R. (1973): Vasopressin: Possible role of microtubules and microfilaments in its action. *Science* 181:347–349.

Taylor, D., and Varela, F.G. (1971): Microtubules and sensory transduction. *Proc. Natl. Acad. Sci. USA* 68:757–760.

Thoenen, H., and Tranzer, J.P. (1968): Chemical sympathectomy by selective destruction of adrenergic nerve endings with 6-hydroxydopamine. *Naunyn-Schmiedbergs Arch. Pharmacol.* 261:271–288.

Tilney, L.G. (1971): Origin and continuity of microtubules. *In: Origin and Continuity of Cell Organelles* (Results and Problems in Cell Differentiation. A Series of Topical Volumes in Developmental Biology. Vol. 2). Reinert, J., and Ursprung, H., eds. Berlin: Springer-Verlag, pp. 222–260.

Ukena, T.E., and Berlin, R.D. (1972): Effect of colchicine and vinblastine on the topographical separation of membrane functions. *J. Exp. Med.* 136:1–7.

Varon, S., Nomura, J., and Shooter, E.M. (1967): Subunit structure of a high-molecular-weight form of the nerve growth factor from mouse submaxillary gland. *Proc. Natl. Acad. Sci. USA* 57:1782–1789.

Weiss, P. (1967): Neuronal dynamics and axonal flow, III. Cellulifugal transport of labeled neuroplasm in isolated nerve preparations. *Proc. Natl. Acad. Sci. USA* 57:1239–1245.

Yamada, K.M., Spooner, B.S., and Wessells, N.K. (1970): Axon growth: Roles of microfilaments and microtubules. *Proc. Natl. Acad. Sci. USA* 66:1206–1212.

Zaimis, E., and Knight, J., eds. (1972): *Nerve Growth Factor and Its Antiserum*. London: Athlone Press of the University of London.

Proc. Natl. Acad. Sci. USA
Vol. 76, No. 10, pp. 5382–5386, October 1979
Neurobiology

Experimental autoimmune model of nerve growth factor deprivation: Effects on developing peripheral sympathetic and sensory neurons

(immunosympathectomy/neuronal development/trophic factor)

PAMELA DOLKART GORIN AND EUGENE M. JOHNSON

Department of Pharmacology, Washington University Medical School, St. Louis, Missouri 63110

Communicated by Oliver H. Lowry, June 19, 1979

ABSTRACT   An experimental autoimmune model of nerve growth factor (NGF) deprivation has been used to assess the role of NGF in the development of various cell types in the nervous system. Adult rats immunized with 2.5S mouse NGF in complete Freund's adjuvant produced antibodies that crossreacted with their own NGF and that were transferred *in utero* to the fetus and in milk to the neonate. Cross-fostering experiments were carried out to separate the effects of exposure to anti-NGF *in utero* from those due to exposure through the milk. Anti-NGF transferred *in utero* and in milk resulted in the destruction of peripheral sympathetic neurons assessed by morphological methods (light microscopy) and biochemical methods (tyrosine hydroxylase activity, choline acetyltransferase activity, and protein content). No effects were observed on the adrenal medulla. Offspring of NGF-immunized females exposed to anti-NGF *in utero* had a decreased protein content in the dorsal root ganglia and were unable to transport ^{125}I-labeled NGF injected in the forepaw to the dorsal root ganglia. These results suggest that a subpopulation of sensory neurons is dependent on NGF for survival during some period of fetal development. This model offers the potential for determining the degree and time of dependence of various cell types on NGF.

Nerve growth factor (NGF) is a protein that acts on peripheral neurons of neural crest origin in both avian and mammalian species (1). Much evidence suggests that NGF is a retrogradely transported trophic factor that regulates the development of immature sympathetic peripheral neurons and the maintenance of mature sympathetic neurons (2–4). Very little is known about the role of NGF for mammalian sensory neurons, although it has been shown that rat dorsal root ganglion (DRG) neurons retain the capability of retrograde axonal transport of NGF throughout postnatal development (5).

One means of assessing the physiological role of NGF on the diverse neuronal populations of the developing mammalian nervous system is to deprive cells of NGF. Because the normal source of NGF is not known, and specific NGF antagonists are not available, the only mechanism of producing a systemic deprivation of NGF is immunological. Previous studies (6–8) have demonstrated that antibodies to NGF can be prepared by repeated injections of animals with NGF derived from mouse. These and subsequent studies, using anti-NGF serum, demonstrated that mammalian sympathetic neurons of the para- and prevertebral ganglia die if deprived of NGF during the neonatal period. Other neural cell types (the short adrenergic neurons innervating the urogenital tract and brown adipose tissue, adrenal medullary chromaffin cells, peripheral sensory neurons of the DRG, and central adrenergic neurons) are not destroyed by anti-NGF serum administered in the neonatal period (9, 10).

The usefulness of antiserum-induced NGF deprivation is limited by problems associated with its repeated administration—e.g., serum sickness. An alternative approach, we have developed an experimental "autoimmune" model of NGF deprivation and have studied the prenatal and postnatal effects of NGF deprivation. The model is "autoimmune" in that rats immunized with 2.5S mouse NGF develop serum antibodies that crossreact with their own NGF and that are transferred to the offspring *in utero* and in milk.

MATERIAL AND METHODS

Animal Treatments. Adult Sprague–Dawley rats (200–250 g) were immunized with 100 μg of 2.5S mouse NGF (11) in complete Freund's adjuvant and were boosted at 4–6-week intervals with 10μg of NGF in complete Freund's adjuvant. Unimmunized rats and rats immunized with cytochrome *c* (Sigma)—a protein with physical properties similar to those of NGF—were used as controls.

Three types of treatment protocols were utilized: (*i*) Passive transfer experiments were carried out to test the crossreactivity of rat serum antibodies raised against mouse NGF with the rats' own NGF. (*ii*) Maternal transfer of anti-NGF *in utero* and through milk was assessed by evaluation of various tissues in offspring born to NGF-immunized females. (*iii*) Cross-fostering experiments were carried out to separate the effects of anti-NGF exposure *in utero* from those due to anti-NGF in milk.

Passive Transfer. In the passive transfer experiments 0.30 ml of sera from NGF-immunized adult rats (titer ≥ 500), sera from control-immunized rats, or sera from unimmunized rats were injected subcutaneously into neonatal rats at postnatal days 1 and 3. Rats were killed at 1 week of age. Superior cervical ganglia (SCGs) were removed for histological and biochemical analysis.

Maternal Transfer. NGF-immunized female rats, cytochrome *c*-immunized female rats, or unimmunized female rats were mated with unimmunized males. Offspring were killed within 12 hr of birth to assess the effects of exposure to anti-NGF *in utero*, and at 1 week or at 8 weeks of age to assess the effects of exposure to anti-NGF both *in utero* and in milk. Blood was obtained for titering. SCGs and adrenals were removed for biochemical analysis, and DRGs were removed for protein determination. SCGs and DRGs were removed for histology.

Cross-Fostering. For the cross-fostering experiments half of a litter born to an NGF-immunized female was exchanged at birth with half of a litter born to an unimmunized or cytochrome *c*-immunized control female. The cross-fostering technique produced two groups of offspring: rats exposed to anti-NGF only *in utero* and rats exposed to anti-NGF only in

---

Abbreviations: SCG, superior cervical ganglion; DRG, dorsal root ganglion; NGF, nerve growth factor.

Neurobiology: Gorin and Johnson

Proc. Natl. Acad. Sci. USA 76 (1979) 5383

milk. These groups were compared to offspring that were born to and nursed by an NGF-immunized female, and to offspring born to and nursed by a control female. Offspring were killed at 2 weeks of age (12 weeks for the retrograde transport experiment). Both SCGs were removed for enzyme analysis and five DRGs at the cervical level (C4–C8) were removed for protein determination.

Titering of Antisera. Serum titers of anti-NGF were monitored, using a modification of the embryonic chicken DRG bioassay (12, 13). Twenty-five microliters of antiserum mixed with NGF (diluted antiserum mixed with an equal volume of 2.5S NGF at 30 ng/ml) was added to 25 μl of chicken plasma (GIBCO), containing three or four DRGs from 9-day chicken embryos. Twenty-five microliters of basal Eagle's medium (1×, 25 mM Hepes buffer, GIBCO), containing kanamycin sulfate (Sigma) at 33 μg/ml and thrombin (Parke, Davis) at 2.5 mg/ml, was then added for a final volume of 75 μl. Titers are defined as being greater than or equal to the reciprocal of the highest serum dilution that blocked the outgrowth of neurites.

Biochemical Analysis. For enzyme measurements, SCGs and adrenals were homogenized in 5 mM Tris·HCl buffer, pH 7.4, containing 0.2% Triton X-100, at a dilution that ensured that the reaction was linear with enzyme concentration and time. Tyrosine hydroxylase (EC 1.14.16.2) activity was measured by a modification of the method of Phillipson and Sandler (14) in the presence of 40 μM tyrosine and 625 μM 6-methyl-5,6,7,8-tetrahydropterine dihydrochloride. Choline acetyltransferase (EC 2.3.1.6) activity was measured by the method of Schrier and Shuster (15) in the presence of 25 mM potassium phosphate, 50 mM choline chloride, 24 μM dithiothreitol, and 10 μM [^{14}C]acetyl-CoA. Proteins were determined by the method of Lowry *et al.* (16) with bovine serum albumin as the standard.

Histological Analysis. SCGs and DRGs were fixed in 10% (vol/vol) formol saline. After dehydration in graded ethanol solutions, ganglia were embedded in paraffin, cut in 7-μm sections, and stained with toluidine blue. Sections from comparable levels were examined under the light microscope for obvious changes in neuronal size or number. No quantitative analyses were performed.

Retrograde Transport. ^{125}I-Labeled NGF (^{125}I-NGF) (1.7 pmol, 3 × 10^6 cpm) was prepared by the lactoperoxidase method (17) and was injected into the forepaw (10 μl) in 12-week-old cross-fostered offspring and offspring of NGF-immunized and control females (see *Animal Treatments*). At 12 hr, the time of peak accumulation (5), animals were killed by decapitation and cervical DRGs C5–C8 were excised on both the ipsilateral and contralateral sides and their radioactivities were measured in a Beckman gamma counter. Both labeled and unlabeled NGF were kindly supplied by Nicholas Costrini and Ralph Bradshaw.

Statistical Methods. The Student's t test for independent groups was used for comparing the means of two groups. When there were more than two groups, analysis of variance was carried out, using either raw data or a logarithmic transformation, depending on which produced homogeneous variances (18).

RESULTS

Passive Transfer. Passive transfer of anti-NGF was demonstrated by the ability of antiserum from adult rats immunized with 2.5S mouse NGF to produce an immunosympathectomy in neonatal rats. SCGs from neonatal rats injected at 1 and 3 days of age with adult rat anti-NGF serum were markedly reduced in size and showed extensive neuronal loss in the SCG at 1 week of age (Fig. 1B). Control antiserum from adult rats

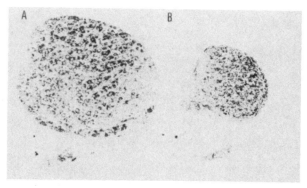

FIG. 1. SCG (×81) of neonatal rats injected with rat anti-cytochrome *c* serum (*A*) or rat anti-NGF serum (*B*). Neonates were injected subcutaneously with 0.3 ml of adult anti-NGF serum (titer ≥500) or anti-cytochrome *c* serum on postnatal days 1 and 3. Neonates were killed by decapitation at 1 week.

immunized with cytochrome *c* produced no morphological effects on neonatal SCG neurons (Fig. 1A).

Tyrosine hydroxylase was also measured in the SCG as an indication of destruction of sympathetic neurons in ganglia. Activity (nmol tyrosine hydroxylated per pair per hour) was 0.30 ± 0.03 ($n = 6$) in 1-week-old animals injected with anti-NGF serum, 4.05 ± 0.09 ($n = 4$) in animals injected with anti-cytochrome *c* serum, and 4.12 ± 0.27 ($n = 5$) in neonates injected with normal rat serum.

Evaluation of the Sympathetic Nervous System of Offspring Born to and Nursed by Female Rats Immunized with NGF. Tyrosine hydroxylase is the rate-limiting enzyme for catecholamine biosynthesis (19) and may be used as an index of maturation of postsynaptic neurons of the SCG and chromaffin cells of the adrenal medulla (20). It has been shown in the mouse SCG that choline acetyltransferase is a valid biochemical index of synapse formation of preganglionic cholinergic neuronal terminals on the principal ganglion cells (20). Tyrosine hydroxylase, choline acetyltransferase, and protein undergo developmental increases after birth in the normal rat SCG, reaching adult levels by 7 to 8 weeks (21). The changes in enzymes and protein seen at the various times are described below for SCG and adrenal. Because there were never significant differences between offspring of unimmunized females and offspring of cytochrome *c*-immunized females, in some cases only one type of control was used. No difference in size, appearance, or vitality was seen in the offspring of animals immunized against NGF or cytochrome *c*.

Tyrosine hydroxylase and choline acetyltransferase activities at birth in the SCGs of offspring exposed to anti-NGF *in utero* were reduced to one-third of those in offspring of control females (Fig. 2 *A* and *B*). Protein levels in the SCG were reduced to less than half of control levels at birth in offspring of NGF-immunized females (Fig. 2C). The decrease in enzyme activities and protein levels at birth in the offspring of NGF-immunized females reflected the marked neuronal atrophy and neuronal loss that were apparent at the light microscopic level (not shown).

Even greater reductions in ganglionic enzyme activities and protein content were observed in offspring of NGF-immunized females killed at 1 week and at 8 weeks of age. Tyrosine hydroxylase activity, choline acetyltransferase activity, and protein levels in the SCG at 1 week and at 8 weeks of age are shown in Fig. 2 *A*, *B*, and *C*, respectively.

Tyrosine hydroxylase activity was determined in the adrenal

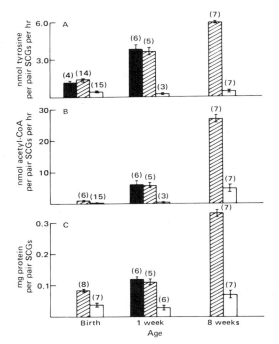

FIG. 2. Tyrosine hydroxylase (*A*), choline acetyltransferase (*B*), and protein levels (*C*) in the SCG of offspring born to and nursed by NGF-immunized or control female rats. Bars represent means ± SEM for offspring of unimmunized control females (solid bars), offspring of cytochrome *c*-immunized females (hatched bars), and offspring of NGF-immunized females (open bars). Number in parentheses at top of bar refers to number of animals in treatment group. In each case, means for the offspring of NGF-immunized rats were significantly different from the means for control groups (*P* < 0.001). There were no significant differences between the two control groups. Anti-NGF titers of offspring of NGF-immunized rats were ≥10 to <50 at birth, ≥50 to <100 at 1 week, and <10 at 8 weeks (4 weeks after weaning). Anti-NGF titers of mothers were ≥500.

glands of animals at birth, at 1 week of age, and at 8 weeks of age. At none of these times was there a difference in enzyme activity in adrenals of animals born to and nursed by anti-NGF producing rats when compared to offspring of either type of control rat (data not shown).

Comparison of Prenatal and Postnatal Effects of Anti-NGF on the Sympathetic Nervous System: Cross-Fostering Experiments. In order to separate the effects of anti-NGF exposure *in utero* from those due to anti-NGF in milk, cross-fostering experiments were carried out. In two different experiments results were similar, and Table 1 contains the pooled data of the two experiments. Significant reductions in tyrosine hydroxylase activity and protein levels in the SCG were seen in rats exposed to anti-NGF only *in utero*, only in milk, and in both situations (Table 1). Serum titers of neonates nursing from NGF-immunized females were higher than those of offspring exposed to anti-NGF only *in utero* (see legend to Table 1). All neonates nursed by control mothers had no serum titers of anti-NGF at 2 weeks.

Comparison of Prenatal and Postnatal Effects of Anti-NGF on Protein Content in the DRG: Cross-Fostering Experiments. In preliminary experiments it was noted that the protein content in DRGs of offspring of NGF-immunized females was significantly lower (35%) than control levels at birth, and it remained significantly lower (22%) in 8-week-old animals.

Table 1. Comparison of prenatal and postnatal effects of anti-NGF in rat SCG: Cross-fostering experiments

Exposure to anti-NGF*		Number in group	Protein,[†] mg per pair SCGs	Tyrosine hydroxylase activity,[†] nmol tyrosine hydroxylated per pair SCGs per hr
In utero	Milk			
−	−	8	0.201 ± 0.011 (100 ± 5%)	4.91 ± 0.30 (100 ± 6%)
+	−	6	0.075 ± 0.013[‡] (37 ± 6%)	1.81 ± 0.37[‡] (37 ± 7%)
−	+	8	0.055 ± 0.006[‡] (27 ± 3%)	0.221 ± 0.033[‡] (5 ± 1%)
+	+	5	0.044 ± 0.010[‡] (22 ± 5%)	0.020 ± 0.020[‡] (0.4 ± 0.4%)

* Anti-NGF titers in offspring at time of sacrifice (2 weeks of age) were <10 for the *in utero* group (≥10 to <50 at birth), ≥100 to <500 for the milk group, and ≥100 to <500 for the *in utero* plus milk group. Anti-NGF titers of NGF-immunized mothers at time of sacrifice of offspring were ≥100 to <1000.
[†] Number in parentheses is the mean ± SEM expressed as percent of control. Results were similar for two different experiments and data within each treatment group were pooled.
[‡] Significant differences (*P* < 0.001) resulted from exposure to anti-NGF *in utero* or in milk.

The separation of effects of anti-NGF exposure *in utero* from those due to anti-NGF in milk on protein content in the DRG of 2-week-old rats cross-fostered at birth is shown in Table 2. Protein levels in the DRG were significantly reduced in both groups exposed to anti-NGF *in utero*. Similar reductions in protein (20–30%) were seen in rats killed at 8 weeks or at 12 weeks (data not shown). The group exposed to anti-NGF in milk alone showed no significant reduction in DRG protein. Serum titers of nursing offspring of NGF-immunized females were higher than those of offspring exposed to anti-NGF only *in utero*, as described previously (Table 1).

Effect of Exposure to Anti-NGF on Retrograde Axonal Transport in the DRG. The decrease in protein content in DRGs from animals exposed to anti-NGF *in utero* suggested the possibility that a population of sensory neurons had not survived. Preliminary experiments were carried out in 8-week-old animals born to and nursed by anti-NGF-producing mothers to determine if these animals retained the ability to

Table 2. Comparison of prenatal and postnatal effects of anti-NGF in rat DRG: Cross-fostering experiments

Exposure to anti-NGF*		Number in group	Protein,[†] mg/DRG
In utero	Milk		
−	−	8	0.047 ± 0.002 (100 ± 5%)
+	−	6	0.035 ± 0.002[‡] (74 ± 2%)
−	+	8	0.043 ± 0.003 (91 ± 6%)
+	+	5	0.033 ± 0.001[‡] (70 ± 2%)

* Anti-NGF titers in offspring at time of sacrifice (2 weeks of age) were <10 for the *in utero* group (≥10 to <50 at birth), ≥100 to <500 for the milk group, and ≥100 to <500 for the *in utero* plus milk group. Anti-NGF titers of NGF-immunized mothers at time of sacrifice of offspring were ≥100 to <1000.
[†] Number in parentheses is the mean ± SEM expressed as percent of control. Results were similar for two different experiments and data within each treatment group were pooled.
[‡] Only *in utero* exposure to anti-NGF resulted in significant differences (*P* < 0.01).

Neurobiology: Gorin and Johnson

Proc. Natl. Acad. Sci. USA 76 (1979)   5385

Table 3. Comparison of prenatal and postnatal effects of anti-NGF on retrograde transport of ^{125}I-NGF in sensory neurons of adult rats: Cross-fostering experiments

Exposure to anti-NGF*		Number in group	Transport,† cpm/four DRGs	
In utero	Milk		Ipsilateral	Contralateral
−	−	8	1637 ± 127	83 ± 18
+	−	7	391 ± 58‡	50 ± 32
−	+	6	1273 ± 94§	80 ± 40
+	+	3	256 ± 83¶	80 ± 61

* At the time of the transport experiment (12 weeks of age) no animals had serum titers of anti-NGF. At time of weaning (4 weeks of age) anti-NGF titers were <10 for the in utero group (≥10 to <50 at birth), ≥100 for the milk group, and ≥100 for the in utero plus milk group. Anti-NGF titers of NGF-immunized mothers at time of weaning were ≥100 to <1000.
† Mean ± SEM of DRGs (C5–C8) from animals injected in the forepaw with 3×10^6 cpm of ^{125}I-NGF (1.7 pmol) and killed 12 hr later.
‡ Significant difference ($P < 0.0001$) resulted from in utero exposure to anti-NGF.
§ Significant difference ($P < 0.05$) resulted from in milk exposure to anti-NGF.
¶ Significant difference ($P < 0.0001$) resulted from exposure to anti-NGF both in utero and in milk.

retrogradely transport NGF in the peripheral sensory ganglia. After it had been determined that these animals no longer had circulating anti-NGF antibodies, ^{125}I-NGF was injected into a forepaw. The animals were killed 12 hr later (time of maximal accumulation), and the radioactivity in ipsilateral and contralateral DRGs (C5–C8) was determined. The accumulation of retrogradely transported ^{125}I-NGF in the ipsilateral DRGs was reduced by 90% (data not shown). The experiment was then repeated in cross-fostered animals in order to assess the relative importance of prenatal and postnatal exposure to anti-NGF. The data in Table 3 demonstrate a pattern of sensitivity to anti-NGF quite different from that seen in sympathetic ganglia (Table 1) but entirely consistent with the DRG protein data in Table 2. Exposure to anti-NGF in utero reduced retrograde transport of ^{125}I-NGF (ipsilateral minus contralateral) by 80–90%, as seen in the preliminary experiment. Despite the much higher titers of anti-NGF achieved postnatally, exposure to anti-NGF in milk alone produced only a small (23%) decrease in retrograde transport of ^{125}I-NGF.

DISCUSSION

Experiments have been reported (22–24) in which attempts have been made to determine the effect of injections of heterologous anti-NGF serum into pregnant mice on the sympathetic nervous systems of the fetus. The results have produced conflicting data and in no case was the titer of antisera in either the mother or offspring determined. Levi-Montalcini and Angeletti (22) failed to see an effect on offspring when heterologous (rabbit) anti-NGF serum was injected into pregnant mice. Administration of the same antiserum to lactating mice resulted in destruction of sympathetic neurons in the suckling offspring. Klingman and Klingman (23, 24) injected heterologous anti-NGF serum into pregnant mice during different periods of gestation and analyzed cell numbers in the SCG and tissue catecholamines in the offspring at 1–7 months of age. The decreases observed were ascribed to in utero transfer of anti-NGF. However, because offspring were evaluated 1–7 months after birth (rather than at birth), and because cross-fostering experiments were not used to exclude the distinct possibility that the effects were due to antibody reaching the neonate through the milk, the conclusions of Klingman and Klingman are subject to doubt.

The work described in this paper utilizes an experimental "autoimmune" model in which 2.5S mouse NGF is administered to rats. The demonstration of passive transfer of homologous serum anti-NGF in rats (Fig. 1) is consistent with a similar demonstration in rabbits in the original paper describing immunosympathectomy (8). The presence of serum titers of anti-NGF that disappear within a few days of birth in cross-fostered animals, histological changes in the SCG, and the reduction in tyrosine hydroxylase activity in the SCG at birth demonstrate that offspring born to NGF-immunized female rats were exposed in utero to anti-NGF (presumably of maternal origin). In general, there was a correlation between serum titer in the mother and amount of tyrosine hydroxylase reduction in the neonate at birth. An exception was one litter (out of nine litters examined) in which there were normal levels of tyrosine hydroxylase activity in the SCGs of the offspring despite a moderate titer (≥100 to <500) in the mother. At no time was anti-NGF activity detected in serum of offspring born to control females. The bioassay used to determine serum titers detects antibodies that react with mouse NGF. The precise titers against rat NGF are not known, because rat NGF is not available. It is possible that a number of subclasses of antibodies directed against mouse NGF are produced by the mother and that the various subclasses differ in their affinity for rat NGF and in their availability to the developing embryo.

Effects of Prenatal and Postnatal Anti-NGF on the Peripheral Sympathetic Nervous System. The failure of tyrosine hydroxylase to reach control levels by 8 weeks indicates that prenatal or neonatal (or both) exposure to anti-NGF results in interference with the normal biochemical development of adrenergic neurons in the SCG. The persistence of reduced tyrosine hydroxylase activity and reduced ganglion size into adulthood, coupled with the histological observations in the SCG at birth, suggest that there is an extensive loss of SCG neurons in offspring born to NGF-immunized females. Morphometric analysis of the SCG is required to exclude the unlikely possibility that neuronal atrophy, rather than neuronal death, accounts for these changes. The failure of choline acetyltransferase to reach control levels by 8 weeks probably represents a permanent retrograde transynaptic effect on presynaptic neurons. Retrograde degenerative changes in preganglionic neurons have been demonstrated in neonatally sympathectomized rats (25–27).

The results of the cross-fostering experiments confirm that rat anti-NGF is transferred both in utero and in milk. The finding of a prenatal period of susceptibility to NGF deprivation for SCG neurons (shown by decreases in tyrosine hydroxylase activity and protein levels at 2 weeks) is consistent with recent in vitro findings with SCG explants from mouse embryos. Coughlin et al. (28) demonstrated that ganglia from 14-day mouse fetuses showed abundant neurite outgrowth and normal developmental increases in tyrosine hydroxylase activity in vitro in the presence of anti-NGF. Ganglia from 18-day fetuses, which showed neurite outgrowth with exogenous NGF, had no neurite outgrowth and reduced levels of tyrosine hydroxylase activity when cultured without exogenous NGF or in the presence of anti-NGF. The finding of transfer of anti-NGF in milk is consistent with the morphological observations of Levi-Montalcini and Angeletti (22) in neonatal mice nursed by mothers injected with rabbit anti-mouse NGF serum. Future fetal studies using the in vivo autoimmune model should be able to determine precisely the onset of NGF dependence in SCG and other peripheral sympathetic neurons and determine unambiguously whether migration, differentiation, and neuronal survival are NGF dependent.

Our finding of normal levels of adrenal tyrosine hydroxylase in offspring exposed to anti-NGF *in utero* and during the first few weeks of postnatal life via mothers' milk suggests that the adrenal is insensitive to anti-NGF. The relative resistance of the adrenal compared to sympathetic ganglia may be due to locally higher concentrations of NGF in the adrenal. It has been shown in organ cultures that mouse adrenal medullary cells are capable of NGF secretion (29). The lack of biochemical evidence of adrenal medullary degeneration in animals exposed to anti-NGF *in utero* is inconsistent with the recent morphological findings of Aloe and Levi-Montalcini (30). These workers injected heterologous anti-NGF into rats at day 17 *in utero* and for the first 8 days of postnatal life and saw degeneration of adrenal medullary cells. It is possible that this discrepancy is due to differences in levels of anti-NGF attained with maternal transfer of anti-NGF vs. exogenous administration of anti-NGF.

Effects of Prenatal and Postnatal Anti-NGF on Peripheral Sensory Neurons. Retrograde axonal transport of ^{125}I-NGF can be used as a functional test for the presence of sensory neurons that are NGF dependent at some stage of development, if it is assumed that the sensory neurons capable of retrogradely transporting NGF (5) are the putative NGF-dependent cells. The present findings that *in utero* exposure to anti-NGF results in a 20–30% decrease in protein levels in the adult DRG and that adult rats exposed to anti-NGF *in utero* have a markedly reduced ability to retrogradely transport ^{125}I-NGF to the DRG suggest that NGF is required for the survival of a subpopulation of DRG sensory neurons in the rat. Definitive proof that cell death occurs will require morphometric analysis of the DRG. The period of susceptibility to anti-NGF (and presumably dependence on NGF) appears restricted to a period prior to birth. This is consistent with findings in the chicken embryo which show that DRG explants require NGF for survival and neurite outgrowth (1). Herrup and Shooter (31) have shown that the disappearance of NGF-stimulated neurite outgrowth *in vitro* between 14 and 16 days of embryonic life is coincident with loss of the ability to bind NGF to specific cell surface receptors in the chicken DRG. Thus a subpopulation of avian sensory neurons appears to be sensitive to NGF *in vitro* only during a circumscribed period of development. A potential role for NGF in the development of sensory neurons in mammals is supported by *in vitro* studies in which dissociated DRGs (but not intact ganglia) from newborn mice and rats show enhanced survival and neurite outgrowth in the presence of NGF (32, 33).

The experimental autoimmune model of NGF deprivation presented in this report should prove to be a useful tool in addressing some of the critical questions concerning the role of NGF in neuronal development. Which cell types are dependent on NGF at any stage of development for survival or maintenance? At what stage in the life of a cell population is NGF required? In addition to elucidating basic trophic mechanisms in neuronal development, the experimental autoimmune model of NGF deprivation may be helpful in elucidating pathophysiological mechanisms in developmental abnormalities of the peripheral nervous system, such as those manifested in familial dysautonomia and the hereditary sensory neuropathies.

The authors thank Mr. Glennon Fox for his excellent technical assistance and Ms. Vapor Robertson for her conscientious care of the animals. The authors also thank Drs. Nicholas Costrini and Ralph Bradshaw for their material and moral support and Drs. Arthur Loewy and John Russell for their many helpful discussions. This work was supported by the National Foundation–March of Dimes, National Institutes of Health Grants HL-20604, and National Institutes of Health Training Grant 5 T32 HL07275. E.M.J. is an Established Investigator of the American Heart Association.

1. Levi-Montalcini, R. & Angeletti, P. U. (1968) *Physiol. Rev.* **48,** 534–569.
2. Mobley, W. C., Server, A. C., Ishii, P. N., Riopelle, R. J. & Shooter, E. M. (1977) *N. Engl. J. Med.* **297,** 1096–1104.
3. Mobley, W. C., Server, A. C., Ishii, D. N., Riopelle, R. J. & Shooter, E. M. (1977) *N. Engl. J. Med.* **297,** 1149–1188.
4. Black, I. B. (1978) *Annu. Rev. Neurosci.* **1,** 183–214.
5. Stoeckel, K., Schwab, M. & Thoenen, H. (1975) *Brain Res.* **89,** 1–14.
6. Cohen, S. (1960) *Proc. Natl. Acad. Sci. USA* **46,** 302–311.
7. Levi-Montalcini, R. & Cohen, S. (1960) *Ann. N.Y. Acad. Sci.* **85,** 324–341.
8. Levi-Montalcini, R. & Booker, B. (1960) *Proc. Natl. Acad. Sci. USA* **46,** 373–384.
9. Levi-Montalcini, R. (1972) in *Immunosympathectomy,* eds. Steiner, G. & Schönbaum, E. (Elsevier, Amsterdam), pp. 55–78.
10. Konkol, R. J., Mailman, R. B., Bendeich, E. G., Garrison, M., Mueller, R. A. & Breese, G. R. (1978) *Brain Res.* **144,** 277–285.
11. Bocchini, V. & Angeletti, P. U. (1969) *Proc. Natl. Acad. Sci. USA* **64,** 787–794.
12. Levi-Montalcini, R., Meyer, H. & Hamburger, V. (1954) *Cancer Res.* **14,** 49–57.
13. Fenton, E. L. (1970) *Exp. Cell Res.* **59,** 383–392.
14. Phillipson, O. T., & Sandler, M. (1975) *Brain Res.* **90,** 283–296.
15. Schrier, B. K. & Shuster, L. (1967) *J. Neurochem.* **14,** 977–985.
16. Lowry, O. H., Rosebrough, N. J., Farr, A. L. & Randall, R. J. (1951) *J. Biol. Chem.* **193,** 265–275.
17. Marchalonis, J. J. (1969) *Biochem. J.* **113,** 299–305.
18. Snedecor, G. W. & Cochran, W. G. (1967) *Statistical Methods* (Iowa State Univ. Press, Ames, IO).
19. Levitt, M., Spector, S., Sjoerdsma, A. & Udenfriend, S. (1965) *J. Pharmacol. Exp. Ther.* **148,** 1–8.
20. Black, I. B., Hendry, I. A. & Iversen, L. L. (1971) *Brain Res.* **34,** 229–240.
21. Thoenen, H., Kettler, R. & Saner, A. (1972) *Brain Res.* **40,** 459–468.
22. Levi-Montalcini, R. & Angeletti, P.U. (1961) *Q. Rev. Biol.* **36,** 99–108.
23. Klingman, G. I. (1966) *Int. J. Neuropharmacol.* **5,** 163–170.
24. Klingman, G. I. & Klingman, J. D. (1967) *Int. J. Neuropharmacol.* **6,** 501–508.
25. Black, I. B., Hendry, I. A. & Iversen, L. L. (1972) *J. Physiol.* **221,** 149–159.
26. Aguayo, A. J., Peyronnard, J. M., Terry, L. C., Romine, J. S. & Bray, G. M. (1976) *J. Neurocytol.* **5,** 137–155.
27. Johnson, E. M., Caserta, M. T. & Ross, L. L. (1977) *Brain Res.* **140,** 1–10.
28. Coughlin, M. D., Boyer, D. M. & Black, I. B. (1977) *Proc. Natl. Acad. Sci. USA* **74,** 3438–3442.
29. Harper, G. P., Pearce, F. L. & Vernon, C. A. (1976) *Nature (London)* **261,** 251–253.
30. Aloe, L. & Levi-Montalcini, R. (1979) *Proc. Natl. Acad. Sci. USA* **76,** 1246–1250.
31. Herrup, K. & Shooter, E. M. (1975) *J. Cell Biol.* **67,** 118–125.
32. Burnham, P., Raiborn, C. & Varon, S. (1972) *Proc. Natl. Acad. Sci. USA* **69,** 3556–3560.
33. Varon, S., Raiborn, C. & Tyszyka, E. (1973) *Brain Res.* **54,** 51–63.

Reprinted from Science, Vol. 206, pp. 1079–1080. 1979

Neuronal Chemotaxis: Chick Dorsal-Root Axons Turn Toward High Concentrations of Nerve Growth Factor

Abstract. *Micropipettes containing 2 to 50 biological units of β nerve growth factor (NGF) were placed near growing axons of chick dorsal-root ganglion neurons in tissue culture. The axons turned and grew toward the NGF source within 21 minutes. This turning response to elevated concentrations of NGF appears to represent chemotactic guidance rather than a general enhancement of growth rate.*

Chemotaxis, the attraction of living protoplasm to a chemical substance, may help guide axons to their target tissues. Several studies in vitro (*1–3*) suggest that β nerve growth factor (NGF), a protein known to enhance axonal outgrowth from dorsal-root and sympathetic ganglia (*4*), is a chemotactic agent. These studies, however, leave unresolved the question of whether NGF actually guides axonal growth or simply enhances the survival or growth rate of axons that happen to be growing near the NGF source. We sought to distinguish between these possibilities by continuously observing the growth cones of chick dorsal-root axons that were exposed to a localized source of NGF. We found that these axons turn and grow toward the NGF source within 21 minutes, even if the background concentration of NGF is sufficient to support survival and rapid axonal growth.

Table 1. Turning response of dorsal-root ganglion axons to NGF.

Concentration of NGF (BU/ml)		Number of axons	
Back-ground	Micro-pipette	Positive response*	No response†
1	50	40	0
1	1	0	40
1	1 (+ BSA‡)	0	5
1	1 (+ FCS§)	0	5
0	1	0	5
1	2	5	0

*Rate of turn, 3.3 ± 0.2 deg/min.　†Rate of turn, 0.01 ± 0.14 deg/min.　‡Bovine serum albumin (0.1 mg/ml) added.　§Fetal calf serum (2.5 μl/ml) added.

Lumbosacral dorsal-root ganglia from White Leghorn chick embryos 7 and 12 days of age were excised and placed onto glass cover slips coated with a mixture of collagen and poly-L-lysine (25:1 by weight). The explants were incubated in air at 34°C in 35-mm plastic petri dishes with nutrient medium similar to Ham's F-12 except buffered with 1,4-piperazinediethanesulfonic acid (Pipes). The medium was supplemented with 5 to 10 biological units (BU) of NGF per milliliter (*5, 6*). After 24 hours, the cover slips were placed in an observation chamber (34°C) and were viewed with an inverted phase-contrast microscope (×750).

A micropipette (tip diameter, 2 to 4 μm) filled with NGF (1 to 50 BU per milliliter of perfusion medium) was used as a localized NGF source. The tip of the micropipette was placed about 25 μm from the tip of a growth cone at approximately 45° to the axon's longitudinal axis (Fig. 1a) and slightly above the surface of the medium. A separate perfusion system added perfusion medium to one side of the observation chamber while continuously removing medium from the opposite side with a vacuum line. This system produced a flow of medium (25 ml/hour) past the axon in a direction opposite to the initial direction of axonal growth. The NGF, flowing from the micropipette at the rate of 1 to 2 μl/hour, was carried along with this background flow, producing a higher concentration of NGF on the side of the growth cone nearest the micropipette (this was initially determined with methylene blue).

Figure 1 shows a dramatic example of

the effect of an NGF concentration gradient on the direction of axonal growth. The five photographs were taken over a 90-minute observation period during which successive repositionings of the NGF-filled micropipette resulted in an almost complete reversal of the axon's original direction of growth. Figure 1a shows the growth cone and the NGF-filled micropipette at the onset of perfusion. As the growing axon gradually turned toward the NGF source, the micropipette was moved to the position shown in Fig. 1b, and the growth cone grew toward the new position. Three subsequent repositionings (Fig. 1, c to e) resulted in a horseshoe-shaped pattern of axon growth (Fig. 1e).

In order to accurately measure the turning response of the axon to NGF, similar experiments were performed in which observation periods of shorter duration (30 minutes) were used and the lateral displacement of the cone tip was measured. Lateral displacement was measured as the shortest distance between the line described by the original axis of the axon and the new position of the growth cone. A lateral displacement of 20 μm within the 30 minutes of observation was considered a positive response (Table 1).

Dorsal-root axons bathed in a background solution containing NGF (1 BU/ml) were exposed to concentrated NGF (50 BU/ml) from a micropipette. All 40 axons tested turned and grew toward the NGF source (Table 1), exhibiting a lateral displacement of 20 μm in 9 to 21 minutes. In control experiments in which the micropipette contained the same concentration of NGF as the background, the axons showed only small random displacements (5 μm or less) toward or away from the micropipette and were scored as no response (Table 1). In ten of these control experiments, growth cones were observed for 2 hours. Lateral axonal displacements were less than 10 μm toward or away from the micropipette. No significant turning or lateral displacement was observed in these control axons even if the pipette was moved in the same pattern as for a positive response. Thus the turning of the axon toward elevated concentrations of NGF is not a response to pipette movement or movement of fluid from the pipette. Nor is the turning response associated with an increase in rate of growth, since the control and experimental axons grew at almost identical rates (88 ± 33 and 85 ± 39 μm/hour, respectively).

The turning response is not just a nonspecific attraction of growing dorsal-root

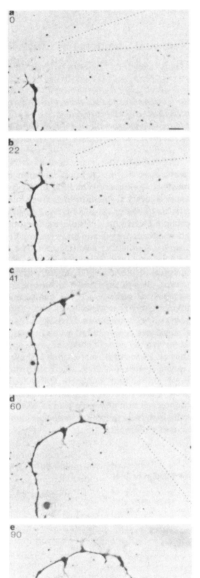

Fig. 1. Sequential photographs of a dorsal-root growth cone bathed in NGF (1 BU/ml) and exposed to an NGF gradient created by outflow from a micropipette containing NGF at 50 BU/ml. Numbers indicate time in minutes after the onset of perfusion by micropipette; dotted lines outline the micropipette in its successive placements. The growth rate for this axon was 72 μm/hour. After 90 minutes, the axon had grown 108 μm and had turned almost 160° relative to its original direction of growth. Scale bar, 10 μm.

axons to any protein source, since axons did not turn toward micropipettes containing bovine serum albumin or fetal calf serum (Table 1). But these axons are very sensitive to even low concentrations of NGF. We observed turning responses (20-μm lateral displacements) of axons toward micropipettes containing as little as 2 BU of NGF per milliliter, which was only 1 BU/ml above the background concentration (Table 1). However, axons did not turn toward a micropipette containing 1 BU of NGF per milliliter when the background contained no NGF.

In summary, chick dorsal-root axons rapidly (in 9 to 21 minutes) alter their direction of growth in response to an extracellular gradient of NGF. This response appears to result from chemotactic guidance rather than general enhancement of growth rate or survival. More extensive experiments are required to determine the relation between this chemotactic response and the previously observed growth of axons toward explants of target tissues or sources of concentrated NGF in longer-term experiments (1–3, 7, 8).

Since all dorsal-root axons that were bathed in low background concentrations of NGF (1 BU/ml) responded to an NGF concentration gradient, the chemotactic response to NGF that we measured does not account for the specificity with which different dorsal-root ganglion axons innervate different peripheral target tissues. Perhaps the response of different axons to NGF has quantitative differences too subtle to be detected. Also, other macromolecules analogous to NGF, or other mechanisms such as contact guidance (9), may help to guide axons and enable them to distinguish among different target tissues.

R. W. GUNDERSEN
J. N. BARRETT

Department of Physiology and Biophysics, University of Miami School of Medicine, Miami, Florida 33101

References and Notes

1. T. Ebendal and C.-O. Jacobson, *Exp. Cell Res.* **105**, 379 (1977).
2. K. A. Charlwood, D. M. Lamont, B. E. C. Banks, in *Nerve Growth Factor and Its Antiserum*, E. Zamis and J. Knight, Eds. (Athlone, London, 1972), pp. 102–107.
3. J. Chambley and J. Dowel, *Exp. Cell Res.* **90**, 1 (1975).
4. R. A. Bradshaw and M. Young, *Biochem. Pharmacol.* **25**, 1445 (1976).
5. W. C. Mobley, A. Scheneker, E. M. Shooter, *Biochemistry* **15**, 5543 (1976).
6. R. Levi-Montalcini and V. Hamburger, *Cancer Res.* **14**, 49 (1954).
7. P. C. Letourneau, *Dev. Biol.* **66**, 183 (1978).
8. M. G. Memesini-Chen, J. S. Chen, R. Levi-Montalcini, *Arch. Ital. Biol.* **116**, 53 (1978).
9. T. Ebendal, *Exp. Cell Res.* **98**, 159 (1976).
10. Supported by NIH grants NS 12207 and NS 07044.

17 September 1979

1080

Brain Research, 150 (1978) 319–331
© Elsevier/North-Holland Biomedical Press

CHARACTERIZATION OF THE RETROGRADE TRANSPORT OF NERVE GROWTH FACTOR (NGF) USING HIGH SPECIFIC ACTIVITY [125I]NGF

EUGENE M. JOHNSON, Jr., ROGER Y. ANDRES and RALPH A. BRADSHAW

Departments of Pharmacology and Biological Chemistry, Washington University Medical School, St. Louis, Mo. 63110 (U.S.A.)

(Accepted November 15th, 1977)

SUMMARY

The process of the retrograde transport of nerve growth factor (NGF) has been recharacterized using a high specific activity preparation of [125I]NGF. Most of the general conclusions reached in the previous studies of Hendry, Thoenen and co-workers have been confirmed. However, significant quantitative differences were noted. Intraocular (anterior eye chamber) administration of [125I]NGF (< 10 ng) resulted in accumulation in the superior cervical ganglia beginning at about 4 h. The ratio of radioactivity in the ipsilateral contralateral ganglia was 15–30:1. Maximal accumulation was seen at about 12 h in the hamster and 16 h in rats. This pattern was quite different from that seen in other tissues. The uptake system from the eye of the rat was saturable (half-maximal at 15 ng) with maximal accumulation of 35–40 pg/ganglion. Systemic administration of [125I]NGF (200 ng) to adult rats resulted in no accumulation in SGG or celiac ganglion prior to 3 h, with subsequent rapid accumulation by 6 h and a rapid fall in radioactivity after 12 h. A similar time course was seen in 5-day-old rats, although the time curve was shifted slightly toward shorter time. The radioactivity in ganglia co-migrated with native NGF by SDS gell electrophoresis. Cytochrome c of comparable specific activity was not transported, and NGF did not stimulate the uptake and transport of cytochrome c. The retrograde transport of [125I]NGF was inhibited by the co-administration of biologically active, but not inactive, oxidized derivatives of NGF.

By any route of administration, a significant percentage of the transported [125I]NGF was found in a purified nuclear fraction of the ganglia. Coupled with previous observations of specific nuclear NGF receptors in embryonic chick and sympathetic ganglia, this suggests that, after internalization and retrograde transport, NGF may directly act on the nucleus to produce at least some of its effects on the responsive cell.

INTRODUCTION

Nerve growth factor (NGF) is an insulin-like protein[5] which induces the morphologic and metabolic maturation of sympathetic and embryonic sensory neurons. The precise mechanism by which it exerts the trophic effects on responsive neurons is not established. Like other polypeptide hormones and growth factors, the first interaction of NGF with its target tissue is the binding to a cell surface receptor[2,6,7,12]. No second messenger system, however, has been found to mediate the ultimate response to the NGF. Recently nuclear binding sites for NGF in responsive neurons have been described[1]. This suggests that at least some of the actions of the growth factor might be mediated by uptake and direct nuclear action.

A specific uptake system for NGF has been described[10,11,18-20]. After injection into the anterior eye chamber of mice or rats, NGF is taken up by the peripheral adrenergic neurons and transported retrogradely to the perikarya of neurons in the superior cervical ganglion.

It has been suggested that the NGF required for survival of the peripheral adrenergic neurons gets there by retrograde transport. Therefore, certain alterations of neuronal function caused by drugs or environmental conditions could ultimately be the consequence of effects on the retrograde transport system for NGF. Specifically, it has recently been proposed that drugs which destroy the sympathetic nervous system (6-hydroxydopamine, guanethidine and vinblastine) do so by preventing the accumulation or utilization of retrogradely transported NGF[13]. Our initial retrograde transport experiments in preparation for the direct testing of this proposal, using high specific activity [^{125}I]NGF prepared by solid phase iodination, yielded data with significant quantitative differences to that previously described. The retrograde transport system was therefore reassessed, and the results reported in this study refine the characterization of the retrograde transport of NGF, and serve as a basis for subsequent investigations in experimentally challenged animals.

MATERIALS AND METHODS

Preparation of labelled proteins

NGF (2.5 S) was prepared by the method of Bocchini and Angeletti[3]. NGF was iodinated by the solid phase (talc) method of Frazier et al.[7] with minor modification. After iodination, the [^{125}I]NGF was eluted with 200 μl of 0.5 N HCl containing 0.1 mg/ml bovine serum albumin (BSA), titrated to neutrality with 10 N NaOH, and used for intraocular administration. For systemic administration this preparation was further diluted with 0.1 mg/ml BSA in 0.1 M potassium phosphate (pH 7.4). Native NGF was added to give the concentration of hormone described in the legends of the appropriate figures.

Specific activities of the [^{125}I]NGF preparations were approximately 50 μCi/μg. Experiments were performed within 48 h of preparation. Preliminary experiments showed that these preparations lose 50% of their binding to membrane preparations within one week. A very similar decrease in accumulation in superior cervical ganglia after intraocular administration was observed.

[^{125}I]cytochrome c was prepared by the method of Greenwood et al.[9].

NGF in which one and two tryptophans were oxidized were prepared by the method described by Frazier et al.[8] based upon the procedure of Spande and Witkop[17].

Treatment of animals

Experiments involving intraocular (anterior eye chamber) administration of [^{125}I]NGF were carried out on male Sprague–Dawley rats (225–250 g) or male Golden Syrian Hamsters (90–110 g). [^{125}I]NGF (5–10 ng, 4–10 × 10^5 cpm) was administered in a volume of 3 μl (hamsters) or 3–5 μl (rat) using a 5 μl Hamilton microsyringe. Intravenous administration of [^{125}I]NGF (200 ng, 2–4 × 10^6 cpm) to adult rats was carried out via indwelling jugular vein cannulae inserted under hexobarbital anesthesia (100 mg/kg) the day prior to the experiment. Systemic administration to neonatal (5-day-old) rats was done by subcutaneous administration of [^{125}I]-NGF (200 ng).

Animals were killed by decapitation and exsanguinated. Tissues were removed and counted in a Beckman Gamma Counter.

SDS gel electrophoresis

Four ganglia, collected 16 h after intraocular administration of [^{125}I]NGF, were homogenized in 100 μl of water containing 1 % SDS and 2 % β-mercaptoethanol. The homogenate was incubated at 100 °C for 5 min and centrifuged (10 min, 5000 × g). The supernatant was electrophoresed (3 mA, room temperature) on a 15 % acrylamide gel in the presence of 0.1 % SDS. The gel was then cut into 2 mm slices which were counted individually. Cytochrome c and bromphenol blue were added as internal markers.

Subcellular fractionation

Subcellular fractionation was carried out by a minor modification of the method of Biessman and Rajewski[4]. Ganglia were homogenized with a closely fitting glass–teflon homogenizer in ice-cold 0.32 M sucrose in 3 mM sodium cacodylate (pH 7.4) containing 1 mM magnesium chloride, 1 % Triton and 10^{-7} M native NGF. An excess of native NGF was included in order to prevent binding of free (cytoplasmic) [^{125}I]-NGF to any structures during homogenization. Triton facilitates lysis of the cells and solubilizes membrane-bound NGF receptors[1]. The homogenate was fractionated by discontinuous sucrose density gradient centrifugation (45 min, 100,000 × g, 0 °C). Material pelleting through 2 M sucrose in 1 mM sodium cacodylate (pH 7.4) containing 1 mM MgCl$_2$ was collected by cutting off the bottom of the tube. The dense, Triton-resistant fraction is made up of nuclear material[4].

RESULTS

Time course of accumulation of radioactivity in various tissues of the adult rat and hamster after unilateral intraocular administration of [^{125}I]NGF

After the injection of 10 ng of [^{125}I]NGF (800,000 cpm) into the left anterior

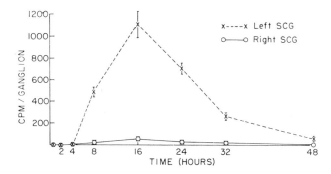

Fig. 1. Time course of radioactivity in superior cervical ganglia after the administration of [^{125}I]NGF (10 ng; 800,000 cpm) into the left anterior eye chamber of adult rats. Values represent the mean $\pm$ S.E.M. of 6–7 animals.

eye chamber of rats, no significant accumulation of radioactivity was seen in either superior cervical ganglion 0.5, 2 or 4 h after injection (Fig. 1). Subsequently radioactivity increased markedly in the ipsilateral ganglia but only slightly in the contralateral ganglia. The ratio of counts in the ipsilateral/contralateral ganglia in several experiments varied between 15–30 to 1. Accumulation reached a maximum about 16 h postinjection, and subsequently decreased at a rate comparable to the rate of accumulation. The pattern seen in other tissues was quite different. Counts in the eye were reduced 66% two hours after injection, indicating rapid removal from the eye (Fig. 2). Counts in the blood and in the contralateral eye were constant between 2 and 4 h postinjection and fell slowly thereafter. Counts in the thyroid rose slowly throughout the 48 h period studied.

In order to determine if a similar pattern would be seen in another species, similar experiments were performed in the hamster (Fig. 3). No radioactivity was observed in either ganglia 3 h after intraocular injection of [^{125}I]NGF. The accumula-

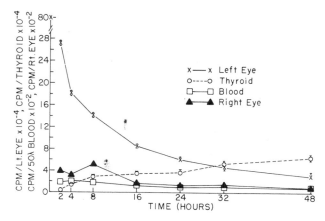

Fig. 2. Time course of radioactivity in several tissues after the administration of [^{125}I]NGF (10 ng; 800,000 cpm) into the left anterior eye chamber of adult rats. Values represent the mean $\pm$ S.E.M. of 6–7 animals.

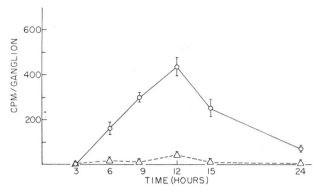

Fig. 3. Time course of radioactivity in superior cervical ganglia (O—O), left; △ --- △, right) after the administration of [^{125}I]NGF (10 ng, 400,000 cpm) into the left anterior eye chamber of hamsters. Values represent the mean ± S.E.M. of 6–7 animals.

tion of radioactivity in the ipsilateral ganglion appeared linear thereafter, reaching a maximum at an earlier time (approx. 12 h) than observed in the rat. The ratio of radioactivity in ipsilateral to contralateral ganglia was 10–20 under these experimental conditions. As in the rat, radioactivity decreased in the ganglia at a rate similar to that of accumulation. Accumulation in other tissues were similar to that seen in the rat (data not shown).

'Saturation' of the NGF uptake mechanism in the anterior eye chamber of the rat

Although it is apparent that after intraocular injection the levels of NGF in the eye are rapidly decreasing and equilibrium conditions are never operative, an experiment was performed to determine the functional 'saturability' and the capacity for accumulation of the system. Varying quantities of native NGF were added to a

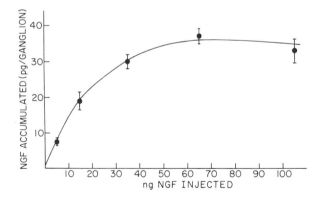

Fig. 4. Saturation of the retrograde transport system in the anterior eye chamber of adult rats. [^{125}I]NGF was injected without or with varying amounts of native NGF. After 16 h the ipsilateral superior cervical ganglion was removed, counted and the amounts of NGF in the ganglia calculated from the specific activity of the injected material. The radioactivity in the contralateral ganglia was insignificant (less than 40 cpm). Values are the mean ± S.E.M. of 7 animals.

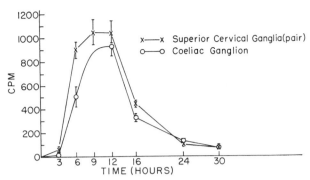

Fig. 5. Time course of radioactivity in superior cervical and coeliac ganglia after intravenous injection of [^{125}I]NGF (200 ng; 2.75 million cpm) to adult rats. Each value represents the mean ± S.E.M. of 5–7 animals.

constant amount of [^{125}I]NGF (6 ng, 500,000 cpm in 5 μl) and injected into the anterior eye chamber (Fig. 4). The system was saturable, with a maximal accumulation of 35–40 pg/ganglion after a single injection of NGF. Half-maximal accumulation was observed with the injection of approximately 15 ng of NGF.

Time course of the accumulation of radioactivity in various tissues after systemic administration of [^{125}I]NGF to adult and neonatal rats

[^{125}I]NGF (200 ng, 2.75 million cpm) was administered to adult rats via indwelling jugular vein cannulae (Fig. 5). The accumulation of radioactivity in superior cervical ganglia and coeliac ganglia showed similar time courses. Little or no radioactivity was seen 3 h after administration. Thereafter radioactivity increased markedly, and leveled off between 9 and 12 h. After 12 h the radioactivity decreased rapidly at a rate similar to that of accumulation. In contrast, total radioactivity in blood decreased very rapidly (Fig. 6) between 3 and 16 h, and more slowly thereafter. The accumulation of radioactivity in the adrenal was much less than in ganglia and decreased steadily during the 3–30 h observation period.

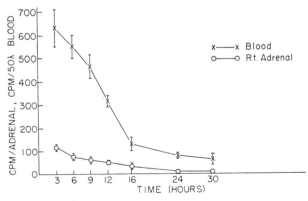

Fig. 6. Time course of radioactivity in blood and adrenals after intravenous injection of [^{125}I]NGF (200 ng; 2.75 million cpm) to adult rats. Each value represents the mean ± S.E.M. of 5–7 animals.

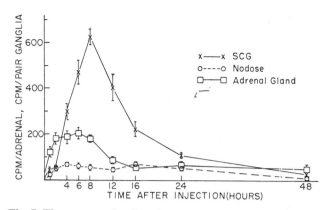

Fig. 7. Time course of radioactivity in superior cervical ganglia, nodose ganglia, and adrenals after subcutaneous injection of [¹²⁵I]NGF (200 ng, 1.84 million cpm) to 5-day-old rats. Each value represents the mean ± S.E.M. of 8 animals.

Subcutaneous administration of [¹²⁵I]NGF to neonatal rats yielded similar results. Radioactivity in adrenals and in the nodose ganglia (Fig. 7) was maximal within two hours, remained stable for about 8 h and subsequently declined slowly. The radioactivity in superior cervical ganglia was very low at two hours (same as in nodose ganglia) and then rapidly increased reaching maximal levels at about 8 h. Thereafter, radioactivity decreased rapidly at a rate similar to the rate of accumulation. The total radioactivity in blood and heart (Fig. 8) peaked at two hours and subsequently declined. Radioactivity in the tail (Fig. 8) did not peak until 6 h and remained relatively constant during the 48-h experiment.

SDS gel electrophoresis of radioactive material in superior cervical ganglia after intraocular administration of [¹²⁵I]NGF

The radioactivity in superior cervical ganglia 16 h after intraocular administration of [¹²⁵I]NGF was analyzed on SDS gels (Fig. 9). The radioactive material comigrated with standards of cytochrome c (indistinguishable from NGF under the conditions of the experiment) or ¹⁴C-labelled NGF prepared by acetylation with [¹⁴C]iodoacetic acid (not shown).

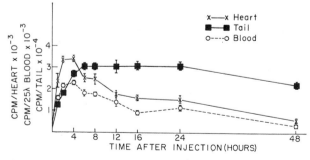

Fig. 8. Time course of radioactivity in heart, blood and tail after subcutaneous injection of [¹²⁵I]NGF (200 ng; 1.84 million cpm) to 5-day-old rats. Each value represents mean ± S.E.M. of 8 animals.

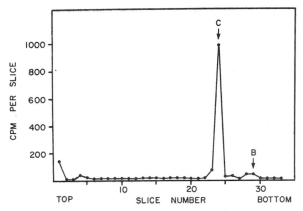

Fig. 9. SDS gel electrophoresis of retrogradely transported [125I]NGF in superior cervical ganglia (see Materials and Methods). Cytochrome c (C) and bromphenol (B) serve as internal markers.

Specificity of the uptake system for NGF

In order to determine the specificity of the uptake for [125I]NGF, two experiments were performed. The uptake of cytochrome c (molecular weight and isoelectric point similar to that of NGF) and the ability of cytochrome c to inhibit the uptake of NGF were determined. The results in Table I show that co-administration of 2.5 μg of cytochrome c does not decrease the accumulation in the superior cervical ganglion of intraocularly administered NGF (100 ng of native NGF decreases accumulation by 80% under these conditions). Intraocular injection of [125I]cytochrome c of similar specific activity results in no accumulation in the ganglia. The co-administration of low (15 ng) or high (2.5 μg) amounts of native NGF does not induce or stimulate the accumulation of [125I]cytochrome c.

Oxidized derivatives of NGF in which one (1-ox) or two (2-ox) of the tryptophans have been oxidized to produce differing degrees of biological inactivation, were co-administered with the tracer [125I]NGF by intraocular injection. The results in Table II show that 1-ox (500 ng) decreased the accumulation of radioactivity in superior

TABLE I

Interaction of NGF and cytochrome c in the process of retrograde transport from the eye to the superior cervical ganglion

The animals were injected in the left anterior eye chamber and killed 24 h later. Values represent mean $\pm$ S.E.M. of 6–7 animals.

Treatment	cpm in ganglion*
[125I]NGF (375,000 cpm)	248 $\pm$ 27
[125I]NGF + 2.5 μg cytochrome c	291 $\pm$ 30
[125I]Cytochrome c (15 ng; 500,000 pcm)	5 $\pm$ 6
[125I]Cytochrome c + 15 ng native NGF	7 $\pm$ 2
[125I]Cytochrome c + 2.5 μg native NGF	2 $\pm$ 6

* Left superior cervical ganglion.

TABLE II

Effect of oxidation of tryptophan residues on the ability of NGF to decrease the accumulation of [^{125}I]-NGF in the superior cervical ganglion after intraocular administration

Values represent mean ± S.E.M. of 7 animals. The animals were killed 16 h after injection.

Addition*	cpm/ganglia	
	Ipsilateral	Contralateral
None	427 ± 31	20 ± 4
500 ng 1-ox NGF	177 ± 8	21 ± 4
500 ng 2-ox NGF	520 ± 20	21 ± 2

* In addition to [^{125}I]NGF (< 10 ng; 220,000 cpm). Oxidized derivatives prepared as described in Materials and Methods.

cervical ganglia by approx. 60%, whereas 500 ng of 2-ox did not reduce accumulation.

Distribution of retrogradely transported [^{125}I]NGF between nuclear and non-nuclear compartments of sympathetic ganglia

In light of the recent report[1] of specific binding of NGF to chromatin from chick embryo dorsal root and sympathetic ganglia, experiments were performed to determine the distribution of retrogradely transported NGF between the nuclear and non-nuclear compartments of the cell. [^{125}I]NGF was administered by intraocular and intravenous injection to adult animals and by subcutaneous injection in neonates. Superior cervical ganglia were taken at the time of peak accumulation determined in the previous experiments. After isolation of nuclei it was found that, by either route of administration (Table III), about 15–30% of the radioactivity was retained in the nucleus. No attempt was made to further define the distribution of the non-nuclear NGF.

TABLE III

Association of retrogradely transported [^{125}I]NGF with the nuclear fraction of superior cervical ganglia

[^{125}]NGF administered as described in Materials and Methods. The animals were killed at the time of peak accumulation. Values represent mean ± S.E.M. of triplicate determinations (4–6 ganglia per experiment).

Age	Route of administration	Total radioactivity (cpm)	Radioactivity in nuclear fraction	
			cpm	Per cent of total
Adult	Intraocular	1755, 1782*	540, 456	31, 26
	Intravenous	3360 ± 260	800 ± 12	24 ± 2
Neonate	Subcutaneous	1248 ± 60	207 ± 25	17 ± 2

* Similar results have been obtained in 3 other experiments.

328

DISCUSSION

The work reported in this paper provides a recharacterization of several aspects of the retrograde transport system for NGF. Using improved methodology the results of Hendry, Thoenen and coworkers[10,11,15,16,18-20] have been refined, and important quantitative differences to earlier work noted (see below). Most of the conclusion of earlier workers, however, have been confirmed.

The quantitative differences noted between our results and the previously reported studies are with regard to time course of NGF accumulation in ganglia, the amounts of NGF required to saturate the anterior eye chamber, and in the ratio of radioactivity in the ipsilateral compared to contralateral ganglion after intraocular administration. The primary difference in methodology lies in the preparation of the [^{125}I]NGF used in the studies. The work here was performed with [^{125}I]NGF prepared by a solid phase method[7] which produced specific activities of approx. 50 μCi/μg, whereas the [^{125}I]NGF used in previous studies had a specific activity of less than 5 μCi/μg. As a result we injected in the eye chamber much less NGF and radioactivity ($<$ 10 ng, $<$ than 0.5 μCi) than in previous studies (for example 3 μg of NGF containing 9 μCi in ref. 16). Since the anterior eye chamber is functionally half-saturated at about 15 ng of NGF (Fig. 4), the amount of material ($<$ 10 ng) used in our experiments more nearly represents tracer amounts of NGF than those used previously (3 μg) which are saturating. This accounts for the difference in results, wherein after intraocular administration of [^{125}I]NGF we observe ratios of radioactivity in the ipsilateral vs. contralateral superior cervical ganglion of 15–30:1, indicating little spillover and subsequent accumulation in the contralateral ganglion. Use of higher amounts of NGF (3 μg) results in significant spillover, and high levels are incorporated in the contralateral ganglion, resulting in ipsilateral:contralateral ratios of 2–3:1. This spillover probably accounts for the difference in the time course of accumulation in the superior cervical ganglion after the intraocular administration of [^{125}I]NGF seen by us (Fig. 1) and that reported previously[16]. That time course[16] is very similar to the time course we see after systemic injection (Fig. 1) and suggests that the previous data represents primarily NGF which had gone into the circulation.

Based on our data we would estimate a velocity of transport of about 3 mm/h (assuming a migration distance of 2 cm from the eye to the ganglion in the rat and the initial appearance in the ganglia at 5 or 6 h, Fig. 1) which is consistent with previous estimates[10,16]. The somewhat shorter time course (Fig. 3) seen in the hamster would yield a similar velocity of transport, and indicates that the velocities of transport in all species now studied (rat, mouse and hamster) are very similar.

A consistent observation in these studies was that the rate of disappearance of [^{125}I]NGF was similar to the rate of appearance, and that this turnover is relatively rapid. Despite this rapid turnover, essentially all of the radioactivity in the ganglia is authentic NGF by molecular weight (ref. 18, Fig. 9) criteria. This indicates that NGF is removed from the cell intact (by release out of the cell or by anterograde transport from the cell body) or that the breakdown products of NGF are excreted from the cell much more rapidly than is native NGF.

Specificity and functional significance of the system

The fact that after systemic administration of [125I]NGF very little radioactivity is in the ganglia initially but rather increases after a lag time of 2–3 h and reaches maximal level at a time (8–10 h) when probably no intact [125I]NGF is still circulating[18] argues strongly for the suggestion[18] that the primary mode of access of NGF to the sympathetic neuron is via uptake and retrograde transport from peripheral parts of the cell.

The results in Fig. 4 and Tables I and II confirm that the NGF uptake system into the cell is specific and saturable. Functional half-maximal saturation in the anterior eye chamber of the rat is produced by approx. 15 ng, which is about an order of magnitude lower than that reported in the mouse[10]. Again, the difference is probably a result of the markedly differing specific activities of [125I]NGF used in the studies.

Intraocular administration of low amounts (15 ng) of cytochrome c of high specific activity resulted in no accumulation of radioactivity in the ganglia and co-administration of NGF did not stimulate the uptake of cytochrome c. This demonstrates that NGF does not induce a general increase in the uptake of proteins from the extracellular environment.

In contrast to native NGF, which competed with [125I]NGF for uptake and reduced accumulation in the ganglion, oxidized NGF (2-ox) was ineffective. The relative effectiveness of the oxidized NGF preparations was consistent with their biological activity in other systems[8]. Our results therefore confirm, and extend by different methods, the conclusions reached by Stoeckel et al.[19] that NGF is specifically taken up by sympathetic neurons and that the binding of oxidized derivatives of NGF parallels biological activity. These results, coupled with the observation (see Methods) that the binding to membrane preparations and the degree of retrograde transport of [125I]NGF preparations decrease at similar rates, suggest that the previously characterized membrane receptors for NGF are involved in the uptake of NGF for subsequent transport.

Comparison of the time courses of the appearance in the eye and superior cervical ganglion after intraocular administration of [125I] NGF

Despite the very rapid decrease in amount of [125I]NGF in the eye after intraocular administration, accumulation in the ganglion appears to increase gradually (Figs. 1 and 3). In the rat, after the administration of 800,000 cpm into the eye, only 40% of the counts (319,000 $\pm$ 31,500, n = 7) remain in the eye 30 min after injection. However, ganglion radioactivity increases almost linearly between 5 and 6 h and 16 h, rather than occurring in a distinctive wave. The linear increase in the hamster is clearly shown in Fig. 3. Three possible explanations for these results are suggested. The first would be that, although NGF is taken up rapidly, almost as a bolus, the retrograde transport occurs at varying rates, the fastest being slightly in excess of 3 mm/h and slowest being less than 1 mm/h.

The second possibility is that the rate of accumulation is constant, despite rapidly decreasing levels in the eye due to negatively co-operative behavior of the NGF receptor responsible for initial binding. Such kinetic behavior has been demonstrated in vitro in isolated plasma membrane preparations[7]. Hence, despite a constantly decreasing amount of [^{125}I]NGF in the eye (due to leaking out of the eye and/or breakdown) the binding affinity constantly increases, thus allowing NGF to be taken up at a nearly constant rate and transported at a constant velocity ($\sim$ 3 mm/h) to the cell body.

A third possibility is that, after NGF is bound to the presynaptic membrane by a time-saturable process, it must be internalized by a time-linear process (pinocytosis). After internalization it is transported again at approx. 3 mm/h back to the cell body. Such a scheme of binding and internalization has been suggested by Norr and Varon[14] in chick embryo dorsal root ganglia.

The second of these alternatives is perhaps favored by the much greater rate of rise of label in the superior ganglia after i.v. administration. This more rapid rise is seen despite the fact that neurons of much more variable length are involved in the total uptake. The administration of 200 ng of NGF systemically would certainly result in a lower concentration of the NGF at receptors than administration of 10 ng into the anterior eye chamber (estimated at 2–5 $\times$ 10^{-8} M, 5–10 ng in 20 μl) thus minimizing the effects of negative co-operativity.

Nuclear binding of NGF. The results of our fractionation experiments indicate that a significant portion of the retrogradely transported NGF is bound to the nucleus. This is not an unexpected result in light of the demonstration of specific NGF receptors on the chromatin of chick embryo dorsal root and sympathetic ganglion cells[1]. These experiments were done in such a way as to preclude contamination with plasma membrane or other membrane receptors which are solubilized by the Triton treatment. These results would suggest that, after internalization and retrograde transport, NGF can directly act on the nucleus to affect the synthesis of specific RNAs involved in specific enzyme synthesis.

These observations and suggestions conflict with the autoradiographic data of Schwab and Thoenen[16] who, after administration of [^{125}I]NGF into the anterior eye (1.26 μg, 24.4 μCi) and submandibular gland (3.78 μg, 73.8 μCi), found labelling in secondary lysosomes, smooth vesicles and endoplasmic reticulum, but no significant labelling in the nucleus of sympathetic neurons in the superior cervical ganglion.

These two experiments were obviously done under very different conditions. The use of amounts of NGF (1.26 μg) which saturate the uptake system (Fig. 4) may result on a different labelling pattern than would be seen under more physiological conditions. This would be especially true if the binding to the nucleus becomes saturated at levels of NGF below the maximum amount which can be accumulated by the cell. Obviously, more work using a variety of methods will have to be carried out to resolve this issue.

ACKNOWLEDGEMENTS

The authors would like to thank Mr. Richard Macia for his excellent technical assistance.

This work was support by the National Foundation, March of Dimes (Basil O'Connor Grant) and by NIH Grants HL20604 and NS10229. Dr. Andres is a fellow of the Swiss National Foundation.

REFERENCES

1 Andres, R. Y., Jeng, I. and Bradshaw, R. A., Nerve growth factor receptors: identification of distinct classes in plasma membranes and nuclei of embryonic dorsal root neurons, *Proc. nat. Acad. Sci. (Wash.)*, 74 (1977) 2785–2789.

2 Banerjee, S. P., Snyder, S. A., Cuatrecases, P. and Green, L. A., Binding of NGF receptor in sympathetic ganglia, *Proc. nat. Acad. Sci. (Wash.)*, 70 (1973) 2519–2523.

3 Bocchini, V. and Angeletti, P. U., The nerve growth factor purification as a 30,000 molecular weight protein, *Proc. nat. Acad. Sci. (Wash.)*, 64 (1969) 787–794.

4 Biessman, H. and Rajewsky, M. F., Nuclear protein patterns in developing and adult brain in ethylnitrosourea-induced neuroectodermal tumors of the rat, *J. Neurochem.*, 24 (1975) 387–393.

5 Frazier, W. A., Angeletti, R. and Bradshaw, R. A., Nerve growth factor and insulin, *Science*, 176 (1972) 482–487.

6 Frazier, W. A., Boyd, L. F. and Bradshaw, R. A., Interaction of nerve growth factor with surface membranes: biological competence of insolubilized nerve growth factor, *Proc. nat. Acad. Sci. (Wash.)*, 70 (1973) 2931–2935.

7 Frazier, W. A., Boyd, L. F. and Bradshaw, R. A., Properties of the specific binding of [125I]nerve growth factor to responsive peripheral neurons, *J. biol. Chem.*, 249 (1974) 5513–5519.

8 Frazier, W. A., Hogue-Angeletti, R. A., Sherman, R. and Bradshaw, R. A., Topography of mouse 2.5 S nerve growth factor. Reactivity of tyrosine and tryptophan, *Biochemistry*, 12 (1973) 3281–3293.

9 Greenwood, F. C., Hunter, W. M. and Glover, J. S., The preparation of 31I-labelled human growth hormone of high specific radioactivity, *Biochem. J.*, 89 (1963) 114–123.

10 Hendry, I. A., Stöckel, K., Thoenen, H. and Iversen, L. L., The retrograde axonal transport of nerve growth factor, *Brain Research*, 68 (1974) 103–121.

11 Hendry, I. A., Stach, R. and Herrup, D., Characteristics of the retrograde transport system for nerve growth factor in the sympathetic nervous system, *Brain Research*, 82 (1974) 117–128.

12 Herrup, K. and Shooter, E. M., Properties of the nerve growth factor receptor of avian dorsal root ganglia, *Proc. nat. Acad. Sci. (Wash.)*, 70 (1973) 3884–3888.

13 Johnson, E. M., Destruction of the sympathetic nervous system in neonatal rats and hamsters by vinblastine: prevention by concomitant administration of nerve growth factor, *Brain Research*, 141 (1978) 105–118.

14 Norr, S. and Varon, S., Dynamic, temperature-sensitivity association of [125I]nerve growth in vitro with ganglionic and non-ganglionic cells from embryonic chick, *Neurobiology*, 5 (1975) 101–118.

15 Paravicini, U., Stoeckel, K. and Thoenen, H., Biological importance of retrograde axonal transport of nerve growth factor in adrenergic neurons, *Brain Research*, 84 (1975) 279–291.

16 Schwab, M. and Thoenen, H., Selective transsynaptic migration of tetanus toxin after retrograde axonal transport in peripheral sympathetic nerves: a comparison with nerve growth factor, *Brain Research*, 122 (1977) 459–474.

17 Spande, T. F. and Witkop, B., Determination of the tryptophan content of proteins with *N*-bromosuccinamide, *Meth. Enzymol.*, 11 (1967) 498–506.

18 Stöckel, K., Guroff, G., Schwab, M. and Thoenen, H., The significance of retrograde axonal transport for the accumulation of systemically administered nerve growth factor (NGF) in the rat superior cervical ganglion, *Brain Research*, 109 (1976) 271–284.

19 Stöckel, K., Paravicini, U. and Thoenen, H., Specificity of the retrograde transport of nerve growth factor, *Brain Research*, 76 (1974) 413–421.

20 Stöckel, K., Schwab, M. and Thoenen, H., Comparison between the retrograde axonal transport of nerve growth factor and tetanus toxin in motor, sensory and adrenergic neurons, *Brain Research*, 99 (1975) 1–16.

Reprinted from Nature, Vol. 286, No. 5768, pp. 25-28, July 3 1980
© Macmillan Journals Ltd. 1980

Nerve growth factors in the rat iris

Ted Ebendal*, Lars Olson†, Åke Seiger† & Kjell-Olof Hedlund*

* Department of Zoology, Uppsala University, Box 561, S-751 22 Uppsala, Sweden
† Department of Histology, Karolinska Institutet, S-104 01 Stockholm, Sweden

Nerve growth factor (NGF) activity was not detected by bioassay in irides killed immediately after excision but NGF appeared within 24 h in living irides placed in culture or grafted to a host eye. Furthermore, sensory and, although less effective, sympathetic denervation of irides in situ led within 10 days to the appearance of NGF activity. In addition, freezing and thawing released a parasympathetic neuronotrophic factor activity from irides.

THE protein nerve growth factor (NGF)[1] has been suggested to mediate trophic influences to sympathetic and sensory neurones from innervated target organs[2]. However, little is known about the distribution of NGF in peripheral tissues to support this concept[3]. Except for some very rich sources of NGF (the male mouse submandibular gland[1], the guinea pig prostate[4]), mammalian tissues are normally inactive when tested as homogenates in the sensitive bioassay based on NGF-susceptible embryonic ganglia[3,5]. We now show that explants of the adult rat iris immediately killed by freezing do not contain NGF at levels detectable by bioassay but that NGF is readily detectable in irides killed by freezing within a day after transfer to a reconstituted collagen gel[6] (compare refs 7, 8) or to the anterior eye chamber of another rat[9]. After re-innervation of the iris transplants, NGF was no longer detectable. Most compelling is the fact that the levels of NGF were also raised in irides *in situ* 10 days after sensory denervation and, although less prominent, 10 days after sympathetic denervation. Furthermore, evidence was obtained for the actions of a parasympathetic, non-NGF, trophic factor released from the rat iris after freezing and thawing. The results support a role for NGF as a signal initiating and directing regenerating sensory and sympathetic fibres in adult mammals and suggest that other trophic factors may fulfil a similar role in other fibre systems.

Effects of culturing on NGF synthesis in the iris

To study the content of NGF, irides of adult Sprague–Dawley rats were excised aseptically and tested in a ganglionic bioassay (Fig. 1). The criterion for NGF activity is an induction of neurite outgrowth in the chick sympathetic and spinal ganglia, which in parallel dishes can be blocked by antiserum to NGF, combined with a lack of fibre response in the ciliary ganglion[6]. Three distinct patterns of neurite outgrowth responses were observed (Fig. 1). Living iris explants taken directly into co-culture with ganglia evoked neurite outgrowth in the sympathetic and spinal

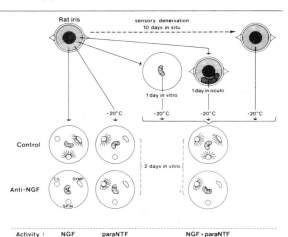

Fig. 1 Schematic representation of the experiments with rat irides and the resulting patterns of neurite growth responses in chick sympathetic (symp), spinal (spin) and ciliary (cil) ganglia. The results are interpreted as evoked by the actions of nerve growth factor (NGF), of a parasympathetic neuronotrophic factor (paraNTF) and of the simultaneous action of these two. Circles represent culture dishes. Irides were from normal rats (left) or from rats in which the trigeminal nerve had been lesioned (sensory denervation, right). For bioassay sympathetic, spinal and ciliary ganglia from 8- to 10-day-old chick embryos were placed surrounding a living or killed (by freezing to −20 °C) half-iris in an 0.3–0.5-mm thick collagen gel in a 35-mm plastic culture dish. The medium of the gel was Eagle's basal medium supplemented with 1% fetal calf serum, penicillin (100 units ml⁻¹) and streptomycin (100 μg ml⁻¹). Parallel dishes received in addition 2–5 μl per ml of specific rabbit anti-mouse-βNGF antiserum[22], levels that readily blocked the activity of 1 biological unit (BU) of NGF. Cultures were incubated at 37 °C with 5% CO_2 in water-saturated air for 2 days and then examined by phase-contrast microscopy.

Table 1 Relative density of neurite outgrowths in chick ganglia

	Without iris explants	With living iris explants	With irides killed after:				
			No special treatment	Culture *in vitro* (1 day)	Grafting *in oculo* (1 day)	Sympathetic denervation *in situ* (10 days)	Sensory denervation *in situ* (10 days)
Sympathetic ganglia							
without anti-NGF	0.0±0.0 (8)	1.0±0.0 (9)	0.3±0.1 (9)	1.0±0.0 (9)	1.0±0.0 (5)	0.6±0.1 (10)	0.9±0.0 (15)
with anti-NGF	0.0±0.0 (8)	0.1±0.0 (8)	0.2±0.1 (8)	0.4±0.1 (5)	0.4±0.1 (5)	0.3±0.1 (7)	0.3±0.1 (11)
Ciliary ganglia	0.0±0.0 (8)	0.1±0.1 (5)	0.7±0.0 (5)	0.8±0.1 (5)	0.8±0.1 (5)	0.8±0.0 (5)	0.7±0.1 (13)

Mean values ± s.e.m. are given. For each group 5 to 15 ganglia (number given in parentheses) were scored for density of outgrowing neurites after 2 days on a blind basis. The scores ranged from 0 (no neurites at all) to 1 (maximum density, fibre halo with circular outline). The scores for the two types of ganglia are not strictly comparable due to differences in neurite morphology. *P* values given in the text refer to rankings of the individual scores evaluated by the Mann–Whitney *U*-test.

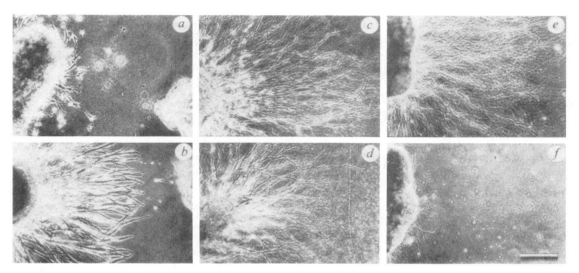

2

Fig. 2 _a_, Sympathetic ganglion (left) combined for 2 days in culture with rat iris (right) immediately killed after extirpation. No neurites emerge from the ganglion. _b_, Ciliary ganglion in the same conditions. In this parasympathetic ganglion extensive formation of thick neurite fascicles (identity controlled by the transmission electron microscope) is elicited by the killed iris explant. _c_, Sympathetic ganglion with dense fibre outgrowth elicited by an iris that had been cultured for 1 day and then frozen–thawed before being tested in the bioassay. _d_, Sympathetic ganglion combined with an iris transplanted to the anterior eye chamber of another rat for 1 day before being killed and tested. _e_, Extensive neurite formation in a sympathetic ganglion evoked by an iris killed 10 days after sensory denervation _in situ_. _f_, Inhibition by anti-βNGF of the neurite outgrowth in the foregoing combination. Phase contrast micrographs. Scale bar, 0.2 mm. See also ref. 13 for low-power darkfield micrographs of total outgrowths elicited by living irides.

ganglia within 20–24 h. Outgrowths developed fully within 2 days (Table 1), were directed mainly towards the living iris explants and had fibre densities resembling those evoked by 0.8 to 1 biological units of NGF (BU)[1]. Anti-NGF nearly completely inhibited these outgrowths (Table 1, $P < 0.01$). Thus it is evident that the living irides in culture release NGF. The ciliary ganglia showed nearly no nerve fibre outgrowth when combined with living iris tissue. In control cultures without irides all three types of ganglia failed to extend neurites[6] (Table 1).

To test whether NGF is present in freshly excised irides or whether it is synthesized _in vitro_, irides were killed by immediate freezing to −20 °C for 1 to 30 days and then thawed. No NGF activity was detected in such iris tissue in the bioassay (Figs 1, 2_a_): in sympathetic ganglia slightly more fibres extended than in controls ($P < 0.05$) but anti-NGF did not significantly (by the _U_-test) reduce this outgrowth (Table 1). On the other hand, killed iris tissue significantly increased formation of neurite bundles in the ciliary ganglia (Fig. 2_b_; Table 1, $P < 0.01$). This stimulation was not abolished by adding anti-NGF, although the antiserum sometimes slightly impaired the response in the ciliary ganglion in this and in the following culture combinations. These results suggest the existence in the iris of a parasympathetic neuronotrophic factor[2] (paraNTF), stimulating the cholinergic neurones of the ciliary ganglion, and being released only after disrupting cells by freezing and thawing. Furthermore, the results show that NGF is not present at detectable levels in the iris _in situ_, but that the iris begins to synthesize NGF when placed in culture.

Effects of freezing and transplantation

To rule out the possibility that the freezing–thawing itself destroys NGF activity in the iris, explanted irides were cultured for 1 day in order to accumulate NGF before being killed. Bioassay demonstrated the same level of NGF activity in these explants as in the living ones (Figs 1, 2_c_; Table 1). Moreover, the ciliary ganglia exhibited dense outgrowths of neurites not significantly different from those evoked by immediately killed

irides (Table 1). Thus these cultures showed a pattern of neurite stimulation that evidently represents the combined activities of NGF and paraNTF (Fig. 1). Anti-NGF inhibited outgrowth of neurites in the sympathetic (Table 1; $P < 0.01$) and spinal ganglia but did not affect outgrowth in ciliary ganglia.

To test whether NGF is produced in the iris only in _in vitro_ conditions, the iris was either transplanted to the anterior eye chamber of another rat, rather than to a culture dish, or was left _in situ_ but subjected either to sympathetic denervation by extirpation of the superior cervical ganglion or to sensory denervation by lesioning the trigeminal nerve[9] (Fig. 1). To prevent appearance of NGF during the subsequent bioassay the irides were killed by freezing before being combined with ganglia (Fig. 1).

After 1 day in the anterior eye chamber the transplanted iris contained the same amount of NGF as iris explants cultured _in vitro_ for 1 day (Fig. 2_d_; Table 1). After 4, 7 and 11 days _in oculo_ the same levels of NGF activity persisted but after 1 month, at which time the iris transplant had become at least sympathetically reinnervated by the host iris[10], NGF activity was no longer detectable. The responses evoked in the ciliary ganglia were the same as those elicited by the other frozen–thawed irides (Table 1).

Role of innervation in NGF synthesis

Experiments with irides denervated _in situ_ show more clearly that the level of NGF is in some way related to the state of innervation. Irides taken for bioassay 10 days after sensory denervation consistently gave dense fibre outgrowths in sympathetic (Figs 1, 2_e_, Table 1; the increase over normal killed irides is significant, $P < 0.01$) and spinal ganglia. The resulting outgrowth could be significantly reduced by anti-NGF (Figs 1, 2_f_, Table 1; $P < 0.01$). Sympathetic denervation for 10 days resulted in a much less although significant ($P < 0.05$) increase in fibre density in sympathetic ganglia (Table 1). That NGF is involved here also is indicated by the significant ($P < 0.05$)

reduction in fibre outgrowth by anti-NGF (Table 1). No NGF was detected 2 or 4 days after denervating the iris *in situ* nor was NGF found 1 month after denervation (at which time some reinnervation is likely to have taken place). Combined sensory and sympathetic denervations gave as high levels of NGF after 10 days as did sensory denervation. For the ciliary ganglia the denervations caused no further increase in fibre density above that evoked by normal killed irides (Table 1).

Sections of the ganglia cut for light microscopy at the end of bioassay add some information on the survival of neurones in response to the irides. In full agreement with the neurite outgrowth response the ciliary ganglion showed excellent neuronal survival after exposure to any iris that had been frozen–thawed (Fig. 3a; 19 ± 1 neurone profiles were found within an area of 0.01 mm^2; mean ± s.e.m. from sections of 5 ganglia) whereas living irides to a less ($P < 0.01$) extent did promote survival of ciliary neurones (Fig. 3b; 5 ± 1 neurone profiles with living irides compared with 1 ± 0 neurone profiles in cultured control ganglia, $P < 0.05$). The outcome for sympathetic ganglia was less expected: here the presence of iris tissue enhanced neuronal survival whether or not outgrowth of neurites occurred (Fig. 3c). The number of neurone profiles was thus 63 ± 4 with normal killed irides, which is not significantly different from the 71 ± 4 neurone profiles found with killed irides plus anti-NGF, whereas neuronal survival was significantly lower ($P < 0.01$) in cultured control ganglia (Fig. 3d; 30 ± 3 neurone profiles). The enhancement may be due to an nonspecific, non-NGF, trophic influence on the neurones exerted by the presence of serum in the explanted irides: thus adding rat serum at 10% by volume resulted in 56 ± 5 neurone profiles. Rat serum, however, totally failed to induce neurite outgrowth in the sympathetic as well as the ciliary ganglia.

The present experiments show that the level of NGF may be raised in a mammalian tissue *in situ* by sensory or sympathetic denervation. The results thus favour the concept that a tissue after denervation during adulthood, and probably also during development, signals with NGF to initiate and attract growing or regrowing sympathetic and sensory nerve fibres[1,2]. This view is also supported by the finding that NGF content falls to undetectable levels concomitant with reinnervation of the iris grafts.

The appearance of NGF in the iris as a result of explantation, transplantation or denervation may be the result of an active response of the iris to increase the production of the factor. Although less plausible, it may also be that the iris is normally drained of the NGF produced in it by retrograde axonal transport[11] to such an extent that the appearance of NGF after, for example, denervation represents an accumulation of the factor rather than an increased production.

The amounts of NGF released from the iris explants that induce a 0.8 to 1 BU response in chick ganglia (Fig. 2c, d, e) can be roughly calculated. The response was evoked only within a zone of about 2 mm around the approximately 5×1 mm half iris in the 0.3–0.5-mm thick gel. Thus the half iris spreads NGF to about 10–20 μl of the gel. If it is assumed[1] that 1 BU corresponds to 5 ng of NGF per ml and that the NGF is evenly distributed, this volume should contain about 40–80 pg. The wet weight of the half iris is about 0.5 mg and thus a reasonable amount of NGF released is of the order of 80–160 ng per g wet weight of cultured or denervated iris tissue. This value is slightly higher than that stated by Johnson *et al.*[8] measuring the release of NGF from irides to a culture medium by radioimmunoassay (RIA). Given the limits of detection of NGF activity for the present bioassay (0.03–0.06 BU)[6], and as we did not detect any NGF activity in initially killed irides, this tissue should release less than 5–10 ng of NGF per g wet weight. Johnson *et al.*[8] stated that the iris initially contains 15–20 ng NGF per g as measured by RIA but this may be an overestimation due to their technique[12]. The present results thus show that the level of NGF is increased by at least one order of magnitude in the positive iris explants.

It is noteworthy that sensory denervation was a much more potent stimulus for the NGF increase *in situ* than sympathetic denervation (Table 1). One possible explanation for this difference may be that the lesioning technique used to obtain sensory denervation also damages a considerable proportion of the sympathetic axons to the iris. This may also explain why a combined sensory and sympathetic denervation was not found more effective in stimulating the production of NGF than was the trigeminal lesion alone. It is also of note that sensory denervation has been shown to cause massive ingrowth of central noradrenergic fibres into the iris from transplants of nucleus locus coeruleus (see ref. 9). Since this nucleus does not respond to NGF[13] the mechanism for this fibre stimulation is, however, unlikely to be a response to the increase in NGF demonstrated here.

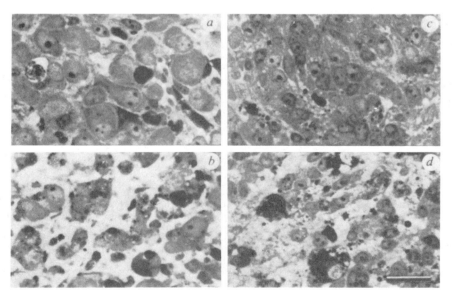

Fig. 3 a, Ciliary ganglion combined with a killed rat iris for 2 days in culture. A high neuronal survival is evident. b, Same but with a living iris explant. A massive death of neurones, also seen in control cultures, is not prevented by the living iris. c, Sympathetic ganglion cultured with an iris killed immediately after extirpation. Despite the addition of anti-βNGF and the fact that no or only few neurites extend from the ganglion (see Fig. 2a'), a markedly good neuronal survival is induced by the iris tissue. d, Sympathetic control ganglion cultured without the presence of iris tissue. Only a few neurones survive in these conditions. For data on neurone survival, see text. Micrographs of toluidine blue-stained 2-μm sections of ganglia fixed in 1.5% glutaraldehyde plus 1.5% paraformaldehyde and embedded in Epon. Scale bar, 20 μm.

A parasympathetic stimulation was evident by irides treated by freezing and thawing, indicating the presence in the iris of trophic factors besides NGF. Similar trophic factors have been found in rat cardiac and skeletal muscle[5,14]. Factors stimulating the ciliary ganglion have also recently been reported in the embryonic chick heart[6,15,16] and chick iris[17,18] as well as in culture medium conditioned by chick heart[19] and muscle cells[20].

Conclusions

Thus two nerve growth stimulating factors, one affecting sympathetic and sensory neurones and the other affecting parasympathetic neurones, were found in rat iris tissue. The present results provide the first demonstration that the level of NGF is raised in a tissue *in situ* as a result of denervation. Our data are in line with the demonstration that immunosympathectomy[1] is brought about by neutralizing endogenous NGF[21] and support the concept of NGF as a messenger between target organs and peripheral neurones in mammals.

This work was supported by the Swedish Medical and Natural Science Research Councils (grants 04X–03185 and B 2021–100, respectively), Magnus Bergvalls Stiftelse and Karolinska Institutets Fonder. We thank Miss Lena Hultgren, Mrs Annika Jordell-Kylberg and Mrs Stine Söderström for technical assistance.

Received 28 January; accepted 29 April 1980.

1. Levi-Montalcini, R. & Angeletti, P. U. *Physiol. Rev.* **48**, 534–569 (1968).
2. Varon, S. S. & Bunge, R. P. *A. Rev. Neurosci.* **1**, 327–361 (1978).
3. Harper, G. P. & Thoenen, H. *J. Neurochem.* **34**, 5–16 (1980).
4. Harper, G. P. *et al. Nature* **279**, 160–162 (1979).
5. Jacobson, C.-O., Ebendal, T., Hedlund, K.-O. & Norrgren, G. in *Control Mechanisms in Animal Cells—Specific Growth Factors* Vol. 1 (Raven, New York, 1980).
6. Ebendal, T. *Devl Biol.* **72**, 276–290 (1979).
7. Harper, G. P., Pearce, F. L. & Vernon, C. A. *Nature* **261**, 251–253 (1976).
8. Johnson, D. G., Silberstein, S. D., Hanbauer, I. & Kopin, I. J. *Neurochemistry* **19**, 2025–2029 (1972).
9. Olson, L., Seiger, Å. & Ålund, M. in *Formshaping Movements in Neurogenesis* (eds Jacobson, C.-O. & Ebendal, T.) 245–256 (Almqvist and Wiksell, Stockholm, 1978).
10. Olson, L. & Malmfors, T. *Acta physiol. scand.* Suppl. **348**, 1–112 (1970).
11. Stoeckel, K., Schwab, M. E. & Thoenen, H. *Brain Res.* **99**, 1–16 (1975).
12. Suda, K., Barde, Y. A. & Thoenen, H. *Proc. natn. Acad. Sci. U.S.A.* **75**, 4042–4046 (1978).
13. Olson, L., Ebendal, T. & Seiger, Å. *Devl Neurosci.* **2**, 160–176 (1979).
14. McLennan, I. S. & Hendry, I. A. *Neurosci. Lett.* **10**, 269–273 (1978).
15. Lindsay, R. M. & Tarbit, J. *Neurosci. Lett.* **12**, 195–200 (1979).
16. Ebendal, T., Belew, M., Jacobson, C.-O. & Porath, J. *Neurosci. Lett.* **14**, 91–95 (1979).
17. Adler, R., Landa, K. B., Manthorpe, M. & Varon, S. *Science* **204**, 1434–1436 (1979).
18. Manthorpe, M., Skaper, S., Adler, R., Landa, K. & Varon, S. *J. Neurochem.* **34**, 69–75 (1980).
19. Helfand, S. L., Riopelle, R. J. & Wessells, N. K. *Expl cell. Res.* **113**, 39–45 (1978).
20. Nishi, R. & Berg, D. K. *Nature* **277**, 232–234 (1979).
21. Banks, B. E. C., Carstairs, J. R. & Vernon, C. A. *Neuroscience* **4**, 1145–1155 (1979).
22. Anundi, H., Rask, L. & Peterson, P. A. in *Formshaping Movements in Neurogenesis* (eds Jacobson, C.-O. & Ebendal, T.) 213–216 (Almqvist and Wiksell, Stockholm, 1978).

Section 7
Other Trophic Interactions

Lømo, T. and R.H. Westgaard. 1976. Control of ACh sensitivity in rat muscle fibers. *Cold Spring Harbor Symp. Quant. Biol. 40:* 263–274.

Rubin, L.L., S.M. Schuetze, C.L. Weill, and G.D. Fischbach. 1980. Regulation of acetylcholinesterase appearance at neuromuscular junctions *in vitro. Nature 283:* 264–267.

Zalewski, A.A. 1969. Combined effects of testosterone and motor, sensory, or gustatory nerve reinnervation on the regeneration of taste buds. *Exp. Neurol. 24:* 285–297.

As discussed in the introduction to the previous section, the effects of NGF are often considered a paradigm for trophic interactions between cells. There are, however, many other examples of trophic interactions, operating in both the anterograde and retrograde directions, in adults as well as in developing animals (see Cowan 1970; Singer 1974; Black 1978; see also Hamburger 1980, reprinted in Section 1). Such interactions can involve long-term effects on cell survival, growth, differentiation, and specific membrane properties.

Perhaps the most intensively studied trophic influence other than NGF is the control of a variety of skeletal-muscle properties by the motor neurons that innervate them (see Harris 1974; Purves 1976). Denervation of adult vertebrate muscle fibers results in dramatic changes in their electrical properties, contractile properties, the distribution of certain membrane proteins, and the fiber's ability to accept innervation. Historically, there has been considerable controversy over how nerves exert this control. Much of the early evidence appeared to favor the notion that motor nerves release a trophic factor that is unrelated either to acetylcholine or to the activity that the transmitter evokes in muscle. The major results supporting this view were the following: (1) The time of onset of fibrillation and supersensitivity to acetylcholine depends on the length of the nerve stump left connected to the muscle after denervation; the longer the stump, the longer it takes for the changes in the muscle to occur, even though the muscle is rendered inactive as soon as the nerve is cut (Luco and Eyzaguirre 1955). It was suggested that the longer nerve stump contained more residual trophic substance and would therefore maintain normal muscle properties for a longer period. (2) Eliminating one of two inputs to frog sartorius muscle fibers does not interfere with nerve-induced muscle contraction but does cause transmitter supersensitivity (Miledi 1960a). Moreover, upon reinnervation, extrajunctional acetylcholine sensitivity may subside before nerve stimulation can elicit muscle contraction (Miledi 1960b). (3) Blockade of axonal transport by local application of colchicine increases acetylcholine sensitivity in normally innervated muscles (Hoffman and Thesleff 1972; Albuquerque et al. 1972). Several candidates for trophic molecules produced by nerves are presently under study (Lentz 1974; Davey et al. 1978; Markelonis and Oh 1979). However, a role for these molecules in the normal development and maintenance of the neuromuscular junction has not been demonstrated.

In spite of this evidence for a neural trophic factor, it became evident by the mid-1970s that muscle activity was certainly capable of influencing the same muscle fiber properties influenced by the postulated trophic agent. Lømo and Rosenthal (1972) found that blockade of nerve impulses with local anesthetics or diphtheria toxin induced muscle atrophy and transmitter hypersensitivity. More importantly, they found that the increase in acetylcholine sensitivity that occurs under these circumstances could be prevented by stimulation of the nerve distal to the region of the block or by direct stimulation of the denervated muscles. Inactivity thus increased extrajunctional sensitivity, whereas muscle activity held it in check. The paradox of denervation effects in the face of the high levels of spontaneous activity (fibrillation) that occur in denervated muscle was resolved when it was found that individual fibers fibrillate only intermittently (Purves and Sakmann 1974). Further work showed that other denervation changes could also be prevented by direct activation of muscle and that the effects of activity depend on the amount and pattern of the stimulation (**Lømo** and **Westgaard** 1975, **1976**). Nerve-induced activity also appears to regulate acetylcholinesterase at newly formed neuromuscular junctions in vivo and in culture (Lømo and Slater 1980; **Rubin, Schuetze, Weill,** and **Fischbach 1980**).

In light of the effects of muscle activity, it was realized that many of the results that had been taken to support the trophic-factor hypothesis might just as well arise from an effect of the degenerating nerve stump that is left after denervation (Cangiano and Lutzemberger 1980). Indeed, both the ability of nerves to sprout and the extrajunctional receptor levels are influenced by products of nerve degeneration, although the effect is relatively small (Jones and Vrbová 1974; Lømo 1976; Brown et al. 1978). At present, then, the weight of opinion favors muscle activity as the primary agent controlling muscle fiber properties. However, chemical signals from nerves do seem likely to be important in normal neuromuscular development; for example, neural agents induce the clustering of acetylcholine receptors (Christian et al. 1978; Podleski et al. 1978; Jessell et al. 1979; see also Section 8).

The differentiation of mammalian skeletal-muscle fibers into slow and fast types is also strongly influenced by innervation. This was shown originally by cross-reinnervation experiments (Buller et al. 1960; Close 1969) and more recently by experiments in which muscle is chronically stimulated (Salmons and Vrbová 1969; Salmons and Sreter 1976; Pette et al. 1976). That a significant part of this influence is a result of the pattern of activity elicited in normal muscle by its innervation was demonstrated by direct stimulation of denervated muscle with different programs of activity (Lømo et al. 1974). These results add further strength to the view that neural activity controls muscle fiber properties.

Another classic trophic interaction is the dependence of a variety of sensory receptors on their innervation (see Werner 1974). For instance, denervation of mature taste buds or lateral line organs results in the degeneration of these sensory receptors (Olmstead 1920; Torrey 1934; Guth 1957). Moreover, when the epithelium of the tongue is reinnervated by certain sensory nerves, the formation of new taste buds is induced (**Zalewski 1969,** 1972). It is not yet clear whether the nerve influences the normal turnover of cells in the tastebud or their differentiation (Beidler and Smallman 1965; Farbman 1971; Guth 1971). A further example of this type of interaction is the control of muscle spindle development. Cutting both motor and sensory nerves to rat intrafusal muscle fibers at birth causes spindles to degenerate. Cutting only the motor input, however, has little effect; therefore, sensory innervation also appears to provide an important trophic support for development of these mechanoreceptors (Zelena 1957; Zelena and Soukup 1973). These interactions may be amenable to study in cocultures of sensory neurons and target cells.

Another aspect of trophism is the determination of neuronal morphology. Since afferents often arrive at the time dendrites are beginning to grow, Ramón y Cajal (1896, 1911) suggested that inputs might initiate and shape dendritic development. Such a trophic interaction would not be surprising, since many different types of neurons have been shown to be adversely affected if their afferent innervation is cut during development (Levi-Montalcini 1949; see also Black 1978). One of the most extensively studied examples of dendrite development is the cerebellar Purkinje cell. The granule cell/parallel fiber input to Purkinje cells can be destroyed or greatly reduced by X-ray irradiation, mutation, viruses, or toxins. Despite such interference, the Purkinje dendrites develop a surprisingly normal shape (see Rakic 1975). Since other inputs to the Purkinje cell are still intact after granule-cell removal, afferents from the climbing fibers (Hamori 1973; but see Sotelo and Arsenio-Nunes 1976) or the locus coeruleus (see Yamamoto et al. 1980) could conceivably be the controlling elements. It has also been suggested, but not proven, that the parallel fiber input controls the shape of the dendritic arbor of the interneurons of the molecular layer of the cerebellum (the basket and stellate cells [Rakic 1972]).

More compelling evidence for an extrinsic influence on dendrite morphology comes from less complex preparations. For instance, when the vestibular input to the axolotl Mauthner cell is removed very early in development, the cell body and axon grow to about their normal sizes, but the medial dendrite is thinner and has fewer branches than controls (Kimmel et al. 1977). Similarly, when the mechanoreceptor input to the cricket giant interneuron is removed, the length of the dendrites is reduced, although the general form of the branching pattern can still be recognized (Murphey et al. 1975). This effect is specific in that two dendrites of a single interneuron can be influenced independently if they are innervated by separate mechanoreceptors. Whether these effects are due to lack of a trophic factor or activity is not clear. However, blocking activity in the mechanosensory structure is sufficient to alter the responsiveness of the cricket giant interneurons (Matsumoto and Murphey 1977). In summary, the differentiation of dendrites may also result in part from a trophic influence arising from a cell's inputs.

Although many of the trophic interactions described here are not well understood, their clarification will probably broaden considerably the concept of trophic interaction based on the apparent function of NGF described in Section 6.

References

Albuquerque, E.X., J.E. Warnick, J.R. Tasse, and F.M. Sansone. 1972. Effects of vinblastine and colchicine on neural regulation of the fast and slow skeletal muscles of the rat. *Exp. Neurol. 37:* 607–634.

Beidler, L.M. and R.L. Smallman. 1965. Renewal of cells within taste buds. *J. Cell Biol. 27:* 263–272.

Black, I.B. 1978. Regulation of autonomic development. *Annu. Rev. Neurosci. 1:* 183–214.

Brown, M.C., R.L. Holland, and R. Ironton. 1978. Degenerating nerve products affect innervated muscle fibres. *Nature 275:* 652–654.

Buller, A.J., J.C. Eccles, and R.M. Eccles. 1960. Interactions between motoneurons and muscles in respect of the characteristic speeds of their responses. *J. Physiol. 150:* 417–439.

Cangiano, A. and L. Lutzemberger. 1980. Partial denervation in inactive muscle affects innervated and denervated fibres equally. *Nature 285:* 233–235.

Christian, C.N., M.P. Daniels, H. Sugiyama, Z. Vogel, L. Jacques, and P.G. Nelson. 1978. A factor from neurons increases the number of acetylcholine receptor aggregates on cultured muscle cells. *Proc. Natl. Acad. Sci. 75:* 4011–4015.

Close, R. 1969. Dynamic properties of fast and slow skeletal muscles of the rat after cross-union. *J. Physiol. 204:* 331–346.

Cowan, W.M. 1970. Anterograde and retrograde transneuronal degeneration in the central and peripheral nervous system. In *Contemporary research methods in neuroanatomy* (ed. S. Ebbesson and W.J.H. Nauta), pp. 217–251. Springer-Verlag, New York.

Davey, B., L.H. Younkin, and S.B. Younkin. 1979. Neural control of skeletal muscle cholinesterase: A study using organ-cultured rat muscles. *J. Physiol. 289:* 501–515.

Farbman, A.I. 1971. Development of the taste bud. In *Handbook of sensory physiology* (ed. L.M. Beidler), vol. 4, pp. 51–62. Springer-Verlag, Berlin.

Guth, L. 1971. Degeneration and regeneration of taste buds. In *Handbook of sensory physiology* (ed. L. Beidler), vol. 4, pp. 63–74. Springer-Verlag, Berlin.

———. 1957. The effects of glossopharyngeal nerve transection on the circumvallate papilla of the rat. *Anat. Rec. 128:* 715–731.

Hamburger, V. 1980. S. Ramón y Cajal, R.G. Harrison, and the beginnings of neuroembryology. *Perspect. Biol. Med. 23:* 600–616.

Hamori, J. 1973. The inductive role of presynaptic axons in the development of postsynaptic spines. *Brain Res. 62:* 337–344.

Harris, A.J. 1974. Inductive functions of the nervous system. *Annu. Rev. Physiol. 36:* 251–305.

Hoffman, W.W. and S. Thesleff. 1972. Studies on the trophic influence of nerve on skeletal muscle. *Eur. J. Pharmacol. 20:* 256–260.

Jessell, T.M., R.E. Siegel, and G.D. Fischbach. 1979. Induction of acetylcholine receptors on cultured skeletal muscle by a factor extracted from brain and spinal cord. *Proc. Natl. Acad. Sci. 76:* 5397–5401.

Jones, R. and G. Vrbová. 1974. Two factors responsible for the development of denervation hypersensitivity. *J. Physiol. 236:* 517–538.

Kimmel, C.B., E. Schabtach, and R.J. Kimmel. 1977. Developmental interactions in the growth and branching of the lateral dendrite of Mauthner's cell (*Ambystoma mexicanum*). *Dev. Biol. 55:* 244–259.

Lentz, T. 1974. Effect of brain extracts on cholinesterase activity of cultured skeletal muscle. *Exp. Neurol. 45:* 520–526.

Levi-Montalcini, R. 1949. The development of the acoustico-vestibular centers in the chick embryo in the absence of the afferent root fibers and of descending fiber tracts. *J. Comp. Neurol. 91:* 209–241.

Lømo, T. 1976. The role of activity in the control of membrane and contractile properties of skeletal muscle. In *Motor innervation of muscle* (ed. S. Thesleff), pp. 289–321. Academic Press, New York.

Lømo, T. and J. Rosenthal. 1972. Control of ACh sensitivity by muscle activity in the rat. *J. Physiol. 221:* 493–513.

Lømo, T. and R.H. Westgaard. 1975. Further studies on the control of ACh sensitivity by muscle activity in the rat. *J. Physiol. 252:* 603–626.

———. 1976. Control of ACh sensitivity in rat muscle fibers. *Cold Spring Harbor Symp. Quant. Biol. 40:* 263–274.

Lømo, T. and C.R. Slater. 1980. Control of junctional acetylcholinesterase by neural and muscular influences in the rat. *J. Physiol. 303:* 191–202.

Lømo, T., R.H. Westgaard, and H.A. Dahl. 1974. Contractile properties of muscle: Control by pattern of muscle activity in the rat. *Proc. R. Soc. Lond. B 187:* 99–103.

Luco, J.V. and C. Eyzaguirre. 1955. Fibrillation and hypersensitivity to ACh in denervated muscle: Effect of length of degenerating nerve fibers. *J. Neurophysiol. 18:* 65–73.

Markelonis, G. and T.H. Oh. 1979. A sciatic nerve protein has a trophic effect on development and maintenance of skeletal muscle cells in culture. *Proc. Natl. Acad. Sci. 76:* 2470–2474.

Matsumoto, S.G. and R.K. Murphey. 1977. Sensory deprivation during development decreases the responsiveness of cricket giant interneurons. *J. Physiol. 268:* 533–548.

Miledi, R. 1960a. The acetylcholine sensitivity of frog muscle fibres after complete or partial denervation.

J. Physiol. 151: 1–23.

———. 1960b. Junctional and extra-junctional acetylcholine receptors in skeletal muscle fibres. J. Physiol. 151: 24–30.

Murphey, R.K., B. Mendenhall, J. Palka, and J.S. Edwards. 1975. Deafferentation slows the growth of specific dendrites of identified giant interneurons. J. Comp. Neurol. 159: 407–418.

Olmstead, J.M.D. 1920. The results of cutting the seventh cranial nerve in Amiurus nebulosus (Lesueur). J. Exp. Zool. 31: 369–401.

Pette, D., W. Müller, E. Leisner, and G. Vrbová. 1976. Time dependent effects on contractile properties, fibre population, myosin light chains and enzymes of energy metabolism in intermittently and continuously stimulated fast-twitch muscles of the rabbit. Pflügers Arch. 364: 103–112.

Podleski, T.R., D. Axelrod, P. Ravdin, I. Greenberg, M.M. Johnson, and M.M. Salpeter. 1978. Nerve extract induces increase and redistribution of acetylcholine receptors on cloned muscle cells. Proc. Natl. Acad. Sci. 75: 2035–2039.

Purves, D. 1976. Long-term regulation in the vertebrate peripheral nervous system. In International review of physiology, neurophysiology II (ed. R. Porter), vol. 10, pp. 125–177. University Park Press, Baltimore.

Purves, D. and B. Sakman. 1974. The effect of contractile activity on fibrillation and extrajunctional acetylcholine-sensitivity in rat muscle maintained in organ culture. J. Physiol. 237: 157–182.

Rakic, P. 1972. Extrinsic cytological determinants of basket and stellate cell dendritic pattern in the cerebellar molecular layer. J. Comp. Neurol. 146: 335–354.

———. 1975. Role of cell interaction in development of dendritic patterns. Adv. Neurol. 12: 117–134.

Ramón y Cajal, S. 1896. Les épines collaterales des cellules du cerveau coloree au bleu de méthyléne. Rev. Trim. Microgr. 1: 5–19.

———. 1911. Histologie du système nerveux de l'homme ēt des vertébrés. A. Maloine, Paris. Reprinted by Consejo Superior de Investigaciones Cientificas, Instituto Ramón y Cajal, Madrid, 1955.

Rubin, L.L., S.M. Schuetze, C.L. Weill, and G.D. Fischbach. 1980. Regulation of acetylcholinesterase appearance at neuromuscular junctions in vitro. Nature 283: 264–267.

Salmons, S. and F.A. Sreter. 1976. Significance of impulse activity in the transformation of skeletal muscle type. Nature 263: 30–34.

Salmons, S. and G. Vrbová. 1969. The influence of activity on some contractile characteristics of mammalian fast and slow muscles. J. Physiol. 201: 535–549.

Singer, M. 1974. Neurotrophic control of limb regeneration in the newt. Ann. N.Y. Acad. Sci. 228: 308–322.

Sotelo, C. and M.L. Arsenio-Nunes. 1976. Development of Purkinje cells in absence of climbing fibers. Brain Res. 111: 389–395.

Torrey, T.W. 1934. The relation of taste buds to their nerve fibers. J. Comp. Neurol. 59: 203–220.

Werner, J.K. 1974. Trophic influence of nerves on the development and maintenance of sensory receptors. Am. J. Phys. Med. 53: 127–142.

Yamamoto, M., V. Chan-Palay, H.W.M. Steinbusch, and S.L. Palay. 1980. Hyperinnervation of arrested granule cells produced by the transplantation of monoamine-containing neurons into the fourth ventricle of rat. Anat. Embryol. 159: 1–15.

Zalewski, A.A. 1969. Combined effects of testosterone and motor, sensory, or gustatory nerve reinnervation on the regeneration of taste buds. Exp. Neurol. 24: 285–297.

———. 1972. Regeneration of taste buds after transplantation with tongue and ganglia grafts to the anterior chamber of the eye. Exp. Neurol. 35: 519–528.

Zelena, J. 1957. The morphogenetic influence of innervation on the ontogenetic development of muscle-spindles. J. Embryol. Exp. Morphol. 5: 283–294.

Zelena, J. and T. Soukup. 1973. Development of muscle spindles deprived of fusimotor innervation. Z. Zellforsch. 144: 435–452.

Reprinted from Cold Spring Harbor Symp. Quant. Biol., Vol. 40, pp. 263–274. 1976

Control of ACh Sensitivity in Rat Muscle Fibers

T. Lømo and R. H. Westgaard*

Institute of Neurophysiology, University of Oslo, Oslo 1, Norway

The effects of denervation and reinnervation on the sensitivity of muscle fibers to acetylcholine (ACh) illustrate in a dramatic way the importance of the nerve for maintaining normal muscular properties. In innervated fibers, only the membrane immediately underneath the nerve terminal is highly sensitive to ACh. Denervation causes the entire membrane to become very sensitive (Axelsson and Thesleff 1959), whereas reinnervation restricts the sensitivity once again to the junctional region. The ACh receptors at the end plate are much more densely packed than the extrajunctional receptors of denervated muscle (Fambrough and Hartzell 1972). The junctional receptors also persist, whereas the extrajunctional ones quickly disappear when denervated muscles are activated by electrical stimulation (Lømo and Rosenthal 1972) or by a foreign nerve innervating the fiber elsewhere (Frank et al. 1975b), a phenomenon perhaps associated with a slower turnover of the junctional receptors (Berg and Hall 1974). Thus the nerve has highly localized effects on the postjunctional membrane distinct from its more generalized effects on the rest of the fiber.

This paper summarizes experiments done in our laboratory aimed at obtaining a better understanding of the mechanisms behind the neural control of ACh sensitivity of muscle. First, experiments will be described which provide strong evidence that the ACh sensitivity of the extrajunctional membrane is directly related to muscle activity per se and not to any "trophic" influence of the nerve, i.e., one which is independent of action potentials in the nerve (Miledi 1963). These experiments, which involved direct electrical stimulation of chronically denervated muscles with controlled amounts and patterns of stimuli, also help to explain why fast and slow muscles normally have different levels of extrajunctional ACh sensitivity (Miledi and Zelená 1966), why limb immobilization (Solandt et al. 1943; Fischbach and Robbins 1971) and spinal cord isolation (Solandt and Magladery 1942; Johns and Thesleff 1961) have little effect on the normal distribution of ACh sensitivity, and why fibrillation does not prevent denervation hypersensitivity.

Second, results are presented which suggest that ACh hypersensitivity may be caused not only by inactivity of the muscle, but also by factors present during the degeneration of nerve terminals. Other results indicate that colchicine, a substance known to block axonal transport (Dahlström 1968; Kreutzberg 1969), in addition may affect the muscle membrane directly.

These findings lead to a reinterpretation of several lines of evidence generally taken to support the concept of neurotrophic control. The lines of evidence in question are the earlier appearance of ACh hypersensitivity, and other signs of denervation, in muscles denervated by cutting the nerve close to, rather than far from, the muscle (Luco and Eyzaguirre 1955; Emmelin and Malm 1965; Harris and Thesleff 1972); the development of ACh hypersensitivity around the degenerating end plate in doubly innervated muscle fibers one of whose nerves has been cut (Miledi 1960b); and the hypersensitivity caused by colchicine in functionally innervated muscle fibers (Hofmann and Thesleff 1972; Albuquerque et al. 1972).

Finally, the idea is presented that the ACh sensitivity at each site along the fiber reflects the outcome of a competitive interaction at these sites between muscle activity that suppresses the sensitivity and various external influences that may induce it. In normal circumstances, muscle activity is probably solely responsible for keeping the extrajunctional sensitivity low, but in experimental or abnormal circumstances, this suppressive influence may be overcome by external factors associated with degenerating nerve terminals, inflammation of adjacent tissue, or colchicine. The high sensitivity at normal end plates may result from a similar, but more intense and prolonged, induction of receptors by the continued presence of the functioning nerve terminal.

EXPERIMENTAL MATERIAL AND PROCEDURE

A main objective in these experiments was to study effects of muscle activity in the absence of accompanying neural influences. Rat soleus muscles were therefore denervated by resection of the sciatic nerve and stimulated directly, through implanted electrodes, 5 or 14 days later, when the nerve terminals had degenerated (Miledi and Slater 1968; Gonzenbach and Waser 1973). A second objective was to find ways of quantitating the effects of different amounts and patterns of imposed muscle activity. By starting the stimulation on day 5 (or 14), when denervation hypersensitivity is fully developed (see Fig. 1), the effectiveness of the stimulation could be assessed in terms of the rate at which it caused the hypersensitivity to disappear. A detailed description of the in vivo stimulation procedures and the subsequent measurements in vitro of the sensitivity of single muscle fibers to electrophoretically applied ACh is given elsewhere (Lømo and Westgaard 1975).

Evidence emerged during these experiments that

* Present address: Sobell Department of Neurophysiology, Institute of Neurology, Queen Square, London WC IN 3 BG, England.

ACh hypersensitivity might be caused by the degeneration of nerve terminals as well as by inactivity of the muscle. We studied this in muscles in which nerve terminals were actively degenerating while muscle activity was maintained by electrical stimulation or through an additional neural input. Double innervation was obtained by transplanting the superficial fibular nerve onto the surface of the soleus and crushing the soleus nerve 3 weeks later. This causes a large number of soleus surface fibers first to become innervated at some distance from the old end plates by the foreign nerve and later to become reinnervated at the old end plates by the regenerating soleus nerve, as described in detail in Frank et al. (1975b).

A different approach was to stop muscle activity and to compare the time course of the subsequent hypersensitivity in muscles with and without degenerating nerve terminals. Active degeneration was avoided by placing an anesthetic cuff around the sciatic nerve (Lømo and Rosenthal 1972), rather than cutting it, or by stimulating a denervated muscle for 15 days and then stopping the stimulation.

RESULTS

Amount and Pattern of Muscle Activity

Denervation causes a roughly synchronous increase in ACh sensitivity along the whole length of mammalian skeletal muscle fibers (Fambrough 1970; Lømo and Westgaard 1975). Direct stimulation of rat soleus muscles from day 5 after the denervation causes the

extrajunctional hypersensitivity to ACh, which is fully developed at this time (Fig. 1, filled circles), to decline at a rate that is critically dependent both on the amount and the pattern of stimuli.

The amount of muscle activity was varied by presenting identical trains of stimuli (10 Hz for 10 s) interrupted by pauses of up to 12 hours so that the overall average frequency ranged from 10 to 0.0023 Hz (Fig. 1). These procedures reduced the extrajunctional sensitivity to 1 mV/nC (within the normal range) within times varying from 5 days (10 Hz mean) to 20 days (0.01 Hz mean). One train (100 stimuli) every 5 hours 33 minutes (0.005 Hz mean) gradually reduced the sensitivity to one-tenth of the denervated control values after 3 weeks of stimulation, whereas one train every 12 hours had no apparent effect. Starting the stimulation on day 14 after the denervation had roughly the same effect as starting it on day 5.

The pattern of activity was varied by changing the timing of a constant number of stimuli presented to the muscle every day (Fig. 2). Stimulation at 100 Hz for 1 second every 100 seconds reduced the sensitivity to 1 mV/nC within 4 days, whereas 10 Hz for 10 seconds every 100 seconds and continuous 1-Hz stimulation required 6 and 10 days, respectively, to bring the sensitivity to the same low levels. The stimulation became much less effective when long pauses (18 hr) alternated with shorter periods (6 hr) of more vigorously imposed activity (10 Hz for 10 s every 25 s).

The differences in rate of decline of ACh sensitivity for each of the stimulation series shown in Figures 1 and 2 were of a high statistical significance ($P < 0.001$,

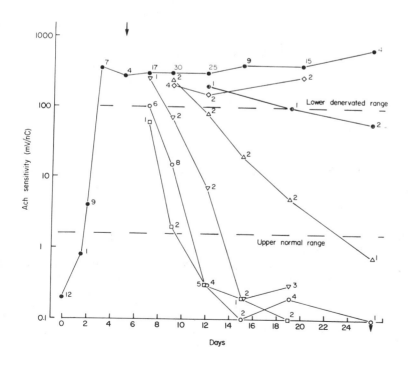

Figure 1. Direct muscle stimulation causes denervation hypersensitivity to ACh to decline at a rate that depends on the number of stimuli. Each symbol gives the median sensitivity of many soleus fibers from a number of soleus muscles (as indicated) measured 2 mm from the Achilles tendon at different days after the denervation. ACh sensitivity in this and subsequent figures is expressed as mV depolarization per nC charge passed through the micropipette containing 3 M AChCl.

(Filled circles) Denervated control fibers. (Open symbols) Fibers stimulated from day 5 after the denervation (arrow) with identical 10-s trains of stimuli at 10 Hz. Each train was interrupted by 0 s (□), 1 min 30 s (○), 16 min 40 s (▽), 2 hr 46 min 30 s (△), 5 hr 33 min 10 s (⊕), or 12 hr (◇), so that the average frequency of stimulation was 10, 1, 0.1, 0.01, 0.005 or 0.0023 Hz, respectively. The interrupted line at 100 mV/nC indicates the lowest ACh sensitivity found in more than 3-day denervated muscles. The interrupted line at 1.6 mV/nC gives the highest sensitivity found in normal fibers. (Reprinted, with permission, from Lømo and Westgaard 1975.)

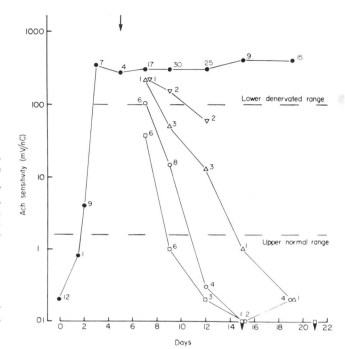

Figure 2. Direct muscle stimulation causes denervation hypersensitivity to ACh to decline at a rate that depends on the pattern of stimuli. The average frequency of stimulation was 1 Hz in each of the four stimulation procedures. Each symbol gives the median sensitivity of many fibers from a number of soleus muscles (as indicated) measured 2 mm from the Achilles tendon at different days after the denervation.

(Filled circles) Denervated control fibers. (Open symbols) Fibers stimulated from day 5 after the denervation (arrow) with 1-s stimulus trains at 100 Hz every 100 s (□), 10-s stimulus trains at 10 Hz every 100 s (○), continuous 1-Hz stimulation (△), or 10-s stimulus trains at 10 Hz every 25 s for 6 hr every 24 hr (▽). The interrupted horizontal lines have the same meaning as in Figure 1. (Reprinted, with permission, from Lømo and Westgaard 1975.)

Wilcoxon two-sample test, Lømo and Westgaard 1975). For most stimulation procedures, the sensitivity of the stimulated fibers eventually became as low as or lower than that of normally innervated fibers. The sensitivity declined at roughly the same rate along the entire length of the muscle fiber, except at the end plate, where the sensitivity remained high and indistinguishable from that of normally innervated fibers.

ACh Hypersensitivity and Degenerating Nerve Terminals

Because most stimulation procedures effectively abolished all denervation hypersensitivity, we were initially surprised to find that stimulation at 10 Hz for 10 seconds every 100 seconds failed to prevent an early rise in hypersensitivity when it was started on the day of denervation. Figure 3 shows that the extrajunctional ACh sensitivity in stimulated and nonstimulated muscles was about equally high on day 4 after denervation, and that only subsequently did the sensitivity fall toward normal levels in muscles stimulated with this pattern. In the first days after denervation, the hypersensitivity was sometimes (2 muscles) much more pronounced around the degenerating end plates than at either end of the fiber (Fig. 4). In two other muscles studied in similar detail, however, the hypersensitivity was more uniformly distributed, and further stimulation experiments are planned to examine this point more thoroughly.

The transient and sometimes local nature of the hypersensitivity just described suggested that the degenerative changes at the end plate might give rise to

an increase in ACh sensitivity which would normally be masked by the generalized increase in sensitivity that results from muscle inactivity after denervation. Therefore we were prompted to look for hypersensitivity around degenerating end plates on muscle fibers whose activity was maintained by a second, intact end plate. This was accomplished by studying dually innervated muscles (see above) after cutting either the soleus nerve or the previously introduced superficial fibular nerve.

When the fibular nerve was cut, a marked hypersensitivity was always present 3 and 7 days later in the proximal part of the soleus, where the end plates associated with this nerve normally occur (Figs. 5A,B and 6A). That points of maximum sensitivity were in fact associated with old fibular nerve end plates was confirmed by subsequent staining for cholinesterase. All these fibers were functionally innervated by the intact soleus nerve, as shown by the presence of miniature end-plate potentials (m.e.p.p.'s) and a high focal ACh sensitivity at the soleus end plates (Figs. 5A and 6A, arrows), by action potentials to stimulation of the soleus nerve, and by a low extrajunctional sensitivity to ACh in the other end of the muscle (Fig. 5B). Seventeen days after cutting the fibular nerve, the surrounding sensitivity had disappeared, leaving only the highly focal junctional sensitivity at the degenerated end plates. For comparison, Figure 6B shows the distribution of sensitivity in a dually innervated soleus fiber with intact fibular and soleus nerves.

We were initially surprised to find that cutting the soleus nerve did not cause a similar hypersensitivity around the degenerating soleus end plates in fibers

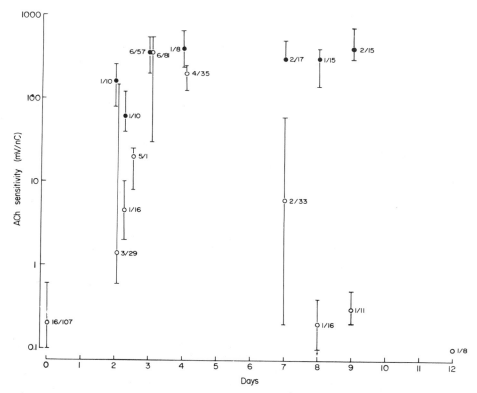

Figure 3. Transient denervation hypersensitivity to ACh in soleus fibers stimulated directly with a "slow" stimulus pattern. Stimulation was 10 Hz for 10 s every 100 s from the time of denervation (abscissa). Each symbol gives the median ACh sensitivity of many fibers at 2 mm from the Achilles tendon. The number of muscles and fibers is indicated. Error bars give the range after the upper and lower 20% of the individual values have been excluded to avoid giving undue weight to occasional very high or low values. The range in subsequent figures is similarly restricted. (○) Denervated and stimulated fibers; (●) denervated control fibers.

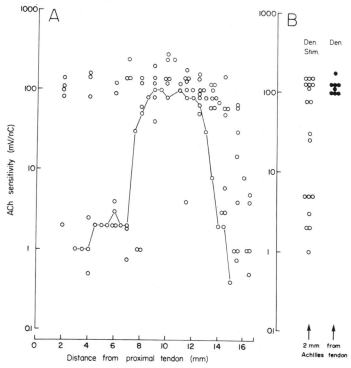

Figure 4. Distribution of ACh sensitivity in soleus fibers after 3 days of denervation and continued stimulation at a "slow" stimulus pattern (10 Hz for 10 s every 100 s). (*A*) Each symbol gives the ACh sensitivity of single soleus fibers at different distances from the proximal tendon. Symbols joined by lines show the sensitivity of a single fiber followed from one end of the fiber to the other. (*B*) ACh sensitivity of denervated stimulated fibers (○) compared with the sensitivity of denervated, unstimulated fibers from the soleus of the opposite leg (●), all fibers tested at 2 mm from the Achilles tendon.

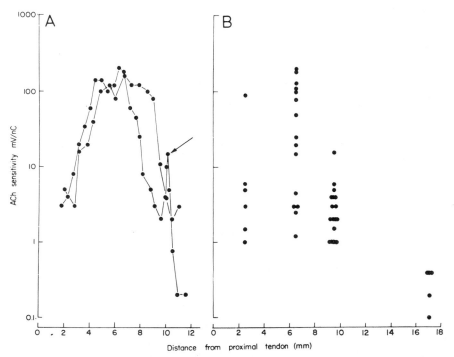

Figure 5. ACh hypersensitivity in soleus fibers innervated by two (the soleus and the foreign fibular) nerves 3 days after cutting the foreign nerve. (A) ACh sensitivity along two surface fibers in the proximal half of the muscle where subsequent staining for acetylcholine esterase revealed large numbers of foreign end plates. Arrow points to the high sensitivity at an intact soleus nerve end plate where m.e.p.p.'s were recorded. (B) ACh sensitivity of single fibers showing the high sensitivity around the degenerating foreign end plates in the proximal half and the low sensitivity in the distal half of the muscle.

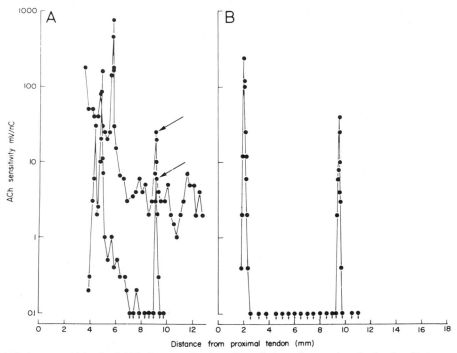

Figure 6. ACh hypersensitivity in doubly innervated soleus fibers 7 days after cutting the foreign fibular nerve (A) and "normal" distribution of sensitivity in a fiber from a muscle with both nerves intact (B). In A, m.e.p.p.'s were recorded only near the sensitive focus in the middle of each fiber (arrows), corresponding to the location of intact soleus end plates. In B, m.e.p.p.'s were recorded from both regions where the sensitivity was high. In this muscle, action potentials were evoked by stimulation of either nerve.

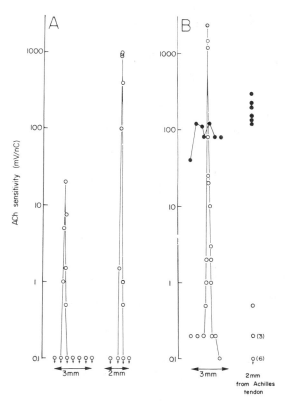

Figure 7. Absence of ACh hypersensitivity around degenerating soleus end plates in fibers whose activity is maintained by an intact foreign fibular nerve input. (A) Examples from two fibers of the essentially normal ACh sensitivity around soleus end plates 3 days after cutting the soleus nerve. The presence of end plates at these spots was verified by staining for acetylcholine esterase at the end of the experiment. (B) Similar preparation 4 days after cutting the soleus nerve. To the left, ACh sensitivity in the soleus end-plate region of a fiber innervated by the fibular nerve (○) and an adjacent fiber not innervated by the fibular nerve (●). To the right, ACh sensitivity at 2 mm from the Achilles tendon in a group of fibers innervated (○) or not innervated (●) by the fibular nerve.

functionally innervated by an intact fibular nerve (Fig. 7). Since the axons in the fibular nerve normally innervate predominantly fast muscle fibers and would be expected to have a different pattern of impulse activity from fibers innervating the slow soleus muscle, it seemed possible that differences in the pattern of impulse activity in the surviving nerve might determine whether or not a spread of ACh sensitivity away from a degenerating end plate would occur. We therefore repeated our previous experiments, in which stimulation of the denervated soleus started at the time of denervation (Figs. 3 and 4), but now with a "fast" stimulus pattern (100 Hz for 1 s every 100 s) rather than a "slow" pattern (10 Hz for 10 s every 100 s). The "fast" stimulus pattern prevented all hypersensitivity around the degenerating end plates (Fig. 8A,B), as did the "fast" nerve (Fig. 7), in sharp contrast to the hypersensitivity developing during a

"slow" stimulus pattern (Figs. 3 and 4) or with a "slow" nerve (Figs. 5A,B and 6A).

If the degeneration of nerve terminals and muscle inactivity both contribute to the hypersensitivity caused by nerve section, then the hypersensitivity following interruption of muscle activity might develop along a different time course in muscles without such nerve degeneration. We tested this by denervating and stimulating the soleus muscle for 15 days with either the "fast" or "slow" pattern referred to above. At day 15, all hypersensitivity was abolished (Figs. 1 and 2), and the process of nerve degeneration was probably complete. When stimulation was stopped on day 15, the subsequent hypersensitivity, which may be attributed to inactivity alone, developed along a time course determined by the type of previous activity (Fig. 9). It appeared considerably later after stimulation with the "fast" pattern than with the "slow" pattern and later with the "slow" pattern than in the opposite control soleus denervated acutely at the time that the stimulation was stopped. It could be argued that hypersensitivity developed along different time courses in all these muscles because their previous level or type of muscle activity was different and not because degenerating nerve terminals were present in the acutely denervated soleus. However, we have preliminary evidence showing that the hypersensitivity develops somewhat earlier if the nerve is cut than if nerve impulse conduction is blocked by a local anesthesia preventing terminal degeneration. Previous results reported by Lømo and Rosenthal (1972) suggested a similar difference.

ACh Hypersensitivity Caused by Colchicine

Colchicine, a drug known to interfere with axonal transport (Dahlstrøm 1968; Kreutzberg 1969) can produce an increase in the ACh sensitivity of normally innervated muscles (Hofmann and Thesleff 1972; Albuquerque et al. 1972; Cangiano 1973; Lømo 1974). This fact has been used to support the view that transport of "trophic" substances along axons is necessary to maintain normal muscle properties (Hofmann and Thesleff 1972; Albuquerque et al. 1972).

However, the effect of colchicine on ACh sensitivity might also result from a direct action on the muscle. To examine this possibility, the effect of colchicine was tested on soleus muscles that had been denervated 10 days previously and whose ACh sensitivity had been kept low by direct stimulation. In the absence of colchicine, the sensitivity of denervated, stimulated fibers (Fig. 10A, striped column) was indistinguishable from normal fibers (Fig. 10A, open columns), except for a few fibers in two of five muscles whose somewhat higher than normal sensitivity may be attributed to inadequate or damaging stimulation. In contrast, a moderate ACh hypersensitivity developed in similarly denervated and stimulated fibers (Fig. 10B, striped columns) as well as in normally innervated fibers (Fig. 10B, open columns) in rats who 4 days previously had

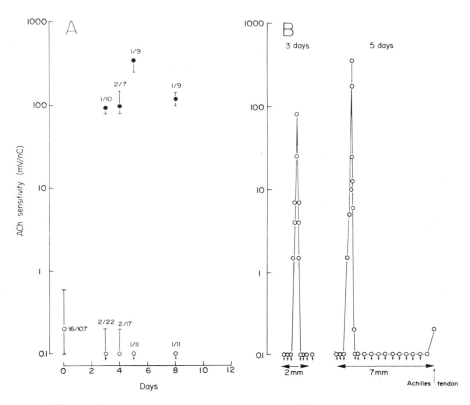

Figure 8. Absence of denervation hypersensitivity in soleus fibers stimulated directly with a "fast" stimulation pattern. Stimulation was 100 Hz for 1 s every 100 s from the time of denervation. (*A*) Each symbol gives the median ACh sensitivity of single fibers measured 2 mm from the Achilles tendon at different times after the denervation. Numbers indicate number of muscles and fibers. (○) Denervated and stimulated fibers; (●) denervated control fibers. (*B*) Examples of the essentially normal ACh sensitivity at a denervated soleus end plate 3 and 5 days after denervation.

received 270 μg of colchicine intramuscularly high in the thigh. A similar hypersensitivity was found in innervated muscles in the leg opposite the injection and in the diaphragm. The hypersensitivity induced by colchicine not only was less marked than the usual denervation hypersensitivity (Fig. 10A, solid columns), it was also transient, as pointed out by Hofmann and Thesleff (1972) and confirmed by Lømo (unpubl. exps.), where 4 and 13 days after a single injection of 270 μg of colchicine (200 g rats), the extra junctional ACh sensitivity was 7.19 ± 3.2 mV/nC (mean $\pm$ s.d., 14 fibers, 2 muscles) and 0.14 ± 0.16 mV/nC (21 fibers, 2 muscles), respectively. It appears that colchicine has a systemic effect that is similar on innervated and stimulated denervated muscles and is therefore independent of its effects on nerves.

DISCUSSION

Control of ACh Sensitivity by Muscle Activity

It is clear from this study that in the absence of any possible "trophic" action of the nerve, direct electrical stimulation of denervated rat soleus muscles causes their sensitivity to ACh to return to normal (and even below normal) levels at a rate that depends critically

on the amount or pattern of activation. Thus brief, high-frequency trains caused the sensitivity to decline much faster than longer low-frequency trains containing the same number of stimuli and repeated at the same frequency. Indeed at the patterns used, 100-Hz stimulation was more effective than 10 times as many stimuli at 10 Hz, and 10-Hz stimulation was about as effective as 10 times as many stimuli at 1 Hz. These results suggest a close coupling between muscle activity and the formation of extrajunctional ACh receptors. Its nature is unknown, but any substance, such as for example calcium, whose free concentration in the fiber varies with the type of muscle activity might be a mediator.

As few as 100 stimuli (10 Hz for 10 s) given every 5 hours 33 minutes or every 2 hours 45 minutes for 3 weeks caused, respectively, a 10- or 100-fold reduction in ACh sensitivity. This may explain the near normal distribution of ACh sensitivity in muscles immobilized by limb fixation (Solandt et al. 1943; Fischbach and Robbins 1969) or spinal cord isolation (Solandt and Magladery 1942; Johns and Thesleff 1961). In these preparations, the level of muscle activity is markedly reduced but probably not completely eliminated.

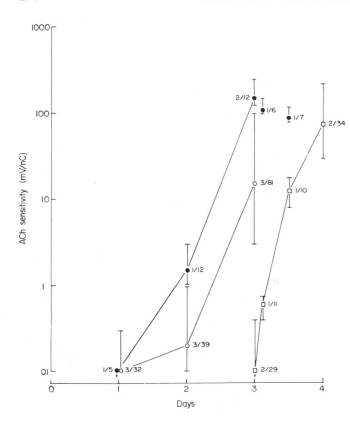

Figure 9. Development of hypersensitivity after cessation of activity in muscles with and without degenerating nerve terminals. Each symbol gives the median ACh sensitivity of single fibers measured 2 mm from the Achilles tendon at different times after cessation of activity. Numbers indicate number of muscles and fibers. (●) Soleus fibers denervated at day 0; (○) soleus fibers denervated and stimulated with a "slow" stimulus pattern (10 Hz for 10 s every 100 s) for the 15 days preceding day 0 when the stimulation was stopped; (□) same as for (○), but stimulation was of the "fast" type (100 Hz for 1 s every 100 s).

"Fast" Vs. "Slow" Patterns of Activity

Brief, high-frequency stimulus trains ("fast" stimulus pattern) induce contractile properties characteristic of fast muscle in denervated slow rat soleus muscles (Lømo et al. 1974) and mimic the effects of reinnervating the soleus with a nerve normally going to a fast muscle (Close 1969). The muscle does not become fast if longer low-frequency stimulus trains ("slow" stimulus pattern) containing the same number of stimuli are used. The "fast" stimulus pattern also appears to keep the formation of ACh receptor more effectively suppressed, since stopping the stimulation of chronically denervated muscles leads to a considerably later development of hypersensitivity when the stimulation is of the "fast" type rather than of the "slow" type (Fig. 9). Thus differences in the pattern of activity in normal fast and slow muscles (Fischbach and Robbins 1971) may explain their different contractile properties as well as their different levels of extrajunctional ACh sensitivity (Miledi and Zelená 1966). The later development of denervation hypersensitivity in fast relative to slow muscles (Albuquerque and McIsaac 1970) is also consistent with this interpretation.

Why Does Fibrillation Not Prevent Denervation Hypersensitivity?

This is a puzzling question since fibrillatory activity is, on the average, relatively high (1 Hz) in mammalian muscles kept in organ culture (Purves and Sakmann

1974), and presumably also in vivo (Belmar and Eyzaguirre 1966). An answer may be provided by the cyclic nature of this activity, with long inactive periods (probably 2–3 days) alternating with shorter periods of relatively intense activity (22–23 hr, Purves and Sakmann 1974). In the present study, one stimulus train (10 Hz for 10 s) every 2 hours 45 minutes was about as effective as 100 times as many stimuli given during a 6-hour period (one train every 25 s) every 24 hours. Evidently long periods without externally imposed activity (18 hr in this example) markedly reduce the effectiveness of the stimulation. This and similar results suggest that the timing of the imposed activity is of crucial importance. During longer periods of inactivity, such as are probably present in denervated fibers, the membrane properties change gradually, and ACh hypersensitivity, fibrillations and other signs of denervation begin to appear after a delay that varies with the type or vigor of the previous activity (see Fig. 9). Purves and Sakmann (1974) found evidence that, to a small extent, fibrillations do suppress ACh hypersensitivity, but as the membrane returns toward normal, the fibrillations stop and the cycle is repeated.

ACh Hypersensitivity Related to Degeneration of Nerve Terminals

Three lines of evidence are presented here suggesting that in addition to the generalized hypersensitivity that results from inactivity, cutting the nerve also induces hypersensitivity by some effect from the

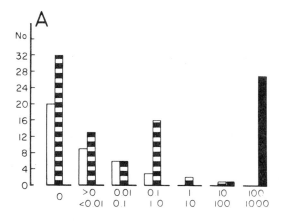

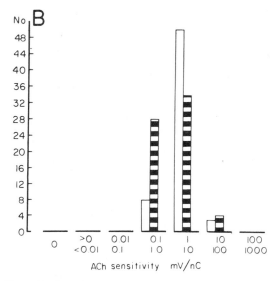

ACh sensitivity   mV/nC

Figure 10. Colchicine causes ACh hypersensitivity of similar magnitude in innervated and denervated, stimulated soleus fibers. (*A*) Control experiments showing the extrajunctional ACh sensitivity of soleus fibers from denervated, stimulated muscles (striped columns), innervated muscles from the opposite leg (open columns) and denervated, unstimulated muscles (solid columns). Denervation lasted 14 days. Stimulation took place from day 1 to day 14 after denervation. (*B*) Similar experiments on rats (approx. 200 g) injected with 270 μg colchicine on day 10, that is 4 days before the ACh sensitivity was tested. The injection was intramuscular, high in the thigh of the stimulated leg. (Reprinted, with permission, from Lømo 1974.)

degenerating nerve terminals. (1) A marked, but transient, hypersensitivity develops after denervation in muscles stimulated directly with a "slow" stimulus pattern (Figs. 3 and 4). (2) A similarly marked and transient hypersensitivity develops in dually innervated soleus fibers around degenerating foreign fibular nerve terminals (Figs. 5 and 6). (3) The hypersensitivity following acute denervation develops considerably faster than the hypersensitivity following the cessation of stimulation of chronically denervated muscles without nerve terminals (Fig. 9). In addition, we have

preliminary evidence that the hypersensitivity occurs faster when impulse activity is stopped by cutting the nerve rather than by placing an anesthetic cuff around the nerve to prevent terminal degeneration (see also Lømo and Rosenthal 1972).

The mechanism that underlies this increase in ACh sensitivity associated with the degenerating nerve terminal is not known. In normally innervated muscle, an intense hypersensitivity can be induced by placing a foreign body (for example, a piece of thread) on the surface of the muscle (Jones and Vrbová 1974; T. Lømo and C. R. Slater, unpubl. obs.). Its time course is similar to that seen in contracting muscles with degenerating nerves, being maximal after about 4 days and absent after more than 10–12 days. It is maximal (up to 1000 mV/nC or more) near the foreign body and may be caused by the inflammatory cells infiltrating that area. Work is now in progress to test the possibility that this hypersensitivity and that around degenerating nerve terminals are related.

Reinterpretation of Evidence for Neurotrophic Control

The results just presented suggest a reinterpretation of certain other results generally taken to support the concept of neurotrophic control. ACh hypersensitivity and other effects of denervation appear later if the nerve is cut far from, rather than close to, the muscle (Luco and Eyzaguirre 1955; Emmelin and Malm 1965; Harris and Thesleff 1972). Since neurally evoked muscle activity stops at the same time in both cases, this delay has been attributed to a continuing release of trophic substances from the longer nerve. However, nerve terminals degenerate earlier if the peripheral nerve stumps are short rather than long (Miledi and Slater 1968). We prefer, therefore, to attribute the earlier appearance of postsynaptic changes with short nerve stumps not to the lack of some trophic influence from the nerve, but to the earlier onset of the terminal degeneration process. The hypersensitivity around degenerating end plates in doubly innervated muscle fibers previously attributed to a lack of neurotrophic influences in that region (Miledi 1960b) can be similarly explained, as has already been suggested by Jones and Vrbová (1974).

Effects of colchicine. The ability of colchicine to increase the ACh sensitivity of normally innervated muscles has been raised as support for the notion of neurotrophic control of muscle properties (Hofmann and Thesleff 1972; Albuquerque et al. 1972). However, the results presented in Figure 10 show that colchicine can raise the extrajunctional ACh sensitivity of muscle fibers by some mechanism not involving axonal transport. The magnitude of the sensitivity increase is similar in denervated, stimulated fibers and in innervated fibers, suggesting that the entire effect of colchicine on ACh sensitivity may be independent of the nerve. The effect appears to be systemic and could be directly on the muscle, but its precise mechanism is unknown.

In a recent study, Kauffman et al. (1974) failed to find any effect of a single injection of colchicine on directly stimulated denervated muscles, and they contrasted this with the hypersensitivity appearing if a silastic cuff containing the same concentration of colchicine is placed around the sciatic nerve. However, with the cuff, there is presumably continuous release of colchicine and a possibility of conduction block by local pressure. As reported by Albuquerque et al. (1972): "with colchicine [in the cuff] the nerve continued to degenerate after 15 days and was progressively replaced by collagen, macrophages and fibroblasts." In contrast, a single injection of colchicine sufficient to cause ACh hypersensitivity has no demonstrable effect on axonal transport (Cangiano and Fried 1974). Other objections are that Kauffman et al. (1974) examined the ACh sensitivity 14 days after injection of colchicine, i.e., after the transient hypersensitivity induced by a single injection has disappeared (Hofmann and Thesleff 1972 and above). At this time, both their colchicine-treated and untreated denervated stimulated muscles were considerably more sensitive than what is usually seen after 4 days (Hofmann and Thesleff 1972; Cangiano 1973; Lømo 1974) when the effect of a single injection is maximal. Since no hypersensitivity is present in effectively stimulated muscles 14 days after denervation (Figs. 1 and 2), their high background sensitivity (approx. 45 mV/nC) was probably caused by ineffective stimulation. Thus these experiments do not invalidate the earlier conclusion that colchicine has effects on the muscle which are not mediated by the nerve (Fig. 10 and Lømo 1974).

Given the evidence for a systemic effect of colchicine on the ACh sensitivity of muscle and the evidence from many different cells for an effect of colchicine on the surface membrane either directly (Wunderlich et al. 1973) or indirectly by an effect on intracellular colchicine binding proteins, possibly microtubules (Berlin et al. 1974; Edelman et al. 1975), it is clearly important that the observations on the effects of colchicine that have been reported in support of the theory of neurotrophic control should be interpreted with great caution.

Other results suggestive of neurotrophic control. First, denervation hypersensitivity appears to decline before neuromuscular transmission is reestablished by regenerating motor axons (Miledi 1960a; Bennett et al. 1973). However since presynaptic block of impulse conduction is often encountered in vitro in the early stages of axon regeneration, it is difficult to rule out that fibers which do not respond to nerve stimulation in vitro and yet have a low sensitivity to ACh are not subject to such block.

Second, cross-innervation with the "fast" fibular nerve has recently been shown largely to prevent the reduction in binding of α-bungarotoxin at denervated soleus end plates that occurs in fibers without such foreign innervation (Frank et al. 1975a). Surprisingly, direct stimulation at 10 Hz did not similarly preserve junctional binding sites, although it suppressed extrajunctional toxin binding. A "fast" stimulus pattern was not tried, however, and it is possible, as mentioned by Frank et al. (1975a), that more adequate stimulation might also preserve junctional binding sites.

Other Membrane Properties Influenced by Muscle Activity

While this paper has emphasized the effect of muscle activity on ACh sensitivity, it is clear that stimulation of denervated muscles restores to normal other properties of the membrane, such as the resting membrane potential (Lømo and Westgaard 1975) and the passive electrical characteristics of the membrane (Westgaard 1975). It also prevents fibrillation (Lømo and Rosenthal 1972; Purves and Sakmann 1974) and largely prevents the formation of synapses with a foreign nerve (Jansen et al. 1973). It appears, therefore, that muscle activity per se controls most, if not all, properties of the non–end-plate part of the muscle membrane.

Control of ACh Sensitivity

It appears from these experiments that direct electrical stimulation and normal innervation have similar effects on the extrajunctional part of the mammalian muscle membrane, and that the muscle activity evoked in each case is their only common feature. Therefore there is no need to postulate any neurotrophic control mechanism to explain the control of this part of the membrane, at least not in mammals. This seems the more reasonable now that several lines of evidence generally taken to support the concept of neurotrophic control (see above) can be given an alternative explanation. At the end plate, however, the nerve has specific and highly localized effects on the muscle membrane that cannot be mimicked by activity. This difference between junctional and extrajunctional parts of the membrane could possibly be accounted for, at least with respect to ACh sensitivity, in the following way: The ACh sensitivity along the entire membrane is seen as reflecting the outcome of competitive interactions in each region along the fiber between two kinds of opposing influences; an activity-linked internal influence that suppresses the sensitivity, and different external influences that may induce it. Evidence is presented here that in abnormal circumstances, the external influences may be factors related to degeneration of nerve terminals, inflammation of adjacent tissue, or effects of colchicine. There is also some evidence that such influences may interact competitively with activity. The hypersensitivity attributed here to degeneration of nerve terminals was seen only during a "slow" activity pattern, evoked either electrically or by the "slow" soleus nerve, and not during a "fast" activity pattern, evoked electrically or by the "fast" fibular nerve. The "fast" stimulus pattern was also more effective in suppressing ACh sensitivity than the "slow" pattern, since it caused denervation hypersensitivity to fall more rapidly during stimulation and to rise more slowly after the stimulation was stopped. Thus both the internal suppressive influence and the external inductive influence probably have graded and opposite effects.

The high local ACh sensitivity at normal end plates suggests that the intact nerve terminal is able to override the suppressive influence of muscle activity at this point, perhaps by a prolonged and highly localized action qualitatively similar to that occurring during inflammation or phagocytosis of nerve terminals during their degeneration. This action might be the result of direct cell contact with the muscle membrane or the release of diffusable substances that induce ACh sensitivity. Such an effect might be called "trophic." However since this term implies "nutritive" and generalized effects, it is arguable how useful this term is to describe something that appears to affect only the synaptic region.

Acknowledgments

We are grateful to Drs. Michael C. Brown, Jan K. S. Jansen and Clarke R. Slater for valuable suggestions.

REFERENCES

ALBUQUERQUE, E. X. and R. J. McISAAC. 1970. Fast and slow mammalian muscles after denervation. *Exp. Neurol.* **26**:183.

ALBUQUERQUE, E. X., J. E. WARNICK, J. R. TASSE and F. M. SANSONE. 1972. Effects of vinblastine and colchicine on neural regulation of the fast and slow skeletal muscles of the rat. *Exp. Neurol.* **37**:607.

AXELSSON, J. and S. THESLEFF. 1959. A study of supersensitivity in denervated mammalian skeletal muscle. *J. Physiol.* **147**:178.

BELMAR, J. and C. EYZAGUIRRE. 1966. Pacemaker site of fibrillation potentials in denervated mammalian muscle. *J. Neurophysiol.* **29**:425.

BENNETT, M. R., A. G. PETTIGREW and R. S. TAYLOR. 1973. The formation of synapses in reinnervated and cross-reinnervated adult avian muscle. *J. Physiol.* **230**:331.

BERG, D. K. and Z. W. HALL. 1974. Fate of alpha-bungarotoxin bound to acetylcholine receptors of normal and denervated muscle. *Science* **184**:473.

BERLIN, R. D., J. M. OLIVER, T. E. UKENA and H. H. YIN. 1974. Control of cell surface topography. *Nature* **247**:45.

CANGIANO, A. 1973. Acetylcholine supersensitivity: The role of neurotrophic factors. *Brain Res.* **58**:255.

CANGIANO, A. and J. A. FRIED. 1974. Neurotrophic control of skeletal muscle of the rat. *J. Physiol.* **239**:31P.

CLOSE, R. 1969. Dynamic properties of fast and slow skeletal muscles of the rat after nerve cross-union. *J. Physiol.* **204**:331.

DAHLSTRØM, A. 1968. Effect of colchicine on transport of amine storage granules in sympathetic nerves of rat. *Eur. J. Pharmacol.* **5**:111.

EDELMAN, G. M., P. G. SPEAR, U. RUTISHAUSER and I. YAHARA. 1975. Receptor specificity and mitogenesis in lymphocyte populations. In *The cell surface in development* (ed. A. A. Moscona), pp. 141–164. John Wiley and Sons, New York.

EMMELIN, N. and L. MALM. 1965. Development of supersensitivity as dependent on the length of degenerating nerve fibers. *Q. J. Exp. Physiol.* **50**:142.

FAMBROUGH, D. M. 1970. Acetylcholine sensitivity of muscle fiber membranes: Mechanism of regulation by motoneurons. *Science* **168**:372.

FAMBROUGH, D. M. and H. C. HARTZELL. 1972. Acetylcholine receptors: Number and distribution at neuromuscular junctions in rat diaphragm. *Science* **176**:189.

FISCHBACH, G. D. and N. ROBBINS. 1969. Changes in contractile properties of disused soleus muscles. *J. Physiol.* **201**:305.

———. 1971. Effects of chronic disuse of rat soleus neuromuscular junctions on post-synaptic membrane. *J. Neurophysiol.* **34**:562.

FRANK, E., K. GAUTVIK and H. SOMMERSCHILD. 1975a. Cholinergic receptors at denervated mammalian motor end-plates. *Acta Physiol. Scand.* **95**:66.

FRANK, E., J. K. S. JANSEN, T. LØMO and R. H. WESTGAARD. 1975b. The interaction between foreign and original nerves innervating the soleus muscles of rats. *J. Physiol.* **247**:725.

GONZENBACH, H. R. and P. G. WASER. 1973. Electron microscopic studies of degeneration and regeneration of rat neuromuscular junctions. *Brain Res.* **63**:167.

HARRIS, J. B. and S. THESLEFF. 1972. Nerve stump length and membrane changes in denervated skeletal muscle. *Nature New Biol.* **236**:60.

HOFMANN, W. W. and S. THESLEFF. 1972. Studies on the trophic influence of nerve on skeletal muscle. *Eur. J. Pharmacol.* **20**:256.

JANSEN, J. K. S., T. LØMO, K. NICOLAYSEN and R. H. WESTGAARD. 1973. Hyperinnervation of skeletal muscle fibres: Dependence on muscle activity. *Science* **181**:559.

JOHNS, T. R. and S. THESLEFF. 1961. Effects of motor inactivation on the chemical sensitivity of skeletal muscle. *Acta Physiol. Scand.* **51**:136.

JONES, R. and G. VRBOVÁ. 1974. Two factors responsible for the development of denervation hypersensitivity. *J. Physiol.* **236**:517.

KAUFFMAN, F. C., J. E. WARNICK and E. X. ALBUQUERQUE. 1974. Uptake of [³H]colchicine from silastic implants by mammalian nerves and muscles. *Exp. Neurol.* **44**:404.

KREUTZBERG, G. W. 1969. Neuronal dynamics and axonal flow. IV. Blockage of intra-axonal enzyme transport by colchicine. *Proc. Nat. Acad. Sci.* **62**:722.

LØMO, T. 1974. Neurotrophic control of colchicine effects on muscle? *Nature* **249**:473.

LØMO, T. and J. ROSENTHAL. 1972. Control of ACh sensitivity by muscle activity in the rat. *J. Physiol.* **221**:493.

LØMO, T. and R. H. WESTGAARD. 1975. Further studies on the control of ACh sensitivity by activity in the rat. *J. Physiol.* **252**:603.

LØMO, T., R. H. WESTGAARD and H. A. DAHL. 1974. Contractile properties of muscle: Control by pattern of muscle activity in the rat. *Proc. Roy. Soc. B.* **187**:99.

LUCO, J. V. and C. EYZAGUIRRE. 1955. Fibrillation and hypersensitivity to ACh in denervated muscle: Effect of length of degenerating nerve fibers. *J. Neurophysiol.* **18**:65.

MILEDI, R. 1960a. Properties of regenerating neuromuscular synapses in the frog. *J. Physiol.* **154**:190.

———. 1960b. The acetylcholine sensitivity of frog muscle fibres after complete or partial denervation. *J. Physiol.* **151**:1.

———. 1963. An influence of nerve not mediated by impulses. In *The effect of use and disuse on neuromuscular functions* (ed. E. Gutmann and R. Hnik), pp. 35–40. Czechoslovac Academy of Sciences, Prague.

MILEDI, R. and C. R. SLATER. 1968. Electrophysiology and electronmicroscopy of rat neuromuscular junctions after nerve degeneration. *J. Physiol.* **169**:289.

MILEDI, R. and J. ZELENÁ. 1966. Sensitivity to acetylcholine in the rat slow muscle. *Nature* **210**:855.

PURVES, D. and B. SAKMANN. 1974. The effect of contractile activity on fibrillation and extrajunctional acetylcholine sensitivity in rat muscle maintained in organ culture. *J. Physiol.* **237**:157.

SOLANDT, D. Y. and J. W. MAGLADERY. 1942. A comparison of effects of upper and lower motor neurone lesions on skeletal muscle. *J. Neurophysiol.* **5**:373.

SOLANDT, D. Y., R. C. PARTRIDGE and J. HUNTER. 1943. The effect of skeletal fixation on skeletal muscle. *J. Neurophysiol.* **6**:17.

WESTGAARD, R. H. 1975. Influence of activity on the passive electrical properties of soleus muscle fibres in the rat. *J. Physiol.* **251**:683.

WUNDERLICH, F., R. MÜLLER and V. SPETH. 1973. Direct evidence for a colchicine-induced impairment in the mobility of membrane components. *Science* **182**:1136.

Reprinted from Nature, Vol. 283, pp. 264–267, 1980
© 1980 Macmillan Journals Ltd.

Regulation of acetylcholinesterase appearance at neuromuscular junctions *in vitro*

Lee L. Rubin*, Stephen M. Schuetze†, Cheryl L. Weill‡ & Gerald D. Fischbach

Department of Pharmacology, Harvard Medical School, 250 Longwood Avenue, Boston, Massachusetts 02115

The appearance of acetylcholinesterase (AChE) at newly formed nerve–muscle synapses depends on synaptic transmission. Synapses form when cultures are grown in the presence of acetylcholine receptor antagonists, but AChE does not accumulate at these synapses. The important component of transmission seems to be muscle activity. Treatment with dibutyryl cyclic GMP mimics muscle activity, directly inducing synaptic AChE appearance.

ACETYLCHOLINE receptors (AChRs) and acetylcholinesterase (AChE) are concentrated at adult motor endplates. The AChR is an integral membrane protein (see ref. 1 for review) restricted to the upper one-third of the postjunctional folds, whereas AChE is a peripheral protein associated with the basal lamina[2] throughout the primary and secondary synaptic clefts[3]. Even though AChRs and AChE are ultimately located at different sites, both molecules begin to accumulate within 24 h of nerve–muscle synapse formation *in vitro*[4–6] and are present in approximately equal numbers at mature junctions [3,7,8]. Therefore, one might suppose that the early AChR and AChE appearance at endplates is regulated in a coordinated way. Certain observations suggest, however, that synaptic AChRs and AChE are influenced quite differently by chronic blockade of synaptic transmission. As AChRs cluster at nerve–muscle contacts when spinal cord–muscle co-cultures are grown in the presence of α-bungarotoxin (α-BTX)[9], this process is independent of synaptic transmission. On the other hand, discrete foci of AChE fail to appear when young chick embryos are injected repeatedly with α-neurotoxin or curare[10,11]. These results have been taken as evidence that receptor antagonists block synapse formation. It is possible, however, that nerve–muscle synapses form in the presence of receptor antagonists (compare refs 12, 13) but that AChE does not accumulate in the absence of synaptic transmission. Data presented here indicate that this, in fact, is the case and, further, that activity of innervated muscle fibres is a crucial parameter regulating the early appearance of AChE at sites of transmitter release. The accumulation of AChRs and of AChE during neuromuscular junction formation is apparently not regulated in exactly the same way. A preliminary account of some of these experiments has been given elsewhere[14].

As AChE accumulates rapidly at newly formed chick nerve–muscle synapses *in vitro*[6], we used this culture system to examine in more detail the influence of synaptic transmission and muscle activity on AChE. Nerve processes emerge from spinal cord explants 10 h after the fragments attach to the culture surface, and synapses form soon after nerve–muscle contact. We have shown previously that AChE can be detected histochemically at some physiologically identified sites of transmitter release within 24 h of the onset of synaptic transmission and that after 4 d of co-culture, AChE reaction product is present at the majority of functional contacts[6]. Synaptic AChE activity was also detected by measuring the time course of synaptic currents recorded with an extracellular electrode. At adult endplates, AChE serves to terminate transmitter action, and this effect is reflected in the rate of synaptic current decay[15–17]. Based on the mean time constant of synaptic current decay ($\bar{\tau}_{syn}$) recorded at 30 °C, synapses formed in culture were arbitrarily divided into

three categories: fast ($\bar{\tau}_{syn} \leqslant 1.8$ ms), intermediate (1.8 ms < $\bar{\tau}_{syn} < 2.6$ ms) and slow ($\bar{\tau}_{syn} \geqslant 2.6$ ms). Whereas 74% of the fast synapses stain for AChE, none of the slow ones stain.

Curare blocks appearance of synaptic AChE

Chick spinal cord explant–muscle co-cultures were prepared as previously described[5,6]. Thin slices cut from the brachial segments of 14-d embryonic cords were added to established muscle cultures. Curare at a final concentration of 50 μM was added to some cultures for 3–4 d beginning at the time of explant addition. Innervated myotubes in control medium twitched vigorously and were continuously active. At 50 μM, curare blocked all synaptic activity and only a few isolated contractions were observed. This high concentration of curare did not block

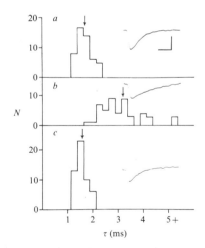

Fig. 1 Histograms of synaptic current decay time constants (τ_{syn}) recorded at 30 °C. Representative synaptic currents recorded with an extracellular microelectrode are shown as insets. Time constants were determined from exponential curves fitted to each synaptic current decay phase with an on-line computer. Arrows above each histogram indicate arithmetic means ($\bar{\tau}_{syn}$). At the control synapse (*a*), $\bar{\tau}_{syn}$ is <1.8 ms, whereas at the synapse formed and maintained in the presence of curare (50 μM for 4 d; *b*), $\bar{\tau}_{syn}$ is >2.6 ms. Both $\bar{\tau}_{syn}$ and the variance of τ_{syn} are increased at the curare-treated synapse, reflecting the lack of synaptic AChE activity[6,17]. After data in *b* were obtained, the culture was placed in control medium without curare and returned to the incubator. Two days later, *c* was obtained by recording at another synapse in the same culture. $\bar{\tau}_{syn}$ and the variance of τ_{syn} were then comparable to control. Calibration bars, 2 ms and 200 μV.

Present addresses: * Department of Neurobiology, Stanford University Medical School, Stanford, California 94305; † Department of Anatomy, Harvard Medical School, 25 Shattuck Street, Boston, Massachusetts 02115; ‡ Department of Neurology, Louisiana State University Medical School, 1542 Tulane Avenue, New Orleans, Louisiana 70112.

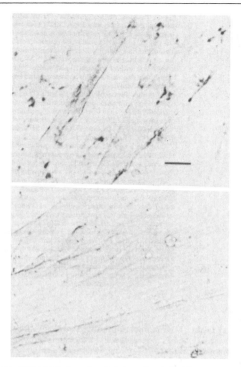

Fig. 2 Bright field view of control (upper) and 50 μM curare-treated (lower) myotubes stained for AChE according to the method of Karnovsky and Roots[32] 4 d after addition of spinal cord explants. Both fields were near (within 300 μm of) the explants. Many patches of reaction product near fine nerve processes (not visible under bright field illumination) are evident on control myotubes. Few, if any, patches are present on curare-treated myotubes. Bar, 100 μm.

the formation of synapses. Spontaneous synaptic activity was detected in most myotubes within 1–2 min of curare washout. In addition, autoradiographs of cultures treated with ^{125}I α-BTX immediately after curare washout showed that AChRs had clustered at sites of transmitter release.

Although synapses formed in the presence of curare, extracellularly recorded synaptic currents decayed relatively slowly (Fig. 1), indicating that AChE did not accumulate at sites of transmitter release. Judging from histograms of τ_{syn} constructed at 97 control and 89 curare-grown synapses (immediately after curare washout), the percentage of fast synapses decreased fivefold, whereas the percentage of intermediate synapses increased twofold and that of slow synapses threefold (Table 1). In the intermediate group, there was a shift towards higher values ($\bar{\tau}_{syn} > 2.2$ ms). The effect of curare was reversible; 1–2 d after cultures were returned to control medium, synaptic currents at most synapses decayed rapidly (Fig. 1).

Prolonged synaptic currents following curare washout were not due to an increase in the mean ACh channel open time. Estimates based on spectra of ACh-induced current fluctuations at control and curare-grown synapses were not significantly different (Table 1).

Histochemical experiments confirmed electrophysiological findings. The number of patches of AChE reaction product on myotubes near spinal cord explants in curare-grown cultures was reduced more than 10-fold compared with control (Fig. 2, Table 1). It cannot be assumed that all AChE patches are located at synapses, so sites of transmitter release were identified by extracellular recording, and then the same sites were relocated after fixation and histochemistry. Reaction

product was evident at 60 of 94 control synapses, but at only 1 of 49 synapses that had formed in the presence of curare. The reversibility of the curare inhibition illustrated above was also confirmed histochemically. Many AChE patches were evident 1–2 d after return to control medium.

Curare at 50 μM did not affect the outgrowth of neurites, but in some cultures the nerve processes were more heavily stained for AChE than in control cultures. Chronic treatment with 2×10^{-8} M α-BTX also eliminated patches of AChE at synapses on innervated myotubes, but did not increase the extent of neuronal staining.

Curare blocks the appearance of 19.5S AChE

Several forms of AChE can be detected by sucrose density gradient centrifugation of extracts prepared from adult muscle (see ref. 18 for review). A high-molecular weight form sedimenting at 16S in rat[19] and 19.5S in chick[20] extracts is present in innervated but not in denervated muscle. With our method of extraction (see Fig. 3 legend), we have never detected 19.5S AChE in chick muscle cultures without added neurones or in spinal cord cultures without target myotubes, nor have we reliably detected 19.5S AChE in spinal cord explant–muscle co-cultures; the number of synapses formed may be too small. However, as shown in Fig. 3a, a 19.5S peak was evident in muscle cultures seeded with a large number of dissociated spinal cord cells (see ref. 21); two other peaks of AChE sedimented at 7S and 11S. In different experiments, the 19.5S peak comprised 5–10% of the total activity. In five experiments, chronic exposure to curare decreased activity in the 19.5S peak at least fourfold (Fig. 3b) without decreasing the total AChE-specific activity (control, 0.314 ± 0.31 μM per min per mg; curare, 0.395 ± 0.5 μM per min per mg). The heavy form of AChE is restricted to the endplate region of innervated rat muscle[19], but it is found in endplate-free regions of innervated chick muscle[20]. Therefore, although a useful marker for the 'innervated state', it is not clear if the 19.5S form accounts for the AChE activity at synapses detected histochemically and electrophysiologically in our cultures.

The appearance of AChE at synapses depends on muscle activity

The effect of curare and α-BTX implies that something in the sequence of events that follow ACh release—ACh binding, ACh-induced increase in membrane conductance, muscle excitation and muscle contraction—is required for the accumulation of synaptic AChE. ACh binding is probably not sufficient; synaptic AChE was drastically reduced by chronic exposure to 10 μM proadifen-HCl (SKF 525A). At this concentration, this local anaesthetic blocks ACh channels, but does not inhibit ACh binding[22]. Subthreshold synaptic conductance changes are probably not sufficient either; the appearance of AChE was substantially suppressed by tetrodotoxin, which blocks action potentials and, thus, impulse-mediated endplate potentials

Table 1 Comparison of control and curare-treated cultures

	$\bar{\tau}_{syn}$ (ms)			AChE patches	τ_0 (ms)
	1.0–1.8	1.8–2.6	> 2.6	(mean ±s.e.)	(mean ±s.e.)
Control (97*)	59.8%	29.9%	10.3%	25.0 ± 2.0 (41†)	1.34 ± 0.08 (4‡)
Curare (89*)	12.4%	56.2%	31.5%	1.9 ± 0.3 (58†)	1.49 ± 0.16 (4‡)

Mean synaptic current decays ($\bar{\tau}_{syn}$) were determined at 30 °C as described in Fig. 1 legend. The number of patches of AChE reaction product (per spinal cord explant) was calculated by counting patches in the vicinity of neurites on undamaged myotubes. No more than 50 patches were counted on myotubes surrounding a single explant, so the control value is an underestimate. ACh channel open times (τ_0) were determined at fast synapses in control cultures and at slow synapses in curare-treated cultures using the technique described by Schuetze *et al.*[32].
 * No. of synapses at which $\bar{\tau}_{syn}$ was determined.
 † No. of explants.
 ‡ No. of synapses at which τ_0 was determined.

Nature Vol. 283 17 January 1980

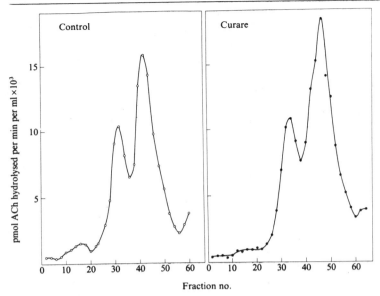

Fig. 3 Sucrose density gradient fractionation of different molecular forms of AChE. Chick muscles were plated at 3×10^5 cells per 60-mm culture dish. On day 3, 6-d embryonic chick spinal cords were dissociated and added ($2-3 \times 10^6$ cells per dish) to the muscle cultures in the presence of 10^{-5} M cytosine arabinoside with or without 50 μM curare. Five days later, three control and three curare-treated cultures were rinsed with Earle's balanced salt solution and the cells were collected by scraping with a Teflon policeman in phosphate-buffered saline containing 0.2 mM EDTA, pH 7.4. The cell suspension was centrifuged at 12,000g for 5 min and resuspended in 1 M NaCl, 0.5% Triton X-100, 0.05 M Tris-HCl, 0.2 mM EDTA and 1 mg ml^{-1} DNase (Sigma), pH 7.3. After 1 h at 0 °C, this suspension was centrifuged at 12,000g for 15 min and the supernatant assayed for protein[34] and AChE activity[35]. An aliquot (approximately 400–600 μg per 125 μl) was layered onto a 5–20% linear sucrose gradient and centrifuged in a Spinco SW41 rotor at 205,000g for 18 h at 4 °C. Sixty 0.25 ml fractions were collected and assayed for AChE by the radiometric method of Potter[36], as modified by Hall[19]. Three peaks of activity sedimenting at 7S, 11S and 19.5S were evident in the control gradient (left). Activity in the 19.5S peak was reduced at least fourfold by curare treatment (right). This figure shows the maximum 19.5S activity found in curare-treated cultures in five different experiments (platings). Gradient markers were alcohol dehydrogenase (4.8S), catalase (11.3S) and β-galactosidase (16S).

(e.p.p.s), but not impulse-independent miniature endplate potentials. Moreover, AChE did not accumulate in low concentrations (3 μM) of curare, which only reduced the mean e.p.p. by 50%.

Although 3 μM curare did not completely block e.p.p.s, most of the synaptic potentials were subthreshold; few innervated fibres were mechanically active. We therefore examined the role of muscle activity in the induction of synaptic AChE by electrically stimulating individual muscle fibres in the presence of curare. Spinal cord–muscle cultures were grown in 50 μM curare, and $\bar{\tau}_{syn}$ was again determined at previously identified sites of transmitter release. Chronic stimulation in the presence of curare significantly decreased τ_{syn} (Fig. 4). Eight synapses at which $\bar{\tau}_{syn}$ was greater than 2.21 ms were studied before and after stimulation (Table 2). Chronic stimulation in the presence of curare significantly decreased $\bar{\tau}_{syn}$ at seven of these synapses to values typical of fast, AChE-positive sites. One other synapse was fast ($\bar{\tau}_{syn} = 1.54$ ms) before stimulation, and its decay constant did not decrease further.

Influence of dibutyryl cyclic GMP on AChE

During these experiments, we found that low concentrations (25–100 μM) of dibutyryl cyclic GMP can reverse the curare inhibition of AChE accumulation. $\bar{\tau}_{syn}$ was determined at 114 synapses in cultures grown in 50 μM curare with dibutyryl cyclic GMP: 64% were fast and only 3.5% were slow. These percentages are comparable to those obtained with untreated control cultures (Table 1). The effect of dibutyryl cyclic GMP was also evident when AChE was assayed histochemically. Reaction product was present at 70% of identified synapses in cultures of curare plus dibutyryl cyclic GMP. Finally, dibutyryl cyclic GMP reversed the curare inhibition of 19.5S AChE assembly (Fig. 5) without increasing the total AChE activity. In six experiments, the ratio of total AChE (control/dibutyryl cyclic GMP treated) was 1.15 ± 0.25 (mean ± s.d.). Dibutyryl cyclic GMP did not 'induce' 19.5S AChE in muscle cells or in spinal cord neurones grown alone. Other agents, including GMP, GTP and dibutyryl cyclic AMP, did not reverse the curare inhibition of synaptic AChE accumulation or assembly of the 19.5S form.

Conclusions

The early accumulation of AChE at newly formed nerve–muscle synapses *in vitro* depends on synaptic transmission. By our physiological and histochemical criteria, the activity of the enzyme is greatly reduced at synapses that form in the presence of curare. Although 19.5S AChE is not restricted to adult chick endplates, it is significant that this form of the enzyme was selectively decreased in curare-blocked cultures.

Of the several events that follow synaptic transmission, muscle activity (electrical and/or mechanical) seems to be the crucial factor, as AChE does accumulate at curare-blocked synapses when innervated myotubes are stimulated directly. Lømo and Slater[23] have also emphasised the role of muscle activity in AChE accumulation at ectopic synapses on adult rat muscle fibres. Weinberg and Hall[24] suggested muscle activity as an explanation for their observation that 16S AChE (and AChE histochemical reaction product) reappears at denervated rat endplates when the denervated muscles are reinnervated at another site. Koenig and Vigny[21] detected 16S AChE in control rat spinal cord–muscle co-cultures but not in inactive cultures grown in the presence of tetrodotoxin[25]. Inadequate muscle activity may explain why no evidence was obtained for AChE activity at nerve–muscle synapses when chick muscle cultures were seeded with a relatively small number of dissociated spinal cord neurones[26]. In this system, innervated myotubes twitch more frequently than uninnervated myotubes, but the overall activity is far less than that observed in innervated myotubes near intact spinal cord explants.

Table 2 Effect of direct muscle stimulation on $\bar{\tau}_{syn}$

Synapse no.	Before	After	% Change
1	2.21 ± 0.70	1.74 ± 0.32	21.3
2	3.09 ± 1.39	1.74 ± 0.39	43.7
3	2.25 ± 0.73	1.35 ± 0.20	40.0
4	3.06 ± 1.04	2.05 ± 0.71	33.0
5	3.19 ± 1.56	1.87 ± 0.49	41.4
6	3.14 ± 0.87	1.75 ± 0.37	44.3
7	2.59 ± 1.15	1.80 ± 0.41	30.5
8	2.42 ± 0.92	2.30 ± 0.65	5.0
9	1.54 ± 0.35	1.51 ± 0.21	1.9

$\bar{\tau}_{syn}$ (±s.d.) was determined from the time constants of decay of at least 20 extracellular potentials recorded at the same synapses in curare-treated cultures before and after direct electrical stimulation of myotubes in the presence of 50 μM curare for 8–12 h at 2–3 Hz and 35–36 °C.

In contrast to the situation with AChE, the clustering of AChRs in the postsynaptic membrane does not depend on activity. Thus, the formation of AChR clusters in the postsynaptic membrane and the accumulation of AChE in the synaptic cleft are not necessariinked. This result does not rule out the possibility that AChE and AChRs are synthesised and transported to the cell surface in a coordinated manner. Muscle activity may simply ensure the anchorage of AChE to the basal lamina of the synaptic cleft.

Muscle activity is probably not the sole determinant of synaptic AChE. Nerve extracts slow the rate of AChE disappearance, measured biochemically, from adult muscle maintained in organ culture[27,28], and saline extracts of central nervous tissue increase total AChE of uninnervated embryonic myotubes in culture[29,30]. Although it is difficult to compare these biochemical estimates of total (intracellular as well as extracellular) AChE with our physiological and histochemical assays, which detect AChE exposed on the cell surface at synapses, our emphasis on the importance of muscle activity is not inconsistent with the notion that synaptic AChE is also regulated by soluble factors supplied by motor nerves. The fact that AChE and AChRs are restricted to sites of transmitter release argues for a local neural influence. Moreover, we have identified AChE-positive and AChE-negative synapses within 500 μm of one another on the same myotube (Fig. 7 in Rubin *et al.*[6]). If both contacts were formed at approximately the same time and if both were exposed to the same degree of muscle activity, some additional factor must be required. Muscle activity may be 'permissive', allowing neuronal factors to exert their effects.

Addition of dibutyryl cyclic GMP to cultures grown in curare mimics the effects of muscle activity on synaptic AChE and on assembly of the 19.5S form of the enzyme. Of interest in this regard is the finding that stimulation of adult skeletal muscle results in an increase in cyclic GMP levels[31]. Neither result demonstrates a necessary connection between activity and cyclic GMP in regulating the appearance of AChE. Perhaps a stronger argument for such a connection could be made if muscle activity and cyclic GMP treatment resulted in phosphorylation of the same muscle proteins.

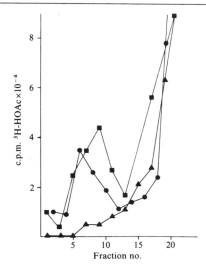

Fig. 5 19.5S AChE appears in spinal cord–muscle cell cultures grown in curare plus dibutyryl cyclic GMP. Cultures were grown without added drugs (●), with 50 μM curare (▲) or with 50 μM curare plus 100 μM dibutyryl cyclic GMP (■). Extracts were prepared and sucrose gradients run, as described in Fig. 3 legend. Only the high-molecular weight region of the gradient is shown. Assembly of 19.5S AChE was nearly completely blocked by curare, but this inhibition was reversed by adding dibutyryl cyclic GMP.

This work was supported by USPHS grant NS 11160, by the Muscular Dystrophy Association of America and by a Helen Hay Whitney Foundation Postdoctoral Fellowship (L.L.R.), an NIH National Research Service Award T32GM07226 (S.M.S.) and a Muscular Dystrophy Association Postdoctoral Fellowship (C.L.W.).

Received 15 February; accepted 31 October 1979.

1. Heidmann, T. & Changeux, J.-P. *A. Rev. Biochem.* **47**, 317–357 (1978).
2. McMahan, U. J., Sanes, J. R. & Marshall, L. M. *Nature* **271**, 172–174 (1978).
3. Salpeter, M. M. *J. Cell Biol.* **32**, 379–389 (1967), **42**, 122–134 (1969).
4. Anderson, M. J., Cohen, M. W. & Zorychta, E. *J. Physiol., Lond.* **268**, 731–756 (1977).
5. Frank, E. & Fischbach, G. D. in *Cell and Tissue Interactions* (eds Lash, J. W. & Burger, M. M.) 285–291 (Raven, New York, 1977).
6. Rubin, L. L., Schuetze, S. M. & Fischbach, G. D. *Devl Biol.* **69**, 46–58 (1979).
7. Barnard, E. A., Wiekowski, J. & Chiu, T. H. *Nature* **234**, 207–209 (1971).
8. Fertuck, H. C. & Salpeter, M. M. *J. Cell Biol.* **69**, 144–158 (1976).
9. Anderson, M. J. & Cohen, M. W. *J. Physiol., London.* **268**, 757–773 (1977).
10. Giacobini, G., Filogamo, G., Weber, M., Boquet, P. & Changeux, J.-P. *Proc. natn. Acad. Sci. U.S.A.* **70**, 1708–1712 (1973).
11. Gordon, T., Perry, R., Tuffery, A. R. & Vrbova, G. *Cell Tissue Res.* **155**, 13–25 (1974).
12. Crain, S. & Peterson, E. R. *In Vitro* **6**, 373 (1971).
13. Cohen, M. W. *Brain Res.* **41**, 457–463 (1972).
14. Rubin, L., Schuetze, S. M., Weill, C. L. & Fischbach, G. D. *Neurosci. Soc. Abstr.*, 374 (1978).
15. Takeuchi, A. & Takeuchi, N. *J. Neurophysiol.* **22**, 395–411 (1959).
16. Kordas, M. *J. Physiol., Lond.* **335**, 317–332 (1972).
17. Katz, B. & Miledi, R. *J. Physiol., Lond.* **231**, 549–574 (1973).
18. Rosenberry, T. L. *Adv. Enzym.* **43**, 103–218 (1975).
19. Hall, Z. W. *J. Neurobiol.* **4**, 343–361 (1973).
20. Vigny, M., Di Giamberardino, L., Couraud, J. Y., Rieger, F. & Koenig, J. *FEBS Lett.* **69**, 277–280 (1976).
21. Koenig, J. & Vigny, M. *Nature* **271**, 75–77 (1978).
22. Cohen, J. B., Weber, M. & Changeux, J.-P. *Molec. Pharmac.* **10**, 904–932 (1974).
23. Lømo, T. & Slater, C. R. in *Synaptogenesis* (ed. Tauc, L.) 9–29 (Naturalia and Biologia, Jouy en Josas, 1976).
24. Weinberg, C. B. & Hall, Z. W. *Devl Biol.* **68**, 631–635 (1979).
25. Koenig, J. & Vigny, M. *Prog. Brain Res.* **49**, 484 (1979).
26. Fischbach, G. D. *Devl Biol.* **31**, 147–162 (1972).
27. Lentz, T. L. *Expl Neurol.* **45**, 520–526 (1974).
28. Younkin, S. G., Brett, R. S., Davey, B. & Younkin, L. H. *Science* **200**, 1292–1295 (1978).
29. Oh, J. H. *Expl Neurol.* **46**, 432–438 (1975).
30. Jessell, T. M., Siegel, R. & Fischbach, G. D. *Proc. natn. Acad. Sci. U.S.A.* (in the press).
31. Nestler, E. J., Beam, K. G. & Greengard, P. *Nature* **275**, 451–453 (1978).
32. Schuetze, S. M., Frank, E. & Fischbach, G. D. *Proc. natn. Acad. Sci. U.S.A.* **75**, 520–523 (1978).
33. Karnovsky, M. J. & Roots, L. *J. Histochem. Cytochem.* **12**, 219–221 (1964).
34. Lowry, O. H., Rosebrough, N. J., Farr, A. L. & Randall, R. J. *J. biol. Chem.* **193**, 265–275 (1951).
35. Ellman, G. L., Courtney, K. D., Andres, V. Jr & Featherstone, R. M. *Biochem. Pharmac.* **7**, 88–95 (1961).
36. Potter, L. T. *J. Pharmac. exp. Ther.* **156**, 500–506 (1967).

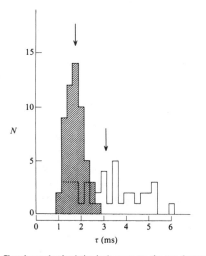

Fig. 4 Chronic muscle stimulation in the presence of curare decreases $\bar{\tau}_{syn}$. This culture was grown in 50 μM curare for 4 d, at which time synaptic current decays (recorded during a brief period of curare washout) at this synapse were prolonged (unshaded histogram). Immediately after the recordings were made, the culture was returned to medium with 50 μM curare, and the innervated myotube was electrically stimulated at 3 Hz for 11 h at 35–36 °C. Immediately after stimulation and curare washout, the same synapse was relocated and a clear decrease in $\bar{\tau}_{syn}$ was observed (shaded histogram). The variance of τ_{syn} was also decreased. All recordings were obtained at 30 °C. Arrows indicate $\bar{\tau}_{syn}$.

Reprinted from Exp. Neurol., Vol. 24, pp. 285–297. 1969
© 1969 Academic Press Ltd.

Combined Effects of Testosterone and Motor, Sensory, or Gustatory Nerve Reinnervation on the Regeneration of Taste Buds

Andrew A. Zalewski [1]

Laboratory of Neuropathology and Neuroanatomical Sciences, National Institute of Neurological Diseases and Stroke, National Institutes of Health, Public Health Service, U. S. Department of Health, Education and Welfare, Bethesda, Maryland 20014

Received February 24, 1969

Taste buds in the rat's vallate papilla degenerate after bilateral glossopharyngeal nerve transection and reappear after unilateral or bilateral nerve regeneration. The present experiment was performed to determine whether they would reappear after unilateral reinnervation by motor (hypoglossal), sensory (auriculotemporal), or different gustatory (chorda tympani, vagus) nerves. Since testosterone treatment causes taste buds to appear in new locations in the normal papilla, additional groups of reinnervated animals were given this hormone. Adult male rats were studied 3 months after nerve regeneration; the hormonally treated animals received 2.0 mg. testosterone daily for 3 weeks before being examined. Buds were found in the trench walls (normal location) after glossopharyngeal, chorda tympani, or vagal reinnervation. In the testosterone-treated animals, buds were also found in new locations, namely the top of the papilla and adjacent to it. No buds were found after denervation, unilateral or bilateral auriculotemporal reinnervation, or unilateral hypoglossal reinnervation, even after testosterone treatment. The results indicate that taste bud regeneration is dependent on a property of gustatory nerves that is not shared by general sensory or motor nerves. The appearance of buds in new sites demonstrates that under appropriate conditions additional regions of tongue epithelium can form taste buds.

Introduction

Taste buds in the rat's vallate papilla degenerate after bilateral glossopharyngeal nerve transection and reappear after unilateral or bilateral nerve regeneration (10, 22). The development and maintenance of taste buds has been attributed to a trophic influence of the gustatory nerve (14). The reappearance of taste buds after reinnervation by the vagus (a gustatory nerve of the pharynx and larynx) but not hypoglossal nerve (7) suggests that taste bud development is dependent on a property of gustatory nerves

[1] The author gratefully acknowledges the surgical assistance of Mrs. Phyllis K. Watson and histological assistance of Mrs. Janina D. Ziemnowicz.

285

that is not shared by motor nerves. The effects of general sensory nerves
on taste bud development have not been reported. The failure of taste buds
to develop after hypoglossal reinnervation could, however, be due to a
quantitatively insufficient trophic influence of motor nerves. The observation that prolonged testosterone treatment of adult male rats causes taste
buds to appear in new locations in the normally innervated papilla indicates
that previously inadequate innervation can effect taste bud development
(21). Could motor or sensory nerves induce taste bud development when
combined with testosterone treatment? The present experiment was performed to determine whether taste buds would reappear in vallate papilla
after reinnervation by motor (hypoglossal), sensory (auriculotemporal),
or different gustatory (chorda tympani, vagus) nerves alone, or after testosterone treatment. In addition, since denervation causes a marked reduction in alkaline phosphatase activity in the surface epithelium adjacent to
the taste buds (19, 20), the effects of the various nerve reinnervations and
hormone treatment on this enzyme were also studied.

Materials and Methods

Osborne–Mendel male rats (175–200g) were anesthetized with chloral
hydrate (400 mg/kg, ip) and the central end of the following nerves anasto-
mosed to the distal glossopharyngeal nerve to effect unilateral reinnervation
of the vallate papilla: (a) glossopharyngeal, (b) vagus, (c) chorda
tympani—lingual nerve trunk (hereafter referred to as chorda tympani
nerve), (d) hypoglossal, (e) auriculotemporal. The nerve ends were apposed within an arterial graft and held in place by the topical applications of
fibrinogen. All unilateral reinnervations were performed on the left side,
and since the taste buds in the vallate papilla are innervated by right and
left glossopharyngeal nerves (6, 8, 17, 19), control groups consisted of (f)
bilateral glossopharyngeal nerve transection, and (g) unilateral (right)
glossopharyngeal nerve transection. The central end of the glossopharyngeal nerve was implanted into adjacent muscle to prevent nerve regeneration. To determine whether the quantity of nerve fibers is critical in taste
bud development, (h) bilateral auriculotemporal nerve reinnervation was
preformed. Finally, since the trophic requirement of a nerve for initiating
the development of taste buds might differ from the requirement for maintaining existing taste buds, a group of animals was prepared (i) in which
the right glossopharyngeal nerve was left intact while the auriculotemporal
nerve was regenerated down the contralateral side. Two weeks before the
papilla was examined, the intact glossopharyngeal was cut (a time sufficient
for denervated taste buds to disappear) leaving regenerated auriculotemporal nerve fibers in contact with fully formed taste buds. If taste buds
were found in this group but not after unilateral or bilateral auriculotem-

poral nerve reinnervation, a function of maintenance distinct from a function of development could be attributed to nongustatory nerves.

Each experimental group consisted of nine animals. Three from each group were studied 3 months after nerve regeneration alone, while three received daily testosterone propionate injections (2.0 mg in 0.1 ml of sesame oil) for 3 weeks before being examined. One control animal from each group received sesame oil alone. In the remaining two animals the regenerated nerve was cut 3 months postoperatively. One animal was studied at 4 or 7 days, and the other 14 days after denervation.

Six-micron frozen sections were prepared and incubated to detect adenosine triphosphatase (16), cholinesterase (5), or alkaline phosphatase (3) activity. Control slides were incubated without added substrate. Details of these procedures have been reported (19). In addition, some sections of the papilla, as well as sections of nerve 1 cm distal to the anastomosis, were stained with PAS-hematoxylin.

Results

Effects of Denervation on the Distribution of Taste Buds. Just as in the normal papilla, taste buds were found in the lower portions of the inner and outer trench walls of the partially denervated (unilateral glossopharyngeal nerve transection) vallate papilla (Fig. 1A). No buds were found on the top of the papilla or area immediately adjacent to it. Beneath the buds a cholinesterase-positive nerve plexus was detected (Fig. 1B), and in the superficial epithelium around the taste buds an alkaline phosphatase reaction was present (Fig. 1C). Control slides incubated without added substrate did not reveal any enzyme activity. A similar distribution of taste buds and nerve fibers was demonstrated with the PAS-hematoxylin stain (Fig. 1D).

Taste buds were absent from the papilla 3 months after total denervation (bilateral glossopharyngeal nerve transection) (Fig. 2A), and no nerve fibers were identified beneath the epithelium (Fig. 2B). Alkaline phosphatase in the superficial epithelium was greatly reduced or absent (Fig. 2C) except in local areas of the trench wall involved in an inflammatory reaction. In these areas an intense reaction was present (Fig. 2D) due to the alkaline phosphatase activity of neutrophilic leucocytes (verified by comparison with peripheral blood films). No inflammatory reaction was present in areas of the papilla normally devoid of taste buds, namely the upper portions of the trench wall or top of the papilla. Despite this localized cellular infiltration the entire epithelium had atrophied and the size of the papilla was reduced.

Effects of Reinnervation on Taste Bud Regeneration. Taste buds were found in the trench walls of the vallate papilla after reinnervation by the glossopharyngeal, chorda tympani, or vagus nerve, but not after reinnerva-

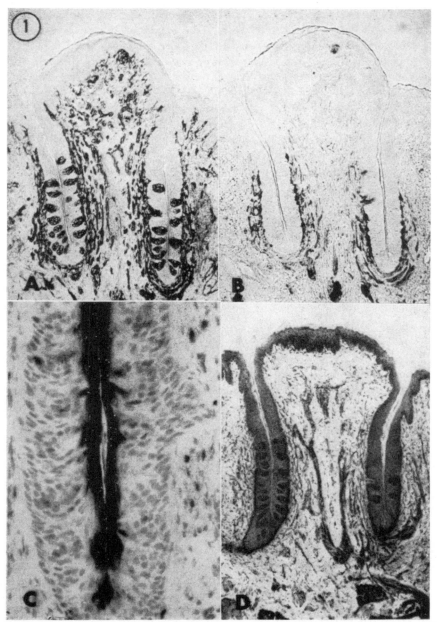

Fig. 1. Partially denervated vallate papilla. A. Adenosine triphosphatase activity of taste bud shows that buds, as in the normal papilla, are present only in the trench walls (×72). B. Beneath the buds, a cholinesterase reaction for nerve fibers is present (×72). C. In the superficial epithelium around the taste buds, an intense alkaline phosphatase reaction is present (×300). D. PAS-hematoxylin stain shows a similar distribution of taste buds and nerve fibers as the enzyme methods (×72).

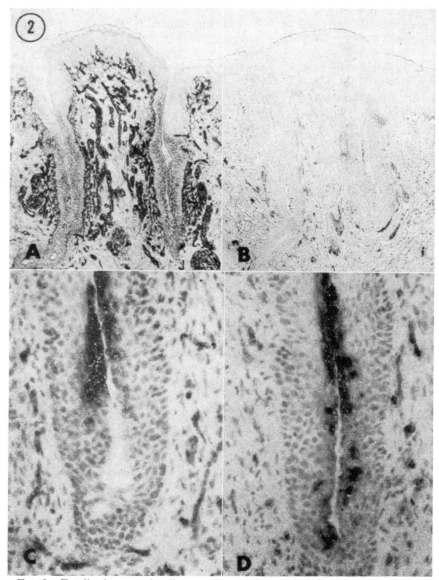

FIG. 2. Totally denervated vallate papilla. A. Adenosine triphosphatase staining reveals the absence of all taste buds (×72). B. Cholinesterase staining demonstrates a lack of nerve fibers beneath the epithelium (×72). C, D. Alkaline phosphatase activity has disappeared in some areas of the trench wall (C), but is intense in regions involved by an inflammatory reaction (D) (×300). A similar effect on alkaline phosphatase activity was present after auriculotemporal or hypoglossal reinnervation, even with testosterone treatment.

tion by the auriculotemporal or hypoglossal nerve. More buds were present after glossopharyngeal (Fig. 3A) than after chorda tympani or vagal reinnervation (Fig. 3B), and they appeared more often and in greater numbers

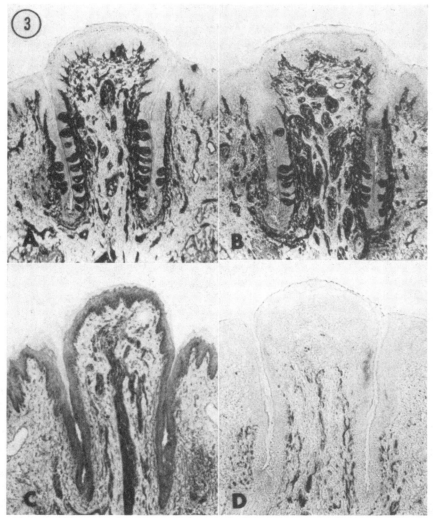

Fig. 3. Reinnervated vallate papilla. A, B. Adenosine triphosphatase reaction reveals that taste buds have reappeared after glossopharyngeal (A) and vagus (B) reinnervation (×72). Note the presence of more buds on the inner rather than outer trench walls. C, D. PAS-hematoxylin and cholinesterase stains (×72). Despite the presence of nerve fibers, no taste buds reappeared after hypoglossal (C) or auriculotemporal (D) reinnervation with testosterone treatment.

in the inner rather than outer trench wall. There was no special preference
of bud regeneration for the left or right trench wall. The regenerated taste
buds extended throughout the width of the epithelium (Fig. 4B) and were
similar in shape, size, and number of cells to normal taste buds (Fig. 4A).
No buds were found on the top of the papilla or area adjacent to it. Nerve
fibers were readily demonstrated beneath the regenerated taste buds by the
PAS and cholinesterase stains. The PAS reacting myelin of the regener-

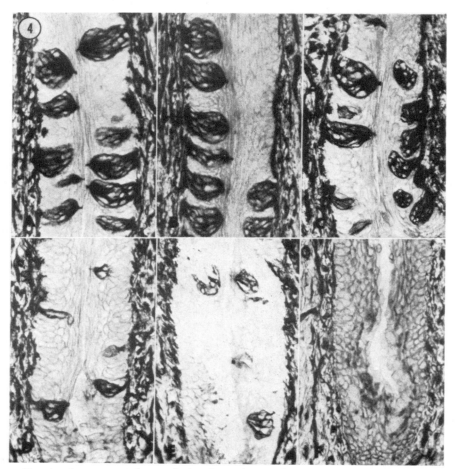

FIG. 4. Appearance of taste buds after reinnervation and subsequent denervation.
A–F. Adenosine triphosphatase reaction (×300). A. Taste buds normally extend
throughout the width of the epithelium. B. Buds after glossopharyngeal reinnervation.
C–E. Buds in various stages of degeneration are seen at 7 days after cutting the regenerated glossopharyngeal (C), chorda tympani (D), and vagus (E) nerves. No
buds were seen 7 days after transection of the regenerated hypoglossal nerve (F).

ated nerves could be traced from the core of the papilla to the basement membrane beneath the buds from which point the unmyelinated cholinesterase positive nerve endings were identified ramifying within the taste buds (2). In some sections, cholinesterase activity was detected beneath the epithelium at the top of the papilla, but no taste buds were found. The distribution of the regenerated auriculotemporal or hypoglossal nerve fibers was similar to that of the aforementioned gustatory nerves, and the failure of taste buds to develop after reinnervation by sensory or motor nerves cannot therefore be attributed to a failure of nerve regeneration (Fig. 3C, D). A qualitative comparison of cross-sections of peripheral nerve (PAS stain) 1 cm distal to the various nerve anastomoses further showed that essentially equal numbers of gustatory and motor or sensory nerve fibers successfully crossed the anastomosis site.

Taste buds were also absent in the group of animals designed to test whether nongustatory nerves (auriculotemporal reinnervation) could perform a function of maintenance rather than initiate development. Two weeks after cutting the intact right glossopharyngeal nerve, all taste buds were absent but a cholinesterase reaction for nerve fibers remained. This reaction represented regenerated auriculotemporal nerve fibers from the left side because after transection of this nerve, the cholinesterase activity disappeared.

In some rats the regenerated glossopharyngeal, chorda tympani, or vagus nerve was cut 3 months postoperatively. Four or 7 days later buds in various stages of degeneration were seen (Fig. 4C–E) and by 14 days no buds remained. This result showed that these nerves alone were responsible for the taste buds that had developed. No buds were seen 4 or 7 days after cutting the auriculotemporal or hypoglossal nerves (Fig. 4F).

Effects of Reinnervation with Testosterone Treatment on Taste Bud Regeneration. As with nerve reinnervation alone, taste buds were found only in the papillae reinnervated by the glossopharyngeal, chorda tympani, or vagus nerve. Even the combined effects of testosterone and bilateral auriculotemporal nerve reinnervation failed to produce taste buds. PAS and cholinesterase staining again showed that in all cases nerve fibers had reached the papilla regardless of whether taste buds had reappeared (Fig. 3C, D). The significant finding, however, was that taste buds appeared in new locations after testosterone treatment of the glossopharyngeal, chorda tympani, or vagally innervated papillae. Taste buds were now found on the top surface of the papilla, or area adjacent to it. Only one or two buds were seen on the top of the partially denervated control papillae, but after nerve regeneration three to six buds were found (Fig. 5A, B). In some instances two buds were seen in the same section, either close together or on opposite sides of the papilla (Fig. 5C). In addition, a single taste bud was found in

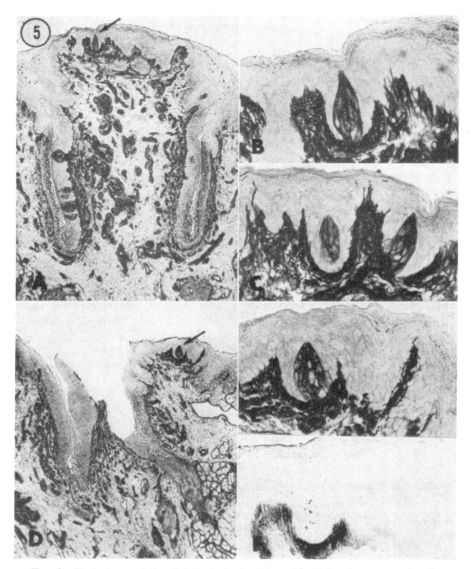

FIG. 5. Testosterone-induced taste buds. A. Adenosine triphosphatase reaction demonstrates the presence of taste buds (arrow) on the top of the papilla after vagus reinnervation with testosterone treatment (×72). B. Same bud as in (A) (×300). C. Same papilla as in (A), but 2 taste buds are present on the top of the papilla (×300). D. A taste bud is present in the epithelium adjacent to the papilla (arrow) after glossopharyngeal reinnervation with testosterone treatment (×72). E. Same bud as in (D) (×300). F. A cholinesterase reaction for nerve fibers is present beneath the epithelium of the testosterone induced taste bud (×300).

the epithelium adjacent to the papilla in one glossopharyngeal and one vagally reinnervated tongue (Fig. 5D,E). In all instances a PAS or cholinesterase reaction could be demonstrated beneath the taste buds in these new sites (Fig. 5F). No taste buds were found in these new areas after combined auriculotemporal or hypoglossal reinnervation and hormone treatment. Similarly no buds were seen anywhere in the testosterone-treated totally denervated papillae. Buds did not appear on the top of the papilla in animals treated with sesame oil alone.

Effects of Reinnervation with Testosterone Treatment on Alkaline Phosphatase Activity. An intense alkaline phosphatase reaction was present in the superficial epithelium only if taste buds had reappeared. Enzyme activity was therefore restored only by gustatory nerve reinnervation. In the auriculotemporal or hypoglossal reinnervated papilla, enzyme activity in the superficail epithelium was greatly reduced, although it was intense in the regions of inflammation (Fig. 2C,D). The nongustatory nerves did not reverse any of the effects of denervation, namely loss of taste buds, atrophy of the papilla, and reduction of alkaline phosphatase activity. Testosterone treatment did not alter the distribution of alkaline phosphatase in the trench walls, and no enzyme was demonstrated in the epithelium above the taste buds found on the top of the papilla. The reason for the failure to demonstrate alkaline phosphatase activity in these new sites is not known since an intense enzyme reaction could be detected over a single taste bud in the trench wall.

Discussion

Taste buds appeared in the vallate papilla after unilateral reinnervation by the glossopharyngeal, chorda tympani, or vagus nerve, but not after reinnervation by the hypoglossal or auriculotemporal nerve. Similar results have been obtained with the glossopharyngeal, vagus, and hypoglossal nerve in the cat (7). Attempts to induce taste bud development by augmenting the number of general sensory fibers reaching the papilla (bilateral auriculotemporal reinnervation), or by combining testosterone treatment with the sensory or motor reinnervation failed. Similarly, general sensory fibers could not subserve a maintenance function on fully formed taste buds. Taste buds disappeared after unilateral auriculotemporal reinnervation of the partially denervated papilla (unilateral glossopharyngeal nerve transection) in which the intact glossopharyngeal nerve was subsequently cut. If general sensory fibers could maintain taste buds some should have persisted after sectioning the glossopharyngeal nerve. The results indicate that taste bud development and maintenance are dependent on a quality of gustatory nerves that is not shared by motor or general sensory nerves.

On the other hand, taste buds in the urodele (newt, salamander) apparently can develop in the absence of the gustatory nerve. Tongue primordia from salamander larvae as well as adult tongue developed taste buds when transplanted to the side of the body (13), orbit (9, 11, 18), or liver (18). The appearance of taste buds in orbital grafts coincided with the arrival of nerve fibers (11), whereas no nerves could be demonstrated in the transplants to the liver (18). The conclusion that taste buds can develop and persist without a gustatory innervation requires further experimental analysis. Taste buds in the urodele have not been studied *in situ* after denervation. It is, therefore, possible that buds in the newt and salamander are not dependent upon any innervation and that their loss immediately after transplantation is a result of the trauma of the operative procedure. It is also possible that in the urodele nongustatory nerves as well as liver could exert a trophic influence on taste buds if the influence is of a common chemical nature. It is significant to note that taste buds did not develop in rat tongue grafts containing dorsal root ganglia when transplanted to the anterior chamber of the eye (4).

Testosterone treatment caused taste bud development in new locations (top of the papilla, area adjacent to it) in the glossopharyngeal (intact or regenerated), chorda tympani, or vagally reinnervated papilla. Testosterone-induced buds on the top of the papilla have been reported in the castrated (1) and normal male (21) animal. Buds have been demonstrated on the top of the papilla in the normal developing newborn (21), but these disappear in the adult; none has been described adjacent to the papilla. It remains to be shown whether these new taste buds developed from ordinary epithelial cells, or whether "cell rests" of previously formed buds were responsible. Buds were found in new locations only after testosterone treatment. None was found in the partially denervated papilla, or after gustatory nerve reinnervation alone. A gustatory nerve–hormone interaction must be involved in forming these new taste buds since no buds were found after hormone treatment of denervated or sensory or motor reinnervated papillaw. Testosterone could exert its effect by increasing the production of trophic factor, or by altering the threshold of peripheral tissue to it. One way the hormone could alter the trophic factor reaching the periphery is by inducing terminal nerve branching. Increased branching of preterminal motor nerve fibers induced by adrenocorticotrophin has been reported (12).

The gustatory nerves that caused taste buds to develop also restored alkaline phosphatase activity in the superficial epithelium around the bud. The fact that activity was present only around the taste bud indicates that the enzyme is in some way associated with the taste cells rather than the stratified squamous epithelial cells. The intense alkaline phosphatase activity in certain areas of the denervated and sensory or motor reinnervated papillae was due to an inflammatory reaction by neutrophilic white blood cells. These inflammatory cells were not observed in a study on the early changes of denervated taste buds (19). Since the leucocytes appeared only after all taste buds had disappeared, inflammation cannot be the important process whereby taste buds are lost. It is unlikely that the alkaline phosphatase activity found in the normal papilla is due to neutrophilic leucocytes because as yet no light- or electron-microscopical study has reported these cells in taste buds.

The results of the present experiment demonstrate that only gustatory nerves can supply the trophic influence required for the development and maintenance of taste buds. It is important, however, to study the endings of the nongustatory nerves to see whether the failure of these nerves to support taste buds could have resulted from their inability to establish connections with the epithelial cells. A comparative study could also reveal the presence or absence of an organelle responsible for the trophic influence (15). Similar studies on the way testosterone causes new regions of tongue to produce taste buds are indicated.

References

1. ALLARA, E. 1952. Sull'influenza esercitata dagli ormoni sulla stattura dell formazioni gustative di mus rattus albinus. *Riv. Biol.* **44**: 209–229.

2. BEIDLER, L. M. 1961. Taste receptor stimulation. *Progr. Biophys. Biophys Chem.* **12**: 107–151.

3. BURSTONE, M. S. 1961. Histochemical demonstration of phosphatases in frozen sections with Naphthal AS-phosphates. *J. Histochem. Cytochem.* **9**: 146–156.

4. FARBMAN, A. I. and M. ZIEGNER. 1968. Differentiation of fetal rat tongue grafts in the anterior chamber of the eye. *Anat. Record* **160**: 347.

5. GOMORI, G. 1952. "Microscopic Histochemistry: Principles and Practice." Univ. of Chicago Press, Chicago, Illinois.

6. GUTH, L. 1957. The effects of glossopharyngeal nerve transection on the circumvallate papilla of the rat. *Anat. Record* **128**: 715–731.

7. GUTH, L. 1958. Taste buds on the cat's circumvallate papilla after reinnervation by glossopharyngeal, vagus, and hypoglossal nerves. *Anat. Record* **130**: 25–37.

8. GUTH, L. 1963. Histological changes following partial denervation of the circumvallate papilla of the rat. *Exptl. Neurol.* **8**: 336–349.

9. MINTZ, B. and L. S. STONE. 1934. Transplantation of taste organs in adult Triturus viridescens. *Proc. Soc. Exptl. Biol. Med.* **31**: 1080–1082.

10. OAKLEY, B. AND F. M. BENJAMIN. 1966. Neural mechanisms of taste. *Physiol. Rev.* **46**: 173–211.

11. PORITSKY, R. L. AND M. SINGER. 1963. The fate of taste buds in tongue transplants to the orbit in the urodele, Triturus. *J. Exptl. Zool.* **153**: 211–218.

12. SHAPIRO, M. S., T. NAMBA, AND D. GROB. 1968. The effect of corticotrophin on the neuromuscular junction. *Neurology* **18**: 1018–1022.

13. STONE, L. S. 1933. Independence of taste organs with respect to their nerve fibers demonstrated in living salamanders. *Proc. Soc. Exptl. Biol. Med.* **30**: 1256–1257.

14. TORREY, T. W. 1934. The relation of taste buds to their nerve fibers. *J. Comp. Neurol.* **59**: 203–220.

15. VAN ARSDALL, C. B., AND T. L. LENTZ. 1968. Neurons. Secretory activity during limb regeneration and induction in the newt. *Science* **162**: 1296–1297.

16. WACHSTEIN, M. AND E. MEISEL. 1957. Histochemistry of hepatic phosphatase at a physiologic pH. *Am. J. Clin. Pathol.* **27**: 13–23.

17. WHITESIDE, B. 1927. Nerve overlap in the gustatory apparatus of the rat. *J. Comp. Neurol.* **44**: 363–377.

18. WRIGHT, M. R. 1964. Taste organs in tongue-to-liver grafts in the newt, Triturus v. veridescens. *J. Exptl. Zool.* **156**: 377–390.

19. ZALEWSKI, A. A. 1968. Changes in phosphatase enzymes following denervation of the vallate papilla of the rat. *Exptl. Neurol.* **22**: 40–51.

20. ZALEWSKI, A. A. 1969a. Role of nerve and epithelium in the regulation of alkaline phosphatase activity in gustatory papillae. *Exptl. Neurol.* **23**: 18–28.

21. ZALEWSKI, A. A. 1969b. Neurotrophic–hormonal interaction in the regulation of taste buds in the rat's vallate papilla. *J. Neurobiol.* **1**: (In press.)

22. ZELENA, J. 1964. Development, degeneration, and regeneration of receptor organs. *Progr. Brain Res.* **13**: 175–211.

Section 8
Synapse Formation

Cohen, M.W., M.J. Anderson, E. Zorychta, and P.R. Weldon. 1979. Accumulation of acetylcholine receptors at nerve-muscle contacts in culture. *Prog. Brain Res.* 49: 335–349.

Sanes, J.R., L.M. Marshall, and U.J. McMahan. 1978. Reinnervation of muscle fiber basal lamina after removal of myofibers. *J. Cell Biol.* 78: 176–198.

Most current information about the morphological and biochemical details of synapse formation comes from work on the vertebrate neuromuscular junction. Among the questions about synaptogenesis that have been explored in muscle are the following: (1) Do uninnervated muscle fibers have specialized regions on their surfaces that are destined to become synaptic sites? (2) Do nerve endings induce postsynaptic specializations? and (3) Do the postsynaptic cells induce differentiation of the presynaptic elements? Additional questions about the selectivity and quantitative regulation of synapse formation are taken up in the subsequent sections (Sections 9 and 11).

The question of whether there are predetermined sites for synapse formation on postsynaptic cells has been examined by studying the distribution of postsynaptic acetylcholine receptors before and during innervation. Diamond and Miledi (1962) first demonstrated that the distribution of receptors on the surfaces of recently innervated embryonic muscle fibers is different from that on adult muscle fibers. Acetylcholine receptors on adult skeletal-muscle fibers in vertebrates are sharply restricted to the subsynaptic region, whereas they can be detected along the entire length of embryonic muscle fibers. Further studies using labeled α-bungarotoxin, a highly specific ligand for acetylcholine receptors, have confirmed this embryonic distribution. Moreover, autoradiographs of muscles treated with labeled bungarotoxin showed that receptors on uninnervated embryonic fibers in culture are often clumped in high-density patches called "hotspots" (Fischbach and Cohen 1973; Sytkowski et al. 1973). Interestingly, acetylcholinesterase, the enzyme that degrades the transmitter, tends to be localized in these same patches (Moody-Corbett and Cohen 1981). Might such receptor clusters induce synapse formation at that point along the muscle surface? Cohen, Anderson, and their collaborators (Anderson and Cohen 1977; Anderson et al. 1977; **Cohen, Anderson, Zorychta,** and **Weldon 1979**), and independently Frank and Fischbach (1979), explored this possibility in experiments in which embryonic muscle fibers were cocultured with appropriate neurons. The processes of the nerve cells did not grow preferentially to receptor clusters but rather caused a reorganization of receptors at points of contact. Receptor reorganization occurs, incidentally, in the absence of muscle activity, which is blocked by unlabeled toxin or curare in the culture medium. This finding has encouraged a search by several groups for an agent derived from nerve that can cause receptor clustering (Christian et al. 1978; Podleski et al. 1978; Burden et al. 1979; Jessell et al. 1979). Finally, neurites from sympathetic or dorsal-root ganglion cells do not cause receptor clusters at points of contact on muscle cells, suggesting that such neural agents may be quite specific (Cohen et al. 1979).

Once nerve-muscle contacts have formed, the surface of the muscle is somehow changed; the surrounding membrane becomes refractory to further innervation (Bennett and Pettigrew 1976; see also Section 11). The cause of this refractoriness in the region surrounding the end plate is not yet known. Certainly, the postsynaptic membrane is very different in composition from extrasynaptic muscle membrane; indeed, even the properties of particular molecules such as acetylcholine receptors and acetylcholinesterase are different in synaptic and nonsynaptic regions (Hall 1973; Fambrough 1979). These differences undoubtedly have something to do with innervation. For example, both the turnover and the properties of acetylcholine receptors are altered when fibers become innervated (Burden 1977a,b; Sakmann and Brenner 1978; Fischbach et al. 1979; Fambrough 1979; Steinbach et al. 1979; Fischbach and Schuetze 1980; Reiness and Hall 1981; Weinberg et al. 1981). Exactly how nerves induce these various changes is not yet clear. Although changes in the properties and distribution of acetylcholine receptors per se are not likely to be the basis of postinnervation refractoriness, similar changes in other membrane components might account for this phenomenon.

The further question of how the growing axon knows when to stop and elaborate the machinery for transmitter release has been explored with a quite different approach. Although axons do not necessarily return to the correct muscle, regenerating axons in adult animals do return quite precisely to the original synaptic sites on denervated muscle fibers (Bennett et al. 1973; Bennett and Pettigrew 1976; Letinsky et al. 1976; see also Raisman 1977). Curious about why old end-plate sites are so attractive, McMahan, Sanes, and Marshall actually rid a portion of a denervated muscle of its myofibers (Marshall et al. 1977; **Sanes, Marshall,** and **McMahan 1978**). Under these conditions, the basal lamina (an extracellular coat of collagen and other material that normally surrounds muscle fibers) remains. Since the enzyme acetylcholinesterase is located largely in basal lamina, the original end-plate site can be identified. By crushing the motor nerve at the same time that muscle fibers were caused to degenerate, these workers could investigate whether regenerating axons still prefer the original synaptic sites in the absence of the postsynaptic muscle cell. The regenerating axons contacted the old sites on the basal lamina ghosts and began to accumulate the organelles characteristic of motor nerve terminals (synaptic vesicles, active zones). Thus, the subsynaptic basal lamina appears to contain molecules that induce axon terminals to elaborate at least some of the specializations found in synaptic endings. The ability to make antibodies that bind specifically to components of basal lamina at synaptic sites should make it possible to identify the relevant molecules (Sanes and Hall 1979; see also Section 10).

Can this general scheme be extended to situations in which the target cells are neurons? Although studies of interneuronal synapses are necessarily less direct, postsynaptic neurons as well as muscle fibers appear to provide cues to the axons seeking to innervate them. For example, preganglionic axons fail to develop significant levels of choline acetyltransferase in the absence of sympathetic ganglion cells (Black et al. 1972; see also Sections 6, 9, and 11). Since this enzyme is characteristic of presynaptic cholinergic terminals, its absence implies that nerve terminals in this system do not differentiate normally in the absence of a postsynaptic signal.

In normal development, the formation of synapses is usually a gradual process, with the functional, biochemical, and morphological characteristics of maturity appearing over days or even several weeks. Thus, even though an influence of nerve on the distribution of acetylcholine receptors in muscle is apparent within a few hours of neural contact (see above), the ultimate pattern of receptors and their adult properties are achieved over a much longer time in early life (see, for example, Diamond and Miledi 1962; Burden 1977a,b; Bevan and Steinbach 1977). One aspect of this gradual change is that the release of transmitter at newly formed synapses is appreciably different from release in maturity. Miniature end-plate potentials are abnormally small and infrequent, and evoked release has a lower quantal content and is more apt to fail altogether (Bennett and Pettigrew 1974; Dennis and Miledi 1974; Dennis 1975; Dennis et al. 1981). In accord with these findings, the attainment of morphological maturity is also gradual (Kelly and Zacks 1969; see also Rees et al. 1976; Pfenninger and Rees 1978). Indeed, when neuromuscular synapses first begin to function, they are hardly recognizable in the electron microscope.

The regulation of acetylcholine receptors by nerves, the instruction provided to regenerating axons by a component of basal lamina, and descriptions of the normal sequence of events during synaptogenesis in vivo only begin to answer the question of how synapses form. Nonetheless, these experiments lead to some important generalizations. From the evidence obtained in muscle, it seems unlikely that specialized sites that attract innervation exist before nerve contact (although clusters of both receptors and acetylcholinesterase are present on uninnervated myofibers). Once formed, however, postsynaptic sites change the surrounding membrane in some way, persist after subsequent denervation, and provide a compelling attraction to regenerating axons. Chemical signals from pre- to postsynaptic cells are also important in synapse formation, as shown by the work on nerve-induced redistribution of acetylcholine receptors. The synapse, then, appears to be the result of a prolonged two-way biochemical conversation during development.

References

Anderson, M.J. and M.W. Cohen. 1977. Nerve-induced and spontaneous redistribution of acetylcholine receptors on cultured muscle cells. *J. Physiol.* 268: 757–773.

Anderson, M.J., M.W. Cohen, and E. Zorychta. 1977. Effects of innervation on the distribution of acetylcholine receptors on cultured muscle cells. *J. Physiol.* 268: 731–756.

Bennett, M.R. and A.G. Pettigrew. 1974. The formation of synapses in striated muscle during development. *J. Physiol.* 241: 515–545.

——. 1976. The formation of neuromuscular synapses. *Cold Spring Harbor Symp. Quant. Biol.* 40: 409–424.

Bennett, M.R., E.M. McLachlan, and R.S. Taylor. 1973. The formation of synapses in reinnervated mammalian striated muscle. *J. Physiol.* 233: 481–500.

Bevan, S. and J.H. Steinbach. 1977. The distribution of α-bungarotoxin binding sites on mammalian skeletal muscle developing *in vivo*. *J. Physiol.* 267: 195–213.

Black, I.B., I.A. Hendry, and L. Iversen. 1972. The role of post-synaptic neurones in the biochemical maturation of presynaptic cholinergic nerve terminals in a mouse sympathetic ganglion. *J. Physiol.* 221: 149–159.

Burden, S. 1977a. Development of the neuromuscular junction in the chick embryo: The number, distribution, and stability of acetylcholine receptors. *Dev. Biol.* 57: 317–329.

——. 1977b. Acetylcholine receptors at the neuromuscular junction: Developmental change in receptor turnover. *Dev. Biol.* 61: 79–85.

Burden, S.J., P.B. Sargent, and U.J. McMahan. 1979. Acetylcholine receptors in regenerating muscle accumulate at original synaptic sites in the absence of nerve. *J. Cell Biol.* 82: 412–425.

Christian, C.N., M.P. Daniels, H. Sugiyama, Z. Vogel, L. Jacques, and P.G. Nelson. 1978. A factor from neurons increases the number of acetylcholine receptor aggregates on cultured muscle cells. *Proc. Natl. Acad. Sci.* 75: 4011–4015.

Cohen, M.W., M.J. Anderson, E. Zorychta, and P.R. Weldon. 1979. Accumulation of acetylcholine receptors at nerve-muscle contacts in culture. *Prog. Brain. Res.* 49: 335–349.

Dennis, M.J. 1975. Physiological properties of junctions between nerve and muscle developing during salamander limb regeneration. *J. Physiol.* 244: 683–702.

Dennis, M.J. and R. Miledi. 1974. Non-transmitting neuromuscular junctions during an early stage of end-plate reinnervation. *J. Physiol.* 239: 3553–570.

Dennis, M.J., L. Ziskind-Conhaim, and A.J. Harris. 1981. Development of neuromuscular junctions in rat embryos. *Dev. Biol.* 81: 266–279.

Diamond, J. and R. Miledi. 1962. A study of foetal and new-born rat muscle fibres. *J. Physiol.* 162: 393–408.

Fambrough, D.M. 1979. Control of acetylcholine receptors in skeletal muscles. *Physiol. Rev.* 59: 165–227.

Fischbach, G.D. and S.A. Cohen. 1973. The distribution of acetylcholine sensitivity over uninnervated and innervated muscle fibers grown in cell culture. *Dev. Biol.* 31: 147–162.

Fischbach, G.D. and S.M. Schuetze. 1980. A postnatal decrease in acetylcholine channel open time at rat endplates. *J. Physiol.* 303: 125–139.

Fischbach, G.D., E. Frank, T.M. Jessell, L.L. Rubin, and S.M. Schuetze. 1979. Accumulation of acetylcholine receptors and acetylcholinesterase at newly formed nerve-muscle synapses. *Pharmacol. Rev.* 30: 411–428.

Frank, E.R. and G.D. Fischbach. 1979. Early events in neuromuscular junction formation *in vitro*. Induction of acetylcholine receptor clusters in the postsynaptic membrane and the morphology of newly formed synapses. *J. Cell Biol.* 83: 143–158.

Hall, Z.W. 1973. Multiple forms of acetylcholinesterase and their distribution in endplate and non-endplate regions of rat diaphragm muscle. *J. Neurobiol.* 4: 343–361.

Jessell, T., R. Siegel, and G.D. Fischbach. 1979. Induction of acetylcholine receptors on cultured skeletal muscle by a factor extracted from brain and spinal cord. *Proc. Natl. Acad. Sci.* 76: 5397–5401.

Kelly, A.M. and S.I. Zacks. 1969. The fine structure of motor endplate morphogenesis. *J. Cell Biol.* 42: 154–169.

Letinsky, M., K. Fishbeck, and U.J. McMahan. 1976. Precision of reinnervation of original postsynaptic sites in frog muscle after nerve crush. *J. Neurocytol.* 5: 691–718.

Marshall, L.M., J.R. Sanes, and U.J. McMahan. 1977. Reinnervation of original synaptic sites on muscle fiber basement membrane after disruption of muscle cells. *Proc. Natl. Acad. Sci.* 74: 3073–3077.

Moody-Corbett, F. and M.W. Cohen. 1981. Localization of cholinesterase at sites of high acetylcholine receptor density on embryonic amphibian muscle cells cultured without nerve. *J. Neurosci.* 1: 596–605.

Pfenninger, K.H. and R.P. Rees. 1978. From growth cone to synapse. Properties of membranes involved in synapse formation. In *Neuronal recognition* (ed. S.H. Barondes), pp. 131–178. Plenum Press, New York.

Podleski, T.R., D. Axelrod, P. Ravdin, I. Greenberg, M.M. Johnson, and M.M. Salpeter. 1978. Nerve extract induces increase and redistribution of acetylcholine receptors on cloned muscle cells.

Proc. Natl. Acad. Sci. 75: 2035–2039.

Raisman, G. 1977. Formation of synapses in the adult rat after injury. *Philos. Trans. R. Soc. Lond. B 278:* 349–359.

Rees, R.P., M.B. Bunge, and R.P. Bunge. 1976. Morphological changes in the neuritic growth cone and target neuron during synaptic junction development in culture. *J. Cell Biol. 68:* 240–263.

Reiness, G.R. and Z.W. Hall. 1981. The developmental change in immunological properties of the acetylcholine receptor in rat muscle. *Dev. Biol. 81:* 324–331.

Sakmann, B. and H.R. Brenner. 1978. Change in synaptic channel gating during neuromuscular development. *Nature 276:* 401–402.

Sanes, J.R. and Z.W. Hall. 1979. Antibodies that bind specifically to synaptic sites on muscle fiber basal lamina. *J. Cell Biol. 83:* 357–370.

Sanes, J.R., L.M. Marshall, and U.J. McMahan. 1978. Reinnervation of muscle fiber basal lamina after removal of myofibers. *J. Cell Biol. 78:* 176–198.

Steinbach, J.H., J. Merlie, S. Heinemann, and R. Bloch. 1979. Degradation of junctional acetylcholine receptors by developing rat skeletal muscle. *Proc. Natl. Acad. Sci. 76:* 3547–3551.

Sytkowski, A.J., Z. Vogel, and M.W. Nirenberg. 1973. Development of acetylcholine receptor clusters on cultured muscle cells. *Proc. Natl. Acad. Sci. 70:* 270–274.

Weinberg, C.R., J.R. Sanes, and Z.W. Hall. 1981. Formation of neuromuscular junctions in adult rats: Accumulation of acetylcholine receptors, acetylcholinesterase, and components of synaptic basal lamina. *Dev. Biol. 84:* 255–266.

Reprinted from Prog. Brain Res., Vol. 49, pp. 335–349. 1979

Accumulation of Acetylcholine Receptors at Nerve-Muscle Contacts in Culture

M.W. COHEN, M.J. ANDERSON *, E. ZORYCHTA ** and P.R. WELDON

Department of Physiology, McGill University, Montreal (Canada)

INTRODUCTION

The subsynaptic membrane at neuromuscular junctions in vertebrate skeletal muscle is specialized to respond to minute quantities of acetylcholine (ACh) and differs in this respect from the rest of the sarcolemma which is much less sensitive to the transmitter substance (Miledi, 1960; Feltz and Mallart, 1971; Dreyer and Peper, 1974; Kuffler and Yoshikami, 1975). This functional specialization reflects the fact that ACh receptors are present in the sub-synaptic membrane in very high density, the order of magnitude being 10,000/ square μm, whereas elsewhere in the sarcolemma their density is about a thousand-fold lower (Barnard et al., 1971; Fambrough and Hartzell, 1972; Hartzell and Fambrough, 1972; Albuquerque et al., 1974; Fambrough, 1974; Fertuck and Salpeter, 1974, 1976; Burden, 1977a; Orkand et al., 1978).Even at relatively early stages of development when muscle fibres have a more sub-stantial density of receptors along their entire length, receptor density is greatest at the developing neuromuscular junction (Diamond and Miledi, 1962; Bevan and Steinbach, 1977) and appears to be as high as at the adult neuro-muscular junction (Burden, 1977a).

To study how ACh receptors become localized in the subsynaptic membrane during formation of the neuromuscular junction we have carried out experi-ments on cell cultures of neural tube (developing spinal cord) and myotomal muscle derived from 1-day-old embryos of the South African frog, *Xenopus laevis*. In this paper we summarize evidence, presented in detail elsewhere (Anderson et al., 1977; Anderson and Cohen, 1977), supporting the following conclusions: the nerve causes ACh receptors to accumulate along paths of nerve-muscle contact; this nerve-induced accumulation of ACh receptors is associated with functional innervation but can occur even when synaptic activ-ity is blocked; it involves a process of redistribution whereby extrajunctional receptors change their location in the sarcolemma and aggregate at sites of nerve-muscle contact. We also present results showing that in contrast to the neural tube two other sources of nerve, sympathetic ganglia and dorsal root

---

* Present address: Neurobiology Department, The Salk Institute, LaJolla, CA (U.S.A.)
** Present address: Department of Pathology, McGill University, Montreal (Canada).

ganglia, do not induce the development of a high receptor density at sites of contact. These results suggest that the triggering of ACh receptor accumulation by neural tube neurites is due to a specific nerve factor.

MATERIALS AND METHODS

All experiments were carried out on cultures of myotomal muscle cells with or without nerve. One-day-old *Xenopus* embryos were skinned and treated with collagenase in order to isolate the myotomes and their associated neural tube from each other and from adjacent tissues. The isolated myotomes were then transferred to a calcium-magnesium-free solution of trypsin-EDTA to dissociate them into single cells or small clusters of cells. These in turn were plated in culture chambers whose floor consisted of a collagen-coated glass coverslip. For mixed cultures containing muscle as well as neural tube, the isolated neural tubes were likewise dissociated into small clusters of cells before being plated. Two other sources of nerve were also used in some cultures: sympathtic ganglia of *Xenopus* juveniles and dorsal root ganglia of *Xenopus* tadpoles. Like the neural tubes, these ganglia were treated with collagenase and with trypsin-EDTA before being added to the culture chambers. This treatment softened the ganglia but did not cause them to dissociate. Depending on their size the ganglia were cultured either whole or in fragments.

Cultures were maintained at room temperature in a medium consisting of L-15 diluted to 60% with water and Holmes' α-1 protein (0.2 μg/ml). For the first day of culture the medium also contained dialyzed horse serum (5%) in order to facilitate adhesion of the cells to the collagen substrate.

The distribution of ACh receptors on cultured myotomal muscle cells was examined by fluorescence and phase contrast microscopy after staining the receptors with fluorescent α-bungarotoxin (Anderson and Cohen, 1974; Anderson et al., 1977). For most experiments tetramethylrhodamine-labelled toxin was used in preference to fluorescein-labelled toxin because it gives brighter staining and fades less rapidly.

Cultures to be examined by electron microscopy were prepared and handled in the same way as described above except that the floor of the culture chamber consisted of a sheet of collagen-coated Aclar rather than glass (see Masurovrsky and Bunge, 1968). The cultures were fixed with 1.5% glutaraldehyde for 30—60 min, post-fixed with 1% osmium tetroxide, stained with 1% aqueous uranyl acetate, dehydrated in a graded series of ethanol, and embedded in Epon 812. Selected areas were sectioned with a Huxley ultramicrotome parallel to the floor of the culture chamber and examined with a Siemens Elsmiskop I electron microscope.

RESULTS

Description of muscle and neural tube cultures

The dissociated muscle cells attach to the collagen substrate and begin to elongate within a few hours after being added to the culture chamber. They begin to acquire striations during the first day and these increase in prominence over the next 3—4 days. During this period most of the yolk granules originally present in the cells are consumed and the cells grow in size, attaining lengths of up to 300 μm, but remain mononucleated. In all of these respects differentiation of the myotomal muscle cells in culture mimics that during the normal development of the embryos (Nieuwkoop and Faber, 1956; Hamilton, 1969; Muntz, 1975).

The growth of neurites and the formation of nerve-muscle contacts in cultures with neural tube was originally described by Harrison (1910) in his pioneering and classical study which firmly established the validity of the neurone theory. Briefly, by one day in culture neurites with active growth cones are seen extending from the neural tube cells. Many have already contacted muscle cells. The neurites may be as much as 2—3 μm in diameter and, as revealed by electron microscopy, are often composed of a few nerve fibres. They continue to grow during the next day in culture but by the third day most growth ceases and neurites begin to retract. As a result, after three days in culture fewer neurites and fewer contacts with muscle cells are seen.

As originally pointed out by Harrison (1910) some of the muscle cells which are contacted by neurites undergo spontaneous contractions whereas all of the non-contacted muscle cells remain quiescent. Muscle contractions can also be evoked by electrical stimulation of the appropriate neural tube cells. Both the spontaneous and neurally-evoked contractions are abolished by curare and by α-bungarotoxin indicating that they are due to cholinergic synaptic transmis-

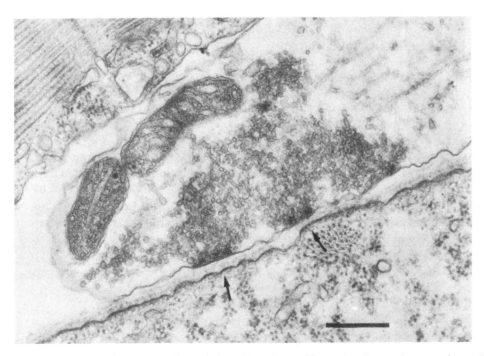

Fig. 1. Nerve-muscle synapse in a 1-day-old culture. Note the dense clusters of vesicles apposed to the axolemma, the basement membrane in the cleft, and the increased electron density of the underlying sarcolemma (arrows). Bar indicates 0.5 μm.

sion. Intracellular recordings have likewise confirmed that the myotomal muscle cells become functionally innervated in mixed cultures (Cohen, 1972).

Electron microscopy indicates that neuromuscular junctions develop in these cultures and that the sequence of development is much the same as during the normal development of the myotomes (see Kullberg et al., 1977). After 2–3 days in culture the nerve-muscle contacts display considerable variability in degree of ultrastructural differentiation. As in vivo, many appear rather immature but a few have the characteristics of relatively mature myotomal neuromuscular junctions, including aggregates of vesicles in close apposition to the junctional axolemma, a prominent basement membrane in the cleft, and a sarcolemma of increased electron density or thickness (Fig. 1).

Accumulation of ACh receptors at sites of nerve-muscle contact

Fluorescent staining of ACh receptors reveals that by 2 days in culture virtually all muscle cells not contacted by nerve have developed patches of high receptor density (see Fig. 5). These patches vary considerably in size, distribution and number. On the whole they appear to increase in size with the age of the culture, but even in 4- and 5-day-old cultures they are rarely more than 20 μm in their largest dimension and never more than 40 μm. The large patches often occur near the ends of the muscle cells or their processes, on the surface in contact with the culture dish. Another common location is in central regions of the cell, on the free surface. In addition to patches of high receptor density autoradiography with ^{125}I-labelled α-bungarotoxin reveals a widespread distribution of receptors whose mean density is some twenty-fold lower than the receptor density in the patches (Anderson et al., 1977). This widespread low density phase of ACh receptors is rather poorly resolved by fluorescent staining.

Quite different patterns of ACh receptor distribution are seen on many nerve-contacted muscle cells (Figs. 2, 3). In 2- and 3-day-old cultures fluorescent staining reveals that over 70% of the contacted cells have regions of high receptor density along the paths of contact (see Table I) and more than half of these cells have no patches of high receptor density elsewhere. The association of high receptor density with paths of nerve-muscle contact is always observed on muscle cells previously identified as being functionally innervated on the basis of spontaneous or neurally-evoked contractions (Anderson et al., 1977). There is considerable variability in the lengths of fluorescent stain along individual paths of nerve-muscle contact but of most interest is the fact that bands of stain sometimes extend for greater distances than the largest patches seen on non-contacted muscle cells. Such examples cannot be explained simply in terms of the neurites having contacted a pre-existing patch of high receptor density. Instead they indicate that the neural tube neurites can induce the development of a high density of ACh receptors at sites of contact.

This conclusion is further supported by experiments in which the patterns of fluorescent stain on individual cells are followed over a period of time. Figure 2 illustrates an example from such an experiment. In this case a 2-day-old culture was stained with fluorescent toxin and then rinsed only mildly so that a low concentration of fluorescent toxin remained in the culture. The first observa-

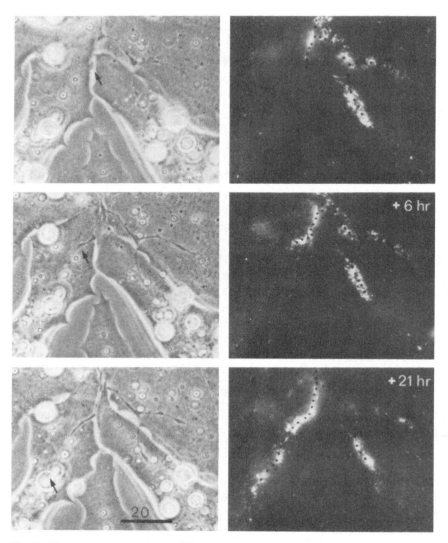

Fig. 2. Changes in the pattern of fluorescent stain on nerve-contacted muscle cells. The culture (2-days-old) was stained and rinsed mildly so that some fluorescent toxin was present throughout the period of observation. The same field was viewed with phase contrast optics (left) and with fluorescence optics (right). Note the neurite growth (arrows) between the first, second (+6 h) and third (+21 h) observations and the corresponding new appearance of fluorescent stain. Also note the loss of fluorescent stain along other paths of nerve-muscle contact. Black dots have been added to the fluorescence micrographs to indicate paths of nerve-muscle contact. Bar indicates 20 μ.

tion, made shortly afterwards, shows a field in which two of the muscle cells are clearly contacted by nerve and have fluorescent stain along the path of contact. A third muscle cell appears to be contacted along its edge and also has stain at this site. The next observation, made 6 h later, shows that the neurite has grown along this third muscle cell and that a high density of receptors has developed along the newly-formed contact. By the time of the third observation, 15 h later, the lengths of this nerve-muscle contact is even greater and, as

372

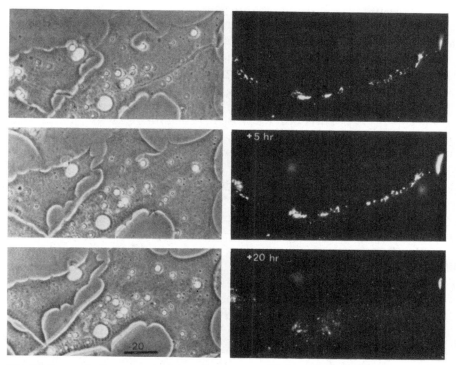

Fig. 3. Loss of fluorescent stain after nerve withdrawal. Procedures were the same as described for Fig. 2. Note that between the first and second (+5 h) observations the neurite withdrew and that by the third (+20 h) observation the fluorescent stain along the original path of nerve-muscle contact had for the most part disappeared. Culture was 2-days-old at the time of the first observation. Bar indicates 20 μm.

before, the region of newly-formed contact has acquired a high receptor density.

In following patterns of stain on nerve-contacted muscle cells one sometimes observes the converse result, the disappearance of fluorescent stain after spontaneous withdrawal of the neurite. Figure 3 shows such an example. The first observation shows a long length of fluorescent stain associated with the path of nerve-muscle contact. The next observation, 5 h later, shows that the neurite has withdrawn but the pattern of fluorescent stain is only marginally altered. However, by the third observation, 15 h later, there is very little stain left along the original path of contact although some new spots of stain have appeared elsewhere on the muscle cell. During the 20 h period in which the observations were made the culture contained a low concentration of fluorescent toxin, as in the experiment of Fig. 2, and no additional fluorescence was observed upon restaining the culture after the third observation.

The results, in addition to emphasizing the role of the nerve in inducing the development of a high receptor density at sites of contact, also raise the possibility that the maintenance of this local high density is initially dependent upon the continued presence of the nerve. However, it is also worth noting that the mere physical presence of the nerve is not a sufficient condition for maintaining the high receptor density. For example, in the experiment of Fig. 2

there was some disappearance of stain along one region of contact (the one on the right hand side) despite the continued presence of the nerve. Such observations suggest, not surprisingly, that the accumulation and maintenance of a high receptor density at sites of contact are dependent upon the state of the neurite and muscle cell.

Receptor accumulation occurs in the absence of synaptic or contractile activity

Myotomal muscle cells can be innervated even when they are cultured in the presence of a concentration (100 μg/ml) of curare which completely obliterates end-plate potentials (Cohen, 1972). Likewise, this high concentration of curare does not prevent the development of long bands of high receptor density along paths of nerve-muscle contact (Anderson et al., 1977). Thus the nerve-induced accumulation of ACh receptors is not triggered by synaptic potentials or muscle contraction or any of the associated changes in membrane permeability. Additional evidence in this regard is that ACh receptors also accumulate at sites of nerve-muscle contact in the presence of 5 μg/ml α-bungarotoxin (see below). This concentration of toxin blocks neurally evoked contraction within 2–3 min and saturates the ACh receptor toxin binding sites within 20 min (Anderson et al., 1977). Since activation of ACh receptors by transmitter must be entirely eliminated under these conditions it is clearly not essential for the nerve-induced accumulation of receptors. Instead these results indicate that the nerve-induced accumulation of receptors is triggered in some other way, by a factor which is either released from the neurites or associated with their surface membrane.

Dependence of receptor accumulation on nerve type

A question of obvious importance is whether all classes of nerve are able to induce accumulation of ACh receptors or whether this induction displays neural specificity. The latter possibility seemed likely in view of the fact that some of muscle cells contacted by NT (neural tube) neurites do not develop a high density of ACh receptors along the path of contact. A simple explanation of this result would be that the neural tube contains different types of nerve cells (see Spitzer, 1976) and that only some of these are competent to induce receptor accumulation. But other explanations, such as variability in the responsiveness of the cultured muscle cells, are not excluded by the observations presented so far. Experiments were therefore undertaken in which two other sources of nerve, sympathetic ganglia (SG) and dorsal root ganglia (DRG) were tested for their ability to induce accumulation of ACh receptors at sites of contact.

Explants of SG were cultured by themselves, usually for 4–6 days, in order to allow them to become firmly attached to the culture dish and to develop a reasonable outgrowth of neurites. Myotomal muscle cells were then plated in the same cultures. The SG neurites continued to grow and over the next 2–4 days contacted many muscle cells (Fig. 4). Explants of DRG adhered and grew more quickly than SG explants so that for these cultures the muscle cells were usually plated at the same time as the DRG explants or within the first 3 days.

342

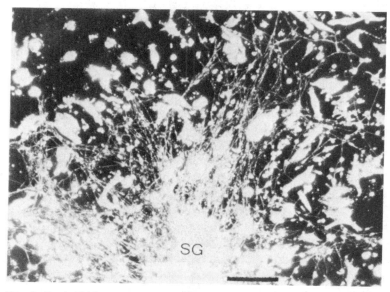

Fig. 4. Dark-field view showing scattered myotomal muscle cells and neuritic outgrowth from an explant of sympathetic ganglion (SG). The ganglion was in culture for 9 days and the muscle cells for 3 days. Bar indicates 300 μm.

In both types of culture ACh receptors were stained with fluorescent α-bungarotoxin and their distribution examined 2–4 days after plating the muscle cells.

In contrast to the muscle cells contacted by NT neurites, most of those contacted by SG or DRG neurites displayed no stain along the path of contact and had patches of stain elsewhere (Fig. 5). In the few examples where some stain was present along the path of contact it was never in the form of a characteristic band of stain as seen on many NT-contacted muscle cells but rather appeared like the patches that occur in non-contacted muscle cells. The results are summarized in Table I. Over 70% of NT-contacted muscle cells had some stain along the path of contact whereas the corresponding value for DRG-contacted muscle cells was 9%, and for SG-contacted cells it was 5%. In addition,

TABLE I

FLUORESCENT STAIN ALONG PATHS OF NERVE-MUSCLE CONTACT

Type of nerve	No. of cultures examined	No. of contacted muscle cells examined	Muscle cells with stain along path of contact (%) *
NT	9	438	73 ± 4
DRG	8	228	9 ± 3
SG	14	414	5 ± 1
SG + NT	6	131 (SG-contacted)	4 ± 3
		249 (NT-contacted)	77 ± 2

* Means and standard errors are based on values obtained in individual cultures.

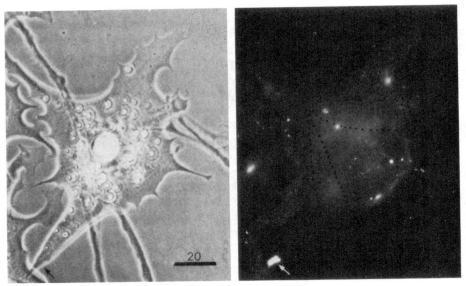

Fig. 5. Pattern of fluorescent stain on a muscle cell contacted by SG neurites. Note the general lack of stain along the paths of nerve-muscle contact. There is instead a bright patch of stain (arrow) near the end of one process of the muscle cell and several other smaller patches elsewhere on the cell. Age in culture; 7 days for SG; 3 days for muscle. Bar indicates 20 μm.

of those NT-contacted muscle cells that did have some stain along the path of contact only 37% had patches of stain elsewhere. In contrast almost all (over 95%) of the SG- and DRG-contacted muscle cells had patches of stain elsewhere even in those cases where there was some stain associated with the contact. These results suggest that SG and DRG neurites do not significantly influence the distribution of ACh receptors on the myotomal muscle cells.

Although it seemed unlikely, it could be argued that the DRG explants and SG explants modify the culture medium in some way which makes the myotomal muscle cells unresponsive to the neurites which contact them. This possibility was tested in cultures of SG explants by adding not only myotomal muscle cells but also neural tube cells. Contacts by NT neurites and SG neurites could easily be distinguished by following the neurites back to their source since SG explants were considerably larger and their neuritic outgrowth much more extensive than NT explants. As summarized in Table I the results obtained with these cultures were similar to those obtained when only one type of nerve explant was present. More than 70% of the NT-contacted muscle cells had stain along the path of contact whereas the corresponding value for SG-contacted muscle cells was only 4%. Clearly the ineffectiveness of SG neurites cannot be explained in terms of some modification of the culture medium. Instead these results indicate that the triggering of ACh receptor accumulation by neural tube neurites is due to a specific factor.

Redistribution of receptors within the sarcolemma contributes
to receptor accumulation

The lateral movement of surface membrane constituents has been well-established in recent years and has been found to contribute to phenomena such as capping whereby multivalent ligands such as antibodies and lectins cause their receptors to aggregate at one pole of the cell (for reviews see Bretscher and Raff, 1975; Edelman, 1976). To study whether the accumulation of ACh receptors at sites of nerve-muscle contact might involve their redistribution within the sarcolemma, experiments were carried out as follows. Myotomal muscle cells were cultured by themselves for 2–3 days and then stained with fluorescent α-bungarotxin. After several rinses the culture medium was replaced with one containing a high concentration (5 μg/ml) of unlabelled toxin and neural tube cells were added to the cultures. By this procedure only those receptors present in the sarcolemma prior to the addition of nerve would be stained, whereas any receptors incorporated into the membrane after the addition of the nerve would not be visible because unlabelled, rather than fluorescent, toxin would be bound to them. Observations were made 1–3 days after adding the neural tube cells. As in freshly stained cultures, a small but statistically significant number of examples were obtained in which the length of stain along paths of nerve-muscle contact was greater than the largest patches on non-contacted muscle cells (Anderson and Cohen, 1977). Accumulation of stained receptors at sites of nerve-muscle contact was also observed directly by following the same cell over a period of about one day (Anderson and Cohen, 1977). These experiments indicate that ACh receptors can change their position in the sarcolemma and aggregate at sites of nerve-muscle contact thereby contributing to the development of a high receptor density.

DISCUSSION

ACh receptors accumulate at sites of nerve-muscle contact in cultures of neural tube and myotomal muscle derived from *Xeonpus* embryos. This accumulation of receptors is induced by the NT neurites and is associated with functional innervation. Since ultrastructurally-differentiated nerve-muscle synapses also develop in these cultures it is most reasonable to assume that they are the sites of function and high receptor density, and that the accumulation of receptors is part of the overall process of neuromuscular synaptogenesis. The lack of effect of SG and DRG neurites on receptor distribution provides additional support that the NT-induced accumulation of ACh receptors is part of the normal process of synapse formation.

Evidence for nerve-induced accumulation of ACh receptors has recently been obtained in other studies as well. Frank and Fischbach (1977) have combined measurements of ACh sensitivity with focal external recordings of synaptic potentials in cultures of pectoral muscle cells and brachial spinal cord derived from chick embryos. By monitoring the same regions over a period of time they have found that new high levels of ACh sensitivity develop at sites of, and as a result of, innervation. Lømo and Slater (1976) have likewise reported nerve-induced development of high ACh sensitivity at ectopic synapses during reinnervation of rat soleus muscle. Also consistent with a process of neural induction is the finding that during normal development of the neuromuscular junction in the rat diaphragm (Bevan and Steinbach, 1977) and in *Xenopus* myotomes (Chow and Cohen, 1977) high densities of ACh receptors develop after the arrival of the growing nerve fibres.

Nerve-induced receptor accumulation occurs even when the receptors are entirely blocked and is therefore not dependent on synaptic or contractile activity or any of the associated changes in membrane permeability. The accumulation must be triggered in some other way, by a factor which is either released from the nerve or associated with its surface membrane. This factor appears to be specific inasmuch as DRG and SG neurites, unlike NT neurites, do not induce receptor accumulation. Furthermore, the rapidity with which receptor accumulation can occur after contact is made between NT neurites and muscle (see Fig. 2) suggests that the factor can act very shortly after the growing neurite comes into close proximity with the muscle cell. This raises the possibility that the triggering factor may participate in one of the primary interactions leading to synapse formation. In this context is should be recalled that skeletal muscle can be innervated not only by motor neurones but also by other cholinergic neurones (Landmesser, 1971, 1972; Bennett et al., 1973; Nurse and O'Lague, 1975; Hooisma et al., 1975; Betz, 1976; Obata, 1977; Schubert et al. 1977) and that at least one class of these "inappropriate" cholinergic neurones (chick ciliary ganglia) appears to be able to trigger receptor accumulation (Betz and Osborne, 1977). It will be of interest in future studies to try to assess further whether all cholinergic neurones have this ability and whether different neurones exhibit different capacities to induce receptor accumulation. The existence of such differences might help explain competitive interactions between different neurones for innervation of a muscle cell, such as occurs during normal development (Redfern, 1970; Bagust et al., 1973; Bennett and Pettigrew, 1974; Brown et al., 1976) and in response to experimental manipulation (Schmidt and Stefani, 1976; Bennett and Raftos, 1977; Yip and Dennis, 1977; Kuffler et al., 1977).

Our studies have indicated that the accumulation of ACh receptors at sites of nerve-muscle contact involves a process of redistribution whereby receptors change their position in the sarcolemma and aggregate at the sites of contact. Additional evidence that ACh receptors are mobile within the sarcolemma has also been provided by Axelrod et al. (1976) in experiments on cultured rat myotubes. These investigators stained ACh receptors with fluorescent α-bungarotoxin and examined the recovery of fluorescence in small areas after bleaching with high intensity excitation. Recovery of fluorescence after bleaching is attributed to the movement of unbleached, fluorochrome-labelled, receptors from adjacent regions into the bleached area. Very little recovery occurred after bleaching receptors within high density patches (hot spots) but significant recovery of fluorescence was observed when regions of lower receptor density were bleached. These results suggest that the receptors within high density patches are for the most part immobile whereas many of these which are present at lower density in the rest of the sarcolemma are mobile (Axelrod et al., 1976). Aggregation of receptors at sites of nerve-muscle contact is likewise most simply accounted for in terms of a loss of mobility.

At adult neuromuscular junctions ACh receptors have a half-life of at least several days (Berg and Hall, 1974, 1975; Chang and Huang, 1975). In contrast, extrajunctional receptors are much less stable and survive with a half-life of about one day (Berg and Hall, 1974, 1975; Chang and Huang, 1975; Devreotes and Fambrough, 1975; Merlie et al., 1976). This difference between extra-junctional receptors is apparent rather early in development; for example, it has been detected in neonatal rat muscle (Berg and Hall, 1975) and in muscle from 3-week-old chicks (Burden, 1977b). Of particular interest is the finding by Burden (1977a) that in muscle from younger chicks junctional receptors have the same short lifespan as extrajunctional receptors. Similar results have also been reported for junctional and extrajunctional receptors on chick myotubes in cultures (Frank and Fischbach, 1977). Despite the short lifespan of the junc-tional receptors in young chick muscle, junctional receptor density is main-tained at the same high level as in the adult and it follows that receptors are added to the subsynaptic membrane at the same rate as they are degraded (Burden, 1977a). Such replenishment could occur by movement of extra-junctional receptors into the subsynaptic membrane or by preferential insertion of receptors directly into the subsynaptic membrane. Neither of these processes is mutually exclusive and both could operate in the formation as well as the maintenance of the high receptor density at sites of innervation.

SUMMARY

Nerve-induced accumulation of ACh receptors has been demonstrated to occur at sites of nerve-muscle contact in cell cultures of neural tube and myo-tomal muscle derived from *Xenopus* embryos. This acculumation of receptors is associated with functional innervation of the muscle cells and presumably occurs at the developing synaptic sites which have been observed in these cul-tures by electron microscopy. The accumulation can occur rapidly, within a few hours after nerve-muscle contact is made, and does not depend on synaptic or contractile activity. It involves a process of receptor redistribution whereby extrajunctional receptors aggregate at the site of contact. The neurites of two other sources of nerve, dorsal root ganglia and synpathetic ganglia, do not cause ACh receptors to accumulate at sites of muscle contact. It is suggested that the ACh receptor accumulation which is induced by neural tube neurites is due to the action of a specific neural factor.

ACKNOWLEDGEMENTS

We thank Mr. V. Vipparti for expert technical assistance. It is also a pleasure to express our gratitude to Professor Stephen Kuffler who introduced one of us some eleven years ago to the study of synapse formation in cultured explants of *Xenopus* neural tube and myotomal muscle. This work was supported by the Medical Research Council of Canada. Personal support (M.W.C.) from the Conseil de la Recherche en Santé du Québec is also gratefully acknowledged.

REFERENCES

Albuquerque, E.X., Barnard, A.E., Porter, C.W., and Warnick, J.E. (1974) The density of acetylcholine receptors and their sensitivity in the postsynaptic membrane of muscle endplates. *Proc. nat. Acad. Sci. (Wash.),* 71, 2818–2822.

Anderson, M.J. and Cohen, M.W. (1974). Fluorescent staining of acetylcholine receptors in vertebrate skeletal muscle. *J. Physiol. (Lond.),* 237, 385–400.

Anderson, M.J. and Cohen, M.W. (1977) Nerve-induced and spontaneous redistribution of acetylcholine receptors on cultured muscle cells. *J. Physiol. (Lond.),* 268, 757–773.

Anderson, M.J., Cohen, M.W. and Zorychta, E. (1977) Effects of innervation on the distribution of acetylcholine receptors on cultured muscle cells. *J. Physiol. (Lond.),* 268, 731–756.

Axelrod, D., Ravdin, P., Koppel, D.E., Schlessinger, J., Webb, W.W., Elson, E.L., Podleski, T.R. (1976). Lateral motion of fluorescently labeled acetylcholine receptors in membranes of developing muscle fibres. *Proc. nat. Acad. Sci. (Wash.),* 73, 4594–4598.

Bagust, J., Lewis, D.M., and Westerman, R.A. (1973) Polyneuronal innervation of kitten skeletal muscle. *J. Physiol. (Lond.),* 229, 241–255.

Barnard, E.A., Wieckowski, J. and Chiu, T.H. (1971) Cholinergic receptor molecules and cholinesterase molecules at mouse skeletal muscle junctions. *Nature (Lond.),* 234, 207–209.

Bennett, M.R. and Pettigrew, A.G. (1974). The formation of synapses in striated muscle during development. *J. Physiol. (Lond.),* 241, 515–545.

Bennett, M.R. and Raftos, J. (1977) The formation and regression of synapses during reinnervation of axolotl skeletal muscles. *J. Physiol. (Lond.),* 265, 261–295.

Bennett, M.R., McLachlan, E.M., and Taylor, R.S. (1973) The formation of synapses in mammalian striated muscle reinnervated with autonomic preganglionic nerves. *J. Physiol. (Lond).* 233, 501–517.

Berg, D.K. and Hall, Z.W. (1974) Fate of α-bungarotoxin bound to acetylcholine receptors of normal and denervated muscle. *Science,* 184, 473–475.

Berg, D.K. and Hall, Z.W. (1975) Loss of α-bungarotoxin from junctional and extrajunctional acetylcholine receptors in rat diaphragm in vivo and in organ culture. *J. Physiol. (Lond.),* 252, 771–789.

Betz, W. (1976) The formation of synapses between chick embryo skeletal muscle and ciliary ganglia grown in vitro. *J. Physiol. (Lond.),* 254, 63–73.

Betz, W. and Osborne, M. (1977) Effects of innervation on acetylcholine sensitivity of developing muscle in vitro. *J. Physiol. (Lond.),* 270, 75–88.

Bevan, S. and Steinbach, J.H. (1977) The distribution of α-bungarotoxin binding sites on mammalian skeletal muscle developing in vivo. *J. Physiol. (Lond.),* 267, 195–213.

Bretscher, M.S. and Raff, M.C. (1975) Mammalian plasma membranes. *Nature (Lond.),* 258, 43–49.

Brown, M.C., Jansen, J.K.S., and Van Essen, D. (1976) Polyneuronal innervation of skeletal muscle in newborn rats and its elimination during maturation. *J. Physiol. (Lond.),* 261, 387–422.

Burden, S. (1977a) Development of the neuromuscular junction in the chick embryo: the number, distribution, and stability of acetylcholine receptors. *Develop. Biol.,* 57, 317–329.

Burden, S. (1977b) Acetylcholine receptors at the neuromuscular junction: developmental change in receptor turnover. *Develop. Biol.,* 61, 79–85.

Chang, C.C., and Huang, M.C. (1975) Turnover of junctional and extrajunctional acetylcholine receptors of rat diaphragm. *Nature (Lond.),* 253, 643–644.

Chow, I. and Cohen, M.W. (1977) Distribution of acetylcholine receptors in developing myotomes of *Xenopus laevis*. *Proc. Canad. Fed. biol. Soc.,* 20, 44.

Cohen, M.W. (1972) The development of neuromuscular connexions in the presence of (+)-tubocurarine. *Brain Res.,* 41, 457–463.

Devreotes, P.N. and Fambrough, D.M. (1975) Acetylcholine receptor turnover in membranes of developing muscle fibers. *J. Cell. Biol.,* 65, 335–358.

Diamond, J. and Miledi, R. (1962) A study of foetal and newborn rat muscle fibres. *J. Physiol. (Lond.),* 162, 393–408.

Dreyer, F. and Peper, K. (1974) The acetylcholine sensitivity in the vicinity of the neuromuscular junction of the frog. *Pflügers Arch. ges. Physiol.,* 348, 273–286.

Edelman, G.M. (1976) Surface modulation in cell recognition and cell growth. *Science*, 192, 218—226.

Fambrough, D.M. (1974) Acetylcholine receptors: revised estimates of extrajunctional receptor density in denervated rat diaphragm. *J. gen. Physiol.* 64, 468—472.

Fambrough, D.M. and Hartzell, H.C. (1972) Acetylcholine receptors: number and distribution at neuromuscular junctions in rat diaphragm. *Science*, 176, 189—191.

Feltz, A. and Mallart, A. (1971) An analysis of acetylcholine responses of junctional and extrajunctional receptors of frog muscle fibres. *J. Physiol. (Lond.)*, 218, 85—100.

Fertuck, H.C. and Salpeter, M.M. (1974) Localization of acetylcholine receptor by ^{125}I-α-bungarotoxin binding at mouse motor endplates. *Proc. nat. Acad. Sci. (Wash.)*, 71, 1376—1378.

Fertuck, H.C. and Salpeter, M.M. (1976) Quantitation of junctional and extrajunctional acetylcholine receptors by electron microscope autoradiography after ^{125}I-α-bungarotoxin binding at mouse neuromuscular junctions. *J. Cell Biol.*, 69, 144—158.

Frank, E. and Fischbach, G.D. (1977) ACh receptors accumulate at newly formed nerve-muscle synapses in vitro. In *Cell and Tissue Interactions* (J.W. Lash and M.M. Burger, Eds.), Raven Press, New York, pp. 285—291.

Hamilton, L. (1969) The formation of somites in *Xenopus*. *J. Embryol. exp. Morphol.*, 22, 253—264.

Harrison, R.G. (1910) The outgrowth of the nerve fibre as a mode of protoplasmic movement. *J. exp. Zool.*, 9, 787—846.

Hartzell, H.C. and Fambrough, D.M. (1972) Acetylcholine receptors: distribution and extrajunctional density in rat diaphragm after denervation correlated with acetylcholine sensitivity. *J. gen. Physiol.*, 60, 248—262.

Hooisma, J., Slaff, D.W., Meeter, E., and Stevens, W.F. (1975) The innervation of chick striated muscle fibres by the chick ciliary ganglion in tissue culture. *Brain Res.*, 85, 79—85.

Kuffler, D., Thompson, W. and Jansen, J.K.S. (1977) The elimination of synapses in multiply-innervated skeletal muscle fibres of the rat: dependence on distance between end-plates. *Brain Res.*, 138, 353—358.

Kuffler, S.W. and Yoshikami, D. (1975) The distribution of acetylcholine sensitivity at the postsynaptic membrane of vertebrate skeletal twitch muscles: iontophoretic mapping in the micron range. *J. Physiol. (Lond.)*, 244, 703—730.

Kullberg, R.W., Lentz, T.L. and Cohen, M.W. (1977) Development of the myotomal neuromuscular junction in *Xenopus laevis*: an electrophysiological and fine-structural study. *Develop. Biol.*, 60, 101—129.

Landmesser, L. (1971) Contractile and electrical responses of vagus-innervated frog sartorius muscles. *J. Physiol. (Lond.)*, 213, 707—725.

Landmesser, L. (1972) Pharmacological properties, cholinesterase activity and anatomy of nerve muscle junctions in vagus-innervated frog sartorius. *J. Physiol (Lond.)*, 220, 243—256.

Lϕmo, T. and Slater, C.R. (1976) Induction of ACh sensitivity at new neuromuscular junctions. *J. Physiol. (Lond.)*, 258, 107P—108P.

Masurovsky, E.G. and Bunge, R.P. (1968) Fluoroplastic coverslips for long term nerve tissue culture. *Stain Technol.*, 43, 161—165.

Merlie, J.P., Changeux, J.P. and Gros, F. (1976) Acetylcholine receptor degradation measured by pulse chase labelling. *Nature (Lond.)*, 264, 74—76.

Miledi, R. (1960) Junctional and extrajunctional ACh receptors in skeletal muscle fibres. *J. Physiol. (Lond.)*, 151, 24—30.

Muntz, L. (1975) Myogenesis in the trunk and leg muscle during development of the tadpole of *Xenopus laevis*. *J. Embryol. exp. Morphol.*, 33, 757—774.

Nieuwkoop, P.D. and Faber, J. (1956) *Normal Table of Xenopus laevis (Daudin)*, 2nd edn., Amsterdam, Nort Holland.

Nurse, C.A. and O'Lague, P.H. (1975) Formation of cholinergic synapses between dissociated sympathetic neurons and skeletal myotubes of the rat in cell culture. *Proc. nat. Acad. Sci. (Wash.)*, 72, 1955—1959.

Obata, K. (1977) Development of neuromuscular transmission in culture with a variety of neurons and in the presence of cholinergic substances and tetrodoxin. *Brain Res.*, 119, 141—153.

Orkand, P.M., Orkand, R.K. and Cohen, M.W. (1978) Acetylcholine receptor distribution on *Xenopus* slow muscle fibres determined by α-bungarotoxin binding. *Neuroscience*, in press.

Redfern, P.A. (1970) Neuromuscular transmission in newborn rats. *J. Physiol. (Lond.)*, 209, 701–709.

Schmidt, H. and Stefani, E. (1976). Reinnervation of twitch and slow muscle fibres of the frog after crushing the motor nerves. *J. Physiol. (Lond.)*, 258, 99–123.

Schubert, D., Heinemann, S., Kidokoro, Y. (1977) Cholinergic metabolism and synapse formation by a rat nerve cell line. *Proc. nat. Acad. Sci. (Wash.)*, 74, 2579–2583.

Spitzer, N.C. (1976) Chemosensitivity of embryonic amphibian neurons in vivo and in vitro. *Proc. 6th Ann. Meet. Soc. Neurosci.*, 2, 204.

Yip, J.W. and Dennis, M.J. (1977) Suppression of transmission at foreign synapses in adult newt muscle involves reduction in quantal content. *Nature (Lond.)*, 260, 350–352.

Reprinted from J. Cell Biol., Vol. 78, pp. 176–198. 1978

REINNERVATION OF MUSCLE FIBER BASAL LAMINA AFTER REMOVAL OF MYOFIBERS

Differentiation of Regenerating Axons at Original Synaptic Sites

JOSHUA R. SANES, LAWRENCE M. MARSHALL, and U. J. McMAHAN

From the Department of Neurobiology, Harvard Medical School, Boston, Massachusetts 02115. Dr. Sanes' present address is the Department of Physiology, University of California, San Francisco, California 94143. Dr. McMahan's present address is the Department of Neurobiology, Stanford University Medical School, Stanford, California 94305.

ABSTRACT

Axons regenerate to reinnervate denervated skeletal muscle fibers precisely at original synaptic sites, and they differentiate into nerve terminals where they contact muscle fibers. The aim of this study was to determine the location of factors that influence the growth and differentiation of the regenerating axons. We damaged and denervated frog muscles, causing myofibers and nerve terminals to degenerate, and then irradiated the animals to prevent regeneration of myofibers. The sheath of basal lamina (BL) that surrounds each myofiber survives these treatments, and original synaptic sites on BL can be recognized by several histological criteria after nerve terminals and muscle cells have been completely removed. Axons regenerate into the region of damage within 2 wk. They contact surviving BL almost exclusively at original synaptic sites; thus, factors that guide the axon's growth are present at synaptic sites and stably maintained outside of the myofiber. Portions of axons that contact the BL acquire active zones and accumulations of synaptic vesicles; thus by morphological criteria they differentiate into nerve terminals even though their postsynaptic targets, the myofibers, are absent. Within the terminals, the synaptic organelles line up opposite periodic specializations in the myofiber's BL, demonstrating that components associated with the BL play a role in organizing the differentiation of the nerve terminal.

KEY WORDS   active zone · basement membrane · neuromuscular junction · synaptogenesis · x-irradiation

From the orderly and specific way in which synapses are formed, it is apparent that the components of the synapse exchange information as synaptogenesis proceeds. Skeletal muscle is a convenient tissue in which to study this interchange; the neuromuscular junction is a relatively simple and accessible synapse, and adult muscle can be reinnervated following damage to the motor nerve. The influence of nerve on muscle is well documented: many properties of the muscle fiber in general (21) and of the postsynaptic membrane in particular (18, 21, 45) are altered by denervation and restored to their original state when the muscle is reinnervated. The nerve terminal not only provides but also receives morphogenetically important information as the neuromuscular junction regenerates. Regenerating axons form contacts precisely at original synaptic sites, making few contacts elsewhere on the muscle fiber's surface (2, 15, 19, 27); the axons differentiate into nerve terminals only when they are within 0.1 μm from the muscle fiber;[1] and synaptic vesicles accumulate above the junctional folds that invaginate the postsynaptic membrane.[1]

The experiments reported here were undertaken as part of a study[1] (27, 31, 44) whose aim is to discover the structures that provide information to regenerating motor nerve terminals, and to determine the types of information that they provide. A sheath of basement membrane, composed of basal and reticular laminae, surrounds each muscle fiber, and the basal lamina (BL) extends through the synaptic cleft of the neuromuscular junction. When muscle fibers are damaged, they degenerate and are phagocytized, but their basement membrane sheaths survive; new myofibers then regenerate within the sheaths (9, 24, 50). We have devised a way to damage and denervate frog muscle in which the orientation of the sheaths is preserved; the sites where synapses had been situated can be identified after both myofiber and nerve terminal are removed (31). By X-irradiating the damaged muscle, we inhibited regeneration of myofibers (32, 42, 52) without blocking the regeneration of the damaged axons. We were therefore able to study the reinnervation of "muscle" in the absence of myofibers.

This paper describes several early steps in the reinnervation of the basement membrane sheaths In the absence of muscle cells, as in their presence, we found that: (a) axons can regenerate to the basement membrane sheaths of the muscle fibers; (b) regenerating axons contact the BL of the sheaths almost exclusively at original synaptic sites; and (c) regenerating axons differentiate into nerve terminals, by morphological criteria, when they reach the original synaptic sites. Further studies revealed that components contained in or connected to the muscle fiber's BL trigger at least some aspects of this differentiation.

---

[1] Rotshenker, S., and U. J. McMahan. Differentiation of regenerating axon terminals at original synaptic sites on frog muscle fibers. Manuscript in preparation.

MATERIALS AND METHODS

The Cutaneous Pectoris Muscles

Experiments were performed on the paired cutaneous pectoris muscles of 5-cm long male frogs (*Rana pipiens*). These thin, flat muscles lie directly beneath the skin of the thorax, and can be exposed for surgery or dissection by cutting and folding back a flap of skin. Each muscle is composed of ~500 muscle fibers and is innervated by a nerve that contains ~25 motor axons (44). The nerve enters the muscle from the lateral edge and courses across its center, in a direction perpendicular to the long axis of the muscle fibers (Fig. 1). Blood vessels enter and run with the nerve. The nerve branches intramuscularly to provide each muscle fiber with a single neuromuscular junction. Most of the neuromuscular junctions are found along nerve branches in the central portion of the muscle, in a 2–3-mm wide band (27).

Damaging and Denervating Muscle

To induce degeneration and phagocytosis of myofibers, a rectangular slab was cut from the muscle on each side of the main nerve trunk, leaving behind a row of damaged muscle fiber segments, a "bridge" (31), extending between groups of undamaged fibers at the medial and lateral edges of the muscle (Fig. 1, right side). Each bridge was 1–1½ mm wide, 3–4 mm long, and contained 250–400 muscle fiber segments. Generally, each bridge bore 50–150 synaptic sites. The numbers of nerve branches and synaptic sites that were

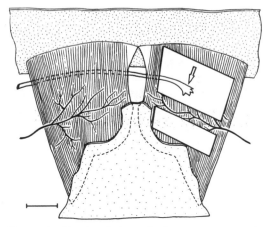

FIGURE 1 Sketch of the paired cutaneous pectoris muscles with attached origin and insertion. The muscle on the left is intact. The nerve enters from the lateral edge. Two rectangular areas have been cut from the muscle on the right, leaving behind a row of muscle fiber segments, a "bridge", between undamaged medial and lateral fibers. In some experiments, a "foreign" nerve (arrow), which normally supplies the forelimb, was implanted near the bridge. Bar, ~3 mm.

preserved could be increased by making the bridge wider, but degeneration of damaged muscle was incomplete if the bridge was much more than 1½ mm wide.

Usually, muscles were denervated by crushing their nerve with fine forceps 1–2 mm from the muscle's lateral edge; reinnervation is prompt following a nerve crush (27). In some experiments, the nerve was cut at the lateral edge of the muscle and a 2-cm long stretch proximal to the cut was evulsed to prevent reinnervation by "native" axons. In these animals, we implanted a "foreign" nerve near the bridge (Fig. 1), and "foreign" axons reinnervated the damaged muscle. The large nerve that supplies the forelimb was cut near the elbow. The central stump was dissected free from its musculature and run under the ipsilateral cutaneous pectoris muscle. The cut end was then laid near the medial edge of the contralateral bridge, where it was held in place with a blood clot.

For all operations, frogs were anesthetized by immersion in 0.1% MS-222 (tricaine methane sulfonate, Ayerst Laboratories, New York) in water. Incisions were closed with 7-0 sutures. Animals were kept at 18°C and were force-fed beef liver twice each week.

X-Irradiation

Frogs were X-irradiated to prevent their damaged muscles from regenerating. Anesthetized frogs were placed ventral side up beneath the source of a Westinghouse Coronado Radiotherapy unit (Westinghouse Electric Corp., Pittsburgh, Pa.). Lead shielding restricted the radiation to a 15-mm wide band (rostral-caudal) centered on the cutaneous pectoris muscles. Radiation was delivered at a rate of 100 rad/min (15 mA, 250 kV, 2 mm Al added filtration, 65 cm from source to center of animal). In a preliminary experiment, we varied the dose of X-rays and the time between muscle damage and irradiation. Doses of 1,600 or 2,000 rads inhibited the regeneration of myofibers almost completely, whereas a 1,200-rad dose was slightly and a 800-rad dose was markedly less effective (Fig. 2a). 1,600- or 2,000-rad doses were equally effective when delivered any time between several hours and 4 days after the muscle was damaged. If, however, irradiation was delayed until 5 days after surgery, some myofibers regenerated during the subsequent few weeks (Fig. 2b). On the basis of these results, we submitted frogs to a 1,600-rad dose, 3 days after surgery in subsequent experiments.

Microscopy

For light and electron microscopy, muscles were fixed in glutaraldehyde (0.8% in 0.06 M phosphate buffer, pH 7.2) for 30–45 min, rinsed in buffer (0.13 M sodium cacodylate, pH 7.2), refixed in osmium tetroxide (1% in 0.11 M cacodylate buffer, pH 7.2), dehydrated in ethanol, rinsed in propylene oxide, and embedded whole in thin (1 mm or less) wafers of Epon. To stain BL for electron microscopy, ruthenium red (Sigma Chemical

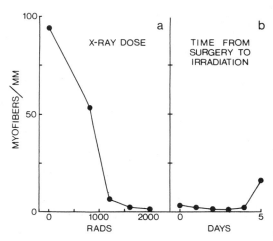

FIGURE 2 X-irradiation inhibits regeneration of myofibers in damaged muscle. Muscles were fixed 16 days after they were damaged and denervated and the number of myofibers per millimeter of bridge length was determined light-microscopically in cross sections. (a) Frogs were irradiated at the indicated dose, 2 or 3 days after surgery. (b) Frogs received a single dose of 1,600 or 2,000 rads at the indicated times after surgery. Each point is the average of counts from two to five bridges. Normal muscles had 80–100 myofibers/mm.

Co., St. Louis, Mo.) was added to the osmium tetroxide fixative, at a final concentration of 0.5 mg/ml (28, 31). To demonstrate cholinesterase (ChE) at neuromuscular junctions, Karnovsky's histochemical stain was applied to the muscle after glutaraldehyde and before osmium fixation (25, 27). In a few experiments, glutaraldehyde fixation was omitted and muscles were treated with a zinc iodide and osmium mixture (27, 30) to impregnate motor nerve terminals.

The Surface of the Muscle
Fiber: Terminology

Electron microscopy of skeletal muscle (49) has revealed that the surface complex of each muscle fiber, the sarcolemma (7), comprises several concentric layers (Figs. 3, 4a, and 5a). The innermost layer, a typical lipid-rich, osmophilic plasma membrane, is coated by a thin, carbohydrate-rich glycocalyx, which can be rendered electron dense by any of a number of stains (40), including the ruthenium red-osmium mixture (28) used in this study. Separated from the glycocalyx by a narrow, electron-lucent gap is the BL, which also stains intensely with ruthenium red. This feltlike layer is 10–15 nm thick and, like the BLs of other tissues (47), it is probably collagenous (12). A reticular lamina of indeterminate width lies just beyond the BL. The reticular lamina contains collagen fibrils embedded in an amorphous matrix; the fibrils but not the matrix are visible in our

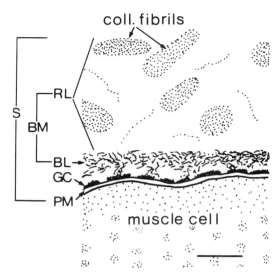

coll. fibrils

muscle cell

FIGURE 3 The surface or sarcolemma (*S*) of a muscle fiber; drawing from an electron micrograph. Cytoplasm of the muscle cell is surrounded by layers of plasma membrane (*PM*), glycocalyx (*GC*), basal lamina (*BL*), and reticular lamina (*RL*) containing collagen fibrils. The BL and RL together compose basement membrane (*BM*). Bar, ~0.1 μm.

electron micrographs. The BL and reticular lamina together are called the basement membrane. In some cases—but not here—the term basement membrane is used to refer to the BL alone, and the term sarcolemma is applied to the plasma membrane alone.

RESULTS

Degeneration of Damaged Muscle and Nerve

MUSCLE: When muscle fibers are damaged as described in Materials and Methods, the myofibers retract and degenerate, but the sheaths of basement membrane that surrounded them are left behind (Fig. 4b). Macrophages invade the sheaths and remove remnants of the disrupted myofibers, including fragments of plasma membrane that adhere to the inner surface of the BL (Fig. 5b). The bulk of the sheath is emptied during the first few days after the muscle is damaged.

If the cut muscle is not damaged further, myofibers regenerate within the surviving basement membrane sheaths (Fig. 4c), laying down a new layer of BL in areas where they do not completely fill the old sheaths (Fig. 5c). By 2 wk after

surgery, nearly all of the sheaths contain regenerating myofibers, and the bridge contracts upon direct electrical stimulation. If, however, the muscle is X-irradiated within a few days of surgery, regeneration is markedly inhibited (Fig. 2). The basement membrane sheaths of the original muscle fibers persist in the irradiated bridge (Figs. 4d and 5d) for at least 5 wk, but myofibers regenerate within only a few of them.

Degeneration and phagocytosis of the damaged muscle continues after X-irradiation, and the sheaths of BL gradually empty (Fig. 4d). 7 days after surgery, <2% of the BL's inner surface is apposed by debris or fragments of plasma membrane (Fig. 6). However, the sheaths never empty completely: mononucleated cells, including macrophages and presumptive myoblasts (9, 24, 39, 46) remain inside the sheaths, and send out long, thin processes that can extend for hundreds of micrometers. These processes, broken during fixation or unidentifiable because of their small size, may account for the small number of plasma membrane fragments that adhere to the BL for several weeks after the bulk of the debris has been removed (Fig. 6).

NERVE: The muscle fiber's BL, but not its reticular lamina, extends through the synaptic cleft at the neuromuscular junction (Fig. 7a). The nerve terminal is capped by processes of a Schwann cell, and the Schwann cell's basement membrane (BL and reticular lamina) fuses with that of the muscle at the edges of the termina. Within the cleft, projections of BL line the junctional folds that invaginate the muscle cell's surface (Fig. 7a). ChE is contained in or connected to the BL of the neuromuscular junction (33); accordingly, in muscles treated with a histochemical stain for ChE, reaction product fills the synaptic cleft (Fig. 7b).

Nerve terminals survive for at least a week in muscles that have been damaged and irradiated but not denervated (Fig. 7c). If, however, the nerve is crushed at the same time that the muscle is cut, nerve terminals degenerate and are phagocytized by Schwann cells, as occurs in denervated but undamaged muscle (6, 35). After a nerve crush near the muscle's edge, virtually all of the terminals are phagocytized within 4 days, and the Schwann cells come to lie directly on the BL of the synaptic cleft (Fig. 7d and e). During the subsequent weeks, Schwann cell processes retract from many of the denervated synaptic sites, as they do in undamaged muscle (27, 35, 45), leav-

SANES, MARSHALL, AND McMAHAN   *Reinnervation of Muscle Fiber Basal Lamina*   **179**

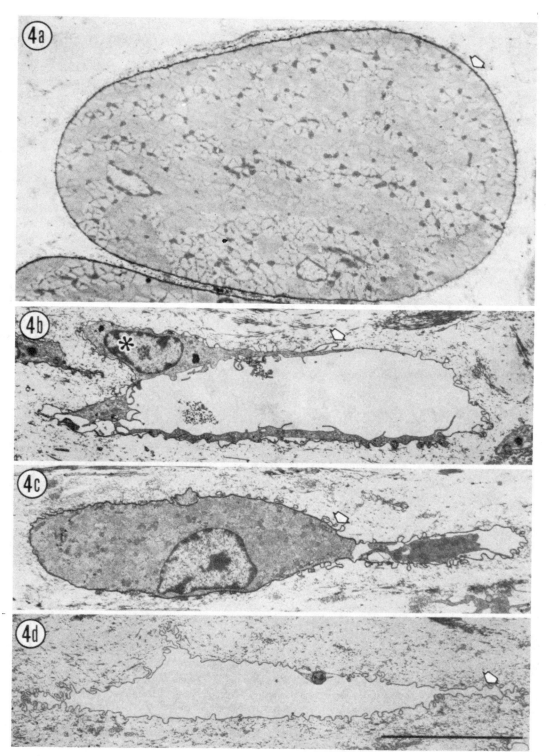

FIGURE 4 Damaged muscle degenerates and then regenerates; x-irradiation prevents its regeneration. Cross sections of muscle fibers and/or their BL sheaths. (*a*) Normal muscle fiber, ensheathed in darkly stained BL. (*b*) 4 days after muscle damage, much of the myofiber has been removed, but its BL survives. A macrophage (*) lies in the lumen of the BL. (*c*) 2 wk after muscle damage, a myofiber has regenerated within the sheath. (*d*) 4 wk after muscle damage and irradiation, the BL sheath remains nearly empty. Arrows indicate regions shown at higher magnification in Fig. 5. Bar, 10 μm.

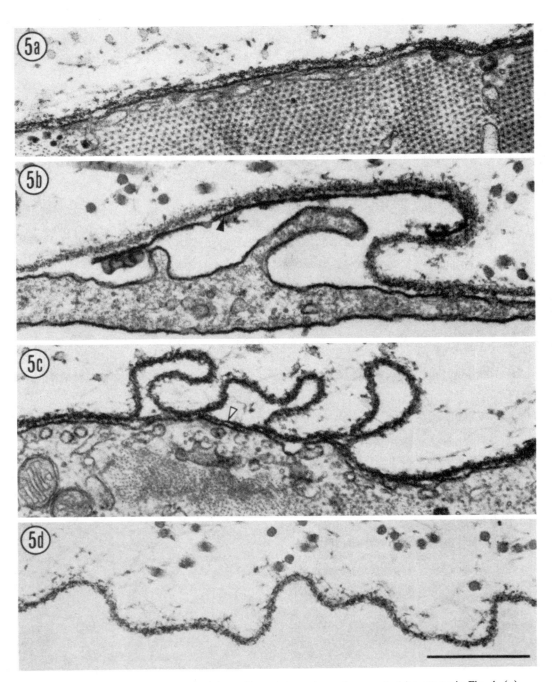

FIGURE 5 BL survives after damaged myofibers degenerate; regions marked by arrows in Fig. 4. (*a*) Undamaged muscle. (*b*) 4 days after muscle damage: a fine process of a macrophage sweeps the inside surface of the BL near a fragment of plasma membrane (arrowhead). (*c*) 2 wk after muscle damage; regenerating myofiber bears new BL (open arrowhead) where it does not fill the surviving BL of the original muscle fiber. (*d*) 4 wk after muscle damage and irradiation; an area of BL free of plasma membrane fragments and debris. Bar, 0.5 μm.

SANES, MARSHALL, AND MCMAHAN   *Reinnervation of Muscle Fiber Basal Lamina*   **181**

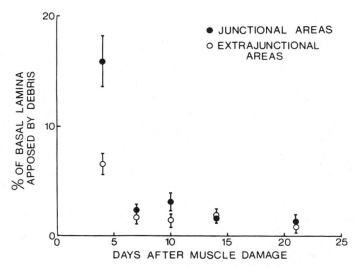

FIGURE 6 Fraction of the inner surface of the myofiber's BL opposed by plasma membrane fragments and amorphous cellular debris, at various times after muscle damage (on day 0) and X-irradiation (on day 3). Electron micrographs of junctional (●) and extrajunctional (○) regions were inspected at × 150,000. Each point shows the mean (±1 SE) of at least 20 samples from two bridges. The average length of BL contained in each sample was 2.7 μm.

ing their BL atop that of the muscle fiber (Fig. 7 f).

Even after the nerve terminal and myofiber have degenerated, several components of the neuromuscular junction persist. As noted above, processes of the Schwann cells directly oppose the BL of the denervated synaptic cleft (Fig. 7 e), and the Schwann cells' BL remains behind even when the processes themselves retract (Fig. 7 f). The projections of BL that extend from the cleft into the junctional folds also survive (Fig. 7 c, e, and f). Finally, histochemically demonstrable ChE remains in the synaptic BL of the bridge for many weeks (Fig. 7 d) (33). These features allow one to recognize synaptic sites on the basement membrane sheaths long after cellular components of the synapse have been removed.

During the first few days after the muscle is denervated and damaged, more debris adheres to the BL of the synaptic cleft than to extrajunctional BL (Fig. 6). The BL of the junctional folds, which could trap membrane fragments or exclude macrophages, might account for this difference. Alternatively, the bonds between BL and plasma membrane may be stronger at the synapse than elsewhere on the muscle fiber. By 1 wk after surgery, however, both junctional and extrajunctional regions of the BL are almost completely clean (Fig.

6). When regenerating axons enter the bridge, as described in the next section, they encounter BL and Schwann cells but few if any remnants of their normal synaptic targets, the myofibers.

Regeneration of Damaged Axons

To determine whether axons regenerate across the bridge, we stimulated the nerve trunk near the lateral edge of the muscle, and looked for contractions in undamaged fibers medial to the bridge (Fig. 1). Stimulation evoked twitches in the medial fibers in 7 of 10 bridges examined 2 wk after nerve crush and muscle damage, and in all of 22 bridges examined a week later (Fig. 8). Thus, the axons were able to grow completely across the region of damage, and to form functional neuromuscular junctions.

The course that the regenerating axons took was studied in preparations stained with zinc iodide and osmium, which impregnates motor nerve terminals and regenerating preterminal axons that have not yet become myelinated (27, 30). Axons generally entered and ran through the bridge in the surviving perineurial tubes of the original axons; the growth of regenerating axons through surviving perineurium is a consistent feature of reinnervation in undamaged muscle following simple nerve crush (19, 27, 48). Within the

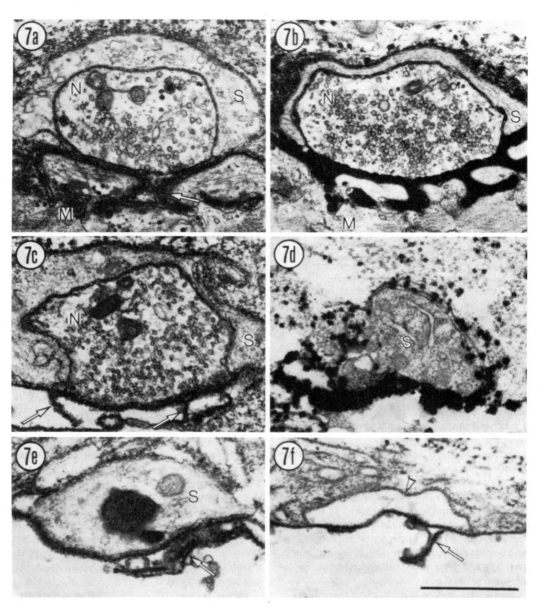

FIGURE 7   Synaptic sites can be recognized in four ways after nerve terminals (N) and myofibers (M) are removed: (i) Projections of BL (arrows) extend into the junctional folds of normal muscle (a) and survive in damaged (c) and damaged, denervated (e, f) muscle after myofibers have been removed. (ii) The electron-dense reaction product that fills the synaptic cleft in normal muscles stained for ChE (b) also stains the BL of the cleft after the muscle is damaged and denervated (d). (iii) Schwann cell processes (S) that cap normal nerve terminals (a, b) phagocytize the terminals after nerve damage and come to lie on cleft BL (d, e). (iv) The BL that surrounds Schwann cell processes (a–e) persists when these processes retract from the synaptic site (arrowhead in Fig. 7f). Specimens were prepared 4 (c, e) or 7 days (d, f) after muscle damage. Bar, 1.0 μm.

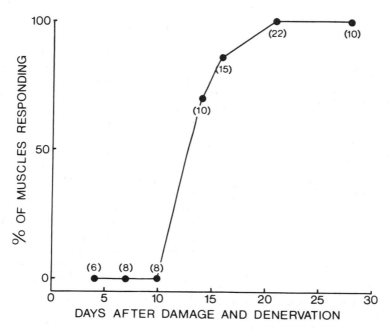

FIGURE 8 Axons regenerate across the bridge after the nerve is crushed. At indicated times after muscle was damaged and denervated (on day 0) and X-irradiated (on day 3), bridges were tested in vitro. The nerve was stimulated electrically near the lateral edge of the muscle and contractions in damaged fibers of the medial edge, across the bridge, were observed through a dissecting microscope (see Fig. 1). Number of bridges tested at each time is shown in parentheses.

bridge, axonal branches left the perineurial tubes to run along the basement membrane sheaths (Fig. 9 b), a pattern similar to that seen at normal (Fig. 9 a) and regenerating (27) neuromuscular junctions. Like axons reinnervating undamaged muscle (27) (although unlike normal terminals), axons often left the sheaths and ran for some distance at an angle to the sheath's long axis (Fig. 9 b) before ending on another sheath or in the connective tissue of the bridge. Thus, in some respects, the bridge was reinnervated in a manner similar to that observed in undamaged muscle.

Nerve terminals in the bridge—i.e., axonal processes closely associated with myofiber BL—were characterized by electron microscopy. Like normal or regenerating nerve terminals in undamaged muscle, terminals in the bridge bear 50-nm diameter agranular synaptic vesicles in a cytoplasmic matrix of relatively low electron density and are coated by a thin glycocalyx that stains intensely with ruthenium red (Figs. 7 a and b, and 10). The terminals varied from ~0.2–1.5 μm in diameter. Some were wrapped in Schwann cell processes which, in turn, lay on the myofiber BL (Fig. 10 a

and b). Others were capped by Schwann cell processes but had a portion of their surface directly apposed to BL (Fig. 10 c). In some cases, two or three terminals lay side-by-side, wrapped or capped by the same Schwann cell process. Finally, terminals frequently lay in the lumen of the BL sheaths (Fig. 10 d). The wide variation in the size of terminals and in the relationships between terminals and Schwann cells seen in the bridge is also characteristic of early stages of reinnervation in undamaged muscle[1] (17, 27, 29, 45). However, the occurrence of terminals within the sheaths is, to our knowledge, unique to the bridge.

Whatever their size or configuration, terminals in the bridge could be distinguished from Schwann cell processes and other cellular elements because they had (a) more 50-nm vesicles, (b) a less electron-dense cytoplasm, (c) a more prominent glycocalyx, and (d) no rough endoplasmic reticulum (Figs. 7 and 10). Our ability to recognize the nerve terminals easily in the electron microscope facilitated quantitative studies of their growth, distribution, and differentiation.

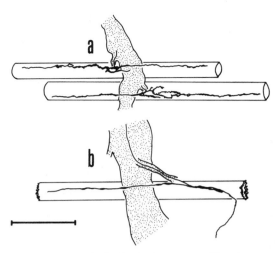

FIGURE 9 Terminal arborizations on myofibers in normal muscle (*a*) and on a basement membrane sheath in a bridge, 4 wk after denervation, muscle damage and X-irradiation (*b*). Camera lucida drawings from whole mounts of zinc iodide/osmium-stained preparations; placement and dimensions of BL in Fig. 9*b* were confirmed by electron microscopy. Axons exit from perineurium (stippled) and run along myofiber (*a*) or its surviving BL (*b*). Like terminals in reinnervated undamaged muscle (21), terminals in the bridge leave BL and continue to grow, while normal terminals end abruptly on the myofiber's surface. Bar, 100 μm.

Precise Reinnervation of Original Synaptic Sites

In vertebrate skeletal muscles (2, 15), including the cutaneous pectoris muscle of the frog (27), reinnervation after a nerve crush is topographically precise: the damaged axons grow back into the muscle and cover a large fraction of the original postsynaptic membrane, while making few contacts elsewhere on the muscle fiber's surface. We have previously shown that this topographic specificity does not require the integrity of the original myofiber for its expression: in unirradiated bridges, regenerating axons contact regenerating myofibers almost exclusively at original synaptic sites on the BL (31). Because irradiation inhibits regeneration of myofibers in the bridge without blocking regeneration of axons, we were able to extend these results.

Our principal finding is that in the absence of muscle, as in its presence, regenerating axons contact the BL almost exclusively at original synaptic sites. This precision is apparent whether one uses the BL of junctional folds (Fig. 10*a* and *c*) or the

ChE of the synaptic BL (Fig. 11) as markers of original sites (31). To quantify the precision of reinnervation, we used ChE-stained preparations. Regions rich in ChE-stained synaptic sites were identified in whole mounts, the appropriate blocks of plastic were cut out, and basement membrane sheaths were cross-sectioned for electron microscopy. In a single section from each block, we counted all of the ChE-stained patches of BL — i.e., original synaptic sites — and noted which were apposed by nerve terminals (or by the Schwann cell processes that enwrapped terminals). We then followed the perimeter of each sheath, searching for terminals that lay (or whose Schwann cell wrapping lay) within 0.1 μm of the BL. We also searched many profiles that did not have ChE-stained patches but were in the vicinity of regenerating axons. Terminals that lay within the lumen of a BL sheath were excluded from this survey because their relationship to the BL was so clearly aberrant.

Fig. 12 shows the extent to which original synaptic sites were reinnervated after a nerve crush. In normal muscles — i.e., muscles that were neither damaged nor irradiated — nearly all of the original postsynaptic membrane was covered by regenerated nerve terminals within a month after the nerve was crushed. In the absence of myofibers — i.e., in muscles that were damaged and irradiated — reinnervation was slower and less complete. Nevertheless, by 3 wk after the nerve was crushed, ~40% of the ChE-stained patches were apposed by nerve terminals (120 of 298 in seven bridges). Thus, a large fraction of the original synaptic sites were reinnervated in the absence of the myofiber. The subsequent decline (3–5 wk after surgery) will be discussed below.

In control experiments, we studied reinnervation of muscles that were either damaged or irradiated (Fig. 12). Myofibers regenerated within 2 wk in unirradiated bridges (Figs. 2 and 4*c*). Reinnervation began at the same rate in these bridges as in undamaged muscle, but did not proceed to completion. Some sites remained uncovered, perhaps because access to them was blocked by connective tissue that built up after surgery; a similar explanation has been advanced to account for the incomplete reinnervation of atrophied mammalian muscle (19). In uninjured, irradiated muscles, myofibers survived without apparent lesion for at least 5 wk (see also reference 38), but reinnervation was delayed by about a week. Among the factors that might account

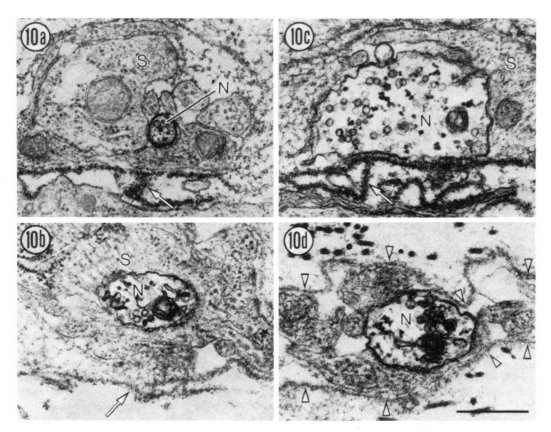

FIGURE 10 Nerve terminals (N) that reinnervate basement membrane sheaths after removal of the myofiber vary in size and in their relationship to the surviving BL. Terminals in Fig. 10a and b are wrapped in Schwann cell processes (S), whereas that in Fig. 10c directly opposes the myofiber's BL. Terminal in Fig. 10d lies within the lumen of the BL sheath (outlined by arrowheads). Terminals in Fig. 10a–c are at original synaptic sites, as shown by BL of junctional folds (arrows). From irradiated bridges fixed 21 days after denervation and muscle damage. Bar, 0.5 μm.

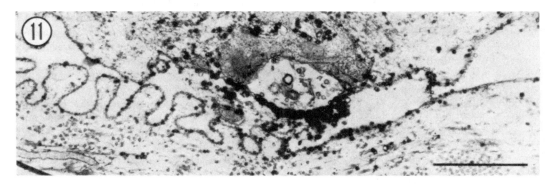

FIGURE 11 Regenerated nerve terminal in an irradiated bridge, 21 days after denervation and muscle damage. Axon has returned to contact BL of original synaptic cleft, marked here by the histochemically demonstratable ChE that it contains. Bar, 1 μm.

for this delay are poor health of irradiated animals, radiation-induced injury of the motoneurons (14), and inhibition of Schwann cell proliferation (10) that helps to repair perineurial pathways after damage to the nerve (20, 53). Thus, the rate and extent to which sheaths are reinnervated in the absence of myofibers can be largely explained by the separate effects of the two procedures that we use to empty the sheaths: cutting the muscle leads to incomplete reinnervation and irradiation induces a delay.

Fig. 13 shows that nearly all of the terminals that contacted the BL did so at original synaptic sites. This precision was observed in normal muscle, in irradiated but undamaged muscle, in unirradiated bridges where new myofibers regenerated within the sheaths, and in irradiated bridges where only a few percent of the sheaths contained myofibers. Most of the terminals that were not at original sites were probably approaching or leaving them — they were generally near ChE-stained patches, and collagen fibrils lay between the terminal (or its Schwann cell sheath) and the BL.

These results suggest that growing axons can reject nonsynaptic BL, a hypothesis that we tested in the following way: a "foreign" nerve was implanted onto the bridge far from the entry of the "native" nerve (Fig. 1) so that regenerating axons would have to grow past long stretches of extrasynaptic BL if they were to reach synaptic sites. 3–4 wk later, the bridges were fixed, stained for ChE to mark original synaptic sites, and cross-sectioned. Electron microscopy revealed that many axonal processes ran through the bridge and some of them approached the basement membrane sheaths. In each of five bridges studied, nearly all of the terminals that were within 0.1 μm of the BL (but were not in the lumen of the sheaths) were situated at ChE-stained sites (Table I). Thus axons contact synaptic BL and reject nonsynaptic Bl when they return to the basement membrane sheaths.

Because the BL is quite clean by the time reinnervation occurs (compare Figs. 6 and 12), it is unlikely that degenerating cellular or membranous remnants of the myofibers account for the precise reinnervation of original synaptic sites. This conclusion gains support from experiments in which we denervated and damaged muscles, delayed reinnervation for up to 2 wk by recrushing the nerve at 4–7-day intervals, and then allowed reinnervation to proceed for 2 or 3 wk. Regener-

ating axons covered as much original synaptic BL (Fig. 14a) and made as few contacts elsewhere on the sheaths (Fig. 14b) when reinnervation was delayed as they did when reinnervation was prompt. The cues used by regenerating axons to find or select original sites must therefore be stable for several weeks after the myofiber is removed.

Differentiation of Regenerating Axons into Nerve Terminals

In normal muscle, the portion of the motor axon that contacts the muscle fiber — i.e., the motor nerve terminal — differs from other portions of the axon in many respects. For example, terminals bear active zones (complexes of membrane-associated organelles, thought to be sites of transmitter release; references 11, 22, 37) and numerous synaptic vesicles, whereas preterminal regions of the axon contain no active zones and relatively few vesicles. When undamaged muscle is reinnervated, axons differentiate into terminals where they approach within 0.1 μm of the muscle fiber's surface[1] (29, 45). Electron microscopic analysis showed that terminals in the bridge (axonal processes associated with myofiber BL) also differentiate, becoming morphologically distinguishable from their parent axons.

In the bridge, the density of synaptic vesicles is much higher in terminals than in preterminal axons (Fig. 15). The accumulation of vesicles in terminals is evident (a) when terminals are compared with a random sample of axonal profiles (Table II A), or (b) when they are compared with any of three morphologically distinguishable classes of axons (myelinating axons within perineurial tubes, unmyelinated axons within perineurial tubes, and unmyelinated axons running through the connective tissues of the bridge outside of perineurial tubes; Table II B). Also, terminals contain fewer neurofilaments and microtubules than do preterminal axons (Fig. 15).

Another sign of the differentiation of nerve terminals in the bridge is that terminal but not preterminal regions of the axons contain active zones. The active zones are characterized by a cytoplasmic density adherent to the inner leaflet of the plasma membrane, and a focal accumulation of synaptic vesicles (Fig. 16b). The densities are elongated and the vesicles that flank them are arranged in rows (Fig. 16c). These features are

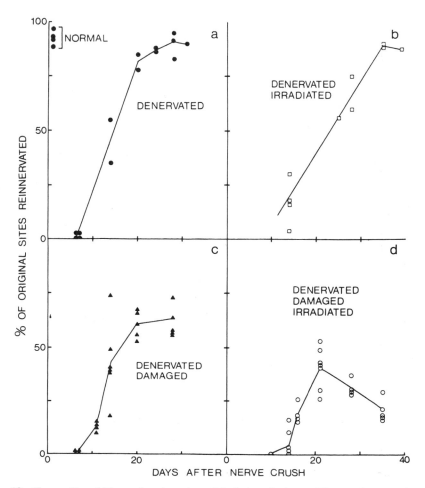

FIGURE 12 Figures 12 and 13 together show that original synaptic sites on BL are reinnervated precisely whether or not myofibers are present. Fig. 12 shows the extent to which original sites, marked by ChE stain, are reinnervated at various times after nerve crush. Each point in Fig. 12a–d represents the percentage of ChE-stained patches apposed by nerve terminals in one muscle or bridge; at least 30 patches were counted in a cross section from each preparation. Lines, drawn through mean of all muscles at each time point in Fig. 12a–d, are redrawn in Fig. 12e for comparison. Four normal muscles were sectioned as controls; >90% of their ChE-stained patches were clearly innervated (a). All other muscles were denervated on day 0. Muscles in Fig. 12c and d were damaged to make bridges at the time of denervation. Muscles in Fig. 12b and d were X-irradiated on day 3.

similar to those revealed when terminals in normal frog muscle are sectioned (Fig. 16a) (11, 22, 37).

A prominent characteristic of normal (5, 34) and regenerated[1] (45) nerve terminals in undamaged muscle is that organelles are asymmetrically distributed within them: synaptic vesicles are concentrated on the side of the terminal that faces the muscle fibers, mitochondria are concentrated on the opposite side, nearer the Schwann cell cap, and active zones are found only on the presynaptic membrane, directly opposite the muscle fiber's surface. Organelles are also asymmetrically distributed within nerve terminals in the bridge. Portions of terminal profiles enwrapped in Schwann cell processes contained no active zones and had fewer vesicles than portions that contacted the myofiber BL (Fig. 10a–c, Table IIC). In terminals that directly apposed the BL of the synaptic cleft, nearly two-thirds of the synaptic vesicles (65 ± 2%, mean ± SE in 52 terminals)

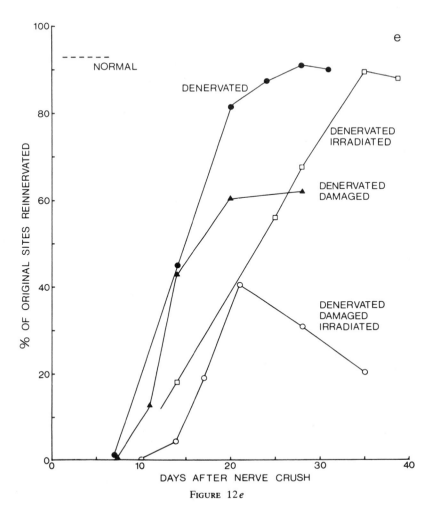

FIGURE 12e

lay in the half of the terminal that faced the cleft (Table II*D*). Mitochondria accumulated in the other side of these terminals—61% (36 of 61 in 52 terminals) lay in the half of the terminal that faced the Schwann cell cap. Furthermore, active zones occurred only on the portion of the nerve terminal's surface that abutted the BL of the myofiber sheath.

Thus, the nerve terminals acquire a normal complement of synaptic organelles and become morphologically polarized in a normal way even when there is no myofiber lying beneath the "presynaptic" membrane. The association of synaptic vesicles and active zones with the BL of the synaptic cleft suggests that components in the BL might play a role in triggering the transformation of the regenerating axon into a nerve terminal.

The next section describes a test of this proposition.

Differentiation of Nerve Terminals is Organized by Basal Lamina

Synaptic vesicles and active zones are not evenly distributed along the length of normal frog motor nerve terminals. Instead, they are associated with junctional folds: there are more vesicles above folds than in between them (5, 34), and the cytoplasmic densities of the active zones lay precisely opposite the mouths of the folds (5, 11). The folds persist in denervated but undamaged muscle for many months (6, 27, 45). When original synaptic sites are reinnervated, vesicles and active zones are once again found associated with

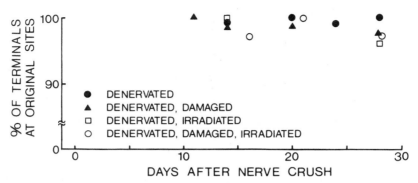

FIGURE 13   Nearly all of the terminals within 0.1 μm of myofiber BL are situated precisely at a ChE-stained patch. Each point represents the summed data from two to five of the preparations presented in Fig. 12; at least 20 cross-sectioned BL sheaths, each bearing one or more ChE-stained patches, were examined in each preparation. In most preparations, nearby sheaths without ChE-stained patches were also surveyed. Symbols as in Fig. 12.

TABLE I

Precise Reinnervation of Original Synaptic Sites in the Bridge by Axons Regenerating from a "Foreign" Nerve

		Axonal processes	
Bridge	Total	Within 0.1 μm of myofiber BL	At original synaptic sites on myofiber BL
1	226	11	11
2	79	12	10
3	136	10	9
4	129	12	10
5	118	8	7
Total	688	53	49

Axonal processes were counted in a single cross section from each of five irradiated bridges fixed 3–4 wk after surgery. 92% (49/53) of the processes that were within 0.1 μm of surviving BL sheaths were situated at the ChE-stained original synaptic sites.

the original synaptic folds.[1] Thus, there must be factors near the folds that organize the differentiation of nerve terminals.

When muscles are cut to make a bridge, the plasma membrane and cytoplasm of the folds are lost. However, as shown above, the projections of BL that extend into the folds survive after the myofibers degenerate (Fig. 7c, e, and f), marking the sites where folds had been; regenerating axons form new terminals directly opposite these sites (Figs. 10 and 15). If factors that organize the differentiation of nerve terminals were located in the BL, one might expect that vesicles and active zones would be preferentially localized above

intersections of cleft and fold BL.

To seek such relationships, we studied cross sections of five bridges that were fixed 3 wk after they were denervated, damaged, and X-irradiated. We collected micrographs that showed nerve terminals directly apposed to the BL of the muscle fiber's sheath and projections of BL whose connection to the sheath lay beneath the terminal. Micrographs that met these criteria (e.g., Figs. 10c and 15b) were analyzed as shown in Fig. 17a. To calculate the density of synaptic vesicles near to and far from intersections of fold and cleft BL, the distance along which the nerve terminal's plasma membrane contacted the myofiber's BL was measured, and all synaptic vesicles situated (entirely or in part) within 100 nm of this membrane were counted. Vesicles within 200 × 100-nm rectangles centered on the intersections (Fig. 17a) were considered to be near intersections whereas those elsewhere in the juxtamembranous strip were classified as far from intersections. To quantify the association of active zones to fold sites, we measured the distance from the midpoint of each active zone's cytoplasmic density to the nearest intersection of fold and cleft BL.

Synaptic vesicles accumulated above the intersections of fold and cleft BL: the density of vesicles was over twice as high within 100 nm of the intersections as elsewhere along the region of contact between nerve and BL (Fig. 17b). Comparison of regions within single cross sections showed that the ratio of vesicle densities near to and far from intersections varied from terminal to terminal (Fig. 17c). However, the mean ratio, 2.9 ± 0.4 to 1 (mean ± SE, n = 84), was signifi-

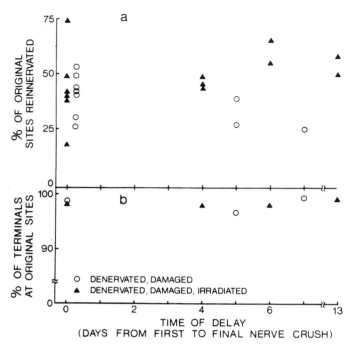

FIGURE 14 Original synaptic sites in the bridge are reinnervated precisely whether or not reinnervation is delayed by repeated nerve crush. Nerve was recrushed at 4–7 day intervals. Bridges were examined 14 (unirradiated bridges, ▲) or 21 days (irradiated bridges, ○) after the final nerve crush. Data was gathered by methods detailed in legends to Figs. 12 and 13.

cantly ($P < 10^{-5}$; Student's t test) greater than the ratio of 1 that would be expected if vesicles were not specifically associated with intersections. The high median ratio (=2; Fig. 17c) provides assurance that the associations we saw did not result from the disproportionate contribution of a small population of terminals with particularly high ratios. Furthermore, even in sections that did not display active zones (see below), the mean ratio was 2.2, significantly >1.

We found a total of 32 active zones in our set of micrographs. The region of contact between BL and terminals with active zones averaged 1.2 μm in length. Intersections of fold and cleft BLs were broadly distributed along this region of contact. If active zones were randomly distributed over this distance, one would expect (from probability theory) a mean distance of nearly 0.4 μm between the center of an active zone's cytoplasmic density and the nearest intersection. Instead, the mean separation was only 81 nm, and 88% (28/32) of the cytoplasmic densities were within 100 nm of an intersection (Fig. 16d). If anything, our measurements overestimate the distance from active

zones to intersections, since some projections of BL may have been damaged or unidentifiable. Furthermore, active zones may have been closer to intersections in adjacent, unexamined sections than to the intersections that we saw.

Thus, the clustering of synaptic organelles that occurs above the mouths of junctional folds when undamaged muscle is reinnervated[1] occurs above intersections of fold and cleft BL when axons reinnervate the bridge. It is therefore difficult to escape the conclusion that components contained in or tightly connected to the BL of the synaptic cleft play a role in organizing the differentiation of the regenerating axon into a nerve terminal.

Fate of Regenerated Nerve Terminals

The experiments described so far demonstrate that axons regenerate to basement membrane sheaths in the bridge and that, once there, they differentiate into nerve terminals. We have not studied bridges after long periods of reinnervation, and we therefore do not know the eventual fate of the nerve terminals. However, the amount of original synaptic surface that regenerating ter-

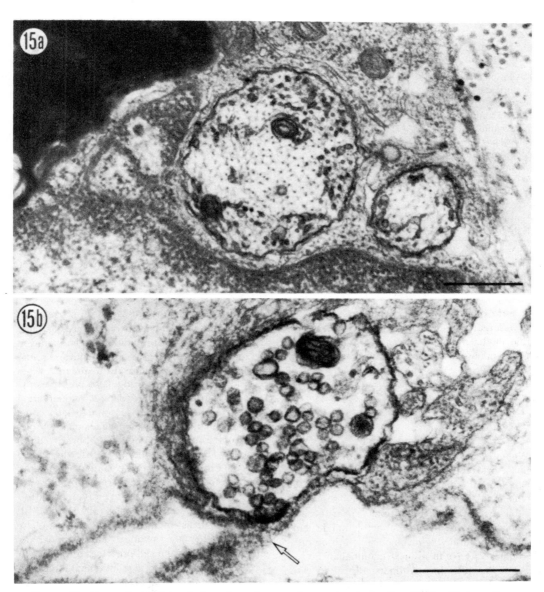

FIGURE 15 Preterminal and terminal portions of axons reinnervating the irradiated bridge 21 days after muscle was damaged and denervated; by morphological criteria, terminals have differentiated. (*a*) Axons in the nerve trunk, wrapped by a Schwann cell, contain many neurofilaments and microtubules but few synaptic vesicles. (*b*) Nerve terminal, apposed to BL of the myofiber sheath, contains numerous vesicles, some of which are focused on an active zone that lies opposite an intersection (arrow) of synaptic cleft and junctional fold BL. Bar, 0.5 μm.

minals cover decreases 3–5 wk after nerve crush, suggesting that some terminals may retract and/or degenerate after they form. Electron microscopy of ChE-stained preparations showed that $41 \pm 4\%$ (mean $\pm$ SE of counts from seven bridges) of the original synaptic BL is reinnervated at 3 wk, 31

$\pm 2\%$ ($n = 4$) at 4 wk, and $20 \pm 3\%$ ($n = 5$) at 5 wk; the difference between 3 and 5 wk is highly significant ($P < .002$; Student's t test). Although the procedures that we use are traumatic, the decline is not simply a consequence of surgery or irradiation, since it was not observed in muscles

TABLE II

Distribution of Synaptic Vesicles in Axons Reinnervating Irradiated Bridges

Region	n	Vesicles/profile	Vesicles/μm^{2*}
A. All axonal profiles			
Preterminal axons	95	6.1 ± 0.8 ⎤	6.7 ± 1.3 ⎤
Terminals	95	17.6 ± 2.2 ⎦	50.0 ± 5.3 ⎦
B. Preterminal axons			
Myelinating	11	18.3 ± 3.3 ⎤	2.2 ± 0.4 ⎦
Unmyelinated, in perineurium	38	5.6 ± 1.0 ⎦	4.7 ± 0.8 ⎦
Unmyelinated, outside of perineurium	46	3.7 ± 0.8 ⎦	9.5 ± 2.5 ⎦
C. Terminals			
Wrapped in Schwann cell process	43	9.5 ± 2.7 ⎤	26.9 ± 4.1 ⎤
Abutting myofiber BL	52	24.2 ± 3.1 ⎦	69.1 ± 8.2 ⎦
D. Terminals abutting myofiber BL			
Half-profiles closest to myofiber BL	52	15.4 ± 1.3 ⎤	81.8 ± 8.6 ⎤
Half-profiles farthest from myofiber BL	52	8.2 ± 1.3 ⎦	52.8 ± 7.6 ⎦

Profiles were selected at random from cross sections through three irradiated bridges fixed 3 wk after denervation and muscle damage. Data is given as mean ± 1 SE for indicated number of profiles. Numbers joined by brackets differ significantly ($P < 0.01$; Student's t test).
* Means of values calculated separately for each terminal.

that were only damaged or irradiated (Fig. 12). This observation suggests that myofibers may play a role in the maintenance and/or maturation of nerve terminals, a hypothesis that we are currently testing.

DISCUSSION

The Bridge of Basement Membrane Sheaths

When we cut the cutaneous pectoris muscle to make a bridge (Fig. 1), the muscle fiber's cytoplasm clumps and retracts, leaving behind the sarcolemmal sheaths of the damaged segments. (In this respect, our observations repeat those of Bowman, who discovered the sarcolemmal sheath in 1840 while studying mechanically injured muscle fibers [7].) As in injured mammalian muscle (9, 24, 39, 46), the myofibers' disrupted cytoplasm and plasma membrane degenerate and are phagocytized in the bridge, but the BL of the sheaths survives. Thus, injury and its sequelae cleave the surface complex of the myofiber between the plasma membrane and the BL (see Fig. 3); we do not know the fate of the glycocalyx.

Muscles can be damaged in many ways, but the bridge is particularly well suited for studies that concentrate on nerve-muscle interactions. Cutting the muscle into short segments results in more uniform and complete degeneration of myofibers than occurs after chemical, thermal, or ischemic injury (4, 9, 13, 24, 39, 46, 50). In contrast to

procedures in which the muscle is excised, minced, and then reimplanted in its bed to insure complete degeneration (9), the orientation of the damaged segments and the integrity of the intramuscular connective tissue are relatively unaffected when the bridge is made. The bridge also preserves the main nerve trunk, which expedites reinnervation after nerve crush (20, 23, 53), and at least some of the vascular supply, which speeds phagocytosis of disrupted myofibers by blood-borne macrophages (9, 39). In addition, because the bridge spans the center of the muscle's innervation band, many synaptic sites are preserved. Synaptic specializations of the basement membrane sheath — ChE (33), BL of junctional folds (13, 31), and BL of Schwann cells — permit identification of these sites even after the myofiber and terminal degenerate and Schwann cell processes retract.

X-irradiation of the bridge inhibits the regeneration of myofibers (32, 42, 52) that would otherwise occur (9, 24, 31) but does not block phagocytosis of damaged nerve and muscle. At the dose we used, irradiation does not prevent regeneration of motor axons, even though the motoneurons that innervate the cutaneous pectoris lie in the thoracic spinal cord and are irradiated along with the bridge.

Precise Reinnervation of Original Synaptic Sites

Axons regenerating to denervated muscle form new neuromuscular junctions precisely at the sites

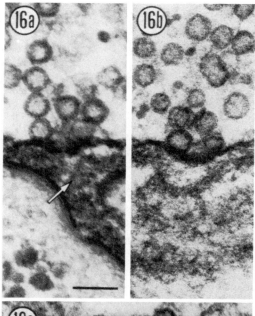

FIGURE 16 Active zones in nerve terminals of the bridge resemble those in normal neuromuscular junctions. (a) Normal muscle. (b, c) Irradiated bridge, 21 days after denervation and muscle damage. Cross-sectioned active zones in Fig. 16a and b show cytoplasmic densities on the plasma membrane flanked by synaptic vesicles that approach the membrane closely. Longitudinally sectioned active zone in Fig. 16c shows vesicles arranged in a row. Cytoplasmic densities of active zones are near intersections (arrows) of synaptic cleft and junctional fold BL, both in normal muscle (a) and in the bridge (c). Bar, 0.1 μm.

of the original synapses where new nerve terminals cover the old junctional folds. Although synapses sometimes form at completely new sites (2, 15), preferential reinnervation of original sites has been documented in mammalian, avian, and amphibian muscles reinnervated by their own or by foreign nerves (1-3, 15, 17, 19, 26, 29, 41, 48). This topographic specificity is nowhere more striking than during reinnervation of frog muscle

after a nerve crush as occurred in this study: regenerating axons cover nearly all of the postsynaptic membrane while making few if any contacts elsewhere on the muscle fiber's surface (Figs. 12 and 13 and reference 27).

One aid to precise reinnervation is provided by tubes of perineurial and Schwann cells that survive in the motor nerve long after damaged axons have degenerated. Regenerating axons often grow through these tubes (19, 20, 23, 27, 41) and (like regenerating sensory axons; see, for example, reference 51) are thus guided to original synaptic sites. However, regenerating axons can unerringly cover long stretches of synaptic surface after they leave the perineurium, lifting off the muscle fiber at the end of the synaptic site (27). Also, axons growing beyond or outside perineurial tubes can "select" and precisely reinnervate original sites (1, 19, 27). Thus, there must be factors at the synaptic site itself that provide cues to regenerating axons.

The nature and precise location of these cues is not known. One attractive possibility has been that the postsynaptic cell—the myofiber—contains the factors that guide reinnervation of original synaptic sites (1, 15, 41). Our results show, however, that the myofiber need not be present for precise innervation of original sites to occur. Myofibers may originally produce (or be required for the production of) factors that make axons prefer original sites, but these factors are present and can be maintained for several weeks outside of the myofibers.

What and where might these factors be? Among the possibilities that remain to be tested are the following: (a) the reticular lamina, which coats extrasynaptic but not synaptic portions of the BL, might act as a mechanical barrier to regenerating axons, shielding them from contact with extrasynaptic areas of the muscle fiber; (b) the basement membrane of the Schwann cell, which forms a tunnel over the synaptic site (Fig. 7f) is certainly not impermeable to axons (19, 27), but it may, like Schwann tubes in the nerve trunk (20), provide mechanical guidance to restrain and/or orient axonal growth; (c) complementary molecules on the surfaces of Schwann cells and axons might provide a basis for recognition by intercellular adhesion, as has been proposed for a variety of neural and nonneural tissues (8, 43); (d) axons may recognize extracellular molecules that are differentially distributed between synaptic and ex-

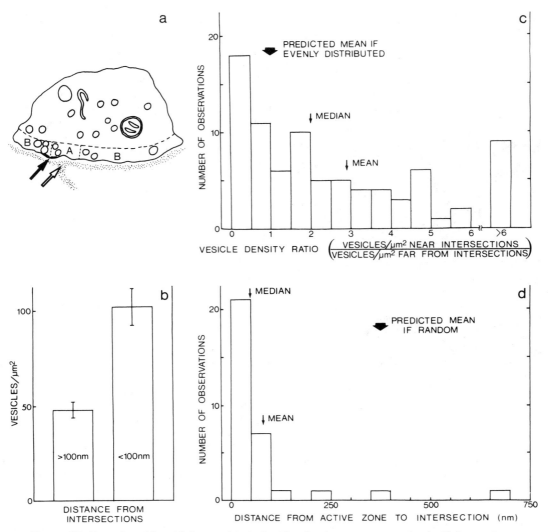

FIGURE 17 Synaptic vesicles and the cytoplasmic densities of active zones are associated with intersections of synaptic cleft and junctional fold BL in the absence of myofibers. (a) Tracing of nerve terminal from 1 of 84 electron micrographs from which data shown in Fig. 17 b–d was collected, to show method of analysis. Micrographs were obtained from five irradiated bridges fixed 3 wk after denervation and muscle damage. (b) Vesicles situated in the 100-nm high strip of nerve terminal cytoplasm nearest the myofiber's BL were counted. Vesicle density (vesicle/μm^2) was calculated separately for areas within 100 nm of interactions between synaptic cleft and junctional fold BL (see A in Fig. 17 a), and for areas farther than 100 nm from intersections (see B in Fig. 17 a). Graph shows mean vesicle density ($\pm$SE) in each of these two areas. (c) Vesicle density ratios (density within 100 nm of intersection/density further than 100 nm from intersection but within the juxtamembranous strip) was calculated separately for each of the 84 terminals. Mean and median ratios are both clearly higher than the mean ratio of 1 that a random distribution would produce. (d) For each of 32 active zones, the distance from the center of the cytoplasmic density (see closed arrow in Fig. 17 a) to the nearest intersection of fold and cleft BL (see open arrow in Fig. 17 a) was measured. Average separation would be nearly 400 nm if active zones were randomly distributed alone zone of nerve terminal-BL contact (see text); in fact, most cytoplasmic densities are <100 nm from an intersection.

SANES, MARSHALL, AND MCMAHAN *Reinnervation of Muscle Fiber Basal Lamina* **195**

trasynaptic regions of the basal lamina. Regenerating axons might be repelled by molecules that are concentrated in extrasynaptic BL, or be immobilized by (i.e., adhere to) molecules (such as ChE [33]) that are concentrated in the synaptic BL.

Differentiation of Nerve Terminals: A Morphogenetic Role for Basal Lamina

Synaptic vesicles accumulate and active zones form in portions of regenerating axons that approach basement membrane sheaths in the bridge. At least by these morphological criteria, axons can differentiate locally into "presynaptic" nerve terminals in the absence of a "postsynaptic" cell. The spatial relationships of synaptic vesicles and active zones in these terminals to extra-axonal structures (e.g., Schwann cells and BL) leave little doubt that extrinsic factors trigger and organize the transformation of axons into nerve terminals.

The differentiation of the nerve terminal is a complex process, and we do not know how many factors are required for its occurrence. Among the cells that might play a role in this differentiation are the Schwann cells that remain at denervated synaptic sites and the unidentified cells — probably including presumptive myoblasts (9, 39, 46) — that lay within the basement membrane sheaths in the bridge. Neurons growing in vitro can be stimulated to differentiate by glial (36) and muscle (16) cells. It is possible that similar trophic interactions occur in the bridge; our results neither demonstrate nor rule out their existence. We have, however, obtained evidence that at least one morphogenetically important factor is located and stably maintained extracellularly, in the BL of the original synaptic cleft.

The involvement of the BL in axonal differentiation is suggested by the observation that synaptic vesicles accumulate preferentially and active zones appear only in portions of terminals that abut the BL of the myofiber sheath. More direct evidence comes from analyzing the distribution of these synaptic organelles along regions of contact between terminals and BL at original synaptic sites. In normal (5, 11, 22, 34, 37) and reinnervated[1] muscles, vesicles and active zones are concentrated directly opposite the mouths of the junctional folds that periodically indent the postsynaptic membrane. After the cytoplasm and plasma membrane of the myofiber have been removed, these sites can be recognized as points where the projections of BL that once lined the folds join the BL of the synaptic cleft. The vesicles and active zones of terminals in the bridge are closely associated with these points (Fig. 17), demonstrating that molecules periodically arranged along the BL of the original synaptic cleft play some role in triggering and/or organizing the differentiation of regenerating nerve terminals. The extracellular location and apparent stability of these molecules is likely to facilitate attempts to isolate them and to elucidate their mechanism of action.

We are grateful to Dr. Henry Kohn for his help with x-irradiation and to Gerald Barry, Grace Burke, Mary Hogan, and Linda Yu for their assistance.

This work was done during the tenure of a Research Fellowship of the Muscular Dystrophy Association (Dr. Marshall) and was supported by U.S. Public Health Service grants NS 70606, NS 12922, NS 02253, and NS 05731.

Received for publication 19 December 1977, and in revised form 23 March 1978.

REFERENCES

1. BENNETT, M. R., E. M. McLACHLAN, and R. S. TAYLOR. 1973. The formation of synapses in reinnervated mammalian striated muscle. *J. Physiol. (Lond.).* **233:**481–500.
2. BENNETT, M. R., and A. G. PETTIGREW. 1975. The formation of neuromuscular synapses. *Cold Spring Harbor Symp. Quant. Biol.* **40:**409–424.
3. BENNETT, M. R., A. G. PETTIGREW, and R. S. TAYLOR. 1973. The formation of synapses in reinnervated and cross-reinnervated adult avian muscle. *J. Physiol. (Lond.).* **230:**331–357.
4. BENOIT, P. W., and P. BELT. 1970. Destruction and regeneration of skeletal muscle after treatment with a local anesthetic, bupivicaine (Marcaine). *J. Anat.* **107:**547–556.
5. BIRKS, R., H. W. HUXLEY, and B. KATZ. 1960. The fine structure of the neuromuscular junction of the frog. *J. Physiol. (Lond.).* **150:**134–144.
6. BIRKS, R., B. KATZ, and R. MILEDI. 1960. Physiological and structural changes at the amphibian myoneural junction, in the course of nerve degeneration. *J. Physiol. (Lond.).* **150:**145–168.
7. BOWMAN, W. 1840. On the minute structure and movements of voluntary muscle. *Philos. Trans. R. Soc. Lond. B. Biol. Sci.* **130:**457–501.
8. BURGER, M. D., R. S. TURNOVER, W. J. KUHNS, and G. WEINBAUM. 1975. A possible model for cell-cell recognition via surface macromolecules. *Philos. Trans. R. Soc. Lond. B. Biol. Sci.* **271:**279–393.
9. CARLSON, B. M. 1972. The regeneration of skeletal

muscle–a review. *Am. J. Anat.* **137**:119–149.

10. CAVANAGH, J. B. 1968. Effects of x-irradiation on the proliferation of cells in peripheral nerve during Wallerian degeneration in the rat. *Br. J. Radiol.* **41**:275–281.

11. COUTEAUX, R., and M. PÉCOT-DECHAVÁSSINE. 1970. Vésicules synaptiques et poches au niveau des "zones actives" de la jonction neuromusculaire. *C. R. Acad. Sci. Ser. D.* **271**:2346–2349.

12. DUANCE, V. C., D. J. RESTALL, H. BEARD, F. J. BOURNE, and A. J. BAILEY. 1977. The location of three collagen types in skeletal muscle. *FEBS (Fed. Eur. Biochem. Soc.) Lett.* **79**:248–252.

13. DUCHEN, L. W., B. J. EXCELL, R. PATEL, and B. SMITH. 1974. Changes in motor end-plates resulting from muscle fibre necrosis and regeneration. A light and electron microscopic study of the effects of the depolarizing fraction (cardiotoxin) of *Dendroaspis jamesoni* venom. *J. Neurol. Sci.* **21**:391–417.

14. FEWINGS, J. D., J. B. HARRIS, M. A. JOHNSON, and W. G. BRADLEY. 1977. Progressive denervation of skeletal muscle induced by spinal irradiation in rats. *Brain.* **100**:157–183.

15. FISCHBACH, G. D. 1974. Some aspects of neuromuscular junction formation. *In* Cell Communication. R. P. Cox, editor. John Wiley & Sons, Inc., New York. 43–66.

16. GILLER, E. L., J. H. NEALE, P. N. BULLOCK, B. K. SCHRIER, and P. G. NELSON. 1977. Choline acetyltransferase activity of spinal cord cell cultures increased by co-culture with muscle and by muscle-conditioned medium. *J. Cell Biol.* **74**:16–29.

17. GOZENBACH, H. R., and P. G. WASER. 1973. Electron microscopic studies of degeneration and regeneration of rat neuromuscular junctions. *Brain Res.* **63**:167–174.

18. GUTH, L., and W. C. BROWN. 1965. The sequence of changes in cholinesterase activity during reinnervation. *Exp. Neurol.* **12**:329–336.

19. GUTMANN, E., and J. Z. YOUNG. 1944. The reinnervation of muscle after various periods of atrophy. *J. Anat.* **78**:15–43.

20. HAFTEK, J., and P. K. THOMAS. 1968. Electron microscope observations on the effects of localized crush injuries on the connective tissues of peripheral nerve. *J. Anat.* **103**:233–243.

21. HARRIS, A. J. 1974. Inductive functions of the nervous system. *Annu. Rev. Physiol.* **36**:251–305.

22. HEUSER, J. E., and T. S. REESE. 1973. Evidence for recycling of synaptic vesicle membrane during transmitter release at the frog neuromuscular junction. *J. Cell Biol.* **57**:315–344.

23. HOLMES, W., and J. Z. YOUNG. 1942. Nerve regeneration after immediate and delayed suture. *J. Anat.* **77**:63–96.

24. HUDGSON, P., and E. J. FIELD. 1973. Regeneration of muscle. *In* The Structure and Function of Muscle. G. H. Bourne, editor. Academic Press Inc., New York. **2**:312–363.

25. KARNOVSKY, M. J. 1964. The localization of cholinesterase activity in rat cardiac muscle by electron microscopy. *J. Cell Biol.* **23**:217–232.

26. LANDMESSER, L. 1972. Pharmacological properties, cholinesterase activity and anatomy of nerve-muscle junctions in vagus-innervated frog sartorius. *J. Physiol. (Lond.).* **220**:243–256.

27. LETINSKY, M. K., G. D. FISCHBECK, and U. J. McMAHAN. 1976. Precision of reinnervation of original postsynaptic sites in muscle after a nerve crush. *J. Neurocytol.* **5**:691–718.

28. LUFT, J. H. 1971. Ruthenium red and violet II. Fine structural localization in animal tissues. *Anat. Rec.* **171**:369–416.

29. LÜLLMAN-RAUCH, R. 1971. The regeneration of neuromuscular junctions during spontaneous reinnervation of the rat diaphragm. *Z. Zellforsch. Mikrosk. Anat.* **121**:593–603.

30. MAILLET, M. 1962. La technique de Champy à l'osmium-ioduré de potassium et la modification de Maillet à l'osmium-ioduré de zinc. *Trab. Inst. Cajal Invest. Biol.* **54**:1–36.

31. MARSHALL, L. M., J. R. SANES, and U. J. McMAHAN. 1977. Reinnervation of original synaptic sites on muscle fiber basement membrane after disruption of the muscle cells. *Proc. Natl. Acad. Sci. U.S.A.* **74**:3073–3077.

32. MASTAGLIA, F. L., R. L., DAWKINS, and J. M. PAPADIMITROU. 1975. Morphological changes in skeletal muscle after transplantation. A light- and electronmicroscopic study of the initial phases of degeneration and regeneration. *J. Neurol. Sci.* **25**:227–247.

33. McMAHAN, U. J., J. R. SANES, and L. M. MARSHALL. 1978. Cholinesterase is associated with the basal lamina at the neuromuscular junction. *Nature (Lond.).* **271**:172–174.

34. McMAHAN, U. J., N. C. SPITZER, and K. PEPER. 1972. Visual identification of nerve terminals in living isolated skeletal muscle. *Proc. Roy. Soc. Lond. B.* **181**:421–430.

35. MILEDI, R. and C. R. SLATER. 1968. Electrophysiology and electronmicroscopy of rat neuromuscular junctions after nerve degeneration. *Proc. R. Soc. Lond. B Biol. Sci.* **169**:289–306.

36. PATTERSON, P. H., and L. L. Y. CHUN. 1974. The influence of non-neuronal cells on catecholamine and acetylcholine synthesis and accumulation in cultures of dissociated sympathetic neurons. *Proc. Natl. Acad. Sci. U.S.A.* **71**:3607–3610.

37. PEPER, K., F. DREYER, C. SANDRI, K. AKERT, and H. MOOR. 1974. Structure and ultrastructure of the frog motor endplate. *Cell Tissue Res.* **149**:437–455.

38. PHILLIPS, T. L., S. BERAK, and G. ROSS. 1972. Ultrastructural and cellular effects of ionizing radiation. *Front. Pediat. Ther. Oncol.* **6**:21–43.

39. PRICE, H. M., E. L. HOWES, and J. M. BLUMBERT. 1964. Ultrastructural alterations in skeletal muscle fibers injured by cold. I. The acute degenerative

changes. *Lab. Invest.* **13:**1279–1302.

40. Rambourg, A., and C. P. Leblond. 1967. Electron microscopic observations on the carbohydrate-rich cell coat present at the surface of cells in the rat. *J. Cell Biol.* **32:**27–53.

41. Ramon Y Cajal, S. 1928. Degeneration and Regeneration of the Nervous System. (Translated and edited by R. M. May, 1959). Hafner Press, New York.

42. Reznik, M., and E. H. Betz. 1967. Influence de l'irradiation locale preálable sur les capacités regénératrices du muscle strié squeltique. *Pathol. Eur.* **2:**69–80.

43. Roth, S. 1973. A molecular model for cell interactions. *Q. Rev. Biol.* **48:**541–563.

44. Rotshenker, S., and U. J. McMahan. 1976. Altered patterns of innervation in frog muscle after denervation. *J. Neurocytol.* **5:**719–730.

45. Saito, A., and S. I. Zacks. 1969. Fine structure observations of denervation and reinnervation of neuromuscular junctions in mouse foot muscle. *J. Bone Jt. Surg. Am. Vol.* **51:**1163–1178.

46. Snow, M. H. 1977. Myogenic cell formation in regenerating rat skeletal muscle injured by mincing. I. A fine structural study. *Anat. Rec.* **188:**181–200.

47. Spiro, R. G. 1972. Basement membranes and collagens. *In* Glycoproteins. A. Gottschalk, editor. Elsevier, Amsterdam. 964–999.

48. Tello, F. 1907. Degeneration et regeneration des plaques motrices après la section des nerfs. *Trav. Lab. Rech. Biol. Univ. Madrid.* **5:**117–149.

49. Uehara, Y., G. R. Campbell, and G. Burnstock. 1976. Muscle and its innervation. Arnold Ltd., London.

50. Vracko, R., and E. P. Benditt. 1972. Basal lamina: the scaffold for orderly cell replacement. *J. Cell Biol.* **55:**406–419.

51. Weddell, G. 1942. Axonal regeneration in cutaneous nerve plexuses. *J. Anat.* **77:**49–62.

52. Williams, R. T., and P. Pietsch. 1965. Time-related inhibition of mammalian muscle regeneration by x-irradiation. *Anat. Rec.* **151:**434.

53. Young, J. Z. 1942. The functional repair of nervous tissue. *Physiol. Rev.* **22:**318–374.

Section 9
Specificity of Neuronal Connections: Selective Synapse Formation

Dennis, M.J. and J.W. Yip. 1978. Formation and elimination of foreign synapses on adult salamander muscle. *J. Physiol.* 274: 299–310.

Purves, D., W. Thompson, and J.W. Yip. 1981. Reinnervation of ganglia transplanted to the neck from different levels of the guinea-pig sympathetic chain. *J. Physiol.* 313: 49–63.

Attardi, D.G. and R.W. Sperry. 1963. Preferential selection of central pathways by regenerating optic fibers. *Exp. Neurol.* 7: 46–64.

Chung, S.-H. and J. Cooke. 1975. Polarity of structure and of ordered nerve connections in the developing amphibian brain. *Nature* 258: 126–132.

Fuchs, P.A., J.G. Nicholls, and D.F. Ready. 1981. Membrane properties and selective connexions of identified leech neurones in culture. *J. Physiol.* 316: 203–223.

Sperry, R.W. 1963. Chemoaffinity in the orderly growth of nerve fiber patterns and connections. *Proc. Natl. Acad. Sci.* 50: 703–710.

Although the term "specificity" is commonly used by developmental neurobiologists, it is not often defined. In general, the term is taken to refer to those mechanisms that lead to the highly stereotyped patterns of connections characteristic of the mature nervous system. In this usage, however, many of the developmental phenomena considered in earlier sections (migration, neuronal differentiation, axon outgrowth) quite properly qualify as mechanisms underlying specificity. Therefore, the phrase "neural specificity" should always be qualified.

An aspect of specificity not considered in previous sections is the mechanism that allows an axon that has reached the vicinity of its target to choose the most appropriate cells from among the potential synaptic partners confronting it. A number of researchers have pursued the problem of selective synaptogenesis in muscle, where several aspects have been addressed. One type of experiment has asked whether each muscle as a whole has some special affinity for its native innervation. Such experiments involve either cutting a nerve carrying innervation to two or more different muscles (Bernstein and Guth 1963; Brushart and Mesulam 1980) or surgically rerouting a foreign motor nerve so that it competes with the native nerve during reinnervation (Weiss and Hoag 1946; Gerding et al. 1977). Both approaches have, for mammalian muscles, given the same result: Different muscles of similar fiber composition show little or no tendency to become preferentially reinnervated by their original motor axons. In some lower vertebrates and invertebrates, however, the situation is quite different in that nerves do show a preference for their original target muscles (Mark 1965; Sperry and Arora 1965; Van Essen and Jansen 1977; see also Section 4). Moreover, this phenomenon is expressed at the level of the synapses, since native axons in some lower vertebrates can compete successfully with foreign ones, even after foreign synapses have become established (Bennett and Raftos 1977; **Dennis** and **Yip 1978**; Bennett et al. 1979). In other vertebrates such competition is not evident, and target cells may remain innervated by native and foreign axons indefinitely (Frank and Jansen 1976; see also Purves 1976). Although this suggests that some lower vertebrate nerves recognize different muscles as such, other explanations are not ruled out. Since peripherally overextended motor axons (or even some normal endings) give way to regenerating axons that have made relatively few synapses (Brown and Ironton 1976; Bixby and Van Essen 1979; Wigston 1980), displacement of the foreign nerve terminals may occur largely on this quantitative basis.

A second class of experiments in muscle asks whether there is selective innervation of functionally different fiber types within a muscle. The axons innervating fast and slow fibers in some amphibian muscles can be separately identified (Kuffler and Vaughan-Williams 1953). When such mixed muscles are reinnervated, both classes of muscle cells are initially contacted by the motor axons that innervated fast muscle fibers (Schmidt and Stefani 1976). However, when slow motor axons (which take longer to regenerate) eventually reach the muscle, they apparently displace the synapses formed by fast axons on slow fibers (Elul et al. 1970; Schmidt and Stefani 1976, 1977; see, however, Miledi and Stefani 1969). In conceptually related experiments, the ability of regenerating axons to distinguish between two muscles with different fiber compositions has been tested (Feng et al. 1965; Hoh 1971, 1975; Bennett and Pettigrew 1976). In general, native nerves appear to prefer their original muscles in these experiments, perhaps because of the different average fiber compositions of the respective targets.

Selective synapse formation has been studied to advantage in another part of the peripheral nervous system, the mammalian sympathetic chain (Purves and Lichtman 1978). Langley first described evidence for selective innervation of autonomic ganglion cells in the 1890s. In adult mammals, the superior cervical ganglion receives innervation from preganglionic nerve cells in seven or eight spinal cord segments (Langley 1892). The axons arising from preganglionic neurons at different rostrocaudal levels do not innervate ganglion cells at random. Rather, those ganglion cells that innervate a particular region of the territory supplied by the ganglion (the eye, for instance) are themselves innervated by preganglionic neurons from a well-defined subset of the spinal segments that provide innervation to the ganglion as a whole (Njå and Purves 1977a; Lichtman et al. 1979, 1980). Moreover, the normal pattern of ganglionic connections is reestablished with considerable fidelity during regeneration (Langley 1897; Njå and Purves 1977b, 1978). Selective reinnervation of two functionally different classes of neurons in a parasympathetic ganglion has also been reported (Landmesser and Pilar 1970). These experiments suggest that some property of ganglion cells and preganglionic axons that varies among neuronal subsets biases the formation of synaptic connections. The idea of such cellular biases has received additional support from the finding that the same set of preganglionic axons responds differently to different sympathetic chain ganglia during synapse formation (**Purves, Thompson,** and **Yip 1981**). This presumably occurs because the cells making up each ganglion are, on average, somewhat different with respect to a property (perhaps related to rostrocaudal position) that influences synapse formation.

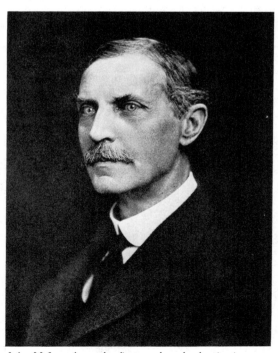

John N. Langley, who first explored selective innervation of target cells.

Historically, the most influential experiments on specificity have been carried out on the central nervous systems of lower vertebrates. In the 1920s, Matthey showed that a newt can see normally again a few weeks after optic-nerve transection (Matthey 1926). Sperry (1943a,b, 1944) and Stone (Stone and Zaur 1940; Stone 1944), working independently, greatly extended these retinotectal studies in the 1940s. Sperry, in particular, asked whether such success represented special affinities between matching retinal and tectal cells or whether recovery represented a functional sorting out of largely random retinal regrowth. To decide between these alternatives, Sperry cut the optic nerve and then rotated the eye 180° (Sperry 1943a,b; Stone 1944). The results of these experiments was that animals behaved as if their visual world had been inverted and shifted left for right, indicating that the retinal ganglion cells had grown back to (approximately) the same tectal cells they contacted originally.

Using the goldfish, **Attardi** and **Sperry (1963)** later provided additional evidence that axons from a particular part of the retina regenerate preferentially to a particular region of the tectum. Their approach was to stain the regenerating retinal axons after surgically removing most of the retina. They found that the regrowing axons took paths in the optic tract that were appropriate to their origin; moreover, rather than spreading out to occupy the whole tectum, the axons ignored large areas of the denervated target and went on to contact the part of the tectum they originally innervated. These widely quoted results have had a profound influence. First, a number of experiments have been done to test whether retinal axons can find their proper destinations in the tectum when their normal routes and arrangements have been distorted (see, for example, Sperry 1943b; Yoon 1973). Even under these abnormal circumstances, axons still show a remarkable ability to locate their original termination sites (see also Section 4). One explanation of this phenomenon might be that regenerating axons recognize a label they originally imparted to the tectum (see Schmidt 1978). Although such labeling may occur, additional factors are clearly involved in establishing the retinotectal map during development (**Chung** and **Cooke 1975,** 1978). Second, a number of experiments have shown that retinotectal preferences are, at least to some degree, flexible. If, for instance, half the goldfish tectum is removed,

then the remaining half will accept regenerating axons from the entire retina (Gaze et al. 1963; Gaze and Sharma 1970; Yoon 1971; Schmidt et al. 1978). Some flexibility of retinotectal connections is also evident during normal development (Chung et al. 1974; Chung and Cooke 1978; Gaze et al. 1979). Finally, the classic experiments on retinotectal specificity stimulated the biochemical experiments described in Section 10. A general problem with the voluminous and sometimes contentious literature on the retinotectal system in recent years is that the relative contributions of the several possible mechanisms of axon guidance and selective synapse formation to the specificity of retinotectal connections are unclear.

Although tectal reinnervation implies (but does not prove) a high level of selective resolution during synapse formation, studies of specificity in the central nervous systems of several invertebrate preparations provide examples of recognition that may be largely unique (see Muller 1979). The advantage of invertebrates in this context is that many neurons can be individually identified from animal to animal. Although some apparently novel synaptic connections are made,

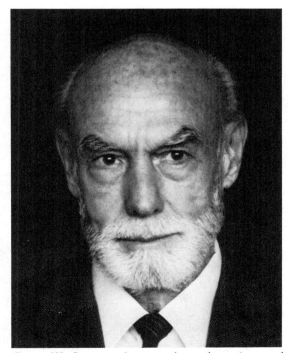

Roger W. Sperry, whose work on the retinotectal system continues to dominate the thinking about specificity in this part of the nervous system.

regeneration of connections between neurons in adjacent leech ganglia occurs reliably at the level of single identified cells (Baylor and Nicholls 1971; Jansen and Nicholls 1972; Wallace et al. 1977; Muller 1979). More recently, the tendency of individual neurons to synapse selectively with one another has been examined using isolated leech neurons in culture (Ready and Nicholls 1979; **Fuchs, Nicholls,** and **Ready 1981**). Clearly, this approach has considerable potential (see, for example, Zipser and McKay 1981).

There is thus reasonable evidence in both the peripheral and central nervous systems that some more or less permanent property of potential synaptic partners is capable of biasing synapse formation. What underlies this bias? Langley (1897) suggested that a chemical component of sympathetic ganglion cells might explain what he called "chemiotaxis"—axons growing more or less randomly throughout the ganglion, exploring the suitability of the cells they happened to contact. This general idea is similar to the better-known chemoaffinity hypothesis put forward by Sperry. Sperry's view (**Sperry 1963**), as Langley's, was that some aspect of the surfaces of pre- and postsynaptic cells led to mutual recognition of appropriate partners. On the basis of his work on the reinnervation of the goldfish tectum (Attardi and Sperry 1963), Sperry suggested that the same mechanism of recognition also allowed growth cones to find appropriate pathways to their targets. This general idea remains the most plausible explanation of selective synapse formation, and recent attempts to provide a biochemical basis for it are described in the next section.

At present, then, studies of the innervation of vertebrate muscle, autonomic ganglia, optic tectum, and the central nervous systems of several invertebrates have begun to provide a detailed phenomenological picture of what to expect of the classes of molecules that are considered candidates for cellular recognition during synapse formation. In vertebrates at least, it appears that such recognition between cells is a relatively weak force that provides a bias rather than the certainty of a lock and key (see Purves and Lichtman 1978). It is also important to bear in mind that recognition is only one aspect of the complex developmental events that produce the specificity characteristic of the mature nervous system.

References

Attardi, D.G. and R.W. Sperry. 1963. Preferential selection of central pathways by regenerating optic fibers. *Exp. Neurol.* 7: 46–64.

Baylor, D.A. and J.G. Nicholls. 1971. Patterns of regeneration between individual nerve cells in the central nervous system of the leech. *Nature 232:* 268–270.

Bennett, M.R. and A.G. Pettigrew. 1976. The formation of neuromuscular synapses. *Cold Spring Harbor Symp. Quant. Biol. 40:* 409–424.

Bennett, M.R. and J. Raftos. 1977. The formation and regression of synapses during reinnervation of axolotl striated muscle. *J. Physiol. 265:* 261–295.

Bennett, M.R., P.A. McGrath, and D.F. Davey. 1979. The regression of synapses formed by a foreign nerve in a mature axolotl striated muscle. *Brain Res. 173:* 451–469.

Bernstein, J.J. and L. Guth. 1963. Non-selectivity in the establishment of neuromuscular connections following nerve regeneration in the rat. *Exp. Neurol. 4:* 262–275.

Bixby, J.L. and D.C. Van Essen. 1979. Competition between foreign and original nerves in adult mammalian skeletal muscle. *Nature 282:* 726–728.

Brown, M.C. and R. Ironton. 1976. Sprouting and regression of neuromuscular synapses in partially denervated mammalian muscles. *J. Physiol. 278:* 325–348.

Brushart, T.M. and M.-M. Mesulam. 1980. Alteration in connections between muscle and anterior horn motoneurons after peripheral nerve repair. *Science 208:* 603–605.

Chung, S.-H. and J. Cooke. 1975. Polarity of structure and of ordered nerve connections in the developing amphibian brain. *Nature 258:* 126–132.

———. 1978. Observations on the formation of the brain and of nerve connections following embryonic manipulation of the amphibian neural tube. *Proc. R. Soc. Lond. B 201:* 335–373.

Chung, S.-H., M.J. Keating, and T.V.P. Bliss. 1974. Functional synaptic relations during the development of the retino-tectal projections in amphibians. *Proc. R. Soc. Lond. B 187:* 449–459.

Dennis, M.J. and J.W. Yip. 1978. Formation and elimination of foreign synapses on adult salamander muscle. *J. Physiol. 274:* 299–310.

Elul, R., R. Miledi, and E. Stefani. 1970. Neural control of contracture in slow muscle fibres of the frog. *Acta Physiol. Lat. Am. 20:* 194–226.

Feng, T.P., W.Y. Wu, and F.Y. Yang. 1965. Selective reinnervation of "slow" or "fast" muscle by its original motor supply during regeneration of mixed nerve. *Sci. Sin. 14:* 1717–1720.

Frank, E. and J.K.S. Jansen. 1976. Interaction between foreign and original nerves innervating gill muscles in fish. *J. Neurophysiol. 39:* 84–90.

Fuchs, P.A., J.G. Nicholls, and D.F. Ready. 1981. Membrane properties and selective connexions of identified leech neurones in culture. *J. Physiol. 316:* 203–223.

Gaze, R.M. and S.C. Sharma. 1970. Axial differences in the reinnervation of goldfish optic tectum by regenerating optic fibres. *Exp. Brain Res. 10:* 171–181.

Gaze, R.M., M. Jacobson, and G. Szekely. 1963. The retino-tectal projection in *Xenopus* with compound eyes. *J. Physiol. 165:* 484–499.

Gaze, R.M., M.J. Keating, A. Ostberg, and S.-H. Chung. 1979. The relationship between retinal and tectal growth in larval *Xenopus:* Implications for the development of retino-tectal projection. *J. Embryol. Exp. Morphol. 53:* 103–143.

Gerding, R., N. Robbins, and J. Antosiak. 1977. Efficiency of reinnervation of neonatal rat muscle by original and foreign nerves. *Dev. Biol. 61:* 177–183.

Hoh, J.F.Y. 1971. Selective reinnervation of fast-twitch and slow-graded muscle fibers in the toad. *Exp. Neurol. 30:* 263–276.

———. 1975. Selective and non-selective reinnervation of fast-twitch and slow-twitch rat skeletal muscle. *J. Physiol. 251:* 791–801.

Jansen, J.K.S. and J.G. Nicholls. 1972. Regeneration and changes in synaptic connections between individual nerve cells in the central nervous system of the leech. *Proc. Natl. Acad. Sci. 69:* 636–639.

Kuffler, S.W. and E.M. Vaughan-Williams. 1953. Small nerve junction potentials. The distribution of small motor nerves to frog skeletal muscle and the membrane characteristics of the fibres they innervate. *J. Physiol. 121:* 289–317.

Landmesser, L. and G. Pilar. 1970. Selective reinnervation of two cell populations in the adult pigeon ciliary ganglion. *J. Physiol. 211:* 203–216.

Langley, J.N. 1892. On the origin from the spinal cord of the cervical and upper thoracic sympathetic fibres, with some observations on white and grey rami communicantes. *Philos. Trans. R. Soc. Lond. B 183:* 85–124.

———. 1897. On the regeneration of pre-ganglionic and post-ganglionic visceral nerve fibres. *J. Physiol. 22:* 215–230.

Lichtman, J.W., D. Purves, and J.W. Yip. 1979. On the purpose of selective innervation of guinea-pig superior cervical ganglion cells. *J. Physiol. 292:* 69–84.

———. 1980. Innervation of neurones in the guinea-pig thoracic chain. *J. Physiol. 298:* 285–299.

Mark, R.F. 1965. Fin movement after regeneration of neuromuscular connections: An investigation of myotypic specificity. *Exp. Neurol. 12:* 292–302.

Matthey, R. 1926. Recuperation de la vue apres

resection des nerfs optiques chez le triton. *C. R. Seances Soc. Biol. 93:* 904.

Miledi, R. and E. Stefani. 1969. Non-selective reinnervation of slow and fast muscle fibres in the rat. *Nature 222:* 569–571.

Muller, K.J. 1979. Synapses between neurones in the central nervous system of the leech. *Biol. Rev. 54:* 99–134.

Njå, A. and D. Purves. 1977a. Specific innervation of guinea-pig superior cervical ganglion cells by preganglionic fibres arising from different levels of the spinal cord. *J. Physiol. 264:* 565–583.

———. 1977b. Re-innervation of guinea-pig superior cervical ganglion cells by preganglionic fibres arising from different levels of the spinal cord. *J. Physiol. 272:* 633–651.

———. 1978. Specificity of initial synaptic contacts made on guinea-pig superior cervical ganglion cells during regeneration of the cervical sympathetic trunk. *J. Physiol. 281:* 45–62.

Purves, D. 1976. Competitive and non-competitive reinnervation of mammalian sympathetic neurones by native and foreign fibres. *J. Physiol. 261:* 453–475.

Purves, D. and J.W. Lichtman. 1978. Formation and maintenance of synaptic connections in autonomic ganglia. *Physiol. Rev. 58:* 821–862.

Purves, D., W. Thompson, and J.W. Yip. 1981. Reinnervation of ganglia transplanted to the neck from different levels of the guinea-pig sympathetic chain. *J. Physiol. 313:* 49–63.

Ready, D.F. and J.G. Nicholls. 1979. Identified neurones isolated from leech CNS make selective connections in culture. *Nature 281:* 67–69.

Schmidt, H. and E. Stefani. 1976. Re-innervation of twitch and slow muscle fibres of the frog after crushing the motor nerves. *J. Physiol. 258:* 99–123.

———. 1977. Action potentials in slow muscle fibres of the frog during regeneration of motor nerves. *J. Physiol. 270:* 507–517.

Schmidt, J.T. 1978. Retinal fibers alter tectal positional markers during the expansion of the half-retinal projection in goldfish. *J. Comp. Neurol. 177:* 279–300.

Schmidt, J.T., C.M. Cicerone, and S.S. Easter. 1978. Expansion of the half retinal projection to the tectum in goldfish: An electrophysiological and anatomical study. *J. Comp. Neurol. 177:* 257–278.

Sperry, R.W. 1943a. Effect of 180 degree rotation of the retinal field on visuomotor coordination. *J. Exp. Zool. 92:* 263–279.

———. 1943b. Visuomotor coordination in the newt (*Triturus viridescens*) after regeneration of the optic nerves. *J. Comp. Neurol. 79:* 33–55.

———. 1944. Optic nerve regeneration with return of vision in anurans. *J. Neurophysiol. 7:* 57–69.

———. 1963. Chemoaffinity in the orderly growth of nerve fiber patterns and connections. *Proc. Natl. Acad. Sci. 50:* 703–710.

Sperry, R.W. and H.L. Arora. 1965. Selectivity in regeneration of the oculomotor nerve in the cichlid fish, *Astronotus ocellatus*. *J. Embryol. Exp. Morphol. 14:* 307–317.

Stone, L.S. 1944. Functional polarization in the retinal development and its reestablishment in regenerating retinae of rotated grafted eyes. *Proc. Soc. Exp. Biol. Med. 57:* 13–14.

Stone, L.S. and I.S. Zaur. 1940. Reimplantation and transplantation of adult eyes in the salamander (*Triturus viridescens*) with return of vision. *J. Exp. Zool. 85:* 243–269.

Van Essen, D.C. and J.K.S. Jansen. 1977. The specificity of re-innervation by identified sensory and motor neurons in the leech. *J. Comp. Neurol. 171:* 433–454.

Wallace, B.G., M.N. Adal, and J.G. Nicholls. 1977. Regeneration of synaptic connexions by sensory neurones in leech ganglia maintained in culture. *Proc. R. Soc. Lond. B 199:* 567–585.

Weiss, P. and A. Hoag. 1946. Competitive reinnervation of rat muscles by their own and foreign nerves. *J. Neurophysiol. 9:* 413–418.

Wigston, D.J. 1980. Suppression of sprouted synapses in axolotl muscle by implanted foreign nerves. *J. Physiol. 307:* 355–366.

Yoon, M.G. 1971. Reorganization of retinotectal projection following surgical operations on the optic tectum in goldfish. *Exp. Neurol. 33:* 395–411.

———. 1973. Retention of original topographic polarity by the 180° rotated tectal reimplant in young adult goldfish. *J. Physiol. 233:* 575–588.

Zipser, B. and R. McKay. 1981. Monoclonal antibodies distinguish identifiable neurones in the leech. *Nature 289:* 549–554.

J. Physiol. (1978), **274**, *pp.* 299–310
With 1 plate and 4 text-figures
Printed in Great Britain

FORMATION AND ELIMINATION OF FOREIGN SYNAPSES ON ADULT SALAMANDER MUSCLE

BY M. J. DENNIS AND J. W. YIP*

*From the Departments of Physiology and Biochemistry,
University of California at San Francisco,
San Francisco, California 94143, U.S.A.*

(*Received 28 April 1977*)

SUMMARY

1. Synapses by flexor nerve were induced on denervated extensor muscle in adult salamander forelimbs. Excitatory potentials evoked by these 'foreign' synapses were at first small but increased to normal amplitude within several weeks, in the absence of correct nerve reinnervation.

2. Upon return of the correct nerve the efficacy of foreign synaptic transmission began to decline. The time of initiation of this decline correlated well with the resumption of correct nerve transmission. The suppression of foreign transmission involved a reduction in mean quantal content of transmitter release.

3. Suppression of foreign synapses was sufficiently thorough that most ceased transmitting entirely. Before reinnervation by the correct nerve 97 % of the extensor muscle fibres received functional foreign synapses while 4–6 months after correct nerve return only 35 % of the fibres retained foreign synapses, with weak transmission.

4. Two lines of evidence indicate that suppressed foreign synapses are lost from the muscle: (*a*) a second correct nerve lesion 6–8 months after the initial denervation produced no significant increase in the proportion of fibres with foreign transmission and (*b*) four muscles which showed complete suppression of foreign transmission were bathed in medium containing horseradish peroxidase (h.r.p.) and the correct nerve was stimulated repetitively. Subsequent histochemical staining for h.r.p. and examination of synapses by electron microscopy revealed that 94 % of the axon terminals had h.r.p. incorporated in vesicles. Thus at least that percentage of all identifiable synapses were from the correct nerve.

5. This ability to eliminate incorrect synapses in favour of correct ones is speculated to be a general characteristic of embryonic nervous systems, which in adulthood is retained by salamanders but lost by most other animals.

INTRODUCTION

Mature neurones and skeletal muscle fibres can be induced through denervation to accept innervation from foreign sources. Whether this foreign innervation remains functional when the correct nerve reinnervates its target is of interest from a developmental point of view. In mammalian skeletal muscle (Bernstein & Guth, 1961;

* Present address: Department of Physiology & Biophysics, Washington University School of Medicine, St. Louis, Mo., U.S.A.

413

Tonge, 1974; Frank, Jansen, Lomo & Westgaard, 1975; Brown, Jansen & Van Essen, 1976) foreign transmission continues unabated upon reinnervation by the correct nerve. The picture is less clear with the teleost fish. Using mostly behavioural criteria, Mark and his collaborators (Marotte & Mark, 1970*a*; Mark & Marotte, 1972) concluded that in cross-innervated extraocular muscles of the carp, the function of foreign synapses was suppressed upon reinnervation by the correct nerve. The absence of degenerating nerve terminals during correct reinnervation led them to propose further that suppressed foreign synapses are morphologically normal but silent (Marotte & Mark, 1970*b*; Mark, Marotte & Mart, 1972). Scott (1975) repeated and extended these experiments on the goldfish but concluded, in contrast, that suppression of foreign synapses did not occur. In addition, Frank & Jansen (1976) found no evidence of foreign synapse suppression with intracellular recording from gill muscles of the perch. A variety of studies in amphibia have indicated a selective preference for correct reinnervation of muscle fibres (Grimm, 1971; Cass, Sutton & Mark, 1973; Fangboner & Vanable, 1974; Hoh, 1971; Schmidt & Stefani, 1976). Moreover, Cass *et al.* (1973), who examined competition between correct and foreign nerve for reinnervation of adult newt muscle, concluded that the suppressed foreign synapses retained their morphological integrity.

In the present study, we have induced cross-innervation of a forelimb extensor muscle in the adult newt and looked for changes in properties of such 'foreign' synapses consequent to correct reinnervation. Our results confirm the finding of Cass *et al.* (1973) that foreign transmission is suppressed upon correct reinnervation. This suppression involves a decline in the quantal content of foreign transmitter release. However, both physiological and morphological evidence suggests that the suppressed synaptic terminals are eliminated from the muscle. Some of these findings have been briefly reported (Yip & Dennis, 1976).

METHODS

Surgical procedures. Adult newts, *Notopthalmus viridescens*, were anaesthetized with tricaine (1/1000 in Ringer solution). The forelimb flexor (humero-antibrachialis) muscle was excised and its nerve displaced laterally to the surface of the extensor (anconeus) muscle. The animals were returned to tanks of tap water and fed weekly with brine shrimp. Two weeks after the initial operation, the correct nerve to the anconeus muscle was crushed in one series of animals and resected in another. In some of these animals, the correct nerve was crushed or resected a second time 6–8 months after the initial nerve lesion.

Physiological recordings. At various times after the correct nerve lesion, the animal was pithed and the entire limb was removed with the third, fourth and fifth nerves. The spinal nerves were dissected through to the inferior and superior brachial nerves, which innervate respectively flexor and extensor musculature in the upper arm (see Grimm, 1971, for further description of innervation pattern). The limb was skinned, pinned on a Sylgard dish with a glass cover-slip bottom and the trunks of the two nerves were drawn into separate suction electrodes. All experiments were performed at room temperature in normal frog Ringer solution of the following composition (in m-mol/l.): NaCl, 120; KCl, 2; $CaCl_2$, 1·8; glucose, 10; HEPES buffer, 4 (pH 7·2).

Intracellular recordings were made using glass micropipettes filled with 4 M-K acetate and having resistances of 50–100 MΩ. The signals were fed through W.P. Instruments M4A amplifiers, 1X gain, and into a Tektronix D11 storage oscilloscope.

The quantal content of foreign nerve transmission was estimated both by the method of failures and from the coefficient of variation of responses (cf. del Castillo & Katz, 1954) evoked by stimulating 200 or more times at a frequency of 0·2 sec^{-1}. There was no significant difference between the values determined for individual fibres by these two methods.

Histological techniques. Active nerve terminals were labelled by stimulating uptake of horseradish peroxidase (h.r.p.) into synaptic vesicle membrane (Heuser & Reese, 1973). The muscle was pinned on Sylgard in a 0·5 ml. chamber and presoaked for an hour in h.r.p. (Worthington 10 mg/ml. normal frog Ringer solution). Equilibration of h.r.p. into the extracellular space was facilitated by squirting the solution on to the muscle with a Pasteur pipette. The nerve of interest was stimulated for 7 min with 10 Hz trains of 1 sec duration at 2 sec intervals. The preparation was then allowed to rest for 3 min. This pattern of stimulation and rest was repeated three times and the muscle allowed to rest in h.r.p. for an hour. The muscle then was extensively washed with frog Ringer solution containing 0-C^{2+}, 10 mM-$MgCl_2$ and 0·5 mM-EGTA. Solutions were changed throughout the wash. The muscle was fixed for 2 hr in a mixture 4 % paraformaldehyde and 2 % glutaraldehyde with 30 mM-HEPES (pH 7·2), left overnight in HEPES buffer, and chopped into slices of 50 μm width. Muscle slices were reacted histochemically with hydrogen peroxide and diaminobenzidine according to the method of Graham & Karnovsky (1966), post-fixed with osmium, embedded in Araldite (Ciba), and thin sections of synapses were obtained randomly throughout the muscles

RESULTS

Properties of normal anconeus fibres. Muscle fibres varied from 2 to 4 mm in length and 20–30 μm in diameter. The resting potentials were in the range of -90 to -110 mV. Spontaneous and evoked e.p.p.s. could be recorded at several sites along the muscle fibre (see also Lehouelleur & Chatelain, 1974 and Dennis, 1975). There was no evidence of electrical coupling between muscle fibres (Dennis, 1975).

To check for multiple innervation, the intensity of stimulus impulses to the nerve was varied in small steps from below threshold to supramaximal. In 120 fibres sampled (eight muscles), twenty-four had a single synaptic input, sixty had two inputs and thirty-six received three inputs. Cholinesterase staining revealed that synapses were distributed at several sites along the length of individual fibres (unpublished observations). Such was also the pattern of innervation of the humero-antibrachialis, the antagonistic flexor muscle whose nerve was used in subsequent cross-innervation studies.

Muscles were checked for inappropriate synaptic inputs by independently stimulating the superior and inferior brachial nerves while recording from single fibres. Of 250 fibres sampled in nine muscles, none received foreign synaptic input.

Innervation of fibres by implanted foreign nerve. About 2 weeks after lesion of the correct nerve, foreign transmission began to appear in some muscle fibres. At this time repeated stimulation of the foreign nerve evoked e.p.p.s of low and variable amplitude, often with intermittent response failures. At longer times after correct nerve lesion the population of fibres innervated by the foreign nerve increased and was virtually complete within one month, provided the correct nerve was kept away. The foreign synaptic responses also increased in magnitude with time, and came to resemble those seen in normally innervated adult fibres; some muscle fibres were multiply-innervated by foreign axons, as indicated by distinct inputs of differing thresholds (Text-fig. 1) and in some the end-plate response was large enough to cause an action potential and twitch.

Decline in quantal content of foreign transmission. Approximately 2–4 weeks after the correct nerve was crushed or 6–8 weeks after it was resected, it began to reinnervate the muscle. The reformed correct synapses rapidly returned to their normal state of suprathreshold transmission (Text-fig. 2A). Conversely, foreign responses evoked subsequent to correct reinnervation were often of low amplitude (Text-fig. 2B) and failures were again frequent. In fibres in which foreign nerve stimulation was so associated with intermittent release failures, the amplitudes of the evoked foreign responses were distributed as predicted by the failures method, using Poisson statistics (cf. del Castillo & Katz, 1954). Furthermore, when the amplitude histogram of these evoked foreign responses was compared to that of the m.e.p.p.s recorded at the same locus, the mean amplitudes of the spontaneous and the unitary evoked events were identical (Text-fig. 3), and were within the normal range (0·5–2·0 mV). Presumably the m.e.p.p.s. in such dually innervated fibres arose from transmitter release by correct as well as foreign terminals. Both the Poisson nature of foreign release and the identity in mean amplitude of spontaneous and foreign-evoked potentials indicate that the small foreign responses seen after correct reinnervation result from a low quantal content, rather than a reduction of quantal unit size or of transmitter sensitivity beneath foreign terminals.

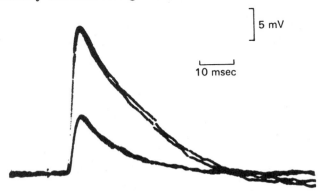

Text-fig. 1. Foreign synaptic responses 45 days after correct nerve resection. The fibre was innervated by two motoneurones as revealed by the increase in response amplitude with increase in the intensity of stimulus impulses to the nerve. Two responses were recorded at each stimulus intensity. No response was obtained from stimulation of the correct nerve.

The quantal content of foreign transmission was estimated in individual fibres at various times after the correct nerve lesion. In both series of animals studied, correct nerve resected and correct nerve crushed, the mean quantal content of foreign transmission declined with time, as illustrated in Text-fig. 4. The initiation of this decline was more rapid following nerve crush than after nerve resection, and was in both situations coincident with the onset of reinnervation by the correct nerve. This suggests that correct reinnervation and foreign suppression are causally related. It should be noted that the data which were used in deriving the mean quantal content at each time point in Text-fig. 4 were taken only from fibres which did show some foreign response. That is, fibres which showed no foreign response ($m = 0$) were not used in calculating the mean. Thus, these figures underestimate the decline in foreign synaptic transmission with time (see below).

At long times after the initial operation there was some regeneration of flexor muscle fibres and these were reinnervated by the flexor nerve. However, such regeneration occurred many weeks after the onset of suppression illustrated in Text-fig. 4. In two muscles where correct reinnervation by chance failed to occur or was sparse, the extent and efficacy of foreign transmission remained high, even 9 months after correct nerve lesion. In both cases the foreign nerve had reinnervated its normal target (flexor) musculature as well.

Decline in extent of foreign transmission. To get another index of the suppression of foreign synapses we asked how the extent of functional foreign innervation changed upon correct reinnervation. At various times after the correct nerve resection, intracellular recordings were made from single muscle fibres and the correct and foreign

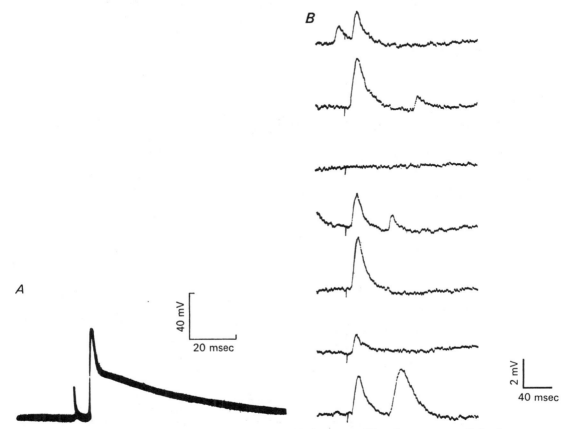

Text-fig. 2. Recordings from a single fibre dually innervated by the correct and foreign nerves, 57 days after the correct nerve resection. *A*, large end-plate response with action potential superimposed evoked by correct nerve stimulation. *B*, consecutive responses to repeated maximal stimulation of the foreign nerve at a frequency of 1 sec⁻¹. A nerve stimulus of constant intensity occurs near the beginning of each sweep, as indicated by the artifact. With some stimuli, the foreign nerve failed to release transmitter (trace 3 from top). Spontaneous potentials appear randomly in several of the traces (1, 2, 4 and 7 from top).

nerves independently stimulated. In ten muscles examined 12–47 days after resection, $97\cdot3 \pm 1\cdot5\%$ of 215 fibres received foreign input, whereas in twenty-nine muscles 57–299 days after resection only 269 of 673 fibres ($39\cdot5 \pm 6\cdot5\%$) had functional foreign input. Thus the extent as well as the efficacy of foreign transmission declined upon reinnervation by the correct nerve, even though the suppression was not always complete.

Second resection of correct nerve 6–8 months after the first. In the light of earlier claims of morphological integrity of suppressed foreign synapses (Mark *et al.* 1972; Cass *et al.* 1973) it was of interest to know the fate of such synapses in our system. To determine whether suppressed foreign synapses could be rapidly reactivated upon loss of correct innervation we resected the correct nerve a second time long after the correct nerve had regenerated (6–8 months after the first resection). In seventeen muscles (383 fibres) sampled 2–20 days after a second correct nerve resection, an average of

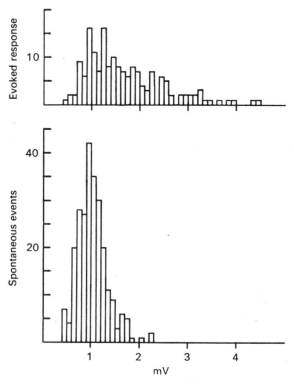

Text-fig. 3. Amplitude histograms of spontaneous (bottom) and foreign evoked (top) responses recorded from a fibre 50 days after correct nerve resection. The foreign nerve was stimulated 294 times with 114 failures. The mean amplitude of the foreign evoked responses = 1·05 mV whilst that of the spontaneous events = 1·08 mV. Stimulation of the correct nerve resulted in an action potential. Medium contained 1·8 mM-Ca^{2+}.

36·2 ± 9·8 % of the fibres had functional foreign inputs. By comparison, in seventeen control muscles (453 fibres), of the same experimental age whose correct nerve had been resected only once 6–8 months earlier, 35·1 ± 7·8 % of the fibres still had some functional foreign innervation. The large standard error of these values reflects the considerable variability encountered from muscle to muscle; in some, no foreign transmission could be detected. The end-plate responses to foreign nerve stimulation were similar in both sets of animals, typically of 1 to several mV amplitude. Thus, foreign transmission did not increase in extent or efficacy, up to 20 days after a second correct nerve resection, at long times after correct reinnervation. Since the initial development of foreign transmission took place in 14–18 days (Text-fig. 4), these results suggest that foreign synapses are not available for reactivation at long times after their suppression. In an initial note (Yip & Dennis, 1976) we erroneously concluded that foreign transmission did increase after a second correct nerve lesion.

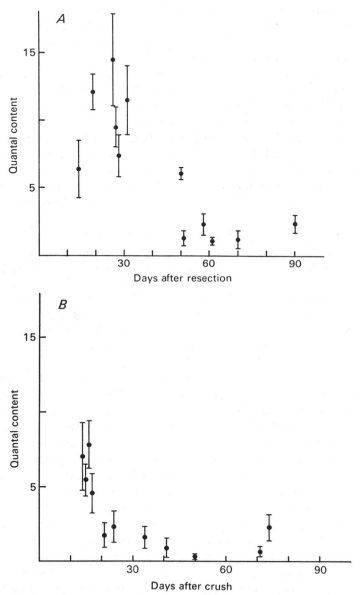

Text-fig. 4. Mean quantal content of foreign nerve release plotted as a function of time after the correct nerve was resected (*A*) and crushed (*B*). Each point is the average of the quantal contents measured in six to ten fibres. Each vertical bar represents the standard error of the mean. Fibres which showed no foreign responses were not used in calculating the mean. Note that the quantal content of foreign transmission becomes higher and remains so longer when the correct nerve is resected.

This error resulted from failure to sample a sufficiently large population of experimental and control muscle fibres.

H.r.p. labelling of active nerve terminals. The best evidence for the existence of morphologically normal but functionless synapses would be a demonstration of their presence by electron microscopy. For this purpose, one would like to be able to distinguish correct from foreign synapses. Cutting the correct nerve so as to use its degeneration products to distinguish it from foreign terminals (Mark *et al.* 1972) is not satisfactory because sprouting of foreign axons might be induced. Therefore, to label correct nerve terminals we made use of the observation of Heuser & Reese (1973) that h.r.p. is taken up by active nerve terminals during vesicle recycling.

To assure ourselves that the technique was applicable in this system, two normal muscles were prepared for h.r.p. experiments, and the correct nerve stimulated as described in Methods. In sixty-one end-plates studied, 95 % were positively labelled as judged by the presence of h.r.p. reaction product on their vesicles. In many of these terminals, more than 50 % of the vesicles were labelled (Pl. 1*A*). This was clearly different from background uptake (Pl. 1*B*), determined in another muscle which was soaked in h.r.p. but not stimulated; here only one or a few vesicles per terminal were labelled.

Normal nerve terminals were characterized by an abundance of clear vesicles, a few with dense cores, mitochondria, occasional neurofilaments, and a thin layer of Schwann cell cytoplasm over their outer surfaces. Terminals were closely apposed to muscle membrane which in some synapses showed well established subsynaptic folds. Their ultrastructure was similar to that reported by Lentz (1969) for the mature newt synapse. Most of the synapses showed only a single nerve ending. Occasionally two or three axon terminals were found apposing a single end-plate, but we do not know whether these were branches of the same axon or were terminals from different motoneurones.

Four cross-innervated muscles which showed no sign of remaining foreign transmission by intracellular recording (125–274 days after correct resection) were prepared for h.r.p. uptake. After correct nerve stimulation 94 ± 3 % of 293 terminals showed positive h.r.p. labelling of their vesicles. To ensure that we were not missing foreign terminals located in a restricted region of the muscle, samples of synapses were taken randomly throughout the muscle; in one case, the long axis of a muscle was cut into three pieces, each was re-embedded and samples taken from each segment. This extent of labelling is like that observed in control experiments on normal muscles (95 %) and suggests that few if any of the synapses on these muscles are foreign. In the absence of physiological signs of foreign innervation following correct re-innervation, foreign terminals are not physically present.

We also studied h.r.p. uptake in two muscles which did not show complete suppression of foreign transmission, 225 and 299 days after correct nerve resection. In these muscles 30 % of the fibres sampled had residual foreign transmission. Upon correct nerve stimulation in h.r.p., 68 % of 150 terminals were labelled, 32 % were not. There was no obvious difference in ultrastructure between labelled and unlabelled terminals.

In one muscle, which by intracellular recording showed no sign of foreign response, 228 days after the initial correct resection the foreign nerve was stimulated in the presence of h.r.p. Of twenty-seven synapses examined all showed no more than background uptake. This negative result served as an additional control against background uptake by unstimulated (in this case, correct) terminals and further supported the conclusion that suppressed foreign terminals are eliminated.

It was of interest to know whether suppression of foreign transmission required direct contact between correct and foreign terminals, especially during the early stages of correct reinnervation when profiles of several terminals are often seen at single end-plates. With this in mind, h.r.p. labelling of the correct nerve was attempted in several muscles at a time when correct reinnervation was in progress. Some of the terminals were labelled and others were not. However, it was not certain that all of these unlabelled terminals were foreign since some of the newly developing correct synapses would be expected not to transmit (Dennis, 1975) due to failure of action potentials to propagate into their terminals (Dennis & Miledi, 1974). Such terminals would not take up h.r.p. To check this possibility we simply denervated and awaited reinnervation of an anconeus muscle, without introducing a foreign nerve. At the time of ongoing reinnervation, the muscle was soaked in h.r.p. and its nerve stimulated as above. Upon examination in EM we here too found multiple axon profiles at single end-plates with some terminals labelled while others were not. Thus, the h.r.p. labelling technique did not permit us to unequivocally distinguish correct from foreign terminals at the time when correct reinnervation was in progress.

DISCUSSION

These results indicate that in adult newt muscle foreign synapses are suppressed as a consequence of correct reinnervation. This suppression involves a decline in the quantal content of transmitter released, with no change in the size of the quantal packets or in the post-synaptic transmitter sensitivity. In most instances this reduction of transmission went to completion and the foreign terminals were eliminated: 35 % of the fibres examined at long times (6–12 months) after correct reinnervation did retain some foreign synaptic function. However, transmission on these fibres too was reduced in that the evoked foreign responses were only a few millivolts in amplitude, in contrast to the suprathreshold foreign responses seen prior to correct reinnervation. Our results do not resolve whether the observed decline in quantal content occurs prior to terminal elimination or whether that decline occurs *as* the terminals are lost.

One would like to know the nature of the signal which initiates the loss of foreign transmission. One possibility is that there is direct contact between foreign and correct terminals which somehow triggers foreign nerve withdrawal. Experiments on errors of innervation made spontaneously during salamander limb regeneration (J. W. Yip & M. J. Dennis, unpublished) indicate that correct and incorrect synapses occur at separate sites on single muscle fibres, and that incorrect synapses are suppressed. This suggests the alternative possibility, that the signal for withdrawal of incorrect synapses is mediated by the target muscle fibre. Such a signal could conceivably involve either a chemical factor released by the target or the pattern of electrical activity of the muscle. Further investigation is necessary before speculation about this mechanism is warranted.

Our conclusion that suppressed synapses are eliminated from the muscle is in striking contrast to the claim of Cass *et al.* (1973) that suppressed synapses are morphologically normal. Two lines of evidence led Mark and his collaborators to believe that there were silent synapses in cross-innervated muscles: (1) the absence of degenerating synapses during correct reinnervation, and (2) the presence of both normal and degenerating synapses several days after a second correct nerve cut. These observations may be explained without invoking the presence of 'silent' synapses. First, upon correct reinnervation, foreign terminals may retract without leaving recognizable degeneration products. Such a mechanism has been indicated in the elimination of polyneuronal innervation of neonatal rat skeletal muscle, in that no morphological signs of synapse degeneration were seen at a time when the number of transmitting synapses was being reduced (Korneliussen & Jansen, 1976). Secondly, the morphologically normal terminals in cross-innervated goldfish fibres observed several days after the correct nerve was cut (Mark *et al.* 1972) may have been those of *functional* foreign synapses: the behavioural test used in that study was not sufficiently sensitive to reveal subthreshold synaptic transmission. More recently, Scott (1975) has questioned whether suppression of foreign transmission occurs at all in goldfish extraocular muscle.

Only 36 % of the muscle fibres examined had functional foreign innervation soon after a second correct nerve resection, 6–8 months after the first. Thus, a second correct nerve lesion produced no significant increase over the 35 % residual foreign transmission seen without a second correct denervation, which was quite distinct from the complete foreign innervation seen after the first correct resection. This indicates that suppressed synapses are not intact. The fact that the residual functional foreign terminals do not sprout to innervate all of the muscle fibres following the second degeneration of correct terminals is somewhat surprising. This may result because the remaining foreign axons are extended beyond their normal scope of innervation and, as a consequence, are not liable to further extension (cf. Brown *et al.* 1976). Such a phenomenon does not, however, seem to be the primary cause of foreign suppression; suppression was well correlated with the time of correct reinnervation, varying according to whether the correct nerve was crushed or resected, regardless of the regeneration and subsequent reinnervation of the normal target of the foreign nerve (m. humero-antibrachialis). Furthermore, in two muscles the correct nerve failed to reinnervate and in those the extent and efficacy of foreign transmission remained high even though the normal target of the foreign nerve was well regenerated and innervated.

Unlike the situation we have described here adult mammalian muscle appears unable to reject foreign innervation once it has been established (Bernstein & Guth, 1961; Frank *et al.* 1975; Brown *et al.* 1976). Urodele amphibia retain in adulthood several embryonic characteristics and in this category perhaps belongs the ability to distinguish foreign from correct synaptic inputs and to suppress the foreign. Consistent with this idea is recent evidence (Yip & Dennis, unpublished) that during newt limb regeneration inappropriate neuromuscular synapses sometimes form but are subsequently removed in favour of the correct ones. Some selectivity in retention of synapses also occurs in adult anuran amphibia. During reinnervation of frog and toad muscles, slow muscle fibres initially receive input from fast motor axons (Schmidt & Stefani, 1976), but this is subsequently replaced by the appropriate slow innervation (Hoh, 1971; Schmidt & Stefani, 1976). Following foreign innervation of the pectoralis muscle of *Xenopus* the original nerve re-establishes synapses, which increase with time in quantal content of evoked transmitter release. When such a junction develops in the same synaptic area as occupied by a foreign axon, the foreign terminal ceases to increase in transmitter output (Haimann, Mallart & Zilber-Gachelin, 1976). This competitive interaction does not occur when correct and foreign terminals are separated by several millimetres. Also upon innervation of ectopically placed frog muscle by two incorrect nerves, there occurs a sorting out of fields such that each nerve synapses with some of the fibres yet with little overlap in the territory of the other nerve (Grinnell, Rheuben & Letinsky, 1977).

The ability of a target cell to distinguish between a variety of presynaptic inputs and eliminate some would be of obvious utility in development and moulding of the central nervous system. The lack of suppression of inappropriate synapses experimentally induced on cells of adult mammals probably results from a loss during maturation of flexibility present in the developing nervous system; such a loss of plasticity with age has been clearly shown in the mammalian visual system (Hubel & Wiesel, 1970). We feel that further examination of normal embryonic development will reveal a mechanism for enhancing the precision of excitable cell interaction such as that described here.

This work was completed in partial fulfilment of the requirements for a Ph.D. degree, to J.W.Y. We would like to thank Greta Fry and Nancy Johnson for their technical assistance and Peter Sargent, Regis Kelly and John Heuser for their comments during the execution of this work. It was supported by N.I.H. Grant no. 5R01 NS10792, and an intramural grant from U.C.S.F.

REFERENCES

BERNSTEIN, J. J. & GUTH, L. (1961). Nonselectivity in establishment of neuromuscular connections following nerve regeneration in the rat. *Expl Neurol.* **4**, 262–275.

BROWN, M. C., JANSEN, J. K. S. & VAN ESSEN, D. (1976). Polyneuronal innervation of skeletal muscle in newborn rats and its elimination during maturation. *J. Physiol.* **261**, 387–422.

CASS, D. T., SUTTON, T. J. & MARK, R. F. (1973). Competition between nerves for functional connections with axolotl muscles. *Nature, Lond.* **243**, 201–203.

DEL CASTILLO, J. & KATZ, B. (1954). Quantal components of the end-plate potential. *J. Physiol.* **124**, 560–573.

DENNIS, M. J. (1975). Physiological properties of junctions between nerve and muscle developing during salamander limb regeneration. *J. Physiol.* **244**, 683–702.

DENNIS, M. J. & MILEDI, R. (1974). Non-transmitting neuromuscular junctions during an early stage of end-plate reinnervation. *J. Physiol.* **239**, 553–570.

FANGBONER, R. F. & VANABLE, J. W. (1974). Formation and regression of inappropriate nerve sprouts during trochlear nerve regeneration in *Xenopus laevis*. *J. comp. Neurol.* **157**, 391–406.

FRANK, E. & JANSEN, J. K. S. (1976). Interaction between foreign and original nerves innervating gill muscles in fish. *J. Neurophysiol.* **39**, 84–90.

FRANK, E., JANSEN, J. K. S., LOMO, T. & WESTGAARD, R. H. (1975). The interaction between foreign and original motor nerves innervating the soleus muscle of rats. *J. Physiol.* **247**, 725–743.

GRAHAM, R. C. & KARNOVSKY, M. J. (1966). The early stages of absorption of injected horseradish peroxidase in the proximal tubule of the mouse kidney: ultrastructural cytochemistry by a new technique. *J. Histochem. Cytochem.* **14**, 291–302.

GRIMM, L. M. (1971). An evaluation of myotypic respecification in axolotls. *J. exp. Zool.* **178**, 479–496.

GRINNELL, A. D., RHEUBEN, M. B. & LETINSKY, M. S. (1977). Mutual repression of synaptic efficacy by pairs of foreign nerves innervating frog skeletal muscle. *Nature, Lond.* **265**, 368–370.

HAIMANN, C., MALLART, A. & ZILBER-GACHELIN, N. F. (1976). Competition between motor nerves in the establishment of neuromuscular junctions in striated muscles of *Xenopus laevis*. *Neurosci. Lett.* **3**, 15–20.

HEUSER, J. E. & REESE, T. S. (1973). Evidence for recycling of synaptic vesicle membrane during transmitter release at the frog neuromuscular junction. *J. Cell Biol.* **57**, 315–344.

HOH, J. F. Y. (1971). Selective reinnervation of fast-twitch and slow-graded muscle fibers in the toad. *Expl Neurol.* **30**, 263–276.

HUBEL, D. H. & WIESEL, T. N. (1970). The period of susceptibility to the physiological effects of eye closure in kittens. *J. Physiol.* **206**, 419–436.

KORNELIUSSEN, H. & JANSEN, J. K. S. (1976). Morphological aspects of the elimination of polyneuronal innervation of skeletal muscle fibres in newborn rats. *J. Neurocytol.* **5**, 591–604.

LEHOUELLEUR, J. & CHATELAIN, A. (1974). Analysis of electrical responses of newt skeletal muscle fibres in response to direct and indirect stimulation. *J. Physiol., Paris* **68**, 615–632.

LENTZ, T. L. (1969). Development of the neuromuscular junction. I. Cytological and cytochemical studies on the neuromuscular junction of differentiating muscle in the regenerating limb of the newt Triturus. *J. Cell Biol.* **42**, 431–443.

MARK, R. F. & MAROTTE, L. R. (1972). The mechanism of selective reinnervation of fish eye muscles. III. Functional, electrophysiological and anatomical analysis of recovery from section of the IIIrd and IVth nerves. *Brain Res.* **46**, 131–48.

MARK, R. F., MAROTTE, L. R. & MART, P. E. (1972). The mechanism of selective reinnervation of fish eye muscles. IV. Identification of repressed synapses. *Brain Res.* **46**, 149–157.

MAROTTE, L. R. & MARK, R. F. (1970a). The mechanism of selective reinnervation of fish eye muscle. I. Evidence from muscle function during recovery. *Brain Res.* **19**, 41–51.

MAROTTE, L. R. & MARK, R. F. (1970b). The mechanism of selective reinnervation of fish eye muscle. II. Evidence from electronmicroscopy of nerve endings. *Brain Res.* **19**, 53–62.

SCHMIDT, H. & STEFANI, E. (1976). Re-innervation of twitch and slow muscle fibres of the frog after crushing the motor nerves. *J. Physiol.* **258**, 99–123.

SCOTT, S. A. (1975). Persistence of foreign innervation on reinnervated goldfish extraocular muscles. *Science, N.Y.* **189**, 644–646.

TONGE, D. A. (1974). Synaptic function in experimental innervated muscle in the mouse. *J. Physiol.* **239**, 968.

YIP, J. W. & DENNIS, M. J. (1976). Supression of transmission at foreign synapses in adult newt muscle involves reduction in quantal content. *Nature, Lond.* **260**, 350–352.

EXPLANATION OF PLATE

PLATE 1

A, cross-section of a normal anconeus end-plate stimulated for h.r.p. uptake as described in text. The nerve terminal, surrounded by a thin layer of Schwann cell cytoplasm, contains synaptic vesicles and a few mitochondria. 48 % of the vesicles contain the electron-dense peroxidase reaction product, indicating that they contain h.r.p.

B, cross-section of a normal anconeus terminal soaked in h.r.p. but not stimulated, to show background uptake. Calibration bar, 0·5 μm.

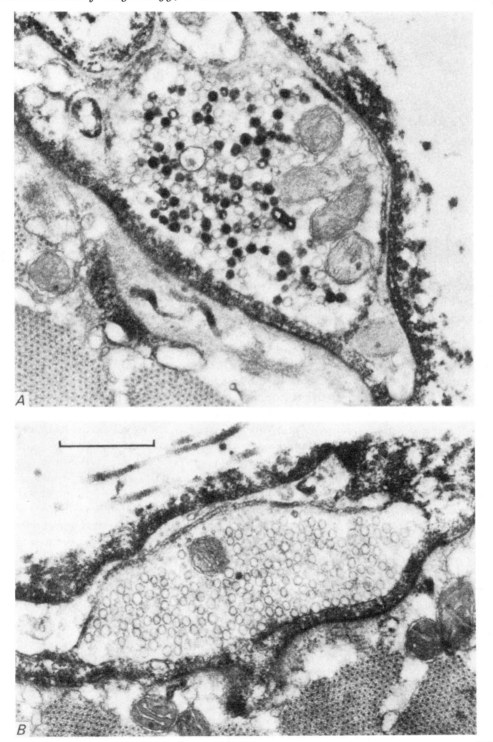

M. J. DENNIS AND J. W. YIP   *(Facing p. 310)*

J. Physiol. (1981), **313**, pp. 49–63

With 1 *plate and* 8 *text-figures*

Printed in Great Britain

RE-INNERVATION OF GANGLIA TRANSPLANTED TO THE NECK FROM DIFFERENT LEVELS OF THE GUINEA-PIG SYMPATHETIC CHAIN

BY DALE PURVES, WESLEY THOMPSON* AND JOSEPH W. YIP†

From the Department of Physiology and Biophysics, Washington University School of Medicine, 660 S. Euclid Avenue, St. Louis, Mo. 63110, U.S.A.

(*Received 17 April 1980*)

SUMMARY

Thoracic and lumbar sympathetic ganglia from donor guinea-pigs were transplanted to the bed of an excised superior cervical ganglion in host animals. Homotopic transplants of superior cervical ganglia served as controls. In this way the same set of preganglionic axons (the cervical sympathetic trunk) was confronted with ganglia from different levels of the sympathetic chain. Re-innervation of the transplants was studied after 3–5 months.

1. Neurones in ganglia transplanted from different levels of the sympathetic chain were re-innervated to about the same over-all degree by the preganglionic axons of the host's cervical sympathetic trunk. Thus, the mean amplitude of post-synaptic potentials, the estimated number of innervating axons, and the number of spinal segments providing innervation to each neurone were similar in transplanted thoracic, lumbar and superior cervical ganglion cells.

2. Neurones in transplanted mid-thoracic ganglia, however, were re-innervated more frequently, and more strongly, by axons arising from more caudal thoracic segments than neurones in transplanted superior cervical ganglia. Stimulation of axons arising from the fourth thoracic spinal segment (T4), for example, elicited post-synaptic potentials that on average were twice as large in transplanted fifth thoracic ganglion cells as in transplanted superior cervical ganglion cells; conversely, axons arising from T1 re-innervated neurones in the superior cervical ganglion about 2–3 times more effectively than fifth thoracic ganglion cells. This difference in the re-innervation of the fifth thoracic and the superior cervical ganglion is in the same direction as (although less pronounced than) the normal difference in the segmental innervation of these ganglia.

3. Transplanted lumbar ganglia were also re-innervated more effectively by relatively caudal segments compared to re-innervated cervical ganglia, but this difference was no greater than that observed for transplanted thoracic ganglia.

4. We conclude that preganglionic axons can distinguish (or be distinguished by) ganglia derived from different levels of the sympathetic chain. Our findings are consistent with the view that ganglion cells have some permanent property that biases the innervation they receive.

* Present address: Department of Zoology, University of Texas, Austin, TX 78712, U.S.A.

† Present address: Department of Physiology, School of Medicine, University of Pittsburgh, Pittsburgh, PA 15261, U.S.A.

INTRODUCTION

The highly specific patterns of neural connexions that characterize the nervous system must arise from a number of different mechanisms, including neuronal differentiation and proliferation, the migration of neurones to a final position, and the guidance of their axons to an appropriate target. A further mechanism of specific connectivity is presumably the ability of axon terminals to form synapses in a selective manner with target cells, contacting those cells which are in some sense correct, while eschewing neighbouring cells within the target that are inappropriate. Although relatively little is known about any of these mechanisms, selective synapse formation has been particularly difficult to study because of the formidable technical problems associated with exploring synapse formation in embryos.

A part of the nervous system in which selective synapse formation has been explored in some detail is the sympathetic chain of adult mammals (see Purves & Lichtman, 1978, for a review). Langley (1892) was the first to observe that stimulation of each ventral root supplying the superior cervical ganglion elicits different end-organ effects, and that these orderly responses to segmental stimulation are re-established upon regeneration of preganglionic fibres (Langley, 1895). Based on these findings, he proposed that preganglionic axons arising from different levels of the spinal cord make preferential connexions with different classes of ganglion cells. The basis of these specific end-organ responses is that each superior cervical neurone is normally innervated by a number of different axons which arise from a contiguous subset of the spinal cord segments that contribute innervation to the ganglion as a whole (Njå & Purves, 1977a; see also Lichtman, Purves & Yip, 1979); when denervated ganglion cells are contacted by regenerating axons, this pattern of innervation is again established (Njå & Purves, 1977b, 1978).

Since there is no obvious way to separate for further investigation the different classes of cells that apparently make up the superior cervical ganglion, it would be of considerable interest if the anatomically separate ganglia of the sympathetic chain also differed from one another with respect to the selective formation of synapses. There is, in fact, some evidence to suggest that the innervation of each ganglion in the sympathetic chain is related to the selective bias observed amongst neurones *within* the superior cervical ganglion. Not only is each ganglion innervated by axons arising from an appreciably different set of spinal segments, but some ganglia are innervated by a relatively restricted subset of the segments whose axons appear to be available to them (Lichtman, Purves & Yip, 1980). In the present work we have explored the selective properties of several different ganglia relative to one another by transplanting cervical, thoracic, and lumbar ganglia to the neck where they become re-innervated by axons of the cervical sympathetic trunk.

Our results show that cervical preganglionic axons can distinguish (or be distinguished by) ganglia transplanted from different levels of the sympathic chain.

METHODS

Transplantation

Mature, inbred guinea-pigs weighing 300–500 g (strain 'Magnum', Biological Systems, Toms River, N.J.) were anaesthesized with pentobarbitone (35 mg/kg, I.P.). In an initial series of

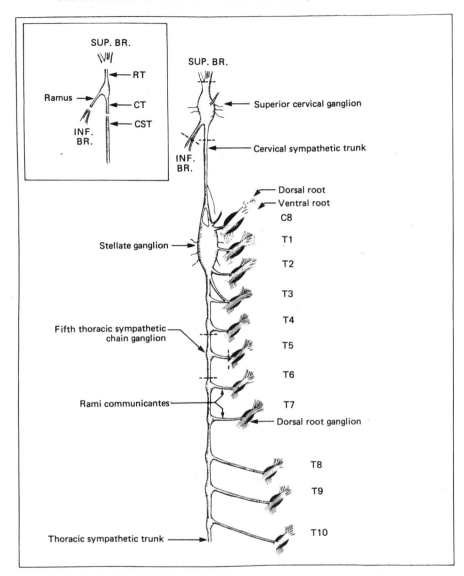

Fig. 1. Diagram of part of the guinea-pig thoracic and cervical sympathetic system used in these experiments (right side shown in ventral view). The ganglia to be transplanted were excised from a donor animal as indicated by the dashed lines. The anastomotic arrangement of implanted fifth thoracic ganglia is shown in the inset. Transplanted superior cervical ganglia were placed in their normal orientation; transplanted lumbar ganglia (not shown) were oriented in the same way as transplanted fifth thoracic ganglia. SUP. BR. = superior post-ganglionic branch; INF. BR. = inferior post-ganglionic branch; RT = rostral sympathetic trunk; CT = caudal sympathetic trunk; CST = pre-ganglionic cervical sympathetic trunk; C8 = eighth cervical segment; T1...T10 = thoracic segments 1–10.

experiments, superior cervical ganglia were removed under sterile conditions from donor animals and transplanted to the position of the excised, right superior cervical ganglion in a host animal of the same sex (in the orientation shown in Fig. 1). In a second series, fifth thoracic ganglia were transplanted from donor animals to the bed of the excised right superior cervical ganglion in a host. In occasional animals the fifth thoracic ganglion was very small; in these instances the fourth or sixth thoracic ganglion was transplanted instead. In a final series of experiments, first lumbar ganglia were transplanted in the same manner. As in transplants from the mid-thoracic level, the L2 or L3 ganglion was sometimes used if L1 was small. In this way, the same set of preganglionic axons was confronted with ganglia transplanted from different rostro-caudal levels of the sympathetic chain.

Electrophysiological examination of transplanted ganglia

After 3–5 months the transplanted ganglia were removed in continuity with the host's cervical sympathetic trunk, thoracic chain, communicating rami, and vertral roots (see Fig. 1); isolated preparations were maintained at room temperature in a bath perfused with oxygenated Ringer fluid (Njå & Purves, 1977a). The ventral roots of the spinal segments that normally contribute axons to the cervical sympathetic trunk (C8–T7) were stimulated with suction electrodes, and the re-innervation of neurones in the transplanted ganglia tested by means of intracellular recording, as in previous experiments (Purves, 1975; Njå & Purves, 1977a, b, 1978). In every neurone impaled we measured the maximum amplitude of the excitatory post-synaptic potential (e.p.s.p.) evoked by individually stimulating the ventral roots C8–T7 and estimated the total number of axons innervating each cell (Purves, 1975; Njå & Purves, 1977a).

Re-innervation of superior cervical ganglia in situ is complete in about 3 months (Njå & Purves, 1977a, 1978), even when the post-ganglionic nerves are also cut (Purves & Thompson, 1979). Thus a 3–5 month inverval between transplantation and the assessment of re-innvervation is probably sufficient to allow establishment of a final pattern. Since in the guinea-pig and other mammals the preganglionic axons in a particular ventral root arise from the corresponding level of the spinal cord (Rubin & Purves, 1980), stimulation of a ventral root activates only those preganglionic axons arising from that spinal segment.

Histological examination of transplanted ganglia

After completion of electrophysiological studies, the transplanted ganglia were treated with Karnovsky's fixative, dehydrated, and embedded in Araldite (Purves, 1975). Semithin sections (1–2 μm) stained with toluidine blue were compared to sections of homologous normal ganglia taken from animals of about the same size. Average cell size was determined with an automated planimeter (Zeiss MOP-3) from outlines of nucleated neuronal profiles drawn with the aid of a camera lucida.

Retrograde labelling with horseradish perioxidase (HRP)

To assess whether peripheral targets had been re-innervated by transplanted ganglion cells, the right eye of three anaesthetized animals was injected with 0·15 ml. HRP solution (10 % w/v in saline, Sigma type VI). After a survival time of 48 hr the transplanted ganglia were removed and fixed; 60 μm frozen sections were treated with tetramethylbenzidine (DeOlmos, Hardy & Heimer, 1978; see also Rubin & Purves, 1980) and counterstained.

RESULTS

Gross and microscopical appearance of transplanted ganglia

Most ganglia looked surprisingly normal 3–5 months after transplantation, and had retained the approximate orientation given them at the time of surgery (Fig. 1). The transplants were, however, only about half as large as their normal homologues. Histological examination showed this shrinkage to result from the death of cells in the interior of transplanted ganglia; thus the surviving neurones formed a rind around a neurone-free central region (Pl. 1; see also Zalewski, 1974). The cells originally in the centre of transplanted ganglia died presumably because of inadequate nutrition prior to revascularization. The size of surviving neuronal somata in the transplants was similar to that of normal ganglion cells (see Pl. 1).

Since mature ganglion cells chronically deprived of target contact lose most of their innervation and degenerate within 3 months (Purves, 1975), it seemed likely that the surviving neurones in transplanted ganglia had sent axons to the periphery. To

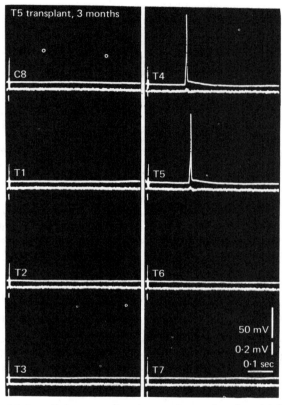

Fig. 2. Example of intracellular recording (upper trace of each pair) from a neurone in a fifth thoracic ganglion transplanted 92 days earlier. Each pair of traces shows response to supramaximal stimulation of the ventral root indicated at the left. A suprathreshold response is elicited by activation of T4 and T5. Lower trace is the compound action potential recorded from the superior post-ganglionic nerve (see Fig. 1). Absence of an appreciable compound action potential to stimulation of ventral roots other than T4 and T5 indicates that the innervation of this transplant was derived primarily from these two segments. Resting potential = -67 mV.

confirm this, HRP was injected into the right eye of three guinea-pigs 5–12 months after transplantation of the fifth thoracic ganglion. Labelled neurones were detected in two of the three ganglia; thus at least some transplanted T5 ganglion cells are able to innervate peripheral targets in locations entirely different from their original targets (see also Purves & Thompson, 1979).

Over-all re-innervation of transplanted ganglia

Neurones in the transplanted ganglia were impaled without difficulty, and showed resting potentials and action potential amplitudes within the normal range (Fig. 2; cf. Purves, 1975). The degree of re-innervation of the transplants was gauged by the percentage of neurones responding to stimulation of one or more ventral roots, the average number of segments contributing innervation to each cell, the number of

TABLE 1. Comparison of the over-all re-innervation of superior cervical, fifth thoracic, and lumbar ganglion cells 3–5 months after transplantation. (means are given ± S.E.)

	Superior cervical ganglion transplants	Fifth thoracic ganglion transplants	Lumbar ganglion transplants
No. of ganglia	36	36	28
No. of neurones impaled	499	491	486
No. of neurones re-innervated	373	354	331
Neurones re-innervated (%)	74·7	72·1	68·1
Mean no. of segments contributing innervation to each neurone	$1·4 \pm 0·1$	$1·3 \pm 0·1$	$1·4 \pm 0·1$
Mean no. of preganglionic axons innervating each neurone	$1·9 \pm 0·1$	$1·6 \pm 0·1$	$2·1 \pm 0·1$
Total mean e.p.s.p. amplitude recorded in each neurone (sum of the segmental responses in mV)	$14·2 \pm 0·6$	$15·0 \pm 0·7$	$14·2 \pm 0·7$

axons innervating each ganglion cell, and the sum of the average e.p.s.p. amplitudes elicited by stimulation of the ventral roots C8–T7. There was no difference in the re-innervation of the ganglia transplanted from different rostro-caudal levels by any of these criteria (Table 1).

Transplanted ganglion cells were, however, contacted by only about a third as many preganglionic axons as superior cervical ganglia re-innervated *in situ* (Njå & Purves, 1977b, 1978), or re-innervated *in situ* after post-ganglionic axotomy (Purves & Thompson, 1979), and by only about one-fifth as many preganglionic axons as normal neurones (Njå & Purves, 1977a). The reasons for the generally weak re-innervation of transplanted ganglion cells are uncertain, but probably include failure of many preganglionic axons to reach the transplant and the lack of attraction between preganglionic axons and ganglion cells during the time that post-ganglionic axons are actually regenerating (Purves & Thompson, 1979). A further difference from normal ganglia was that post-synaptic potentials recorded in the neurones of particular transplanted ganglia were often elicited at about the same threshold and with the same latency, suggesting that a single regenerated axon had made synaptic contact with many of the cells in the transplant. Normally only a small percentage of the total number of ganglion cells is innervated by a particular axon (D. J. Wigston and D. Purves, unpublished). This difference is presumably due to the smaller number of neurones and innervating axons in the transplants.

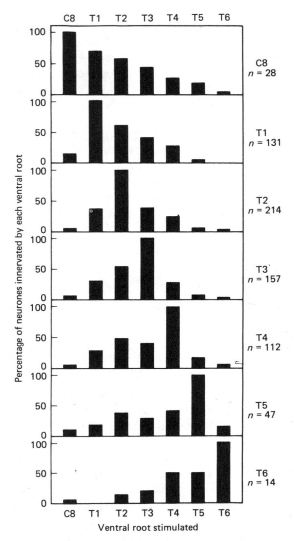

Fig. 3. Likelihood of other segments innervating neurones receiving synapses from particular spinal levels. Each histogram is based on all the neurones in transplanted superior cervical ganglia innervated by a particular ventral root (indicated to right). Selective re-innervation (see text) is apparent, even though this must be impeded by the failure of appropriate axons to reach the transplant in many instances, and by the generally less effective re-innervation by preganglionic axons arising from the more caudal segments represented in the cervical trunk (Njå & Purves, 1977b). Only one cell of 499 was re-innervated by preganglionic axons arising from T7.

Selective re-innervation of transplanted superior cervical ganglion cells

An important question is whether the re-innervation of transplanted ganglia continues to reflect the selective mechanisms that operate during re-innervation *in situ*. It might be, for example, that the period of poor nutrition that precedes revascularization abolishes selectivity, or that selectivity cannot be expressed in the face of the generally weak re-innervation that characterizes transplants. In fact, the overall weakness of innervation to the transplants made it difficult to use contiguity of segmental origin as a measure of selectivity during re-innervation (see Njå & Purves, 1977 a, b, 1978). We could, however, ask if neurones innervated by axons from a relatively rostral segment (C8, for example) were appreciably different in their

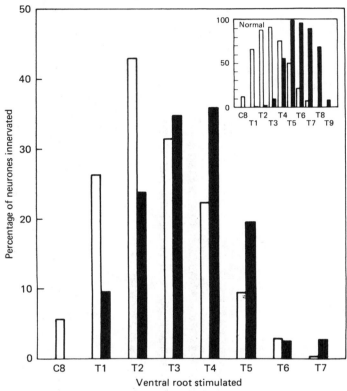

Fig. 4. Percentage of neurones in transplanted superior cervical ganglia (open bars; $n = 499$) and transplanted fifth thoracic ganglia (filled bars; $n = 491$) re-innervated by preganglionic axons arising from the different spinal segments. Inset (redrawn from Lichtman *et al.* 1980) shows the segmental innervation of these two ganglia in normal animals.

predilection for innervation from other segments compared to neurones innervated by axons arising from a relatively caudal segment (T6, for example). As in normal (Njå & Purves, 1977a) and re-innervated superior cervical ganglia (Njå & Purves, 1977b), transplanted superior cervical neurones innervated by axons arising from rostral segments showed a higher probability of being co-innervated by axons from adjacent rostral segments; conversely, neurones innervated by axons arising from relatively caudal segments showed a higher probability of being co-innervated by axons arising from adjacent caudal segments (Fig. 3). Thus, selective mechanisms are still able to influence the re-innervation of transplanted ganglion cells.

Re-innervation of transplanted ganglia by preganglionic axons arising from different levels of the thoracic spinal cord

(a) *Comparison of the segmental re-innervation of superior cervical and fifth thoracic ganglia.*

Although the over-all degree of re-innervation of ganglion cells transplanted from different rostro-caudal levels was similar, there was a difference in the segmental

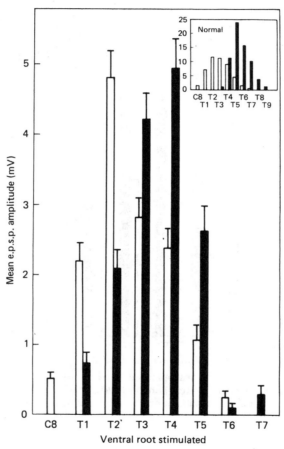

Fig. 5. Mean amplitude ($\pm$s.e.) of synaptic responses elicited by stimulation of each ventral root in transplanted superior cervical (open bars; $n = 499$) and fifth thoracic ganglion cells (filled bars; $n = 491$) after 3–5 months. A similar result was obtained if the estimated number of innervating axons from each segment was used as the index of re-innervation. Inset shows amplitude distribution in normal ganglia (from unpublished observations of J. W. Lichtman, D. Purves and J. W. Yip).

origin of the axons that best re-innervated homo- and heterotopic transplants. Thus, fifth thoracic ganglion cells tended to be re-innervated more strongly by axons arising from relatively caudal thoracic segments; conversely, control superior cervical transplants were better re-innervated by relatively rostral segments. This difference was apparent whether the criterion of re-innervation was simply the number of neurones contacted by axons arising from each ventral root (Fig. 4), the average e.p.s.p. amplitude elicited by stimulation of each ventral root (Fig. 5), or the distribution of those ventral roots supplying the strongest (dominant) innervation to each ganglion cell (Fig. 6).

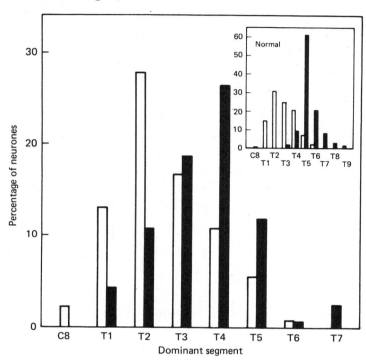

Fig. 6. Fraction of neurones in transplanted cervical and thoracic ganglia dominated by innervation arising from different ventral roots using e.p.s.p. amplitude as the criterion of segmental dominance. Open bars = transplanted superior cervical ganglion cells ($n = 499$); filled bars = transplanted fifth thoracic neurones ($n = 491$). Inset (redrawn from Njå & Purves, 1977 *a*, and Lichtman *et al*. 1980) shows distribution of dominant segments in these two ganglia in normal animals.

The caudally shifted re-innervation of transplanted fifth thoracic ganglia might reflect the influence of selective synapse formation observed *within* transplanted superior cervical ganglia. Alternatively, the caudally shifted segmental pattern might be due to a relative failure of rostral axon regeneration. When we compared the strength of T1 and T4 innervation to those cells in the fifth thoracic transplants that received contacts from *both* these segments it was apparent that the fifth thoracic ganglion cells preferred T4 innervation even when T1 innervation was available (Table 2). This suggests that the tendency of transplanted fifth thoracic ganglion cells to be re-innervated by the more caudally derived axons in the sympathetic trunk is due to some quality of the transplanted ganglion cells rather than to a systematic failure of rostral axons to reach the heterotopic transplants.

TABLE 2. Comparison of innervation from T1 and T4 preganglionic axons to those neurones in transplanted thoracic and lumbar ganglia receiving contacts from *both* these segments. Means are given ± S.E.)

Fifth thoracic ganglion cells receiving innervation
from both T1 and T4 ($n = 15$)

	T1	T4
Mean e.p.s.p. amplitude (mV)	3·0 ± 0·7	13·3 ± 2·8
Mean no. of axons	1·1 ± 0·1	1·7 ± 0·2
Mean depolarization/axon (mV)	2·8 ± 0·6	8·0 ± 1·2

Lumbar ganglion cells receiving innervation
from both T1 and T4 ($n = 27$)

	T1	T4
Mean e.p.s.p. amplitude (mV)	8·5 ± 1·5	7·3 ± 1·6
Mean no. of axons	1·4 ± 0·1	1·4 ± 0·1
Mean depolarization/axon (mV)	6·0 ± 1·2	5·4 ± 1·3

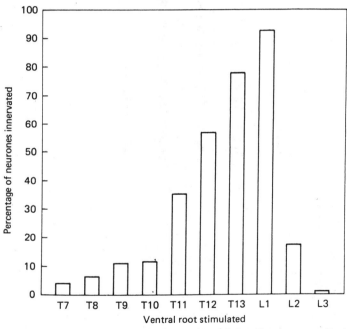

Fig. 7. Percentage of neurones ($n = 199$) in normal first lumbar ganglia innervated by preganglionic axons arising from different spinal segments.

(b) *Segmental re-innervation of transplanted lumbar ganglia*

These results with mid-thoracic transplants raise the question of whether a ganglion transplanted from a still more caudal level of the sympathetic chain might cause an even greater bias during re-innervation. We thus undertook another series of experiments in which a lumbar ganglion was transplanted to the neck.

Impalements of 199 neurones in the first lumbar ganglion from thirteen unoperated animals showed that this ganglion *normally* receives innervation from axons arising from T7–L2, the largest contribution arising from the corresponding spinal cord segment, L1 (Fig. 7). Thus the first lumbar ganglion normally shares little or no preganglionic innervation with the superior cervical ganglion. A somewhat smaller number of segments ($3 \cdot 1 \pm 0 \cdot 1$) and axons ($8 \cdot 0 \pm 0 \cdot 3$) innervated normal L1 neurones compared with normal fifth thoracic ganglion cells (Lichtman *et al.* 1980), or superior cervical ganglion cells (Njå & Purves, 1977*a*).

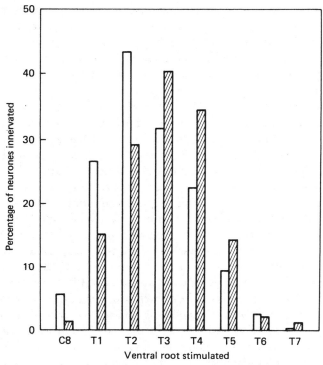

Fig. 8. Percentage of neurones in transplanted lumbar ganglia (crosshatched bars, $n = 486$) re-innervated by preganglionic axons from different spinal levels compared with the re-innervation of transplanted superior cervical ganglia (open bars; redrawn from Fig. 4). The segmental origin of the innervation to transplanted lumbar ganglia is shifted caudally compared to the innervation of transplanted superior cervical ganglia, but no more so than the innervation of transplanted mid-thoracic ganglia (cf. Fig. 4).

The segmental distribution of innervation to *transplanted* lumbar ganglia was also shifted caudally compared with transplanted superior cervical ganglia (Fig. 8), but no more so than the segmental origin of innervation to transplanted fifth thoracic ganglia (cf. Fig. 4). Thus this more caudal ganglion did not lead to re-innervation by more caudally derived axons than a mid-thoracic ganglion. In spite of this, transplanted lumbar ganglia did not appear to be entirely equivalent to mid-thoracic ganglia. For example, those lumbar ganglion cells innervated by *both* T1 and T4 axons, unlike fifth thoracic neurones, did not show a clear preference for T4 axons (Table 2). This somewhat paradoxical finding suggests that while most transplanted lumbar ganglion cells prefer relatively caudal axons, *some* also attract T1 axons; a possible explanation of this result is considered in the Discussion.

DISCUSSION

The major finding of these experiments is that a given set of regenerating axons, the preganglionic fibres in the cervical sympathetic trunk, is able to distinguish (or be distinguished by) ganglia transplanted from different levels of the sympathetic chain. Although the neurones in the various transplanted ganglia were re-innervated to about the same over-all degree, cervical trunk axons arising from upper thoracic segments were more effective in re-innervating the superior cervical ganglion than thoracic or lumbar ganglia. Conversely, axons arising from the more caudal thoracic levels represented in the cervical trunk were more effective in re-innervating thoracic and lumbar ganglia.

Nearly a century ago, Langley (1895) proposed that the innervation of ganglion cells might be influenced by a 'chemiotactic' affinity between particular ganglion cells and preganglionic axons arising from different levels of the spinal cord. This idea, expressed in a more general form by Sperry (1963), has come to be called the chemoaffinity hypothesis of specific neuronal connectivity. Because the discrimination made by cervical trunk axons is in the same direction as the normal segmental difference in the innervation of the superior cervical and more caudal ganglia, average chemical differences between these anatomically distinct neuronal populations may explain our results. Several other factors, however, must be considered.

First, the segmental origin of the innervation of the heterotopic ganglion transplants is abnormal, presumably because the pool of axons available to them is quite different from the pool that would be available at their normal level in the sympathetic chain. For example, some fifth thoracic ganglion cells are normally contacted by axons arising from T8–T10, which do not run as far rostral as the cervical trunk (Lichtman *et al.* 1980). Moreover, there are fewer axons from T5–T7 (which normally provide most of the innervation to the fifth thoracic ganglion) in the cervical sympathetic trunk than in the mid-thoracic preganglionic nerves (see, for example, Rubin & Purves, 1980). The cervical sympathetic trunk is therefore incapable of fully restoring the normal segmental innervation of the fifth thoracic ganglion. This may explain the fact that the normal difference in the average innervation of the superior cervical ganglion and fifth thoracic ganglion is about two to three segments, while after transplantation the average difference is only about $1\frac{1}{2}$–2 segments (see Figs. 4–6). The same argument of course applies to transplanted lumbar ganglia. In sum, the final pattern of innervation established in the transplants is probably a compromise between selective criteria and the compatibility of those axons which are available (see also Lichtman *et al.* 1980).

Secondly, one might expect the innervation of a particular ganglion (or ganglion cell) to reflect not only preference for axons arising from a particular segmental level, a phenomenon which appears to be based on the *positional* attributes of the pre- and post-synaptic cells (Lichtman *et al.* 1980), but on functional modality as well. The three ganglia we have examined are presumably made up of neurones that are substantially different in this regard. While functions like piloerection are almost

438

certainly represented in each ganglion, other functions such as pupillary dilatation, cardioacceleration, and the control of various viscera must be distributed unevenly along the sympathetic chain. Thus, it is quite possible that preganglionic innervation arising from a particular level might be unattractive to a transplanted ganglion cell on positional grounds, but be attractive according to some functional criterion. A conflict of this sort might explain why those transplanted lumbar cells innervated by both T1 and T4 showed a roughly equal preference for these axons (Table 2), while the ganglion as a whole preferred caudal to rostral preganglionic innervation (Fig. 8).

Finally, it is possible that something other than (or in addition to) selective synapse formation contributes to the bias we have observed. Since each transplanted ganglion was accompanied by a short stump of preganglionic nerve (see Fig. 1), regenerating axons could conceivably have responded to guidance cues provided by degenerating preganglionic axons or axon terminals (or non-neural cells), rather than to synaptogenic cues provided by the ganglion cells themselves. Differences in the size of the transplanted ganglia (see Fig. 1 and Lichtman *et al.* 1980) might also have influenced re-innervation in some systematic way.

The simplest explanation of the results of ganglion transplantation, however, and the one most consistent with our previous findings (Njå & Purves, 1977*a*, *b*, 1978; Purves & Thompson, 1979; Lichtman *et al.* 1980), is that each ganglion cell has some permanent quality that selectively influences the innervation it receives. The finding that this quality is, on average, different in at least some of the ganglia that make up the sympathetic chain may allow a further analysis of the basis of selective synapse formation.

We are grateful to J. W. Lichtman for much helpful discussion, to R. I. Hume, D. A. Johnson, E. Rubin, J. R. Sanes and D. J. Wigston for critical comments, and to E. C. E. Gordon for valuable assistance. This work was supported by U.S.P.H.S. grant NS-11699, a grant from the Muscular Dystrophy Association of America, and Training Grant T32-NS-07071 to W. Thompson.

REFERENCES

DeOlmos, J., Hardy, H. & Heimer, L. (1978). The afferent connections of the main and accessory olfactory bulb formations in the rat: an experimental HRP study. *J. comp. Neurol* **181**, 213–244.

Langley, J. N. (1892). On the origin from the spinal cord of the cervical and upper thoracic sympathetic fibres, with some observations on white and grey rami communicantes. *Phil. Trans. R. Soc.* **183**, 85–124.

Langley, J. N. (1895). Note on regeneration of pre-ganglionic fibres of the sympathetic. *J. Physiol.* **18**, 280–284.

Lichtman, J. W., Purves, D. & Yip, J. W. (1979). On the purpose of selective innervation of guinea-pig superior cervical ganglion cells. *J. Physiol.* **292**, 69–84.

Lichtman, J. W., Purves, D. & Yip, J. W. (1980). Innervation of sympathetic neurones in the guinea-pig thoracic chain. *J. Physiol.* **298**, 285–299.

Njå, A. & Purves, D. (1977*a*). Specific innervation of guinea-pig superior cervical ganglion cells by preganglionic fibres arising from different levels of the spinal cord. *J. Physiol.* **264**, 565–583.

Njå, A. & Purves, D. (1977*b*). Re-innervation of guinea-pig superior cervical ganglion cells by preganglionic fibres arising from different levels of the spinal cord. *J. Physiol.* **272**, 633–651.

Njå, A. & Purves, D. (1978). Specificity of initial synaptic contacts on guinea-pig superior cervical ganglion cells during regeneration of the cervical sympathetic trunk. *J. Physiol.* **281**, 45–62.

Purves, D. (1975). Functional and structural changes in mammalian sympathetic neurones following interruption of their axons. *J. Physiol.* **252**, 429–463.

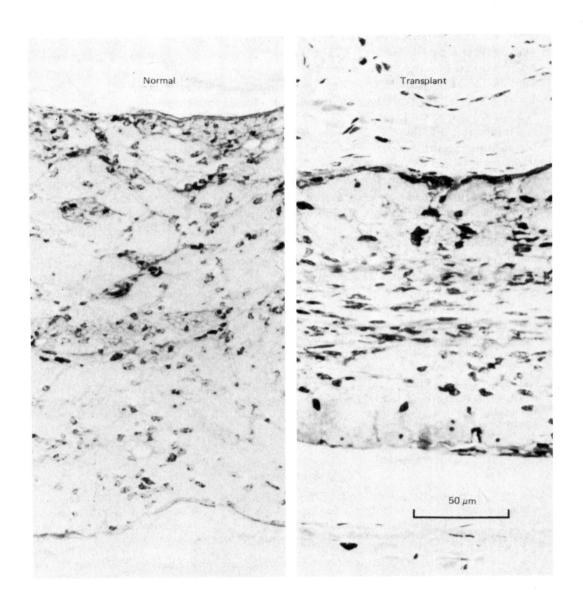

D. PURVES, W. THOMPSON AND J. W. YIP

(Facing p. 63)

PURVES, D. & LICHTMAN, J. W. (1978). Formation and maintenance of synaptic connections in autonomic ganglia. *Physiol. Rev.* **58**, 821–861.

PURVES, D. & THOMPSON, W. (1979). The effects of postganglionic axotomy on selective synaptic connexions in the superior cervical ganglion of the guinea-pig. *J. Physiol.* **297**, 95–110.

RUBIN, E. & PURVES, D. (1980). Segmental organization of sympathetic preganglionic neurons in the mammalian spinal cord. *J. comp. Neurol.* **192**, 163–174.

SPERRY, R W. (1963). Chemoaffinity in the orderly growth of nerve fiber patterns and connections. *Proc. natn. Acad. Sci. U.S.A.* **50**, 703–709.

ZALEWSKI, A. A. (1974). Trophic functions of neurons in transplanted neonatal ganglia. *Expl Neurol* **45**, 189–193.

EXPLANATION OF PLATE

Typical histological appearance of a normal fifth thoracic ganglion (left), and a fifth thoracic ganglion 3–5 months after transplantation (right). Normal neurones are evenly distributed throughout the thickness of the ganglion; after transplantation, neurones are present near the ganglion surface, but are absent in its centre. Sections are from the mid-region of each ganglion: the dorsal surface is uppermost.

Reprinted from Experimental Neurology
Copyright © 1963 by Academic Press Inc.

Volume 7, Number 1, January 1963
Printed in U. S. A.

Experimental Neurology **7**, 46-64 (1963)

Preferential Selection of Central Pathways by Regenerating Optic Fibers

Domenica G. Attardi and R. W. Sperry[1]

Division of Biology, California Institute of Technology, Pasadena, California

Received September 28, 1962

The time-course and general features of optic nerve regeneration in goldfish were followed in sections prepared at spaced intervals between 3 and 67 days after nerve section. Differential route and destination preferences of fibers from different parts of the retina were then tested by removing specific portions of the retina in combination with complete section of the optic nerve. With the dorsal half of the retina destroyed, surviving ventral fibers became segregated beyond the nerve scar and selectively entered the medial tract to connect with dorsal tectum. Conversely, when dorsal retina remained intact, the regenerating fibers filled selectively the lateral tract and the ventral tectum. Fibers from the posterior (temporal) hemiretina invaded the anterior portion of the tectum and did not extend into the posterior regions. Conversely, those from the anterior hemiretina bypassed the anterior zones to innervate the posterior tectum. Fibers from the center of the retina, after reaching the parallel layer within the tectum, bypassed the plexiform layer in the margin to connect only in the central zone. The plexiform layer in the marginal zones was innervated only when fibers were available from the peripheral retina. The results furnish direct microscopical evidence for the orderly selective termination of optic fibers in the brain centers. They also demonstrate a remarkable and unexpected (presumably chemotactic) selectivity in the tendency of different retinal fiber groups to choose and to follow specific central pathways en route to their synaptic destinations. The thesis that specific chemical affinities govern the formation and maintenance of neuronal associations is extended on the basis of the present results to include the patterning of central fiber pathways.

Introduction

Regeneration of the severed optic nerve in fishes and amphibians leads, under optimal conditions, to good recovery of visual function (21).

[1] This investigation was supported in part by the Frank P. Hixon Fund and by a PHS research grant (M3372) from the National Institute of Mental Health, Public Health Service. A brief presentation of the results was made at the 1960 Fall meetings of the American Physiological Society (3).

46

442

The perception of color, directionality, movement and pattern as well as visual acuity have all been shown to be recovered at a high level approximating that of normal vision. Further, visual discrimination habits involving color, brightness and pattern, learned by fishes prior to section of the optic nerve are reinstated by the regeneration process and in cichlids, *Astronotus ocellatus*; these have been found to exhibit interocular transfer and to survive the combined ablation of forebrain plus cerebellum (1, 2).

The collected evidence including histological observations and mapping data obtained with localized tectal lesions (16-21) was taken to indicate that the regenerating fibers re-establish their central connections on an orderly plan that systematically reduplicates the original topographic projection of the retina on the tectum in accordance with the projection pattern characteristic of the species. It has been suggested that the establishment of this topographic projection may be regulated by specific chemical affinities between matching loci in retinal and tectal fields respectively, the affinities being established by embryonic differentiation gradients that sweep over retina and tectum early in development, first, along the rostrocaudal axis and then the dorsoventral axis.

Extension of the experiments into early embryonic stages has brought more direct evidence for the presence of at least the two main retinal gradients and for the respective timing of their establishment (22, 23). Recent mapping of retinally evoked electrical potentials in the tectum of anurans following optic nerve regeneration by Gaze (4, 5) and by Lettvin, Maturana and associates (12, 13) has brought further support for the inference that the regenerating optic axons achieve selective reconnection with their original loci of termination.

A question long at issue in the foregoing is whether the experimental data including the electrophysiological maps might not be accounted for without assuming any orderly regeneration of central connections. It has been pointed out that certain coding-decoding schemes might in theory account for all the observed behavioral data without the assumption of anything more than a randomized reconnection (11). The available data could also be accounted for in terms of the resonance principle of Weiss (24), which was designed expressly to explain organized function within randomized networks, and in networks deranged by surgery and misregeneration.

Neither the lesion nor the electrical mapping studies have been decisive on this question, in part because of uncertainty as to whether the observed scotomata and the tectal potentials reflect presynaptic or postsynaptic effects. Postsynaptic activity could yield the orderly maps obtained after a purely haphazard regrowth if something caused the resultant synapses to be functionally effective only within the appropriate loci. This might be the case, for example, in the above resonance or coding schemes. The exact source of the tectal potentials is considered uncertain by Gaze (4-6), while Maturana and his colleagues (14) favored the terminal arborizations of the optic axons as the probable origin. In the latter case the possibility of random meandering and widespread arborization is not excluded. The electrical studies of Gaze (6) and Jacobsen (8) have suggested the possibility of a scheduled timing of fiber ingrowth and the presence of an early diffuse nonlocalized phase of regeneration that subsequently may or may not be transformed into a systematized topographic organization. They have also pointed out another complicating factor in the presence of a previously unrecognized projection of each retina to the ipsilateral as well as to the contralateral tectum (7). The overlapping ipsilateral projection is not in register with the main contralateral projection.

The following was undertaken in the hope that some of the above and other uncertainties about the regeneration process might be clarified. The experiments, started in 1958, were undertaken on the supposition that the sectioned optic fibers probably remain fortuitously scrambled in regeneration until they regain the plexiform layer of the tectum, an inference drawn from earlier results on the frog (21). It thus proved something of a surprise to find evidence of highly discriminative, presumably chemotactic, differences among the regenerating fiber groups enabling them to select and to follow preferentially their own original pathways en route to their specific terminal stations.

Materials and Procedure

Most of the experiments were carried out on goldfish, *Carassia aurata*, about 5 to 9 cm in standard length. Selected aspects of the work as mentioned in context below were repeated in the cichlid, *Astronotus ocellatus*, in which the visual system is more highly developed. Results in the two species were essentially the same; the following text applies principally to the goldfish unless otherwise indicated.

Normal Anatomy with Reference to the Regeneration Problem. The main retinal projection to the optic tectum in the goldfish is diagrammed in Fig. 1. The optic nerves cross completely at the chiasm so that each eye connects to the contralateral optic lobe. Before entering the midbrain tectum the primary optic tract divides into two main bundles, the medial and lateral optic tracts. These course along the medial and lateral circumference of the optic lobe, respectively, giving off fibers all along the periphery which they turn radially into the optic tectum where they run in a superficial parallel layer to reach their local synaptic zones.

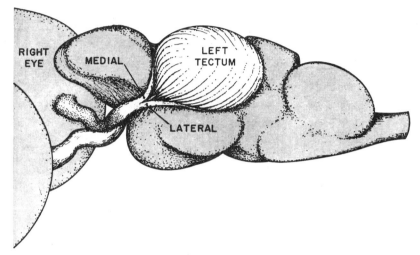

FIG. 1. Schematic drawing of goldfish optic system showing division of main optic tract into medial and lateral bundles and their relations with midbrain tectum.

The medial tract, as shown below, consists of fibers arising in the ventral part of the retina. The fibers spread fanlike into the dorsal portion of the tectum from its medial border. Conversely, the fibers of the lateral tract arise in the dorsal retina and spread from the ventral border of the lobe into its ventral and lateral areas.

Along the circumference of the tectum small bundles of fibers separate from the main medial and lateral tracts to enter the tectum where they then proceed in a relatively straight, roughly parallel course toward the center of the optic lobe. Fibers originating in the posterior (temporal) quadrants of the retina are destined for the anterior or rostral quadrants of the optic lobe and accordingly they leave the main tracts earlier, whereas those from the anterior (nasal) retina remain in the tracts until they reach the posterior regions of the tectum.

After the fibers have run their course in the superficial parallel layer of the tectum they exit from this layer by dipping centrally into an underlying plexiform layer. In accordance with the principle of topographic correspondence between retina and tectum, fibers arising from the outer periphery of the retina exit from parallel to plexiform layers abruptly after entering the tectum. Whereas those from more and more central points along a given retinal radius successively delay their entrance into the plexiform layer until reaching correspondingly more central zones of the tectum.

Thus the normal central course of the optic fibers is so laid out that, in effect each regenerating optic axon finds itself confronted by a kind of multiple Y-maze. In order to return to the tectum by its own original pathway, a given regenerating axon must first select correctly the medial or the lateral tract. After that comes a continuous series of decision points along the circumference of the tectum at each of which the fiber can either turn radially into the parallel layer of the tectum or continue to push ahead tangentially in the main tract. Upon entering the parallel layer of the tectum, each fiber again meets a series of choice points as it advances from periphery to center wherein it can either dip downward into the plexiform layer or continue to grow on farther centrally within the parallel layer.

Finally, after entering the plexiform layer the different types of retinal fibers must again select presumably the proper tectal units for appropriate patterns of synapsis, not only with reference to tectal topography and directionality in vision but also with respect to other dimensions of physiological specificity. For example, fibers for red, blue, green, and yellow, those for luminous flux, the "on", "on-off" and "off" fibers, and perhaps other specialized detector types (11–14), must each form its own characteristic pattern of tectal linkages after arrival at the correct locus of the tectal map. Within the plexiform layer it can be seen that the fibers begin to bifurcate and the branches get thinner than the parent fiber, lose their myelin, and no longer run parellel, but course erratically in all directions, eventually to synapse with tectal neurons.

Experimental Plan. In a first group of thirty-nine goldfish one optic nerve was severed in order to study the time-course of optic fiber regeneration in sections prepared at spaced intervals varying between 3 and 67 days after nerve section. In cases with fully regenerated nerves, the fiber pattern within the nerve, tracts, and in the parallel and plexus layers of the tectum were compared with those of normal fish.

In a second group of seventy-four fishes, removal of a large sector of one retina was combined with section of the optic nerve of the same side in order to determine the course taken by the fibers regenerating from the remaining intact retinal areas, as follows:

(a) Ventral-dorsal series. The ventral (or, in other cases, the dorsal) half of one retina was removed and the optic nerve of the same side completely severed. As a control in some cases, the opposite nerve was sectioned as well.

(b) Anterior-posterior series. The anterior (or the posterior) half of one retina was removed and the optic nerve of the same or both sides completely severed.

(c) Central-peripheral series. A partial or complete peripheral ring of retina was removed and one or both optic nerves severed.

Many of the operated fish yielded little or no information owing to inadequate differentiation of the stain, poor placement or excessive extension of the retinal lesion, inadequate regeneration, poor plane of section, and other factors encountered in the early exploratory procedures. Further cases were prepared in each series until a convincing mass of evidence was obtained. The described results represent a composite impression drawn from the total but based largely on the several best cases in each series. In most cases the histology was checked at 17 to 25 days after nerve section, though a few were taken earlier and later for special purpose.

Surgical Procedure. The surgery was performed out of water under a stereoscopic microscope. The fish were anesthetized in a 0.5% solution of tricaine methanesulphonate (MS 222 Sandoz Chemical Co.) in conditioned tap water. The anesthetized fish was wrapped in a wet cloth and placed in a plasticene mold to hold it in the desired position. Anesthesia was maintained during surgery by dropping a dilute solution of tricaine over the gills.

The nerve section was performed within the orbit. The approach was posterodorsal with the eyeball tilted anteroventrally. The nerve was severed fairly close to the eyeball at about one-fourth of its length to the chiasma. The nerve was cut and broken with finely pointed forceps leaving intact only a small strand of the outer dural sheath. This remnant of the outer sheath was left to hold the nerve stumps close together and to serve as a bridge for the regenerating fibers.

The retinal lesions were made in different ways. In the earlier cases the retina was approached through the pupil after cutting the cornea and lifting the lens. The area of retina to be removed was pinched and teased with fine forceps after which the fragments were delicately sucked away. The lens was then replaced and the shreds of the cornea rejoined.

In the majority of cases, the retina was approached by making a cut along more than a half of the border of the anterior face of the eyeball with fine scissors. The front part of the eyeball with the attached lens was then lifted and the whole retina clearly exposed. In a few of these the portion of retina to be removed was cut away together with the external layers of the eyeball. In most, however, an incision was made through only the retinal layer with the sharpened edge of a fine wire loop, thus separating the selected part of the retina from the adjacent portions without injury to the outer membranes. Care was taken to avoid damage to the peripapillar area. The isolated sector of retina was then removed with fine forceps. In practice this latter became the preferred method and most of the results described below were obtained with this technique.

Histology. At sacrifice the retinal lesions were checked. Under deep anesthesia, the eyeball was opened and the retina examined in the living state with the stereomicroscope.[2] Afterward the cranium was opened and the whole head quickly immersed in abundant fixative (18 parts of 80% ethanol, 1 part acetic acid, 1 part formalin). A few hours later, the brain with the optic nerves and eyes attached was carefully dissected free and placed for 24 to 48 hours in fresh fixative. The fixed brains were then embedded in paraffin, serially sectioned at 15μ, and the sections stained with the Bodian protargol method. In most cases, the normal fibers stained black with this method while the newly regenerated fibers acquired an intense pink or reddish hue. The contrast seemed to be enhanced by increasing the prescribed amount of protargol until the pH approached 8.8 and by reducing the amount of copper to about 0.25 gr.

Observations

Time-course and General Features of Optic Nerve Regeneration. The speed of the regeneration process, as judged from the time required for recovery of visual function (14 to 18 days in *Carassius*; 25 to 35 days in *Astronotus*) was found to vary in relation to various factors such as

[2] It is of incidental interest that extensive regeneration of the ablated retinal areas was found to be well underway in many cases. Further details of this retinal regeneration are left for another study.

the size and age of the fish, the season, and the degree of hemorrhage and displacement of the cut stumps. The following times indicate a rough summer-season average for goldfish 5 to 9 cm long.

At 3 to 4 days after nerve section, the whole distal segment of the optic nerve and the two bundles, medial and lateral, into which the optic nerve divides before entering the tectum, appear to be degenerated. Within the tectum, the two main bundles are completely degenerated up to the point at which the fibers spread into the parallel optic layer. Within the retinic layers of the tectum, however, signs of fiber degeneration are not yet noticeable at this time. It is known that the process of elimination of the retinic fibers of the cortex is a relatively slow one (10). In the proximal segment of the severed optic nerve also there were signs in many cases of some retrograde degeneration due perhaps to surgical trauma, such as stretching of the nerve and of the retinal artery which were difficult to avoid.

At 4 to 7 days after section, the optic fibers have started to regenerate and have become mixed and entangled in a dense and swollen neuromatous growth between the two nerve stumps. Here one cannot recognize any orderly pattern of regeneration, although the possibility that the fibers tend to segregate cannot be ruled out. As soon as the entangled regenerated fibers have reached the central stump of the severed nerve, they take again a grossly parallel alignment. Where the fibers emerge from the scar one can observe a progressive rearrangement; the fibers gather in groups becoming more and more conspicuous. In most cases, when the regenerated nerve reaches the point of separation into medial and lateral bundles the fibers destined for one or the other tract seem to have gathered in advance toward the corresponding lateral or medial side. Sometimes one sees small bundles of fibers transferring from one nerve sector to another just before the point of bifurcation.

At 10 to 12 days after nerve section the regenerated fibers start to reinnervate the optic lobe. Small groups of fibers exit from each bundle at different points along the circumference of the lobe and enter the tectum to course in the superficial parallel layer. This layer is markedly thicker in the proximity of the bundles, along the inner and ventral borders of the optic lobe, and becomes progressively thinner toward the central areas of the cortex. Already fibers may be seen leaving the parallel layer to enter the underlying plexiform layer particularly in the border regions.

At 14 to 18 days after nerve section, when visual function is being re-

instated, the plexiform layer formed by the regenerated fibers is visible
in all areas of the optic tectum. The layer as a whole is markedly thicker
and the fiber bundles are more richly interwoven than in the normal
tectum as can be seen in Fig 2. Also the distinction between parallel and
plexiform layers is less clear.

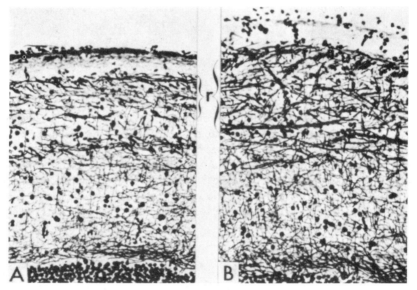

FIG. 2. Sections through corresponding parts of normal (A) and reinnervated
(B) tectum of goldfish 16 days after section of one optic nerve. Layers with retinal
fibers are indicated at r. Bodian stain; 160 ×.

The regenerated fibers were clearly distinguishable from the normal
ones for several weeks after recovery of vision, not only by the reddish
hue that they assumed with the modified Bodian stain, but also by their
structure and their interrelationships. The normal optic fibers, which are
myelinated in the nerve and in the parallel layer of the cortex and
unmyelinated in the plexus layer, appear when stained by the above
method, as black, well-individualized filaments. The regenerated fibers,
on the other hand, which are not yet myelinated when vision returns,
are packed together in the nerve in small bundles within which single
fibers are not clearly distinguishable. In the optic layers of the cortex the
bundles of regenerated fibers appear thicker, often ribbon-shaped, and
not well individualized (Fig. 2).

During the following weeks the regenerated fibers undergo a slow process of maturation toward the normal aspect. They become better individualized as the myelin sheath is forming, assuming then a filamentous, normal appearance. This process does not take place simultaneously in the whole fiber, but proceeds from the nerve cell in the retina toward the terminal arborization.

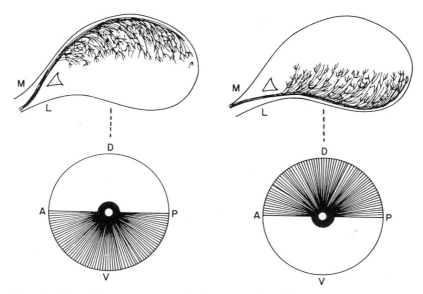

FIG. 3. Schematic representation of the regeneration fiber patterns obtained with nerve section and ablation of dorsal or ventral hemiretina, respectively.

Selectivity of Regeneration. Ventral-dorsal series. The first set of experiments was aimed at determining whether the fibers regenerating from the ventral or dorsal half of the retina would show any preference to enter the medial or, respectively, the lateral optic tract. The results for this series are schematically summarized in Fig. 3. When the dorsal half of the retina was removed and the optic nerve of the same side severed, the remaining fibers originating in the ventral half of the retina regenerated and were found to enter the medial bundle. The route of the lateral bundle was left empty with the exception of a few fibers that presumably originated mainly in the zone immediately adjacent to the papilla in the dorsal retina, which was intentionally left intact during the surgery. The retinic parallel and plexiform layers were restored in the dorsal tectum only. Conversely, when the ventral half of the retina was

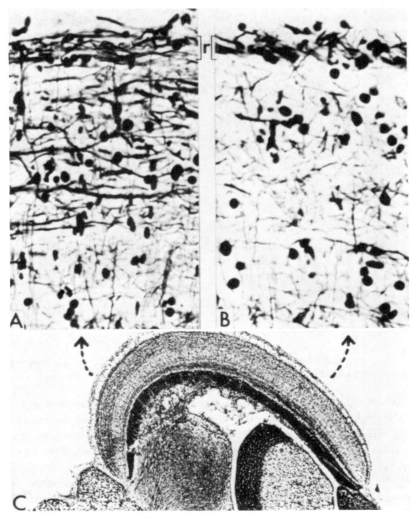

FIG. 4. Cross section of goldfish optic lobe (C) following optic nerve regeneration with ventral hemiretina ablated; details from the reinnervated ventral zone (A) and from the dorsal zone lacking regenerated fibers (B). The level of the parallel retinic layer is indicated at r. Bodian stain; A and B, 360 ×.

removed, nearly all of the regenerated fibers were found to enter the lateral bundle, and only the ventral half of the cortex was reinnervated.

In each case the one half of the tectum showed an abundant supply of regenerated fibers both in the parallel and plexus layers, whereas the other half appeared generally void of regenerated fibers (Fig. 4). The border between the empty and reinnervated halves of the cortex was not abrupt but was fairly distinct, especially in *Astronotus*. More exact

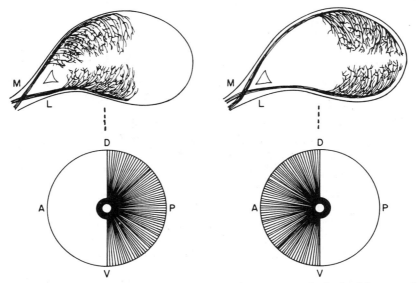

Fig. 5. Schematic representation of regeneration patterns obtained with removal of anterior (nasal) or posterior (temporal) hemiretina, respectively.

determinations along this line must be left for further study with different procedures.

In some cases the two types of retinal lesion were made in the same animal, i.e., a ventral removal was made in one eye and a dorsal removal in the other and both optic nerves sectioned. Under these conditions the double reverse effects were evident and easily compared in the same transverse sections.

Anterior-posterior series. The second set of experiments was designed to test for preference on the part of the regenerating fibers for the point of entrance into the tectum along its circumference. The results are schematically summarized in Fig. 5.

When the posterior half of the retina was removed and the nerve of
the same side severed, the regenerating fibers arising from both ventral
and dorsal quadrants of the anterior retina split into two groups, one
of which entered the medial and the other the lateral bundle. Within both

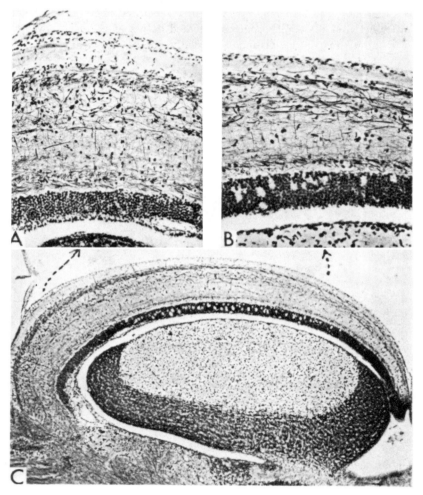

FIG. 6. Sagittal section of goldfish tectum (C) showing selective reinnervation
of posterior zone following ablation of temporal hemiretina. Enlarged details from
anterior (A) and posterior (B) sectors show plexiform layer to be absent in
anterior region but richly developed posteriorly. Bodian stain; A and B, 170 ×.

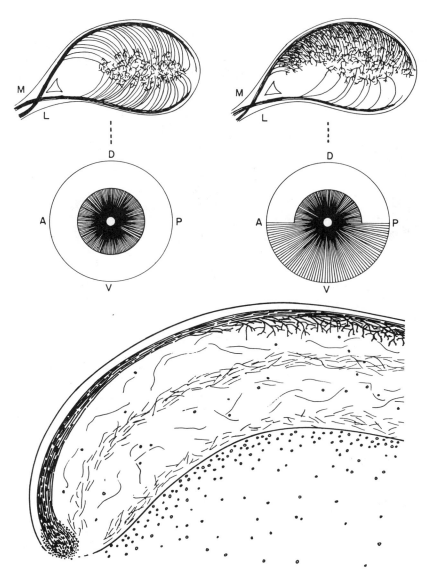

FIG. 7. Type of regeneration patterns obtained with removal of peripheral retina.
Below: Enlarged detail of the result as viewed in a transverse section of tectum.

tracts the bulk of the fibers were found to remain in the bundle until they approached the posterior regions of the tectum. A few fibers were evident anteriorly in the parallel layer but they passed through without entering the plexus layer. The plexiform layer was formed only in the posterior of the tectum (Fig. 6).

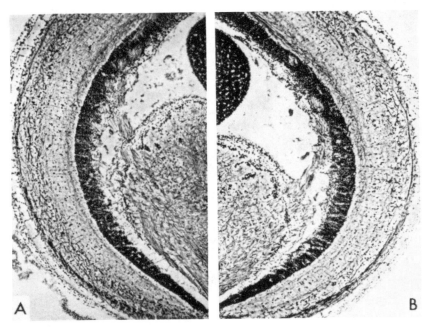

FIG. 8. Cross sections of ventral region of reinnervated right and left optic lobes. A, complete reinnervation with no retinal lesion; B, selective by-passing of plexiform layer in marginal zone (lower half of photo) after removal of dorsal periphery of retina. Bodian stain; 68 ×.

In the other fishes in which the anterior portion of the retina was excised and the nerve severed, the fibers similarly split into two groups, one of which entered the medial and the other the lateral tract. However, in these the fibers from both tracts entered and reinnervated the anterior regions of the tectum and did not extend back into the posterior regions in either the parallel or plexiform layers.

Radial series. The third set of experiments was designed to determine whether the regenerating fibers after their entry into the parallel layer of the cortex, would show any preference in entering the underlying plexiform layer. The results are schematically summarized in Fig. 7.

In this series the peripheral retina was first removed from just the dorsal half and the same or both optic nerves were severed. In these fishes the regenerating fibers coming from the intact ventral retina entered the medial bundle and reached their terminations throughout the dorsal part of the tectum. The fibers coming from the central peripapillar portion of the dorsal retina, on the other hand, after running through the lateral bundle, entered the parellel layer of the cortex but remained in this layer until they arrived at the central zone of the tectum. Thus the marginal part of the ventral tectum contained a parallel layer but the plexiform formation was absent (Fig. 8).

When a complete peripheral ring of retina was removed, leaving intact only the center of the retina, the regenerating fibers entered the tectum through both the medial and lateral bundles, but in neither case after entering the tectum did the fibers descend into the plexiform layer until they had reached the central zone. The entire margin of the optic lobe was thus by-passed by these fibers arising from the central retina.

Discussion

The foregoing provides direct microscopical confirmation of earlier deductions that the regenerating optic axons reconnect selectively in matching loci of the tectal field to restore an orderly topographic projection of the retina upon the tectum. In addition the findings disclose for the first time an unexpectedly high degree of specificity in the choice of central pathways taken by the fibers en route to their terminal stations. The results would appear to dispel any remaining doubts that the growing optic fibers are destination-bound. They appear to be not only rather specifically destination-bound, but also definitely inclined to follow particular routes to their respective destinations.

It would seem most probable that the selective growth along specific central routes by the different fiber types is chemotactic in nature and is based on biochemical specificities, presumably similar to or identical with those we have inferred to be operative in the formation and maintenance of functional synapses. The same set of anteroposterior and dorsoventral gradients in retina and tectum needed to explain the topographic reconnection pattern would be sufficient to account also for the orderly tract and radiation formations observed.

In addition it would seem likely that the various extraneuronal elements in and immediately around the nerve routes, must also possess distinctive chemical properties. For example, the opposite walls of the main nerve trunk just before its bifurcation into medial and lateral tracts may differ sufficiently to favor an advance segregation of fibers into medial and lateral bundles. We may imagine any growing fiber tip to be continuously testing its surroundings as it advances, by extending and retracting a number of microfilaments along the surrounding cellular surfaces in all directions. Most of these scouting filaments are then withdrawn in favor of the one that finds the substrate most favorable and the extension of which also is most in accord with the intrinsic individual growth properties of the given fiber.

Our thesis that specific chemical affinities govern neuronal synapsis (1–3, 15–21) may be extended on the basis of the present findings to include the patterning of central fiber pathways. Not only the details of synaptic association within terminal centers, but also the routes by which the fibers reach their synaptic zones would seem to be subject to regulation during growth by differential chemical affinities. This becomes essentially a chemotactic interpretation and takes us a long way from the prevailing doctrine of the 1920's, and 30's which held that nerve fiber outgrowth and termination is basically nonselective, with chemotropic and electrical factors seemingly ruled out in favor of mechanical contact guidance. The well-demonstrated importance of mechanical factors (25) is not to be minimized, but the present evidence suggests a reconsideration of some of the more ancient ideas of chemotaxis, chemotropism, neurotropism and of chemical selectivity in general in the guidance of nerve fiber growth and connection particularly within the central nervous system.

We found no indication in these fishes of an early nonselective phase of regeneration. Selectivity was already evident with respect to choice of medial and lateral tracts and the invasion of the tectum as early as 12 days after nerve section. The possibility of initial diffuse and excessive growth of fibers with subsequent elimination of the more devious and circuitous branches remains to be considered; however, with reference to the local terminal growth on microscopical dimensions within the plexiform layer.

References

1. ARORA, H. L. 1959. *Ann. Repts. Biol., Psychobiol. Sect., Caltech.* **1956-60**.
2. ARORA, H. L., and R. W. SPERRY. 1958. Studies on color discrimination following optic nerve regeneration in cichlid fish, *Astronotus ocellatus. Anat. Record* **131**: 529.

3. ATTARDI, D. G., and R. W. SPERRY. 1960. Central routes taken by regenerating optic fibers. *Physiologist* **3**: 12.

4. GAZE, R. M. 1958. The representation of the retina on the optic lobe of the frog. *Quart. J. Exptl. Physiol.* **43**: 209-214.

5. GAZE, R. M. 1959. Regeneration of the optic nerve in *Xenopus laevus*. *Quart. J. Exptl. Physiol.* **44**: 290-308.

6. GAZE, R. M. 1960. Regeneration of the optic nerve in Amphibia. *Intern. Rev. Neurobiol.* **2**: 1-40.

7. GAZE, R. M., and M. JACOBSON. 1962. The projection of the binocular visual field on the optic tecta of the frog. *Quart. J. Exptl. Physiol.* **47**: 273-280.

8. JACOBSON, M. 1961. Recovery of electrical activity in the optic tectum of the frog during early regeneration of the optic nerve. *Proc. Roy. Soc. Edinburgh*, B **28**: 131-137.

9. KOPPANYI, T. 1955. Regeneration in the central nervous system of fishes, pp. 3-19. *In* "Regeneration in the Central Nervous System," Wm. F. Windle [ed.]. Thomas, Springfield, Illinois.

10. LEGHISSA, S. 1955. La struttura microscopica e la citoarchitettonica del tetto ottico dei pesci teleostei. *Z. Anat. Entwicklungsgeschichte* **118**: 427-463.

11. LETTVIN, J. L., H. MATURANA, W. H. PITTS, and W. S. McCULLOCH. 1959. How seen movement appears in the frog's optic nerve. *Federation Proc.* **18**: 90.

12. LETTVIN, J. Y., H. R. MATURANA, W. S. McCULLOCH, and W. H. PITTS. 1959. What the frog's eye tells the frog's brain. *Proc. Inst. Radio Engrs.* **47**: 1940-1951.

13. MATURANA, H. R., J. Y. LETTVIN, W. S. McCulloch, and W. H. PITTS. 1959. Evidence that cut optic nerve fibers in a frog regenerate to their proper places in the tectum. *Science* **103**: 1409-1710.

14. MATURANA, H. R., J. Y. LETTVIN, W. S. McColloch, and W. H. PITTS. 1960. Anatomy and physiology of vision in the frog (*Rana pipiens*). *J. Gen. Physiol.* **43**: 129-175.

15. SPERRY, R. W. 1941. The effect of crossing nerves to antagonistic muscles in the hind limb of the rat. *J. Comp. Neurol.* **45**: 1-19.

16. SPERRY, R. W. 1942. Re-establishment of visuomotor coordinations by optic nerve regeneration. *Anat. Record* **84**: 470.

17. SPERRY, R. W. 1944. Optic nerve regeneration with return of vision in anurans. *J. Neurophysiol.* **7**: 57-69.

18. SPERRY, R. W. 1945. Restoration of vision after crossing of optic nerves and after contralateral transplantation of eye. *J. Neurophysiol.* **8**: 15-28.

19. SPERRY, R. W. 1948a. Orderly patterning of synaptic associations in regeneration of intracentral fiber tracts mediating visuomotor coordination. *Anat. Record* **102**: 63-75.

20. SPERRY, R. W. 1948b. Patterning of central synapsis in regeneration of the optic nerve in teleosts. *Physiol. Zoöl.* **21**: 351-361.

21. SPERRY, R. W. 1955. Functional regeneration in the optic system, pp. 66-76. *In* "Regeneration in the Central Nervous System," W. F. Windle [ed.]. Thomas, Springfield, Illinois.

22. STONE, L. S. 1960. Polarization of the retina and development of vision. *J. Exptl. Zoöl.* **145**: 85-95.

23. SZEKELY, G. 1954. Zur Ausbildung der lokalen funktionellen Spezifität der Retina. *Acta Biol. Acad. Sci. Hung.* **5**: 157-167.

24. WEISS, P. 1936. Selectivity controlling the central-peripheral relations in the nervous system. *Biol. Rev.* **11**: 494-531.

25. WEISS, P. 1960. Nervous system: Neurogenesis, pp. 346-401. *In* "Analysis of Development." B. H. Willier, P. A. Weiss, and V. Hamburger [eds.]. Saunders, Philadelphia.

Reprinted from Nature, Vol. 258, pp. 126–132. 1975
© 1975 Macmillan Journals Ltd.

Polarity of structure and of ordered nerve connections in the developing amphibian brain

Shin-Ho Chung & Jonathan Cooke

National Institute for Medical Research, London NW7 1AA, UK

Tectal polarity for retinal connections remains reversible long after the anatomical pattern of neural structures has been determined. Cells in the diencephalon seem to control this polarity. Following certain embryonic operations, the diencephalon developed behind the tectum. In such cases, the polarity of the retino-tectal projection was reversed.

THE amphibian retino-tectal projection has been widely used for studying the mechanisms governing selective nerve connections. One important fact which has emerged from the study of this system is that critical events occuring early in ontogeny determine the axial polarity of the retina with respect to its connections to the tectum, the primary visual centre. When an eye in a stage 32 *Xenopus*[1] is rotated by 180°, cells in the original anterior pole of the retina connect to the posterior pole of the tectum, as they would have done if left undisturbed, and the animal's visual world is accordingly rotated by 180°. If a similar operation is performed some 7 h earlier (Stage 28 in *Xenopus*), the animal develops normal visuo-tectal connections[2–5], because of repolarisation of the eye in the orbit.

It has been conjectured[6] that an equivalent determination of axial polarity occurs within the tectum, to which retinal cells later connect through their optic nerve fibres. The time of tectal polarisation is not known, for the only attempted rotation experiments on the tectum comparable with those on the embryonic eye did not give clear results[7]. If such tectal polarisation does take place, it is likely that the information for this, whatever its nature, may originate from a local group of cells, as has been demonstrated for the control of spatial patterns of cellular differentiation early in embryonic development[8,9].

Here we report briefly on the results of an investigation directed at these questions. Our findings indicate that such polarising information can originate from a group of cells outside the tectum, namely, those which are subsequently to form the diencephalon. They also suggest that tectal cells do not acquire permanent positional labels before optic innervation. Detailed reports, including autoradiographic studies of histogenesis and electrophysiological evidence for the presence of normal synapses in rotated tecta, will be presented elsewhere.

Embryonic operation

The presumptive midbrain regions of 83 embryonic *Xenopus* were cut out and replaced after rotation by 180°. Most of the operations were carried out at stages 21–24, or approximately 22–26 h after fertilisation, with some at stage 37, some 24 h before the optic nerve reaches the tectum[10,11]. No differentiation is detectable among cells of the neural tube until midway between these two periods, but earlier work on another species[12] has shown that even well before stage 20 the neural rudiment is a mosaic of regions, each with a strong tendency to develop into a particular part of the brain. We confirmed that this situation obtains also in *Xenopus* by examining embryonic brains following rotation of small pieces in neural plate stages.

The dorsal diencephalon (thalamus) and adjoining optic tecta develop from a dorsal section, some 15 to 20 cells square as counted directly through the dissecting microscope, of the stage 22 neural tube (Fig. 1). By varying the anterior–posterior levels of the cuts, but attempting to rotate in each case a similar sized piece, we were able to produce brains with different spatial arangements of these anatomical parts.

Owing to elastic forces resulting from morphogenetic movements and cellular differentiation, the operation on the brain rudiment of stage 37 larvae is difficult. Nevertheless, we have succeeded in mapping two animals after rotating tectal structure at this stage.

We used several criteria for assessing operations as successful. First, we checked visually whether the cut tissue remained in place 48 h after operation. Second, we observed gross derangements of brain anatomy in cases where the rotated tissue had healed properly, and confirmed this in serial histological sections. Finally, when we carried out control experiments in which the cut piece of neural tube was discarded, we observed two classes of results from those animals surviving until metamorphosis. In one class of animals, regeneration had given rise to brain structure and retino-tectal connections indistinguishable from those of unoperated animals, and the other showed atectal brains with forebrain grossly enlarged and the diencephalon joining the brainstem.

Normal visual map in spite of rotated tectal tissue

Following the operation, only 10 animals failed to establish good retino-tectal connections. From the remaining animals, 63 electrophysiological maps of the direct optic projection to the contralateral tecta were obtained during metamorphic climax, using procedures detailed elsewhere[10]. For clarity, only one or two of the several rows of electrode positions plotted are shown for each map presented here. The brains and their associated maps fell into three main categories, which we now discuss in turn.

A parasagittal section of the normal brain is shown in Fig. 2a. The diencephalon (D) is seen immediately in front of the midbrain, with its single tectum (T). Figure 2b shows a comparable section of a brain where we believe the anterior part of the tectal precursor had been rotated. Viewed from the dorsal surface, a pair of tecta were clearly identifiable on each side, separated by the indentation and blood vessels seen at the tecto-diencephalic junction in the normal animal. In brain sections of such animals, tectal histogenesis can often be seen to progress from this new junction, forwards in anterior tectum and backwards, as normally[10], in the posterior. As the recording electrode was moved successively backward from the anterior pole of the anterior tectum to the posterior pole of the posterior tectum, positions in the visual field from which electrical responses could be evoked also shifted from the anterior pole to the posterior pole. Note that, throughout, we use the terms anterior and posterior in relation to the animal's present body axis, rather than any original polarity of tissue in the embryo. Figure 3a shows the visuo-tectal map

A full account of this study is given in Chung and Cooke, *Proc. R. Soc. Lond. B 201:* 335–373 (1978).

obtained from one such animal, a histological section of which is exhibited in Fig. 2b. Similar anatomy and map were observed from two animals whose tectal rudiment had been rotated at stage 37 (Fig. 3b). Thus the array of

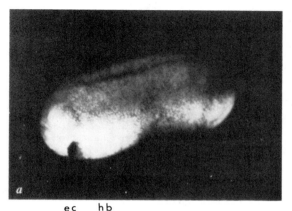

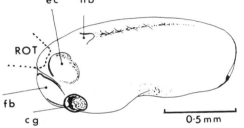

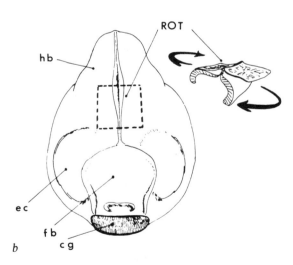

Fig. 1 Embryonic operation. *a*, Photomicrograph and *camera lucida* drawing of a stage 24 *Xenopus* embryo. Embryos were staged according to the tables of Nieuwkoop and Faber[1]. Operations were performed with sharpened tungsten needles and hair loop, in two-thirds strength Niu Twitty solution brought to *p*H 7.1 with diluted HCl. On the drawings, the heavy dashed line marks the limits of tissue reversed in a typical operation. *b*, Drawing of the head from anterior-dorsal aspect at stage 24. ec, Eyecup; hb, hind-brain; cg, cement gland; fb, forebrain vesicle; ROT, rotated piece of neural tube and overlying epidermis.

retinal fibres ignores the anatomical consequences of operation to produce a normal, single map with respect to the visual field and animal's body axis, by distributing itself across the two tecta. We therefore conclude that tectal tissue itself, rather than having assumed a fixed axial polarity for selective nerve connections, remains subject to overriding influences from outside the tectum until at least some 13 h after the equivalent retinal polarity is irrevocably determined[2-5].

In many animals of the present category, particularly those where the new junctional groove and blood vessels were conspicuous between the anterior and posterior tecta, the path of the optic nerve was altered. Instead of entering the tectum at its anterior border[13], the optic nerve now invaded both tecta from the position of the new intervening groove. Evidence for this is threefold. First, massive responses with large receptive fields were obtained at the junction point, instead of at anterior poles of both tectum and visual field as in normal animals[10]. Second, we observed instances in which both the anterior pole of the anterior tectum and posterior pole of the posterior one were electrically silent. Finally, histological preparations of certain animals clearly show ascent of fibres between the two tecta. We therefore believe that factors normally guiding these fibres to the tectum are distinctive to the diencephalon–midbrain junction, which has been transferred posteriorly in these operations. Regardless of the trajectory of the optic nerve, incoming fibres treated the two tecta as one and distributed themselves with correct order and polarity, thereby showing that control of the direction of innervation and of progressive tectal differentiation are quite independent of the polarity of the visuo-tectal map.

Reversal of visual maps related to position of diencephalon

When the positions of cuts, at operation, were brought forward by only some 5–10 cells in the neural tube, the diencephalic structure (epithalamus, thalamus and hypothalamus) developed behind the tectum, rather than in front (Fig. 4a and b). Thus a small group of precursor cells, at stage 24, are determined as diencephalic; they form the diencephalon even when moved to a position adjacent to hind-brain precursor cells. The anterior pole of the tectum in such animals was joined directly to the telencephalon, whereas normally the diencephalon is interposed between these two structures (compare Fig. 4a and b). A typical visuo-tectal map obtained from one such animal is shown in Fig. 4c. In contrast to a normal map, the anterior visual field was now represented in the posterior pole of the tectum, and the posterior in the anterior pole; the visuo-tectal map was completely reversed.

The medio–lateral polarity, unlike the anterior–posterior one, was not reversed. As in normal animals, fibres stemming from the ventral part of the retina (namely, those subserving the superior visual field, as the lens inverts the image) positioned themselves more medially than those from the dorsal retina. Because the original operation was symmetrical about the animal's midline, we do not expect, and indeed have never found, any reversal in the medio–lateral axis of maps.

Following the version of the operation just discussed, 13 animals developed two separate tecta on each side, separated by the diencephalon (Fig. 5a). This presumably occurred because of inevitable variability in the operation, whereby in these cases some tectal precursor tissue had been left unrotated posteriorly.

A parasagittal section of such an animal shows clearly that the infundibular recess and hypothalamic nuclei lie directly below the level at which the two tecta join, and the cellular mass constituting the dorsal and ventral thalamic nuclei is interposed between the tecta (Fig. 5a). In trans-

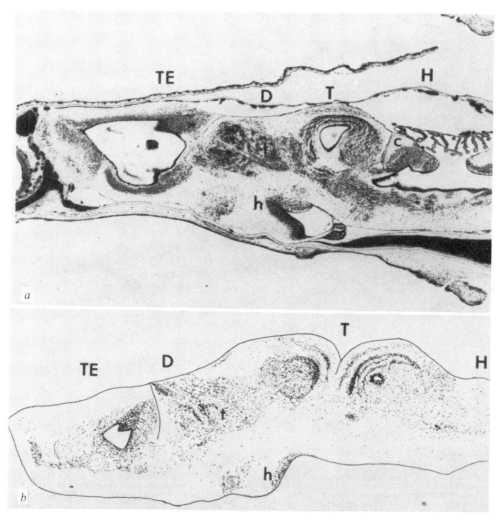

Fig. 2 Parasagittal sections of brains from (*a*) normal and (*b*) experimental tadpoles at stage 66. To make the rearranged structures more apparent, we have selected parasagittal sections throughout, although detailed anatomy is best followed in serial transverse sections. Because the experimental (*b*) animal was one also treated for ³H-autoradiography, a *camera lucida* drawing is given since the visual appearance of the tectum is not comparable with the control (*a*) or with subsequent sections shown. TE, Telencephalon; D, diencephalon; T, tectum; H, hind-brain; h, hypothalamic nuclei; t, thalamus; c, cerebellum.

verse sections, not shown here, different diencephalic nuclei, including those of the epithalamus, can be identified more clearly. The pattern of visuo-tectal map in these animals showed that a complete visual field was represented in each tectum. The polarity of the map in the anterior tectum was reversed, whereas that of the posterior tectum was normal (Fig. 5*b*). Thus, the population of incoming fibres distributed themselves across the two tecta, those originating from the posterior part of the retina occupying, as in the normal brain, that tectal tissue adjacent to diencephalon.

In several animals, an extra diencephalon developed anterior to the tecta, in addition to the one between the two tecta. Embryologically, such an anomaly would be expected if some diencephalic cells were left *in situ* and some were translocated, and both groups then regulated to give complete structures. The anterior tectum, situated between the two diencephalons, showed two superimposed maps with opposing polarity, as illustrated in Fig. 6. When the recording electrode was at the most anterior pole of this

tectum, responses could be elicited both from the far anterior and far posterior parts of the visual field. Similar responses could be obtained from the posterior pole of this tectum. Two ordered series of symmetrical pairs of responses were then obtained as the electrode positions advanced along the intervening tectum. Such overlapping projections of opposing polarity indicate that each diencephalon can exert its own polarising influence on the intervening tectum, independently of the other.

Implications for selective nerve connections

Several inferences can be made from our study about the mechanisms governing formation of selective nerve connections. The most general conclusion we can draw from our findings, without recourse to any specific notions previously advanced, is that polarity for selective nerve connections within tissues remains labile long after that for the anatomical pattern of the brain as a whole is fixed. The possibility remains, however, that the same positional

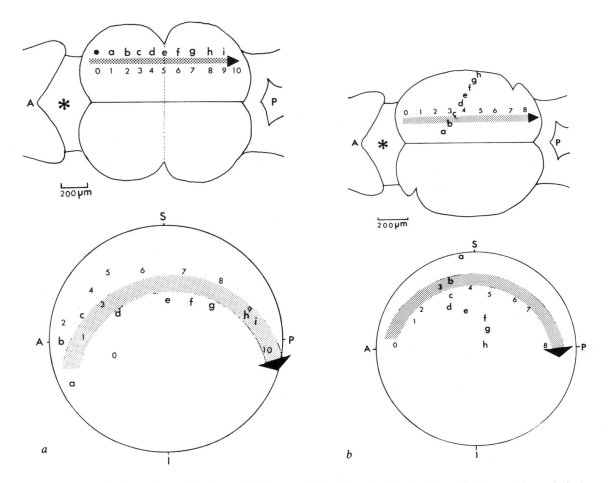

Fig. 3 Normal visual map after rotation of *a*, neural tube at stage 24 and *b*, tectal rudiment at stage 37. The map (*a*) was obtained from the animal whose histological section is displayed in Fig. 2*b*. All animals discussed in this paper were mapped between stages 62 and 66. Many rows of electrode positions were tested, but for the sake of simplicity, we show in this and following figures the results for only one or two rows. Positions in particular rows are either numbered or lettered consecutively, and positions in the visual field from which responses were obtained are then shown. Overall polarity of rows is shown for quick inspection by broad shaded arrows. Asterisks indicate the location of the diencephalic structure. A, Anterior; P, posterior; S, superior; I, inferior.

signal[9] is involved first in morphological determination and subsequently in establishing axial reference for selective nerve connections. The nature of such signals and of the cellular responses to them remain unknown. Nevertheless, our findings provide a basis for experimental attack on these problems in developing nervous systems.

Our results also suggest that a group of cells other than the tectal precursors can organise axial information within the developing tectum for incoming optic nerve fibres. These cells appear to be some or all of those which are determined to form the diencephalic structure itself. This conclusion is strengthened by results of the first category of animals (Figs 2, 3 and 4). Polarity of visuo-tectal maps in these animals was normal, although tissue normally situated at the very junction of diencephalon and tectum had been transferred posteriorly. The diencephalon thus may act in a way quite analogous to an embryonic organiser, in that each of them controls an axial polarity in surrounding tissue. In the case of the diencephalon, the polarity is that for the retino-tectal connections. Classical organisers, on the other hand, control anatomical patterns of cellular differentiation in surrounding embryonic tissues[9,14,15]. It is relevant to note

here that the organiser for the axial pattern of the whole body during amphibian development is a small group of cells at the dorsal lip of the blastopore, which later form the anterior mesoderm[8,14,15]. This mesoderm then induces in overlying ectoderm the formation of the forebrain rudiment, of which the diencephalon is the central part. An obvious test for the hypothesis of diencephalic organiser is to transplant a presumptive diencephalon alone as a graft behind the presumptive tectum of the host. Our preliminary results from a series of such animals are conforming with our expectation.

Several models have been proposed for the formation of ordered retino-tectal connections during development[8,16–18]. Before trying to evaluate these models, one has to ask a fundamental question: how much information is encoded in each tectal cell? Maximum information is assigned to each tectal cell if each possesses a uniquely labelled positional code[6]. On the other hand, the minimum possible information is assigned to the tectum if there is only one reference point within or outside it, to align properly the projection of incoming fibres, and no positional memory is encoded in individual tectal cells[16].

464

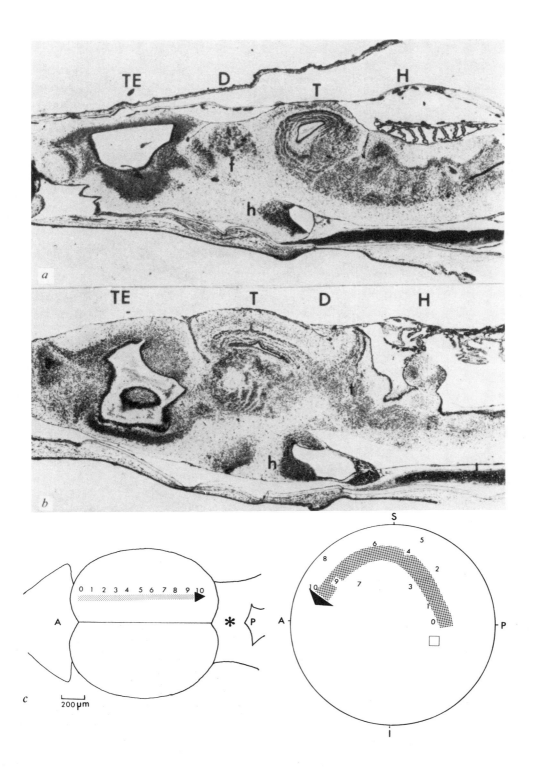

Fig. 4 Reversed visual map with diencephalon situated behind the tectum. Comparable parasagittal sections of *a*, normal and *b*, experimental animal (operated at stage 24). *c*, Reversed visuo-tectal map across the single tectum. The map and the histological section (*b*) were obtained from the same animal. From the electrode positions 2, 3, 4, 5, 6 and 8, responses could also be elicited by stimulating the visual field marked by the square. We can offer no plausible explanation for this anomaly. See Figs 2 and 3 for legend and abbreviations.

465

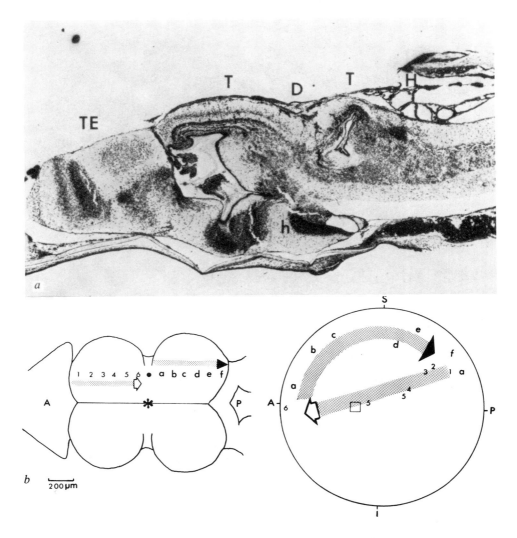

Fig. 5 Transposition of the diencephalon to lie between anterior and posterior tecta (operation at stage 24). *a*, Parasagittal section. *b*, Visuo-tectal map showing complete reversal for the anterior tectum and normal representation in the posterior tectum. The map and the histological section were obtained from the same animal. From the electrode positions 2, 4 and 6, responses could also be elicited by stimulating the visual field indicated by the square. See Figs 2 and 3 for legend and abbreviations.

Our present results show that positional labelling within tectal cells, if such ever occurs, can be overridden at least until stage 37 (Fig. 3*b*). Since functioning synapses are present by stage 45 in normal tadpoles[19], any positional labels having significance in ordering connections must have been acquired within the intervening period. Because the tectal rudiment at such stages is fragile and sticky, we have not succeeded in eliminating this possibility. The observation of dual projection patterns with opposed polarity (Fig. 6), across the same tissue, nevertheless makes it difficult to suppose that tectal cells possess unique labels before optic innervation.

Our results are equally consistent with a theory which requires no positional memory in tectal cells. If we assume that, in addition to a reference point in the nervous system, there is a mechanism whereby optic nerve fibres can preserve, on the tectum, the spatial contiguity of their origin in the retina, a wide range of experimental data

including ours can be accounted for. The idea that mechanisms other than graded chemical labelling may be used by the nervous system in maintaining spatial contiguity, has been advanced previously. Lettvin's notion (cited in Chung[16]), for instance, is based on the fact that dendritic trees of retinal ganglion cells arborize extensively and interdigitate with neighbouring ones. Two fibres arising from adjoining retinal ganglion cells are, therefore, likely to exhibit a temporal contiguity in their discharge patterns, and such a coincidence in firing can, in principle at least, be used for maintaining spatial relations between the fibres. An alternative notion, advanced by Goodwin and Cohen[20], makes use of a signalling system arising from oscillatory metabolic processes in assigning positional codes to retinal and tectal elements, which then match up. In both of these models, each tectal element need not be uniquely labelled in order to establish ordered connections with retinal fibres. An underlying assumption in these

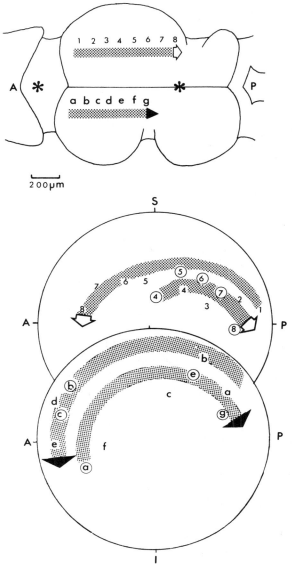

Fig. 6 Visuo-tectal maps obtained from tecta lying between 2 sets of diencephalic structure (operation at stage 24). Two superimposed ordered maps of the visual field with opposed polarity across the tectum, are seen on each side of the brain. Two circles represent the right and left visual fields. See text. For legend and abbreviations, see Fig. 3.

models is that fibres compete to achieve optimal matching with the available post-synaptic sites[17,18]. Whether such models reflect physical reality remains to be investigated.

Experiments involving tectal rotation in adult *Xenopus*[21] and goldfish[22,23] as well as transplantation studies on the *Rana catesbiana* tectum[24,25], suggest that the situation in the adult brain may differ from that during development. For instance, when tissues from one part of the adult tectum were interchanged with those from another part, they appeared to retain memory of their previous position in 13 cases[25], whereas no such information was retained in 14 other cases[24]. The conditions in which these two occur must first be ascertained.

A final evaluation of the two classes of theory we have outlined must, however, await further investigations. We propose that before tectal cells are innervated by optic nerve fibres, they possess no positional memory, and axial information for incoming optic fibres originates from a polarising structure located in the diencephalon. If it can be shown either that critical events occurring between stages 37 and 45 irrevocably label tectal cells, or that a properly aligned map can be established in a developing tectum *in vitro* without diencephalic tissue, then our theory, in its simplest form, will have proved to be wrong.

We thank M. L. Errington and S. J. Caidan for technical assistance.

Received August 13; accepted October 10, 1975.

1 Nieuwkoop, P. D., and Faber, J., *Normal Tables of* Xenopus laevis (*Daudin*) (North-Holland, Amsterdam, 1956).
2 Stone, L. S., *Proc. Soc. exp. Biol. Med.*, **57**, 13–14 (1944).
3 Székely, G., *Acta biol. Acad. Sci. Hung.*, **5**, 157–167 (1954).
4 Jacobson, M., *Devl Biol.*, **17**, 202–218 (1968).
5 Hunt, R. K., and Jacobson, M., *Proc. natn. Acad. Sci. U.S.A.*, **70**, 507–511 (1973).
6 Sperry, R. W., *J. comp. Neurol.*, **79**, 33–55 (1943); *J. Neurophysiol.*, **7**, 57–70 (1944).
7 Crelin, E. S., *J. exp. Zool.*, **120**, 547–577 (1952).
8 Spemann, H., *Embryonic Development and Induction* (Hafner, New York, 1967).
9 Wolpert, L., *J. theor. Biol.*, **25**, 1–48 (1969).
10 Gaze, R. M., Keating, M. J., and Chung, S. H., *Proc. R. Soc.*, **B185**, 301–330 (1974).
11 Chung, S. H., Stirling, R. V., and Gaze, R. M., *J. Embryol. exp. Morph.*, **33**, 915–940 (1975).
12 Jacobson, C.-O., *J. Embryol. exp. Morph.*, **7**, 1–21 (1959).
13 Potter, H. D., *J. comp. Neurol.*, **144**, 269–284 (1972).
14 Cooke, J., *J. Embryol. exp. Morph.*, **28**, 27–46 (1972); *ibid.*, **30**, 283–300 (1972).
15 Cooke, J., *A. Rev. Biophys. Bioengng*, **4**, 185–217 (1975).
16 Chung, S. H., *Cell*, 3, 201–205 (1974).
17 Gaze, R. M., and Keating, M. J., *Nature*, **237**, 375–378 (1972).
18 Prestige, M. C., and Willshaw, D. J., *Proc. R. Soc.*, **B190**, 77–98 (1975).
19 Chung, S. H., Keating, M. J., and Bliss, T. V. P., *Proc. R. Soc.*, **B187**, 449–459 (1974).
20 Goodwin, B. C., and Cohen, M. H., *J. theor. Biol.*, **25**, 49–107 (1969).
21 Levine, R. L., and Jacobson, M., *Expl Neurol.*, **43**, 527–538 (1974).
22 Sharma, S. C., and Gaze, R. M., *Arch. Ital. Biol.*, **109**, 357–366 (1971).
23 Yoon, M. G., *J. Physiol., Lond.*, **233**, 573–588 (1973).
24 Jacobson, M., and Levine, R. L., *Brain Res.*, **88**, 339–345 (1975).
25 Jacobson, M., and Levine, R. L., *Brain Res.*, **92**, 468–471 (1975).

467

J. Physiol. (1981), **316**, pp. 203–223
With 4 *plates and* 13 *text-figures*
Printed in Great Britain

MEMBRANE PROPERTIES AND SELECTIVE CONNEXIONS OF IDENTIFIED LEECH NEURONES IN CULTURE

By PAUL A. FUCHS, JOHN G. NICHOLLS and DONALD F. READY*

From the Department of Neurobiology, Stanford University School of Medicine, Stanford, CA 94305, U.S.A.

(*Received 17 September 1980*)

SUMMARY

1. Individual, identified neurones, dissected from the central nervous system of the leech and maintained in culture for several weeks, sprouted processes and formed synaptic connexions.

2. The action potentials of isolated touch (T), pressure (P), nociceptive (N) cells and Retzius cells resembled those of their counterparts *in situ*, enabling them to be recognized unambiguously. Their input resistances were approximately 4 times greater than those of corresponding cells within the animal. In T, P and N cells trains of impulses were followed by a pronounced after-hyperpolarization, as in the animal.

3. In certain cells, notably the L motoneurones, membrane properties became altered in culture. The current–voltage relation showed novel rectification and action potentials became much larger.

4. Numerous neurites often extended for hundreds of micrometres from isolated neurones and ended in typical growth cones. Electron micrographs revealed that many fine axons were braided together to form thicker fascicles. Frequently, the processes were orientated between two neighbouring cells rather than at random. The fine structure of the cytoplasm, nucleus and organelles in cultured cells resembled those of their counterparts *in situ*. The glial cell that normally surrounds the neurones was, however, absent.

5. Pairs of Retzius cells in culture usually became coupled electrically after about 6 days. Similarly L motoneurones became coupled *in vitro*. These junctions allowed current to pass in both directions and resembled those seen in the animal.

6. Selective connexions were made by certain types of cells. Thus, P sensory neurones did not become coupled with Retzius cells but did develop electrical connexions with L motoneurones, as in the animal.

7. Novel synaptic interactions not obvious in the animal could appear in culture. Retzius and L cells became electrically coupled and, in some instances where electrical coupling between Retzius cells failed to develop, chemically mediated inhibitory potentials became apparent.

8. Isolated, identified leech neurones not only survive but regenerate processes and are capable of forming selective connexions in culture. The ability to define interactions between isolated pairs of cells offers the opportunity to explore in detail problems relating to synapse formation and cell–cell recognition.

* Present address: Department of Biology, Princeton University, Princeton, NJ 08540, U.S.A.

INTRODUCTION

Following a lesion to the central nervous system (C.N.S.) neurones of lower vertebrates and invertebrates are able to regenerate synaptic connexions with sufficient accuracy to restore function (Gaze, 1970; Anderson, Edwards & Palka, 1980). Although a number of mechanisms, such as axonal guidance and timing, may play a part in enabling the regenerating axons to find their correct targets, some form of cell–cell recognition is presumably involved in the final selection of the appropriate post-synaptic cell (Sperry, 1963).

A considerable simplification for studying the mechanism and specificity of synapse formation can be achieved by working with neural tissue in culture, where greater control is possible over the cells and their environment (Crain, 1976; Varon & Bunge, 1978; Banker & Cowan, 1979). Preparations used for such studies include explants of brain containing heterogeneous populations of neurones and glia, neurones dissected from the C.N.S., or peripheral ganglia and muscle fibres maintained in culture. In the present experiments we have dissected individual identified nerve cells from the C.N.S. of the leech and maintained them in culture. These neurones, which can be isolated by a simple mechanical procedure avoiding exposure to enzymes, offer distinct advantages for studying the selectivity of synapse formation. In the highly stereotyped ganglia of the leech a variety of sensory cells, interneurones or moto-neurones have been identified, and the properties of the chemical and electrical synapses between them have been extensively studied (Muller, 1979). Thus, many different types of nerve cells can be kept alive in culture singly, in pairs or in groups and compared with their counterparts in the ganglion.

Our aims have been first to compare the membrane properties and fine structure of the isolated cells with those in the animal and second to examine the synaptic interactions that develop when cells are cultured together. Will cells form synapses in culture at random or selectively? If selective connexions are formed, how will these compare with the pattern of connexions seen in the animal? To approach these problems single identified cells can be placed repeatedly next to one another to determine the frequency and efficacy with which connexions are formed and to explore the range of compatible synaptic partners.

Isolated cultured leech neurones may also provide simplified preparations for studying the development of synapses and mechanisms of synaptic transmission. Within the C.N.S. of the leech, as in other invertebrates, experiments on these problems are complicated by the fact that synapses occur in the neuropile at a distance from the cell body. Hence, intracellular recordings made from the soma do not faithfully mirror the synaptic potentials; by the same token currents injected into the presynaptic cell body to modulate transmitter release or to spread through electrotonic junctions between coupled cells are attenuated and distorted at the terminals. In addition, the synapses are inaccessible for direct exploration by techniques such as ionophoretic application of drugs or transmitters, and sites of contact between cells are buried in a tangle of processes, complicating anatomical studies. In culture cells can be placed in direct contact and it may therefore be possible to develop synaptic connexions in which one can more fully analyse the anatomy, physiology and pharmacology of regenerated synapses between neurones.

The present study shows that isolated leech neurones survive, maintain normal resting and action potentials, sprout and form electrical and chemical connexions in culture. One example of preferential connexions has been observed. A brief account of some of these observations has been reported elsewhere (Ready & Nicholls, 1979).

METHODS

Dissection

Single cells were removed from the nervous system in a series of steps illustrated in Pl. 1 *A*. After opening the connective tissue capsule and washing away the glia (Kuffler & Potter, 1964; Nicholls & Kuffler, 1964), a fine nylon loop (Ethilon nylon monofilament, 13 μm in diameter, from Ethicon

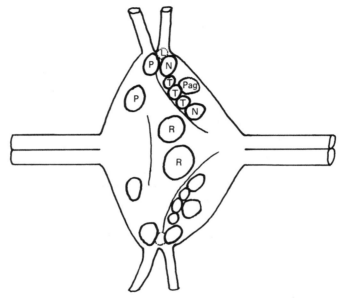

Fig. 1. Drawing of a leech ganglion in which the individual identified neurones used in these experiments are labelled. T, P, and N are the touch, pressure and nociceptive sensory cells, respectively, R is the large paired Retzius cell and L is the longitudinal motoneurone. Pag is the anterior pagoda cell, the function of which is unknown.

Corp., Somerville, N.J.) was slipped over the cell's soma, tied tightly around the initial process and the cell pulled away from the ganglion (Sargent, 1977). After 10 min the neurone was freed by shaking gently or by snapping the thread and transferred to the dish by a fine suction pipette with a constriction. After plating, the cultures were left for 1 hr at room temperature before being moved to the incubator. This gave time for cells to stick tightly to the dish bottom.

Certain cells such as the Retzius and P sensory neurones could be recognized unambiguously by visual inspection and were isolated under a dissection microscope set up in a laminar flow hood. N and T sensory cells, AE and L motoneurones and anterior pagoda cells were identified by recording intracellularly before isolation (Fig. 1). When cells were isolated under non-sterile conditions they were transferred through several drops of sterile medium before plating. Cell bodies, which were translucent before isolation, became white and opaque for a few hours before recovering their normal appearance.

Culture of single cells

Fig. 1 shows the positions in a typical leech ganglion of the various cells used for these experiments. Identified cells were cultured in 35 mm plastic tissue culture dishes (Falcon no. 3001) containing 2–3 ml. of medium (Leibowitz 15 plus 2% fetal calf serum (Gibco), 100 μg/ml. gentamycin (Schering Corp., Kenilworth, N.J.) and 0·6% glucose; 100 u./ml. mycostatin (Gibco) was added in some cases. To provide a sticky substrate, dishes were coated with rat-tail collagen (Bornstein, 1958) to which polylysine (1·0 mg/ml. in 0·1 M-sodium borate buffer, pH 8·2) was covalently bound using glutaraldehyde. Cells were positioned either as closely apposed pairs (Pl. 1 *B*) or at a distance from one another (Pl. 2 *B* and Fig. 11). They usually adhered immediately. Cultures were prepared under sterile conditions in a laminar flow hood. Usually about twenty pairs of cells were placed in each dish. The cultures were maintained at 20 °C in a humid incubator and the medium was changed once a week.

Electrical recording

Glass electrodes (Haer ultratip capillary tubing) of 15–30 MΩ resistance filled with 4 M-potassium acetate were used to record from cultured cells. The recording techniques were conventional (Wallace, Adal & Nicholls, 1977).

Light microscopy

Cultured cells were photographed on a Leitz Diavert, using phase contrast optics.

Electron microscopy

The cultures were washed with leech saline adjusted with glucose to the osmolarity of Leibowitz 15 (as were all succeeding solutions: 380 m-osmole) then fixed in 0·8% glutaraldehyde (in 0·1 M-phosphate buffer, pH 7·2) for 1 hr. Cells were post-fixed in osmium tetroxide (1% in phosphate buffer) 1 to 2 hr, stained with uranyl acetate (1% in 0·2 M-acetate buffer), dehydrated and embedded in Epon. After hardening, the Epon wafer containing the cells was separated from the tissue culture dish by repeated immersion in liquid nitrogen. Small blocks of plastic containing the cell or cells of interest could then be cut out and sectioned. Sections were stained with lead, then examined and photographed on a Phillips 201 electron microscope.

RESULTS

Growth and structure of isolated neurones

Freshly isolated leech neurones adhering to the polylysine–collagen substrate appeared rounded, with no sign of the large process that had been ligated close to the cell body during the dissection. After about 5 days in culture a number of fine sprouts began to appear around the perimeter of the cells. Unlike their counterparts in the ganglion, which are unipolar, isolated leech neurones appeared to initiate neurite outgrowth at numerous points on the soma. Pl. 2 *A* and *B* show the development of branches in isolated cells over several days. The neurites tended to track along each other, producing braided fascicles which grew approximately 10 to 20 μm in length per day. When two isolated cells were cultured within 50–200 μm of one another, many of the neurites spanned the area between the cells, as shown in Pl. 2 *B* and Fig. 11. This characteristic appearance was often obvious by about 1 week. It is not clear whether fibres grew preferentially from cell to cell, or whether those fibres that contacted another cell were more likely to survive and acted as guides for others to follow. Single cells cultured on their own usually showed a more randomly orientated distribution of processes (Pl. 2 *A*). No systematic differences were observed in the arborization of neurites produced by Retzius cells, sensory cells or motoneurones cultured with like cells or with dissimilar cells. The extent of sprouting shown by isolated cells plated on polylysine over collagen varied unpredictably from dish to dish. In some dishes the cells survived but all of them failed to grow. In others, most of the cells would sprout, while the usual pattern was of successful sprouting by some cells but not others.

For more detailed examination of structure, Retzius cells in culture were compared with their counterparts *in situ*. Three weeks after isolation cytoplasmic components including mitochondria, rough endoplasmic reticulum, bundles of fine fibrillar material 0·5 μm in diameter and lysosomes appeared normal (Gray & Guillery, 1963; Coggeshall & Fawcett, 1964). Moreover the distribution of organelles into zones containing predominantly rough endoplasmic reticulum or mitochondria, Golgi bodies and lysosomes was preserved in cultured cells. Scattered throughout the cytoplasm were characteristic dense-core vesicles, 90 nm in diameter, resembling those described in normal Retzius cells containing serotonin (Rude, Coggeshall & Van Orden, 1969). Clear vesicles of smaller diameter (45 nm) were also found in the cytoplasm. Accumulations of both vesicle types were occasionally found in short processes that projected from the cell soma. A degenerative change occasionally seen in the cytoplasm was a roughly spherical region a few micrometres in diameter filled with irregular membranous debris, including occasional myelin figures. Moreover, the Golgi system appeared more extensive in cultured cells, perhaps in association with synthesis required for growth of processes.

A major difference between cultured and normal Retzius cells was the absence of glia. Within the ganglion, the soma of the Retzius cell is surrounded by one of the large 'packet' glial cells that invaginate the surface creating a trophospongium. During the isolation of a neurone the packet glial cell which surrounds the soma is destroyed, leaving only a coating of glial membranes and cytoplasm (Kuffler & Nicholls, 1966); in culture this was shed over the first few days, forming a small layer of debris around the cell (seen in Pl. 2). Frequently the cells cleaned this debris from a zone around their perimeter, suggesting activity by filopodia (Albrecht-Buehler, 1980). Also adherent to isolated cells were a number of small satellite cells that resembled fibroblasts and microglial cells (Gray & Guillery, 1963; Coggeshall & Fawcett, 1964). In culture some of these satellite cells often migrated a short distance from the neurone, while others remained on the cell body. They could survive for many days especially when the medium was changed frequently, but they did not divide extensively. After 3 weeks in culture the periphery of the cell was indented and irregular with intervening smooth areas. Most of the surface of the neurone was bare and in direct contact with the medium, except for regions in apposition to the occasional small satellite cells or other neurites.

The projections of Retzius cells that contacted the dish extended and branched into a profusion of neurites ranging in diameter from 0·1 to 1 μm (most being between 0·3 and 0·5 μm: Pl. 3). As shown in Pl. 3, growth cones exhibiting numerous spike-like extensions and thin membrane sheets occurred at the leading edge of outgrowing neurites. Neurites were attached to the substrate at numerous points along their length. Like the cell bodies, the processes were not ensheathed by glia (Pl. 3 C and Pl. 4). The fine structure of the neurites appeared normal. Most contained longitudinally orientated neurotubules, as well as mitochondria and an extensive system of smooth endoplasmic reticulum. Occasionally, axons also contained fibrillar

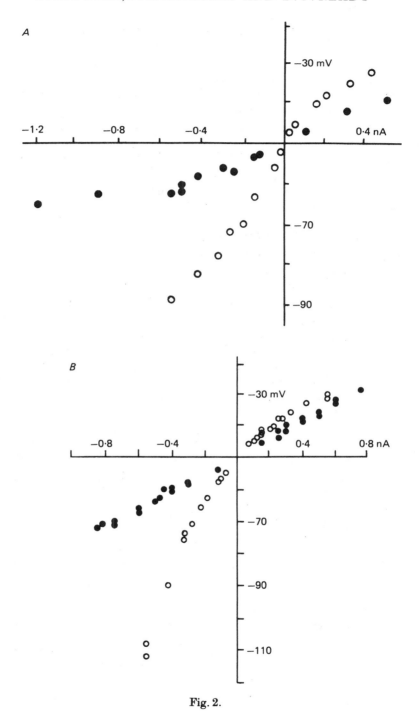

Fig. 2.

bundles up to 0·5 μm in diameter. Dense-core vesicles were dispersed throughout the length of most processes, while the smaller clear vesicles were found in numerous clusters containing from tens to hundreds of vesicles. Both types of vesicles were often observed at sites of contact with the substrate (Pl. 4).

A striking feature of Retzius cell neurites was the presence of varicosities along their length. These swellings occurred irregularly along processes at intervals of several micrometres, particularly in regions not directly in contact with the substrate. In phase contrast they appeared as dark swellings on the fascicles (Pl. 3). Typically, the varicosities were about 1 μm in diameter and 2 μm in length and contained concentrations of both clear and dense-core vesicles, as well as mitochondria and smooth endoplasmic reticulum (Pl. 4). In the animal comparable varicosities (colloquially named 'dingleberries') are normally seen on the processes of Retzius cells in the periphery and within the ganglion (Muller & McMahan, 1976; Muller, 1979).

Electrical properties of isolated neurones

Immediately after a cell had been isolated it became depolarized and the input resistance fell to a low value. Recovery of the membrane properties occurred within 1 hr. For example, in one Retzius cell the resting potential was -50 mV and the input resistance was 22 MΩ immediately before isolation. Twenty minutes after it had been tied off the resting potential was -12 mV and the input resistance only 8 MΩ. Within the next 10 min this cell recovered its normal resting potential and the input resistance had increased to 30 MΩ. After 60 min the input resistance was 72 MΩ.

The input resistance of cultured cells continued to increase for several days. In one series of experiments the average input resistance for four Retzius cells *in situ* was $20·7 \pm 3·0$ (s.e.m.) MΩ (normal Retzius cell input resistance can be as high as 30 MΩ). After 3 days in culture the average input resistance for these four cells was 129 ± 36 MΩ, with the highest value recorded being 240 MΩ. Since isolating a cell for culture entails removal of all its processes, one would expect such increases from the reduction in surface area alone. Furthermore, single isolated Retzius cells in culture were no longer electrically coupled to the contralateral Retzius cell as *in situ* and this could also increase the input resistance. In addition, we cannot rule out a possible increase in the specific membrane resistance of isolated cells as a factor.

The passive electrical properties of Retzius cells and sensory cells were in general

Fig. 2. *A*, voltage responses of cultured and normal Retzius cells plotted as a function of current injected through an intracellular electrode. Both cells were held at -50 mV resting potential with hyperpolarizing d.c. current. The normal Retzius cell (filled circles) was from the second ganglion of the leech nerve cord. Results from a Retzius cell isolated for 8 days are shown by open circles. The shape of the curve is similar for both cultured and normal Retzius cells, showing decreased resistance in both the depolarizing and hyperpolarizing directions. The input resistance (slope at the origin) of the normal Retzius cell was 21 MΩ, that of the cultured cell 120 MΩ. Measurements were made using two intracellular electrodes. *B*, voltage response of cultured and normal L motorneurones plotted as function of injected current. The L cell *in situ* (filled circles) showed a linear current–voltage relation; its input resistance was 25 MΩ. In culture L cells showed a marked change in the shape of the current–voltage relation, as well as an increase in input resistance. The cultured L cell (open circles) had an input resistance of 50 MΩ in the depolarizing direction, and 150 MΩ in the hyperpolarizing direction. Measurements were made using one electrode using a bridge circuit.

comparable with those recorded from each type of cell *in situ*, except for the increase in resistance. The steady-state current–voltage relationship for cultured (open circles) and normal (filled circles) Retzius cells is shown in Fig. 2*A*. Apart from a difference in slope the two relations are similar in form. L motoneurones, however, developed novel characteristics in culture (Fig. 2*B*). *In situ* the current–voltage relation was

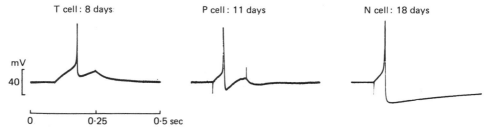

Fig. 3. Action potentials of T, P, and N cells after several days in culture. Each cell was from a different culture. The resting potential was −60 mV for the T cell, and −50 mV for the P and N cells. The characteristic shape of the action potential in each cell was similar to that recorded from homologous cells in the ganglion.

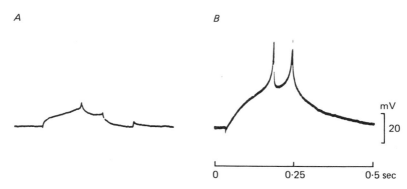

Fig. 4. Action potentials recorded from L motoneurones in the ganglion (*A*) and after culture for 10 days (*B*). Resting potential of the cultured L cell was −80 mV; the normal L cell was held at −82 mV with injected d.c. current. Depolarizing current pulses produced small (5 mV) responses in the normal L cell. Depolarization of cultured L cell produced an impulse of 30 mV, considerably larger than any responses seen in normal L cells.

linear over a large range, but in culture, in addition to the increase in slope near the origin, the curve showed a resistance increase with hyperpolarization and a resistance decrease with depolarization. This rectification was similar to that seen in T, P and N cells *in situ* (Baylor & Nicholls, 1969*a*) and in culture.

The resting potentials of various types of cultured cells were often larger than those reported for their normal counterparts *in situ*, which are usually about −40 to −50 mV. For isolated T, P and N sensory cells the values ranged from −50 to −70 mV; for cultured Retzius cells the range was −50 to −60 mV, but since the cells often fired upon penetration it was difficult to assess resting potentials accurately. The highest resting potentials were recorded from cultured L motoneurones: −80 to −100 mV, compared with −40 mV *in situ*.

The action potentials of isolated T, P and N cells were indistinguishable from those of their counterparts in the ganglion (Fig. 3). In addition, since they retained their characteristic features indefinitely in culture, the impulses provided a reliable and convenient confirmation of the identity of the cell. Similarly, Retzius cells in culture had action potentials that appeared unchanged. In contrast, cultured L cells showed changes. After about 10 days in culture the action potentials could be as large as 30 mV in amplitude, about 6 times larger than those of L cells *in situ* (Fig. 4). The ionic basis of these action potentials is not known. Presumably the soma of the islolated L cells became more excitable, since large action potentials were observed in neurones that had not sprouted.

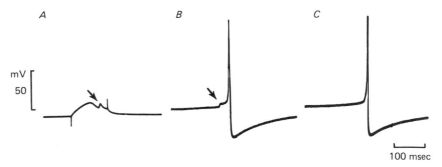

Fig. 5. Responses to depolarizing current in an N sensory cell cultured for 21 days. This cell had lengthy processes. In *A* the cell was held at −80 mV with injected current and a superimposed depolarizing pulse caused small spikes to appear, although the soma itself did not fire. In *B* the cell was allowed to depolarize to a resting level of −65 mV. Now a depolarizing current pulse elicited a full action potential from the soma, but it was preceded by a small prepotential, similar in amplitude to the 'axon' spike seen in *A*. Presumably the processes can be brought to threshold before the soma and initiate the action potential. *C* shows an impulse initiated in the soma when the N cell was further depolarized. These results suggest that, as in the ganglion, the processes are electrically excitable.

Outgrowth of processes seemed not to affect electrical excitability of the soma; the action potentials of cells which had sprouted did not obviously differ from those which had not. Indirect evidence suggested, however, that the membrane of the newly grown processes was electrically excitable. First, depolarizing pulses applied to cultured N cells that had sprouted gave rise to small, fast depolarizing potentials characteristic of axon spikes that failed to invade the soma (Fig. 5 *A*). Second, d.c. depolarization of N cells and various other types of cells also gave rise on occasion to full-sized action potentials preceded by small prepotentials (resembling those seen in N cells within the ganglion). This suggested that activity in the processes had initiated the soma spike (Fig. 5 *B*).

Additional evidence for the maintenance of normal concentration gradients and electrical properties by isolated cells is provided by Fig. 6. Trains of impulses in cultured sensory cells were followed by a prolonged after-hyperpolarization, resembling that seen in normal ganglia. There the mechanism underlying the potentials has been shown to be an electrogenic sodium pump and a prolonged increase in potassium conductance mediated by calcium entry (Jansen & Nicholls, 1973).

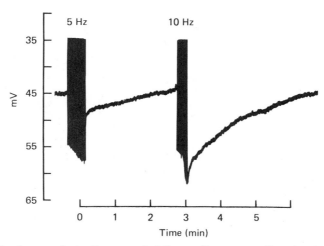

Fig. 6. After-hyperpolarization recorded from a P sensory cell maintained for 24 days in culture. Action potentials at 5 and 10 Hz were followed by a prolonged slow hyperpolarization similar to that seen *in situ*.

Electrical connexions of isolated cells

The development of electrical connexions in culture was followed by recording from various pairs of identified cells known to be coupled *in situ*. For example, the two Retzius cells in each ganglion are coupled by non-rectifying junctions, as are the two L motoneurones (Hagiwara & Morita, 1962; Stuart, 1970). The structure and location of these junctions within the neuropile are not known. In contrast, certain neurones are connected by rectifying electrical junctions. Thus, depolarization of T or P sensory neurones spreads to L motoneurones, but hyperpolarization does not (Nicholls & Purves, 1970); and in the course of these experiments (see below) similar but weak rectifying coupling was also seen between N and L cells *in situ*.

To test for coupling *in vitro*, pairs of cells were plated in direct apposition as in Pl. 1 *B*. All of the cells were from an individual leech, but no attempt was made to combine cells with their original partners. Under these conditions Retzius cells usually became coupled to each other, as shown in Fig. 7. Similar results were obtained with pairs of L cells. As in the animal, both the Retzius and L cell connexions were non-rectifying (Hagiwara & Morita, 1962; Stuart, 1970). The efficacy of coupling was variable; occasionally, the coupling ratio approached 1 but in other instances the cells were weakly coupled or uncoupled (see below). Close apposition of cell pairs facilitated the formation of such connexions since pronounced outgrowth of processes did not always occur. However, cells at a distance from one another were also able to form electrical connexions by way of processes (Fig. 7).

Other identified leech nerve cells were able to form synapses in culture. The development of electrical coupling between sensory and motor neurones in culture was of particular interest since these cells are involved in reflexes that have been extensively studied in the leech. In culture, as in the animal, P sensory cells and L motor neurones became electrically coupled when placed next to one another. Moreover the spread of current showed clear rectification, resembling properties of

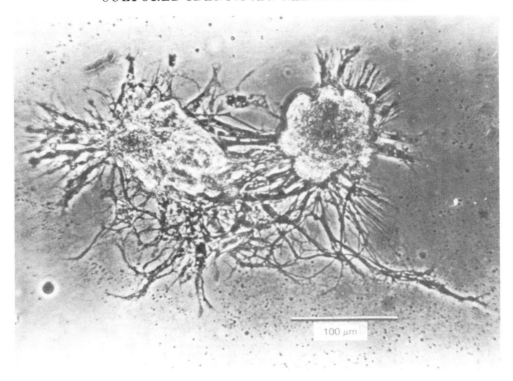

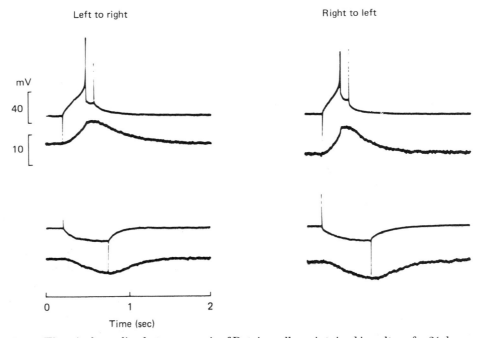

Fig. 7. Electrical coupling between a pair of Retzius cells maintained in culture for 21 days.

these connexions within the ganglion. Depolarizing current spread from the P cell to the L cell with 2 to 3 times greater efficacy than hyperpolarizing current, and hyperpolarizing current spread more effectively from the L cell to the P cell. Fig. 8 shows that N sensory cells and L motoneurones also became electrically coupled with similar rectification in culture. It was this finding that prompted re-examination of

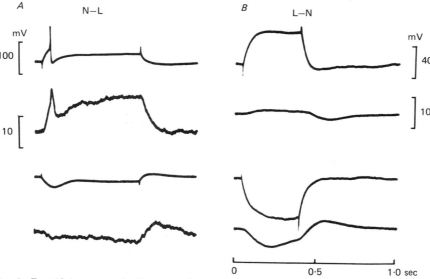

Fig. 8. Rectifying spread of current between an N cell and and L cell in culture. *A*, depolarizing current spread more effectively than hyperpolarizing current from the N cell to the L cell. *B*, conversely, hyperpolarizing current spread more effectively from the L cell to the N cell. The lower record in *A* shows that the N cell became transiently depolarized following the hyperpolarizing current pulse, giving rise to a clear depolarization of the L cell. Hyperpolarizing currents were used to maintain the resting potential of the N cell at −55 mV and that of the L cell at −100 mV. Electrical coupling between closely apposed N and L cells was usually found after about 10 days in culture. Similar rectification was observed between pairs of P and L cells that became coupled in culture.

the N to L synapse in the ganglion, where weak but definite rectifying coupling was observed for the first time, in addition to the more pronounced chemical coupling previously described by Nicholls & Purves (1970: see also Fig. 13). Such asymmetry in current flow between sensory cells and L motoneurones in culture and in the ganglion could result from rectification of the junctional membranes, the non-junctional membranes or both. (Rectification of the current–voltage relation in a cultured L cell is shown in Fig. 2*B*.)

The frequency with which electrical synapses developed varied from preparation to preparation. Out of more than 100 apposed Retzius cell pairs in which both neurones showed resting potentials of greater than −40 mV and overshooting action potentials, about 50 % became electrically coupled. It will be shown below that several pairs of the uncoupled cells showed clear signs of chemical synaptic transmission. Fewer experiments were made with L motoneurones since they were more difficult to isolate and maintain in culture. Nevertheless, seven out of nine pairs of L cells that did survive showed pronounced electrical coupling (5:1 or better). Out of twenty healthy, closely apposed N or P to L cell pairs, fifteen pairs became coupled.

Selectivity of electrical connexions formed in culture

To test whether isolated cells form connexions randomly or specifically with some targets but not others, combinations of Retzius cells, L motoneurones and P sensory cells were placed in close apposition. In one type of experiment, illustrated in Pl. 1 *B*, the cells were paired as follows:

1. Retzius cells with other Retzius cells;
2. Retzius cells with P sensory cells;
3. P sensory cells with P sensory cells.

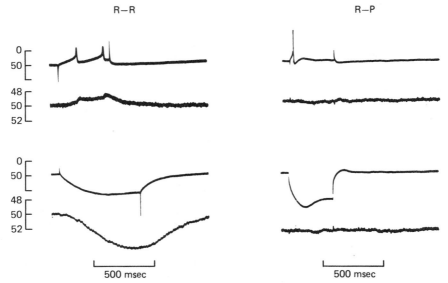

Fig. 9. Specificity of formation of electrical coupling by Retzius cells in culture. After 24 days in culture pairs of closely apposed Retzius cells (R–R) were found to be electrically coupled. In the same culture dish closely apposed pairs of Retzius and P cells (R–P) were not electrically coupled.

In five dishes maintained for 12–24 days, seventeen out of twenty-four pairs of Retzius cells became electrically coupled. Not a single instance of coupling was found between Retzius with P cells (twenty-two pairs) or P cells with P cells (eight pairs). The results of one such experiment are illustrated in Fig. 9. On the other hand, as described above, P cells did become coupled to L cells. The failure of P cells and Retzius cells to form electrical synapses therefore suggests that the development of connexions in culture is not an indiscriminate process but depends on some form of inherent cell–cell recognition.

A related but separate question is whether the connexions formed in culture mirror those seen in the animal. The results described above show that isolated cells are strikingly similar to their counterparts *in vivo*, both in the pattern of connexions and in the properties of the junctions. At the same time, certain differences become apparent in culture. For example, isolated Retzius cells became coupled to L cells (Fig. 10), a connexion one cannot discern in the ganglion by passing current. And P cells did not become coupled to P cells in culture, although there is evidence of weak

R to L   L to R

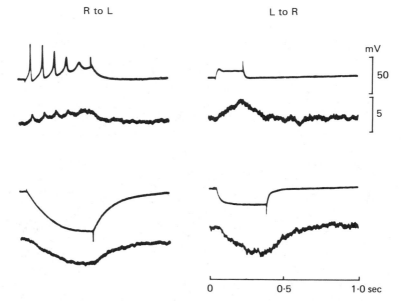

Fig. 10. Electrical coupling between a Retzius cell (R) and an L motoneurone (L) maintained in culture for 9 days. The resting potential of the Retzius cell was −50 mV, that of the L cell −40 mV. These cells were closely apposed. Coupling of this type is not readily discernible in the ganglion.

coupling in the ganglion. The possible reasons for such apparent discrepancies, which seem hardly surprising, are discussed below.

Chemically mediated synaptic interactions

Chemical interactions between cultured cells were observed far less frequently than electrical connexions. However, in certain pairs of Retzius cells, where electrical coupling was weak or absent, impulses or depolarization of one cell evoked slow hyperpolarizing potentials in the other (Fig. 11). The cells shown in Fig. 11 were some distance apart but similar responses were also seen in closely apposed cells. The long latency and time course of the hyperpolarizing potentials suggested the involvement of a chemical transmitter. This was confirmed by experiments such as that illustrated in Fig. 12, where the slow hyperpolarizing potential was reversed by hyperpolarization of the post-synaptic cell. These Retzius cells were not coupled electrically; when cells were coupled, it was not possible to determine whether inhibitory post-synaptic potentials were present, owing to the masking effect of the action potential undershoots.

In the ganglion the dominant synaptic interaction between N sensory and L motoneurones is chemical, with only a weak electrical component. In culture most N to L pairs failed to demonstrate a chemical connexion, although they became coupled electrically (see Fig. 8). In one pair of cells, however, electrical coupling was not obvious and action potentials in the N cell gave rise to clear depolarizing potentials in the L cell (Fig. 13). Unlike electrical coupling, this excitatory post-synaptic potential was labile and when thirty such responses were averaged, an 8·5

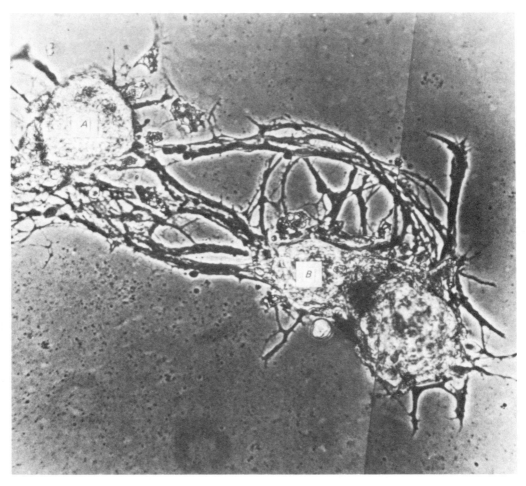

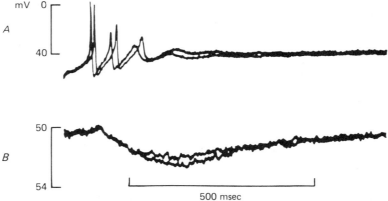

Fig. 11. Action potentials in one Retzius cell (*A*) Gave rise to hyperpolarizing responses in its neighbour (*B*) after 22 days in culture. These cells were only weakly coupled electrically. Impulses arose at the end of a hyperpolarizing pulse (not shown). Two sweeps are superimposed. Note the abundance of processes running from cell to cell, with fewer processes orientated randomly.

msec delay occurred between the peak of the presynaptic spike and the initiation of the excitatory post-synaptic potential, suggesting that this response was chemically mediated. However, without additional direct tests the mechanisms of transmission between these two cells remains less certain than the electrical connexions seen more frequently between isolated N and L cells.

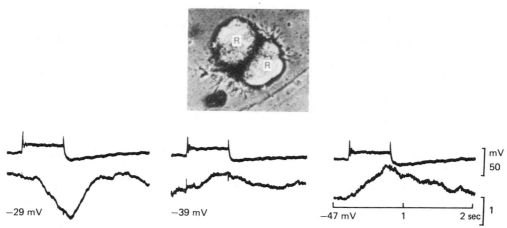

Fig. 12. Reversal of the slow chemical hyperpolarizing response in a Retzius cell after 18 days in culture. Here again prolonged depolarization of one Retzius cell gave rise to a slow hyperpolarization in its neighbour. Hyperpolarization of the post-synaptic cell caused a reversal of sign of this response. The membrane potential of the post-synaptic cell is given at the left of each trace (assessed by passing d.c. current through the bridge circuit of an intracellular electrode).

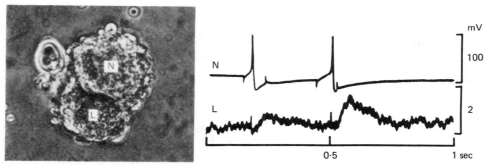

Fig. 13. After 6 days in culture action potentials in an N sensory cell gave rise to depolarizing responses in a closely apposed L motoneurone which had the appearance of chemical synaptic potentials. When thirty such responses were measured an average delay of 8.5 ± 3.7 msec from peak of the spike to the foot of the response was obtained.

DISCUSSION

Membrane properties and growth of isolated neurones

Torn from their normal surroundings and placed in a foreign environment, leech neurones survive well for several weeks. During the first days, in the absence of glia or normal blood, the neurones not only recover but sprout and form electrical and chemical connexions. In addition, the fine structure of the isolated cells continues to appear normal, and even after several weeks in culture there is still a striking similarity between the membrane properties of isolated T, P and N sensory cells and Retzius cells and those of their counterparts *in situ*. Hence, the cultured cells preserve their unique sets of membrane conductances and maintain a roughly normal distribution of intracellular ions. Indirect evidence further suggests that for several types of cells the abundant new processes that sprout from a cell are able to generate impulses without changing the current–voltage characteristic of the cell body. This raises the possibility that newly formed membrane may have ionic conductance channels similar to those of the cell body.

In contrast, certain neurones show novel membrane properties in culture. When L motoneurones are isolated for several days, their resting potential increases, pronounced rectification with hyperpolarizing current developed and large impulses can be evoked in the soma. These changes suggest an increase in excitability of a normally inexcitable cell, similar to those observed following axotomy of insect and crayfish neurones (Pitman, Tweedle & Cohen, 1972; Goodman & Heitler, 1979; Kuwada, Hagiwara & Wine, 1979).

The increase in input resistance observed in cultured cells presumably occurs owing to the detachment of the cell from its processes and from other neurones with which it is coupled in the ganglion. The geometry of isolated leech neurones without sprouts makes it feasible to estimate the specific membrane resistance (R_m), since the soma is approximately spherical and isopotential for current–voltage measurements. For a spherical cell with an input resistance of 200 MΩ, of radius 40 μm, R_m would be 40000 Ω cm^2. Even higher values of R_m, 100000 Ω cm^2, are obtained from measurements of the prolonged membrane time constant, assuming $C_m = 1$ μF cm^{-2} (see Fig. 10). This discrepancy may arise because convolutions of the surface membrane seen in electron micrographs of cultured cells tend to make the effective surface area larger than that estimated from the radius. In any event, these values are considerably higher than those found for squid axons and are comparable to those in barnacle photoreceptors and *Aplysia* neurones (Graubard, 1975). At present we have no direct information about R_m of leech neurones *in situ*, but there also the length constant is large, suggesting high value (Frank, Jansen & Rinvik, 1975).

Formation of electrical connexions

The electrical synapses seen in culture resemble those in the animal in many respects. The appropriate cells can become coupled with properties that are appropriate with respect to rectification. The efficacy of Retzius to Retzius coupling in culture can be as high as 1:1, although in general coupling is less than that observed *in situ*. Synchrony of spiking, which is common in the animal, rarely occurs between pairs of cultured cells. The long time constant for coupling of cultured cells may account for some of this drastic attenuation of the action potentials. In our preparations cells are usually placed close to one another to facilitate the formation of connexions (Pl. 1 *B*). Hence the coupling ratios reflect the properties of the junction more directly than those measured in the animal, where spread of current is attenuated to a variable extent along processes within the neuropile. Presumably, then, the lower ratios observed in culture reflect a lower efficacy of coupling; this in turn may be due to a smaller area of contact or to higher resistance junctions. The sites and structures of junctions that enable current to flow from cell to cell are not known in the animal or in culture. Although in theory specialized structures giving rise to high extracellular resistance could contribute, gap junctions or related membrane specializations seem more likely to account for coupling at the non-rectifying and rectifying synapses observed both in culture and in the animal.

We do not yet know how the time for which cells are kept in culture influences the properties and numbers of junctions. The first evidence of coupling appears at about 6 days in culture; however, transient junctions might have been formed and disrupted earlier. And at longer periods of several weeks further changes may develop.

Formation of chemical synapses in culture

We found chemical synapses between cells in culture only rarely, possibly as a result of our culture conditions. Moreover the synaptic potentials were small in view of the great increase in input resistance of isolated cells. Transmitter synthesis may be reduced or arrested, although the large numbers of normal dense-core and clear vesicles seen in electron micrographs of cultured Retzius cells suggest that transmitter synthesis continues *in vitro*. The slow hyperpolarizing potentials that developed between these cells might be the result of diffuse release rather than the formation of specialized pre- and post-synaptic structures. Another cause may be a failure to develop appropriate receptors in the membrane of regenerated neurites or to accumulate them at sites of transmitter release from the presynaptic terminal. It also seems likely that conditioning factors normally present in the blood or substrate are absent from our medium and that adding them or using higher density cultures would facilitate the formation of chemical synapses between the isolated cells that are bathed in a relatively large volume of fluid (O'Lague, MacLeish, Nurse, Claude, Furshpan & Potter, 1976).

Selectivity of connexions

One goal of the present experiments has been to develop a preparation in which questions concerning the specificity of neuronal connexions can be examined. Our first concern, therefore, has been whether isolated leech cells in culture form connexions according to fixed rules or randomly. Clearly some degree of selectivity exists for the formation of electrical synapses in culture, since certain connexions formed in culture parallel those found *in situ*. On the other hand the coupling of Retzius cells with L motoneurones and the inhibitory chemical connexions occasionally seen between Retzius cells have not been described in normal ganglia. It is possible that the strong electrical coupling between Retzius cells in the ganglion masks a weak inhibitory chemical synapse. At the same time, using electrical techniques to demonstrate connexions between neurones in the ganglion may be an indecisive criterion to apply. The electrical coupling between N sensory cells and L motoneurones is ordinarily not obvious in the face of the more pronounced chemical synaptic transmission between these cells. Conversely, it is now known that demonstrable electrical coupling between cells in the leech ganglion can be mediated not only by direct contact but also by a third interposed cell (Muller & Scott, 1979). Thus leech neurones in culture may demonstrate a pattern of cell–cell recognition which only appears to be different from that of their counterparts *in situ*.

For a number of reasons novel connexions are to be expected in culture: (1) neurones *in vitro* have been deprived of numerous cues that may influence the way in which they form connexions, such as growth along one tract or another; (2) it is reasonable to expect differences in the mechanisms used by immature cells to find their targets during development and those used by mature neurones during regeneration; (3) mechanical barriers present in the ganglion but not in culture might deny cells access to each other (for example, in the ganglion the processes of Retzius and L cells might always be kept apart by layers of glia); and (4) a cell's specific affinities may be relative rather than absolute and might change after isolation. Indeed, although leech neurones within the ganglia generally re-form their connexions with a high degree of precision (Wallace *et al.* 1977; Muller, 1979) novel interactions are observed after lesions have been made in the c.n.s. (Jansen, Muller & Nicholls, 1974) and when whole ganglia are maintained in culture (Wallace *et al.* 1977).

The selective formation of connexions by isolated neurones in our experiments must depend on inherent properties of the cells rather than on factors such as access to synaptic sites or competition. The present experiments set the stage for testing the ability of a particular cell to form synapses with a wide variety of potential targets and for defining cellular mechanisms involved in setting up a hierarchy of specificities. With two cells directly in contact and in the absence of a complex neuropile, the chemical and electrical synapses formed in culture also appear favourable for biophysical studies on intercellular movement of ions and small molecules, as well as transmitter release and chemoreception.

This work was supported by U.S.P.H.S. Grant No. 11544 and by a Grant from the March of Dimes for which we are most grateful. D. Ready was supported in part by U.S.P.H.S. Training Grant No. NS 07158-01. P. Fuchs was supported by fellowships from the N.S.F. and N.I.H. We wish to thank Miss Lyn Lazar for valuable technical assistance, and Drs D. Baylor, S. Blackshaw, B. Wallace and Miss L. Henderson for their contributions to the work and to this manuscript. We owe a particular debt to Mr R. B. Bosler, who has generously supplied advice through the years and who recently showed us new procedures for making micro-electrodes far more effective than any we had before.

REFERENCES

ALBRECHT-BUEHLER, G. (1980). Navigation of non-neuronal cells. In *The Role of Intercellular Signals*, ed. NICHOLLS, J. G., pp. 75–96. Berlin: Dahlem Konferenzen.

ANDERSON, H., EDWARDS, J. S. & PALKA, J. (1980). Developmental neurobiology of invertebrates. *A. Rev. Neurosci.* **3**, 97–139.

BANKER, G. A. & COWAN, W. M. (1979). Further observations on hippocampal neurons in dispersed cell culture. *J. comp. Neurol.* **187**, 469–494.

BAYLOR, D. A. & NICHOLLS, J. G. (1969*a*). After-effects of nerve impulses on signalling in the central nervous system of the leech. *J. Physiol.* **203**, 571–589.

BAYLOR, D. A. & NICHOLLS, J. G. (1969*b*). Chemical and electrical synaptic connexions between cutaneous mechanoreceptor neurones in the central nervous system of the leech. *J. Physiol.* **203**, 591–609.

BORNSTEIN, M. D. (1958). Reconstituted rat-tail collagen used as a substrate for tissue cultures on coverslips on Maximow slides and in roller tubes. *Lab. Invest.* **7**, 134–137.

COGGESHALL, R. E. & FAWCETT, D. W. (1964). The fine structure of the central nervous system of the leech, *Hirudo medicinalis. J. Neurophysiol.* **27**, 229–289.

CRAIN, S. M. (1976). *Neurophysiologic Studies in Tissue Culture.* New York: Raven Press.

EDWARDS, J. S. & PALKA, J. (1971). Neural regeneration: delayed formation of central contacts by insect sensory cells. *Science, N.Y.* **172**, 591–594.

FRANK, E., JANSEN, J. K. S. & RINVIK, E. (1975). A multisomatic axon in the central nervous system of the leech. *J. comp. Neurol.* **159**, 1–13.

GAZE, R. M. (1970). *Formation of Nerve Connections*. New York & London: Academic Press.

GOODMAN, C. S. & HEITLER, W. J. (1979). Electrical properties of insect neurones with spiking and non-spiking somata: normal axotomized and colchicine-treated neurones. *J. exp. Biol.* **83**, 95–121.

GRAUBARD, K. (1975). Voltage attenuation within *Aplysia* neurons: the effect of branching pattern. *Brain Res.* **88**, 325–332.

GRAY, E. G. & GUILLERY, R. W. (1963). An electron microscopical study of the ventral nerve cord of the leech. *Z. Zellforsch. microsk. Anat.* **60**, 826–849.

HAGIWARA, S. & MORITA, H. (1962). Electronic transmission between two nerve cells in the leech ganglion. *J. Neurophysiol.* **25**, 721–731.

HODGKIN, A. L. & RUSHTON, W. A. H. (1946). The electrical constants of a crustacean nerve fibre. *Proc. R. Soc.* B **133**, 144.

JANSEN, J. K. S., MULLER, K. J. & NICHOLLS, J. G. (1974). Persistent modification of synaptic interactions between sensory and motor nerve cells following discrete lesions in the central nervous system of the leech. *J. Physiol*, **242**, 298–305.

JANSEN, J. K. S. & NICHOLLS, J. G. (1973). Conductance changes, an electrogenic pump and the hyperpolarization of the leech neurones following impulses. *J. Physiol.* **229**, 635–665.

KUFFLER, S. W. & NICHOLLS, J. G. (1966). The physiology of neuroglial cells. *Ergebn. Physiol.* **27**, 1–90.

KUFFLER, S. W. & POTTER, D. D. (1964). Glia in the leech central nervous system: physiological properties and neurone–glia relationship. *J. Neurophysiol.* **27**, 290–320.

KUWADA, J. Y., HAGIWARA, G. C. & WINE, J. J. (1979). Increased electrogenicity of crayfish neurones following axotomy: investigations of the signal and mechanisms. *Neurosci. Abstr.* **5**, 251.

MULLER, K. J. (1979). Synapses between neurones in the central nervous system of the leech. *Biol. Rev.* **54**, 99–134.

MULLER, K. J. & CARBONETTO, S. T. (1979). The morphological and physiological properties of a regenerating synapse in the C.N.S. of the leech. *J. comp. Neurol.* **185**, 485–516.

MULLER, K. & MCMAHAN, U. J. (1976). The shapes of sensory and motor neurones and the distribution of their synapses in the ganglia of the leech: a study using intracellular injection of horseradish peroxidase. *Proc. R. Soc.* B **194**, 481–499.

MULLER, K. J. & SCOTT, S. (1979). Direct electrical synaptic connection is mediated by an interneuron. *Neurosci. Abstr.* **5**, 744.

NICHOLLS, J. G. & KUFFLER, S. W. (1964). Extracellular space as a pathway for exchange between blood and neurones in the central nervous system of the leech: ionic composition of glial cells and neurons. *J. Neurophysiol.* **27**, 645–671.

NICHOLLS, J. G. & PURVES, D. (1970). Monosynaptic chemical and electrical connexions between sensory and motor cells in the central nervous system of the leech. *J. Physiol.* **209**, 647–667.

O'LAGUE, P. H., MACLEISH, P. R., NURSE, C. A., CLAUDE, P., FURSHPAN, E. J. & POTTER, D. D. (1975). Physiological and morphological studies on developing sympathetic neurons in dissociated cell culture. *Cold Spring Harb. Symp. quant. Biol.* **40**, 399–407.

PITMAN, R. M., TWEEDLE, C. D. & COHEN, M. J. (1972). Electrical responses of insect central neurons: augmentation by nerve section or colchicine. *Science, N.Y.* **178**, 507–509.

READY, D. F. & NICHOLLS, J. G. (1979). Identified neurones isolated from leech CNS make selective connexions in culture. *Nature, Lond.* **281**, 67–69.

RUDE, S., COGGESHALL, R. E. & VAN ORDEN, III, L. S. (1969). Chemical and ultra-structural identification of 5-hydroxytryptamine in an identified neuron. *J. cell Biol.* **41**, 832–854.

SARGENT, P. B. (1977). Synthesis of acetylcholine by excitatory motoneurones in central nervous system of leech. *J. Neurophysiol.* **40**, 453–460.

SPERRY, R. W. (1963). Chemoaffinity in the orderly growth of nerve fiber patterns and connections *Proc. nat. Acad. Sci. U.S.A.* **50**, 703–710.

STUART, A. E. (1970). Physiological and morphological properties of motoneurones in the central nervous system of the leech. *J. Physiol.* **209**, 627–646.

VARON, S. S. & BUNGE, R. P. (1978). Trophic mechanisms in the peripheral nervous system. *A. Rev. Neurosci*, **1**, 327–361.

WALLACE, B. G., ADAL, M. N. & NICHOLLS, J. G. (1977). Sprouting and regeneration of synaptic connexions by sensory neurones in leech ganglia maintained in culture. *Proc. R. Soc.* B **199**, 567–585.

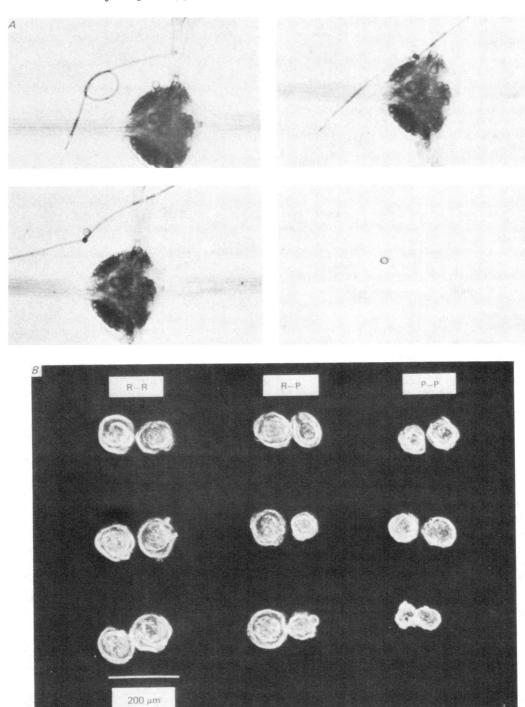

P. A. FUCHS, J. G. NICHOLLS AND D. F. READY

(*Facing p.* 222)

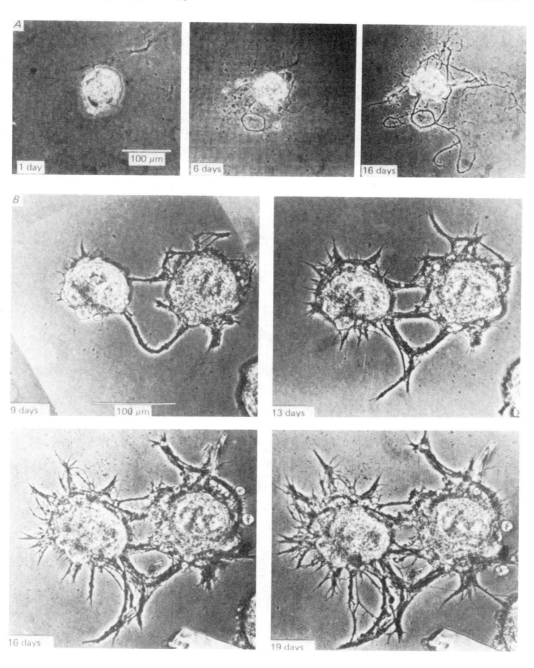

P. A. FUCHS, J. G. NICHOLLS and D. F. READY

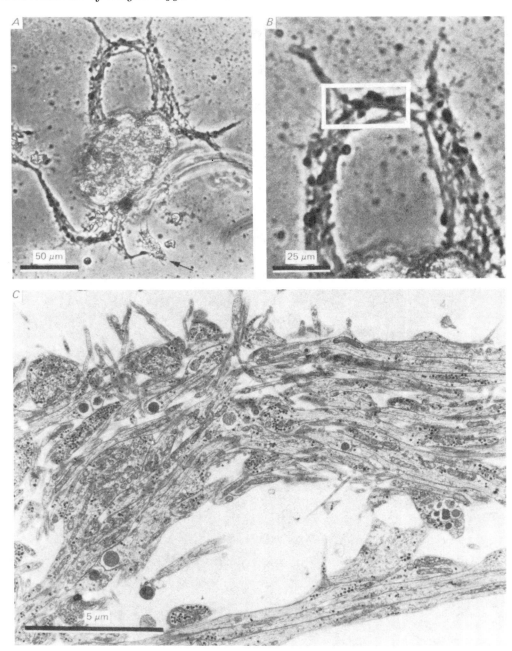

P. A. FUCHS, J. G. NICHOLLS AND D. F. READY

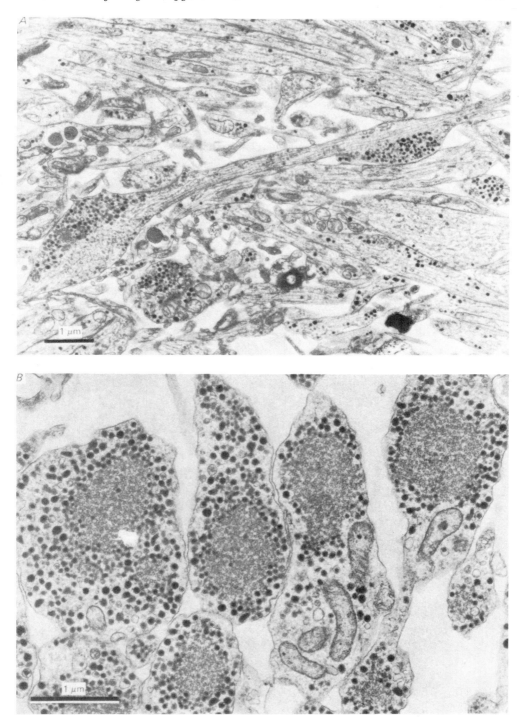

P. A. FUCHS, J. G. NICHOLLS AND D. F. READY

PLATE 1

A, Dissection of a single N sensory cell body (diameter 60 μm) from a leech ganglion. *B*, the disposition of pairs of cells in a typical culture. Pairs of Retzius cells (R–R) were apposed in the left column, Retzius to P sensory cell pairs (R–P) in the middle column, and P to P cell pairs (P–P) in the right column. Such close apposition of the cells was often used to facilitate the formation of connexions.

PLATE 2

A, growth of an isolated anterior 'pagoda' cell over 16 days. Processes, often consisting of bundles of fine axons, could extend 20 μm per day or more, becoming thickened with time. *B*, growth of processes of two Retzius cells maintained in culture for 19 days. Processes appear to run predominantly between the two cells, rather than in all directions equally (see also Fig. 11).

PLATE 3

Light and electron micrographs of a single Retzius cell cultured for 25 days. The area of outgrown processes indicated in panel *B* was sectioned parallel to the surface of the dish shown in *C*. The arrow in *A* indicates a growth cone.

PLATE 4

A, varicosities in the processes of a Retzius cell after 25 days in culture. *B*, accumulations of clear and dense-core vesicles in projections of Retzius cell near the dish bottom, cut parallel to the surface of the dish.

Reprinted from the PROCEEDINGS OF THE NATIONAL ACADEMY OF SCIENCES
Vol. 50, No. 4, pp. 703–710. October, 1963.

CHEMOAFFINITY IN THE ORDERLY GROWTH OF NERVE FIBER PATTERNS AND CONNECTIONS*

BY R. W. SPERRY

DIVISION OF BIOLOGY, CALIFORNIA INSTITUTE OF TECHNOLOGY

Communicated July 29, 1963

In early observations on the outgrowth and termination of nerve fibers, it appeared that different fiber types must be guided to their respective end organs and other connection sites by selective chemical or electrical forces. Explanatory terms like chemotaxis, chemotropism, galvanotaxis, and neurotropism were commonly employed by Cajal[7] and others early in the century. These selectivity concepts later came under attack, especially during the 1930's and 40's when the application of more analytic experimental approaches to the mechanics of nerve growth seemed to rule out the presence of either chemical or electrical selectivity in favor of a predominantly mechanical interpretation.[34, 37]

The numerous examples of apparent selectivity described earlier, as well as the developmental patterning of the central nerve tracts and fiber systems in general, we came to believe, were more properly and correctly explained on a mechanical basis, particularly in terms of the orienting effects of mechanical stresses on tissue ultrastructures and the resultant formation of submicroscopic systems of mechanical guide lines in the colloidal matrix of the growing medium.

At the height of this antiselectivity movement I was led, from evidence indirect and partly behavioral, to postulate again in 1939 a form of chemical selectivity in nerve growth even more extreme in some respects than in the earlier proposals. The hypothesis,[18–24] in brief, suggested that the patterning of synaptic connections in the nerve centers, including those refined details of network organization heretofore ascribed mainly to functional molding in various forms, must be handled instead by the growth mechanism directly, independently of function, and with very strict selectivity governing synaptic formation from the beginning. The establishment and maintenance of synaptic associations were conceived to be regulated by highly specific cytochemical affinities that arise systematically among the different types of neurons involved via self-differentiation, induction through terminal contacts, and embryonic gradient effects.

Coming at a time when "instinctive" was still a disreputable term in most scientific quarters, and when concepts of nerve growth were strongly dominated by the mechanical theory, this seemed a long shot at first and hardly less wild than some of the opposing interpretations of the day like the "resonance principle"[32, 33] that it was proposed to replace. When tested experimentally, however, study after study through the 1940's[18–24, 29] yielded results that fit nicely. In brief, whenever central fiber systems were disconnected and transplanted or just scrambled by rough surgical section, regrowth always led to orderly functional recovery and under conditions that precluded re-educative adjustments. The functional outcome was always *as if* the scrambled fibers somehow unsorted themselves in regeneration and managed to "home in" on their original and proper central nerve terminals.

It seemed a necessary conclusion from these results that the cells and fibers of the brain and cord must carry some kind of individual identification tags, presumably

703

cytochemical in nature, by which they are distinguished one from another almost, in many regions, to the level of the single neuron; and further, that the growing fibers are extremely particular when it comes to establishing synaptic connections, each axon linking only with certain neurons to which it becomes selectively attached by specific chemical affinities.

This chemoaffinity theory included additional features such as the application of morphogenetic gradients in retinal, cutaneous, vestibular, and other systems to explain their orderly topographic projection and central representation, the patterning of central neurotization by peripheral induction, neuronal specification through synaptic contact, and related principles of growth and differentiation as applied to the specialized problems in the functional organization of neuronal connections in neurogenesis.[23-26] It carried previous conceptions of nerve specificity to a new order of refinement and put on a prefunctional chemical basis the ordering of the brain networks for inherited components in behavior.

Taken as a whole, the scheme offered an explanation of the developmental patterning of central nervous organization that seemed to have distinct advantages over alternative concepts applied previously, like "disuse atrophy," "neurobiotaxis," "mechanical contact guidance," "bioelectric fields," "autonomous differentiation of resonance scores," and "stimulogenous fibrillation." The chemoaffinity interpretation also fitted nicely with related developments in animal behavior and ethology on the one hand, and in experimental embryology and genetics on the other to bring together a number of loose concepts into a systematic approach to the inheritance and development of behavior patterns.

In spite of the attractions and the considerable supporting data, there have always been a number of persisting objections and gaps in the evidence to prevent our accepting the hypothesis completely. In the first place, we had never actually seen growing nerve fibers bypass a series of empty neuron slots to settle on their own proper terminals. This always had to be inferred indirectly, mainly from behavioral evidence. Moreover, this same behavioral evidence could be accounted for in other terms without recourse to all the postulated chemical affinities and without the assumption of selective reconnection—by schemes involving certain physiological coding and resonance phenomena that could operate in randomized nerve nets. The "resonance principle" of Weiss,[32, 33] which had remained for nearly 20 years the favored explanation of related phenomena produced by peripheral nerve derangements, was just such a scheme in which the growth of synaptic connections was conceived to be completely nonselective, diffuse, and universal in downstream contacts. Nothing in the evidence, including the postregenerative mapping data from electrical[9, 15] and lesion[21] studies on the optic tectum, could be considered critical in deciding between these alternatives; direct histological evidence was needed to settle the questions involved.

The chemoaffinity interpretation also met objections on the grounds that there are not enough distinct chemical labels available in the embryo. The scheme requires literally millions, and possibly billions, of chemically differentiated neuron types, each distinguishable from all others on the same side of the midsagittal plane. Each half of the nervous system is presumed to be a chemical mirror map of the other. This labeling problem, plus the further task of interconnecting in precise detail all the postulated millions of chemically specific neuron units into functionally adaptive brain circuits, also seemed prohibitive from the standpoint of information theory because of a supposed lack of enough "bits of information" within the zygote to handle all the developmental decisions involved in building a brain on this plan.

Evidence obtained recently seems to provide a direct experimental answer to such objections. This has come in the past few years from histological studies started in 1958 on the optic system of fishes, in which I was joined in 1959–1960 by Dr. Attardi,[4, 5] and in the past year and a half by Dr. Arora.[1, 2] In brief, we think we have finally man-i

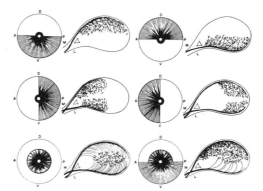

Fig. 1.—Diagrammatic reconstructions of regeneration patterns formed in optic tracts and tectum by fibers originating in different retinal halves, as indicated (after Attardi and Sperry[4, 5]).

aged to demonstrate quite directly by histological methods the postulated selectivity in nerve growth and synaptic formation. The new evidence shows that fibers arising from different parts of the retina preferentially select separate central pathways as they grow into the brain, and that they eventually find, and connect with, specific predesignated target zones in the midbrain tectum.

In these experiments, the main optic trunk was severed in a rough manner to enhance the inevitable scrambling among the hundreds of thousands of constituent fibers. The corresponding eye was then opened, and half of the retina was removed (as indicated in Figs. 1, 2, and 3) in order that the course and termination of the remaining fibers from the intact half-retina might be differentiated histologically. A summary of the results from the different types of cases is presented in Figure 1. As shown in the diagrams, removal in separate cases of the *top* half of the retina, the *bottom* half, the *front*, the *back*, or the *outer* peripheral hemiretina resulted, respectively, in quite different and consistently distinctive regeneration patterns. At each of the successive forks in the system of trails leading back to their tectal destinations, the various fiber groups made different and correct choices.

Of special interest are those cases in which the regenerating fibers, in order to

Left Tectum

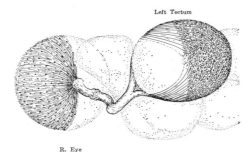

R. Eye

Fig. 2.—Following ablation of temporal retina and optic nerve section, regenerating optic fibers grow through extensive stretches of the semidenervated anterior tectum, but form synaptic layer and connections only in posterior tectum.

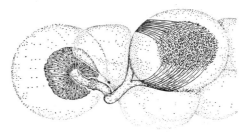

Fig. 3.—Fibers from center of retina grow through denervated peripheral zone of tectum without establishing plexiform layer and synaptic connections until they reach central zone.

reach their own synaptic zones, were obliged to first grow through and across non-terminal sectors of optic tectum. This was true when the posterior half-retina was removed, and the fibers from the anterior hemiretina, particularly those of the medial tract, had to cross large stretches of the partially denervated anterior half of the tectum without forming synaptic linkages (Fig. 2). In this situation the regenerated fibers remained in the superficial parallel layer and coursed straight through without branching or synapsis to bypass the whole population of potential terminal neurons that lay empty and readily accessible all through the front half of the tectum.

Something similar occurred when the peripheral part of the retina was removed (Fig. 3). In these cases, all the regenerating fibers, in order to reach their proper synaptic zones in the center of the tectum, were obliged to grow from the outer tectal border across the denervated peripheral zone. Here again they remained confined to the superficial parallel layer passing straight through without synapsis. Only within the central zone of the tectum did these fibers from the central retina ramify and form the deeper synaptic layer.

It is evident that optic fibers advancing along the same central channels grew very differently depending on their retinal origins. On reaching a given point in the peripheral tectum, for example, one fiber type dipped centrally and ramified in the deeper plexiform layer to form connections among the neuronal elements of the immediate vicinity, whereas other fibers in the same position continued to grow right on through and beyond these same free, denervated neurons, bypassing them and many others for varying distances, until the fiber tips reached the appropriate tectal zone that matched their retinal origin. With the mechanical conditions of the growing medium identical for these different fiber types, and with other factors like timing, rate of growth, and functional feedback seemingly eliminated,[21, 23, 24] the systematic variance in the course and termination seems most reasonably explained on the basis of specific chemoaffinities between the different optic fibers and the elements encountered in growth. Studies still in progress show that, when the main medial and lateral tracts in these fish are freed and surgically interchanged in the brain where they approach the tectum, the displaced fiber bundles promptly recross in growth to regain their proper channels.[2] Fiber bundles, deflected still farther centrally at the edge or within the tectum, tend to form new short-cut pathways in the parallel layer oriented in a direction in which no optic fibers would ordinarily grow in the given region.[1] We also find that fibers from neighboring points in the retina tend to segregate at the first opportunity within the nerve scar and may remain thus segregated through the chiasma and all the way to the tectum.

It is apparent from the results that not only the synaptic terminals, but also in these fishes the route by which the growing optic fibers reach those terminals, is selectively determined, presumably on the basis of similar or identical chemoaffinity factors. From direct observation and photography of living nerve fibers,[17] it is known that, as the growing tip advances, it continuously sends out a spray or flare of rapidly elongating and retracting microfilaments that extend outward into the surrounding front in all possible directions (Fig. 4). The above evidence suggests that factors more chemical than mechanical determine which of the various microfilament probes will preponderate at each point to set the course of growth. The results lead us to what is essentially a chemotactic view of nerve outgrowth, though without the "distance action" imputed in some definitions of chemotaxis. The general principle of contact guidance is assumed to apply here as it always has in any chemical, electrical, or mechanical theory of nerve growth since about 1913 when Harrison made it clear that nerve fibers are able to grow only in contact with surfaces, never freely into or across fluid spaces.[14]

There remains the problem of explaining the topographic plan inherent in the "homing behavior" of the optic fibers that is responsible for the neat maplike projection that is laid down among retino-tectal connections. For this, I still go back

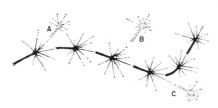

Fig. 4.—Schematic representation of sequential steps in chemotactic guidance of a growing nerve fiber. A spreading flare of microfilaments constantly reaches out in front of the advancing fiber tip testing the surroundings in all directions. The critical factors determining which microfilaments will prevail to set the course of growth would appear from present evidence to be mainly chemical. Numerous alternative possible paths, as represented at A, B, and C, are open and mechanically feasible at each point but fail to develop because of differential chemical attraction.

to my initial interpretation[19, 23] proposing an orderly cytochemical mapping in terms of two or more gradients of embryonic differentiation that spread across and through each other with their axes roughly perpendicular. These separate gradients successively superimposed on the retinal and tectal fields and surroundings would stamp each cell with its appropriate latitude and longitude expressed in a kind of chemical code with matching values between the retinal and tectal maps. The inversion of the retinal map on the tectum suggests complementary relations in the affinity forces involved in linking corresponding points in the two fields. Similar inversions in other systems point to general use of complemental gradient values in synapsis. The same set of cytochemical factors extended from the ganglion cells of the retina into the microfilament flare at the tip of the growing optic axons and also stamped on the optic pathways could be utilized for guiding the respective fiber types into their separate proper channels at each of the numerous forks or decision points which they encounter as they make their way back through what essentially amounts to a multiple Y-maze of possible pathways. The final course laid down by any given fiber reflects the history of a continuous series of decisions based on differential affinities between the various advance filaments that probe the surroundings ahead and the diverse elements that each encounters.

Prediction that the nasotemporal (anteroposterior) gradient might be shown to be fixed separately and prior to the dorsoventral gradient,[21] has since been confirmed in the experiments of Székely[31] and Stone.[30] These and other embryological studies with correlated electrical analyses by Gaze[10] and his associates give further credence to the gradient interpretation. Apparent discrepancies in the recent report of Burgen and Grafstein[6] are instructive regarding the dynamics of gradient organization, but require no change in the basic hypothesis. We have been able to show in behavioral studies that the discrimination of color and brightness, like the perception of directionality and spatial factors in vision, also undergoes an orderly restoration in optic nerve regeneration.[3] This means that additional specification of the optic fibers is required to assure the appropriate tectal linkages for the different types of color and luminosity fibers. The same would seem to be true for the "on," "off," and "on-off" classes of optic fibers in order to explain the observed orderly recovery of optokinetic responses and of learned pattern discriminations.

Those familiar primarily with the visual system of man or other mammals may see objections in the foregoing interpretation. The partial crossing of fibers in the mammalian chiasma gives difficulty; and worse, the fact that the *nasal* half-retina of one eye terminates in close register with the *temporal* half-retina of the other eye in primates may look at first like a direct contradiction. Actually, with the incorporation of certain minor developments that we assume must have taken place in the course of evolution, the same gradient hypothesis works nicely also for the mammals, including man. First, we must postulate that fibers from the temporal pole of the retina and gradually from the whole temporal half-field have evolved a

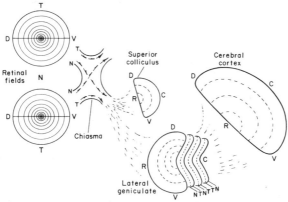

FIG. 5.—Schematic diagram indicating possible application of chemoaffinity interpretation to genesis of mammalian visual system (see text). Axial labeling of gradients for brain centers is highly tentative as the effective embryonic gradients underlying their topographic differentiation remain uncertain. D·V: dorsoventral gradient; N·T: nasotemporal; R·C: rostrocaudal.

lateral growth affinity that prevents their crossing in the chiasma region. Secondly, keeping the dorsoventral axis as before to mark latitude in the retinal field, we may postulate that in mammalian evolution the *nasotemporal* gradient came to be replaced by the *radial* gradient for topographic labeling. This would give the required cytochemical correspondence for functionally identical points in nasal and temporal half-fields (see Fig. 5); it would also leave the differential nasal-temporal and analogous matching properties in the centers for determining decussation, laterality, layered projection, and related features of the mammalian system associated with stereoscopic vision and retinal rivalry, that in themselves have always been puzzling from the standpoint of neurogenesis. At present the possibility cannot be excluded that the decussation patterns in the optic chiasma are determined mechanically in development in combination with rate and timing of fiber ingrowth. However, previous attempts to explain chiasma formation on a mechanical basis[8] have run into difficulties that appear to be more easily resolved on the chemoaffinity plan.

There is reason to think, from the evidence available,[16, 23-25, 29] that the above principles, as outlined here for the visual system, apply to the patterning of pathways and connections in the vertebrate nervous system in general, though it is to be expected that their manifestation will be found to vary in form and degree in different species and in different parts of the system. A considerable backlog of supporting observations suggestive of chemotaxis has accumulated during the last two decades, but has not been emphasized owing to the prevailing unpopularity of anything suggestive of neurotropism and chemical guidance. With the demonstration of chemotactic regrowth in the optic system leaving little room for further doubt of the selectivity effects,[4] the way seems cleared for retrospective reassessment of some of the earlier observations with an increased recognition of the importance of selective chemoaffinity in nerve growth and connection in general.[13]

Extension of chemoaffinity concepts to the growth of fiber patterns and connections in the peripheral nervous system may require brief comment at this point, since it is in reference to peripheral nerve growth and regeneration that the strongest evidence has been gathered in support of earlier impressions that nerve outgrowth and termination are basically nonselective. Furthermore, many of the observations indicating absence of selectivity in peripheral nerve regeneration remain in good standing.[11, 35-37] On the other hand, there are exceptions where peripheral innervation is clearly selective, and other cases where it appears to be more selective than not.[11, 12, 22, 23] Though it must thus remain for the present partly a matter of emphasis, it may nevertheless be worthwhile to caution here that, in the changing total picture as we now see it, the established examples of indiscriminate nerve outgrowth and termination begin to look more and more as if they might represent the exceptions rather than the general rule.

* The work was supported by a U.S. Public Health Service grant (M3372) and the F. P. Hixon fund of the California Institute of Technology. A shortened version of the material was presented at the annual meeting of the American Association of Anatomists in Washington, D.C., April 1963.

[1] Arora, H. L., *Anat. Record*, **145**, 202 (1963).

[2] Arora, H. L., and R. W. Sperry, *Amer. Zool.*, **2**, 389 (1962).

[3] Arora, H. L., and R. W. Sperry, *Dev. Biol.*, **7**, 234 (1963).

[4] Attardi, D., and R. W. Sperry, *Physiol.*, **3**, 12 (1960).

[5] Attardi, D., and R. W. Sperry, *Exptl. Neurol.*, **7**, 46 (1963).

[6] Burgen, A. S. V., and B. Grafstein, *Nature*, **196**, 898 (1962).

[7] Cajal, Santiago Ramon Y., *Studies on Veretebrate Neurogenesis*, trans. L. Guth (Springfield, Illinois: Charles C Thomas, 1960).

[8] Ferreira-Beirutti, Pedro, *Proc. Soc. Exptl. Biol. Med.*, **76**, 302 (1951).

[9] Gaze, R. M., *Intern. Rev. Neurobiol.*, **2**, 1 (1960).

[10] Gaze, R. M., M. Jacobson, and G. Székely, *J. Physiol.*, **165**, 484 (1963).

[11] Guth, Lloyd, *Physiol. Revs.*, **36**, 441 (1956).

[12] Guth, Lloyd, *Exptl. Neurol.*, **4**, 59 (1961).

[13] Hamburger, Viktor, *J. Cellular Comp. Physiol.*, **60**, 81 (1962).

[14] Harrison, R. G., *J. Exptl. Zool.*, **17**, 521 (1914).

[15] Maturana, H. R., J. Y. Lettvin, W. S. McCulloch, and W. H. Pitts, *Science*, **103**, 1409 (1959).

[16] Miner, N. M., *J. Comp. Neurol.*, **105**, 161 (1956).

[17] Pomerat, C. M., *Anat. Record*, **145**, 371 (1963).

[18] Sperry, R. W., *J. Comp. Neurol.*, **75**, 1 (1941).

[19] Sperry, R. W., *Anat. Record*, **84**, 470 (1942).

[20] Sperry, R. W., *J. Comp. Neurol.*, **79**, 33 (1943).

[21] Sperry, R. W., *J. Neurophysiol.*, **8**, 15 (1945).

[22] Sperry, R. W., *Quart. Rev. Biol.*, **20**, 311 (1945).

[23] Sperry, R. W., in *Handbook of Experimental Psychology*, ed. S. S. Stevens (New York: Wiley and Sons, 1950), chap. 7.

[24] Sperry, R. W., *Growth*, **10**, 63 (1950).

[25] Sperry, R. W., in *Biochemistry of the Developing Nervous System*, ed. H. Waelsch (New York: Academic Press, 1955), p. 74.

[26] Sperry, R. W., in *Developmental Basis of Behavior and Evolution*, ed. Ann Roe and G. G. Simpson (Yale University Press, 1958).

[27] Sperry, R. W., *Anat. Record*, **145**, 288 (1963).

[28] Sperry, R. W., and N. Deupree, *J. Comp. Neurol.*, **106,** 143 (1956).

[29] Sperry, R. W., and N. M. Miner, *J. Comp. Neurol.*, **90,** 403 (1949).

[30] Stone, L. S., *J. Exptl. Zool.*, **145,** 85 (1960).

[31] Székely, G., *Acta Biol. Acad. Sci. Hung.*, **5,** 157 (1954).

[32] Weiss, Paul, *Naturwiss.*, **16,** 626 (1928).

[33] Weiss, Paul A., *Biol. Rev.*, **11,** 494 (1936).

[34] Weiss, Paul A., in *Principles of Development* (New York: Henry Holt and Co., 1939), part 4.

[35] Weiss, Paul, in *Analysis of Development*, ed. B. H. Willier, P. A. Weiss, and V. Hamburger (Philadelphia: Saunders, 1960), pp. 346–401.

[36] Weiss, Paul, and Ann Hoag, *J. Neurophysiol.*, **9,** 413 (1946).

[37] Weiss, Paul, and A. Cecil Taylor, *J. Exptl. Zool.*, **95,** 233 (1944).

Section 10
Surface Molecules
and Cell-Cell Recognition

Gottlieb, D.I., K. Rock, and L. Glaser. 1976. A gradient of adhesive specificity in developing avian retina. *Proc. Natl. Acad. Sci.* **73:** 410–414.

Buskirk, D.R., J.-P. Thiery, U. Rutishauser, and G.M. Edelman. 1980. Antibodies to a neural cell adhesion molecule disrupt histogenesis in cultured chick retinae. *Nature* **285:** 488–489.

Trisler, G.D., M.D. Schneider, and M. Nirenberg. 1981. A topographic gradient of molecules in retina can be used to identify neuron position. *Proc. Natl. Acad. Sci.* **78:** 2145–2149.

Since the mechanism of recognition during axon outgrowth (Section 4) and selective synapse formation (Section 9) probably depends, in part, on surface interactions between cells, a number of investigators have applied recent advances in the techniques of immunology, cell biology, and genetics to the problem of isolating and studying cell-surface molecules. Although this effort has been under way for several years, it is safe to say that the molecular basis of the preferences expressed by axons during growth and synapse formation will remain a difficult area for some time. Two particular problems are the nature of the assay used for the purification of candidate molecules and the identification of the precise role(s) a candidate molecule plays. For example, surface molecules may be important not only in axonal outgrowth and the initial recognition of an appropriate target, but also in competition and reorganization of presynaptic endings, in the development of pre- and postsynaptic specializations, and in the maintenance of final relationships (see Sections 4, 8, 9, and 11).

Because synapse formation per se cannot be assayed by present biochemical techniques, and since the relevant electrophysiological and microscopic methods are time-consuming and largely qualitative, other less direct measures of intercellular "recognition" have been sought. One approach has been to study the adhesion of cells dissociated from various parts of the embryonic nervous system (Gottlieb and Glaser 1980). Under appropriate conditions, dissociated cells from a given tissue form aggregates (Holtfreter 1964) and, in general, cells from particular regions of the brain tend to aggregate preferentially with each other (Garber and Moscona 1972). In pursuit of the basis of this phenomenon, a protein has been purified that specifically stimulates the formation of large aggregates of retinal cells (Hausman and Moscona 1979). Plasma membranes from homologous cells can prevent such intercellular adhesions, and a small membrane protein thought to be responsible for this inhibition has also been purified and partially characterized (Jakoi and Marchase 1979). A more specific sort of adhesion is evident when cells from different areas of the retina are tested: Cells from different retinal regions also adhere to one another preferentially. Indeed, there is a gradient of adhesive specificity, so that ventral retinal cells bind more avidly to dorsal cells than to other ventral retinal cells (**Gottlieb, Rock, and Glaser 1976**). In addition to this sort of evidence for a retinal gradient, a monoclonal antibody has recently been produced that binds in a dorsal-ventral gradient across the embryonic chick retina (see below).

In light of the specificity of retinotectal connections (Section 9), it is particularly interesting that cells dissociated from the ventral retina adhere preferentially to dorsal tectal halves, whereas dorsal retinal cells prefer ventral tectal halves (Barbera et al. 1973). Similar results have been obtained using monolayers of tectal cells rather

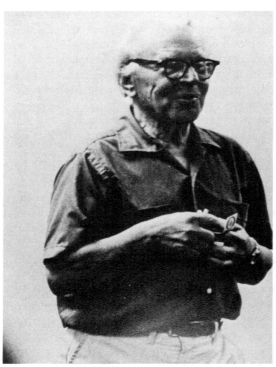

Johannes Holtfreter, whose studies of cell aggregation initiated modern attempts to define the molecular basis of cell recognition.

than intact tectal halves (Gottlieb and Arington 1979; see also Bonhoeffer and Huf 1980; Halfter et al. 1981). A glycosyltransferase and a ganglioside may be involved in this adhesion, and a gradient of ganglioside-binding activity on the tectal surface has been reported (Roseman 1970; see also Marchase 1977). Although specific adhesion molecules in the retina and the tectum may well be important in the development of these systems, the role of such molecules in axon outgrowth and synapse formation is still unclear.

Another way to identify molecules involved in cellular interactions is by immunological methods. These techniques have the advantage of providing a means of interfering with a particular molecule during development, as demonstrated by the use of NGF-antiserum (see Section 6). A recent series of experiments using this approach involves an antiserum that interferes with cell adhesion; this antibody has been used to purify a large protein termed cell adhesion molecule (CAM) (Thiery et al. 1977). CAM is present on the cell surface, and antibodies to it interfere not only with cell adhesion, but also with the formation of neurite bundles and histogenesis in cultured chick retinas (Rutishauser et al. 1978; **Buskirk, Thiery, Rutishauser, and Edelman 1980**). CAM is found throughout the nervous system, although not in other tissues. Given this evidence, it seems more likely that the molecule is involved in the growth and cohesion of axons than in axon guidance or in the selective formation of synaptic connections.

The specificity of the immunological approach has been much increased by the monoclonal antibody technique. Monoclonal antibodies are particularly useful for studying surface antigens present in low amounts. For example, "hybridoma" antibodies have been found that bind selectively to different classes of retinal cells (Barnstable 1980) and to individual identified neurons (Zipser and McKay 1980). Moreover, such antibodies can inhibit the development of certain neuronal functions with a high degree of selectivity (Chun et al. 1980). One of the most intriguing studies using monoclonal antibodies has demonstrated the existence of a molecule in chick retina that is distributed in a dorsoventral gradient (**Trisler, Schneider, and Nirenberg 1981**). Such a gradient is consistent with the idea that surface properties are important in the retinotectal preferences described in the preceding section and could also provide an explanation of the aggregation studies outlined above. It is not yet known whether the antigen identified by this antibody plays a role in the retinotectal specificity, but this work shows that molecules can be identified whose distribution suggests a function in the encoding of positional information.

In addition to integral surface-membrane components, molecules in the extracellular matrix may also mediate intercellular recognition. Matrix material contains a mixture of incompletely characterized glycosaminoglycans and, in the electron microscope, appears as a somewhat amorphous coating around and between cells in both the peripheral and central nervous systems. As described in Section 8, the matrix material at the end plates of muscle fibers (subsynaptic basal lamina) influences motor axons to reinnervate their original synaptic sites (Marshall et al. 1977) and to differentiate synaptic specializations at that point (Sanes et al. 1978, reprinted in Section 8). In principle, antibodies to basal lamina (see Sanes and Hall 1979) could be used to determine which components of the basal lamina are responsible for these phenomena, and to investigate the role of the basal lamina in the original innervation of muscle during development.

Extracellular recognition molecules also appear to be involved in certain neuron-glia interactions. Studies using nerve grafts, cell culture, and mutant mice have shown that axonal signals are important in the differentiation of Schwann cells. For example, axons appear to specify whether or not the Schwann cells that invest them are to make myelin (Aguayo et al. 1976a,b; Weinberg and Spencer 1976). Myelination is correlated with axonal diameters of 1 μm or greater, and it may be that Schwann cells also influence the diameter sizes of the axons they surround (Raine et al. 1981). The results of a variety of in vitro experiments support the idea of such reciprocal interactions between neurons and glial cells. Thus, axon plasma membranes contain an agent that stimulates Schwann-cell mitosis (Salzer et al. 1980; Hanson and Partlow 1980), and a diffusible Schwann-cell mitogen is also found in the pituitary and other brain regions (Brockes et al. 1980). Finally, Schwann cells contribute to the synthesis of matrix material that surrounds axons (Bunge et al. 1980). It seems likely that a combination of soluble, matrix, and membrane molecules coordinates the neuron–Schwann-cell relationship.

In general, these molecular studies of cellular recognition are at an early stage. As intriguing as these observations are, it will probably be some time before strong links can be forged between the phenomenology of axon outgrowth and synapse formation described in previous sections and the biochemical studies described here.

References

Aguayo, A.J., L. Charron, and G.M. Bray. 1976a. Potential of Schwann cells from unmyelinated nerves to produce myelin: A quantitative ultrastructural and radiographic study. *J. Neurocytol.* 5: 565–573.

Aguayo, A.J., G.M. Bray, L.C. Terry, and E. Sweezey. 1976b. Three dimensional analysis of unmyelinated fibres in normal and pathologic autonomic nerves. *J. Neuropathol. Exp. Neurol.* 35: 136–151.

Barbera, A.J., R.B. Marchase, and S. Roth. 1973. Adhesive recognition and retinotectal specificity. *Proc. Natl. Acad. Sci.* 70: 2482–2486.

Barnstable, C.J. 1980. Monoclonal antibodies which recognize different cell types in the rat retina. *Nature* 286: 231–235.

Bonhoeffer, F. and J. Huf. 1980. Recognition of cell types by axonal growth cones *in vitro*. *Nature* 288: 162–164.

Buskirk, D.R., J.-P. Thiery, U. Rutishauser, and G.M. Edelman. 1980. Antibodies to a neural cell adhesion molecule disrupt histogenesis in cultured chick retinae. *Nature* 285: 488–489.

Brockes, J.P., G.E. Lemke, and D.R. Balzer. 1980. Purification and preliminary characterization of a glial growth factor from the bovine pituitary. *J. Biol. Chem.* 255: 8374–8377.

Bunge, M.B., A.K. Williams, P.M. Wood, J. Uitto, and J.J. Jeffrey. 1980. Comparison of nerve cell and nerve cell plus Schwann cell cultures, with particular emphasis on basal lamina and collagen formation. *J. Cell Biol.* 84: 184–202.

Chun, L.L.Y., P.H. Patterson, and H. Cantor. 1980. Preliminary studies on the use of monoclonal antibodies as probes for sympathetic development. *J. Exp. Biol.* 89: 73–83.

Garber, B.B. and A.A. Moscona. 1972. Reconstruction of brain tissue from cell suspensions. II. Specific enhancement of aggregation of embryonic cerebral cells by supernatant from homologous cell cultures. *Dev. Biol.* 27: 235–243.

Gottlieb, D.I. and C. Arington. 1979. Patterns of adhesive specificity in the developing central nervous system of the chick. *Dev. Biol.* 71: 260–273.

Gottlieb, D.I. and L. Glaser. 1980. Cellular recognition during neural development. *Annu. Rev. Neurosci.* 3: 303–318.

Gottlieb, D.I., K. Rock, and L. Glaser. 1976. A gradient of adhesive specificity in developing avian retina. *Proc. Natl. Acad. Sci.* 73: 410–414.

Halfter, W., M. Claviez, and U. Schwarz. 1981. Preferential adhesion of tectal membranes to anterior embryonic chick retina neurites. *Nature* 292: 67–70.

Hanson, G.R. and L.M. Partlow. 1980. A comparison of two factors affecting the proliferation of nonneuronal (glial) cells in vitro. *Brain Res.* 192: 371–381.

Hausman, R.E. and A.A. Moscona. 1979. Immunological detection of retina cognin on the surface of embryonic cells. *Exp. Cell Res.* 119: 191–204.

Holtfreter, J. 1964. Tissue affinity, a means of embryonic morphogenesis. In *Foundations of experimental embryology* (ed. B.H. Willier and J.M. Oppenheimer), pp. 186–225. Prentice Hall, New York.

Jakoi, E.R. and R.B. Marchase. 1979. Ligatin from embryonic chick neural retina. *J. Cell Biol.* 80: 642–650.

Marchase, R.B. 1977. Biochemical investigations of retinotectal adhesive specificity. *J. Cell Biol.* 75: 237–257.

Marshall, L.M., J.R. Sanes, and U.J. McMahan. 1978. Reinnervation of muscle fiber basement lamina after removal of myofibers. Differentiation of regenerating axons at original synaptic sites. *J. Cell Biol.* 78: 176–198.

Raine, C.S., H. Wisniewski, and J. Prineas. 1969. An ultrastructural study of experimental demyelination and remyelination. II. Chronic experimental allergic encephalomyelitis in the peripheral nervous system. *Lab. Invest.* 21: 316–327.

Roseman, S. 1970. The synthesis of complex carbohydrates by multiglycosyltransferase systems and their potential function in intercellular adhesion. *Chem. Phys. Lipids* 5: 270–297.

Rutishauser, U., W.E. Gall, and G.M. Edelman. 1978. Adhesion among neural cells of the chick embryo. IV. Role of the cell surface molecule CAM in the formation of neurite bundles in cultures of spinal ganglia. *J. Cell Biol.* 79: 382–393.

Salzer, J.L., R.P. Bunge, and L. Glaser. 1980. Studies of Schwann cell proliferation. III. Evidence for the surface localization of the neurite mitogen. *J. Cell Biol.* 84: 767–778.

Sanes, J. and Z.W. Hall. 1979. Antibodies that bind specifically to synaptic sites on muscle fiber basal lamina. *J. Cell Biol.* 83: 357–370.

Sanes, J.R., L.M. Marshall, and U.J. McMahan. 1978. Reinnervation of muscle fiber basal lamina after removal of myofibers. Differentiation of regenerating axons at original synaptic sites. *J. Cell Biol.* 78: 176–198.

Thiery, J.-P., R. Brackenbury, U. Rutishauser, and G.M. Edelman. 1977. Adhesion among neural cells of the chick embryo. II. Purification and characterization of a cell adhesion molecule from neural retina. *J. Biol. Chem.* 252: 6841–6845.

Trisler, G.D., M.D. Schneider, and M. Nirenberg. 1981. A topographic gradient of molecules in retina can be used to identify neuron position. *Proc. Natl.*

Acad. Sci. 78: 2145–2149.

Weinberg, H.J. and P.S. Spencer. 1976. Studies on the control of myelinogenesis. II. Evidence for neuronal regulation of myelin production. *Brain Res. 113:* 363–378.

Zipser, B. and R. McKay. 1980. Monoclonal antibodies distinguish identifiable neurones in the leech. *Nature 289:* 549–554.

Proc. Nat. Acad. Sci. USA
Vol. 73, No. 2, pp. 410–414, February 1976
Biochemistry

A gradient of adhesive specificity in developing avian retina

(neural retina/cell–cell adhesion/neuronal recognition/embryonal gradients)

DAVID I. GOTTLIEB, KENNETH ROCK, AND LUIS GLASER

Department of Biological Chemistry, Division of Biology and Biomedical Sciences, Washington University, St. Louis, Missouri 63110

Communicated by Oliver H. Lowry, November 24, 1975

ABSTRACT   Cell–cell adhesion was examined in the developing chick neural retina. A dorsoventral gradient of adhesive specificity in dissociated cells was detected which exhibits a complementarity such that the highest cell–cell affinities are exhibited between cells derived from the extremes of the gradient. If a nasotemporal gradient exists it must exhibit significantly lower cell–cell affinity. The relevance of these findings to pattern formation in the nervous system is discussed.

There is now an extensive body of literature demonstrating tissue specific cell–cell adhesion by dissociated embryonal cells. In most instances homologous cells adhere to one another far more rapidly than to heterologous cells (1–4). This is not universally true, since we have demonstrated a case where heterologous binding of brain cells from different brain regions occurs more rapidly than homologous binding (5). Taken together, these cell–cell binding experiments provide strong evidence for the existence of tissue specific cell–cell receptors. Additional evidence for this class of receptors comes from experiments that show that purified plasma membranes will bind selectively to embryonal cells (6–8), and that active and specific binding components can be extracted from these plasma membranes (9).

The functional role of embryonic cell–cell receptors is obscure. While it is reasonable to assume that they play an important role in determining the arrangement of cells in tissues, direct evidence for this point is lacking. Suggestive evidence that cell–cell receptors are important during early development in the mouse has recently been obtained using t mutants (10, 11).

One way of investigating the role of cell–cell receptors in the developing brain would be to study regional variations in cell–cell affinity in detail to determine if patterns of adhesive specificity could be correlated with developmentally significant patterns. Gradients of either soluble effectors or of surface properties have been postulated to be of importance in embryonal development in general (for example, see refs. 12–15). Specifically in the case of the neural retina, the highly ordered pattern of retinotectal connections could be explained (12, 15, 16) if both the retina and the tectum had two sets of mutually complementary adhesive gradients on cell surfaces, one set of gradients in the dorsal-ventral direction and the other in the anterior-posterior direction.

To facilitate this sort of study, we have developed a variation of the cell adhesion assay of Walther *et al.* (4) which is capable of measuring the adhesive specificity of relatively small numbers of embryonal brain cells shortly after they are removed from the embryo (5). In this assay, radioactive probe cells are incubated with a confluent monolayer of cells and the rate of adhesion of the radioactive probe cells to the monolayer is determined. Using this assay, we have demonstrated that there is a strong gradient of adhesive specificity running along the dorsal to ventral axis of the developing chick retina. It is likely that the gradient features a sort of

complementarity such that cells at either extreme of the gradient show highest affinity for cells at the opposite extreme. While it would be premature to assume that this gradient is directly related to retinotectal specificity, we demonstrate for the first time the existence of a gradient of the appropriate type on the surface of retinal cells. It should be clear, however, that in these experiments we are measuring a property of a majority of the retinal cells and not only of the ganglion cells, which are the cells that project to the tectum. Indeed it is not clear that the ganglion cells, which are no more than a small percentage of the retinal cells, participate in the gradient.

MATERIALS AND METHODS

Embryonic Material. Embryonated mycoplasma-free white leghorn eggs obtained from Spafas were incubated at 37.5° for the indicated number of days.

Preparation of Retinal Cell Suspension for Forming Monolayers. Appropriate portions of the retina from 9- or 12-day-old embryos were dissected and dissociated by the standard procedure of this laboratory to yield a suspension of viable cells consisting mostly of single cells and small clumps (6, 7). Briefly, four retinal halves were incubated at 37° for 15 min in 4 ml of calcium- and magnesium-free Hanks' solution (Grand Island Biological) containing 10% heat inactivated (30 min at 56°) chicken serum. The tissue was gently triturated at intervals with a pasteur pipette. After 15 min crude trypsin (Difco 1:250) was added to a final concentration of 600 μg/ml, DNase I (Sigma) to a final concentration of 25 μg/ml, and the tissue was incubated at room temperature for 30 min with trituration every 5 min. Sedimentation for 5 min at 25° at unit gravity removed all large clumps. Viability was judged by trypan blue exclusion and was greater than 95% for suspensions from the 9-day retina and greater than 90% for suspensions from the 12-day retina. The dissociation of the tissue is carried out in the presence of serum and is a relatively gentle procedure.

Preparation of ^{32}P-Labeled Single Cells (Probe Cells). Appropriate portions of one or two retinae were dissected and labeled by incubating the triturated tissue in 5 ml of Dulbecco's modified Eagle's medium (17) + 10% heat inactivated chicken serum with the addition of 500 μCi of carrier-free $H_3{}^{32}PO_4$. After shaking at 100 rpm in a 25-ml erlenmeyer flask for 3 hr at 37° in a New Brunswick G76 shaker, the tissue was transferred to the same medium without isotope and incubated for an additional hour to wash out free radioactivity. Single cell suspensions were prepared from the labeled tissue by standard methods (6, 7) including a low-speed sedimentation (9 × g) to remove clumps of cells. This procedure results in cells having a specific radioactivity of about 0.02–0.10 cpm per cell. In a typical experiment, on the order of 5 × 10^4 cells are bound, giving about 5 × 10^3

410

Biochemistry: Gottlieb *et al.*

Proc. Nat. Acad. Sci. USA 73 (1976)   411

cpm. During the course of the experiments about 10% of the counts in cells leaks into the supernatant. This quantity is measured in each experiment and used in the computation of cell binding. Control experiments show that leaked radio-activity does not label the monolayers significantly (5).

Formation of Monolayers and Cell Adhesion Assays.
Retinal suspensions were used to form monolayers on deriviatized glass by a miniaturized modification of the method described by us previously (5). In these assays smaller vials were used (surface area 1.7 cm²) as opposed to 5 cm² in the original method. About 3.0×10^6 cells were used per vial, about 1.5 times the number necessary for confluency. To the monolayer were added 1.5×10^5 radioactive cells in 0.3 ml of Ca^{++}-Mg^+-free Hanks' solution containing 0.5% bovine serum albumin and the vials were incubated for the indicated times at 120 rpm and 37° in a New Brunswick G76 shaker. At the end of the incubation the monolayers and adhering cells were washed with 4 ml of the Hanks' solution and dissolved in 0.3 ml of 1% Triton X-100. After addition of 3.5 ml of 3a70 counting fluid (Research Products International), the radioactivity was determined in a scintillation counter. Evidence that probe cell adhesion is to the cells in the monolayer and that there is no transfer of radioactive soluble material is presented in ref. 5.

Orientation of Dissection. The choroid fissure served as an internal landmark for the various dissections.

RESULTS

Patterns of Specific Adhesion in 9-Day Retina. Monolayers and labeled probe cells were prepared from both the dorsal and ventral halves of the 9-day retina by dissecting the retina along a line roughly perpendicular to the choroid fissure. During the dissection, care was taken to trim away and discard a small strip on either side of the bisecting cut to avoid any possible overlap between dorsal and ventral halves. Monolayer adhesion assays were then carried out in reciprocal combinations, with the results illustrated in Fig. 1. It can be clearly seen that dorsal probe cells have a higher binding rate to ventral than to dorsal monolayers. Ventral probe cells show the converse behavior, having a higher binding rate to dorsal than to ventral monolayers. This pattern is highly reproducible, and has been seen in all four separate experiments that were performed. It is also worth pointing out that even though heterologous binding is clearly preferred over homologous, the rate of homologous binding is still substantial, being about ½ to ⅓ the rate of heterologous binding. The results illustrated in Fig. 1 are compatible with either a gradient of adhesive affinity along the dorsal to ventral axis or with a binary division of the retina into dorsal and ventral halves, each with a characteristic affinity over its entire extent. Evidence that the affinities follow a gradient will be presented below in experiments on the 12-day retina. It should be pointed out that in this assay there are 20 times more cells in the monolayer than there are radioactive probe cells. Since the monolayer cells are in large excess, the simplest interpretation of the differences in rate of adhesion observed in Fig. 1 would be that they represent fairly large differences in the number of adhesive sites in each monolayer for each type of cell; thus the dorsal half of the retina would have more adhesive sites for ventral cells than for dorsal cells. However, we do not know the relative contribution to this assay of the number of sites compared to the affinity of the sites, and a change in either of these parameters could account for the data in Fig. 1.

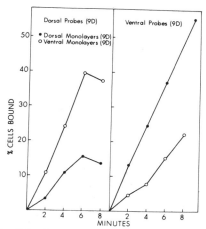

FIG. 1.   Cell–cell binding characteristics of dorsal and ventral 9-day neural retinal cells. *Left panel:* Radioactive probe cells prepared from dorsal neural retina are tested for their ability to bind to monolayers prepared from either dorsal or ventral neural retina. *Right panel:* The reciprocal experiment to the one shown in the left panel. Ventral probes are tested for their ability to bind to monolayers prepared from dorsal and ventral neural retina. In both cases, heterotypic binding is more rapid than homotypic binding. The same cell populations are tested in both experiments. In this and other figures, D is used as abbreviation for day.

Since retinotectal specification is thought to involve two sets of gradients at right angles to each other (12, 15, 16), we looked for differences in cell–cell adhesion between cells obtained from the anterior and posterior halves of the retina. In these experiments the retina was divided into anterior and posterior halves by a cut at right angles to the one in the previous experiment, i.e., roughly parallel to the choroid fissure. Reciprocal monolayer binding assays were performed on probe cells and monolayer cells prepared in this fashion. The results, illustrated in Fig. 2, show that these populations of cells are virtually indistinguishable. Therefore, using this assay we cannot detect a second gradient of adhesive specificity at right angles to the first one we described. A number of experiments were performed in which the retina was cut at a 45° angle from the lines of the previous two experiments. In these experiments, the results seemed intermediate between the results of Fig. 1 and Fig. 2 in that cells showed appropriate recognition but with lower difference in binding rates.

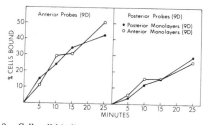

FIG. 2.   Cell–cell binding characteristics of anterior and posterior 9-day neural retinal cells. The experimental conditions are identical to those used in Fig. 1, but radioactive anterior and posterior neural retinal cells were tested for their ability to bind to the corresponding monolayers. No significant difference was observed in binding to the two types of monolayer.

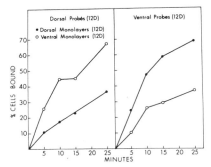

FIG. 3. Cell–cell binding characteristics of dorsal and ventral 12-day neural retinal cells. The experimental design is as in Fig. 1. The left panel shows that cells obtained from the dorsal neural retina adhere more rapidly to a monolayer prepared from ventral neural retinal cells. The right panel shows that ventral probe cells have the opposite behavior.

Patterns of Adhesive Specificity in 12-Day Retina. A number of cell surface specificities change during development (7, 9, 11). We have, therefore, examined the adhesive specificity of cells from the 12-day-old neural retina. At 12 days the retina is considerably larger than at 9 days, and this makes it easier to obtain single cells and cell monolayers from very small portions of the retina. In the first set of experiments, the retina was again divided into dorsal and ventral halves. The results in Fig. 3 show that cells from dorsal and ventral half-retinae show binding affinities that are analogous to those of their 9-day counterparts. This is also a highly reproducible result, and the adhesive differentials between 12-day dorsal and ventral cells appear qualitatively to be at least as great as those between 9-day dorsal and ventral cells. We also performed experiments in which the 12-day retina was divided into anterior and posterior halves and found no significant difference in adhesive behavior between cells of the anterior and posterior halves.

The results with both the 9-day and the 12-day retina are consistent with two models. The first is a dorsal to ventral gradient of adhesive specificity spanning the full extent of the retina. The second would have the retina divided into two specific fields, dorsal and ventral, with each field having a homogeneous arrangement of adhesive determinants. We have done experiments on the 12-day retina that favor the first possibility. In these experiments, the retina was divided into six equatorial strips along the dorsoventral axis. Cell suspensions were prepared from each strip and used to make monolayers. Radioactively labeled probe cells were prepared from the most dorsal and most ventral strips. Since limitations of material made full kinetic assays difficult, the relative binding of probe cells to the different monolayers was determined in duplicate at a single time point (20 min). The results shown in Fig. 4 indicate that dorsal probe cells have a uniformly low affinity for the three most dorsal strips, but an increasing affinity for progressively ventral strips across the midline. Ventral probe cells exhibit the converse behavior. One aspect of these results is clear-cut. There seems to be a gradient of adhesive affinity for a particular type of probe cell in the opposite hemisphere of the retina. However, the gradient appears to level off in the homologous half, and this feature has been consistently observed in all experiments. If a continuous gradient is present, then we would have to assume that limitations in the monolayer method do not allow us to measure differences in the rate of

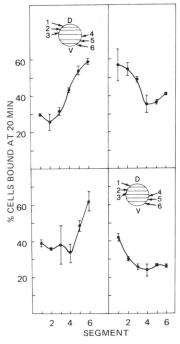

FIG. 4. Dorsal-ventral gradient in adhesive specificity in the 12-day neural retina. The top and bottom panels represent separate but identical experiments which are presented separately because of the difficulty in averaging data of this type. For each experiment retinae were divided into six segments, as indicated by the inset. Radioactively labeled probe cells were prepared from the most dorsal and most ventral strips (1 and 6 in insert). Monolayers were prepared from each of the strips and dorsal and ventral probe cells were tested for their ability to bind to these monolayers. Binding at 20 min was measured in duplicate for each combination. The extremes of the bars at each time point represent the duplicate experiments. Dorsal probe cells (left) show increasing affinity for more ventral monolayers. Ventral probe cells (right) show the opposite behavior.

binding of cells to monolayers prepared from cells adjacent to the region from which the probe cells were obtained. A difference in the rate of adhesion of cells to a monolayer can arise in a number of ways: (*i*) because there is a change in the number of adhesive sites on the cells; (*ii*) because the affinity of the adhesive sites is different; and (*iii*) because the topography of the sites on the cell surface is different. These are not mutually exclusive alternatives, and may each contribute differently to the overall adhesion rate along the gradient.

Although the results presented in Fig. 4 indicate that a gradient of adhesive affinities exists across the dorsoventral axis of the retina, a more detailed and quantitative analysis of this issue appears warranted. For technical reasons it was easiest to measure in replicate experiments the adhesion of probe cells from the extreme dorsal and ventral portions of the retina to paired sets of monolayers obtained either from segments 1 and 2 or segments 5 and 6 of the retina (Fig. 4). The results shown in Table 1 show that cells from segment 1 (extreme dorsal) prefer to bind to monolayers prepared from segment 6 rather than segment 5, but cannot distinguish monolayers prepared from segments 1 and 2. Conversely, cells

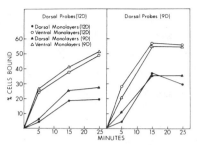

FIG. 5. Cross recognition of 9- and 12-day retinal adhesive determinants. Dorsal probe cells obtained from 12-day neural retina (*left panel*) and 9-day neural retina (*right panel*) were tested for their ability to bind to monolayers prepared from 9- and 12-day dorsal and ventral neural retinal cells. In each case the dorsal probe cells adhere preferentially to ventral monolayers prepared from either 9-day neural retina or from 12-day neural retina.

prepared from segment 6 (extreme ventral) prefer to bind to monolayers prepared with cells from segment 1, over those of segment 2, but show no preference between monolayers prepared from cells in segments 5 and 6. These results substantiate two features of the results of Fig. 4, namely, that there appears to be no graded adhesive preference within the homotopic retinal half but that there is a gradient of adhesive affinity in the opposite half.

Finally, we were curious to see if the recognition elements were the same on 9-day and 12-day cells. Fig. 5 shows the results of experiments in which dorsal probe cells were prepared from 9- and 12-day retinae and tested against dorsal and ventral monolayers from 9- and 12-day retinae. The results show that 9-day probe cells can distinguish between

dorsal and ventral cells of both the 9- and 12-day retina, and that 12-day dorsal probe cells have the same ability.

DISCUSSION

The present results clearly show a gradient of cell–cell affinity along the dorsoventral axis of the developing chick retina. Taken at face value, the results show that affinities are arranged so that the highest affinity is shown between cells at the extremes of the gradient. It is interesting to note that Barondes (15) and Marchase *et al.* (16) propose a model with just such properties to account for retinotectal binding specificity. They propose that the retina has dorsoventral gradients of two complementary cell surface receptors, such that if the dorsal cells have an excess of one complementary ligand, the ventral cells have an excess of the other complementary ligand. They then suggest that identical gradients exist in the tectum; therefore, an axon derived from the dorsal portion of the retina would bind preferentially to a ventral portion of the tectum, etc. A second gradient at right angles, i.e., anterior-posterior, of similar type would then be adequate to explain retinotectal specificity in two dimensions.

Our assays suffer from a technical limitation that should be discussed. The cells forming monolayers are in contact with one another, and it is therefore possible that receptors on adjacent cells are interacting on the monolayer. If cell–cell receptors are mobile, it is conceivable that a process analogous to capping of antigens in lymphocytes is occurring. If the major determinants were for self-recognition, i.e., dorsal-dorsal and ventral-ventral, these might be neutralized by self-interaction on the monolayer, leaving minor components as the only determinants able to react. We have tried to perform experiments on "diluted" monolayers in

Table 1. Binding of retinal cells to monolayers prepared from different areas of the retina

	Dorsal probe cells					Ventral probe cells				
	5:Monolayer		6:Monolayer			5:Monolayer		6:Monolayer		
Exp.	cpm	% Binding	cpm	% Binding	Ratio 6/5	cpm	% Binding	cpm	% Binding	Ratio 5/6
1	1457(2)	48.5	1864(2)	62	1.28	1090(2)	27.6	1045(2)	26.9	1.04
2	3044(2)	53.9	3320(2)	58.9	1.19	2255(2)	36.5	2556(2)	41	0.88
3	2599(4)	50.9	3376(4)	66.1	1.29	—	—	—	—	—
4	1229(2)	54	1534(3)	68	1.24	1109(3)	28	1080(3)	27	1.02
5	1024(3)	30	1644(3)	48	1.60	600(3)	17.5	585(3)	16.5	1.02
6	1021(3)	67	1226(3)	80.5	1.20	418(3)	28.3	388(3)	26.3	1.07
				Average	1.30 ± 0.13				Average	1.006 ± 0.06

	1:Monolayer		2:Monolayer			1:Monolayer		2:Monolayer		
	cpm	% Binding	cpm	% Binding	Ratio 2/1	cpm	% Binding	cpm	% Binding	Ratio 1/2
7	1675(2)	29.7	1472(2)	26.1	0.87	3495	56.6	3104	54.7	1.03
8	1171(2)	39.0	1075(2)	35.8	0.92	1659	42.3	1192	30.2	1.40
9	543(3)	14.4	633(3)	16.8	1.16	1194	57.6	718	34.6	1.66
10	447(3)	20.7	455(3)	21.1	1.01	668	46.0	511	35.0	1.31
			Average	0.99 ± 0.11					Average	1.35 ± 0.22

The experiments were carried out as described in Fig. 4. In Exps. 1–6 are shown data for the binding of dorsal probe cells obtained from the extreme dorsal area of the retina (area 1, Fig. 4), and ventral probe cells obtained from the extreme ventral area of the retina (area 6, Fig. 4) to monolayers prepared from areas 5 and 6 (Fig. 4) of the retina. Exps. 7–10 show the binding of similar probe cells to monolayers obtained from areas 1 and 2 of the retina. The figures in parentheses represent the number of monolayers that were used in each experiment. Exps. 1, 2, 7, and 8 are the same as those in Fig. 4. The incubation time in Exps. 1, 2, 7, and 8 was 20 min, and was 11 min on all other experiments. All experiments carried out to date are shown. The difference in binding of dorsal cells to monolayers obtained from areas 5 and 6, and of ventral cells to monolayers obtained from areas 1 and 2 differ significantly at the 0.01 level of confidence when tested by Student's *t* test or by paired comparison (18). The average of the data is shown together with the standard error of the mean.

which the adhering cells are plated at low density or are mixed with non-sticky cells such as red cells to exclude this last possibility. However, the results of these efforts have not been precise enough to determine if cell–cell interaction on the monolayer influences the results. Thus, while our experiments unambiguously detect a gradient, it is conceivable that the form of the gradient is influenced by self-interaction on our monolayers. Although we favor a continuous gradient as the most reasonable interpretation of our results, it is also possible that a limited number of discrete changes in affinity could account for these observations.

Gradients have been implicated in at least two important processes during the development of the nervous system. First, there are clear-cut gradients of *neurogenesis* in several developing brain regions, including the retina (19, 20). One fact argues strongly against the gradient we have described being a reflection of the neurogenetic gradient. The gradient of neurogenesis in the retina begins at the fundus of the retina and proceeds towards its margin (19, 20) and although the point hasn't been studied explicitly, it is likely that growth proceeds equally along the dorsal-ventral and anterior-posterior axes of the retina. If the adhesive gradient we have described were a reflection of a neurogenetic gradient, we would expect to find a similar anterior-posterior gradient, while in fact, we do not. We have recently been informed by Dr. M. Jacobson of unpublished results in his laboratory which show that in the frog retina there is a dorso-ventral developmental gradient, such that cells in the dorsal region of the retina go through their last cell division before ventral cells. If a similar gradient exists in the chick retina, it would be of obvious significance to the interpretation of our results.

Data showing that retinotectal binding can mimic the retinotectal axonal projection under certain circumstances (16, 21) favor the interpretation that the retinal gradient is related to specific synapse formation. The failure to find a second gradient perpendicular to the first argues against such an interpretation, since if synaptogenesis is to be explained by such gradients, two perpendicular gradients are required. However, it is conceivable that our methods are too insensitive to detect a second gradient, and the fact that the anterior-posterior gradient in the frog retina is determined before the dorsal-ventral gradient suggests that the two might have different physical bases (22). In spite of the multiple interpretations of the experiments, the finding of a gradient of adhesive specificity in the dorsal-ventral axis of the retina is of great importance since it establishes a gradient of surface specificity in this organ which seems to parallel functional developmental parameters.

This work was supported by U.S. Public Health Service Grant GM-18405 and NSF Grant BMS 75-22638. D.I.G. was supported by Grant NS 10943 and K.R. by a summer fellowship from the University of Rochester. We would like to thank Dr. Thomas Woolsey for critically reading the manuscript, and Dr. M. Jacobson for unpublished results from his laboratory.

1. Roth, S. (1968) *Dev. Biol.* **18**, 602–631.
2. Roth, S. & Weston, J. (1967) *Proc. Nat. Acad. Sci. USA* **58**, 974–980.
3. Roth, S., McGuire, E. J. & Roseman, S. (1971) *J. Cell Biol.* **51**, 525–535.
4. Walther, B. T., Ohman, R. & Roseman, S. (1973) *Proc. Nat. Acad. Sci. USA* **70**, 1569–1573.
5. Gottlieb, D. I. & Glaser, L. (1975) *Biochem. Biophys. Res. Commun.* **63**, 815–821.
6. Merrell, R. & Glaser, L. (1973) *Proc. Nat. Acad. Sci. USA* **70**, 2794–2798.
7. Gottlieb, D. I., Merrell, R. & Glaser, L. (1974) *Proc. Nat. Acad. Sci. USA* **71**, 1800–1802.
8. Merrell, R., Gottlieb, D. I. & Glaser, L. (1975) in *Neuronal Recognition*, ed. Barondes, S. (Plenum Press, New York), in press.
9. Merrell, R., Gottlieb, D. I. & Glaser, L. (1975) *J. Biol. Chem.* **250**, 5655–5659.
10. Artz, K., Bennett, D. & Jacob, F. (1974) *Proc. Nat. Acad. Sci. USA* **71**, 811–814.
11. Artz, K. & Bennett, D. (1975) *Nature* **256**, 545–547.
12. Sperry, R. W. (1963) *Proc. Nat. Acad. Sci. USA* **50**, 703–710.
13. Crick, F. H. C. & Lawrence, P. A. (1975) *Science* **189**, 340–347.
14. Lawrence, P. A., Crick, F. H. C. & Munro, M. (1972) *J. Cell Sci.* **11**, 815–853.
15. Barondes, S. H. (1970) in *The Neurosciences Second Study Program*, ed. Schmitt, F. O. (Rockefeller University Press, New York), pp. 747–760.
16. Marchase, R. B., Barbera, A. J. & Roth, S. (1975) "A molecular approach to retino-tectal specificity," from "*Cell Patterning,*" in *Ciba Symposium* (Elsevier, Amsterdam), Vol. 29, pp. 315–327.
17. Dulbecco, R. & Freeman, G. (1959) *Virology* **12**, 185–196.
18. Daniel, W. W. (1971) in *Biostatistics* (J. Wiley & Sons, New York), pp. 124 and 165.
19. Coulombre, A. J. (1955) *Am. J. Anat.* **96**, 153–189.
20. Kahn, A. J. (1973) *Brain Res.* **63**, 285–290.
21. Barbera, A., Marchase, R. B. & Roth, S. (1973) *Proc. Nat. Acad. Sci. USA* **70**, 2482–2486.
22. Jacobson, M. (1968) *Dev. Biol.* **17**, 202–218.

Reprinted from Nature, Vol. 285, No. 5765, pp. 488-489, June 12 1980
© Macmillan Journals Ltd., 1980

Antibodies to a neural cell adhesion molecule disrupt histogenesis in cultured chick retinae

Daniel R. Buskirk, Jean-Paul Thiery*, Urs Rutishauser
& Gerald M. Edelman†

The Rockefeller University, 1230 York Avenue, New York, New York 10021
*CNRS et Collège de France, Institute d'Embryologie, 49 bis, av. de la Belle Gabrille, 94130 Nogent-sur-Marne, France
†To whom correspondence should be addressed

Cell-surface proteins are believed to have important roles in cell–cell interactions during brain development, particularly in such processes as cellular adhesion, neurite outgrowth and synapse formation[1–4]. The chick neural cell adhesion molecule, CAM, is a cell-surface protein specific to the nervous system and has been implicated in cell adhesion among cells and neurites of the developing retina and brain[5–8]. Previous studies have shown that F(ab') fragments of antibodies directed against CAM inhibit the *in vitro* aggregation of cells obtained from 9-day embryonic chick retina. The specific antibody fragments also reduce the diameter of neurite fascicles that grow out from cultured dorsal root ganglia, apparently by blocking side-to-side adhesion between the neurites. In addition, anti-CAM antibodies alter the appearance of histotypic patterns in retinal cell aggregates maintained in culture for several days[7]. We now demonstrate that the antibodies can disrupt histogenesis of the developing retina in organ culture, strengthening the notion that the cell–cell adhesion properties mediated by CAM are involved in the normal development of histological layers in the chick retina.

In the chick, cell and plexiform layers of the central portion of the retina are formed between the sixth and ninth days of embryonic life[9,10]. Although many cells have left the mitotic cycle by day 6 (ref. 9), all remain in a single nuclear or 'matrix' layer. Retinae dissected from White Leghorn embryos on day 6 and placed in organ culture for 3 days undergo histogenesis similar to that which occurs *in vivo*, as can be seen in Fig. 1. To achieve uniformity of developmental stage, all retinal fragments were dissected from the region surrounding the choroid fissure. Pigment epithelium clinging to the neural retina was largely removed; any remaining pieces of epithelium seem not to have altered the progress of development. Retinal fragments were placed with their vitreous side down on 13-mm Millipore filters, 1.2 μm pore size, that had been wetted with medium, and were cultured on the stainless steel grid of a Falcon organ culture dish. In all experiments the medium was Dulbecco's modified Eagle's medium, supplemented with 1/10 volume of heat-inactivated fetal calf serum (Microbiological Associates). The anti-CAM sera were obtained from rabbits injected with purified CAM as described earlier[5], and control antisera were obtained from unimmunized rabbits. F(ab') fragments prepared from the antibodies were dissolved in the tissue culture medium to a concentration of 1 mg ml^{-1}. All cultures were carried out for 3 days at 37 °C in an atmosphere of 5% CO_2, and the retinae were then fixed either in Bouin's fixative for paraffin embedding or for 1 h in 2% glutaraldehyde in phosphate-buffered saline in preparation for embedding in Epon 812.

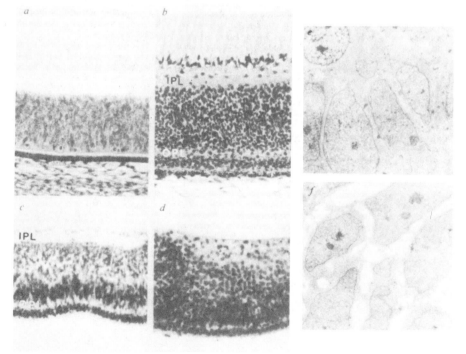

Fig. 1 *a, b* Represent *in vivo* chick retinae at 6 and 9 days of embryonic age, respectively. Retinae are from the central, most differentiated area of the retinae. The scleral side of the retinae, containing the photoreceptor cells, is shown towards the bottom in these photographs; in both photographs the pigment epithelia and scleral tissue can be seen lying below the neuroretina. In *b* the outer and inner plexiform layers are clearly visible. *c, d* Are chick retinae that have been in organ culture for 3 days following their dissection from the embryo on day 6. The retina shown in *c* was cultured in the presence of F(ab') antibody fragments from unimmunized rabbits, and that in *d* in the presence of antibodies to the cell adhesion molecule CAM. Although the cultured retinae are thinner and not as fully developed as *in vivo* 9-day retinae, the histological layers can be clearly identified and mark a significant differentiation from the 6-day stage. The retinae cultured in the presence of anti-CAM showed identifiable but disrupted histological layers which do not have the sharp boundaries between adjacent layers characteristic of both the *in vivo* and the cultured control retinae. Ganglion cells, at the top of the photographs, form neat rows in the *in vivo* and control retinae, but are scattered in the retina treated with anti-CAM. The light micrographs are ×650. *e, f* Are electron micrographs of cell bodies on the vitreous side of the nuclear layer of retinae cultured in the presence of non-immune and anti-CAM F(ab'), respectively. Note that the cells in the control retina show large areas of membrane apposition and small areas of extracellular space, whereas the retina cultured with antibodies to CAM shows large areas of extracellular space and few areas of cell–cell contact. Electron micrographs are ×5,800.

511

Tissues cultured in the presence of anti-CAM showed both disorder in the pattern of histological layers and an increase in the extracellular space surrounding the cell perikarya. In contrast, retinae cultured in the presence of antibodies from unimmunized rabbits developed in a manner analogous to retinae in vivo.

Paraffin sections of retinae cultured with non-immune serum (Fig. 1) revealed that, during the 3 days of culture, the initially rather uniform nuclear layer had developed distinct histological layers resembling the retina of a 9-day-old embryo. Inner and outer plexiform layers were clearly visible, as were the layers of photoreceptor cell bodies and cells believed to be ganglion cells. The photoreceptor cells had buds which mark the first stage in the development of the inner segments. The substantial layer of ganglion cells found in the in vivo 9-day retina was not observed, however, in the cultured retinae. Other workers studying the differentiation of chick retinae transplanted to the chorioallantoic membrane also observed a deficiency of ganglion cells, and attributed this to a failure to make tectal connections[11]. It is also possible that the cells observed along the vitreous edge of cultured retinae represent displaced ganglion cells which during the normal course of development are migrating back to the nuclear layer[12,13].

Retinal tissues cultured in the presence of anti-CAM displayed several additional alterations which sharply reduced the resemblance to normal retina. The ganglion cells, normally arranged in an even layer along the vitreous edge of the retina, were less organized and were found scattered throughout the inner plexiform layer. In control retinae, cells within the nuclear layer could be divided into two layers based on cell shape, the outermost consisting of bipolar and horizontal cells and the layer towards the vitreous side of the nuclear layer corresponding to the amacrine cells. In the retinae exposed to anti-CAM (Fig. 1e), these layers were not clearly distinguishable, suggesting that the distribution of specific cell types had been altered. More definitive evidence on the exact arrangement and morphological differentiation of specific cell types will require additional studies using Golgi staining techniques.

Electron microscopy of the anti-CAM-treated tissues revealed differences in the packing of cells in the nuclear layer. In the tissue cultured with anti-CAM F(ab′) fragments, large extracellular spaces surrounded the cell bodies of the nuclear layer. The extracellular spaces in the retinae cultured without anti-CAM F(ab′) were similar to those observed in sections of in vivo 9-day retinae. This difference was observed in all tissues sectioned, including those which had differentiated poorly during the culture period. It resembles changes previously seen in histotypic aggregates that were similarly treated[7]. The possibility that this difference is a consequence of increased susceptibility of the anti-CAM-treated retinae to shrinkage during processing has not been ruled out completely, but

seems unlikely in view of the normal appearance of cytoplasmic ultrastructure in the treated retinae. This question is being investigated directly through the measurement of extracellular space by horseradish peroxidase diffusion and staining techniques.

As judged by dense haematoxylin staining, necrotic cells were present in both untreated cultured retinae and those treated with anti-CAM. Approximately 1% of the cells in the treated retinae were pycnotic at day 9, and about 0.1% of the untreated retinal cells also seemed to be pycnotic. The amount of total cell loss during the 3-day period is not known, but both control and anti-CAM retinae were thinner than in in vivo 9-day retinae.

The present results extend the previous studies on CAM by demonstrating that antibodies against CAM disrupt the internal development of a tissue never subjected to mechanical dissociation. The observed increase in the extracellular space and the concomitant decrease in regions of cell–cell contact are consistent with the interpretation that CAM is a cell adhesion molecule. Because the individual cells in the anti-CAM-treated retinae were morphologically similar to those in the control tissues, it seems that the effects are not simply a consequence of changes in the developmental pathway of individual cells. This conclusion is supported by the ability of the anti-CAM-treated retinae to form some histological layers which, although altered, could be directly identified with layers in the normal retina. It seems, then, that the processes necessary for the differentiation of cell types and the formation of plexiform layers may occur unimpeded by the presence of anti-CAM. Nonetheless, the observation of misplaced ganglion cells and the apparent mixing of cell types in the nuclear layer suggests that, during the 6–9-day period of embryonic retinal development, cell–cell interactions mediated by CAM are important in achieving the appropriate arrangement of cells in nervous tissue.

This work was supported by PHS grants HD-09635 and AI-11378, and a grant to J.-P.T. from the Délégation Générale de la Recherche Scientifique et Technique.

Received 11 February; accepted 10 April 1980.

1. Brown, J. C. Expl Cell Res. 69, 440–442 (1971).
2. Santala, R., Gottlieb, D. I., Littman, D. & Glaser, L. J. biol. Chem. 252, 7625–7634 (1977).
3. Stallcup. W. B. Brain Res. 126, 475–486 (1977).
4. Mahler. H. R. in Complex Carbohydrates of Nervous Tissue (eds Margolis, R. U. & Margolis, R. K.) 165–184 (Plenum, New York, 1979).
5. Brackenbury, R., Thiery, J.-P., Rutishauser, U. & Edelman. G. M. J. biol. Chem. 252, 6835–6840 (1977).
6. Thiery, J-P., Brackenbury, R., Rutishauser, U. & Edelman, G. M. J. biol. Chem. 252, 6841–6845 (1977).
7. Rutishauser, U., Thiery, J-P., Brackenbury, R. & Edelman, G. M. J. Cell Biol. 79, 371–381 (1978).
8. Rutishauser, U., Gall, W. E. & Edelman, G. M. J. Cell Biol. 79, 382–393 (1978).
9. Kahn, A. J. Devl Biol. 38, 30–40 (1974).
10. Mishima, H. & Fujita, H. Albrecht v. Graefes Arch. Ophthal. 206, 1–16 (1978).
11. McLoon, S. C. & Hughes, W. F. Brain Res. 150, 398–402 (1978).
12. Hinds, J. W. & Hinds, P. L. J. comp. Neurol. 197, 277–300 (1978).
13. Heaton, M. B., Alvarez, I. M. & Crandall, J. E. Anat. Embryol. 155, 161–178 (1979).

Proc. Natl. Acad. Sci. USA
Vol. 78, No. 4, pp. 2145–2149, April 1981
Biochemistry

A topographic gradient of molecules in retina can be used to identify neuron position

(cell membrane/antigen/embryo/synapses/hybrid cells)

G. David Trisler, Michael D. Schneider, and Marshall Nirenberg

Laboratory of Biochemical Genetics, National Heart, Lung, and Blood Institute, National Institutes of Health, Bethesda, Maryland 20205

Contributed by Marshall Warren Nirenberg, December 24, 1980

ABSTRACT   A monoclonal antibody was obtained that binds to cell membrane molecules distributed in a topographic gradient in avian retina. Thirty-five-fold more antigen was detected in dorsoposterior retina than in ventroanterior retina. Most of the antigen was associated with the synaptic layers of the retina. Less antigen was detected in cerebrum, thalamus, cerebellum, and optic tectum, but little or none was found in non-neural tissues tested. The antigen was found on most or all cell types in retina, and the concentration of antigen found is a function of the square of the circumferential distance from the ventroanterior pole of the gradient toward the dorsoposterior pole. Thus, the antigen can be used as a marker of cell position along the ventroanterior–dorsoposterior axis of the retina.

Topographic relationships between retina ganglion neurons are conserved, forming point-to-point representations of the retina, when ganglion neurons synapse in tectum or certain other regions of brain. Thus, the retina is a favorable model system for studying the formation of synaptic circuits. However, the molecular basis for spatial order has not been defined. Sperry (1) hypothesized that two orthogonal gradients of molecules on retina ganglion neurons and corresponding gradients of complimentary molecules in the optic tectum might determine the specificity of synaptic connections between retina and tectum neurons. Other mechanisms proposed include adhesive interactions between migrating neurites, myelination of bundles of axons, and formation of extracellular channels by glia to guide axons in appropriate directions (2).

Antibodies provide a means of identifying surface molecules and reactions required for neural function (3–7). Rabbit antiserum to clonal retina hybrid cells was used to detect an antigen with a restricted domain in retina (8).

Our objective was to detect cell surface molecules with topographic specificity in the retina, as candidates for neuronal recognition molecules. Monoclonal antibodies were obtained by fusing P3X63 Ag8 mouse myeloma cells (9) with spleen cells from mice immunized with small portions of dorsoposterior or ventral chicken embryo retina. A hybridoma antibody was obtained that binds to cell membrane molecules that are distributed in a dorsoposterior → ventroanterior gradient in retina.

RESULTS

The rationale for the experiments is shown in Fig. 1. Spleen cells from mice immunized with small portions of dorsoposterior or ventral neural retina from the left eyes of 14-day chicken embryos were fused with P3X63 Ag8 mouse myeloma cells, and the binding of hybridoma antibody to cultured cells from the sector of the retina used for immunization was compared with

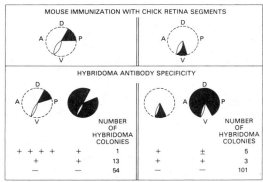

FIG. 1.   (*Upper*) Hybridoma cell lines were derived from mice immunized with cells mechanically dissociated from dorsoposterior (*Left*) or ventral (*Right*) retina from the left eyes of 14-day White Leghorn chicken embryos (*Gallus gallus*) (sections labeled 4 and 1, respectively, in Fig. 2). Symbols, A, D, P, and V correspond to anterior, dorsal, posterior, and ventral, respectively. The choroid fissure, through which axons exit or enter the retina, shown extending from the ventroanterior margin of the retina, was used as a landmark for dissection. Female BALB/c mice were injected intraperitoneally at 0, 7, and 14 days with 8×10^6 retina cells in 0.4 ml of Dulbecco's phosphate-buffered saline and intravenously with 2×10^6 cells in 0.1 ml of the saline. On day 17, 10^8 dissociated spleen cells from each mouse were fused (10) with 2×10^7 P3X63 Ag8 mouse myeloma cells. After fusion, the cells were suspended with 5×10^6 spleen cells from a mouse that had not been immunized in 50 ml of medium A. [Medium A is selective medium D20SHAT of Berzofsky *et al.* (11) except that it contains 10% fetal bovine serum, 1 μM aminopterin, 2 milliunits of insulin per ml, and each nonessential amino acid at 0.1 mM.] Cells were added to 96-well plates (Falcon) (186,000 cells per 74 μl of medium A per well), incubated at 37°C in a humidified atmosphere of 10% CO_2/90% air, and fed additional medium A (0.1 ml per well) on the 5th and 10th days of incubation. (*Lower*) To identify hybridomas synthesizing antibodies to regional antigens in retina, cells from the portion of 12-day chicken embryo retina (left eye) used for mouse immunization, or the rest of the retina, were dissociated with trypsin and collagenase, and transfer plates (12) were inoculated with 1.2×10^6 of the cells per well. Cells were cultured for 2 days in 90% Eagle's minimal essential medium/10% fetal bovine serum; the medium was replaced with 50 μl of medium conditioned by hybridoma cells, and plates were incubated for 30 min at 37°C. Each well was washed three times with 150 μl of solution B (1 mg of pigskin gelatin per ml of phosphate-buffered saline) at 4°C. Each cell monolayer was incubated for 30 min at 37°C with 50 μl of solution B containing 1.6 nM rabbit ^{125}I-labeled F(ab')$_2$ antibody fragment [^{125}I-F(ab')$_2$] directed against mouse IgG heavy and light chains (9799 cpm) and 500 μg of bovine serum albumin. Cells were washed as above, and bound radioactivity was determined. F(ab')$_2$ (Cappel) was purified on a mouse IgG-Sepharose 4B column and iodinated with mono-^{125}I Bolton–Hunter reagent (Amersham) (13).

binding to cells from the remainder of the retina. Cultured retina cells were used to increase the probability of detecting antibodies directed against cell surface molecules. Sixty-eight of

672 wells inoculated contained hybridoma colonies derived from a mouse immunized with dorsoposterior retina cells. One cell line (14H3) synthesized antibody that bound more to dorsoposterior retina cells than to cells from the rest of the retina, whereas 13 hybridoma antibodies bound equally to cells from both portions of retina. Antibodies to retina were not detected with 54 additional cell lines. Hybridoma colonies derived from a mouse immunized with ventral retina cells were detected in 109 of the 672 wells plated. Five antibodies of the 87 tested bound somewhat more to cells from ventral retina than to cells from the rest of the retina, and 3 antibodies bound equally. Thus, 14% of the 155 hybridoma cell lines examined synthesize antibodies to retina; however, only one antigen was detected, termed TOP for toponymic (i.e., a marker of position), with an asymmetric distribution, more abundant in dorsoposterior retina than in the remainder of the retina.

Distribution of TOP Molecules in Retina. Retinas from right or left eyes of chicken embryos were cut into eight sections as shown in Fig. 2, and cells from each section were assayed for $[^{125}\text{I-F(ab')}_2\cdot\text{anti-TOP antibody}\cdot\text{TOP antigen}]$ complexes. Bilaterally symmetrical gradients of TOP were found in retina from right and left eyes. The highest concentrations of antigen detected were in dorsoposterior or dorsal retina and the lowest, in ventroanterior or ventral retina. Little $^{125}\text{I-F(ab')}_2$ bound to

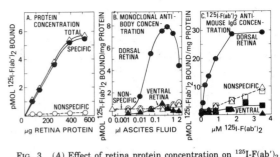

FIG. 3. (A) Effect of retina protein concentration on $^{125}\text{I-F(ab')}_2$ binding in the presence of anti-TOP antibody ($\triangle$) or P3X63 Ag8 antibody ($\bigcirc$). $\bullet$, $^{125}\text{I-F(ab')}_2$ bound specifically. (B) Effect on hybridoma antibody (ascites fluid) concentration on $^{125}\text{I-F(ab')}_2$ binding. Solid symbols, specific binding of $^{125}\text{I-F(ab')}_2$ due to anti-TOP antibody; open symbols, nonspecific binding with P3X63 Ag8 antibody. $\bullet$, $\bigcirc$, Dorsal retina, sections 4 and 5; $\blacktriangle$, $\triangle$, ventral retina, sections 1 and 8. Reaction mixtures contained 220 nM $^{125}\text{I-F(ab')}_2$ (3.68×10^{-3} μCi/pmol). (C) Effect of concentration of rabbit $^{125}\text{I-F(ab')}_2$ anti-mouse IgG. Solid symbols, specific $^{125}\text{I-F(ab')}_2$ binding; open symbols, nonspecific binding to cells from dorsal retina ($\bullet$, $\bigcirc$) or ventral retina ($\blacksquare$, $\square$, $\blacktriangle$, $\triangle$).

retina cells when antibody to TOP was omitted or was replaced with P3X63 Ag8 antibody. Other hybridoma antibodies including A2B5 (6) bound equally to cells from different regions of retina (not shown).

Assay Conditions. The effects of varying retina protein, hybridoma antibody, or $^{125}\text{I-F(ab')}_2$ anti-mouse IgG are shown in Fig. 3. Specific binding of $^{125}\text{I-F(ab')}_2$ was proportional to retina protein in the range 65–300 μg of protein (Fig. 3A). Half-maximal and maximal specific binding of $^{125}\text{I-F(ab')}_2$ to dorsoposterior retina cells were obtained with 1:1350 and 1:100 dilutions of ascites antibody to TOP, respectively; higher concentrations of antibody to TOP reduced specific $^{125}\text{I-F(ab')}_2$ binding (Fig. 3B). Specific $^{125}\text{I-F(ab')}_2$ binding to ventral retina was low; however, the concentrations of anti-TOP antibody required for half-maximal and maximal specific binding did not differ greatly from those found with dorsal retina. Thus, no obvious difference was detected in the affinity of the antibody for antigen in dorsal and ventral retina. Nonspecific binding of $^{125}\text{I-F(ab')}_2$ to retina cells was low at all concentrations of P3X63 Ag8 antibody tested. The antibody to TOP was identified as an IgG1 with κ light chains (not shown). Half-maximal and maximal specific binding of $^{125}\text{I-F(ab')}_2$ were obtained with approximately 0.5 and 2 μM $^{125}\text{I-F(ab')}_2$, respectively, both to dorsal and ventral retina cells (Fig. 3C). Nonspecific $^{125}\text{I-F(ab')}_2$ binding in the presence of P3X63 Ag8 ascites antibody was proportional to $^{125}\text{I-F(ab')}_2$ concentration and was not saturating at 3.52 μM, the highest $^{125}\text{I-F(ab')}_2$ concentration tested.

Geometry of the Gradient. The retina grows by accretion of concentric rings of neurons at the periphery; thus, central retina is the oldest portion of the retina and peripheral retina is the youngest. To determine whether the antigen gradient is a polar gradient that rotates around the center of the retina with uniform antigen concentration along any arc from center to periphery or is a circumferential gradient extending from dorsoposterior to ventroanterior retina, left retinas of 14-day chicken embryos were cut into eight central and eight peripheral sections (Fig. 4A) which were assayed for TOP. A 35-fold gradient of antigen was found extending from dorsoposterior to ventroanterior margins of the retina aligned parallel to the long axis of the choroid fissure.

As shown in Fig. 4B, strips of retina extending from the dorsoposterior to ventroanterior margins, or perpendicular to this axis from anterior to posterior margins, were removed and each

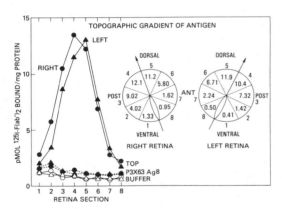

FIG. 2. Gradients of TOP molecules in retina from right ($\bullet$) and left ($\blacktriangle$) eyes of 14-day chicken embryos. $\bullet$—$\bullet$ and $\blacktriangle$—$\blacktriangle$, anti-TOP antibody; $\bullet$----$\bullet$ and $\blacktriangle$----$\blacktriangle$, P3X63 Ag8 antibody; $\bigcirc$—$\bigcirc$ and $\triangle$—$\triangle$, buffer B without antibody to TOP. Values shown within appropriate sections of retina are pmol of $^{125}\text{I-F(ab')}_2$ specifically bound per mg protein (i.e., pmol of $^{125}\text{I-F(ab')}_2$ bound in the presence of anti-TOP antibody minus pmol of $^{125}\text{I-F(ab')}_2$ bound in the presence of P3X63 Ag8 antibody). The assay conditions for TOP antigen used in this and subsequent experiments, except where stated, were as follows. Each retina was cut into eight sections as shown. Retina cells were mechanically dissociated in phosphate-buffered saline at 4°C by trituration (10 times) with a 200 μl micropipette tip (Medical Laboratory Automation), and 100 μl of a cell suspension (usually 160 μg of protein; range, 50–250 μg) was added to each well of polyvinyl chloride 96-well V-bottom plates (Dynatech) treated with solution B. Cells were centrifuged at 1300 $\times$ g for 5 min at 4°C and supernatant solutions were decanted. Each pellet was washed three times in solution B at 4°C (150 μl each wash), suspended in 50 μl of an antibody solution containing 1.0 μl of ascites fluid in solution B (except where specified), and incubated for 30 min at 4°C. Retina cells were washed three times as above, suspended in 50 μl of solution B containing 440 nM rabbit $^{125}\text{I-F(ab')}_2$ (5–10 $\times 10^4$ cpm) and 500 μg of bovine serum albumin, and incubated at 4°C for 30 min, unless otherwise specified. Pellets were washed three times as described above, wells were separated, and radioactivity was determined. Each value shown is the mean of two or three determinations. Protein was determined by a modification of the method of Lowry *et al.* (14).

Biochemistry: Trisler *et al.*

Proc. Natl. Acad. Sci. USA 78 (1981)   2147

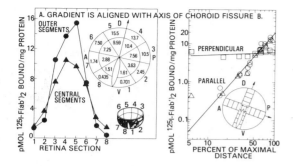

FIG. 4. Geometry of the TOP gradient in 14-day chicken embryo retina. Specifically bound ^{125}I-F(ab')$_2$ (pmol/mg of protein) is shown on the ordinate in *A* and *B* and within the appropriate segment of retina tested in *A*. (*A*) Each retina (left eye) was cut into eight 45° sections (7.25 mm in length from the center to periphery of retina) and each was divided into central (4.9 mm) and outer (2.35 mm) segments. (*B*) Demonstration that TOP concentration detected depends on the square of distance from the ventroanterior margin of the retina. Percentage of maximal circumferential distance is shown on the abscissa; 100% corresponds to 14.5 mm. △, Strips of retina from ventroanterior (0%) to dorsoposterior (100%) retina margins, 14.5 × 2.5 mm, were removed from eight retinas (left eyes), and each was cut into nine segments (1.6 × 2.5 mm) as shown; each segment was assayed for TOP antigen. □, Strips of retina from dorsoanterior (0%) to posterior (100%) margins of the retina perpendicular to the choroid fissure were prepared and assayed as above. ○, Data from *A*. The length of the arc from the ventral pole of the gradient to the center of each segment was calculated by assuming the retina to be a hemisphere and using equations for spherical triangles.

was cut into nine pieces which were assayed for antigen. The concentration of TOP molecules detected varied continuously and logarithmically with the logarithm of distance along the circumference of the retina from the ventroanterior pole of the gradient to the dorsoposterior pole, with a slope of 2. In contrast, little or no change was detected in retina cells along a perpendicular axis from anterior to posterior margins of the retina. The data are described somewhat better by a power function than by a logarithmic function, but a logarithmic function has not been ruled out.

The concentration of [^{125}I-F(ab')$_2$·anti-TOP antibody·TOP antigen] complex detected is described by the relationship:

$$[\text{TOP complex}] = \text{distance}^2.$$

Thus, cell position along a ventroanterior–dorsoposterior axis of retina can be identified by the concentration of TOP detected:

$$D_x = D_{max} (F_x/F_{max})^{0.5}$$

in which [TOP complex] is the fraction of maximal pmol of ^{125}I-F(ab')$_2$ specifically bound per mg of protein, F_x/F_{max}, and distance is the fraction of maximal circumferential distance from the ventroanterior to the dorsoposterior poles of the gradient, D_x/D_{max}. Under the conditions used, F_{max} is 20 pmol of ^{125}I-F(ab')$_2$ bound specifically per mg of protein and D_{max} is 14.5 mm. Thus, the calculated mean position in retina of cells that bind 5 pmol ^{125}I-F(ab')$_2$ specifically per mg protein is 7.25 mm from the ventroanterior pole of the gradient, which agrees well with the experimental values.

Autoradiography and Immunofluorescence. Autoradiography revealed most antigen in dorsoposterior chicken embryo retina in the inner and outer synaptic layers of the retina (Fig. 5 *A* and *B*). The antigen was detected in lesser amounts on the soma of most, or all, cell types in dorsoposterior retina. Little antigen was detected in ventroanterior retina (Fig. 5 *C* and *D*). Similar results were obtained by immunofluorescence (not shown). All cells mechanically dissociated from 8-day chicken embryo dorsoposterior retina exhibited punctate ring fluorescence. All cells from middle retina also were fluorescent, but less intensely than dorsoposterior retina cells. At each location, no obvious heterogeneity in cell population was seen. No fluorescent cells were detected in ventroanterior retina, although low levels of TOP were detected in ventroanterior retina by ^{125}I-F(ab')$_2$ binding.

Expression of Antigen During Development. The concentration of TOP antigen detected was higher in dorsoposterior retina than in ventroanterior retina at every age tested from the 4-day embryo through the adult (Fig. 6*A Inset*), and the axis and polarity of the gradient did not change during development (Fig. 6*A*). The concentration of antigen detected in the dorsal half of the retina increased 3-fold between the 4th and 12th days of embryonic development and then decreased slightly in the adult. Antigen concentration detected in ventral retina did not vary with development. The amount of protein per retina and

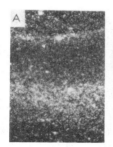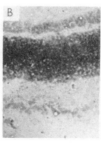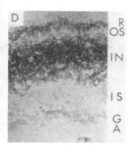

FIG. 5. Autoradiographs of 14-day chicken embryo retina. (*A* and *B*) Dark-field (*A*) and phase-contrast (*B*) views of dorsal retina. In *A*, some silver grains over cell soma in the inner nuclear layer appear dim due to staining of cells by toluidine blue. (*C* and *D*) Dark-field (*C*) and phase-contrast (*D*) views of ventral retina. R, photoreceptor layer; OS, outer synaptic layer; IN, inner nuclear layer; IS, inner synaptic layer; G, ganglion cell layer; A, ganglion cell axon layer. (×630.) Outer halves of 14-day chicken embryo dorsal or ventral retina were immersed in liquid Freon and then in liquid nitrogen and were cut in sections 16 μm thick. Each section was incubated with antibody to TOP or P3X63 Ag8 antibody (ascites fluid diluted 1:50 with solution B) for 45 min at 4°C, washed six times (15 min) with solution B (50 μl per wash), incubated with 50 μl of solution B containing 20 μg of fluorescein conjugate of rabbit IgG anti-mouse IgG (Cappel) for 45 min at 4°C, and washed as above. For autoradiography, each section was incubated with 50 μl of solution B containing 440 mM ^{125}I-F(ab')$_2$ (1 × 10^5 cpm) and 500 μg of bovine serum albumin for 30 min at 4°C, washed as above, and coated with NTB-2 nuclear track emulsion (Kodak). Slides were exposed in the dark (22 days) at 4°C in the presence of a dessicant and stained with 0.02% toluidine blue.

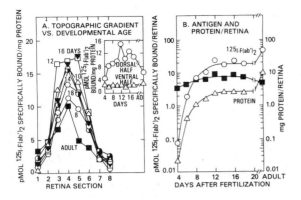

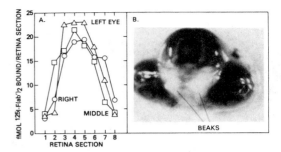

FIG. 6.   TOP antigen in chick retina as a function of developmental age. (A) Each retina (left eye) was cut into eight sections as shown in Fig. 2. Symbols and days *in ovo* are: ○, 8; △, 10; □, 12; ○, 14; ▼, 16; ◐, 18; and ■, adult. (*Inset*) ^{125}I-F(ab')$_2$ bound specifically is shown on the ordinate; days *in ovo* and adult (AD) are shown on the abscissa. ○, dorsal half of retina (sections 3–6); △, ventral half of retina (sections 1, 2, 7, and 8). Data for retina from 4- and 6-day embryos are shown only in *Inset*. (B) ○, ^{125}I-F(ab')$_2$ bound specifically per retina; △, protein per retina; ■, ordinate represents pmol ^{125}I-F(ab')$_2$ bound specifically per mg of protein.

TOP antigen detected per retina increased 470- and 620-fold, respectively, between the 4-day embryo and the adult; the amount of antigen detected per mg of protein remained relatively constant (Fig. 6B). These results show that a gradient of TOP molecules is formed early in retina development, during the period of active neuroblast proliferation and neuron genesis, and that the gradient is maintained after neuron genesis ceases.

Tissue Specificity. Highest concentrations of TOP antigen detected were in regions of the nervous system derived from prosencephalon (forebrain): retina > cerebrum > thalamus (Table 1). Low levels of antigen were found in dorsal and ventral retina pigment epithelium, optic nerve, optic tectum, and cerebellum; little or no antigen was detected in heart, liver, kidney, or cells from blood.

Chicken Embryo with an Ectopic Eye. During the course of these studies, a chicken embryo with three eyes was found (Fig. 7). The third eye was situated in the middle of the forehead, facing in a dorsoanterior direction. Retinas from right, middle, and left eyes contained gradients of TOP molecules with normal polarity and alignment with the choroid fissure.

Table 1.   Distribution of TOP antigen in chicken tissues

	^{125}I-F(ab')$_2$ specifically bound, pmol/mg protein	
Tissue	14-day embryo	Adult
Dorsal neural retina	12.0	7.70
Ventral neural retina	1.08	2.70
Cerebrum	3.30	3.12
Thalamus	2.13	—
Optic nerve	—	0.58
Optic tectum	0.15	—
Cerebellum	0.23	0.46
Dorsal retina pigment epithelium	0.26	—
Ventral retina pigment epithelium	0.25	—
Heart, liver, kidney, or blood cells	0.002–0.055	

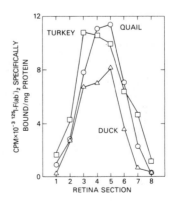

FIG. 7.   (A) TOP antigen gradients in retinas from the right (○), middle (□), and left (△) eyes of a 14-day chicken embryo with three eyes. Total ^{125}I-F(ab')$_2$ bound per retina section is shown. Reaction mixtures contained 2.38 nM ^{125}I-F(ab')$_2$. (B) Frontal view of head of embryo. The third eye is situated on the forehead facing in a dorsoanterior direction. The embryo had two pairs of beaks, two brains in one head, and one body.

Thus, a gradient of TOP antigen was generated with normal orientation in the supernumerary eye despite the abnormal orientation of the eye in the embryo.

Species Specificity. Gradients of TOP molecules with similar orientation and symmetry were detected in turkey, quail, and duck embryo retina, 17, 15, and 16 days after fertilization, respectively (Fig. 8). ^{125}I-F(ab')$_2$ concentrations in reaction mixtures were low (0.074–0.26 nM); thus, bound ^{125}I-F(ab')$_2$ also was low. With 440 nM ^{125}I-F(ab')$_2$, 7.5 pmol of ^{125}I-F(ab')$_2$ bound specifically per mg of dorsoposterior quail retina protein, comparable to chicken retina. The antigen was not detected in retina of goldfish, *Xenopus laevis*, *Rana pipiens*, or Fisher rats (not shown).

Properties of TOP Antigen. A dorsal→ventral gradient of GM$_2$ ganglioside molecules (II^{3}NeuAc-G$_g$Ose$_3$Cer) in chicken embryo retina has been postulated but not detected (15). Bovine brain gangliosides (10–10,000 μM) did not inhibit the binding of anti-TOP antibody to retina (not shown). Rabbit antisera to mono-, di-, and trisialogangliosides (gift of C. Alving) bound to retina; however, a ganglioside gradient was not detected.

FIG. 8.   TOP gradients in retina from Japanese quail (○), *Coturnix coturnix japonica* (15-day embryo); White Pekin duck (△), *Anas platyrhynchos* (16-day embryo); and turkey (□), *Meleagris gallopavo* (17-day embryo). The eggs hatch 17, 28, and 28 days after fertilization, respectively. ^{125}I-F(ab')$_2$ concentrations and μCi/pmol were as follows: quail, 0.26 nM, 0.90 μCi/pmol; duck, 0.074 nM, 2.92 μCi/pmol; and turkey, 0.078 nM, 2.38 μCi/pmol.

Table 2. Effect of trypsin or heat on TOP antigenicity

			^{125}I-$F(ab')_2$ bound specifically to retina cells	
	Treatment of retina cells			
Exp.	0–30 min	30–40 min	cpm	%
1	Control	+ Trypsin inhibitor	1700	100
	Trypsin	+ Trypsin inhibitor	93	6
	Trypsin + trypsin inhibitor	—	1803	106
2	4°C, 30 min		1607	100
	100°C, 30 min		132	8

Inactivation of TOP retina molecules in 14-day chicken embryo dorsal retina by trypsin or heat. In Exp. 1, retina cells were incubated for 30 min at 37°C, in phosphate-buffered saline alone or with 11 μM trypsin (crystallized three times, Worthington) or with 11 μM trypsin inactivated with 12 μM soybean trypsin inhibitor (Worthington), and then for 10 min in soybean trypsin inhibitor. TOP ascites fluid was diluted 1:1000; 1.86 nM ^{125}I-$F(ab')_2$ (90.5 nCi/pmol) was used. In Exp. 2, TOP and P3X63 Ag8 antibodies were diluted 1:100; 1.82 nM ^{125}I-$F(ab')_2$ (96.9 nCi/pmol) was used.

TOP antigenicity was lost upon incubation at 100°C or by incubation with trypsin (Table 2). All TOP antigenicity in retina cell homogenates was recovered from the 100,000 × g particulate fraction; soluble antigen was not detected (not shown).

DISCUSSION

Fusion of spleen cells from a mouse immunized with dorsoposterior chicken embryo retina with P3X63 Ag8 mouse myeloma cells yielded a line of hybridoma cells that synthesizes antibody to molecules that are distributed in a topographic gradient in the retina. At least 35-fold more antigen was detected in dorsoposterior than in ventroanterior retina. The antigen was found by autoradiography in highest concentration in 14-day chicken embryo retina on neurites in the inner and outer synaptic layers. The antigen was found by immunofluorescence on most, or all, cells from dorsoposterior and middle portions of 8- and 14-day chicken embryo retina. These results suggest that antigen molecules are distributed in the retina on the basis of cell position, rather than cell type.

Neurons in dorsal and ventral retina differ in several ways. For example, *Xenopus* retina is composed of at least three clonal domains (16). One cell on each side of the 16-cell embryo gives rise to dorsal retina, another cell gives rise to middle retina, and a third cell gives rise to cells that migrate across the midline of the embryo and form ventral retina on the opposite side. In addition, dorsal retina ganglion neurons synapse in ventral tectum, whereas ventral retina ganglion neurons synapse in dorsal tectum (1, 17, 18), establishing a continuous, point-to-point retino-tectal map.

Neurons are generated in chicken embryo retina between the 2nd and 12th days after fertilization; central retina is the oldest portion of the retina, and peripheral retina is the youngest. The concentration of TOP molecules detected in dorsoposterior retina increased as the diameter of the retina increased, and it varied with cell position at every stage tested, from the 4-day embryo through the adult, suggesting that the gradient of TOP is established as neurons and glia (and possibly their precursors) are generated in retina. Proliferation of clonal populations of cells with different genotypes in mosaic mice results in radial patterns of cells in neural retina and retina pigment epithelium (19); whether the gradient of TOP molecules is due to clonal inheritance remains to be determined.

Dorsal and ventral retina cells also differ in adhesive specificity—i.e., cells from dorsal retina adhere preferentially to cells from ventral retina or tectum and vice versa (20–22). However, the properties of TOP molecules differ from those reported for preferential adhesion of dorsal retina cells and for retina adhesion factors such as cognin (4), CAM (5), and ligand and agglutinin (23).

The dorsoposterior portion of chicken or pigeon retina contains a fovea, 3- to 5-fold more amacrine synapses than ventral retina (24), and a relatively high concentration of red droplets in photoreceptor cells and functions as a binocular visual field for pecking (25). Thus, dorsoposterior retina differs from other portions of retina in embryologic development, migration of cells and axons across the midline of the embryo, synapse specificity, adhesive specificity, and function.

The results suggest that a gradient of TOP molecules is formed by a gradient of cells which have different numbers of antigenic TOP molecules depending on cell position in the retina. No evidence was found for topographically distributed differences in antigen affinity for antibody or in the proportion of cells expressing antigen. Variation in antigen accessibility has not been excluded. The mechanism of generating and maintaining the gradient of TOP, highly ordered with respect to the axis of the retina, remains to be determined.

The function of TOP molecules has not been determined. However, since TOP antigen concentration detected is continuously graded and distributed on the basis of cell position not cell type, our working hypothesis is that TOP molecules play a role in the coding of positional information in the retina.

1. Sperry, R. W. (1963) *Proc. Natl. Acad. Sci. USA* **50**, 703–710.
2. Silver, J. & Sidman, R. L. (1980) *J. Comp. Neurol.* **189**, 101–111.
3. Goldschneider, I. & Moscona, A. A. (1972) *J. Cell Biol.* **53**, 435–449.
4. Hausman, R. E. & Moscona, A. A. (1979) *Exp. Cell Res.* **119**, 191–204.
5. Thiery, J.-P., Brackenbury, R., Rutishauser, U. & Edelman, G. M. (1977) *J. Biol. Chem.* **252**, 6841–6845.
6. Eisenbarth, G. S., Walsh, F. S. & Nirenberg, M. (1979) *Proc. Natl. Acad. Sci. USA* **76**, 4913–4917.
7. Barnstable, C. J. (1980) *Nature (London)* **286**, 231–235.
8. Trisler, G. D., Donlon, M. A., Shain, W. G. & Coon, H. G. (1979) *Fed. Proc. Fed. Am. Soc. Exp. Biol.* **38**, 2368–2373.
9. Köhler, G. & Milstein, C. (1975) *Nature (London)* **256**, 495–497.
10. Galfre, G., Howe, S. C., Milstein, C., Butcher, G. W. & Howard, J. C. (1977) *Nature (London)* **266**, 550–552.
11. Berzofsky, J. A., Hicks, G., Fedorko, J. & Minna, J. (1980) *J. Biol. Chem.* **255**, 11188–11191.
12. Schneider, M. D., & Eisenbarth, G. S. (1979) *J. Immunol. Methods* **29**, 331–342.
13. Bolton, A. E. & Hunter, W. M. (1973) *Biochem. J.* **133**, 529–539.
14. Lowry, O. H., Rosebrough, N. J., Farr, A. L. & Randall, R. J. (1951) *J. Biol. Chem.* **193**, 265–275.
15. Marchase, R. B. (1977) *J. Cell Biol.* **75**, 237–257.
16. Hirose, G. & Jacobson, M. (1979) *Dev. Biol.* **71**, 191–202.
17. Hamdi, F. A. & Whitteridge, D. (1954) *Quant. J. Exp. Physiol.* **39**, 111–119.
18. McGill, J. I., Powell, T. P. S. & Cowan, W. M. (1966) *J. Anat.* **100**, 5–33.
19. Sanyal, S. & Zeilmaker, G. M. (1977) *Nature (London)* **265**, 731–733.
20. Barbera, A. J., Marchase, R. B. & Roth, S. (1973) *Proc. Natl. Acad. Sci. USA* **70**, 2482–2486.
21. Gottlieb, D. I., Rock, K. & Glaser, L. (1976) *Proc. Natl. Acad. Sci. USA* **73**, 410–414.
22. Cafferata, R., Panosian, J. & Bordley, G. (1979) *Dev. Biol.* **69**, 108–117.
23. Rutz, R. & Lilien, J. (1979) *J. Cell Sci.* **36**, 323–342.
24. Yazulla, S. (1974) *J. Comp. Neurol.* **153**, 309–324.
25. Galifret, Y. (1968) *Zeitschrift für Zellforschung* **86**, 535–545.

Section 11
Synapse Elimination: Rearrangement of Synaptic Connections in Early Life

Brown, M.C., J.K.S. Jansen, and D. Van Essen. 1976. Polyneuronal innervation of skeletal muscle in newborn rats and its elimination during maturation. *J. Physiol.* 261: 387–422.

Lichtman, J.W. 1977. The reorganization of synaptic connexions in the rat submandibular ganglion during post-natal development. *J. Physiol.* 273: 155–177.

Hubel, D.H., T.N. Wiesel, and S. LeVay. 1977. Plasticity of ocular dominance columns in monkey striate cortex. *Philos. Trans. R. Soc. Lond. B* 278: 377–409.

In addition to those mechanisms that lead to the establishment of transmission between qualitatively correct pre- and postsynaptic cells, an additional problem must be solved during synapse formation. Each postsynaptic cell must be innervated by a number of synapses and axons appropriate to its intended function. How does this quantitative apportionment of synaptic connections occur?

Considerable insight into this problem has been provided by studies of developing muscle. Anatomists had long remarked on the different appearance of the neuromuscular junction in neonatal and mature muscles (Tello 1917; Boeke 1932). Little attention was paid to this observation until Redfern (1970) showed, by electrophysiological means, that skeletal-muscle fibers in neonatal mammals are innervated differently from adult cells. In general, adult muscle fibers are innervated by a single axon. Intracellular recordings from muscle fibers in neonatal animals, however, show a postsynaptic response that is characteristically complex; discrete steps in the synaptic potential elicited by increasing the strength of motor-nerve stimulation indicate innervation by several axons with different thresholds (Redfern 1970; Bagust et al. 1973; Bennett and Pettigrew 1974; Letinsky 1974; **Brown, Jansen,** and **Van Essen 1976**). Morphological, electrophysiological, and pharmacological studies have shown that these initial synaptic contacts on each neonatal fiber are located at approximately the same place, the site of the mature end plate (Bennett and Pettigrew 1974, 1976; Brown et al. 1976; Riley 1976, 1977; Korneliussen and Jansen 1976). This comparison of adult and neonatal innervation shows that some initial synapses must have been eliminated.

These and other studies at different postnatal ages (see Bixby and Van Essen 1979) make it clear that the elimination of the redundant axon terminals occurs gradually, the mature one-on-one pattern being established a few weeks after birth. This change apparently does not involve neuronal death (see Section 5), since the number of motor neurons remains unchanged throughout this period (Brown et al. 1976). A similar process of synapse elimination is also evident during reinnervation of adult muscle (McArdle 1975; Benoit and Changeux 1978).

A postnatal elimination of some initial contacts is not limited to muscle, but also occurs at interneuronal synapses. The simplest neuronal system in which synapse elimination has been studied is the submandibular ganglion of the rat (**Lichtman 1977**, 1980). The cells in this parasympathetic ganglion are similar to skeletal-muscle fibers in that most of them are innervated by a single preganglionic axon in maturity. At birth, however, each neonatal ganglion cell is innervated by an average of five different axons. As in muscle, the initial convergence of several axons on each target cell is reduced to the adult one-on-one pattern over the first few weeks of life. Synapse elimination has also been observed in the superior cervical ganglion of the hamster (Lichtman and Purves 1980) and in the ciliary ganglion of the rabbit (Johnson and Purves 1981). Since most adult neurons in these ganglia remain innervated by a number of different axons, synapse elimination is not limited to those target cells that are ultimately innervated by only a single axon. In the rabbit ciliary ganglion, as in the neuromuscular system, the pre- and postsynaptic populations are stable during the period when many of the initial synaptic contacts are lost; thus, cell death does not appear to play a role in this phenomenon.

An important and somewhat paradoxical finding in these autonomic preparations is that synapse elimination occurs in the face of a net increase in the overall number of synaptic contacts (boutons) made with the target neurons (Lichtman and Purves 1980; Smolen and Raisman 1980; Johnson and Purves 1981; Lichtman 1977). This suggests that the underlying feature of what is generally called synapse elimination is not the elimination of synapses per se, but a rearrangement of synaptic connections that alters the number of different axons that innervate each cell.

Such early synaptic rearrangements may also be characteristic of the central nervous system. Electrophysiological experiments using the cere-bellum of newborn rats suggest that Purkinje cells are initially innervated by several different climbing fibers, all but one of which are lost over the first few weeks of postnatal life (Crepel et al. 1976; Mariani and Changeux 1981). In the spinal cord, contacts initially present on the axon hillock of motor neurons are also lost in early life (see, for example, Conradi and Skoglund 1969). Rearrangement of synaptic connections has also been described in the developing retinotectal system of lower vertebrates (see Section 9). The most striking example, however, comes from studies of the developing visual cortex (Wiesel and Hubel 1963, 1965; Hubel and Wiesel 1965, 1970, 1972; **Hubel, Wiesel,** and **LeVay 1977;** Rakic 1977; LeVay et al. 1978; Shatz and Stryker 1978). In adult cats and some species of monkey, cortical neurons in layer IV of the primary visual cortex are segregated into columns dominated alternately by the right eye and the left eye. At birth, however, or in late embryonic life, there is considerable overlap of adjacent ocular-dominance columns. Both anatomical and electrophysiological evidence suggest that the progressive definition of ocular-dominance columns involves the elimination of some initial synaptic connections.

What sort of mechanism underlies these developmental rearrangements of synaptic connections? To some degree, the process may reflect an intrinsic tendency of the innervating cells to withdraw a portion of their terminal arborization (Brown et al. 1976); however, this would not explain the pattern of innervation found in skeletal muscles and in some autonomic ganglia. Most workers in this field now seem to agree that competition between different axons is a central feature of synaptic rearrangement. Evidence for this in the peripheral nervous system is the one-on-one pattern in muscle and some autonomic ganglia, together with the finding that elimination proceeds less vigorously when the number of axons innervating a muscle is reduced by partial denervation (Betz et al. 1980; see, however, Brown et al. 1976). The fact that ocular-dominance columns develop in the frog tectum when implantation of a third eye causes two sets of axons to innervate a region normally innervated by axons from a single eye also supports the competitive view (Law and Constantine-Paton 1981). The basis of the competition, however, remains obscure. It seems likely that a trophic factor provided by the target is an essential ingredient (see Section 6), but positive feedback mediated by a trophic agent does not, by itself, explain all of the observations (see Purves and Lichtman 1980). Competition is also related to neural activity. Thus, chronically paralyzing motor nerves with a local anesthetic or otherwise decreasing activity slows the progress of the competition (Benoit and Changeux 1975, 1978; Riley 1978; Thompson et al. 1979), whereas stimulation has the reverse effect (O'Brien et al. 1977).

The importance of activity is also indicated by the dramatic effects of monocular deprivation on the segregation of ocular-dominance columns (Hubel et al. 1977): If one eye is made less active than the other (by occlusion, for example), the cortical afferents subserving the nondeprived eye do not retract as they normally would. What is particularly interesting about the effects of monocular deprivation is that the timing of activity among the competing inputs appears to be more important than simply the overall level of activity of different axons. Hubel and Wiesel (1965) have thus proposed that axons whose

neural activities are synchronous compete less vigorously than those whose inputs fire out of step with one another. Recent experiments have suggested that the diffuse adrenergic innervation of the visual cortex also plays a role in monocular deprivation (Kasamatsu and Pettigrew 1976, 1979; Kasamatsu et al. 1979), an effect conceivably related to the different patterns of activity observed in sleeping and awake animals (Livingstone and Hubel 1981).

In addition to activity, the geometry of postsynaptic neurons appears to influence the number of different axons that ultimately innervate them. Thus, in autonomic ganglia there is a strong correlation in maturity between the dendritic complexity of individual ganglion cells and the number of innervating axons (Purves and Hume 1981). Ganglion cells without dendrites are innervated by a single axon, whereas neurons with dendrites are innervated by a number of different axons proportional to the complexity of the dendritic arbor. Since in at least some ganglia the geometry of the target cells is largely established before the postnatal rearrangement

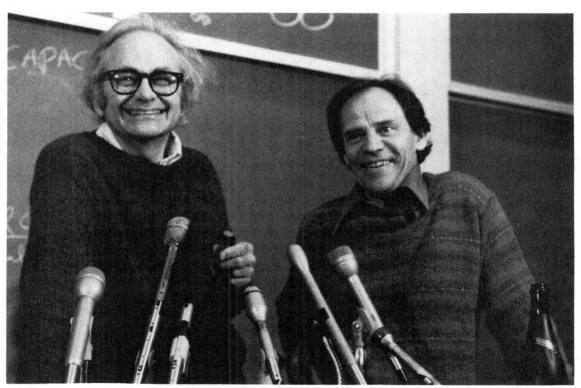

David H. Hubel and Torsten N. Wiesel, who showed that neural connections in the brain are normally rearranged during a critical period in newborn mammals and that this process can be modified by an animal's early experience.

521

of innervation is complete, the final number of axons that innervate a neuron is apparently regulated to some degree by postsynaptic geometry (Hume and Purves 1981). In muscle as well, competition between two axons innervating the same cell may depend on the geometrical arrangement of the competitors, in this case the distance between them (Bennett and Pettigrew 1976; Kuffler et al. 1977, 1980). These findings suggest that the spatial arrangement of synapses on postsynaptic cells plays an important part in their competitive interaction.

All told, rearrangements of the initial pattern of synaptic connections occur in many regions of the developing nervous system. In those neuronal systems where this phenomenon can be studied in detail, elimination of some initial contacts involves the focusing of an increasing number of synapses from each axon onto a smaller number of target cells. Synapse elimination appears to be competitive and seems to be a means of regulating the number of different axons that innervate each target cell. The major result of this phenomenon, then, is quantitative, rather than qualitative, accuracy.

References

Bagust, J., D.M. Lewis, and R.A. Westerman. 1973. Polyneuronal innervation of kitten skeletal muscle. *J. Physiol. 229:* 241–255.

Benoit, P. and J.-P. Changeux. 1975. Consequences of tenotomy on the evolution of multi-innervation in developing rat soleus muscle. *Brain Res. 99:* 354–358.

———. 1978. Consequences of blocking the nerve with a local anaesthetic on the evolution of multi-innervation at the regenerating neuromuscular junction of the rat. *Brain Res. 149:* 89–96.

Bennett, M.R. and A.G. Pettigrew. 1974. The formation of synapses in striated muscle during development. *J. Physiol. 241:* 515–545.

———. 1976. The formation of neuromuscular synapses. *Cold Spring Harbor Symp. Quant. Biol. 40:* 409–424.

Betz, W.J., J.H. Caldwell, and R.R. Ribchester. 1980. The effects of partial denervation at birth on the development of muscle fibres and motor units in rat lumbrical muscle. *J. Physiol. 303:* 265–279.

Bixby, J.L. and D.C. Van Essen. 1979. Regional differences in the timing of synapse elimination in skeletal muscles of the neonatal rabbit. *Brain Res. 169:* 275–286.

Boeke, J. 1932. Nerve endings, motor and sensory. In *Cytology and cellular pathology of the nervous system* (ed. W. Penfield), vol. 1, pp. 243–315. Hoeberg, New York.

Brown, M.C., J.K.S. Jansen, and D. Van Essen. 1976. Polyneuronal innervation of skeletal muscle in newborn rats and its elimination during maturation. *J. Physiol. 261:* 387–422.

Conradi, S. and S. Skoglund. 1969. Observations on the ultrastructure of the initial motor axon segment and dorsal root boutons on the motoneurons in the lumbrosacral spinal cord of the cat during postnatal development. *Acta Physiol. Scand.* (Suppl.) *333:* 53–76.

Crepel, F., J. Mariani, and N. Delhaye-Bouchaud. 1976. Evidence for a multiple innervation of Purkinje cells by climbing fibers in the immature rat cerebellum. *J. Neurobiol. 7:* 567–578.

Hubel, D.H. and T.N. Wiesel. 1965. Binocular interaction in striate cortex of kittens reared with artificial squint. *J. Neurophysiol. 28:* 1041–1059.

———. 1970. The period of susceptibility to the physiological effects of unilateral eye closure in kittens. *J. Physiol. 206:* 419–436.

———. 1972. Laminar and columnar distribution of geniculo-cortical fibers in the macaque monkey. *J. Comp. Neurol. 146:* 421–450.

Hubel, D.H., T.N. Wiesel, and S. LeVay. 1977. Plasticity of ocular dominance columns in monkey striate cortex. *Philos. Trans. R. Soc. Lond. B 278:* 377–409.

Hume, R.I. and D. Purves. 1981. Geometry of neonatal neurones and the regulation of synapse elimination. *Nature 293:* 469–471.

Johnson, D.A. and D. Purves. 1981. Postnatal reduction of neural unit size in the rabbit ciliary ganglion. *J. Physiol. 318:* 143–159.

Kasamatsu, T. and J.D. Pettigrew. 1976. Depletion of brain catecholamines: Failure of ocular dominance shift after monocular occlusion in kittens. *Science 194:* 206–209.

———. 1979. Preservation of binocularity after monocular deprivation in the striate cortex of kittens treated with 6-hydroxydopamine. *J. Comp. Neurol. 185:* 139–162.

Kasamatsu, T., J.D. Pettigrew, and M. Ary. 1979. Restoration of visual cortical plasticity by local microperfusion of norepinephrine. *J. Comp. Neurol. 185:* 163–182.

Korneliussen, H. and J.K.S. Jansen. 1976. Morphological aspects of the elimination of polyneuronal innervation of skeletal muscle fibres in newborn rats. *J. Neurocytol. 5:* 591–604.

Kuffler, D.P., W. Thompson, and J.K.S. Jansen. 1977. The elimination of synapses in multiply-innervated skeletal muscle fibres of the rat: Dependence on distance between end-plates. *Brain Res. 183:* 353–358.

———. 1980. The fate of foreign endplates in cross-innervated rat soleus muscle. *Proc. R. Soc. Lond. B 208:* 189–222.

Law, M.I. and M. Constantine-Paton. 1981. Anatomy and physiology of experimentally produced striped tecta. *J. Neurosci. 1:* 741–759.

Letinsky, M.S. 1974. The development of nerve muscle junctions in *Rana catesbeiana* tadpoles. *Dev. Biol. 40:* 129–153.

LeVay, S., M.P. Stryker, and C.J. Shatz. 1978. Ocular dominance columns and their development in layer IV of the cat's visual cortex: A quantitative study. *J. Comp. Neurol. 179:* 223–244.

Lichtman, J.W. 1977. The reorganization of synaptic connexions in the rat submandibular ganglion during post-natal development. *J. Physiol. 273:* 155–177.

———. 1980. On the predominantly single innervation of submandibular ganglion cells in the rat. *J. Physiol. 302:* 121–130.

Lichtman, J.W. and D. Purves. 1980. The elimination of redundant preganglionic innervation to hamster sympathetic ganglion cells in early post-natal life. *J. Physiol. 301:* 213–228.

Livingstone, M.S. and D.H. Hubel. 1981. Effects of sleep and arousal on the processing of visual information in the cat. *Nature 291:* 554–561.

Mariani, J. and J.-P. Changeux. 1981. Ontogenesis of olivocerebellar relationships. I. Studies by intracellular recordings of the multiple innervation of Purkinje cells by climbing fibers in the developing rat cerebellum. *J. Neurosci. 1:* 696–702.

McArdle, J.J. 1975. Complex end-plate potentials at regenerating neuromuscular junctions of the rat. *Exp. Neurol. 49:* 629–638.

O'Brien, R.A.D., R.D. Purves, and G. Vrbová. 1977. Effect of activity on the elimination of multiple innervation in soleus muscles of rats. *J. Physiol. 271:* 54P.

Purves, D. and R.I. Hume. 1981. The relation of postsynaptic geometry to the number of presynaptic axons that innervate autonomic ganglion cells. *J. Neurosci. 1:* 441–452.

Purves, D. and J.W. Lichtman. 1980. Elimination of synapses in the developing nervous system. *Science 210:* 153–157.

Rakic, P. 1977. Prenatal development in the visual system in the rhesus monkey. *Philos. Trans. R. Soc. Lond. B 278:* 245–260.

Redfern, P.A. 1970. Neuromuscular transmission in new-born rats. *J. Physiol. 209:* 701–709.

Riley, D.A. 1976. Multiple axon branches innervating single endplates of kitten soleus myofibers. *Brain Res. 110:* 158–161.

———. 1977. Spontaneous elimination of nerve terminals from the endplates of developing skeletal myofibers. *Brain Res. 134:* 279–285.

———. 1978. Tenotomy delays the postnatal development of the motor innervation of the rat soleus. *Brain Res. 143:* 162–167.

Shatz, C.J. and M.P. Stryker. 1978. Ocular dominance in layer IV of the cat's visual cortex and the effects of monocular deprivation. *J. Physiol. 281:* 267–283.

Smolen, A. and G. Raisman. 1980. Synapse formation in the rat superior cervical ganglion during normal development and after neonatal deafferentation. *Brain Res. 181:* 315–323.

Thompson, W., D.P. Kuffler, and J.K.S. Jansen. 1979. The effect of prolonged, reversible block of nerve impulses on the elimination of polyneuronal innervation of new-born rat skeletal muscle fibers. *Neuroscience 4:* 71–81.

Tello, J.F. 1917. Genesis de las terminaciones nerviosas motrices y sensitivas. *Trab. Lab. Invest. Biol. Univ. Madr. 15:* 101–199.

Wiesel, T.N. and D.H. Hubel. 1963. Single cell responses in striate cortex of kittens deprived of vision in one eye. *J. Neurophysiol. 26:* 1003–1017.

———. 1965. Comparison of the effects of unilateral and bilateral eye closure on cortical unit responses in kittens. *J. Neurophysiol. 28:* 1029–1040.

J. Physiol. (1976), **261**, *pp.* 387–422
With 2 plates and 13 text-figures
Printed in Great Britain

POLYNEURONAL INNERVATION OF SKELETAL MUSCLE IN NEW-BORN RATS AND ITS ELIMINATION DURING MATURATION

By M. C. BROWN,* J. K. S. JANSEN and D. VAN ESSEN†

From the Institute of Physiology, University of Oslo, Karl Johans Gate 47, Oslo 1, Norway

(*Received 27 February 1976*)

SUMMARY

1. The events taking place during the elimination of polyneuronal innervation in the soleus muscle of new-born rats have been studied using a combination of electrophysiological and anatomical techniques.

2. Each immature muscle fibre is supplied by two or more motor axons which converge on to a single end-plate. There was no sign of electrical coupling between muscle fibres receiving multiple synaptic inputs. By the end of the second week after birth virtually all muscle fibres are innervated by only a single motor axon.

3. The average tension produced by individual motor units, measured in terms of the percentage of the total muscle twitch tension, declined dramatically during the first 2 weeks after birth. During this period there was no significant change in the number of motor neurones innervating the soleus muscle. Thus, the disappearance of polyneuronal innervation reflects a decrease in the number of peripheral synapses made by each motor neurone.

4. The decline in motor unit size was delayed, but not ultimately prevented, by the early surgical removal of all but a few motor axons to the soleus muscle. This procedure also caused a delay in the removal of polyneuronal innervation involving the remaining motor units.

5. Following a crush of the soleus nerve in neonatal animals, regenerating axons usually returned to the original end-plates. Polyneuronal innervation was extensive at early stages of re-innervation and it disappeared during the second week after birth just as in normal muscles.

6. Cross-innervation of neonatal muscles by an implanted foreign nerve caused a rapid disappearance of cholinesterase at denervated original

* Present address: University Laboratory of Physiology, Parks Road, Oxford.
† Present address: Department of Anatomy, University College London, Gower Street, London WC 1.

end-plates and in most fibres prevented re-innervation by the original nerve. In the small proportion of fibres that did become innervated through both the foreign and original nerves the end-plates were more than 1 mm apart, and both foreign and original nerve end-plates could persist indefinitely.

7. Many cross-innervated fibres received multiple inputs through the foreign nerve. Some foreign end-plates were separated by distances ranging up to 1 mm. Polyneuronal innervation through the foreign nerve was completely eliminated during maturation but over a slightly longer period than in normal muscles. Apparently the elimination process can act over a distance up to but not much more than 1 mm.

8. These observations suggest that there are several factors influencing the elimination of redundant inputs in immature muscles. Individual motor neurones appear to have an inherent tendency to withdraw the majority of their original complement of peripheral terminals. The determination of which particular synapses are to survive, however, seems to be made in the periphery by a selection among all the synapses that innervate a limited region of each muscle fibre. There may be a competitive interaction among synapses in which those belonging to smaller motor units are less likely to be eliminated, thereby leading to a relatively uniform size of the motor units in the soleus.

INTRODUCTION

Mature mammalian skeletal muscle is innervated in a remarkably simple way by its motor axons, in the sense that each muscle fibre is supplied by only a single axon terminal situated approximately midway along the length of the fibre. It thus came as a surprise when Redfern (1970) demonstrated that the end-plate potentials (e.p.p.s) of muscle fibres from newborn rats consisted of several discrete components, indicating that each muscle fibre initially receives an input from several motor axons. During the first few weeks after birth multiple innervation disappears and the adult pattern of single innervation of each muscle fibre is achieved. These observations have been confirmed and extended by Bennett & Pettigrew (1974a); Bagust, Lewis & Westerman (1973) have shown that a similar phenomenon occurs in kitten muscles.

The accessibility of muscles even in neonatal animals to experimental procedures such as micro-electrode recording, partial denervation, re-innervation, and cross-innervation has made it possible to ask a variety of questions concerning the process of synapse elimination. For example, where are the synaptic terminals located? What factors determine the time at which synapses disappear: is it related specifically to the age of the muscle, the motor neurone, or the synapse? Does synapse elimination involve only terminals situated very close to one another, or can the interaction take place between spatially separated terminals? Do immature fibres show a preference for retaining innervation from their original nerve supply rather than from a foreign nerve? In addition to providing answers to some of these and related questions, our results give clues to the control mechanisms involved in producing the end result of one and only one synapse per muscle fibre. Some of the observations have been presented in preliminary communications (Brown, Jansen & Van Essen 1975, 1976).

METHODS

Physiological recordings. Experiments were made on the soleus and diaphragm muscles of rats of different ages, starting as early as the first day after birth. We refer to muscles from animals under 2 weeks of age as immature, because up until that time they retain a pattern of innervation clearly different from that seen in the adult. For physiological recordings the muscle and its motor nerve supply were isolated, pinned out in a small chamber coated with transparent Sylgard resin, and perfused at room temperature with a well-oxygenated Ringer solution of the following composition (in mM): NaCl, 137; KCl, 5; $CaCl_2$, 10; $MgCl_2$, 1; glucose, 11; Tris Cl, 10; buffered to pH 7·4. The high Ca in the solution improved the stability and quality of micro-electrode penetrations. Intracellular recordings were made using glass micro-electrodes filled with 4 M K-acetate and having resistances of 20–60 MΩ. Using dark-field illumination it was possible to resolve individual muscle fibres even in the small immature muscles. Nerves were stimulated through glass-tipped suction electrodes. In many experiments the muscle was curarized by adding just enough D-tubocurarine (0·5–2 μg/ml.) to block nerve-evoked contractions. In experiments involving iontophoresis of acetylcholine (ACh) the ACh was delivered from a micropipette filled with 1 M ACh having a resistance of 200–400 MΩ. A backing current of 1–3 nA was used to minimize the desensitization of ACh receptors.

Measurement of motor unit tension. In one series of experiments we counted the total number of motor axons supplying the soleus muscle and the tension generated by individual motor units. The nerve supply to the soleus muscle was dissected free all the way back to spinal roots L5 and L4. The preparation was then transferred to a chamber having two compartments separated by a thin plastic partition. The soleus nerve was placed through a slot in the partition, and the proximal tendon of the muscle was pinned to the bottom of the chamber close to the partition. The distal tendon was connected by fine surgical thread to a sensitive strain gauge. Activity in the soleus nerve was monitored by recording differentially from the two compartments, which were perfused independently. Each ventral root was split into several filaments that were stimulated individually. The splitting was continued until each filament contained at most four, and usually only one or two soleus motor axons. We occasionally saw action potentials in the soleus nerve not followed by measurable tension changes in the muscle, but these were discounted because they were presumably either from γ motor axons or from gastrocnemius motor axons extending unusually far into the soleus nerve. For direct stimulation current pulses were passed between coarse electrodes placed on opposite sides of the muscle. In the course of most experiments there was an unexplained slow and parallel decline of 10–30 % in the tensions produced by direct muscle stimulation and by maximal stimulation of the nerve. When this occurred the individual motor unit tensions were expressed as a percentage of the original total. The decline in muscle tension, whatever its cause, would have only a slight effect on our estimates of *average* motor unit size. It might, however, seriously affect our measurements of the total range in motor unit size if the over-all tension decline involved large losses by only a few motor units. This seems unlikely, though, as small motor units were encountered even in experiments where little or no tension loss was seen and also at early stages of the other experiments, before the tension decline had set in.

Histological techniques. End-plate cholinesterase was stained using the procedure of Karnovsky (1964). Muscles were prefixed for 10–15 min in a solution containing 2·5 % glutaraldehyde, 2 % paraformaldehyde, and 0·1 M cacodylate buffer at pH 7·5. They were then incubated in the staining solution at room temperature for 30 min, fixed in the same fixative solution for 1–24 hr, and stored in H_2O. The distribution of end-plates throughout the muscle could be seen easily in whole mount preparations viewed under a dissecting microscope. In order to count the number of end-plates on individual fibres we found it necessary to tease out single fibres over the entire region where cholinesterase was visible in the whole mount. Fibres were dissected free with the aid of electrolytically sharpened tungsten needles and fine dissecting forceps. Each fibre was placed in Aquamount under a cover-slip and viewed at high power in order to resolve individual end-plates and to ensure that only a single fibre had been isolated.

Nerve terminals and their preterminal axons were stained using the zinc iodide–osmium technique (Akert & Sandri 1968). Muscles were incubated 16–18 hr in the staining solution and washed in H_2O for at least 2 hr. Frozen sections of 30 μm thickness were cut parallel to the length of the muscle and mounted in Aquamount. The staining of nerve terminals was more consistent in the diaphragm than in the soleus muscle, presumably because the diaphragm is a much thinner sheet of muscle.

Surgical procedures. Operations were carried out under ether anaesthesia, usually on the first or second day after birth. The soleus muscle was denervated by crushing the nerve next to its entry into the muscle and cross-innervated by placing the superficial branch of the fibular nerve on to the proximal surface of the muscles. The effectiveness of the nerve crush in completely interrupting the original nerve supply was demonstrated by showing that at early stages (up to a week after the operation) most muscle fibres were still denervated, and that those which were innervated had end-plate potentials with abnormally long latencies owing to the slower conduction velocity of regenerated axons. Furthermore, cross-innervation, which did not occur when the original nerve was left intact, took place just as effectively after a nerve crush as after a cut. Nerve crushes were preferred for most experiments because re-innervation took place more quickly and reliably than after a nerve cut.

In one series of experiments the soleus muscle was partially denervated between day 3 and day 7 after birth by cutting ventral root L5, which contains all but a few of the motor axons supplying the muscle. The root was cut either within or just outside the spinal column. Most animals survived the operation but since it was not possible to recognize the nerve roots individually during the operation L5 was successfully cut and L4 left undamaged in only nine animals out of more than fifty upon which we operated.

RESULTS

Normal neonatal muscle

The compound end-plate potential

In muscles taken from animals less than 10 days old virtually all muscle fibres receive synaptic inputs from several motor axons. Text-fig. 1 shows, for example, an intracellular recording from a fibre in a

5-day-old soleus muscle paralysed with curare. By grading the strength of the stimulus to the nerve it was possible to demonstrate three distinct components of the e.p.p. The nerve was stimulated twice in each of the six superimposed traces in the Text-figure. The first stimulus was varied in strength, progressively recruiting one, two and then three discrete inputs; the second stimulus was kept supramaximal to indicate the degree of variability in maximal e.p.p. amplitude from one trial to the next. The

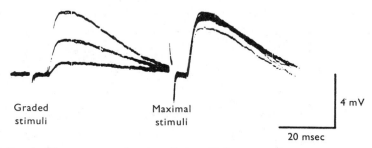

Text-fig. 1. The compound e.p.p. Intracellular recording (a.c.) from a soleus muscle fibre of a 5-day-old rat. The soleus nerve was stimulated twice during each of six superimposed sweeps. The first shock was graded in strength, while the second was kept supramaximal. Each of the three different e.p.p. components was recruited at sharply defined threshold levels. The muscle was paralysed with D-tubucurarine, 1 μg/ml.

different components of the e.p.p. invariably had very similar rise times which were as short as 2 msec when the recording electrode was situated focally. Often all of the components had a similar amplitude, as in Text-fig. 1, but occasionally their sizes differed by as much as a factor of ten. These observations are in basic agreement with those of Redfern (1970) and of Bennett & Pettigrew (1974a), except that Bennett & Pettigrew occasionally saw e.p.p. components having different time courses in muscles examined before the end of gestation.

Absence of electrical coupling between muscle fibres

One simple explanation for the presence of several components in the e.p.p. is that immature muscle fibres might be electrically coupled to one another, a phenomenon which has been demonstrated in regenerating salamander muscle (Dennis, 1975) and in developing amphibian muscle (Blackshaw & Warner, 1976). In the rat the coupling would have to be strong in order to account for the equality in rise times and similarity in amplitudes of the different components of the e.p.p. We were not, however, able to detect any signs of coupling between immature muscle fibres in extensive surveys of several muscles examined in the first 2 weeks after birth. When two adjacent muscle fibres were impaled with separate micro-electrodes, current injected into one fibre never caused a measurable potential change in the neighbouring fibre, even when the stimulus was sufficient to set up an action potential in the first fibre. This result rules out any widespread electrical coupling in the immature soleus muscle, but a more restricted alternative, that of coupling within small groups of muscle fibres, remained a possibility if one supposed that most of the fibres within a group were too small to be clearly resolved in the dissecting microscope. We therefore carried out other experiments to elucidate the pattern of innervation of neonatal muscle fibres.

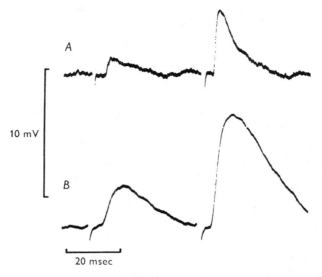

Text-fig. 2. The effect of prostigmine on the compound e.p.p. *A*, rapidly rising and decaying e.p.p.s (single component on left, double on right) in the absence of prostigmine in a 10-day muscle paralysed with curare, 1 µg/ml. *B*, slowly rising and decaying e.p.p. components recorded from the same fibre several minutes after applying prostigmine, 2×10^{-6} g/ml.

Multiple innervation of single end-plate sites

Staining of a neonatal soleus muscle for cholinesterase reveals that the end-plates are distributed along a narrow band that lies roughly midway along the length of the muscle, just as is found in adult muscles. In whole mounts and in sectioned material, it is difficult to tell whether adjacent spots of cholinesterase are on the same or on neighbouring fibres. Lubinska & Zelená (1966) found, however, only a single spot of cholinesterase on single muscle fibres teased from the new-born rat diaphragm. We have confirmed this point for the immature soleus muscle (Pl. 1 *B*).

We tested for the possibility that some synapses might lack end-plate cholinesterase altogether by examining the effects of prostigmine on the time course of e.p.p.s in partially curarized muscles. In the experiment illustrated in Text-fig. 2 the application of prostigmine (2 μg/ml.) to the bathing solution more than doubled the rise times and amplitudes of both the low-threshold e.p.p. component elicited by the first stimulus and the maximal e.p.p. evoked by the second stimulus. Prostigmine had a similar effect on all components of the e.p.p. in every muscle fibre tested, indicating that there is cholinesterase associated with all of the synapses present in immature muscles. Since only one spot on each fibre stains for cholinesterase, it is likely that all its terminals are situated at this one end-plate.

Further evidence for convergent innervation from several motor axons came from examining muscles whose nerve terminals had been stained using the zinc iodide–osmium technique. In well-stained sections from immature muscles (both the soleus and the diaphragm) it was usually possible to see two or more axons leading into each end-plate (Pl. 1*A*, arrows). In older muscles examined 20 or more days after birth, when physiological signs of multiple innervation have virtually disappeared, there was only one axon supplying each end-plate. These observations, which are in agreement with those made by Bennett & Pettigrew (1974*a*) on silver-stained muscles, provide strong support for the idea that each end-plate initially receives an input from several motor axons. Strictly speaking, though, the anatomical evidence is not by itself conclusive because we were not able to trace the preterminal axons to each fibre far enough back towards the main nerve to be certain that they were no branches of the same parent axon.

Our final piece of evidence concerning the distribution of synapses in immature muscles comes from experiments in which localized application of ACh from a micropipette was used to set an upper limit to the separation between synapses on each fibre. The principle of the experiment was to see whether desensitization of the ACh receptors over a small region of a muscle fibre had an equal effect on all components of the e.p.p. The recording micro-electrode was first inserted into a muscle fibre near the synaptic region in a curarized muscle and multiple components of the e.p.p. were demonstrated by the paired stimulation technique described above (Text-fig. 3*A*). The ACh micropipette was then moved in small steps along the fibre until a spot was found having a moderately high sensitivity to ACh ($\geqslant 10$ mV/nC in the presence of curare, $1-2 \times 10^{-6}$ g/ml.). At this point a steady positive current of 1–5 nA through the ACh pipette invariably caused a large reduction or even a complete abolition of all components of the e.p.p. (Text-fig. 3*B*). Such a parallel reduction of all components of the e.p.p. was seen in every experiment. The ACh application also caused a steady conductance change and membrane depolarization (Text-fig. 3, lower traces), both of which would contribute indirectly to the reduction in e.p.p. amplitude. The membrane potential always remained well below the reversal potential for the e.p.p., however, even during ACh applications that completely abolished the e.p.p.; moreover, considerable reductions in e.p.p. amplitude could be obtained by ACh applications that depolarized the membrane by only a few milli-volts. It is clear, therefore, that the parallel effects of ACh application on all components of the e.p.p. must have resulted primarily from a direct desensitization of ACh receptors at the end-plate.

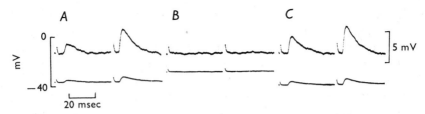

Text-fig. 3. Desensitization of end-plate receptors by ACh iontophoresis. *A*, compound e.p.p. from a 10-day-old curarized soleus muscle fibre. High gain, a.c. records above; low gain, d.c. records below. *B*, all components of the e.p.p. were abolished during steady iontophoretic application of ACh to the end-plate region. *C*, both e.p.p. components recovered completely several seconds after the cessation of ACh ionophoresis. Preparation curarized, 1 μg/ml.

Careful positioning of the ACh pipette was necessary in order to obtain this desensitizing effect. Movements of the pipette by 30–40 μm in either direction along the length of the fibre or over to adjacent fibres greatly reduced or abolished the effect. Although the spatial resolution provided by the technique as we used it was somewhat coarser than the dimensions of an end-plate or the diameter of an immature muscle fibre, it is neverthe-less sufficient to demonstrate that all of the synapses on an immature muscle fibre are situated within about 50 μm of one another.

The elimination of polyneuronal innervation

The percentage of muscle fibres receiving more than one synaptic input declined rapidly during the second week after birth. Text-fig. 4 shows the results from twenty-six muscles examined between the second and nine-teenth day after birth. At least twenty fibres from each muscle were tested for multiple inputs in the manner illustrated in Text-fig. 1. During the 5 day period from day 10 to 15 the percentage of fibres having multiple inputs dropped from 91 % (forty of forty-four) fibres to 2·5 % (one of forty fibres). The incidence of fibres having three or more components was clearly higher during the first week after birth than in the second week, but we did not examine this point systematically because the fluctuations in maximal e.p.p. amplitude (which were usually greater than that shown in Text-fig. 1) often made it difficult to determine exactly how many components were present. The elimination of multiple synaptic inputs

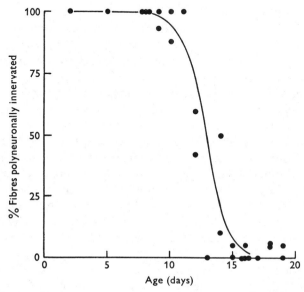

Text-fig. 4. Percentage of soleus muscle fibres innervated by more than one axon at different ages, determined from intracellular recordings in curarized muscles. At least twenty fibres were examined in each muscle. Three or more e.p.p. components were seen in many fibres, especially at early ages, suggesting that the loss of extra synapses may be well under way before day 10. Continuous line drawn by eye to fit the observations.

thus appears to be an ongoing process that starts sometime during the first week after birth and continues until the end of the second week (see also Bennet & Pettigrew, 1974a and Text-fig. 6 below). After this time we found a low level of multiple innervation remaining for a few days, but even this must eventually disappear (see Jansen & Van Essen, 1975).

During the period when multiple synaptic inputs were being eliminated there was no sign that significant numbers of muscle fibres became transiently denervated. Once the recording micro-electrode was placed in a region where focal e.p.p.s. could be recorded it was usually possible to record long sequences of twenty or more fibres all having normal e.p.p.s with one or more components. In the few cases where one or more fibres showing no response to nerve stimulation were encountered it was possible to attribute the change either to a sudden shift in the location of the end-plates or to a widespread block in neuromuscular transmission. This result suggests that if there is a period of transient denervation during the maturation of the muscle, it either involves very few fibres or else lasts for a very short time before the fibre disappears or is re-innervated.

Number and size of motor units

The removal of hyperinnervation during maturation could be associated with the complete loss of whole motor neurones, by a reduction in the number of peripheral terminations made by each motor neurone, or by some combination of the two. Degeneration of presumptive motor neurones is a well known phenomenon during early stages of development (Hughes, 1968; Landmesser & Pilar, 1974), and Bennett & Pettigrew (1974a) suggested that this might explain the elimination of synapses during the early post-natal period. The question was settled by determining the size and the total number of motor units supplying the soleus muscle at different ages. On account of the rapid growth of the muscle during maturation, motor unit size is defined operationally as the percentage of the total muscle twitch tension produced by that unit. Since fibre diameters are relatively uniform in the soleus the tension measurements should provide a reasonable indication of the percentage of muscle fibres innervated by each motor unit.

In order to count the total number of soleus motor units, the muscle was dissected free along with its nerve supply all the way back to the spinal cord and mounted in a chamber that allowed impulse activity in the soleus nerve and tension in the muscle to be recorded while small filaments of the ventral roots were stimulated electrically (see Methods). We found that the total number of motor units remained virtually constant throughout the period when polyneuronal innervation was being eliminated. This number was between twenty-one and twenty-five for the seven muscles between 3 and 42 days of age for which we obtained complete counts. There was no significant difference in the number of motor units for the three muscles examined before day 10 (mean 22·7 units) and the four muscles examined after that time (mean 23·5 units). A few motor units may have been missed in some of the preparations; in fact, our value for mature muscle is slightly lower than the estimates of others based on *in vivo* tension measurements (28–30 units; Close, 1967) or fibre counts in deafferented motor nerves (thirty-two α motor axons; Gutman & Hanzlíková, 1966). Nevertheless, it is unlikely that we missed a much greater number of units in younger than in older rats and we therefore conclude that the number of motor units to the soleus stays relatively constant after birth.

In contrast to the constancy of the number of motor units, there were dramatic changes in motor unit size shortly after birth. Text-fig. 5, for example, shows a single motor unit from an immature muscle that generated a tension greater than one fifth of the total muscle tension. Text-fig. 5*B* is a recording from the soleus nerve at a fast sweep speed to demonstrate that the stimulus activated only a single soleus motor axon. Text-fig. 5*A* shows, at a much slower sweep speed, the tension generated by the

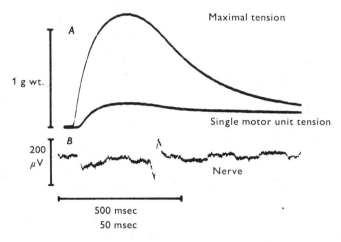

Text-fig. 5. Measurement of motor unit size in an immature muscle. *A*, shows the tension generated in the soleus muscle of a 3-day-old rat by stimulation of a single ventral root filament and, for comparison, the tension produced by maximal stimulation of the whole nerve. *B*, shows, at a fast sweep speed, the unitary action potential recorded *en passage* from the soleus nerve (see Methods) after stimulation of the ventral root filament. Note the very slow time course of the contraction, which is characteristic of immature muscle.

single motor unit and, for comparison, the total muscle tension produced by maximal stimulation of the nerve. (Direct electrical stimulation of the muscle also produced the same maximal tension.)

Our observations on motor unit tensions are summarized in Text-fig. 6, which gives the relative tension of the motor units in ten different muscles as a function of the age of the animal. The tensions are displayed as percentages of the total twitch tension evoked by direct stimulation of the muscle. Each vertical line represents the observations in one animal, and the mean values (filled circles) as well as the values for individual units (horizontal lines) are presented for each muscle. Tension measurements were included only for the lowest threshold unit in each ventral root filament because there was, as expected, non-linear summation of tension values when more than one unit was stimulated. The open circles show the average tension that would be expected if there were no multiply inner-

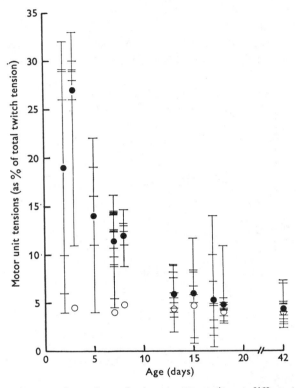

Text-fig. 6. Size and number of soleus motor units at different ages. Each vertical line represents observations on one animal. The ordinate gives the size of motor units expressed as their percentage of the maximal twitch to direct stimulation. Filled circles (●) give the mean size of motor units in each muscle; horizontal lines indicate the individual measurements for the lowest-threshold motor unit in each ventral root filament. Open circles (○) show the average motor unit size one would expect in the absence of poly-neuronal innervation [$100 \times$ (total number of units^{-1})]. In three muscles (2, 5 and 17 days) this value is not given because a partial nerve block in the region of the ventral roots prevented completion of the motor unit count.

vated fibres. This value, obtained simply by taking the inverse of the total number of motor units, was between 4 and 5 % for the seven muscles for which complete motor unit counts were available.

Text-fig. 6 shows that motor units were about five times larger at early times (mean 23 % at days 2 and 3) than at later times (mean 5·1 % at days 15–18 and 4·4 % at day 42). This reduction in motor unit size is large enough to account entirely for the disappearance of polyneuronal innervation in immature muscles. In fact, the average degree of polyneuronal innervation estimated from the motor unit measurements (obtained by taking the ratio of the filled circle to the open circle values for each muscle), is about five at days 2 and 3. An average value of five synapses per fibre is higher than either we or Bennett & Pettigrew (1974*a*) obtained by counting the number of e.p.p. components in individual fibres but the discrepancy is not surprising in view of the inherent inaccuracies in each type of estimate. A safe conclusion would be that there are many separate synaptic inputs to each neonatal muscle fibre, each one of which is capable of activating the muscle fibre by itself.

It is interesting that there was considerably more scatter in the size of motor units throughout the period of maturation than in adult muscles. The total range was about a factor of three in the one adult muscle we examined and in the larger sample of motor units obtained by Close (1967), whereas the range was about tenfold in several of the immature muscles. At all ages there were some motor units that were within the range seen in the adult.

In the 15- and 17-day-old muscles a few of the motor units were actually smaller than any seen in the adult. It is possible that the tension values were spuriously low owing to an axonal conduction block or to a failure in synaptic transmission. This explanation seems unlikely, however, because the maximal indirect and direct twitches were equal and in the same muscles there were still other motor units larger than those seen in the adult. If the tension measurements provide a reasonably accurate measure of motor unit size in terms of numbers of muscle fibres innervated, then the results suggest that at a time when almost all polyneuronal innervation has been eliminated, some readjustments in motor unit sizes remain to be completed.

Modifying the time course of synapse removal

The effects of partial denervation

If one could remove all but a few of the motor axons to the soleus muscle shortly after birth, a reduction in size of the remaining ones would have to take place at the expense of leaving some fibres completely denervated. *A priori* it seemed plausible that this might influence or even reverse the normal reduction in motor unit size. The experiment was performed by sectioning the lower of the two ventral roots supplying the soleus muscle. The remaining root (L4) usually contains at least one and sometimes as many as nine soleus motor axons. The operation was carried out successfully on nine animals. They were examined between days 15 and 43 after birth. The results were quite striking: partial denervation, on the one hand, delayed the normal reduction in motor unit size and even the elimination of polyneuronal innervation; on the other hand, it did not seem to prevent the eventual shrinkage of motor units to approximately their normal adult size.

Five muscles with five to nine remaining motor units were examined between days 15 and 17, just after the time when most polyneuronal innervation normally has been eliminated. The histogram in Text-fig. 7

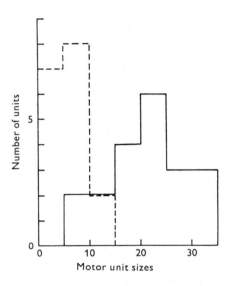

Text-fig. 7. Motor unit sizes at intermediate times after partial denervation. Continuous lines: motor unit sizes, determined from tension measurements (as in Text-fig. 6), of twenty motor units in five muscles examined 15–17 days after birth following partial denervation on day 3–5 (three on day 3, one each on days 4 and 5). In each animal there were between four and nine motor units in the remaining ventral root (L4) but tension measurements were not obtained for all of these. Dashed lines: motor unit sizes in two normal soleus muscles aged 15 and 17 days (from Text-fig. 6).

shows the tensions generated by twenty of the motor units remaining in these five muscles. The sizes of seventeen units from two normal muscles of comparable age are shown for comparison. The mean size of the motor units from the partially denervated muscles (20 %) was much larger than that of the normal muscles (5·6 %) and was, in fact, very close to the mean size of motor units at the time of the initial operation (21 %; results from days 3 and 5 in Text-fig. 6). The abnormally large motor units did not appear to result simply from hypertrophy of innervated muscle fibres or to atrophy of the denervated ones. The muscles were not noticeably atrophic and they generated a normal tension to nerve stimulation. In addition, cross-sections of two of the muscles showed that they contained close to the normal number of muscle fibres (2500–2900) having relatively uniform diameters. Thus, it appears that the motor units remaining after partial denervation innervated a much larger number of muscle fibres than they normally would have at this age.

There were two other obvious abnormalities in the partially denervated muscles examined between days 15 and 17. The first was that the twitch contractions to stimulation of single motor units fatigued very rapidly, even during stimulation at frequencies as low as 0·5–1 Hz. After a few stimuli the twitch tension was often less than half of its initial value, after which it remained stable. In normal muscles there was little tension decrement even during stimulation at rates of 2–3 Hz. The rapid fatigue in the partially denervated muscles was not related to an impairment in the contractile properties of the muscle as there was no fatigue during direct muscle stimulation. A likely explanation for the fatigue is that transmission at many synapses was only marginally above threshold and was readily brought below threshold by repetitive stimulation.

The other abnormality in this group of partially denervated muscles was that there was extensive polyneuronal innervation remaining 2 weeks after the operation. We recorded e.p.p.s. having more than one component in about half of the innervated fibres in each muscle (range 22–65 % in five muscles). This was not a general 'systemic' consequence of the operation, because in every experiment we found that polyneuronal innervation in the control soleus muscle from the opposite leg had been reduced to its normal level of 5 % or less.

The situation was quite different in muscles examined at later times after partial denervation. The clearest illustration of this came from a muscle partially denervated four days after birth and examined on day 33. There were only two motor axons supplying the soleus muscle through the intact ventral root and the muscle itself had atrophied considerably. A cross-section of the muscle, shown in Pl. 2*B*, revealed that a minority of the muscle fibres, 321 in all, had escaped atrophy and were actually larger than normal. The other fibres were very small and difficult to resolve individually. For comparison, Pl. 2*A* shows the relative uniformity of fibre diameters in a normal muscle of similar age. We found no multiply innervated fibres during a micro-electrode survey of the partially denervated muscle after it was curarized. Hence, a reasonable estimate of motor unit sizes can be obtained by assuming that the very small fibres in the muscle were all denervated and then simply dividing up the number of larger fibres in accordance with the relative sizes of the motor unit tensions. The two motor units in this muscle contributed 40 and 60 % to the total muscle tension, suggesting that they innervated approximately 130 and 190 muscle fibres, respectively. These values are about 4 and 6 % of the total of approximately 3000 fibres found in normal muscles (Chiakulas & Pauly, 1965; Frank, Jansen, Lømo & Westgaard, 1975). A similar estimate was obtained indirectly by comparing the absolute values of the motor unit tensions obtained from normal muscles of comparable age. The total twitch tension from the partially denervated muscle was about 15 % of that from normal muscles of a similar age (1·2 g wt. *vs.* 6·9–10 g wt. for five normal 4–6-week-old muscles), and the individual motor unit tensions were roughly 6 and 9 % of the normal total. Thus, even without a correction for the effects of the obvious hypertrophy of innervated muscle fibres, the tension measurements support the suggestion that the number of muscle fibres innervated by each motor unit was closer to the mean value in normal adult muscle, than to the mean value at the time of the initial operation or after 2 weeks of partial denervation. Owing to the large scatter in individual motor unit sizes in immature muscles, however, it is not possible to conclude that these particular motor units had actually decreased in size, as opposed to starting out small and not expanding.

Similar results were obtained for two of the three other muscles examined 4–6 weeks after partial denervation. One of these, partially denervated on day 7 and examined on day 43, had two remaining motor units and 408 large fibres visible in a cross-section of the muscle. The individual motor unit tensions were approximately equal in amplitude (Text-fig. 8A: upper record, one motor unit; lower record, both motor units) but they were several times larger in absolute value than those in a normal muscle of the same age, owing in part to the hypertrophy of the innervated fibres. The total tension produced by stimulating the nerve close to the muscle (Text-fig. 8B) was no larger than that from combined stimulation of the two motor units, indicating that there were no other large motor units in the nerve. Moreover, the tension from direct muscle stimulation was the same as the nerve-evoked tension, suggesting that non-innervated fibres (presumably all the atrophied ones) contributed little to the total muscle tension. A low level of multiple innervation was found in this muscle (four of twenty fibres tested). Accordingly, the estimated size of each motor unit, based on the muscle fibre counts and allowing for 20 % of the large fibres being doubly innervated, was about 245 fibres, or 8 % of the normal total. In another muscle, partially denervated on day 7 and examined on day 41, only one surviving motor unit was counted (plus a few very small motor units that had regenerated through the cut nerve); we estimated that it innervated 280 muscle fibres, or 9 % of the normal total.

Finally, one muscle having six surviving motor axons was examined at a slightly earlier time (31 days *vs.* 33, 41 and 43 days); it had not under-gone changes as extensive as in the other muscles. A cross-section of the muscle appeared normal, with no hypertrophied fibres and no obvious population of small, presumably denervated fibres. The motor unit tensions were all between 12 % and 16 % of the total for the five units for

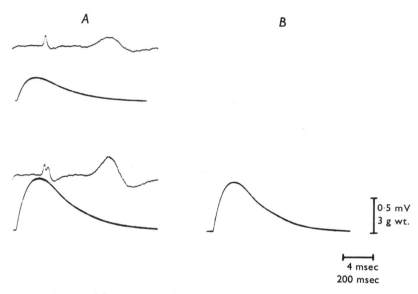

Text-fig. 8. Two remaining motor units in a 43-day-old soleus muscle partially denervated by extraspinal section of L5 on day 7. *A*, records of nerve impulses (upper traces, fast sweep speed) and twitch tensions (lower traces, slow sweep speed) after stimulation of the intact ventral root. Low intensity stimuli activated a single soleus motor axon (upper records); maximal stimuli activated only two motor axons (lower records). The slow wave in the right half of the nerve records is an artifactual pick-up of the gross muscle action potential. *B*, the maximal twitch to stimulation of the whole soleus nerve near the muscle. Note that the tension is no larger than that from activating just the two motor units in *A*. The maximal twitch to direct stimulation was the same as the maximal nerve-evoked twitch. There were 408 large fibres counted in a cross-section of this muscle.

which individual measurements were obtained. The larger size of the motor units in this muscle, compared to those seen in the three preceding examples, might have been a chance occurrence, or it might be related to the younger age of the muscle or to the fact that it happened to have a larger number of surviving motor units.

These results are summarized in Text-fig. 9, which compares the motor unit sizes for the four muscles partially denervated for 4–6 weeks (continuous lines) with those seen around the time of the initial operation (days 3, 5 and 7, dashed lines). The mean size of motor units was considerably lower in the partially denervated muscles (10·6 *vs.* 15·9 %), especially if one considers only the three muscles with an obvious mixture of hypertrophied and atrophied fibres (hatched area, mean 7 %), excluding the remaining muscle (dotted area) on the grounds that its histological uniformity suggests that it might still have been in a transitional state.

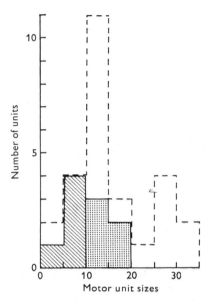

Text-fig. 9. Histogram of unit sizes at late times after partial denervation. Hatched area: motor unit sizes for five units in three soleus muscles examined at 33, 41 and 43 days after birth following partial denervation at 4, 7 and 7 days, respectively. The estimates were based on counts of large, non-atrophied muscle fibres seen in histological cross-sections, expressed as a percentage of the normal value of 3000 fibres. Dotted area: motor unit sizes, based on tension measurements for five units in a muscle partially denervated on day 4 and examined on day 31. Dashes lines: histogram of motor unit sizes for twenty-six motor units in three normal muscles aged 3, 5, and 7 days (from Text-fig. 6).

In any event, whether or not the one muscle is excluded from the sample, the results are consistent with a genuine shrinkage of motor units during maturation after partial denervation. They are not conclusive, however, owing to the relatively large scatter in motor unit sizes and to the uncertainties that result from comparisons involving two different methods for measuring motor unit sizes (tension measurements and muscle fibre counts). We conclude that, at the very least, there is no widespread sprouting of axon collaterals to take over large numbers of denervated fibres after partial denervation in immature rats. To the contrary, it is probable that some motor units are not able to maintain their original complement of peripheral synapses even though some muscle fibres consequently are stripped of their remaining inputs.

Re-innervation and cross-innervation of immature muscle

By examining the events that occur during re-innervation of the immature soleus muscle by its original nerve and cross-innervation by a foreign nerve it has been possible to study several questions that would be difficult or impossible to investigate in a normal muscle. For example, we were interested in whether newly formed terminals can take part in the process of synapse elimination, whether interactions between synapses situated at a distance from one another can lead to the elimination of one of them and whether there is any selectivity in the choice of which synapses are to survive and which are to be removed.

Re-innervation by the original nerve

Re-innervation of the immature soleus muscle occurred relatively quickly and completely following a crush of the nerve just at its entry into the muscle. Substantial contractions to nerve stimulation were seen within a week following denervation on the first or second day after birth. By days 11–12 more than half of the muscle had been re-innervated, as assessed by micro-electrode surveys of superficial muscle fibres and by comparing nerve-evoked and direct muscle tensions (three experiments). Three weeks after birth re-innervation was nearly complete (80–100 % in two experiments); muscle cross-sections taken at this time showed a normal number of muscle fibres having relatively uniform diameters, indicating that there had not been a loss or severe atrophy of large numbers of fibres.

During the first two weeks of re-innervation many muscle fibres were innervated by more than one motor axon. In some muscles as many as 80–90 % of the re-innervated fibres had e.p.p.s with more than one component. Text-fig. 10 shows the time course of elimination of polyneuronal innervation in the re-innervated muscles. Most of the synapses that were eliminated during days 10–15 were presumably formed during the preceding week when re-innervation was taking place most rapidly and were therefore much younger than synapses in normal muscles, which are formed in the final week of gestation (Bennett & Pettigrew 1974a). It is remarkable how closely the decline in multiple innervation followed that seen in normal muscles (dashed line, taken from Text-fig. 4). The elimination process seemed to run its normal course even though the synapses it acted upon were about half their normal age.

In the great majority of fibres examined in the re-innervated muscles all components of the e.p.p. had similar rapid time courses, just as in normal immature muscles. This indicated that they were all associated with end-plate cholinesterase, and that they were relatively close to one another. Occasional e.p.p.s. had components of clearly different rise times, suggesting that they might be spatially separated. In order to examine the spatial

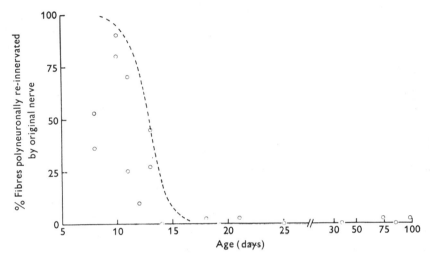

Text-fig. 10. Incidence of multiple innervation during re-innervation by the soleus nerve. Each point shows the percentage of re-innervated fibres in which more than one e.p.p. component was detected. At least twenty fibres were sampled in each muscle. The soleus nerve was crushed next to its entry into the muscle on the first or second day after birth. Some muscles had also been cross-innervated through the fibular nerve but these measurements were made in parts of the muscle well away from the zone of foreign innervation. Note that very occasional multiple inputs were seen even at long times after birth. The interrupted line shows the time course of elimination of multiple inputs in normal muscles (from Text-fig. 4).

distribution of synapses more, closely we looked at the disposition of cholinesterase in single muscle fibres isolated from the re-innervated muscles. All of the end-plates were situated in the vicinity of the original end-plate band, presumably because the regenerating axons were guided there along the old nerve branches. Most fibres had only a single end-plate, even in muscles where the majority of fibres were multiply innervated. For example, in one 10-day-old re-innervated muscle, eighteen of twenty fibres tested physiologically were multiply innervated, whereas only eight out of twenty-one fibres isolated from the same region of the muscle had more than one end-plate. Thus, it is likely that some of the regenerating axons converged on to the same end-plate site, just as in normal immature muscle. This site is probably the original end-plate present before denervation but this is not certain in view of the lability of end-plate cholinesterase in immature fibres (see below). The presence of some multiple cholinesterase spots (twenty-five double sites and two triple sites in ninety-two fibres from six muscles aged 10 to 21 days) suggests that not all axons returned exactly to the old end-plates and that some fibres might have been innervated at more than one location. It was difficult, however, to estimate the frequency of occurrence of distributed end-plates because of the problem in knowing whether the old end-plate had been re-innervated, whether it was present but still denervated, or whether it had been eliminated. A better understanding of the spatial distribution of newly-formed synapses came from examining muscles that had been cross-innervated by a foreign nerve in a region well outside the original end-plate zone.

Cross-innervation by a foreign nerve

Cross-innervation of the immature soleus muscle took place only after disruption of the original nerve supply, just as in adult muscle (Elsberg 1917; Jansen, Lømo, Nicolaysen & Westgaard, 1973). In three new-born rats the superficial branch of the fibular nerve was transplanted on to the soleus muscle without interrupting the original nerve. At the time of the final experiment, nineteen days after birth, there were no contractions to stimulation of the foreign nerve in any of the muscles, even though the nerve had grown extensively over the surface of the muscle; nor were any sub-threshold e.p.p.s detected in the one muscle where a micro-electrode survey was made. In contrast, innervation by the foreign nerve took place readily when the soleus nerve was cut or crushed. As in the adult (Frank *et al.* 1975) the foreign nerve never took over more than about a third of the muscle, even when re-innervation was delayed by cutting or re-secting the original nerve.

Two types of polyneuronal innervation involving the foreign nerve were seen. Some fibres received separate inputs from the foreign and original nerves, while other fibres received more than one input through the foreign nerve alone. These two forms of polyneuronal innervation will be considered separately, since our methods for testing for them differed slightly and, more importantly, because there was a striking difference in the persistence of the two types of multiple innervation during maturation.

The interaction between foreign and original nerves

The extent of innervation by each nerve was assayed by recording action potentials and e.p.p.s. intracellularly from a series of superficial muscle fibres, noting whether each fibre was innervated by one, both or neither nerve. Twenty-one muscles were examined at times ranging from 8 to 99 days after soleus nerve crush and fibular nerve implant. The usual result from this survey was that the foreign nerve tended to innervate only the

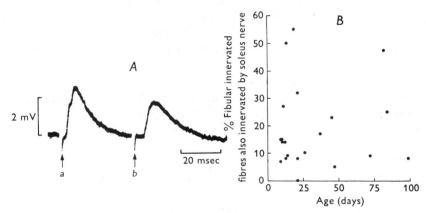

Text-fig. 11. Dual innervation of individual soleus muscle fibres by both original and transplanted foreign (fibular) nerve. *A*, intracellular record of end-plate potentials to both soleus nerve stimulation (*a*) and fibular nerve stimulation (*b*) from a 9-day-old animal in which the superficial fibular nerve was transplanted and the soleus nerve crushed 8 days before. *B*, percentage of cross-innervated fibres that were also re-innervated by the original nerve in muscles of different ages. The initial operation was performed at days 1 or 2 in all animals. Each point represents the observations in one soleus muscle in which at least twenty cross-innervated muscle fibres were examined.

lateral one third to one half of the muscle, and in this region very few fibres had in addition been re-innervated by the original nerve. Fibres in the medial half of the muscle were innervated only by the soleus nerve. In the border region between the two territories many fibres received an input from both nerves. Text-fig. 11*A* shows an example of a fibre with a dual input from the two nerves, taken from a 9-day-old muscle. Stimulation of the soleus nerve evoked an e.p.p. having two components with slightly different latencies and stimulation of the fibular nerve evoked an e.p.p. of similar amplitude.

As an index of the frequency of dual innervation by the two nerves we determined what percentage of muscle fibres innervated by the foreign nerve had in addition an input from the original nerve. Text-fig. 11 *B* shows the results for twenty-one muscles in which ten to fifty fibres with foreign innervation were examined in each muscle. The percentage of dually innervated fibres varied over a wide range but it did not appear to change significantly with time. The average percentage for muscles under 25 days of age (19·5 %) is not significantly different from that for older muscles (18 %), nor was there a significant difference if any other age was chosen as the dividing point. The particular values obtained for the percentage of dually innervated fibres in each muscle may not be very accurate owing to the sampling problems that arose because these fibres tended to lie in a narrow strip between the foreign and original nerve territories. Nevertheless, the results demonstrate that substantial numbers of fibres with both foreign and original nerve synapses can be found at all ages, and that there is no dramatic reduction in their incidence as a function of time.

It is surprising that the majority of fibres innervated by the foreign nerve never became re-innervated through the original nerve. The failure to re-innervate cross-innervated muscle fibres in the immature animals was not due simply to a lowered over-all capacity for regeneration by the soleus nerve, because in the absence of the foreign nerve the soleus nerve was capable of completely re-innervating its muscle, as mentioned above. It thus seems that the presence of foreign innervation can inhibit re-innervation of old end-plates in immature rats.

The separation between foreign and original synapses on dually-innervated fibres was determined by staining the muscle for end-plate cholinesterase. In all but one experiment the region of foreign end-plates was in the proximal part of the muscle, well away from the original end-plate band, just as is seen in adult soleus muscles after cross-innervation (Frank *et al.* 1976). The minimal separation between the original end-plate band and the closest foreign end-plates was at least 1 mm and usually more. In the one exceptional case the foreign nerve had grown directly into the original end-plate region and made synapses there. It is perhaps significant that this was the one muscle in which we did not find any fibres receiving an input from both foreign and original nerves.

There was usually a sharp transition in the appearance of the original end-plate band just at the border between foreign and original nerve territories. The band was continuous and of normal appearance in the re-innervated zone while it was much less dense and consisted of scattered isolated end-plates in that part of the muscle which was cross-innervated by the foreign nerve. Examination of single, isolated fibres confirmed that the original end-plate cholinesterase had often completely disappeared from cross-innervated fibres. On those fibres which had both foreign and original end-plates the distance between them was, as expected, always 1 mm or more.

The disappearance of the cholinesterase at the original end-plates was not simply a consequence of the end-plate itself not being re-innervated. Following simple denervation of neonatal muscles cholinesterase remains at the original end-plate for at least a month (Lubinska & Zelená 1966). In contrast, we found that the cholinesterase at denervated end-plates on fibres innervated elsewhere by a foreign nerve disappeared entirely within about a week. A clear illustration of this came from a 13-day-old muscle in which the fibular nerve had been implanted on the first day after birth and the soleus nerve cut far enough from the muscle to prevent re-innervation by the time of the final experiment. In the region of the muscle innervated by the foreign nerve only scattered end-plates were visible in the original end-plate band, whereas outside the region of cross-innervation the old denervated end-plates appeared in the whole mount as a continuous dense band of cholinesterase. Isolation of individual fibres teased from the cross-innervated region of the muscle demonstrated that seven out of eight fibres having foreign nerve end-plates had completely lost their original end-plates; the one fibre having both foreign and original end-plates presumably had been cross-innervated for a shorter time than the others. We did not investigate in detail the time required for foreign innervation to suppress cholinesterase at the original end-plate but it is clear that the process cannot take much more than a week. The lability of end-plate cholinesterase indicated by this experiment might be related to the inability of regenerating soleus nerve axons to re-innervate most cross-innervated muscle fibres.

Polyneuronal innervation through the foreign nerve

At early times after cross-innervation, graded stimulation of the fibular nerve showed that many muscle fibres were innervated by more than one foreign motor axon. Two lines of evidence indicate that many of the foreign synapses on multiply innervated fibres were situated at an appreciable distance from one another. First, the different components of the e.p.p. often had clearly different time courses. For example, in the fibre illustrated in Text-fig. 12A a low intensity stimulus (left) to the fibular nerve elicited an e.p.p. with a rise time of about 12 msec, while a stronger stimulus (right) evoked an additional component whose rise time was 5 msec. A likely explanation for the difference in time course is that the two synapses were located at different distances from the recording micro-electrode.

More direct evidence for spatially separated end-plates came from examining the distribution of cholinesterase on individual fibres isolated from the region of foreign innervation. Many fibres had two distinct end-plates separated by distances of up to 1 mm; an example of a fibre having two end-plates about 150 μm apart is shown in Pl. 2C (arrows). A few fibres had three separate end-plates in the region of the fibular nerve, and on one fibre five closely spaced but distinct end-plates were found. Multiple fibular end-plates were seen in more than a quarter of the fibres isolated from four cross-innervated muscles between 10 and 13 days old (thirty out of 107 fibres). In the same four muscles the incidence of polyneuronal innervation estimated physiologically was about one fibre in three (twenty-eight of seventy-nine fibres). This suggests that most but perhaps not all polyneuronal innervation mediated by the foreign nerve occurs at spatially separate synapses.

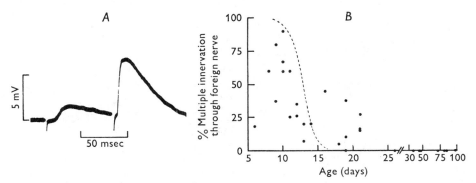

Text-fig. 12. Polyneuronal innervation by a foreign nerve. A, multiple e.p.p. components evoked by fibular nerve stimulation in a 19-day-old soleus muscle cross-innervated on day 2. Low intensity stimuli (left) produced a small e.p.p. with rise time about twice as long as that of the higher threshold component (right). B, percentage of foreign innervated fibres in which more than one e.p.p. component was detected during graded stimulation of the foreign nerve. Each point gives the results for one muscle in which at least ten and usually twenty or more cross-innervated fibres were examined. The interrupted line shows the time course of synapse elimination in normal muscles (from Text-fig. 4).

All physiological signs of polyneuronal innervation through the foreign nerve eventually disappeared in the cross-innervated muscles. Text-fig. 12B shows the time course of elimination of multiple innervation as determined physiologically with intracellular recordings. Each point represents the observations in one muscle and gives the percentage of fibres with more than one input from the fibular nerve. The incidence of polyneuronal innervation was quite high up to about the tenth day after birth, with 80 % or more multiple innervation in some muscles. The disappearance of multiple innervation initially was similar to that seen in normal muscles (dashed line) but a substantial percentage of the multiple inputs persisted for about a week longer than normal. The delay in removal of extra inputs was not due simply to the initial surgical interference with the muscle because there was no significant prolongation of the synaptic elimination process during re-innervation by the original nerve (Text-fig. 10). No physiological signs of multiple innervation through the foreign nerve remained in muscles examined 25 days or more after birth (135 fibres in eight muscles). Thus the process that leads to the elimination of convergent inputs in normal muscles evidently is able to act in muscle fibres where the synapses are spatially distributed.

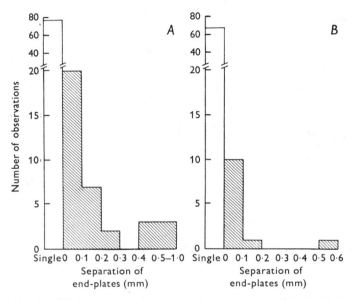

Text-fig. 13. Histograms of the separation between multiple foreign end-plates in cross-innervated soleus muscles. Open column shows the number of fibres having only a single end-plate in the region of foreign innervation. Hatched columns indicate the separation between multiple foreign end-plates. *A*, there were thirty fibres (out of 108) in the four young muscles (10–13 days) having more than one foreign end-plate; two of these had three and five end-plates, respectively, which were included in the histogram according to the distance to their nearest neighbour. *B*, none of the fibres from the three older muscles (77–99 days) had more than two foreign end-plates.

In order to see whether there was an elimination of multiple end-plates corresponding to the disappearance of polyneuronal synaptic inputs we isolated single muscle fibres from the region of foreign innervation in several muscles that had been cross-innervated for long periods (11–14 weeks) and compared the results with those obtained from younger muscles (10–13 days). It was surprising to find that despite a clear reduction in the incidence of spatially separated end-plates compared with that seen in younger muscles, there was still a substantial number of fibres that retained more than one foreign end-plate. Text-fig. 13 shows histograms of the distance between multiple foreign end-plates in young muscles (*A*) and in older muscles (*B*). Almost all of the double end-plates that persisted in the older muscles were within 100 μm of one another (e.g. Pl. 2*D*), whereas many of the end-plates in the younger muscles were separated by distances up to 1 mm. The reduction in the incidence of end-plates separated by more than 100 μm provides evidence that the process of synapse elimination can work on synapses that were sufficiently mature to have induced the incorporation of cholinesterase at a new end-plate.

DISCUSSION

The location of synapses on immature muscle fibres

The argument that each immature muscle fibre receives a direct and convergent input from more than one motor neurone depends upon several lines of evidence, none of which is by itself conclusive. Our electrophysiological experiments show that all of the synaptic inputs to any particular fibre are at most about 50 μm apart (from the desensitizing effects of iontophoretically applied ACh), and that all of the synapses must be associated with end-plate cholinesterase (from the effects of prostigmine on e.p.p. time course). Since there is only one cholinesterase spot per immature muscle fibre, it follows that either the multiple inputs all converge on to a single end-plate, or that there is strong electrical coupling between neighbouring fibres whose end-plates are immediately adjacent to one another. We found no sign of widespread electrical coupling between immature muscle fibres, although the possibility was not excluded that there might be coupling within small groups of fibres linked closely enough to appear as a single fibre in the dissecting microscope. On the other hand, each end-plate in an immature muscle is supplied by several preterminal axons and all but one of these disappear during maturation. Although we could not show directly that each preterminal branch belonged to a different motor axon, it seems very likely that the multiple preterminal axons are the anatomical basis for the presence of several e.p.p. components in each immature muscle fibre. Finally, it is clear that the multiple synaptic inputs demonstrated by graded stimulation of the nerve do not come about because of a division of each motor axon into several separate branches that subsequently converge on to the same set of muscle fibres. This is because the tensions produced by stimulating individual motor units in ventral root filaments are so large that there must inevitably be a large overlap in the innervation of different motor units. We therefore conclude, in agreement with Redfern (1970) and Bennett & Pettigrew (1974a) that there is genuine polyneuronal innervation in immature skeletal muscles of the rat. In muscles that are only a few days old all muscle fibres receive at least two inputs and estimates of the average degree of multiple innervation range from about three (Bennett & Pettigrew, 1974a) to about five (Text-fig. 6, above). It is remarkable that all of the inputs are crowded into an area that is smaller than an end-plate on an adult muscle fibre, yet each synapse is able to excite the muscle fibre on its own. Presumably the efficiency of transmission is related in part to the higher input resistance of smaller muscle fibres.

Polyneuronal innervation has also been seen in the soleus muscle of kittens (Bagust *et al.* 1973), suggesting that it may be a widespread or even universal event in the maturation of mammalian skeletal muscle. The extent of hyperinnervation which exists in new-born animals will, however, presumably vary according to the degree of maturity at birth. It will be interesting to know whether in a particular species the loss of polyneuronal innervation occurs synchronously in all muscles, as is the case for the soleus and diaphragm muscles of the rat.

The elimination of synapses during normal maturation

During the period when polyneuronal innervation disappears the number of motor axons to the soleus muscle remains constant, while the average size of motor units decreases severalfold. The elimination of multiple innervation and the reduction in motor unit size conceivably might come about by muscle fibres dividing in such a way as to leave only one synapse on each fibre. Chiakulas & Pauly (1965) have shown that there may be an increase of about 50 % in the number of soleus muscle fibres after the first post-natal week. They suggest that the new fibres originate from myoblasts rather than from division of pre-existing fibres but even if some division took place it would be quantitatively insufficient to account fully for the loss of multiple innervation. Hence, it is evident that many terminals must eventually disappear by undergoing either degeneration or retraction. H. Korneliussen (personal communication) found no obvious signs of terminal degeneration in electron micrographs of synapses from immature muscles, suggesting that simple retraction of extra synapses is the more likely alternative. It would be interesting to know whether e.p.p. components that are particularly small relative to other components on the same fibre, or which have a particularly long latency following nerve stimulation (e.g. Fig. 2 in Redfern, 1970) might be in the process of being eliminated but it is difficult to see how to test these possibilities directly. There are numerous other changes in muscle and motor nerve properties that take place during the time that neuromuscular connexions are maturing. In addition to growing in length and cross-sectional area the muscle develops fast, or slow contractile properties, or both (Close, 1964), and the nerve becomes myelinated and gains in conduction velocity. It is not yet known whether the removal of multiple innervation is specifically dependent on any of these changes.

The total spread of motor unit sizes within a given muscle was considerably greater in young animals than in the adult, with a few motor units being within the adult range at all ages we examined. This suggests that the shrinkage of motor units does not come about simply by the synchronous loss by each motor neurone of a fixed percentage of its peripheral terminals. Either there must be considerable variability in the times at which different motor units reach their peak size, or else some motor units never become much larger than their eventual adult size. In either case, it appears that at any given time the elimination process acts predominantly on the terminals of the largest motor units. This could come about if the terminals of small motor units somehow had a selective advantage over the terminals of larger ones. One can imagine, for example, that as a motor neurone gradually lost some of its synapses it might be able to supply its remaining terminals with some material or quality that improved their chances for survival.

Synapse elimination following partial denervation

The removal of all but a few motor axons to the soleus muscle leaves the remaining neurones with the opportunity to innervate large numbers of muscle fibres while facing only minimal competition at the level of peripheral synaptic interactions. One might expect to find that whatever residual polyneuronal innervation was present would be removed normally, while the remaining motor units would either remain constant in size or even expand by sprouting on to neighbouring denervated fibres. It thus came as a surprise to find that partial denervation resulted, on the one hand, in a delay in the removal of polyneuronal innervation among surviving motor units and that, on the other hand, a reduction in motor unit size nevertheless eventually took place.

It is puzzling that multiple innervation should persist on some muscle fibres just because most of the motor input to the muscle has been removed. The delay might be an indirect effect of the surgical interference within the spinal cord but this seems unlikely because multiple innervation disappeared with its normal time course in the control soleus muscle on the opposite side. A more interesting possibility is that the delay might be related to the large size of the remaining motor units: for example, if the

14-2

maturation of synaptic terminals proceeded more slowly in larger motor units and if the process of synapse elimination on each fibre did not begin until the favoured terminal reached a certain absolute, rather than relative maturity, then one would expect partial denervation to delay the removal of multiple innervation.

The eventual reduction in motor unit size that took place after partial denervation was usually associated with gross hypertrophy of the remaining innervated fibres and atrophy, or at least failure to grow, of the denervated fibres. Many motor units were closer to their normal adult level than to their mean initial size; this happened too frequently to be accounted for by a chance selection of small motor units at the time of the initial operation. Moreover, it is difficult to account for the shrinkage simply in terms of the elimination of residual multiple innervation, since small motor units were seen in muscles having only one or two motor units left. Hence it seems likely that the withdrawal of synapses can continue even though many previously innervated fibres actually become denervated.

It is not surprising that there should be a natural limit to how many muscle fibres a motor neurone can innervate. What is interesting, though, is that there should be an actual reduction in the upper limit of motor unit size during maturation. This might come about if the total synaptic area that a motor neurone could supply grew more slowly than the mean area of individual end-plates. Presumably the natural tendency of each motor unit to reduce its initial size plays a major role in the elimination of hyperinnervation. It cannot be the sole mechanism involved, however, because there must be some way of insuring that each muscle fibre ends up with one and only one synapse.

There is no inconsistency between the occurrence of axonal sprouting after partial denervation of adult muscles (Edds, 1953; Guth, 1962) and our failure to detect sprouting of immature motor units. The lack of sprouting in immature muscles is presumably related to the large initial size of motor units. The existence of an upper limit to motor neurone size is entirely compatible with a moderate degree of sprouting in the adult. Our results suggest that the limiting size of mature motor units might be substantially larger (i.e. a factor of two or so) than their normal adult size.

The relative uniformity in adult motor unit sizes seen in the soleus muscle is not found in other muscles such as the fast-twitch extensor digitorum longus, where there is about a tenfold range in size (Close, 1967). It would be interesting to know whether this greater variability is related to larger inherent differences among fast motor neurones.

The elimination of synapses after re-innervation and cross-innervation

Multiple innervation through regenerated axons of the original nerve disappeared with a time course similar to that seen in normal muscles. This shows that the process of synapse elimination is not heavily influenced by either the age of the terminals involved or the period of muscle inactivity before re-innervation took place. The lack of an effect is remarkable in view of the delay in the removal of hyperinnervation following several other procedures that might seem to be less disruptive to the synapses involved. For example, partial denervation leads to a prolonged innervation overlap among motor units that were not directly affected by the operation. In addition Benoit & Changeux (1975) have shown that tenotomy causes a delay in the removal of polyneuronal innervation, and we have seen a similar effect following the injection of botulinum toxin into immature muscles (M. C. Brown, J. K. S. Jansen and D. Van Essen, unpublished observations).

The events that took place during cross-innervation by a foreign nerve differed in several important respects from those that occurred during re-innervation and during the maturation of normal muscles. Firstly, many synapses on fibres multiply innervated through the foreign nerve were situated at separate sites up to 1 mm apart. Distributed synapses were never seen in normal muscles, and were probably not the most common form of multiple innervation during re-innervation. Presumably, the difference between re-innervation and cross-innervation is that regenerating axons from the original nerve tend to be guided back to the surviving old end-plates. Secondly, a moderate level of polyneuronal innervation through the foreign nerve persisten through the third week after birth. That these multiple inputs were eventually eliminated means that the interactions leading to synapse elimination can act over considerable distances. The delay in synapse removal suggests that the process might take longer when the synapses are some distance apart. Indirect support for this comes from the observation that there was a higher incidence of fibres having e.p.p. components with different rise times in the 2–3-week-old cross-innervated muscles than in the younger ones.

The final major difference seen after foreign innervation was that some multiple end-plates persisted indefinitely in cross-innervated muscles. This came about in two distinct ways: some fibres received separate functional inputs from the foreign and original nerves; while other fibres had two closely spaced end-plates in the region of foreign innervation, even though they had only one input that could be demonstrated physiologically. The distance between synapses from the foreign and original nerves was always 1 mm or more, suggesting that the degree of separation between synapses may determine whether one of them will be eliminated. If distance is indeed an important factor, then the basis for synapse elimination cannot be a process that affects the entire muscle fibre equally, such as the action potential or contractile activity.

It is interesting that the distance of about 1 mm suggested by the present experiments is similar to the spacing between synapses in slow muscles of the adult chicken. The development of the adult pattern of innervation in the chicken appears to come about by a selective elimination of synapses which initially are more closely spaced than in the adult (Bennett & Pettigrew, 1974 *b*). Slow muscles in the chicken do not conduct action potentials and it has been suggested that the decremental spread of synaptic potentials might be involved in determining the spacing between synapses (Gordon, Perry, Tuffery & Vrbová, 1974). This cannot, however, be the sole explanation for mammalian skeletal muscles, which conduct action potentials throughout the period when synapse elimination takes place.

The persistence of double esterase-stained end-plates in the region of foreign innervation appears to be quite a different phenomenon than the dual innervation through foreign and original nerves that was seen in the same muscles. Foreign and original end-plates on the same muscle fibre remained functional indefinitely, whereas we never saw physiological signs of inputs from more than one foreign motor axon at long times after cross-innervation. If there were functional synapses at both foreign end-plates, they must both have belonged to the same parent axon. This is an intriguing possibility, because it suggests that a muscle fibre is not inherently resistant to maintaining more than one closely-spaced end-plate, provided that they are all supplied by one axon. The key to protection of multiple synapses from elimination might be the synchrony in the patterns of synaptic activity, or it might be some other specific factor common to all terminals of a particular motor neurone.

Differences between immature and adult muscle

There are several important differences in the events that take place during re-innervation and cross-innervation of immature *vs.* adult muscles. Perhaps the most striking are the changes at the original end-plate region. Our results show that immature, cross-innervated muscle fibres, but not fibres which are simply denervated, lose the cholinesterase at the original end-plate quickly and completely. Associated with this is a loss in most cross-innervated fibres of the ability to accept re-innervation by the original nerve. In adult cross-innervated soleus muscle fibres the original end-plate properties are much more stable. The intensity of cholinesterase staining declines but never disappears and original end-plates will accept re-innervation for many weeks in spite of foreign innervation of the same fibres (Frank *et al.* 1975).

The degree of polyneuronal innervation seen at various stages of re- and cross-innervation is also different for immature and adult rats. Multiple innervation was seen in only a small percentage (10–15 %) of fibres examined in the first week of re-innervation of the adult rat diaphragm (Jansen & Van Essen, 1975). It is not known whether the multiple inputs were spatially distributed and whether they would eventually be removed. In adult cross-innervated muscles, polyneuronal innervation through the foreign nerve occurs commonly, even many months after the operation (Frank *et al.* 1975). However, recent experiments by T. Lømo and C. R. Slater and by H. Sommerschild (personal communications) suggest that there is a removal of closely spaced foreign synapses even in the adult rat.

Possible mechanisms of synapse elimination

The elimination of peripheral synapses could in principle be controlled by a variety of different mechanisms involving any combination of the three cell types present at the neuromuscular junction: neurones, Schwann cells and muscle fibres. Our results serve to restrict the number of acceptable hypotheses by specifying more explicitly the conditions under which synapse elimination can or cannot take place. The most important restraints are the following: (1) the end result of maturation is invariably that each muscle fibre is innervated by a single motor axon; (2) during normal maturation there are never a substantial number of muscle fibres that are completely denervated but after partial denervation withdrawal of terminals continues even though some muscle fibres consequently are left without innervation; (3) terminals from small motor units are more likely to survive than those of larger units; (4) the elimination process has a restricted range: it can act over distances of hundreds of microns but not over millimetres.

The elimination of synapses does not appear to be a random process, either in the sense that a particular motor neurone loses a randomly selected proportion of its terminals (since this would lead to transient denervation of many fibres), or in the sense that on each muscle fibre there is a random choice of which terminal is to survive (since terminals of smaller units survive preferentially). Instead, there seems to be some sort of competition among the synapses on each fibre. It may be of interest to speculate on the cellular mechanisms that might operate in a way consistent with these restraints.

Selection by Schwann cells. Since all of the terminals on a normal immature muscle fibre are crowded into a single end-plate, it is possible to imagine that a single Schwann cell, or row of Schwann cells, could select one of the terminals to be the survivor. This could be accomplished by the myelination of only one preterminal axon, providing that the remaining unmyelinated axons were eventually withdrawn. The selection of which axon to myelinate could be made on the basis of some quality such as axon diameter, in which case the smaller motor units might attain a selective advantage simply because their terminals become larger. The myelination hypothesis cannot, however, account for the events related to the elimination of spatially separated end-plates in any simple way.

Interactions between nerve terminals. The elimination process might involve interactions only between the nerve terminals co-existing on a fibre, without any direct participation of the muscle fibre or of Schwann cells. The interactions might take the form of one terminal physically crowding out the others, or of a biochemical signal passing from one terminal to the others to induce the withdrawal of synapses. In either case this type of hypothesis suffers from the same disadvantage as the myelination hypothesis, in that it is difficult to explain direct and specific interactions between terminals separated by hundreds of microns.

Interactions directly involving the muscle fibre. In order to account for the elimination of distributed inputs in seems necessary to invoke some type of signal passing from the muscle fibre to the synapses upon it. It is not clear what the nature of the communication between muscle and nerve could be. There might, for example, be a signal from the muscle that actively induced the removal of unwanted terminals. A different type of explanation is that synapses might compete for some substance, provided in limited amounts by the muscle fibre and needed for the survival of the synapse. The persistence of distant multiple synapses might then reflect the limits over which synapses could compete for this hypothetical substance.

It is evident that we are now at the stage of understanding only a few of the rules of the process whereby neuromuscular connexions reach their mature state. These rules serve to restrict the types of mechanisms that could control the elimination of synapses but as yet they provide only indirect hints concerning the specific cells and intercellular signals involved. A major impetus behind the elimination process seems to be a natural inability of the motor neurone to maintain more than a fraction of its original complement of synapses. The choice of which synapses are to be removed results from a competitive interaction between all of the synapses within a limited distance on each muscle fibre. The nature of the competition is still not known but it is probably geared to favour the survival of terminals from smaller motor units and it appears to involve a signal from muscle to nerve.

We thank Mr Håvard Tønnesen for invaluable technical assistance. Drs Eric Frank, Terje Lømo and Wesley Thompson have all given good advice at various stages. D.V.E. was supported by a Helen Hay Whitney fellowship. M.C.B. was European exchange fellow of the Royal Society.

REFERENCES

AKERT, K. & SANDRI, C. (1968). An electron-microscopic study of zine iodide-osmium impregnation of neurons. I. Staining of synaptic vesicles at cholinergic junctions. *Brain Res.* **7**, 286–295.

BAGUST, J., LEWIS, D. M. & WESTERMAN, R. A. (1973). Polyneuronal innervation of kitten skeletal muscle. *J. Physiol* **229**, 241–255.

BENNETT, M. R. & PETTIGREW, A. G. (1974a). The formation of synapses in striated muscle during development. *J. Physiol.* **241**, 515–545.

BENNETT, M. R. & PETTIGREW, A. G. (1974b). The formation of synapses in re-innervated and cross-innervated striated muscle during development. *J. Physiol.* **241**, 547–573.

BENOIT, P. & CHANGEUX, J.-P. (1975). Consequences of tenotomy on the evolution of multiinnervation in developing rat soleus muscle. *Brain Res.* **99**, 345–358.

BLACKSHAW, S. W. & WARNER, A. E. (1976). Low resistance junctions between mesoderm cells during development of trunk muscles. *J. Physiol.* **255**, 209–230.

BROWN, M. C., JANSEN, J. K. S. & VAN ESSEN, D. (1975). A large-scale reduction in motor neurone peripheral fields during post-natal development in the rat. *Acta physiol. scand.* **95**, 3–4A.

BROWN, M. C., JANSEN, J. K. S. & VAN ESSEN, D. (1976). Polyneuronal cross-innervation of the immature rat soleus muscle. *Acta physiol. scand.* **96**, 20A.

CHIAKULAS, J. J. & PAULY, J. E. (1965). A study of postnatal growth of skeletal muscle in the rat. *Anat. Rec.* **152**, 55–61.

CLOSE, R. (1964). Dynamic properties of fast and slow skeletal muscles of the rat during development. *J. Physiol.* **173**, 74–95.

CLOSE, R. (1967). Properties of motor units in fast and slow skeletal muscles of the rat. *J. Physiol.* **193**, 45–55.

DENNIS, M. (1975). Physiological properties of junctions between nerve and muscle developing during salamander limb regeneration. *J. Physiol.* **244**, 683–702.

EDDS, M. V., JR (1953). Collateral nerve regeneration. *Q. Rev. Biol.* **28**, 260–276.

ELSBERG, C. A. (1917). Experiments on motor nerve regeneration and the direct neurotization of paralyzed muscles by their own and by foreign nerves. *Science, N.Y.* **45**, 318–320.

FRANK, E., GAUTVIK, K. & SOMMERSCHILD, H. (1976). Persistence of junctional acetylcholine receptors at mammalian neuromuscular synapses following dener-vation. *Cold Spring Harb. Symp. quant. Biol.* **40**, 275–281.

FRANK, E., JANSEN, J. K. S., LØMO, T. & WESTGAARD, R. H. (1975). The interaction between foreign and original motor nerves innervating the soleus muscle of rats. *J. Physiol.* **247**, 725–743.

GORDON, T., PERRY, R., TUFFERY, A. R. & VRBOVÁ, G. (1974). Possible mechanisms determining synapse formation in developing skeletal muscle of the chick. *Cell & Tissue Res.* **155**, 13–25.

GUTH, L. (1962). Neuromuscular function after regeneration of interrupted nerve fibres into partially denervated muscle. *Expl Neurol.* **6**, 129–141.

GUTMAN, E. & HANZLIKOVÁ, V. (1966). Motor unit in old age. *Nature, Lond.* **209**, 921–922.

HUGHES, A. F. W. (1968). *Aspects of Neural Ontogeny*, pp. 249. London: Lagos Press.

JANSEN, J. K. S., LØMO, T., NICOLAYSEN, K. & WESTGAARD, R. H. (1973). Hyperinnervation of skeletal muscle fibres: dependence on muscle activity. *Science, N.Y.* **181**, 559–561.

JANSEN, J. K. S. & VAN ESSEN, D. (1975). Re-innervation of rat skeletal muscle in the presence of α-bungarotoxin. *J. Physiol.* **250**, 651–667.

KARNOVSKY, M. (1964). The localization of cholinesterase in rat cardiac muscle by electron microscopy. *J. Cell Biol.* **23**, 217–232.

LANDMESSER, L. & PILAR, G. (1974). Synaptic transmission and cell death during normal ganglionic development. *J. Physiol.* **241**, 737–749.

LUBINSKA, L. & ZELENÁ, J. (1966). Formation of new sites of acetylcholine esterase activity in denervated muscles of young rats. *Nature, Lond.* **210**, 39–41.

REDFERN, P. A. (1970). Neuromuscular transmission in new-born rats. *J. Physiol.* **209**, 701–709.

EXPLANATION OF PLATES

PLATE 1

A, multiple preterminal axons (arrows) to single end-plates in an 8-day-old rat diaphragm stained with zinc iodide–osmium. The muscle fibres, which run horizontally in the photograph, stain lightly and are not easily resolvable.

B, single end-plate stained for cholinesterase on a fibre isolated from a 6-day-old soleus muscle.

PLATE 2

A, cross-section from the middle of a 32-day-old normal soleus muscle, stained with Toluidine blue.

B, cross-section of a 33-day-old soleus muscle partially denervated since day 4. There were 321 large fibres in this muscle, which was innervated by only two motor axons. The scale applies to *A* and *B*.

C, multiple foreign end-plates on a cross-innervated muscle fibre. The fibre was isolated from a 13-day-old cross-innervated muscle after staining for cholinesterase. Two end-plates are visible at a separation of about 150 μm.

D, double foreign end-plates on an isolated fibre from a 72-day-old cross-innervated muscle stained for cholinesterase. No fibres with multiple foreign e.p.p. components were seen in this muscle.

A

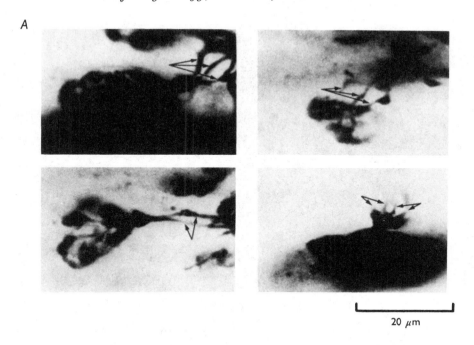

20 μm

B

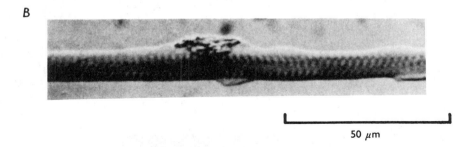

50 μm

M. C. BROWN, J. K. S. JANSEN AND D. VAN ESSEN   *(Facing p. 422)*

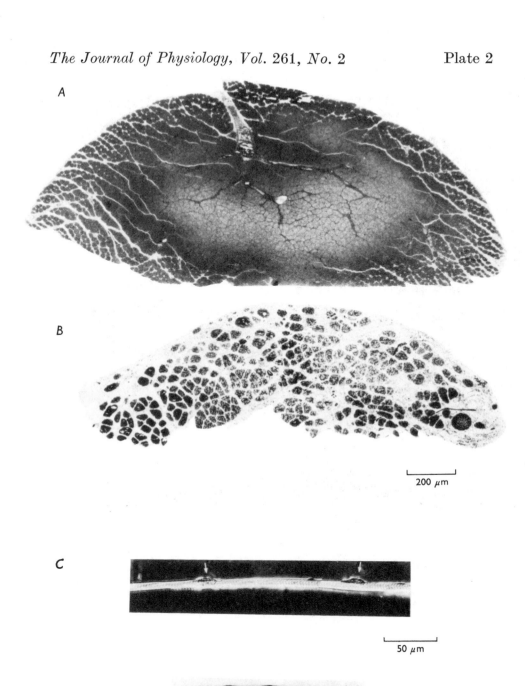

M. C. BROWN, J. K. S. JANSEN AND D. VAN ESSEN

J. Physiol. (1977), **273**, *pp.* 155–177
With 5 plates and 9 text-figures
Printed in Great Britain

THE REORGANIZATION OF SYNAPTIC CONNEXIONS IN THE RAT SUBMANDIBULAR GANGLION DURING POST-NATAL DEVELOPMENT

By JEFF W. LICHTMAN

From the Department of Physiology and Biophysics, Washington University School of Medicine, St Louis, Missouri, 63110 U.S.A.

(*Received 14 April 1977*)

SUMMARY

1. The innervation of neurones in the submandibular ganglion of neonatal and adult rats has been studied with intracellular recording, and light and electron microscopy.

2. Intracellular recordings from neurones in isolated ganglia from adult animals showed that about 75 % of the ganglion cells are innervated by a single preganglionic fibre.

3. However, multiple steps in the post-synaptic potential (about five on average) were elicited in ganglion cells from neonatal animals by graded stimulation of the preganglionic nerve. The same result was obtained when the preganglionic fibres were stimulated at their emergence from the brainstem, indicating that neonatal neurones are innervated by several different preganglionic nerve cells.

4. The number of preganglionic fibres innervating individual ganglion cells gradually decreased during the first few weeks of life, and by about 5 weeks each ganglion cell was generally contacted by a single preganglionic axon.

5. Synapses were made on short protuberances in the immediate vicinity of the neuronal cell bodies in both neonatal and adult ganglia as shown by staining presynaptic boutons with the zinc-iodide osmium method, injection of horseradish peroxidase into ganglion cells, and electron microscopical examination.

6. Electron microscopical counts of synaptic profiles per ganglion cell perimeter showed that the number of synaptic contacts made on ganglion cells actually increased during the first few post-natal weeks, when the number of axons innervating each neurone was decreasing.

7. These results show that in the rat submandibular ganglion there is a reorganization of neuronal connexions during the first few weeks of life which results in a transition from multiple to generally single innervation of ganglion cells.

INTRODUCTION

The ways in which nerve cells establish and maintain synaptic connexions with one another are largely unknown. The rules that govern these processes must account not only for the specificity of neuronal connexions, but also for the numerical balance of presynaptic endings and post-synaptic sites. Some of the principles underlying this balance have been suggested by studies of the developing neuromuscular junction (Redfern, 1970; Bagust, Lewis & Westerman, 1973; Bennett & Pettigrew, 1974, 1975, 1976; Brown, Jansen & Van Essen, 1976). A general feature of the developing neuromuscular junction appears to be transient multiple innervation of individual end-plates, with subsequent elimination of a portion of the synaptic contacts initially formed. In most mammalian muscles this process results in each adult muscle fibre being contacted by a single motor nerve terminal. Since synapse elimination can occur without a reduction in the number of motor units in mammalian muscle (Brown *et al.* 1976), the transition from multiple to single innervation probably involves the rearrangement of innervation, rather than the death of presynaptic cells. The aim of the present work was to examine whether a similar rearrangement of synaptic connexions occurs between developing neurones. The submandibular ganglion of the rat was chosen because preliminary experiments showed it to be remarkably simple in organization, most neurones being innervated in maturity by a single preganglionic axon.

The results of intracellular recording during the first few days of post-natal life show that immature ganglion cells are innervated by multiple preganglionic axons. As at the neuromuscular junction, there is a gradual decline in the number of presynaptic axons contacting each post-synaptic cell, leading to the establishment of the adult pattern of generally single innervation within about a month of birth. The similarity of the process of synapse elimination in developing mammalian muscle and in the immature submandibular ganglion suggests that this may be a general feature of neural ontogeny.

METHODS

Dissection

Twenty-six female albino rats (Wistar strain) 1–35 days of age and seventeen young adult animals (8–14 weeks of age, 160–220 g) were anaesthetized with chloral hydrate (0·35 gm/kg, I.P.) and perfused through the heart with mammalian Ringer fluid (Liley, 1956). A ventral mid line incision was made in the neck, and the submandibular and major sublingual glands and their ducts were freed by blunt dissection to the disappearance of the ducts beneath the mylohyoid muscle (Text-fig. 1 A). This muscle was cut to expose the ducts rostrally to the point at which the lingual nerve crosses them from the lateral side. The ducts, lingual nerve and connective tissue between them, were removed from the animal and placed in oxygenated Ringer fluid.

The triangular connective tissue sheet between the ducts and the lingual nerve contains a number of neurones which innervate the salivary glands, and is subsequently referred to as the submandibular ganglion (Text-fig. 1 *B*) (see also below).

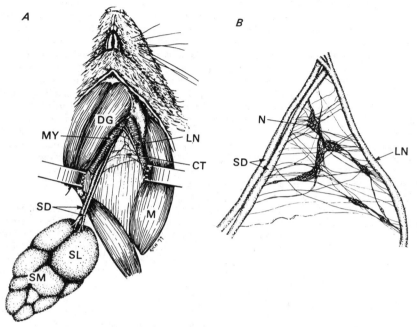

Text-fig. 1. The submandibular ganglion of the rat (left ganglion, ventral aspect). *A*, the ganglion cells, which innervate the submandibular (SM) and sublingual (SL) salivary glands, lie in a thin connective tissue sheet (CT) beneath the mylohyoid muscle (MY) (which has been cut between the digastric (D) and masseter (M) muscles). The connective tissue sheet is bordered by the lingual nerve (LN) laterally, and the salivary ducts (SD) medially. *B*, when the connective tissue between the lingual nerve (LN) and the salivary ducts (SD) is removed and examined at higher magnification, clusters of neurones (N), can be seen within the sheet. The preganglionic axons enter the sheet in many small branches from the lingual nerve. These branches run either directly to the salivary ducts, or through the clusters of ganglion cells. The post-ganglionic axons follow the salivary ducts to the salivary glands.

In four 3-week-old rats the preganglionic fibres were dissected proximally to their emergence from the brainstem in the nervus intermedius. The submandibular ganglion was denervated in five additional adult rats by cutting the chorda tympani near the medial side of sphenoid spine 4–10 days before removing the ganglion.

Recording methods

Ganglia were pinned out in a small chamber (vol. = 0·5 ml.) perfused with oxygenated Ringer fluid at a rate of approximately 2 ml./min, and viewed with an inverted differential interference contrast microscope (Biovert, Reichert) through a cover-slip 0·1 mm thick which formed the bottom of the recording chamber. The lingual nerve and salivary ducts were taken into close fitting glass suction electrodes for stimulation with single pulses (0·5–1·0 msec, 10–100 V).

Impalements of ganglion cells were made with glass micro-electrodes bent at a 75° angle within a few millimetres of their tips to allow easy movement within the working distance of the microscope condenser (7 mm). Electrodes were filled with 0·5 M potassium citrate, and had resistances of 80–120 MΩ. In all experiments the Ca^{2++} concentration of the bathing fluid was increased from 2 to 8 m-mole/l. to improve the stability of intracellular recordings. Impalements were facilitated by passing brief pulses of hyperpolarizing current through a bridge circuit in series with the recording electrode. Only neurones giving action potentials of 60 mV or more in response to intracellular injection of depolarizing current were included in the results.

The number of discrete steps in the excitatory post-synaptic potential (e.p.s.p.) in response to graded stimulation of the preganglionic nerve was taken as a measure of the number of preganglionic fibres innervating each cell. Counting the number of steps was often easier if action potentials superimposed on the synaptic response were eliminated by passing depolarizing current through the recording electrode to initiate a spike; the synaptic response was then timed so that it occurred during the refractory period of the directly elicited action potential (see Text-fig. 4, for example). Although generally reliable, estimates of the number of fibres innervating a neurone obtained by this method were subject to several uncertainties. For example, if a fibre making a large synaptic contribution was activated at a low intensity of stimulation, a small synaptic potential from another axon with a higher threshold could be obscured because of shunting. That this sometimes occurred was evident from antidromic stimulation of fibres making *en passant* synaptic contacts. A further difficulty with this method was that the latency of e.p.s.p.s often decreased as the strength of stimulus increased. Presumably this occured because the action potential was initiated closer to the point of recording. As a consequence, changes in latency could not be used as a criterion of additional recruitment, and fibres with the lowest threshold often appeared to be the most slowly conducting (see, for example, Text-figs. 4B and 5C). These deficiencies would lead to an underestimate of the number of axons innervating a neurone, but would not affect the observation that the complexity of the synaptic response changed markedly with age.

Anatomical methods

(a) *Zinc-iodide osmium staining.* Preganglionic boutons were stained with a mixture of zinc-iodide and osmium tetroxide (Maillet, 1962). Ganglia from nine neonatal (1–35 days old), and eleven young adult rats were incubated overnight in the staining solution, dehydrated in graded ethanol solutions, cleared in xylene, and mounted in synthetic mounting medium (Fisher Preservaslide) on glass slides.

(b) *Intracellular injection of horseradish peroxidase.* Twenty-eight neurones in adult ganglia and twenty-four in neonatal ganglia were pressure-injected with horseradish peroxidase (type VI, Sigma, St Louis) and stained with benzidine dihydrochloride. The procedure used was similar to that of Muller & McMahan (1976) with the following modifications. To ensure a stable and agranular reaction product (the brown reaction product; Straus, 1964), ganglia fixed in glutaraldehyde were immersed in a 2 % benzidine dihydrochloride solution in 0·01 M-Tris maleate buffer (pH 7·4) at room temperature. One drop of 3 % H_2O_2 was added after 10 min. When the injected cells were blue-brown, the ganglia were washed in distilled water, and dehydrated at room temperature by passage through graded ethanol solutions.

This procedure usually removed the granular blue reaction product which formed initially. The tissue was cleared in xylene and mounted whole in Preservaslide under a cover-slip. The cells and their processes were traced with the aid of a camera lucida.

(c) *Measurements of cell area.* To determine the size of ganglion cells at different ages, semi-thin sections (1 μm) of ganglia from 2-day-old, 2- to 3-week-old and adult rats were stained with toluidine blue. The sections were taken from the blocks prepared for ultrastructural examination (see below). The perimeters of 100 nucleated neuronal profiles from each age group were traced by camera lucida using an oil-immersion objective ($\times$ 1200), and the area of each profile calculated by a computer-assisted planimeter (Cowan & Wann, 1973).

(d) *Electron microscopy.* Thirty-two additional ganglia from twenty-two neonatal and ten young adult rats were pinned in dishes with Sylgard resin bottoms, and immersed in half strength Karnovsky fixative (Karnovsky, 1965) for 30 min. The ganglia were transferred to full strength fixative for an hour, and were then post-fixed in 2 % osmium tetroxide in cacodylate buffer at pH 7·2 for an additional 3 hr. Following dehydration in graded ethanol solutions, the ganglia were imbedded in Araldite (Ciba). Thin sections were mounted on 200-mesh grids, and stained with lead citrate and uranyl acetate.

The number of synaptic profiles per cell perimeter was taken as an index of the relative number of profiles contacting cells at different ages. Synapse counts were made only on cell perimeters which contained a nuclear profile and were entirely within a grid square. Neurones whose perimeters bordered closely upon other neurones were avoided, since in these cases it was sometimes difficult to assign synapses to one cell or the other. To be counted as a synapse, a profile had to show pre- and post-synaptic membrane thickenings, and presynaptic agranular vesicles focused on a presynaptic membrane specialization (see Pl. 3).

To compare the size of presynaptic elements from neonatal and adult ganglia, fifty randomly chosen synaptic profiles from ganglia in 2-day-old rats, and fifty profiles from adults were photographed and printed at a total magnification of 48,900. The cross-sectional area of the presynaptic terminals and the extent of the pre- and post-synaptic membrane thickenings were measured by a computer assisted planimeter.

RESULTS

The preparation

The anatomy of the parasympathetic innervation of the mammalian submandibular and sublingual salivary glands has been briefly described by a number of workers (Langley, 1890; Szentágothai, 1957; Snell, 1958; McMahan & Kuffler, 1971). In the rat, about half of the ganglion cells which innervate the glands are located in the thin connective tissue sheet defined here as the submandibular ganglion (Text-fig. 1 B), while the remainder are grouped along the salivary ducts, or occasionally within the submandibular gland itself (Snell, 1958). The preganglionic axons orginate in the superior salivatory nucleus and run in the nervus intermedius, facial nerve, chorda tympani, and lingual nerve from which they enter the connective tissue sheet by way of numerous small branches. Within the sheet the preganglionic nerves branch extensively. Many of the branches run through clusters of ganglion cells, while others course directly to the

6

ducts. The ganglion usually consists of three to ten clusters, each containing from five to about 250 neurones (Text-fig. 1 *B* and Pl. 1). Occasional neurones occur in isolation.

Individual nerve cell bodies and adjacent Schwann cell nuclei were easily seen with differential interference contrast optics. The clusters of ganglion cells are often one cell thick (Pl. 1) and their arrangement is in many ways similar to certain parasympathetic ganglia of amphibians (McMahan & Kuffler, 1971; McMahan & Purves, 1976). Ganglion cells were

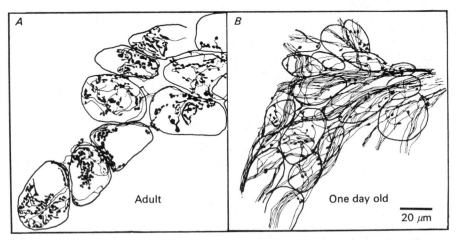

Text-fig. 2. Camera lucida drawings of groups of neurones from the submandibular ganglion stained with zinc-iodide osmium. *A*, the cell bodies of neurones in adult ganglia show numerous boutons in apparent contact with the neuronal surface. The boutons are variable in shape, size and location on the cell bodies. Photomicrographs of single focal planes of three neurones stained with zinc-iodide osmium are shown in Pl. 2*A*, *B*, *C*. *B*, neonatal ganglia stained with zinc-iodide osmium show relatively few boutons, but an abundance of fine fibres (see Pl. 2*D*, *E*).

generally the same in size and appearance; this argued against the presence of interneurones ('small intensely fluorescent' cells) found in some parasympathetic and sympathetic ganglia in both mammals and lower vertebrates (Siegrist, Dolivo, Dunant, Foroglou-Kerameus, De Ribaupierre & Rouiller, 1968; Mathews & Raisman, 1969; Williams & Palay, 1969; McMahan & Purves, 1976). The absence of interneurones containing dense core vesicles was confirmed by electron microscopy (see below).

To determine the distribution of preganglionic boutons on the neurones, ganglia were stained with zinc-iodide osmium. In adult ganglia, dense pleomorphic boutons were observed on the surface of many neurones (Text-fig. 2*A*; Pl. 2*A–C*). The fibres interconnecting the boutons were often quite thick, making it difficult to estimate the number of individual endings on some cells. On cells where counts could be made, the number of boutons ranged from 25 to 80 with mean of 44 per neurone (n = 110). This number is relatively large: in the mudpuppy cardiac ganglion there are an average of 22 boutons per cell (McMahan & Purves, 1976), and an average of only 12 per cell in the parasympathetic ganglion of the frog atrial septum (McMahan & Kuffler, 1971). There was no indication that boutons contacted nerve cells other than in the immediate vicinity of the cell body.

Electron microscopical examination of the ganglion showed that the population of neurones was homogeneous by ultrastructural criteria, although Schwann cells and connective tissue cells were also present. Synapses on ganglion cells were usually on small fingers of cytoplasm within a few microns of the cell body surface (Pl. 3). Profiles of presynaptic boutons in adult ganglia contained densely packed, agranular vesicles about 50 nm in diameter, as well as a few dense core vesicles up to 150 nm in diameter, and numerous mitochondria (Pl. 3 *A*, *B*). These profiles resemble cholinergic preganglionic terminals in other autonomic ganglia (see for example, Taxi, 1965). Gap junctions, which occur between parasympathetic ganglion cells in some lower vertebrates (McMahan & Purves, 1976) were not seen in the submandibular ganglion. However, symmetrical desmosome-like junctions were observed between some neurones; these resembled junctions seen in other autonomic ganglia (Gabella, 1972).

The anatomy of the submandibular ganglion as demonstrated by zinc-iodide osmium staining and electron microscopy suggested that the nerve cells do not have an extensive dendritic aborization. To confirm this, neurones were injected with horseradish peroxidase. Cells visualized in this way had few if any large dendrites, but numerous smaller processes extended from the perikaryon and the initial portion of the axon (Text-fig. 3, Pl. 4). It is likely that most of the presynaptic profiles seen in electron microscopical sections contacted these short processes. Horseradish peroxidase injections failed to demonstrate axonal branching beyond the initial segment, even though postganglionic axons could often be followed for long distances (Text-fig. 3; see also Pl. 5 and below). The short processes extending from the initial portion of the axons were probably not postganglionic collaterals (see the next section).

Intracellular recordings from adult neurones

In general, the electrophysiological properties of submandibular neurones are similar to those of other mammalian autonomic cells which have been studied with intracellular recording (see, for example, Blackman, Crowcroft, Devine, Holman & Yonemura, 1969). Action potentials elicited

6-2

by depolarizing current injection through the recording micro-electrode, or by ortho- or antidromic stimulation, had amplitudes of 60–114 mV; resting potentials ranged from −40 to −73 mV, and input resistances were between 55 and 200 MΩ.

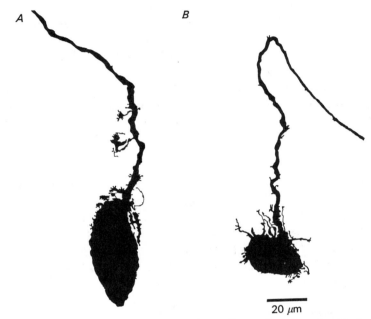

20 μm

Text-fig. 3. Camera lucida drawing of ganglion cells injected with horse-radish peroxidase. *A*, an adult neurone showing numerous small processes extending from the cell body and the initial portion of the axon. The axon could be followed out of this field for distance of several hundred microns, and remained unbranched. *B*, ganglion cell from a 1-week-old rat. The cellular geometry of immature ganglion cells was similar to that of adult neurones; the axon of this neurone and other immature cells also remained unbranched as far as they could be followed. Pl. 4*A* and *B* show single focal planes of these same neurones.

In the majority of adult neurones, a single suprathreshold excitatory post-synaptic potential (e.p.s.p.) was elicited by graded stimulation of the lingual nerve (Text-fig. 4*A*). Changes in the strength, duration, or polarity of the stimulus did not alter the amplitude or shape of the post-synaptic potential. In twenty-seven of 121 adult neurones impaled (22 %), a second e.p.s.p. was observed, and in four neurones (3 %) a third could be seen. These additional e.p.s.p.s were subthreshold in all but two cases (Text-fig. 4*B*). Thus, although adult neurones were sometimes innervated by more than one preganglionic fibre, suprathreshold innervation from a single axon was the rule.

Stimulation of the nerve fibres which run with the salivary ducts also elicited e.p.s.p.s., as well as antidromic action potentials, in many ganglion cells. Antidromic action potentials were distinguished from regenerative responses arising from synaptic activation by collision with directly initiated action potentials. To see if ganglion cells received innervation from sources other than the preganglionic fibres (for example, from post-

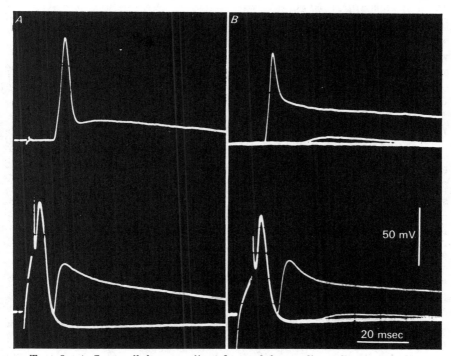

Text-fig. 4. Intracellular recordings from adult ganglion cells. *A*, recording from a singly innervated neurone. Upper trace: stimulation of the lingual nerve (at artifact) elicited a suprathreshold synaptic response. Resting potential was -50 mV. Lower trace: Same neurone as in *A*. In order to observe the e.p.s.p. without the regenerative response, depolarizing current (5 msec pulse) was injected through the recording electrode to initiate an action potential; the synaptic response was timed so that it occurred during the refractory period of the directly elicited action potential (two traces superimposed). A unitary e.p.s.p. such as this was observed in 75% of adult neurones. *B* recording from a multiply innervated neurone. Upper trace: gradually increasing the stimulus to the lingual nerve elicited two steps with separate thresholds in the synaptic response. The smaller synaptic potential was well below threshold (three traces superimposed). Resting potential was -44 mV. Lower trace: one large and one very small e.p.s.p. were seen when the synaptic response was timed so that it occurred in the refractory period of a directly elicited action potential; this was typical of multiply innervated adult ganglion cells (three traces superimposed).

ganglionic axon collaterals or afferents arising in the salivary glands), ganglia from five animals were denervated by cutting the chorda tympani, and examined 4–10 days later when the preganglionic fibres had degenerated. In neurones impaled in these ganglia there was no response to stimulation of the lingual nerve, and stimulation of the nerve fibres that run with the salivary ducts elicited only antidromic action potentials. Thus ganglion cells appear to be innervated solely by preganglionic fibres arising from the lingual nerve, some of which make *en passant* contacts and run on to synapse with other neurones along the salivary ducts or in the salivary glands. Antidromic stimulation confirmed the results of orthodromic stimulation: in the majority of neurones in which e.p.s.p.s. could be elicited by stimulating the salivary ducts, a single suprathreshold e.p.s.p. was observed.

Intracellular recordings from neonatal neurones

Although neonatal neurones were more difficult to impale, action potential amplitudes, resting potentials, and input resistances were similar to those of adult neurones. However, the results of graded preganglionic stimulation of neonatal ganglion cells were quite different than those obtained in adults. Complex e.p.s.p.s were invariably elicited in neonatal neurones by gradually increasing the strength of lingual nerve stimulation (Text-fig. 5). The amplitude, shape, and latency of the synaptic response changed in discrete steps as the stimulus strength was increased and often more than one of the steps in the synaptic response gave rise to an action potential (Text-fig. 5B, D).

The estimated number of steps in the e.p.s.p.s. was greatest during the first week of life (range 3–7, mean = $4 \cdot 7 \pm 1 \cdot 1$ (S.E. of mean), $n = 60$), and gradually decreased thereafter (Text-fig. 6). By the fifth post-natal week the number of steps was similar to that in neurones from adult ganglia (range 1–3, mean = $1 \cdot 3 \pm 0 \cdot 5$, $n = 50$).

Multiple steps in the synaptic response of neonatal neurones are presumably due to several preganglionic axons innervating each cell. However, other explanations are possible. For instance, complex e.p.s.p.s. might occur if neonatal neurones were electrically coupled. Electrotonic junctions have been demonstrated between immature muscle fibres (Kelly & Zacks, 1969; Dennis & Ort, 1976; Blackshaw & Warner, 1976), and between adult parasympathetic neurones in the mudpuppy (McMahan & Purves, 1976; Roper, 1976). To examine the possibility of electrical coupling in the submandibular ganglion, adjacent neurones were impaled using two independent electrodes, and current was injected into one cell while recording from the other. Weak electrical coupling was observed between some pairs of neurones in both neonates and adults. There was, however, at least a fiftyfold attenuation of the potential in coupled neurones. This degree of coupling is far too small to account for the complex e.p.s.p.s observed in young animals. The apparent absence of gap junctions between ganglion cells in electron microscopical sections (see above) is consistent with the failure to demonstrate strong electrical coupling.

Multiple steps in the post-synaptic response might also be due to branches of the same preganglionic axon arising above the point of lingual nerve

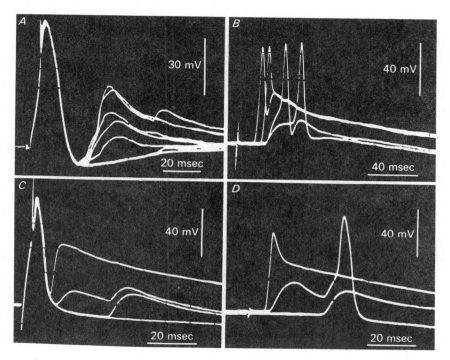

Text-fig. 5. Intracellular recordings from neonatal ganglion cells. *A*, neurone from a 7-day-old rat. Gradually increasing the preganglionic stimulus stength elicited multiple steps with different thresholds in the post-synaptic response. In this tracing, the synaptic response was timed so that it occurred during the refractory period of a directly elicited action potential which eliminated the superimposed regenerative responses. At least six separate steps can be observed (seven traces superimposed). Resting potential was − 41 mV. *B*, neurone from a 14-day-old rat. In this cell, graded stimulation to the lingual nerve elicited 4 post-synaptic responses with different thresholds. Two were just at threshold and two were suprathreshold (four traces superimposed). Resting potential was − 46 mV. *C*, neurone from a 20-day-old rat showing a decrease in the complexity of the synaptic response. There are three discrete steps with separate thresholds and latencies (four traces superimposed). Resting potential was − 48 mV. *D*, intracellular recording from same neurone as *C*. Two of the steps in the synaptic response gave rise to action potentials.

stimulation. To explore this possibility, the preganglionic fibres were stimulated at their emergence from the brainstem in the nervus intermedius. In four ganglia from 3-week-old rats, stimulation of the nervus intermedius produced complex synaptic responses composed of discrete steps with separate thresholds. This result was indistinguishable from the response to lingual nerve stimulation. Thus neonatal neurones are innervated by

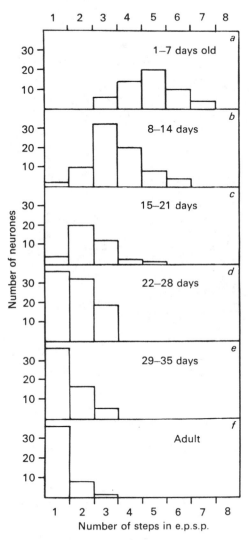

Text-fig. 6. Histogram of the number of innervating fibres estimated from number of steps in the synaptic response recorded in neurones from birth to 35 days of age (*a–e*). The number of steps in fifty adult neurones is shown in *f*.

several different fibres emerging from the brainstem. In two experiments, suction electrodes were applied to both the nervus intermedius and to the lingual nerve just proximal to the ganglion. Every e.p.s.p. step elicited by stimulation of the nervus intermedius was also observed when the lingual nerve was stimulated. Therefore once a preganglionic fibre emerges from the brainstem it probably sends only one preterminal branch to a neurone. Axonal branches arising within the brainstem and contacting the same ganglion cell cannot be ruled out, but this seems unlikely.

Finally, multiple steps in the e.p.s.p.s of neonatal neurones could occur if postganglionic axon collaterals made synapses with other ganglion cells as occurs, for example, in the cardiac ganglion of the mudpuppy (McMahan & Purves, 1976; Roper, 1976). It was difficult to denervate neonatal ganglia and to rule out axon collaterals by subsequent antidromic stimulation as in adult ganglia (see above). However, horseradish peroxidase injections of ganglion cells from 1-week-old animals demonstrated that the post-ganglionic axons resembled those in adult ganglia: aside from several short processes arising from the initial segment, they remained unbranched as far as they could be followed (Pl. 5).

In summary, electrical coupling of ganglion cells, multiple branches from individual preganglionic fibres, and recurrent axon collaterals are probably not responsible for the multiple steps in the post-synaptic responses recorded in neurones from young animals. Rather, each nerve cell appears to be innervated by several preganglionic neurones at birth, this number gradually decreasing during the first 5 weeks of life.

Anatomical aspects of synaptic reorganization

Ganglia from neonatal rats were similar in appearance to adult ganglia. Intracellular injection of horseradish peroxidase showed the cellular geometry to be similar as well. Although the twenty-four peroxidase injected ganglion cells from 1-week-old rats were generally smaller than the twenty-eight adult neurones injected, most had many short processes ($< 5\ \mu$m), as adult cells (Text-fig. 3B and Pl. 4B and 5). A few neonatal neurones had occasional longer, thicker processes (for example cell 3 in Pl. 5) which were not observed in adult ganglia. It is possible that the retraction of these somewhat larger dendrites could result in a decrease in the number of axons innervating a ganglion cell. Most injected neurones, however, did not have large processes during the early post-natal period when all the cells are multiply innervated.

Although the cellular geometry of neonatal and adult ganglion cells was generally the same, the arrangement of preganglionic boutons stained with zinc-iodide osmium on neonatal neurones differed considerably from the

arrangement in adults (Text-fig. 2 and Pl. 2). In neonatal ganglia surprisingly few boutons were observed, and unlike adult ganglia, numerous
fine fibres were stained. The difference in the staining pattern of neonatal
and adult ganglia suggested that each neonatal neurone received a smaller
number of synaptic contacts, although many more axons appeared to be
available. The paucity of boutons in neonatal ganglia could, however, be
due to the method itself. That this technique is to some degree capricious
is shown by the presence of some ganglion cells without any impregnated
boutons in many zinc-iodide osmium preparations.

To quantitate the relative number of synaptic contacts received by
neonatal and mature ganglion cells, synapses were counted in electron
microscopical sections of neonatal and adult ganglia. The number of synaptic profiles per cell perimeter was lower in 2-day-old rats than in 2- to
3-week-old or adult rats, but there was no significant difference in the
number of synapses contacting two 3-week-old neurones and the number
contacting adult ganglion cells (Text-fig. 7). The actual difference in the
number of synapses per cell in 2-day-old and more mature rats may be
larger than suggested by the results shown in Text-fig. 6 because the
cross-sectional area of ganglion cells increased roughly threefold between
birth and maturity (Text-fig. 8). Thus, assuming presynaptic profiles of
constant size, a larger fraction of the total number of synapses per cell would
be counted on each perimeter in ganglia from young animals. Measurements
from electron micrographs showed that the cross-sectional area of presynaptic profiles and the length of the presynaptic specilization in fact were
relatively constant between birth and maturity. The mean cross-sectional
area of fifty presynaptic profiles from 2-day-old ganglia was 0.99 ± 0.10 μm^2,
compared with 1.01 ± 0.13 in adult ganglia ($n = 50$). The average length of
the presynaptic specialization was 0.55 ± 0.04 μm in the 2-day-old ganglia,
and 0.50 ± 0.03 in adults. Thus during post-natal development the number
of synapses made on individual ganglion cells increases while the number
of preganglionic axons contacting each neurone decreases.

Ultrastructural study also indicated that individual synaptic profiles from
2-day-old rats differed from those in older animals in that the presynaptic profiles were less densely packed with vesicles and mitochondria
(Pl. 3C and D). This appearance is generally similar to immature profiles
described in other autonomic preparations (Brenner & Johnson, 1976;
Landmesser & Pilar, 1972). Degenerating nerve terminals (usually characterized by increased affinity for osmium, aggregation of vesicles, auto-
phagic vacuoles, and lysosomes – Hámori, Láng & Simon, 1968) were
occasionally seen in both neonatal and adult ganglia, but were not more
prevalent in developing ganglia. The absence of degeneration may mean
that elimination of synapses occurs through the gradual resorption of

terminals, as may occur at the developing neuromuscular junction (Korneliussen & Jansen, 1976; see, however, Rosenthal & Taraskevich, 1977). Preganglionic cell death, however, cannot be ruled out.

As in adult ganglia, the synaptic profiles in 2-day-old rats contacted small fingers of cytoplasm in the immediate vicinity of the cell bodies. Multiple

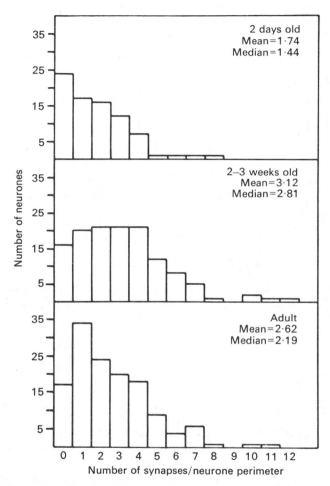

Text-fig. 7. Distribution of the number of synapses per neurone perimeter from 2-day-old, 2- to 3-week-old and adult rats. The median (and 95 % confidence interval; Noether, 1973) for 2-day-old rats was 1·44 (0·93–1·94), for 2- to 3-week-old rats 2·81 (2·33–3·39), and for adult rats 2·19 (1·71–2·69). The difference in the number of synapses per neurone perimeter between 2-day-old rats and either the 2- or 3-week-old or adult rats was highly significant ($P < 0.001$; Wilcoxon two-tailed test). The difference between the 2- to 3-week-old rats and adults was not significant ($P < 0.05$).

JEFF W. LICHTMAN

synaptic contacts innervating the same post-synaptic specilization were not observed. This suggests that presynaptic axons probably do not share the same post-synaptic sites during the period of multiple innervation, as occurs at the developing neuromuscular junction (Bennett & Pettigrew, 1974; Brown *et al.* 1976).

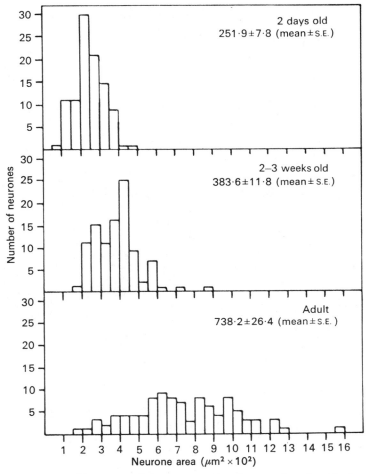

Text-fig. 8. Histogram of the cross-sectional areas of one hundred nucleated ganglion cell profiles from 2-day-old, 2- to 3-week-old and adult rats. The mean cell cross-sectional area increased about threefold from birth to maturity. The greater variance of the areas of adult neurones suggests that some cells increase in size much more than others.

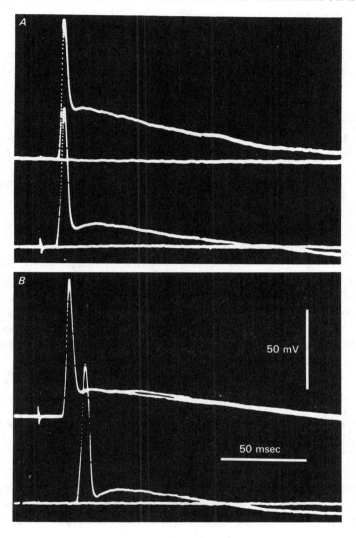

Text-fig. 9. Simultaneous recordings from a pair of adult ganglion cells. *A*, upper and lower traces are intracellular recordings from two nearby ganglion cells innervated by the same preganglionic fibre. At one stimulus strength neither cell fires; however, a slight increase in the stimulus to the lingual nerve elicits suprathreshold post-synaptic responses in both cells. Cells innervated by the same preganglionic fibre always failed together when the stimulus was adjusted to threshold levels, and had nearly identical latencies. *B*, a pair of adjacent neurones innervated by separate preganglionic fibres. At one stimulus strength the cell monitored in the upper trace fires, while the other cell (lower trace) does not. Increasing the stimulus strength elicited a post-synaptic potential in the cell monitored in the lower trace; its latency was also different from the post-synaptic potential elicited in the other cell. Two traces are superimposed in both *A* and *B*.

The arrangement of innervation within clusters of ganglion cells

As the number of fibres innervating each ganglion cell decreases during development, one of the fibres contacting a neurone becomes its dominant source of innervation. By simultaneously impaling pairs of ganglion cells in a cluster, it was possible to determine whether or not a single preganglionic fibre 'captured' not only individual neurones, but entire clusters of cells. Two cells were considered innervated by the same preganglionic axon if the post-synaptic potentials elicited in the ganglion cells appeared at exactly the same stimulus strength, had the same latency (± 0·5 msec), and always failed together when the stimulus was adjusted to threshold levels (Text-fig. 9 *A*, *B*).

In these experiments one electrode remained in a 'reference' cell, while the other electrode successively impaled nearby neurones. With each new impalement, the pair was tested to see if the same preganglionic fibre innervated both cells. In 4 of 25 clusters studied in adult ganglia, all the cells recorded from in the cluster were innervated by a single preganglionic fibre. Most of the clusters, however, were innervated by two to eight different fibres. Although preganglionic fibres usually innervated multiple neurones within a cluster, neighbouring ganglion cells were not necessarily captured by the same preganglionic fibre; rather, adjacent cells were often innervated by different axons.

DISCUSSION

The results of this study show that during the first post-natal month there is a gradual reorganization of the innervation in the rat submandibular ganglion. At birth each ganglion cell is innervated by several (three to seven) preganglionic fibres, while by 5 weeks of age most of the neurones are innervated by a single axon. Synaptic reorganization during development is probably a widespread phenomenon. Muscle fibre endplates in amphibia (Letinsky, 1974; Bennett & Pettigrew, 1975), birds (Bennett & Pettigrew, 1974) and mammals (Redfern, 1970; Bagust *et al.* 1973; Bennett & Pettigrew, 1974; Brown *et al.* 1976) are transiently innervated by multiple motor axons during development. There is also some evidence for synapse elimination during the development of connexions within the central nervous system (Conradi & Skoglund, 1970; Ronnevi & Conradi, 1974; Delhaye-Bouchaud, Crepel & Mariani, 1975; Crepel, Mariani & Delhaye-Bouchaud, 1976).

In the submandibular ganglion, as at the neuromuscular junction, synapse elimination is not haphazard: the majority of synaptic contacts from all but one axon innervating a neurone are usually removed. The transition from multiple to predominantly single innervation of ganglion cells could occur because preganglionic neurones are dying, or because the peripheral connexions of a stable number of preganglionic neurones are reorganized. Preganglionic cell death has been suggested as a cause of the loss of synapses during embryonic development in the chick ciliary ganglion (Landmesser & Pilar, 1974, 1976). However, presynaptic cell death seems a less likely mechanism in post-natal life since in most vertebrates the major phase of neural loss is embryonic (Glücksmann, 1951; Cowan, 1973). Moreover, Brown *et al.* (1976) have shown that the elimination of polyneuronal innervation from muscle fibres in early post-natal life occurs without a change in the number of motor axons innervating rat soleus muscle.

Although a similar mechanism may underlie synapse elimination in the developing submandibular ganglion and at the neuromuscular junction, an important difference between the innervation of muscle fibres and submandibular ganglion cells is the location of the presynaptic terminals. On each neonatal muscle fibre innervation is confined to the endplate where several axons share the same post-synaptic site (Bennett & Pettigrew, 1974; Brown *et al.* 1976; see also Rotshenker & McMahan 1976). In contrast the post-synaptic sites on ganglion cells are spatially separate, and each of these is apparently occupied by only one preganglionic axon terminal. Yet in maturity each submandibular ganglion cell, as each mammalian skeletal muscle fibre, is generally innervated by a single dominant axon. Thus the total number of spatially separate post-synaptic sites on a ganglion cell appears to be functionally equivalent to a single endplate during the process of synapse elimination.

The mechanism of synapse elimination is not understood. The experiments of Brown *et al.* (1976) suggest that during the development of the neuromuscular junction there is an intrinsic tendency for presynaptic fibres to retract since synapse elimination occurs even when the number of innervating axons is drastically reduced by partial denervation. In the submandibular ganglion, the number of fibres innervating each ganglion cell decreases while the number of synapses per cell is increasing. This argues against an intrinsic tendency for each preganglionic neurone to reduce the number of synaptic contacts it makes during development: assuming a constant number of preganglionic axons and ganglion cells, the total number of synapses made by each preganglionic neurone must increase during the period of synapse elimination.

Some competitive interaction among the multiple axons initially innervating each post-synaptic cell seems likely. Elimination of synapses in the developing submandibular ganglion might be explained if preganglionic fibres compete for a limited amount of trophic substance associated with the post-synaptic cell: growth and increased uptake of a factor by one axon might result in the local regression of terminals of other axons as they receive a smaller and smaller share of the trophic agent. A trophic dependence of adult ganglionic synapses on some property of the post-synaptic cells might also explain collateral sprouting after partial denervation (Murray & Thompson, 1957), and the reversible loss of synapses following post-ganglionic axotomy (Matthews & Nelson, 1975; Purves, 1975; Njå & Purves, 1978). Additional mechanisms, however, probably would be required to explain why each ganglion cell tends ultimately to be innervated by a single preganglionic axon.

I am grateful to Dr Dale Purves for advice and encouragement during the course of this work. I also thank Dr A. Njå for helpful discussions, Dr C. C. Hunt for the loan of the differential interference contrast microscope, and Drs J. Szentágothai and U. J. McMahan who provided helpful descriptions of the dissection at the outset of the project. J. Arndt and W. De Palma provided skillful technical assistance. This work was supported by U.S.P.H.S. Grant no. NS 11699 to Dr Purves, a grant from the Muscular Dystrophy Associations of America and N.I.H. Training Grant GM 02016.

REFERENCES

BAGUST, J., LEWIS, D. M. & WESTERMAN, R. A. (1973). Polyneuronal innervation of kitten skeletal muscle. *J. Physiol.* **229**, 241–255.

BENNETT, M. R. & PETTIGREW, A. J. (1974). The formation of synapses in striated muscle during development. *J. Physiol.* **241**, 515–545.

BENNETT, M. R. & PETTIGREW, A. G. (1975). The formation of synapses in amphibian striated muscle during development. *J. Physiol.* **252**, 203–239.

BENNETT, M. R. & PETTIGREW, A. G. (1976). The formation of neuromuscular synapses. *Cold Spring Harb. Symp. quant. Biol.* **40**, 409–424.

BLACKMAN, J. G., CROWCROFT, P. J., DEVINE, C. E., HOLMAN, M. E. & YONEMURA, K. (1969). Transmission from preganglionic fibres in the hypogastric nerve to peripheral ganglia of male guiniea-pigs. *J. Physiol.* **201**, 723–743.

BLACKSHAW, S. W. & WARNER, A. E. (1976). Low resistance junctions between mesoderm cells during development of trunk muscles. *J. Physiol.* **255**, 209–230.

BRENNER, H. R. & JOHNSON, E. W. (1976). Physiological and morpological effects of post-ganglionic axotomy on presynaptic nerve terminals. *J. Physiol.* **260**, 143–158.

BROWN, M. C., JANSEN, J. K. S. & VAN ESSEN, D. (1976). Polyneuronal innervation of skeletal muscle in newborn rats and its elimination during maturation. *J. Physiol.* **261**, 387–422.

CONRADI, S. & SKOGLUND, S. (1970). Observations on the ultrastructure of the initial motor axon segment and dorsal root boutons on the motoneurons in the lumbrosacral spinal cord of the cat during post-natal development. *Acta physiol. scand.* **78**, suppl. 333, 53–76.

COWAN, W. M. (1973). Neuronal death as a regulative mechanism in the control of cell number in the nervous system. *Development and Aging in the Nervous System*, ed. ROCKSTEIN M. E. & SUSSMAN, M. L., pp. 19–41. New York: Academic Press.

COWAN, W. M. & WANN, D. F. (1973). A computer system for the measurement of cell and nuclear sizes. *J. Microscopy* **99**, 331–348.

CREPEL, F., MARIANI, J., & DELHAYE-BOUCHAUD, N. (1976). Evidence for a multiple innervation of purkinje cells by climbing fibres in the immature rat cerebellum. *J. Neurobiol.* **7**, 567–578.

DELHAYE-BOUCHAUD, N., CREPEL, F. & MARIANI, J. (1975). Mise en évidence d'une multi-innervation temporaire des cellules de Purkinje du cervelet par les fibres grimpantes au cours du développment chez le rat. *C. r. hebd. Séanc. Acad. Sci., Paris* **281**, 909–912.

DENNIS, M. J. & ORT, C. A. (1976). Physiological properties of nerve-muscle junctions developing *in vivo. Cold Spring Harb. Symp. quant. Biol.* **40**, 435–442.

GABELLA, G. (1972). Fine structure of the myenteric plexus in the guinea-pig ileum. *J. Anat.* **111**, 69–97.

GLÜCKSMANN, A. (1951). Cell deaths in normal vertebrate ontogeny. *Biol. Rev.* **26**, 59–86.

HÁMORI, J., LÁNG, E. & SIMON, L. (1968). Experimental degeneration of the preganglionic fibres in the superior cervical ganglion of the cat. *Z. Zellforsch. mikrosk. Anat.* **90**, 37–52.

KARNOVSKY, M. J. (1965). A formaldehyde gluturaldehyde fixative of high osmolarity for use in elecron microscopy. *J. cell. Biol.* **27**, 137 A.

KELLY, A. M. & ZACKS, S. I. (1969). The histogenesis of rat intercostal muscle. *J. cell. Biol.* **42**, 135–153.

KORNELIUSSEN, H. & JANSEN, J. K. S. (1976). Morphological aspects of the elimination of polyneuronal innervation of skeletal muscle fibres in newborn rats. *J. Neurocytol.* **5**, 591–604.

LANDMESSER, L. & PILAR, G. (1972). The onset and development of transmission in the chick ciliary ganglion. *J. Physiol.* **222**, 691–713.

LANDMESSER, L. & PILAR, G. (1974). Synaptic transmission and cell death during normal ganglionic development. *J. Physiol.* **241**, 737–749.

LANDMESSER, L. & PILAR, G. (1976). Fate of ganglionic synapses and ganglion cell axons during normal and induced cell death. *J. cell Biol.* **68**, 357–374.

LANGLEY, J. N. (1890). On the physiology of the salivary secretion. *J. Physiol.* **11**, 123–158.

LETINSKY, M. (1974). The development of nerve-muscle junctions in *Rana catesbeiana* tadpoles. *Devl Biol.* **40**, 129–153.

LILEY, A. W. (1956). An investigation of spontaneous activity at the neuromuscular junction of the rat. *J. Physiol.* **132**, 650–666.

MAILLET, M. (1962). La technique de Champy á l'osmium-ioduré de potassium et la modification de Maillet á l'osmium-ioduré de zinc. *Trab. Inst. Cajal Invest. biol.* **54**, 1–36.

MATTHEWS, M. R. & NELSON, V. (1975). Detachment of structurally intact nerve endings from chromatolytic neurones of the rat superior cervical ganglion during depression of synaptic transmission induced by post-ganglionic axotomy. *J. Physiol.* **245**, 91–135.

MATTHEWS, M. R. & RAISMAN, G. (1969). The ultrastructure and somatic efferent synapses of small granule-containing cells in the superior cervical ganglion. *J. Anat.* **105**, 255–282.

MCMAHAN, U. J. & KUFFLER, S. W. (1971). Visual identification of synaptic boutons on living ganglion cells and of varicosities in post-ganglionic axons in the heart of the frog. *Proc. R. Soc. B.* **177**, 485–508.

MCMAHAN, U. J. & PURVES, D. (1976). Visual identification of two kinds of nerve cells and their synaptic contacts in a living autonomic ganglion of the mudpuppy (*Necturus maculosus*). *J. Physiol.* **254**, 405–425.

MULLER, K. J. & McMAHAN, U. J. (1976). The shapes of sensory and motor neurones and the distribution of their synapses in ganglia of the leech. A study using intracellular injection of horseradish peroxidase. *Proc. R. Soc. B.* **194**, 481–499.

MURRAY, J. G. & THOMPSON, J. W. (1957). The occurrence and function of collateral sprouting in the sympathetic nervous system of the cat. *J. Physiol.* **135**, 133–162.

NOETHER, G. E. (1971). *Introduction to Statistics – A Fresh Approach*, pp. 106–110. Boston: Houghton Mifflin.

NJA, A. & PURVES, D. (1978). The effects of nerve growth factor and its antiserum on synapses in the superior cervical ganglion of the guinea-pig. *J. Physiol.* (In the press.)

PURVES, D. (1975). Functional and structural changes of mammalian sympathetic neurones following interruption of their axons. *J. Physiol.* **252**, 429–463.

REDFERN, P. A. (1970). Neuromuscular transmission in new-born rats. *J. Physiol.* **209**, 701–709.

RONNEVI, L. O. & CONRADI, S. (1974). Ultrastructural evidence for spontaneous elimination of synaptic terminals on spinal motoneurons in the kitten. *Brain Res.* **80**, 835–839.

ROPER, S. (1976). An electrophysiological study of chemical and electrical synapses on neurones in the parasympathetic cardiac ganglion of the mudpuppy *Necturus maculosus*: evidence for intrinsic ganglionic innervation. *J. Physiol.* **254**, 427–454.

ROSENTHAL, J. L. & TARASKEVICH, P. S. (1977). Reduction of multiaxonal innervation at the neuromuscular junction of the rat during development. *J. Physiol.* **270**, 299–310.

ROTSHENKER, S. & McMAHAN, U. J. (1976). Altered patterns of innervation in frog muscle after denervation. *J. Neurocytol.* **5**, 719–730.

SIEGRIST, G., DOLIVO, M., DUNANT, Y., FOROGLOU-KERAMEUS, C., DE RIBAUPIERRE, Fr. & ROUILLER, Ch. (1968). Ultrastructure and function of the chromaffin cells in the superior cervical ganglion of the rat. *J. Ultrastruct. Res.* **25**, 381–407.

SNELL, R. S. (1958). The histochemical appearances of cholinesterase in the parasympathetic nerves supplying the submandibular and sublingual salivary glands of the rat. *J. Anat.* **92**, 534–543.

STRAUS, W. (1964). Factors affecting the cytochemical reaction of peroxidase with benzidine and the stability of the blue reaction product. *J. Histochem. Cytochem.* **12**, 462–469.

SZENTÁGOTHAI, J. (1957). Zum elementaren bau der interneuronalen Synapse. *Acta anat.* **30**, 827–841.

TAXI, J. (1965). Contribution à l'étude des connexions des neurones moteurs du système nerveux autonome. *Annls Sci. nat.* **7**, 413–674.

WILLIAMS, T. H. & PALAY, S. C. (1969). Ultrastructure of the small neurone in the superior cervical ganglion. *Brain Res.* **15**, 17–34.

EXPLANATION OF PLATES

PLATE 1

Neurones in the living submandibular ganglion viewed with differential interference contrast optics (× 880). Cellular details of the ganglion are readily visible. The nuclei and nucleoli (N) of the neurones are apparent, as are numerous nerve fibres (F). Schwann cells surround the neurones; their nuclei (SN) often cap the neurone cell bodies. The three neurones in this photomicrograph are part of a cluster of about fifteen cells.

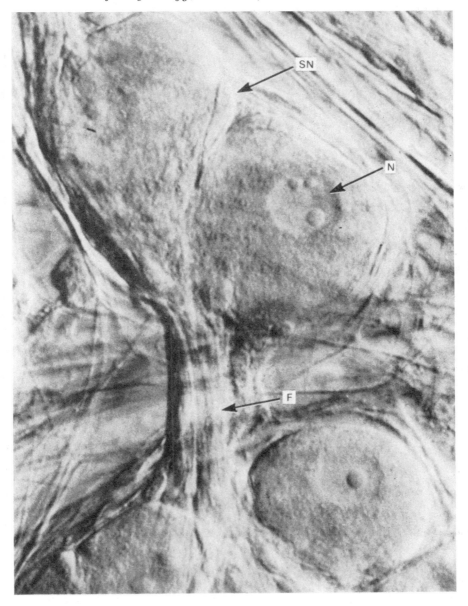

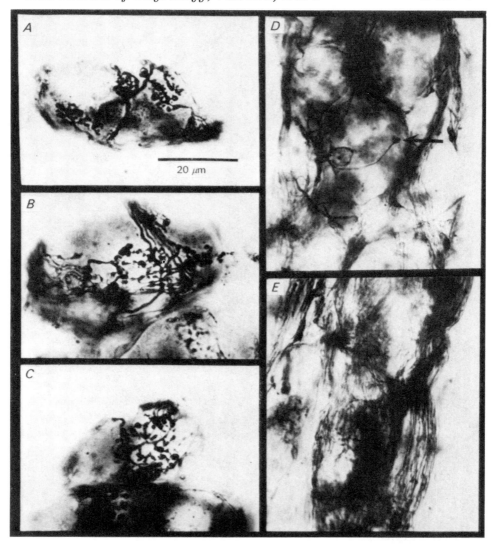

20 μm

J. W. LICHTMAN

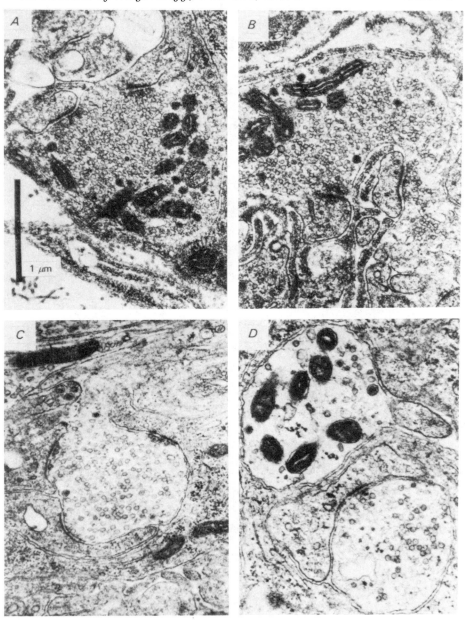

J. W. LICHTMAN

The Journal of Physiology, Vol. 273, No. 1   Plate 4

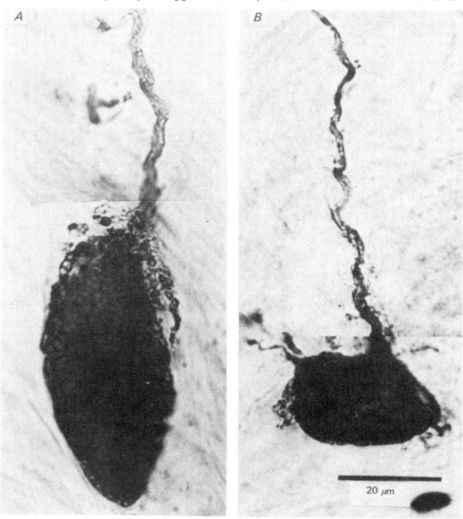

J. W. LICHTMAN

The Journal of Physiology, Vol. 273, No. 1   Plate 5

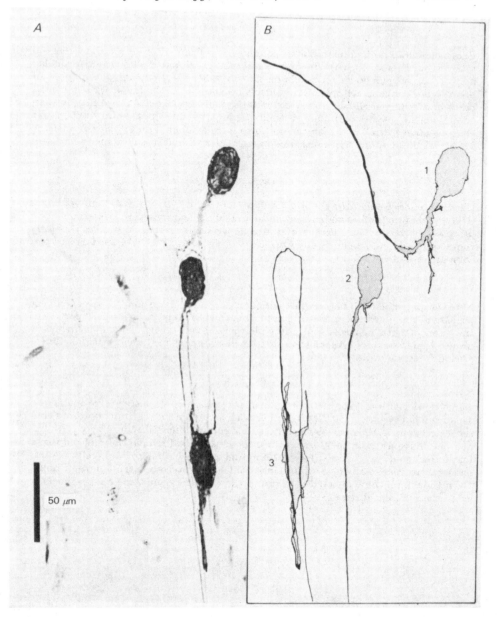

50 μm

J. W. LICHTMAN

PLATE 2

Photomicrographs of submandibular ganglion cells from adult (*A–C*) and 1-day-old rats (*D* and *E*) stained with zinc-iodide osmium. *A*, *B* and *C* show the pericellular network of preganglionic terminals on three adult cells. Counting the number of boutons per ganglion cell was often difficult because of the thickness of the terminal parts of the preganglionic fibres. Neonatal ganglia appeared quite different than adult ganglia treated with this method. Before the third post-natal week, fewer boutons (arrow in *D*) and many more fibres were evident than in older animals. A dense reticulum of fine fibres obscured much of the cellular detail on many neonatal cells (*E*).

PLATE 3

Electron micrographs of synaptic profiles from adult (*A*, *B*) and 2-day-old rats (*C*, *D*). Synaptic profiles on both neonatal and adult neurones were located on small processes within a few microns of the cell perimeter. Neonatal profiles generally contained fewer mitochondria and were less densely packed with vesicles (for example, compare *A* and *B* to *C* and *D*).

PLATE 4

Neurones injected with horseradish peroxidase from adult (*A*) and a 1-week-old rat (*B*). Many small protuberances originate from the cell body and the initial portion of the axon of both neonatal and adult neurones (see Text-fig. 3 for camera lucida drawings of these cells). Axons show no branches other than the short protuberances arising from the initial segment.

PLATE 5

Three neurones injected with horseradish peroxidase in a cluster of about fifteen cells from a 1-week-old rat (*A*), together with a camera lucida drawing of the cells separated from each other so that the axons can be followed more easily (*B*). The neurones have no axon collaterals within the cluster, and remain unbranched for as far as they could be followed (several hundred microns). Unlike adult cells, several neonatal neurones had one or more somewhat larger processes (cell 3, for example). Even though all three injected cells run to the salivary glands, their axons initially extend in different directions.

Phil. Trans. R. Soc. Lond. B. **278**, 377–409 (1977)   [377]
Printed in Great Britain

Plasticity of ocular dominance columns in monkey striate cortex

By D. H. Hubel, T. N. Wiesel and S. LeVay
Department of Neurobiology, Harvard Medical School,
25 Shattuck Street, Boston, Massachusetts 02115, U.S.A.

[Plates 1–12]

Ocular dominance columns were examined by a variety of techniques in juvenile macaque monkeys in which one eye had been removed or sutured closed soon after birth. In two monkeys the removal was done at 2 weeks and the cortex studied at $1\frac{1}{2}$ years. Physiological recordings showed continuous responses as an electrode advanced along layer IV C in a direction parallel to the surface. Examination of the cortex with the Fink–Heimer modification of the Nauta method after lesions confined to single lateral-geniculate layers showed a marked increase, in layer IV C, in the widths of columns belonging to the surviving eye, and a corresponding shrinkage of those belonging to the removed eye.

Monocular lid closures were made in one monkey at 2 weeks of age, for a period of 18 months, in another at 3 weeks for 7 months, and in a third at 2 days for 7 weeks. Recordings from the lateral geniculate body showed brisk activity from the deprived layers and the usual abrupt eye transitions at the boundaries between layers. Cell shrinkage in the deprived layers was moderate – far less severe than that following eye removal, more marked ipsilaterally than contralaterally, and more marked the earlier the onset of the deprivation. In autoradiographs following eye injection with a mixture of tritiated proline and tritiated fucose the labelling of terminals was confined to geniculate layers corresponding to the injected eye. Animals in which the open eye was injected showed no hint of invasion of terminals into the deprived layers. Similarly in the tectum there was no indication of any change in the distribution of terminals from the two eyes.

The autoradiographs of the lateral geniculates provide evidence for several previously undescribed zones of optic nerve terminals, in addition to the six classical subdivisions.

In the cortex four independent methods, physiological recording, transneuronal autoradiography, Nauta degeneration, and a reduced-silver stain for normal fibres, all agreed in showing a marked shrinkage of deprived-eye columns and expansion of those of the normal eye, with preservation of the normal repeat distance (left-eye column plus right-eye column). There was a suggestion that changes in the columns were more severe when closure was done at 2 weeks as opposed to 3, and more severe on the side ipsilateral to the closure. The temporal crescent representation in layer IV C of the hemisphere opposite the closure showed no obvious adverse effects. Cell size and packing density in the shrunken IVth layer columns seemed normal.

In one normal monkey in which an eye was injected the day after birth, autoradiographs of the cortex at 1 week indicated only a very mild degree of segregation of input from the two eyes; this had the form of parallel bands. Tangential recordings in layer IV C at 8 days likewise showed considerable overlap of inputs, though some segregation was clearly present; at 30 days the segregation was much more advanced. These preliminary experiments thus suggest that the layer IV C columns are not fully developed until some weeks after birth.

Two alternate possibilities are considered to account for the changes in the ocular dominance columns in layer IV C following deprivation. If one ignores the above evidence in the newborn and assumes that the columns are fully formed at birth, then after eye closure the afferents from the normal eye must extend their territory, invading the deprived-eye columns perhaps by a process of sprouting of terminals. On the other hand, if at birth the fibres from each eye indeed occupy all of layer IV C, retracting to form the columns only during the first 6 weeks or so, perhaps by a process of competition, then closure of one eye may result in a competitive disadvantage of the terminals from that eye, so that they retract more than they would normally. This second possibility has the advantage that it explains the critical period for deprivation effects in the layer IV columns, this being the time after birth during which retraction is completed. It would also explain the greater severity of the changes in the earlier closures, and would provide an interpretation of both cortical and geniculate effects in terms of competition of terminals in layer IV C for territory on postsynaptic cells.

INTRODUCTION

Physiological experiments in cats and monkeys visually deprived from a young age indicate a certain amount of plasticity in central-nervous pathways, especially at the cortical level. The nature of this plasticity is unclear. Connections present at birth can certainly be made non-functional as a result of deprivation, but whether there are actual morphological changes is not known. Neither is it known whether deprivation can lead to abnormal connections, either through sprouting or by the pathological persistence of connections that exist at birth and normally disappear postnatally.

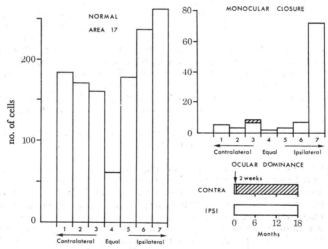

FIGURE 1. Ocular dominance histograms in normal and monocularly deprived macaque monkeys. Histogram on the left is based on 1256 cells recorded from area 17 in normal adult and juvenile rhesus monkeys. Cells in layer IV C are excluded. Histogram on the right was obtained from monkey no. 3 of the present series; the right eye was closed from 2 weeks to 18 months, and recordings were then made from the left hemisphere. Shading in histogram indicates cells with abnormal responses. (Cells in group 1 are driven exclusively from the contralateral eye, those in group 7 exclusively from the ipsilateral, group 4 cells are equally influenced, and the remaining groups are intermediate.)

In cats and monkeys deprived of vision in one eye by lid suture early in life, the cells in area 17 come to be strongly dominated by the eye that remained open (Wiesel & Hubel 1963, 1971; Baker, Grigg & von Noorden 1974). This is illustrated in figure 1 (left), an ocular dominance histogram from a series of experiments in normal adult monkeys, and (right) in a histogram from a monkey deprived by monocular suture at 2 weeks of age for a period of 18 months. The takeover by the good eye at the expense of the bad seems to be due largely to competition between the two eyes, since closing both eyes produces effects that are far milder than would be predicted if the binocular closure were equal to the sum of two monocular closures (Wiesel & Hubel 1965). The idea that competition is involved was borne out by the effects of monocular deprivation on geniculate responses, since here the physiological changes are rather mild, possibly because at this stage the inputs from the two eyes are largely kept separate, anatomically and physiologically, with little chance for competition. There is, to be sure, considerable cell shrinkage throughout the layers connected to the closed eye, except for the monocular crescent representation, but this may be secondary to a deterioration, through competition, of terminals in the cortex, and not a direct result of a lessening of input from the deprived eye (Guillery & Stelzner 1970; Guillery 1972a).

In the macaque monkey, binocular convergence in area 17 is delayed beyond what are probably the first and second synaptic stages (Hubel & Wiesel 1968). Cells representing both these stages, with concentric receptive fields and 'simple' fields, are located in layer IV and are perhaps confined to that layer. The bulk of the geniculate afferents terminate in the deep part of layer IV (layer IV C), where they segregate themselves into a series of roughly parallel alternating stripes, one set connected to the left eye, the other to the right. Given the apparent lack of convergence of input from the two eyes onto single cells in layer IV, we were anxious to learn whether monocular deprivation would result in a redistribution of the afferent terminals to layer IV, or whether the boundaries would prove to be relatively immutable, as they seem to be in the lateral geniculate body. From the outset, in our studies of monocular deprivation in monkeys, we had been struck by the normality of the cortex in Nissl stains, and particularly by the absence of any hint of bands of cell atrophy in layer IV C to parallel the marked cell shrinkage in the deprived geniculate layers. This suggested that the geniculate and cortical layers were reacting in a very different way to deprivation.

We began by recording from layer IV C in monocularly deprived monkeys (lid sutured or enucleated). In addition to the technique of physiological recording there now exist three independent morphological methods for demonstrating ocular dominance columns (Hubel & Wiesel 1972; Wiesel, Hubel & Lam 1974; LeVay, Hubel & Wiesel 1975), and we were anxious to use these in examining the deprived cortex. It turned out that the physiological and the three anatomical methods all revealed very marked abnormalities, with clear evidence for an expansion of one set of columns at the expense of the other set. We also studied the distribution of geniculo-cortical terminals at birth, to learn whether the increase in the size of the columns corresponding to the open eye involved the formation of new connections or a regression of connections present at birth.

METHODS

Ten macaque monkeys were used, of which 9 were rhesus (*Macaca mulatta*) and one, no. 7, a pig-tailed macaque (*M. nemestrina*). The procedures used in these animals are summarized in table 1. Two monkeys had one eye removed at 2 weeks of age; three had the lids of one eye sutured at 2 days–3 weeks of age, and four served as controls. Results from one of the normal monkeys (no. 6) have already been published (Wiesel, Hubel & Lam 1974). In another control (no. 7), a 4½-year-old adult, the right eyelids had been sutured at 2½ years of age, and reopened 6 months later; behavioural testing showed no visual defects in the eye that had been sutured, and this animal was therefore assumed, for our purposes, to be normal.

TABLE 1

no.	identifying nos. and dates	pages	figs.	procedure	age when procedure done	age studied	physiology	Nauta	autoradiography	reduced silver
eye removals:										
1	LM 50, 19 June 1972		2, 4b, 6, 7	eye removal (rt)	2 weeks	19 months	×	×	—	—
2	LM 57, 17 Jan. 1974		3	eye removal (rt)	2 weeks	18 months	×	×	—	—
lid closures										
3	LM 58, 23 Apr. 1974 157		1, 8a, 9, 11 14–18	lid closure (rt)	2 weeks	18 months	×	×	× (normal eye inj.)†	×
4	202, 23 Dec. 1974		8b, 10, 19–21, 27	lid closure (rt)	3 weeks	3 weeks / 7 months	at 3 weeks / at 7 months	—	× (deprived eye inj.)† / —	—
5	201		22	lid closure (rt)	2 days reopened 7 weeks	7 months	—	—	× (deprived eye inj.)†	×
controls										
6	197, 28 Aug. 1973 (W. H. & L.)		—	normal	—	juvenile	—	—	× (left eye inj.)‡	—
7	186, 21 Aug. 1974		12, 13	late lid closure (rt)	2½ years reopened 3 years	4¼ years	—	—	× (rt eye inj.)†	×
8	209, 30 Jan. 1975		—	normal	—	juvenile (LGB cell size)	—	—	—	—
9	230		23–25	normal	left eye inj. at 1 day	1 week	—	—	× (left eye inj.)§	—
10	243, 30 Oct. 1975		26	normal	—	8 days	×	—	—	—

† 1 mCi L-proline [2,3-³H(N)], S.A. 30–50 Ci/mmol, and 1 mCi L-fucose [6-³H], S.A. 10–15 Ci/mmol, in 100 µl normal saline.
‡ 1.5 mCi proline and 1.5 mCi fucose.
§ 2 mCi fucose.

The lids of an infant monkey are surprisingly translucent; measurements showed that they attenuate light by about 0.5 log units. The lid tissue is nevertheless cloudy enough to prevent any dark-light contours from falling on the retinas.

Brains were examined by one or more of four procedures:

(1) *Nauta method* (Hubel & Wiesel 1972). In some animals electrolytic lesions were placed with microelectrodes in single laminae of the lateral geniculate nucleus; the brains were perfused four days later, cut in frozen section at 30 μm and stained by the Nauta–Fink–Heimer–Wiitanen method (Wiitanen 1969).

(2) *Autoradiography* (Wiesel *et al.* 1974). In six monkeys, one eye was injected with 2.0 mCi of a mixture of tritiated proline and tritiated fucose or with tritiated fucose alone. The brains were perfused 14 days later, and 25 μm thick frozen sections were prepared for autoradiography.

(3) *Liesegang stain* (Le Vay *et al.* 1975). Other sections were examined by a reduced-silver stain, which has been shown to reveal ocular dominance columns in layer IV in normal juvenile or adult monkeys.

In conjunction with these special morphological procedures, every fourth section was stained by a Nissl method (Cresyl Violet), and also some of the autoradiographs were counterstained for Nissl substance. Cell size was determined in the lateral geniculate and in layer IV of the cortex by measuring cross sectional areas of neuronal somata in which nucleoli were visible. Planimetry was done on the profiles traced in camera lucida, using an *X-Y* tablet.

(4) *Neurophysiology*. Finally, most of these animals were recorded from. In the monkeys used for Nauta-degeneration studies, the geniculate lesions were placed by electrophysiological monitoring of the electrode position. On these occasions we also looked for possible abnormalities in the responses, and for any signs of spread of influence of the open eye beyond its normal territory. In the cortex, recordings were made at an acute angle to the surface, usually at 30–40°. Because of the gentle convex curvature of the exposed part of area 17, the electrode tended to become more and more tangential as it advanced, so that if ideally positioned it took a course precisely tangential to layer IV or V (see figure 3). This usually required several attempts, with the electrode either first missing layer IV completely or traversing it at too steep an angle to allow the recording of more than one eye-dominance shift. Each shift was marked by an electrolytic lesion (1 μA × 1 s; d.c., electrode negative). Recording procedures were otherwise the same as described previously (Hubel & Wiesel 1968).

RESULTS: PART I. EYE REMOVAL

In the first two monkeys of the present series one eye was enucleated rather than lid-sutured in order to maximize the likelihood of producing changes in the cortical columns. In retrospect such a drastic operation was not necessary, but it provided an opportunity to compare the effects of enucleation and eye closure. In these two animals the Nauta–Fink–Heimer was the only anatomical method used.

Lateral geniculate body

Physiology

Recordings were made in the lateral geniculate bodies of the two eye-enucleated monkeys (nos. 1 and 2), primarily in order to position the electrode for making electrolytic lesions in the normal and deafferented layers, but also to learn whether the deafferented layers had been invaded by fibres from the normal eye. Without this knowledge it was obviously difficult to interpret any possible changes in the cortex.

In the geniculate contralateral to the normal eye, entrance of the electrode into the most dorsal layer was indicated by rich unit activity and brisk responses to visual stimulation. This persisted for about 0.5 mm; the electrode then suddenly entered a virtually silent region, with no hint of responses to stimulation of the normal eye and almost no spontaneous activity. As the electrode was further advanced a region of rich activity with brisk responses was again suddenly encountered, and was followed, again, by a silent region. This sequence of events of course reflected the passage of the electrode first through a normal layer, then through a deafferented one, and so on, as expected from the well-known layering pattern of the geniculate. The position of the electrode in a given layer was later verified histologically. The results suggest that there was no significant reinnervation of cells in the deafferented layers by terminals from the normal eye.

Histology

As expected from previous studies (Minkowski 1920; Matthews, Cowan & Powell 1960) there was profound transneuronal atrophy of cells in the deafferented layers. This can be seen in figure 2, plate 1, for monkey 1, whose right eye was removed at 2 weeks and the brain examined at 18 months. The results of measurements of the cross sectional areas in the normal and deprived layers in the eye-removal and eye-sutured monkeys are given in table 2; the ratio of areas in the two sets of layers (average of the two sides) was 2.80 for monkey no. 1 and 1.86 for no. 2, the large values in both cases reflecting the severity of the atrophy. (We have no explanation for the difference in these values.) The atrophy was uniform through the entire thickness of each deprived layer, with an abrupt transition from atrophic to normal at the boundaries between layers supplied by opposite eyes. This by itself suggests an absence of any extensive reinnervation of the deprived layers by the remaining eye. Both physiological and anatomical results thus indicate that enucleation shortly after birth caused a permanent deafferentation of the corresponding geniculate layers, with no extensive sprouting between layers.

DESCRIPTION OF PLATE 1

FIGURE 2. Coronal sections through lateral geniculate bodies of monkey no. 1, whose right eye was removed at 2 weeks, and the brain examined at 19 months. Brain embedded in celloidin; cresyl violet stain.

FIGURE 3. Electrode track in a tangential penetration through the left striate cortex of monkey no. 2; right eye removed at 2 weeks and the recordings made at 18 months. The electrode passed antero-posteriorly through layer IV C for a total of 3.7 mm, during which responses were continuously obtained from the remaining (left) eye. Cresyl violet. Anterior is to the right; parasagittal section. Circle at end of track indicates electrolytic lesion.

FIGURE 4. Dark-field photographs of Nauta–Fink–Heimer stained striate cortex in monkeys following lesions confined to a single geniculate layer. (*a*) Normal monkey, following lesion in layer 6 of the left geniculate. (monkey no. 12 in Hubel & Wiesel 1972; cf. figure 5 of present paper and Figures 7–10 in Hubel & Wiesel 1972). (*b*) 19-month-old monkey in which right eye was removed at 2 weeks (monkey no. 1 of present paper.) Lesion was in layer 3 of left geniculate, this layer being innervated from the remaining (normal) eye; cf. figure 6. Each photograph includes white matter, near the bottom, but does not quite reach layer I above. In *a* the band of degeneration in IV C is about equal in width to the gap between. In *b* the gap between bands is ill defined and smaller than the band to the right.

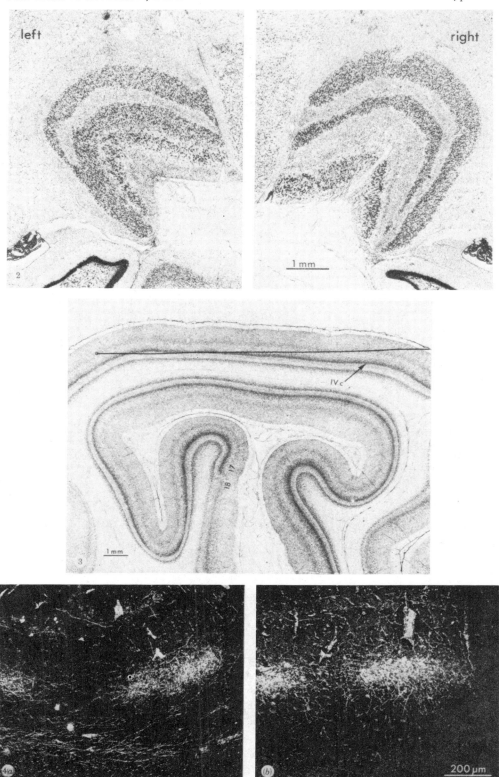

FIGURES 2–4. For description see opposite.   *(Facing p.* 382)

Striate cortex

Physiology

In the normal macaque monkey striate cortex the geniculate afferents associated with the two eyes are segregated as they terminate in the IVth layer in such a way that cells innervated by the left and right eyes form parallel alternating bands about 400 μm wide. This is the basis for the ocular dominance columns, regions in which one or other eye dominates, and which are most sharply defined in layer IV C but extend through all layers of the cortex. Thus in a typical tangential penetration the electrode moves from a region in which one eye gives the best

TABLE 2. COMPARISONS OF GENICULATE CELL SIZES AND OF CORTICAL COLUMN AREAS

			(lateral geniculate body 50 cells/layer)				cortex. ratio of column areas‡
monkey no.	side	layer	mean area μm²	s.d. μm²	ratio‖	significance†	
1. rt. eye removal	L	6	*51*§	12	2.65	< 0.01	
		5	135	36			
	R	6	159	33	2.94	< 0.01	
		5	*54*	14			
2. rt. eye removal	L	6	*91*	15	1.87	< 0.01	
		5	170	33			
	R	6	171	28	1.84	< 0.01	
		5	*93*	12			
3. rt. eye closure	L	6	*128*	31	1.44	< 0.01	2.77
		5	·184	45			
	R	6	150	29	1.48	< 0.01	—
		5	*108*	28			
4. rt. eye closure	L	6	*156*	33	1.26	< 0.01	1.60
		5	197	46			
	R	6	184	37	1.20	< 0.01	1.97
		5	*154*	36			
7. 'control' (late closure right eye)	L	6	*196*	42	1.04	N.S.	
		5	188	39			
	R	6	229	53	1.18	< 0.01	1.05
		5	*194*	48			
8. control	L	6	*268*	68	1.04	N.S.	
		5	258	68			
	R	6	248	70	1.12	< 0.02	
		5	*280*	54			

† Welch test.   ‡ Swollen/shrunken (see table 3).   § Right eye layer italics.   ‖ Larger/smaller.

responses to another in which the other eye dominates. In the IVth layer the cells are strictly monocular and their segregation according to eye input is very sharp; consequently transitions here are extremely abrupt. If there is any overlap at all, the regions must be 25 μm or less. In all our normal material we have seen no difference in widths of bands innervated by the contralateral as opposed to the ipsilateral eye: in the binocular part of area 17 (i.e. outside the representation of the temporal crescents) the two eyes seem to make almost exactly equal contributions. This equality is doubtless related to the symmetry suggested by the left histogram of figure 1, in which groups I–III are about as well represented as groups V–VII.

In the enucleated animals we were mainly interested in learning whether any changes had taken place in this arrangement of layer IV C ocular-dominance bands. If not, then in a tangential penetration one should expect an alternation between silent regions and regions of responsiveness to the remaining eye, as was found in the lateral geniculates of these animals. The results, in fact, were very different. Figure 3, plate 1, shows the reconstruction of a long (13.3 mm) tangential penetration through the striate cortex of monkey no. 2. In the layers above IV all of the cells encountered responded normally to stimulation of the remaining (left) eye. This was not entirely unexpected, since normally the majority of these cells are binocularly innervated. What was more surprising was to find that the cells in layer IV responded well to left-eye stimulation over the entire 3.7 mm during which the electrode was in that layer (3.0 mm entering the cortex, and 0.7 mm leaving). The recordings were typical for layer IV C, showing rich background activity, responsive cells with centre-surround receptive fields, and no clear tendency for the cells to prefer oriented line stimuli. There were no silent areas, only some waxing and waning of the evoked activity as the electrode advanced, perhaps more than is seen normally.

In the other eye-removal monkey (no. 1), the two penetrations in area 17 gave results that were consistent with this in showing continuous responses through the entire extent of layer IV C. The angle to the surface was too steep and the distance traversed in layer IV therefore too short to permit any conclusions to be drawn from this animal alone, but taken together, the results from monkeys nos. 1 and 2 suggested an expansion of the territory occupied by the columns of the normal eye at the expense of the set corresponding to the enucleated eye. One might, of course, explain the continuous IVth layer activity by supposing that the electrode had approached this layer in a direction almost parallel to the borders separating the bands, and had stayed in a single left-eye band throughout the entire penetration. In many previous tangential penetrations in normal monkeys we have never, in fact, recorded so long a sequence of cells dominated by one eye. In any case, the anatomical results to be described below rule out such an explanation.

Morphology

An apparent disappearance of ocular-dominance stripes in layer IV C, in physiological recordings, could conceivably be due not to a takeover by the good eye, but rather to a simple dropping out (i.e. death) of the cells in these stripes, with either an absolute shrinkage of cortex to half its surface area or a spreading out of the remaining layer IV C cells together with an associated thinning of the layer. A routine examination of the morphology of the striate cortex using a Nissl stain failed to show any hint of such changes (figure 3); the total extent of the striate cortex was normal, there was no obvious reduction in thickness or cell density in any of the layers, and layer IV C appeared uniform along its horizontal extent, with cells of normal size. In short, any reorganization had taken place in such a way as to leave no trace in routine histology.

In a previous study in normal monkeys the ocular dominance stripes in layer IV were visualized and reconstructed in serial sections by making lesions restricted to single laminae in the lateral geniculate body and later staining the cortex for degenerating terminals by a modified Nauta method (Hubel & Wiesel 1972). In any one section in these normal monkeys there were patches of terminal degeneration interrupted by equally wide patches with no degenerating terminals. Figure 4a, plate 1, shows an example of the cortical degeneration pattern in a normal monkey after a small lesion restricted to the most dorsal geniculate layer. Regions of layer IVC containing terminals are sharply delineated from the terminal-free gaps, which are bridged by only an occasional degenerating afferent axon running between one zone of degenerating terminals and another. Figure 5 shows a serial reconstruction of the entire, necessarily relatively small, area of cortex containing degenerating terminals, to illustrate the characteristic striped pattern of normal ocular dominance columns, each with a width of about 400 µm (Hubel & Wiesel 1972, Figs. 8 and 10).

Similar single-layer lesions were made in both enucleated animals. Figure 4b shows the result of a geniculate lesion in layer 3 of monkey no. 1, on the left side, ipsilateral to (and innervated by) the normal eye. In contrast to what was found in the normal animals, the

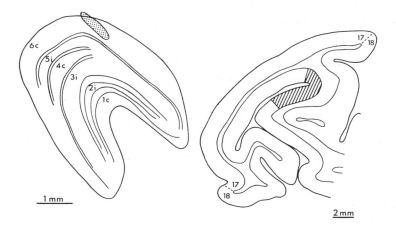

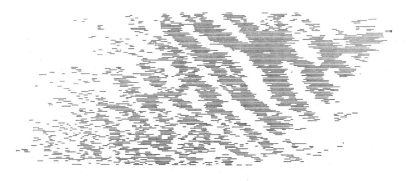

1mm

FIGURE 5. Normal monkey. Reconstruction of cortical area of Nauta degeneration, made from 121 serial parasagittal sections. The projection site in area 17, shaded in the drawing on the upper right, corresponds to the layer 6 geniculate lesion on the upper left. Each interrupted horizontal line in the reconstruction is derived from a single cortical section, by graphically straightening the shaded part of the mushroom shaped calcarine cortex, and tracing the regions of degeneration (cf. figure 4a). When these lines are assembled the result is a surface view of layer IV C bands, which appear as roughly parallel stripes separated by equal-size gaps, with a repeat distance of about 0.8 mm (Hubel & Wiesel 1972, monkey no. 12, Figures 8–10).

terminals in the cortex were distributed over virtually the entire region receiving input from the area of the lesion. Within this region there were variations in the density of degeneration, but gaps free of degenerating endings were only occasionally seen and were usually ill-defined and small, only a fraction of the size of the terminal-free gaps seen normally. A typical gap is shown in figure 4b. Except for the waxing and waning and the small gaps in terminal degeneration, the picture was reminiscent of the continuous degeneration seen after a lesion in a normal monkey involving two adjacent dorsal layers (Hubel & Wiesel 1972).

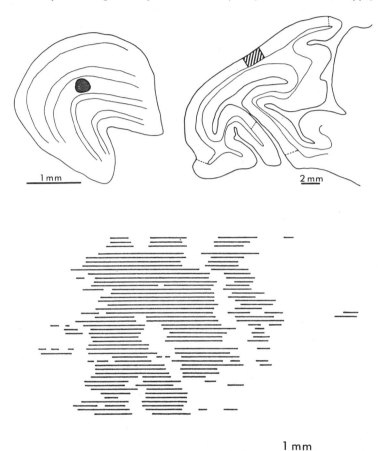

FIGURE 6. Reconstruction of an area of terminal degeneration similar to that of figure 5, but in a 19-month-old monkey (no. 1) in which the right eye was removed at 2 weeks. Lesion in layer 3 of the left lateral geniculate, supplied by the left (normal) eye. Compared with figure 5, the regions of degeneration in the reconstruction are mostly much wider and the gaps narrower, the repeat distance being unchanged.

A serial reconstruction of the entire region of terminal degeneration associated with this lesion, in monkey no. 1, is shown in figure 6. No attempt has been made to illustrate the variation in terminal density; the regions free or almost free of degenerating fragments have simply been shown as gaps. A striped pattern is strongly suggested, with a drastic narrowing of one set of stripes and a probable widening of the other. The combined widths of the expanded and shrunken columns, assuming a 30 % shrinkage in processing the tissue, is roughly 800 µm, a value close to the normal (see below).

Lesions in this monkey were also made in geniculate layer 6 on the side contralateral to the enucleated eye, i.e. a deafferented layer. The resulting degeneration in the cortex was very weak, and was confined to small narrow patches separated by wide regions with no degeneration. The picture was thus the complement of that observed after a lesion in a layer corresponding to the surviving eye. A reconstruction of one of these projection areas is shown in figure 7.

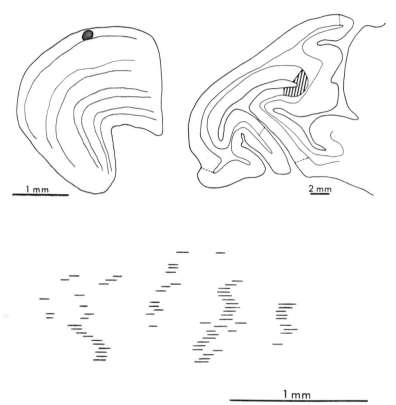

FIGURE 7. Reconstruction similar to that of figure 6 and in the same monkey, following a lesion in a deafferented geniculate layer (no. 6 on the left side). Now the areas of degeneration are shrunken and the gaps widened.

Very similar results were found in monkey no. 2 both for normal layer lesions and for deafferented layer lesions.

Thus in both the recordings and the Nauta degeneration studies it was as though the geniculate afferents serving the normal eye had invaded and virtually taken over the layer-IV territory of the enucleated eye. As Part II shows, similar results were found in animals with prolonged lid suture. Part III, however, will present evidence that casts doubt upon the notion of an invasion of one region by another, at least in any literal sense.

27-2

PART II. MONOCULAR LID SUTURE

In three monkeys (table 1, nos. 3–5) the lids of one eye were sutured closed in the first few weeks of life. Nos. 3 and 4 were expressly prepared to examine the results of long standing deprivation. No. 5 was part of a study on the time course of sensitivity to deprivation: an eye was closed from 2 days to 7 weeks and then reopened, and the animal was examined at 7 months. This monkey is mentioned in the present paper as a further illustration of monocular deprivation effects, because there is little likelihood that the reopening of the eye had any influence on the outcome.

Four control animals (nos. 6–10) are included: nos. 6 and 7 provide examples of normal cortical autoradiography; no. 7 (also part of the time-course study) had a six month period of monocular closure at $2\frac{1}{2}$–3 years, but no abnormalities were found in a variety of behavioural tests; no. 8 was used for determination of normal geniculate cell size; nos. 9 and 10 represent a preliminary study of eye dominance columns in newborn and very young monkeys.

For the animals with eye closure two new methods were available for demonstrating ocular dominance columns, besides physiological recording and Nauta degeneration. These were, first, transneuronal autoradiography (Wiesel, Hubel & Lam 1974), in which radioactive compounds are injected into one eye and the cortex later examined autoradiographically for label transported up to layer IV of the striate cortex. The second method depends on preparing of sections tangential to layer IV C with a reduced-silver stain (LeVay *et al.* 1975). The four methods – physiological recording, Nauta degeneration, autoradiography, and reduced-silver stain – are entirely independent, relying as they do on a nerve fibre's ability to conduct impulses and on synaptic integrity, on degeneration following injury, on axonal transport, and on the ability of certain fibres to take up a particular stain.

Lateral geniculate body

Physiology

In monkeys with monocular eye closure one could observe responses from the deprived geniculate layers to stimulation of the eye that had been closed – something that was obviously impossible in the eye removal animals. Lateral-geniculate recordings were made only in monkey no. 3, in the course of making lesions for the Nauta degeneration studies. About a dozen cells were recorded from the deprived layers: these seemed to have normal receptive field properties, giving vigorous responses to stimulation with small spots. Transitions from normal to deprived layers and back, as judged by responses, were abrupt, with no hint in the deprived layers of any driving from the normal eye. The sample of unit recordings was obviously too small and our examination too cursory to permit any conclusions except that there were no gross physiological abnormalities, and no signs of invasion of the deprived layers by the fibres from the normal eye.

Histology: Nissl studies

Nissl stained sections through the lateral geniculate bodies of monkeys nos. 3 and 4 showed moderate pallor and shrinkage in the layers corresponding to the deprived eye. These results are thus similar to those seen by Headon & Powell (1973). Not surprisingly, the changes were far less marked than those following eye removal. The black and white photomicrographs of figure 8, plate 2, are perhaps deceptive, however, since they show the changes much less vividly than would be expected from simple inspection of the sections at low power, perhaps because

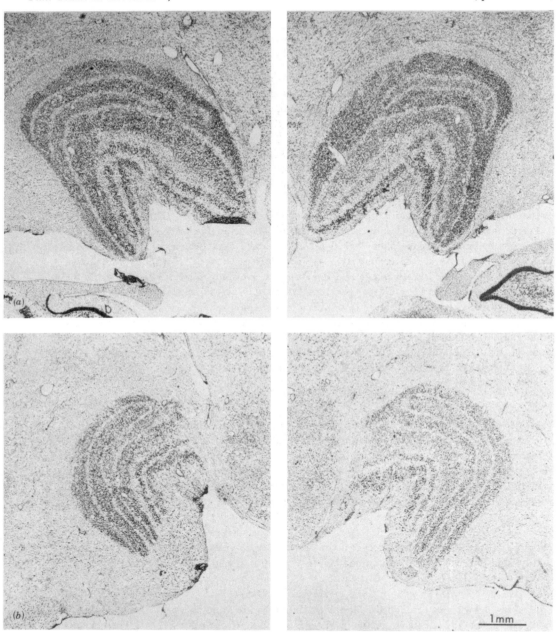

FIGURE 8. Coronal Nissl-stained sections through lateral geniculates of (*a*) Monkey no. 3, right eye closed at
2 weeks for 18 months. (*b*) Monkey no. 4, right eye closed at 3 weeks for 7 months. Note that the atrophy of
the layers receiving input from the closed eye is more marked on the ipsilateral (right) side and more marked
in *a* than in *b*. Cresyl violet; frozen sections.

(Facing p. 388)

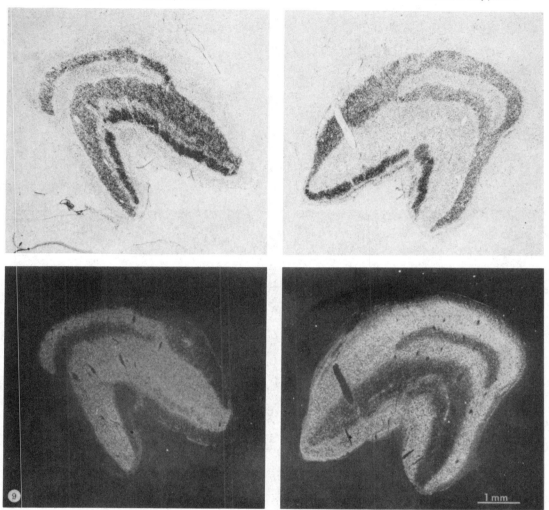

FIGURE 9. Autoradiographs of geniculates from monkey no. 3 (right eye closed at 2 weeks for 18 months) following injection of label into *left* (normal) eye. Coronal sections. Upper half, light-field, counterstained with cresyl violet. Lower half, dark-field of same sections. Note the band of label between classical layers 3 and 2, in the dark-field picture on the right (compare figure 24, layer *d*).

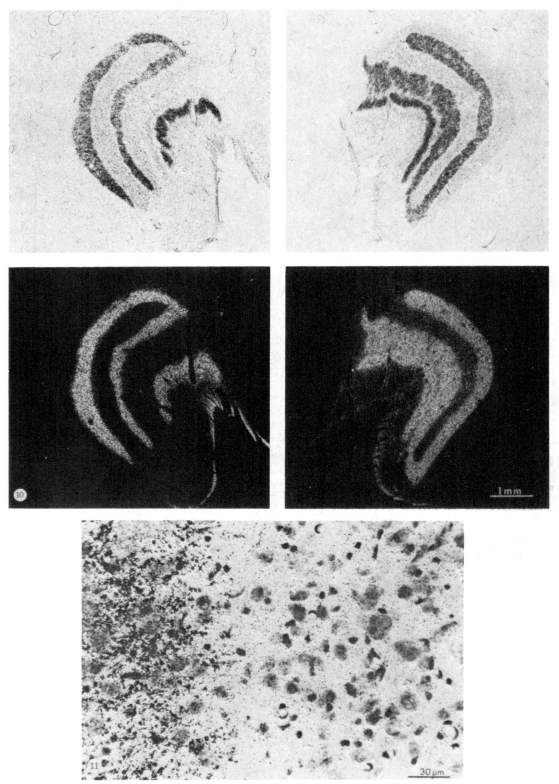

Figures 10 and 11. For description see opposite.   *(Facing p.* 389)

the colours help bring out the differences in staining between normal and deprived layers. Measurements of cell size are given in table 2: the ratio of cross sectional areas in presumably normal *vs.* deprived layers was 1.46 : 1 for monkey no. 3 and 1.23 : 1 for no. 4. This is to be compared with an average of 2.33 : 1 for the two eye-removal monkeys.

That the deprivation effects were more severe in monkey no. 3 than in no. 4 can be seen both in figure 8 and in the cell measurements. In the cortex, as described below, the effects were likewise more severe in monkey no. 3. These differences could either be related to the week's difference in the time of eye closure or to the difference in duration of closure. Other results in the cortex of deprived and newborn monkeys suggest, however, that in eye closures lasting more than a few months the time of closure is more important than the duration.

In both of these eye sutured animals (nos. 3 and 4) the geniculate changes were most marked on the side ipsilateral to the suture – indeed, in the contralateral sections of monkey no. 4 (figure 8) it is not easy to see the changes at all. A similar asymmetry was seen by Headon & Powell (1973). Curiously, no difference between the sides showed up in the cell measurements, perhaps again because mild effects are expressed more in cell pallor than in shrinkage. A difference in susceptibility of the two sides, with more severe effects ipsilaterally, has been observed in many monkeys besides those of the present series. It also occurs in the cortical columns (see below), and there seems to be little doubt that it is genuine. (The interpretation of the apparently significant difference in a control monkey (table 2, no. 7), in cell sizes of layers 5 and 6 on the right side, is not clear.)

In describing the differences in cell size in the various pairs of layers it has been tacitly assumed that it is shrinkage in the closed-eye layers that produces the disparity. Whether there is an enlargement of cells in the normal-eye layers is difficult to determine because of the large variations in average cell size from one brain to the next, related possibly to small differences in technique. Obviously this is a question of some interest, given the increase in width of the corresponding cortical columns, to be demonstrated below.

Histology: autoradiography

In monkeys nos. 3, 4 and 5 one eye was injected with radioactive label. The resulting autoradiographs in the lateral geniculate bodies are illustrated in darkfield, in figure 9, plate 3, for monkey no. 3 and figure 10, plate 4, for no. 4. There was heavy labelling of the appropriate layers, even in monkey no. 4, whose closed eye had been injected. In both animals the label in the layers corresponding to the non-injected eye was only slightly above background levels. This is well seen in figure 11, plate 4, a higher power light-field photomicrograph from the geniculate of monkey no. 3 (normal eye injected). Here the deprived layer, to the right, showed none of the grain clumps which indicate the positions of the optic nerve terminals belonging to

---

DESCRIPTION OF PLATE 4

FIGURE 10. Autoradiographs from geniculates of monkey no. 4 (right eye closed at 3 weeks, for 7 months) following injection of label into *right* (lid-sutured) eye. Upper half, light field; lower half, dark field, of same sections. Counterstained with cresyl violet.

FIGURE 11. Higher power light-field view of right lateral geniculate of monkey no. 3 (compare figure 9). Layer 6 (the most dorsal layer) is to the left, layer 5 to the right, with the relatively cell sparse interlaminar leaflet between. Note the abrupt fall-off in grains, particularly in the large clumps of grains presumably representing terminals, at the boundary between layer 6 and the leaflet, indicating a lack of any noticeable invasion of the deprived layer by terminals from the normal eye.

the injected eye. Thus the autoradiography gave no indication of transgression of terminals beyond the normal boundaries. Obviously this was important in interpreting possible changes in the cortical columns.

A consistent finding in these autoradiographs of the lateral geniculate body was an accumulation of grains in several regions besides the classical 6 layers. In figure 9 one can see a bilateral accumulation of grains in a narrow band between layers 2 and 3, best seen on the left in light field, and on the right in dark field. Also there is a band of grains of contralateral origin ventral to layer 1 on the right, best seen in light field, and a clump of ipsilateral origin near the hilum, interrupting and lying ventral to layer I (left, dark field). Higher power examination suggested that the grains were mostly in terminals rather than in fibres. These additional inputs to the geniculate were not seen at more caudal levels (figure 9). They are discussed further in Part III, where similar aggregations are described in a normal newborn animal.

Superior colliculus

The distribution of optic-nerve terminals from the two eyes in the superior colliculus takes a very special form (Hubel, LeVay & Wiesel 1975). In the superficial grey, where the bulk of the input ends, the contralateral terminals tend to make up a continuous band whose lower half frequently contains cavities, and whose lower border is irregular and scalloped. The ipsilateral terminals tend to form a row of clumps which are concentrated at a level matching these holes and scallops; thus they appear to be embedded in the deep part of the contralateral input. Towards the foveal representation the ipsilateral input also comes close to the surface, in patches that appear to alternate with the contralateral input. On the whole the contralateral input probably exceeds the ipsilateral, and while the extent to which the two overlap is not clear anatomically, recordings indicate that the two eyes are not kept entirely separate.

We were curious to learn whether the eye closures had produced any changes in this patchy distribution of terminals, and especially whether there were signs of an expansion of the territory of one eye or contraction of that belonging to the other. Autoradiographs showed no hint of any changes: as in the geniculates, the distribution of terminals was normal in monkeys nos. 3 and 4. In sections counterstained with cresyl violet an examination of cells showed no hint of shrinkage or change in cell packing density in regions which from the autoradiography were known to receive input from the closed eye. Thus from the anatomical studies the superior colliculi seemed to be normal. We have not made recordings in the colliculi of deprived monkeys.

Striate cortex

Control monkeys (nos. 6 and 7): morphology

The brains of monkeys nos. 3, 4 and 7 were cut in tangential sections in the region of the exposed striate cortex (the operculum). Brains of monkeys nos. 3, 4, 6 and 7 were also cut in sections that were either parasagittal or in a plane tipped back 45° from the coronal; in most places they were roughly perpendicular to cortex, and passed through the calcarine fissure. We begin by showing autoradiographs of presumably normal cortex (monkeys nos. 6 and 7) following injection of one eye.

The transverse section from monkey no. 7, shown in figure 12a, plate 5, is perpendicular to the occipital operculum (i.e. to the exposed surface of the occipital lobe) and to part of the underlying calcarine fissure: almost all of the cortex in this section is striate, ipsilateral to the injected eye. Layer IV as expected shows a series of patches rich in label (brightly glowing in this

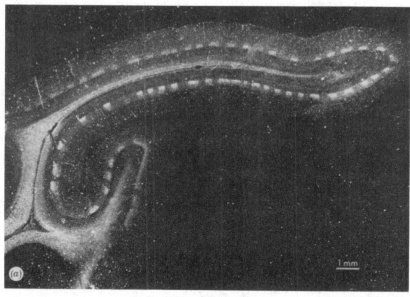

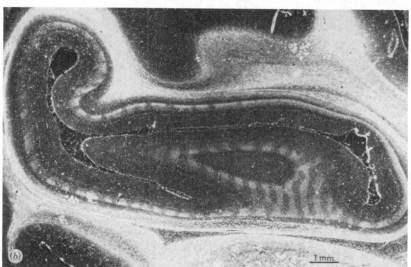

FIGURE 12. Dark-field autoradiographs of striate cortex in normal adult monkeys following right-eye injection of radioactive fucose-proline mixture 2 weeks before. (*a*) Transverse section through right striate cortex, perpendicular to occipital operculum, in a plane normal to the sagittal, tipped back from coronal by about 45°. Labelled bands can be clearly made out in layer IV C. In the finger-like gyrus, the opercular cortex above and the superior bank of the calcarine fissure below are separated by a brightly labelled continuous band; this represents the optic radiations. (The lower bank of the calcarine fissure has fallen away.) Medial is to the right. (Monkey no. 7.) (*b*) Parasagittal section through the buried calcarine cortex contralateral to the injected eye; most of the cortex is cut in a plane perpendicular to the layers, but one fold is intersected tangentially, and here the layer IV C columns are seen as parallel bands. The upper tier in layer IV A can just be made out in most places. The stretch of continuous label in layer IV C in the upper right part of the ring represents the temporal crescent. Anterior is up and to the right; the operculum would be just to the left of the figure. (Monkey no. 6.)

(*Facing p.* 390)

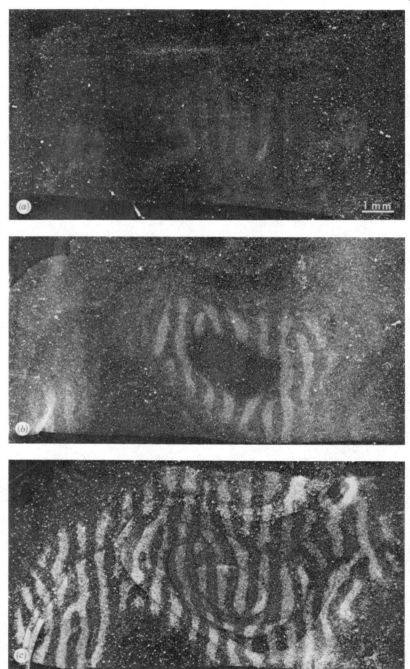

FIGURE 13. Normal monkey (no. 7). Autoradiographs taken in dark field, of tangential sections through the dome shaped exposed surface of the right occipital lobe (operculum), ipsilateral to the injected (right) eye. The section shown in (*a*) passes tangential to layer IV C, which is seen as a series of light stripes, representing the labelled right-eye columns, separated by gaps of the same width representing the left eye. (*b*) is some 160 μm deeper than *a*, passing tangential to layer V and showing layer IV C as a ring of dark and light stripes into which the oval of *a* can be fitted. (*c*) is a reconstruction made by fitting together eight parallel sections including those of *a* and *b*. Anterior is up, medial to the left.

darkfield photograph) interrupted by label free gaps. In this figure about 56 pairs of columns can be counted.

Figure 12*b* shows a parasagittal section through the calcarine fissure of monkey no. 6, contralateral to the injected eye. Layer IVC is cut in most places transversely, forming a large irregular ring surrounding a smaller one, again with patches of label separated by gaps as in figure 12*a*. To the lower right the two rings join, and here IVC is cut tangentially, forming parallel stripes arranged in an oval (as occurs in figure 13). The upper right part of the outer ring of layer IVC in the figure is continuously labelled: this is the temporal crescent representation, with input entirely from the far peripheral temporal visual field of the contralateral eye.

TABLE 3. ESTIMATION OF COLUMN AREAS

monkey no.	hemi-sphere	eye injected	eye closed	combined width μm	ratio†	shrinkage deprived columns (%)	ratio‡	shrinkage deprived columns (%)
3 (157)	left	left	right	892	2.24	38	2.77	47
4 (202)	left	right	right	817	1.45	18	1.60	23
	right	right	right	831	1.61	23	1.97	33
7 (186) ('control')	right	right	(right)§	848	1.05	—	1.05	—

† Determined from small regular patches within reconstruction.
‡ Determined from virtually the entire reconstructions (figures 13, 15, 20).
§ Closed at aged 2½ years for 6 months, probably without effect.

Tangential sections through the operculum ipsilateral to the injected eye of monkey no. 7 are shown in figure 13, plate 6. The opercular cortex is dome shaped, and a plane of section that is tangential to a particular layer shows that layer as a circular patch or oval; deeper planes of section show the layer as an annulus. The section of figure 13*a* just grazed layer IVC, which appears as an oval region of alternating dark and light stripes, surrounded by the more superficial layers. Figure 13*b* is taken at a slightly deeper level, and layer IVC appears as a ring made up of stripes, surrounding the deeper layers and surrounded by the more superficial ones.

Successively deeper sections through the operculum produced larger and larger IVC rings. By photographing every second or third section, cutting out layer IVC in each and superimposing them, it was possible to reconstruct the columns over a considerable area. The result is shown in figure 13*c*. The pattern is highly regular, with a tendency for the stripes to intersect the 17–18 border at a 90° angle. This border is near the top of figure 13*c*, where the stripes end abruptly.

In this reconstruction, for comparisons with the deprived animals, calculations were made to determine the repeat distance for columns, i.e. the combined width of a left-eye column and an adjacent right-eye column. For this purpose we traced a number of regular roughly rectangular portions of the reconstruction, each containing an even number of stripes, between four and eight, avoiding areas where stripes forked or terminated. The two long edges of the block were chosen so that they fell along stripe borders. The areas of the blocks were determined by weighing. By dividing the area of each block by the total length of column pairs (number of pairs × length of block) one could estimate the repeat distance. Table 3 shows the results for monkey no. 7 and also for eye-closed monkeys nos. 3 and 4 (see below). The repeat distance for monkey no. 7 was 848 μm.

The relative areas occupied by the two sets of columns were estimated from the reconstruction of figure 13*c* by tracing the borders, cutting apart the two sets, and weighing them. The difference in weight amounted to 5 %, the contralateral set exceeding the ipsilateral (table 3, ratio‡). This difference is probably not significant. Similar determinations were made from the selected regular blocks described above, with a difference again of 5 % (table 3, ratio†). This figure agrees well with a similar comparison made previously using the reduced silver method in another monkey (LeVay *et al.* 1975). Thus the anatomy and physiology both suggest that in the binocular representation of striate cortex the contributions of the two eyes are about equal.

Monkey no. 3: physiology

In this monkey the right eye was closed from 2 weeks to age 18 months. The left eye was then injected. A week later 5 lesions were made in the right lateral geniculate body for Nauta studies. A week after that, finally, four penetrations were made in a direction almost parallel to the layers, in an effort to have long traverses through layer IV so that points of eye transition could be noted and marked with electrolytic lesions. In two of the penetrations (nos. 2 and 3) the tilt was sufficient so that more than one eye transition occurred in layer IV.

As expected from the eye-removal results and from previous work in cats, the great majority of cells were strongly dominated by the normal eye. In the layers outside of IV only about one-fifth of cells were influenced from the deprived eye, many of these weakly but with the normal orientation specificity. The ocular dominance histogram from this monkey has already been shown in figure 1. (A detailed account of the physiological properties of the cells in these animals will be presented elsewhere.)

In layer IV C, on the contrary, there were periods in which the activity was dominated strongly or completely by the deprived eye. The transitions from dominance by one eye to dominance by the other were as abrupt as in normal monkeys. In regions of domination by the deprived eye the responses seemed, surprisingly, to be quite normal, with the usual briskness and lack of any orientation specificity. These regions were nevertheless all distinctly shorter than those in which the normal eye dominated. Both the micromanipulator readings and the

---

DESCRIPTION OF PLATE 7

FIGURE 14. Reconstruction of two penetrations, P_2 and P_3 through the left striate cortex in monkey no. 3. Both penetrations were almost tangential to the surface, aimed in a roughly mediolateral direction through the operculum and placed 1 mm apart. (Autoradiographs and reduced-silver sections from the same region are shown in figures 15 and 17.) At the top are shown the reconstructions made from micrometer depth readings. Dots numbered 1–6 represent lesions made in layer IV while withdrawing the electrode, at the points of passing from one eye's territory to that of the other eye. L and R indicate the dominant eye where only one eye evoked responses: R(L) means that the right eye dominated but the left evoked a lesser response from the multiunit activity. Middle portion shows a cresyl-violet stained tangential section roughly in the plane of the penetrations, passing through the centre of lesion 6 and almost through the centres of 1 and 5. No. 6 is clearly in layer IV C, as were 1, 2 and 5, when the appropriate sections were examined. Lower section, a reduced-silver fibre stain (LeVay *et al.* 1975), passing through the centre of lesion 4 and just missing the centre of 3. Both are at the border of layers IV B (which contains most of the densely-staining line of Gennari) and IV C. This section is not ideally placed to show the columnar banding: a more superficial section at lower power appears in figure 17.

FIGURE 15. This figure is the counterpart of figure 13, in monkey no. 3, whose right eye was closed from age 2 week to 18 months. Left hemisphere operculum: (*a*) is tangential to layer IV C, (*b*) is 200 μm deeper, and (*c*) is the result of cutting and pasting 9 such sections, representing a total depth of 900 μm. Label in IV C, representing input from the normal eye, is in the form of swollen bands which in places coalesce, obliterating the narrow gaps which represent the columns connected to the closed eye. The thin, almost continuous belt of label in the upper tier (IV-A) is seen in all three parts. The six dots in (*c*) represent the positions of the six lesions of figure 14, identified on neighbouring cresyl-violet or reduced-silver sections and superimposed on the autoradiographs. The lesions are clearly at or close to the column boundaries.

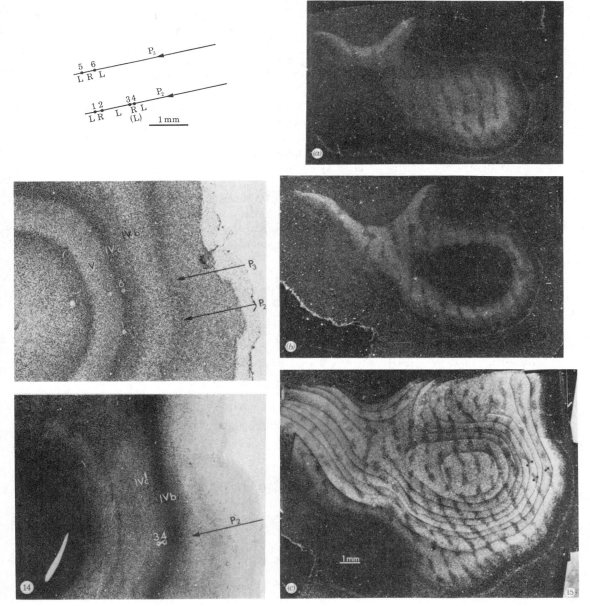

FIGURES 14 AND 15. For description see opposite.

(*Facing p.* 392)

613

histological reconstruction showed that the spans in the left (normal) eye regions were 2–3 times as long as the spans in the right-eye regions. This is illustrated in figure 14a, plate 7, which shows the relation between penetrations 2 and 3, and the lesions made at the transition points. Both penetrations were made in the left hemisphere, from medial to lateral. The lesions were made on withdrawing the electrode so that the points of transition could be checked – hence the order of the lesion numbers. Figure 14b shows a Nissl-stained section almost in the plane of the penetrations and thus almost parallel to the surface, passing through the centre of lesion 6 and just missing the centres of 1 and 5. Appropriate sections through their exact centres demonstrated that lesions 1, 2, 5 and 6 were all well within layer IVC, and that lesions 3 and 4 were at the border between IVB and IVC, as seen in the fibre-stained section of figure 14c.

Throughout all of the left-eye (nondeprived) columns no activity could be evoked from the right (deprived) eye. In the right-eye dominated columns weak but clearly audible responses could be heard in the span between lesions 3 and 4. This is not surprising, given that these lesions were made on the IVB–IVC border, since in normal animals the eye segregation in layer IVB is not as strict as in layer IVC. In the deeper right (deprived) eye segments (1–2 and 5–6) the left eye was silent.

In summary, there were small regions within layer IV in which cells were actively driven and strongly dominated by the deprived eye, in contrast to the virtual absence of influence of that eye in the upper layers. Within layer IVC there was a striking and consistent difference in the distances the electrode travelled in the two sets of columns.

Monkey no. 3: morphology

Two neighbouring opercular sections are shown in figure 15a and b, plate 7, and a reconstruction from nine neighbouring sections including these two is shown in figure 15c. Confirming the results of the recordings, the labelled columns (normal eye) are very much wider than normal, and the gaps (closed eye) are very much narrower. Comparing figures 13 and 15 it is evident that the repeat distance – the combined widths of two neighbouring columns, one from each eye – is roughly the same in the two animals. Measurements made as described above for monkey no. 7 showed a combined width (repeat distance) of 892 μm, as opposed to 848 μm for the control (table 3). (Unlike the millimetre scales on the illustrations, which refer to distances on the microscopic slides, these figures have been calculated from the histology by assuming a 30% shrinkage. This is only a rough estimate based on reconstructions of electrode tracks in other animals, but the comparison is valid, provided the brains have shrunk roughly equally.) The fact that the repeat distance was apparently unchanged in monkey no. 3 is consistent with the conclusion that the expansion of one set of columns is complemented by a contraction of the other. In addition to being reduced in width the deprived columns were pinched off at irregular intervals of a millimetre or so.

The relative areas occupied by the labelled columns and the gaps were estimated by the methods outlined above for the normal. Taking the entire reconstruction and cutting apart the left-eye and right-eye regions the result was a ratio of 2.77:1 for labelled columns to unlabelled ones, as compared with 1.05:1 for the normal (table 3, ratio‡). The ratio from selected regular blocks, calculated as for monkey no. 7 (table 3, ratio†), was lower, amounting to 2.24:1. The lower ratio presumably resulted partly from the omission of pinched off areas, in selecting these blocks.

We found that electrolytic lesions of the rather miniscule size necessary to mark the points of transition from one eye to the other, in the physiological recordings, were impossible to identify in dark-field autoradiographs. They were easily found, however, in the Nissl and reduced-silver sections that were interspersed between the autoradiographs (see figure 14), so that comparison of adjacent sections made it possible to determine their precise position on the autoradiographs, with respect to the column boundaries. These are marked in figure 15c.

An autoradiograph through the calcarine fissure (figure 16, plate 8) likewise showed gaps, between labelled regions, that were markedly shrunk and in places almost obliterated. The section is taken from the side ipsilateral to the closed eye. Though it is difficult to compare the severity of shrinkage on the two sides, given the difference in planes of section, our impression from this and other examples is that deprivation effects were more marked on the side ipsilateral to the closed eye (compare figures 21a and 21b).

The reduced-silver stains gave results that faithfully paralleled the autoradiographs and the physiology. The bands corresponding to columns in layer IV could be seen only in tangential or very oblique sections, and were seen best at very low power in the upper part of IV C, just beneath the line of Gennari. In figure 17, plate 8, an alternation of wide (W) and narrow (N) dark bands can easily be seen. The narrow bands were clearly identified as corresponding to the deprived columns, and the wide bands to the non-deprived, by noting their positions with respect to the lesions in penetrations 2 and 3, and to the columns as shown in the autoradiographs.

Another abnormality observed in the reduced-silver sections was the appearance of broad pale bands (P) in layer V, where normally no banding is visible. These bands, which stand out clearly in the central part of figure 17, were in register with the set of shrunken ocular dominance columns just above, in layer IV C. Similar bands could be seen, though less clearly, in

---

DESCRIPTION OF PLATE 8

FIGURE 16. Monkey no. 3; right eye closed from 2 weeks to 18 months. Left eye injected. Dark-field autoradiograph through right calcarine cortex. Over the mushroom, label representing input from the contralateral (normal) eye has almost obliterated the gaps, representing the deprived eye, and greatly narrowed them even where they are best preserved, in the dorsal stem. Anterior is up and to the right.

FIGURE 17. Monkey no. 3. Reduced-silver stained section parallel to those of figure 15, and 40 μm deep to the section of figure 15b. The Gennari Line, layer IV B, appears as the most densely stained black ring. Dark bands corresponding to the layer IV C columns are best seen in the most superficial part of IV C, i.e. just deep to IV B or the Gennari Line – in this section just inside the dark ring. These bands are alternatingly wide (W) and narrow (N). In autoradiographs neighbouring this section, such as the one shown in figure 15b, the labelled (bright) columns were found to correspond precisely to the wide bands and the unlabelled (dark) gaps to the narrow bands. Still further inside the Gennari ring is a prominent light area, the cell-dense part of layer IV C; within this is layer V, with its pale bands (P) in register with the narrowed dark bands of IV C (N).

FIGURE 18. Monkey no. 3. The results of making a lesion in the right lateral geniculate nucleus, confined to layer 3, a layer corresponding to the closed eye. The lesion and electrode track are shown in the cresyl-violet section in a. The resulting Nauta degeneration was deep in the calcarine fissure, no more than one or two small patches occurring in any one section. One such patch of terminals is shown in the dark field photograph in c. The next section to this was dipped for autoradiography, with the result shown in b: here layer IV C is almost continuously labelled except for a narrow gap at the knee where the calcarine stem joins the mushroom. Sections b and c were superimposed, and in d the region showing Nauta degeneration is indicated by white, in the autoradiograph. The two regions match precisely, except that the Nauta degeneration appears only in bottom half of IV C (IV C β), as expected following a parvocellular geniculate lesion.

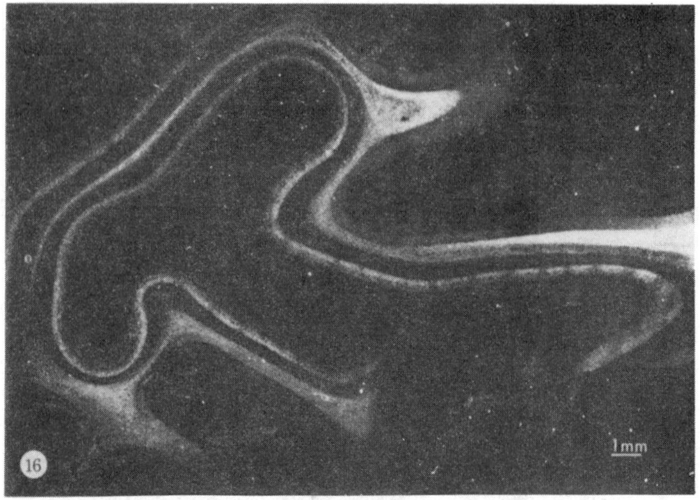

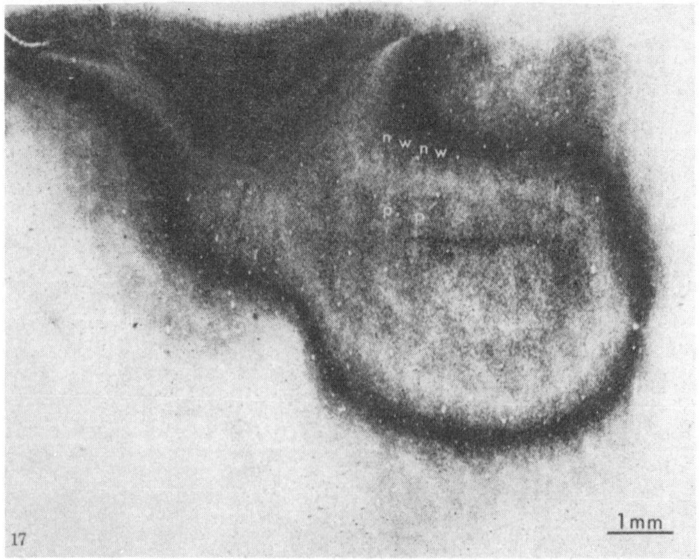

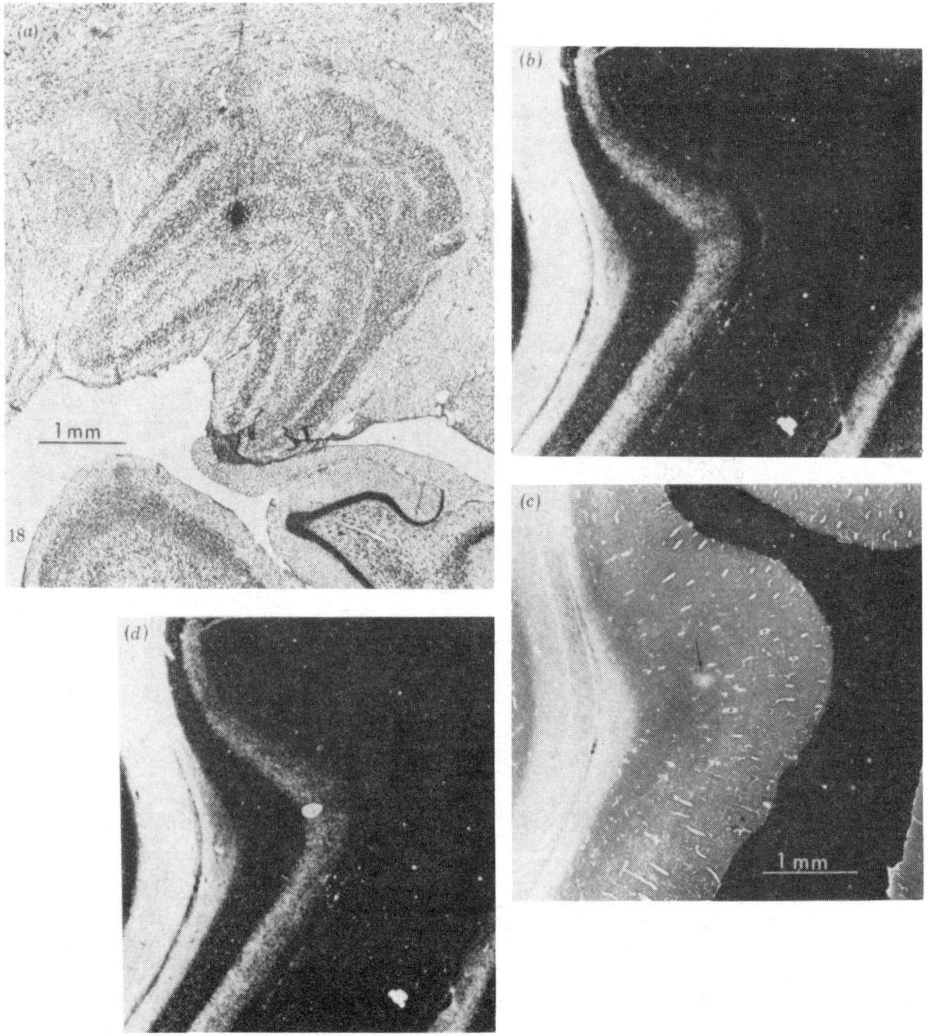

FIGURES 16–18. For description see opposite.

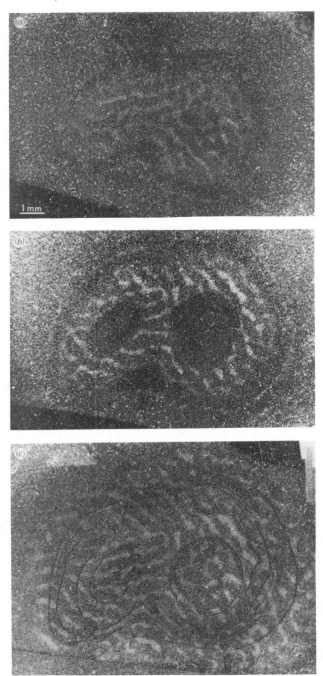

FIGURE 20. This is the counterpart of figures 13 and 15, for monkey no. 4; right eye closed at 3 weeks, until age 7 months; right eye injected. Dark-field autoradiographs of right occipital operculum. (*a*) tangential to layer IV C; (*b*) 120 μm deeper than *a*, tangential to layer V and intersecting it twice because of dimple in cortex. (*c*) reconstruction made up of 7 sections including *a* and *b*; total depth 640 μm. The labelled columns, corresponding to the closed eye, are markedly shrunken.

layer III. Close inspection of layer V showed that within the pale bands the tangential fibres were of abnormally fine calibre. The tangential fibre plexus of layer V consists largely of collaterals of the descending axons of layer III pyramidal cells (Spatz, Tigges & Tigges 1970; Lund & Boothe 1975). These observations thus suggest a deterioration of descending connections between layers III and V within the deprived-eye columns.

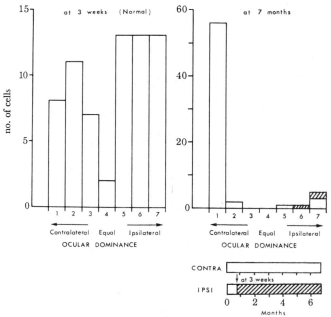

FIGURE 19. Ocular dominance histograms from striate cortex of monkey no. 4, at 3 weeks, when the right eye was closed, and in a second recording session at age 7 months. The histogram at 3 weeks (right hemisphere) is similar to the adult histogram (figure 1). After the deprivation the histogram is as expected strikingly abnormal, and almost identical to that of monkey no. 3 (see figure 1). Here four penetrations were made, three on the right side and one on the left. 'Ipsilateral' refers to domination by the right (deprived) eye. Shading in histogram indicates cells with abnormal responses.

Finally, we were anxious to determine the degree of overlap (if any) between the widened and the apparently narrowed columns of this animal. The recordings, as described above, indicated that the deprived-eye columns were reduced, and no activity was evoked from the deprived eye in the normal-eye columns in layer IV C, suggesting that there was little or no overlap. Autoradiographs from normal-eye injections by themselves could obviously prove nothing about the width of the stripes corresponding to the closed eye, and we wished to confirm morphologically the impression from the physiology-plus-lesions (figure 14, 15c) that the gaps in the autoradiographic picture did actually represent the deprived-eye columns. Two studies in which deprived eyes were injected support this contention (see below), but for more direct evidence Nauta studies were made in monkey no. 3, and the results were correlated with the results of the autoradiography.

Five geniculate lesions were made in the hemisphere ipsilateral to the removed eye, 1 each in layers 1, 3, and 4, and two lesions in layer 6, and for three of these lesions the corresponding regions of degenerating terminals in the cortex were found. Figure 18a, plate 8, shows a lesion in geniculate layer 3, which receives input from the closed eye, and figure 18c (lower right) a Nauta-stained section from the corresponding region in the calcarine fissure. A single focus of degenerating terminals is conspicuous deep in layer IVC (arrow). This could be followed in neighbouring sections, and represented a wormlike structure 150 μm wide, extending some 400 μm in a direction normal to the plane of the section.

An autoradiograph made from the section immediately neighbouring that of figure 18c is shown in figure 18b. The gap between labelled columns corresponds precisely to the region of terminal degeneration (figure 18d), providing a welcome mutual confirmation of the two methods. The fact that the space taken by degenerating fibres in the Nauta section and the size of the gap in the autoradiograph were roughly the same suggests, as had the recordings, that there was little if any overlap between the inputs from the normal and abnormal eyes.

Figure 18d shows that the terminal degeneration in layer IV following this dorsal-layer geniculate lesion was confined to the deeper half of layer IVC (IVCβ), in agreement with what was found in a previous study (Hubel & Wiesel 1972). The radioactive label following eye injection of course occupied the full thickness of IVC, since both dorsal and ventral geniculate layers were involved in the transport.

The remaining lesions were made in geniculate layers corresponding to the open eye. In all of these the corresponding degeneration in the cortex resembled that found in the eye-removal monkeys (figure 6) and was present only in portions of layer IVC which, in the autoradiographs, were occupied by silver grains.

Monkey no. 4: physiology

The right striate cortex of this monkey was recorded from twice, at 22 days, at which time the right eye was sutured closed, and then at 7 months, after just over 6 months of deprivation. On the first occasion 66 cells were recorded in two penetrations. The ocular dominance histogram was entirely normal by adult standards, as may be seen by comparing the histogram from these two penetrations (figure 19) with that of figure 1 for the normal adult. The results of this recording session will be described in more detail in Part III.

The ocular-dominance histogram at 7 months is shown to the right in figure 19. Four penetrations were made, all tangential. Again, cells from layer IVC are not included. (We wished to study layer IV in detail, and therefore recorded as many cells as possible from it. The inclusion of these cells would have greatly increased the number of cells in groups 1 and 7.) The pronounced effects of the eye closure on the upper and lower layers is obvious, as can be seen by comparing the two parts of the figure.

DESCRIPTION OF PLATE 10

FIGURE 21. Monkey no. 4, dark field autoradiographs through calcarine cortex, (a) contralateral to the closed, injected eye, (b) ipsilateral to the injected eye Note that the deprived columns are more severely shrunken on the ipsilateral side. The temporal-crescent representation is very conspicuous in a, and seems not to be affected at all.

FIGURE 22. Monkey no. 5; right eye closed at 2 days for a period of 7 weeks, then reopened up to the age of 7 months, when the right eye was injected and the brain examined 2 weeks later. Dark-field autoradiograph, transverse section through ipsilateral calcarine fissure. Labelled columns are markedly reduced in width in layer IVC, but comparatively intact in the upper tier, IVA.

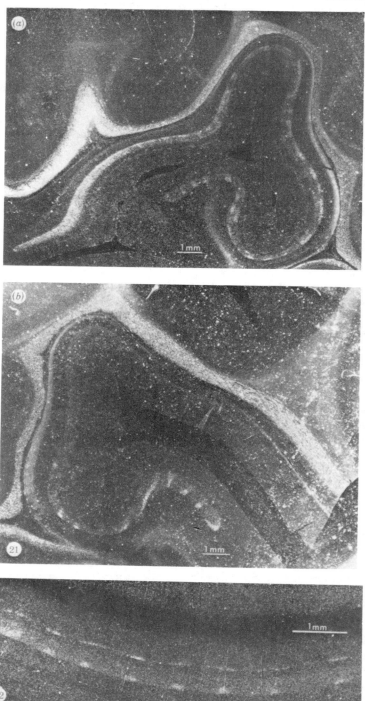

FIGURES 21 AND 22. For description see opposite.　　　*(Facing p.* 396)

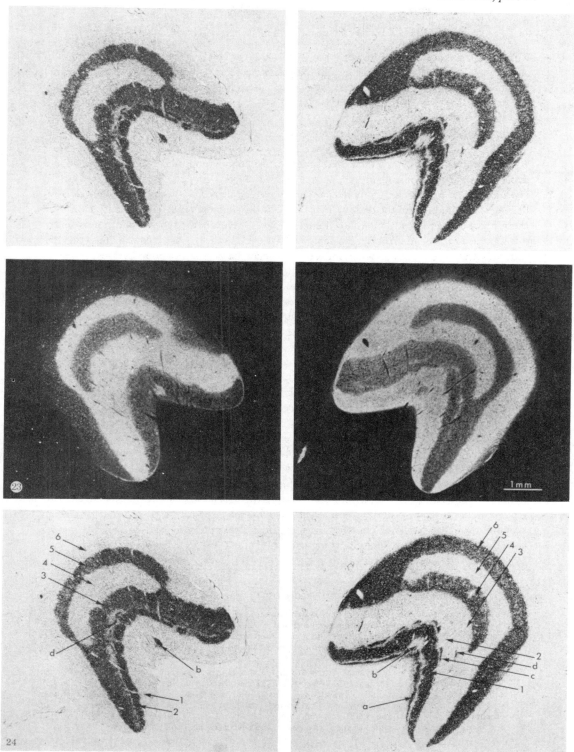

FIGURES 23 AND 24. For description see opposite.

In all four penetrations the activity recorded from layer IV C was strictly monocular, and in one of these penetrations the positions of six lesions made at the points of transition matched the column boundaries as revealed in subsequent autoradiography (compare figure 15c).

Monkey no. 4: morphology

This monkey differed from monkey no. 3 in that the deprived (right) eye, rather than the normal one, was injected. Also the eye was closed at 3 weeks instead of 2, and the closure lasted 7 months rather than 18 (see table 1). Sections of the operculum ipsilateral to the injected and deprived eye are shown in figure 20, plate 9. Part *a* shows a single section which just grazed layer IV C, and *b* shows a slightly deeper section cutting layer V in two places, presumably reflecting some dimpling of the cortex; here IV C has the shape of an 8. These sections form the central part of the reconstruction shown in figure 20c. Cutouts of the two sets of columns on this side showed a ratio of areas, normal to deprived, of 1.97:1 (table 3). On the contralateral side this ratio was 1.60:1, suggesting, as in monkey no. 3, that the side ipsilateral to the closed eye was the more severely affected.

The calcarine cortex of the two hemispheres is shown in figure 21, plate 10, contralaterally (A) and ipsilaterally (B); again there is a suggestion that in the ipsilateral hemisphere the labelled columns are narrower than in the contralateral. In addition one can see that the deep part of layer IV C (IV Cβ) is labelled much more heavily than the superficial. This difference is seen in normal monkeys, but seems more pronounced here, while it might be taken to mean that the IV Cα component is more susceptible than IV Cβ to deprivation effects, the results in monkey no. 3 (see figure 16) suggest, if anything, the very reverse. In the geniculate, furthermore, there was no indication that the magnocellular layers, which correspond to IV Cα, were more atrophic than the parvocellular. This is in agreement with the findings of Headon & Powell (1973).

In figure 21a, plate 10, a long continuous expanse of layer IV label can be seen over the anterior stem of the calcarine fissure in the region known to represent the part of the visual field temporal periphery that is visible only to one eye (temporal crescent). This label is at least as heavy as in any of the shrunken deprived-eye columns elsewhere on the same slide, and occupies as extensive an area of cortex as it does in the normal monkey. It thus seems that the temporal-crescent representation is little affected by the deprivation procedure. This again supports the suggestion that the effects of monocular deprivation depend on competition between the two eyes rather than simple disuse.

DESCRIPTION OF PLATE 11

FIGURE 23. Normal newborn monkey (no. 9). Autoradiographs of lateral geniculate bodies. The left eye was injected at 1 day of age and the brain examined at 1 week. Upper part, light field, lower, dark field. The label in the layers corresponding to the right, non-injected eye is denser than the background but is in fibres rather than terminals. Several layers other than the six classical ones can be identified; these are indicated in figure 24.

FIGURE 24. Monkey no. 9; same as light-field part of figure 23. Nine regions of input have been identified. In addition to the two classical magnocellular layers, 1 and 2, and the four parvocellular (dorsal) layers, 3, 4, 5, and 6, one can see two thin leaflets *a* and *c*, both contralaterally supplied, the one dorsal to 1 and the other ventral to it; a thin leaflet *d*, sandwiched between the dorsal four and the ventral two classical layers, and probably receiving input from both eyes; and finally a clump of label *b* (ipsilaterally supplied) between *a* and 1, which shows up as a labelled region on the left, and a label-free space on the right.

In this monkey the reduced-silver sections showed no banding, perhaps because the animal was too young. (The method has so far been successful only in animals a year or more old.) No geniculate lesions were made, and consequently no Nauta preparations were available.

Monkey no. 5 (201): Morphology

This animal is included as a second example of monocular closure with deprived eye injected. The right eye was closed at 2 days and opened at 7 weeks, and the animal lived up to an age of 7 months. A more complete description of this monkey will be given as part of a separate paper on duration of the sensitive period and extent of recovery. The opercular autoradiographs were unsatisfactory, showing almost no label, probably because of uneven distribution of the injected material in the eye. A part of the calcarine cortex was labelled, however, and is shown in transverse section in figure 22, plate 10. We include this monkey here because it forms an almost exact complement to monkey no. 3 (figure 16), with the deprived eye injected instead of the normal. Again, as in monkey no. 4, layer $IVC\alpha$ seems more severely affected than $IVC\beta$, in apparent contradiction to what was seen in monkey no. 3.

TABLE 4. CELL DENSITY AND SIZE, MONKEY NO. 3, LAYER $IVC\beta$, R.H.†

column type	density (cells/ 2500 μm²)	mean area (μm²)	(s.d.)	significance (Welch test)
normal	31	48	8.9	N.S.
deprived	30	48	11.1	
normal	33	50	11.8	p < 0.05
deprived	23	41	10.7	
normal	22	54	12.9	N.S.
deprived	37	54	14.6	
normal	29	50	9.6	N.S.
deprived	26	49	8.4	
total:	(cells/ 10 000 μm²)			
normal	115	50		N.S.
deprived	116	49		

† 4 pairs of samples from normal and deprived columns. Each consists of all the neurones in a 2500 μm² square in the middle of the column and the middle of the layer.

Gross anatomy and Nissl studies

In monkeys nos. 1–4, there was no obvious change in the extent or overall shape of the striate cortex. No measurements were made of the total area of striate cortex, but the occipital lobes were not grossly shrunk as would be expected if half of the columns had been reduced to a fraction of their normal size; the extent of striate cortex in Nissl-stained sections, moreover, appeared quite normal. This strongly suggests that the shrinkage of one set of columns was compensated for by an expansion of the other set, supporting the conclusion already reached from measurements of the repeat distance. For the same reason it is unlikely that one set simply failed to grow following the eye closure. Indeed, if the differences in column width in monkey no. 3 had been due to a failure of one set to grow, the striate cortex of a 2 week old monkey would have been about one-third its adult size. Far from this, comparisons between newborn and adult show that the newborn brain is closer to 80 % of the adult size.

In marked contrast to the lateral geniculates, the Nissl-stained cortex in all of the experimental monkeys appeared normal. In particular, layer IV C gave no hint of any fluctuations in thickness, cell size or cell density, to parallel the changes seen in the autoradiography or degeneration studies. Measurements of cell density and cell size were made in monkey no. 3 to learn whether any minor variations, too subtle to be seen by mere visual inspection under the microscope, might be present. In an autoradiographic section counterstained for Nissl substance, squares were selected in the middle of four normal-eye columns, midway between the borders, and these were compared with squares similarly centred in the neighbouring deprived-eye columns. Each square measured 50 μm × 50 μm. The locations of column boundaries were determined directly from the autoradiography by examining the same slide under dark-field illumination. Table 4 shows the results of these measurements: no significant differences were seen in cell density or cell size.

PART III. NEWBORN MONKEYS

An interpretation of the findings just described depends heavily on a knowledge of the state of the ocular dominance columns at the time an eye was closed or removed. Some preliminary studies were therefore made on three very young monkeys. The first of these (no. 9) was studied anatomically following eye injection; the second and third were recorded from, the second (no. 10) at 8 days and the third (no. 4) at 22 days.

Monkey no. 9: autoradiography

This monkey was injected in the right eye with 2.0 mCi of tritiated fucose the day after it was born. Though we normally allow 14 days for transport, the animal died of a respiratory infection at 6 days and was perfused probably less than an hour after death.

The geniculates seemed to be fully developed by adult standards. The layers corresponding to the injected eye were heavily labelled, as shown in figure 23, plate 11. On each side the three layers corresponding to the uninjected eye showed some label in excess of background, perhaps somewhat more than was seen in monkeys nos. 3 and 4. Comparisons are difficult, however, given the large amount of label injected relative to the size of the eye or the monkey's weight, the use of fucose alone instead of a fucose-proline mixture, the differences in the time allowed for transport, and a number of other variables that could not be completely controlled.

In addition to the six classical layers, figure 23 shows four subsidiary groups of terminations. These are labelled in figure 24, plate 11. From ventral to dorsal they consist of: (1) a thin layer *a* ventral to layer 1, contralaterally supplied, and separated from most of 1 by a thin label-free gap. (2) A clump of label *b* near the hilum, supplied ipsilaterally and sandwiched between *a* and layer 1. This is seen as a small aggregation of label on the left, and its position is marked by a space on the right. (3) A thin leaflet *c* just dorsal to layer 1, contralaterally innervated; and, like, *a*, separated from layer 1 by a label free gap. (4) A thin leaflet *d* sandwiched between layers 2 and 3, contralaterally innervated so that it stands out clearly between these two, especially in dark-field illumination (figure 23, lower right). This layer is probably also ipsilaterally innervated as shown in light field (see also figure 9). *c* and *d* appear to be joined in some sections by bands of label that pass through layer 2. Layers *a*, *b* and *d* are also shown in figure 9. *a* and *b* probably correspond to the single lamina 'S', described by Campos-Ortega & Hayhow (1970), and thought by them to receive only ipsilateral innervation.

The findings in the striate cortex came as a surprise. At first glance no columns were evident at all. Sections cut in the parasagittal plane through the calcarine fissure contralateral to the injected eye showed almost continuous moderately dense label in layer IV C. This is shown in figure 25 a, plate 12. The minor fluctuations in density of layer IV label were hard to evaluate in these sections and we were tempted to dismiss them until we examined tangential sections through the dome of the mushroom of the calcarine fissure on the ipsilateral side (figure 25 b). Though the parallel bands in the central oval region through IV C are faint their regularity is very clear, with a repeat distance of about 700 µm, or 20 % less than our value for the normal adult. Even in the regions of minimum label the density is considerably higher than outside IV C. It is difficult to compare the sides ipsilateral and contralateral to the injected eye because of differences in the planes of section, but our impression is that the fluctuations in density were more marked ipsilaterally.

There are two possible explanations for this result. The first is that label may have leaked from the path originating in the injected eye to the non-injected path. The geniculates would be the most likely site of spillover. Some leakage of this sort may indeed occur in the normal adult, as is shown in figures 12 and 13 by the above-background levels in the gaps between labelled columns. It may be that any such leakage is more serious in the newborn. The second possibility is that the columns are indeed not fully formed at birth, the full extent of layer IV being occupied by terminals from the two eyes, with only minor but regular variations in density representing the precursors of the columns.

Monkeys nos. 10 and 4: physiology

One obvious method for resolving this impasse was to record from a newborn monkey. No. 9, unfortunately, died before recordings could be made. No. 10 was not injected, but was recorded from at 8 days of age, having been in a normally lit nursery up to that time.

Four penetrations were made in monkey no. 10, in area 17 of the left hemisphere. They were made very obliquely so as to explore as great a span of layer IV C as possible. The reconstruc-

---

DESCRIPTION OF PLATE 12

FIGURE 25. Newborn monkey, no. 9, Autoradiographs in dark field. (a) Transverse section through calcarine fissure and operculum on the right side, contralateral to the injected eye. Label is virtually continuous, both in the fissure and over the convexity, though there is some suggestion of fluctuations in density over the dorsal calcarine stem. (The part of this stem furthest to the left is probably the temporal crescent representation, where one expects continuous label; compare figure 21 a.) Anterior is up and to the left. (b) Tangential section through operculum of left occipital lobe (ipsilateral to the injected eye). Section passes deep to the outer convexity, and cuts the buried mushroom-like calcarine convexity, grazing layer IV C which appears as an oval near the centre. Throughout this area levels of label are well above background, but there is nevertheless a definite regular banding with a periodicity of about 0.7 mm. 1–2 mm outside of the oval is a ring of label formed by the optic radiations. Still further out is a continuous double ring of label in layers IV C α and β of the outer exposed convexity.

FIGURE 26. Reconstructions of four penetrations made in striate cortex of an 8-day-old monkey (left hemisphere). The object was to explore as long an extent of layer IV C as possible, determining how much binocular mixing was present. Circles indicate points at which electrolytic lesions were made. The lower diagram indicates, on the left, the ocular dominance of the multiunit activity in layer IV C. The right hand portion, with smaller dots, indicates ocular dominance of the cells in the upper layers, in the early parts of the penetrations. The points are pooled from all four penetrations, preserving the cortical position of each recording site. In the region explored, obviously the contralateral (right) eye dominated in the portions to the left and right and the ipsilateral eye dominated in the middle. For the left hand region the input was almost exclusively contralateral; in the middle region, however, there was considerable mixing of inputs from the two eyes. In adult monkeys virtually no mixing is found in layer IV C.

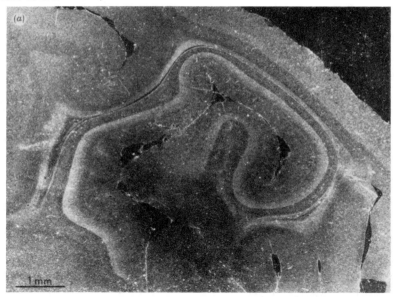

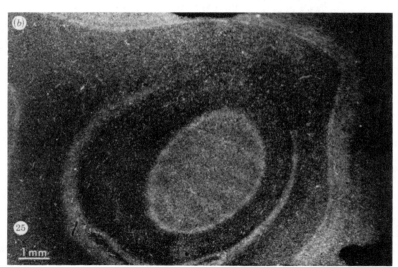

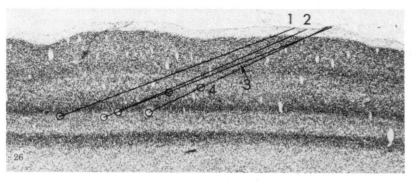

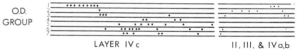

FIGURES 25 AND 26. For description see opposite.   (*Facing p.* 400)

tion of these penetrations is shown in figure 26, plate 12, with the ocular dominance of the cells indicated below. Points to the left of the gap in the diagram indicate units or unit clusters in layer IV C. The smaller dots, to the right of the gap, indicate cells in the upper layers. Our main concern was of course to learn whether single cells or local groups of cells in IV C were fed from one eye or from both.

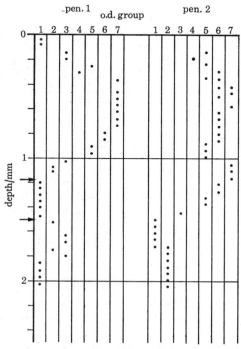

FIGURE 27. Ocular dominance in two penetrations made at 45° through right striate cortex of a normal 3-week-old monkey (no. 4, first recording, compare figure 19). Penetration 1 passed through layer IV C in the region indicated by the arrows; this activity was strictly monocular. There are clear regular fluctuations in ocular dominance, just as is found in adult monkeys.

The first penetration was normal by adult standards: in the layers above IV C most cells had sharp orientation specificity and most were driven from both eyes, one or other being preferred. The contralateral eye dominated at first, then came a span of about 1 mm in which the ipsilateral eye dominated, and finally, in IV C, all cells had unoriented fields and were activated from the contralateral eye only. In the other three penetrations, binocular cells similarly prevailed in the upper layers, but in IV C a variable amount of binocular input was also found. Thus in penetrations 2 and 3 the ipsilateral eye dominated but the contralateral contributed weakly or moderately throughout the traverse through IV C, while in penetration 4 the two eyes were almost equal. These observations refer mostly to the unresolved multiunit activity, since single units are hard to resolve in IV C. Nevertheless, there were in layer IV C several clear examples of binocularly driven cells with no preferred orientation. In this monkey, then, layer IV C showed the usual variation in eye emphasis, but much more binocular mixing than we have ever found in juvenile or adult monkeys.

A recording was also made in monkey no. 4 at 3 weeks of age, up to which time both eyes had been normally exposed. (After the recording the monkey was resurrected and the right eye was sutured closed.) In this animal the results were very similar to those previously obtained in the adult, and are illustrated in figure 27. In both penetrations (each at about 45°) binocularly driven cells were present in abundance above and below layer IV C, with the normal swings in dominance from eye to eye. The short passage through layer IV C in penetration 1 (between arrows) showed monocular influence only, but a subsequent experiment in a 3-week-old monkey has indicated a lack of complete segregation in this layer; another at 6 weeks suggests that by then segregation is virtually complete. (These experiments are part of a separate study on the time course of columnar development.)

Thus early in life layer IV C probably contains a mixture of inputs from the two eyes, perhaps at most points along its length; by 3 weeks, on the other hand, segregation seems to be fairly well advanced but probably still not complete.

DISCUSSION

The chief finding of the present study concerns the effects of early eye removal or monocular lid closure on the ocular dominance stripes in layer IV C. Deprivation in the first few weeks of life resulted in a change in the relative sizes of the two sets of stripes, with a shrinkage of stripes receiving input from the deprived eye and a correponding expansion of those with input from the normal eye.

In discussing the nature of these changes a number of possibilities can be quickly dispensed with. The first of these is the notion that in the shrunken columns the reduction is only apparent: that in the areas invaded by the normal-eye terminals, the terminals from the deprived eye remain but are non-functional. The concept of non-functional synapses in the nervous system is not unheard of, the best established example probably being botulinum poisoning at the nerve-muscle junction. In the present experiments, given the variety of techniques we have used to demonstrate the abnormalities, one would have to suppose in this model not only that the synapses were physiologically non-functional, but that the fibres did not degenerate after geniculate lesions in such a way as to show up with Nauta–Fink–Heimer methods, did not transport materials normally, and were not revealed with reduced silver stains. Such an interpretation thus seems most improbable.

Secondly, we must consider the idea that there is not only an abnormal distribution of terminals in layer IV, but also a change in the territory occupied by each entire band, cells and all. This could only happen if the cell packing density deviated markedly from normal, increasing in the shrunken columns and decreasing in the expanded ones, or if cells died in large numbers in one set and proliferated in the other. But a fluctuation in packing density of the magnitude necessary to fit the changes in width that we see can be ruled out by direct counts (table 4), while cell proliferation ceases altogether in the cortex 2 months before term (Rakic 1974), and a cell death sufficient to equalize the cell counts would produce a radical drop in cell numbers which in fact does not occur.

Thirdly, there is a possibility that the brain of the newborn monkey is much smaller than that of the adult, and that the columns in area 17 are present at birth and also correspondingly smaller. The disparity in column size would then arise if the columns connected to the deprived eye simply failed to grow. It appears, however, that in overall size the striate cortex increases very roughly 20% after birth – it certainly does not double or triple in area as would be required to explain the discrepancies in column width. Consistent with this, the columns in the newborn show a periodicity not very different from that of the adult, to judge from direct anatomical (figure 25b) and physiological (figures 26 and 27) observations. Finally, there is the finding that in the deprived animals the columns associated with the open eye are larger than normal, and the combined width of a left eye–right eye pair is unchanged. None of this would be consistent with an explanation based on failure to grow.

With these possibilities out of the way, a discussion of the pathogenesis of the changes due to deprivation hinges strongly on a knowledge of the state of the columns at birth. If one assumes that in the newborn monkey (or within a few days of birth) the geniculocortical fibres have already taken up their final positions in the form of clearly defined parallel IVth-layer stripes, then it is hard to avoid the conclusion that in the final state one set of terminals has extended its territory, possibly by sprouting, while the other set has retracted. If sprouting were involved here it would be of some interest. Although a number of examples of sprouting have been reported, all of them were brought about by a destructive deafferentation of one source of input to a structure. In the present series even eye enucleation amounts to a lesion one synapse away from the site of the changes, and the eye closures involve no direct destruction of any neural tissue. If the changes in layer IV are indeed produced by sprouting and retraction the result is in marked contrast to what is seen in the geniculate or colliculus, for there we have no hint of invasion of terminals from the normal eye into the deprived or deafferented territory. This may simply be a matter of timing with respect to normal developmental events, since it is known that in enucleated cats there is no invasion of afferents into a deprived geniculate layer unless the enucleation is done in the first week after birth (Kalil 1972; Guillery 1972b). Even then the invasion is modest and occurs only near the laminar borders; that it occurs at all is probably related to the immaturity of the cat visual system at birth, compared with that of the monkey.

Up to the time when we saw the results of autoradiography in the newborn, described in Part III, we regarded a sprouting of terminals as the strongest contender in explaining the cortical changes. Our previous physiological recordings in young monkeys (Hubel & Wiesel 1974) had actually tended to support the idea that ocular dominance columns were present at birth. By the second day, for example, there was a clear grouping of upper-layer, mostly binocular, cells according to ocular dominance, and in an animal with both eyes closed up to 3 weeks there was an almost complete segregation of eye inputs even in the upper and lower layers, reminiscent of the picture obtained with artificial strabismus. Tangential penetrations were not used in either of these animals, however, so that no clear idea was obtained of the state of affairs in layer IVC.

In the present paper both the physiological recordings and the anatomy in monkeys in the first week or so of life strongly suggest that the sets of terminals associated with the two eyes have arrived at layer IVC but have not yet separated themselves out completely into distinct bands. There is, to be sure, a clear banding visible in the autoradiographs in tangential sections (monkey no. 9, figure 25b), but these are produced by mild fluctuations in levels of label, rather than a series of abrupt rises and falls from maximum to minimum and back. The physiology in monkey no. 10 confirmed this mixing of inputs, though there was perhaps more segregation than would have been expected from the autoradiographic picture.

The notion that the columns are not fully formed at birth in this species can at present be

28-2

only rather tentative; what is still needed is a set of injections and recordings at various ages in the first 6 weeks. But our results so far receive support from the findings of Rakic (1976 *a*, *b*), in foetal monkeys in which one eye was injected with radioactive label at different times during gestation. At 6 weeks before term label was present in IV C but appeared uniform, with no hint of columns. Three weeks before term there were fluctuations in label density that were only barely discernable on visual inspection of transverse sections, but were clearly confirmed by grain counts. As with our eye-injection results, one must keep in mind the possibility of leakage of label in the geniculate.

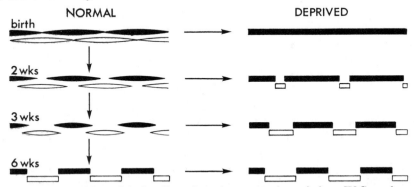

FIGURE 28. Scheme that might explain the effects of eye closures on columns in layer IV C, on the assumption that the segregation of the eyes is not complete until some weeks after birth. The thick dark lines represent the terminations of geniculate afferents in layer IV C corresponding to one eye; the open lines, the terminations from the other eye. In each, the width is intended to represent the presumed density of the terminals. At birth there is some periodic and regular variation in density (figure 25 *b*): it is unlikely that the minimum is zero, as the drawing suggests, and in any case the fluctuations are probably different in different parts of the striate cortex. In this scheme we suppose that competition normally occurs between the eyes, with the weaker input at any given point declining and the stronger being fortified. The result is a progressive retraction as the sparse terminals die out entirely. For purposes of the drawing we assume that the retraction process has the time course illustrated and that it takes about 6 weeks; again, the exact time course is far from clear.

If the columns do, as it were, crystallize out only in the few weeks before and after term, the process presumably occurs by a retraction of the two sets of terminals. One may imagine that in any areas occupied by both sets of terminals there is a competitive mechanism in which the weaker set at any point tends to regress. Given such an unstable equilibrium, the normal end result of any initial inequalities would be a complete segregation of terminals. Such a model for the normal development, based on competition, is illustrated schematically in the left half of figure 28. In this figure the terminals dominated by one eye in layer IV C are blackened, and the other set is represented by open areas. (Obviously the two sets should be superimposed, but are shown one under the other for clarity.) The thickness of these representations suggests the relative density of label at each point along IV C. If we suppose that at birth there exist some mild periodic out-of-phase fluctuations (which may be less than portrayed here) the density of the weaker inputs at any point will decline, with consequent production of a series of ever widening gaps until all overlap is eliminated.

On this model for the normal development, the deprivation results in layer IV can be predicted. One has only to assume that lack of use of a set of terminals puts them at a competitive disadvantage which transcends that related to mere numbers, so that at any point along IV C the terminals from the opposing normal-eye set take over, provided they have not already retracted. This is illustrated in the right half of figure 28. Where no competition is possible, because the other set has already disappeared (or in the case of the temporal crescent representation, where only one set was present from the beginning – see figure 21 *a*) the deprived sel survives and is apparently intact. The end result of the deprivation thus depends on the amount of overlap that still existed at the time of eye closure or removal.

It should be emphasized that the details of figure 28, such as the ages assigned to the four illustrated stages of development or the amount of fluctuation of label density at birth, should not be taken literally. We do *not* know, for example, that closure of an eye from birth produces a complete takeover by the open eye. The illustration merely provides, at present, the best fit with the results from the few deprivation and control monkeys available (nos. 1–5, and 9 and 10). We are still uncertain of the variation to be expected from one animal to the next, even under experimental conditions that are as similar as possible.

One advantage of the scheme of figure 28 is that it removes some of the mystery connected with the 'critical period' – the period of susceptibility to monocular deprivation. At least as far as layer IV is concerned the flexible state would, by this model, involve not some kind of ill-defined vulnerability to insult, or capacity for nerve-terminal proliferation, but merely the period of development from birth to the final consolidation of the columns.

If the idea of a post-natal retraction of inputs is correct, it would be interesting to know whether there are consistent differences in the timing of the process, in different parts of area 17 (for example, foveal *vs.* more peripheral representations) and, in a given hemisphere, between terminals belonging to the ipsilateral and contralateral eyes. As far as laterality is concerned, deprivation effects have consistently been more severe in the hemisphere ipsilateral to the eye that was closed; this has been true both for the shrinkage of cortical columns and the attendant geniculate atrophy (see also Headon & Powell 1973). On the model of figure 28 this would be readily explained if it were found that the fibres from the contralateral eye were slower in retracting than their counterparts from the ipsilateral. We have fragmentary hints that this may indeed be so, since in the layer IV C recordings from monkey no. 10 (figure 26) at 8 days the contralateral eye had already gained exclusive possession of some territory in IV C, whereas the ipsilateral eye had not. On the competition model a closure of the contralatera eye would find ipsilateral terminals available only in the designated ipsilateral territory; a closure of the ipsilateral eye would find terminals from the contralateral eye available to take over everywhere. The autoradiography (figure 25) tended to support this idea, although comparisons were difficult since the planes of section in the two hemispheres were different.

The model of course says nothing about changes in connections beyond layer IV C. That such changes almost certainly occur is shown by the scarcity in deprived animals of cells in layers outside IV that can be influenced from the closed eye, a scarcity more severe than would be expected from the extent to which deprived stripes in IV C are spared, and the relative normality of responses within those stripes. (We were, in fact, surprised when we first recorded from layer IV C to find any significant number of cells responsive to the deprived eye.) Also it is clear that monocular deprivation can produce changes in the ocular dominance of cells outside layer IV when closures are done well beyond 6 weeks – effects are seen as late as 4 months and possibly even later, if an eye is closed for a long enough time. We have some indication, from reduced silver stains, that such late deprivation leaves the layer IV band widths unchanged. Thus eye-dominance changes in higher order cells may have to be explained in terms of competition between different groups of afferents for territory on a single postsynaptic cell, as has been proposed previously (Wiesel & Hubel 1965). Indeed, an important reason for doing the present experiments was a curiosity to learn what would happen in layer IV C, where competition between eyes on a single-cell level seemed impossible. This is in contrast to the situation in the cat, in which the physiology suggests that there is a direct convergence of geniculate afferents from the two eyes on cortical cells. It now appears that the mechanisms for the layer-IV changes in the monkey could also involve competition, since before the columns are fully formed terminals from the two eyes may likewise converge on single cells in that layer. The presence of a few resolvable binocular cells in layer IV C of monkey no. 10 (at 8 days) tends to support this, although we admittedly have no guarantee that the particular cells we recorded received direct input from the geniculate. The question would have to be resolved by intracellular or morphological (EM) techniques. In any case, it is probably easier to imagine competition between afferents for territory on a single cell than a competition between entire columns or large groups of afferents.

Since the notion of competition between eyes is now a dominant one in visual deprivation, and a recurring theme in the present paper, it may be useful to review some of the evidence in its favour. It was originally suggested to account for the surprising finding that binocular deprivation in cats produced defects in cortical cell responses that were far milder than predicted from monocular closures (Wiesel & Hubel 1965). This seemed to rule out simple disuse as a mechanism for the unresponsiveness of cells when one eye was deprived. In 1970 Guillery & Stelzner observed that in the geniculate of monocularly deprived cats the part of layer A representing the temporal crescent did not show the same defect in cell growth as the rest of this layer: a possible explanation advanced to explain this was competition between the two eyes, with a sparing of the part of the geniculate in which there could be no competition. Since convergence of input from the two eyes occurs first (for all practical purposes) in the cortex, it was suggested that the cell shrinkage in the geniculate might reflect a failure of axon terminals to compete effectively for synaptic surface of cortical cells. Subsequent experiments have strengthened this idea: (1) In cats deprived of vision in one eye, focal retinal lesions in the open eye produced a protection from deprivation effects, of just those geniculate cells whose competition had been removed (Guillery 1972a). (2) Behavioural tests after monocular deprivation showed relatively normal responses to visual cues in the temporal crescent of the deprived eye (Sherman 1973). (3) Sherman, Guillery, Kaas & Sanderson (1974), finally, showed that focal retinal lesions in the eye that remained open protected the closed eye from defects in behavioural and cortical-cell responses in the corresponding part of the visual field.

To this accumulated evidence the present paper has added the anatomical observation that the temporal-crescent input to the monkey cortex is largely spared on the side opposite to the closed eye, compared to the severe effects on cortical columns in the binocular part of area 17. One would expect also to see a sparing of the corresponding geniculate cells, as is found in the cat, but for this problem parasagittal sections would probably be necessary. In a study of the geniculate in monocularly deprived monkeys, von Noorden, Middleditch & Crawford (1975) saw no sparing in the monocular segment representation.

It is worth noting, in this context, that in the foetal eye-injection experiments of Rakic (1976a, b) the optic afferents both to the geniculates and to the superior colliculi occupied their entire targets for an extended period between their first arrival and their eventual segregation into layers (geniculates) or clumps (colliculi). In both targets segregation occurred during the middle period of gestation and was apparently complete by birth. A similar process, then, may well take place in geniculate, colliculus and cortex, though in the cortex it seems to occur later, and to be still incomplete at birth. This would suggest that the apparent reluctance of optic terminals in geniculate and tectum to extend their territory in monocular deprivation is a reflection of the complete segregation of the terminals at birth: the deprivation simply comes too late to produce an effect.

Though direct proof is still lacking, there are strong indications that the formation of ocular dominance columns does not require visual experience, even though some of the formation takes place postnatally and can be rendered abnormal by binocular closure. At present there are two kinds of evidence for this: (1) the autoradiographs at and before birth, i.e. the bands seen on tangential sections (figure 26 b) or the fluctuations in grain counts 21 days before term (Rakic 1976 b); and (2) physiological recordings at 4 weeks in monkeys with both eyes closed at birth (Wiesel & Hubel 1974), where layer IV was not examined carefully, but extreme eye segregation was present in the layers outside IV, and therefore, a fortiori, in IV. We have examined one macaque dark raised to an age of 6 weeks, and found the responses in layer IV C to be strictly monocular. What is still needed is autoradiography after eye injection in a monkey dark reared, or with both eyes sutured, for the first six weeks or more.

The model involving mutual competition to explain the normal process of post-natal IVth layer segregation presupposes some initial inequality that starts the process. It would be most interesting to know what causes this, and what forces lead to a pattern of parallel lines roughly 0.4 mm apart. If the model is correct it must explain the obliteration of the deprived columns at irregular intervals along the bands, seen in cases of early eye closure (see figure 15), and hinted at in the eye-removal reconstructions (figure 6). Perhaps the process begins at multiple foci along the future bands and spreads in two directions forming line segments which then join similar segments, while simultaneously widening. (On a sprouting model one is tempted to conclude that the obliteration of columns here and there reflects an instability in the columns when they shrink beyond some limiting width.)

An intriguing problem arises from a consideration of the topographic representation of the visual field upon layer IV C (Hubel, Wiesel & LeVay 1974). This topography is detailed enough so that in crossing a single eye-dominance column one can observe a precisely corresponding displacement of receptive fields through the visual field. A displacement of equal magnitude, but in the visual field as seen by the other eye, takes place when the next column is crossed. The representations seem to be interlaced, so that on crossing a boundary between columns the receptive fields in the second eye jump back to about the midpoint of the territory just traversed in the first eye. All of this means that the magnification (mm/deg) across a column must be one-half that along its length. What happens, then, when two neighbouring columns are distorted, one compressed and the other expanded? How do the magnifications change during development? Answers to these questions may lead to a deeper understanding of the developmental mechanisms by which topographic representations arise.

Finally, one may ask again whether there is any benefit to the animal in having a critical period of postnatal flexibility. Does a virtual doubling of the IVth layer territory devoted to one of the eyes in any way improve the capabilities of that eye? Until behavioural tests can be made this question must be left open, but one would hardly expect to find an improvement in acuity, which is presumably limited by such things as the optics of the eye, the inter-receptor spacing, and the number of bipolar and ganglion cells. If an eye is lost early in life a number of cortical cells are clearly kept in use rather than being allowed to lie fallow, but how this helps the animal, if it does at all, is a complete mystery.

We wish to thank Claire Wang, Gail Grogan and Sharon Mates for histological assistance, and Carolyn Scott for help with photography.

Supported by National Institutes of Health Grants EY00605 and EY00606, The Esther A. and Joseph Klingenstein Foundation, Inc. and The Rowland Foundation, Inc.

REFERENCES (Hubel, Weisel & LeVay)

Baker, F. H., Grigg, P. & von Noorden, G. K. 1974 Effects of visual deprivation and strabismus on the response of neurons in the visual cortex of the monkey, including studies on the striate and prestriate cortex in the normal animal. *Brain Res.* **66**, 185–208.

Campos-Ortega, J. A. & Hayhow, W. R. 1970 A new lamination pattern in the lateral geniculate nucleus of primates. *Brain Res.* **20**, 335–339.

Guillery, R. W. 1972*a* Binocular competition in the control of geniculate cell growth. *J. Comp. Neur.* **144**, 117–130.

Guillery, R. W. 1972*b* Experiments to determine whether retinogeniculate axons can form translaminar collateral sprouts in the dorsal lateral geniculate nucleus of the cat. *J. Comp. Neur.* **146**, 407–420.

Guillery, R. W. & Stelzner, D. J. 1970 The differential effects of unilateral lid closure upon the monocular and binocular segments of the dorsal lateral geniculate nucleus in the cat. *J. Comp. Neur.* **139**, 413–422.

Headon, M. P. & Powell, T. P. S. 1973 Cellular changes in the lateral geniculate nucleus of infant monkeys after suture of the eyelids. *J. Anat. (Lond.)* **116**, 135–145.

Hubel, D. H., LeVay, S. & Wiesel, T. N. 1975 Mode of termination of retinotectal fibers in macaque monkey: an autoradiographic study. *Brain Res.* **96**, 25–40.

Hubel, D. H. & Wiesel, T. N. 1968 Receptive fields and functional architecture of monkey striate cortex. *J. Physiol., Lond.* **195**, 215–243.

Hubel, D. H. & Wiesel, T. N. 1972 Laminar and columnar distribution of geniculo-cortical fibers in the macaque monkey. *J. Comp. Neur.* **146**, 421–450.

Hubel, D. H., Wiesel, T. N. & LeVay, S. 1974 Visual field representation in layer IVC of monkey striate cortex. *Soc. Neurosci., 4th Annual Meeting (Abstracts)* 264.

Kalil, R. E. 1972 Formation of new retino-geniculate connections in kittens after removal of one eye. *Anat. Rec.* **172**, 339–340.

LeVay, S., Hubel, D. H. & Wiesel, T. N. 1975 The pattern of ocular dominance columns in macaque visual cortex revealed by a reduced silver stain. *J. Comp. Neur.* **159**, 559–576.

Lund, J. S. & Boothe, R. G. 1975 Interlaminar connections and pyramidal neuron organisation in the visual cortex, area 17, of the macaque monkey. *J. Comp. Neur.* **159**, 305–334.

Matthews, M. R., Cowan, W. M. & Powell, T. P. S. 1960 Transneuronal cell degeneration in the lateral geniculate nucleus of the macaque monkey. *J. Anat.* **94**, 145–169.

Minkowski, M. 1920 Über den Verlauf, die Endigung und die zentrale Repräsentation von gekreuzten und ungekreuzten Sehnervenfasern bei einigen Säugetieren und bei Menschen. *Schweiz. Arch. Neur. u. Psychiat.* **6**, 201–257.

Rakic, P. 1974 Neurons in rhesus monkey visual cortex: systematic relation between time of origin and eventual disposition. *Science, N.Y.* **183**, 425–427.

Rakic, P. 1976*a* Prenatal genesis of connections subserving ocular dominance in the rhesus monkey. *Nature, Lond.* (in the press).

Rakic, P. 1976*b* Prenatal development of the visual system in the rhesus monkey. *Phil. Trans. R. Soc. Lond.* B **278**, 245–260 (this volume).

Sherman, S. M. 1973 Visual field defects in monocularly and binocularly deprived cats. *Brain Res.* **49**, 25–45.

Sherman, S. M., Guillery, R. W., Kaas, J. H. & Sanderson, K. R. 1974 Behavioral, electrophysiological and morphological studies of binocular competition in the development of the geniculo-cortical pathways of cats. *J. Comp. Neur.* **158**, 1–18.

Spatz, W. B., Tigges, J. & Tigges, M. 1970 Subcortical projections, cortical associations and some intrinsic interlaminar connections of the striate cortex in the squirrel monkey (*Saimiri*). *J. Comp. Neur.* **140**, 155–174.

von Noorden, G. K., Middleditch, P. R. & Crawford, M. L. J. 1975 Disuse or abnormal binocular interaction in the etiology of amblyopia. *Proc. A.R.V.O.* p. 79.

Wiesel, T. N. & Hubel, D. H. 1963 Single-cell responses in striate cortex of kittens deprived of vision in one eye. *J. Neurophysiol.* **26**, 1003–1017.

Wiesel, T. N. & Hubel, D. H. 1965 Comparison of the effects of unilateral and bilateral eye closure on cortical unit responses in kittens. *J. Neurophysiol.* **28**, 1029–1040.

Wiesel, T. N. & Hubel, D. H. 1971 Long-term changes in the cortex after visual deprivation. *Proceedings of the International Union of Physiological Sciences.*

Wiesel, T. N. & Hubel, D. H. 1974 Ordered arrangement of orientation columns in monkeys lacking visual experience. *J. Comp. Neur.* **158**, 307–318.

Wiesel, T. N., Hubel, D. H. & Lam, D. N. K. 1974 Autoradiographic demonstration of ocular-dominance columns in the monkey striate cortex by means of transneuronal transport. *Brain Res.* **79**, 273–279.

Wiitanen, J. T. 1969 Selective silver impregnation of degenerating axons and axon terminals in the central nervous system of the monkey (*Macaca mulatta*). *Brain Res.* **14**, 546–548.

Section 12
Maintenance and Modifiability of Synaptic Connections in the Adult Nervous System

Brown, M.C. and R. Ironton. 1977. Motor neurone sprouting induced by prolonged tetrodotoxin block of nerve action potentials. *Nature* **265:** 459–461.

Diamond, J., E. Cooper, C. Turner, and L. Macintyre. 1976. Trophic regulation of nerve sprouting. *Science* **193:** 371–377.

Wernig, A., M. Pécot-Dechavassine, and H. Stöver. 1980. Sprouting and regression of the nerve at the frog neuromuscular junction in normal conditions and after prolonged paralysis with curare. *J. Neurocytol.* **9:** 277–303.

Are the synaptic connections present at the end of what might be loosely considered the period of development immutable, or are they susceptible to further modification? Several lines of evidence indicate that synaptic connections are, in fact, actively maintained throughout life. A corollary is that patterns of connections can be modified to some degree in maturity. Thus, the pattern of connectivity achieved during development is best regarded as a balance.

Support for the idea that synaptic connections represent an equilibrium that must be maintained comes partly from studies of sprouting by intact nerves in the adult nervous system. The most thoroughly studied stimulus for sprouting is partial denervation: If a portion of the innervation to a neural target is destroyed, the remaining axon terminals proliferate and form new synapses with the denervated target cells. This sequence of events has been observed in skeletal muscle, sensory innervation of skin, autonomic ganglia, spinal cord, and brain (see Edds 1953; Raisman and Field 1973; Cotman and Nadler 1978; Roper and Ko 1978; Diamond and Jackson 1980; Brown et al. 1981; Tsukuhara 1981). Partial denervation, however, is not the only way to produce this proliferation of axon terminals and novel synaptic connections. In muscle, sprouting also occurs when neuromuscular transmission is blocked by botulinum toxin (Duchen and Strich 1968), when muscles are paralyzed by chronic local nerve block (**Brown** and **Ironton 1977**), or when the muscle surface is irritated by a variety of exogenous agents or by the products of nerve degeneration (Hoffman 1951; Jones and Vrbová 1974; Brown et al. 1978). Finally, sprouting of cutaneous nerves can be induced by blocking axoplasmic transport in the axons innervating adjacent skin (**Diamond, Cooper, Turner,** and **Macintyre 1976**).

Does a common mechanism underlie these various sprouting stimuli? One possibility, based on what is known of trophic influences (and of the biological role of NGF in particular; see Section 6) is that sprouting is a response to agents secreted by target cells. The gist of this idea is that when target cells are denervated, they continue to secrete (or perhaps increase their secretion of) a trophic agent; whereas this agent would normally be taken up (or otherwise neutralized) by the innervating axons, following partial denervation it becomes available as a stimulus to the remaining intact axons which therefore sprout. Of course, positive feedback arising from an agent secreted by target cells is not the only plausible explanation of sprouting. An alternative idea is that axons actively inhibit each other from sprouting under normal circumstances (Diamond et al. 1976). However, the demonstration that some targets do provide a trophic signal to their innervation (Section 6) makes the idea of a chemical feedback from the target an attractive explanation. In this conception, the effects of postsynaptic cell activity (or the lack of it), of inflammation, and of blocked axonal transport reflect the influence of these conditions on the production, secretion, and/or uptake of the putative chemical signal. Even if the notion of trophic feedback is correct, though, other influences are almost certainly involved. For example, Diamond and his collaborators have shown that sensory axons from salamander and rat cutaneous nerves sprout more vigorously within their proper dermatome than into adjacent dermatomes (Diamond et al. 1976; Diamond and Jackson 1980; Jackson and Diamond 1981; Macintyre and Diamond 1981), a phenomenon perhaps related to the role of positional information in axon guidance (see Section 4).

A quite different body of evidence indicates that the terminal arborizations of axons are also capable of contracting in maturity. For example, if the axonal links between sympathetic ganglion cells and their peripheral targets are interrupted, most of the synaptic contacts made on the ganglion cells by preganglionic axons are withdrawn (Matthews and Nelson 1975; Purves 1975, 1976; Brenner and Johnson 1976; Njå and Purves 1978). When the ganglion cells regenerate their peripheral axons, the synaptic contacts on the ganglion cells are restored; if, on the other hand, peripheral regeneration is prevented, then the synapses normally present on the ganglion cells

are not reestablished (Purves 1975). A similar retrograde influence on the synaptic contacts made on cells whose axons have been interrupted has also been observed in parasympathetic ganglia, spinal motor neurons, and brainstem nuclei (see Watson 1974; Purves and Njå 1978). It therefore seems likely that this retrograde loss of synapses in reaction to target removal is also a fairly general one.

Despite superficial differences, the retraction of the terminal arborizations from the surfaces of neurons cut off from their normal targets is probably related to sprouting. Indeed, the loss of contacts from injured neurons may represent the reverse of the process that augments terminal arborizations after partial denervation. According to this idea, neurons, like muscle cells, secrete trophic agents on which their innervation depends (see Purves 1977). When a neuron's connection with its target is interrupted, its own production or secretion of a trophic material may be reduced temporarily. Conversely, when peripheral connectivity is restored, production or secretion is resumed and synapses are regained. Although speculative, this trophic view of synapse loss in maturity is again consistent with what is known of trophic interactions in development (see Section 6); it simply postulates the persistence in the adult nervous system of the trophic dependencies that are more obvious at early stages. It is quite possible, for instance, that the same signals required for the initial survival of neurons are later important in a more local way to maintain axon terminals. Certainly, mature sympathetic neurons retain some sensitivity to NGF (see Levi-Montalcini and Angeletti 1968; Njå and Purves 1978). Additional support for the idea that there is a reciprocal relationship between sprouting and retrograde synapse loss after axotomy is the so-called pruning effect that has been observed after early destruction of parts of the projection of the mammalian optic tract. When a portion of a neuron's arborization is removed, sprouting is elicited in the residual arbor (Schneider 1973). Whatever the particular mechanism underlying these synaptic changes in maturity, the fact that the terminal arborizations of axons can either extend (sprout) or contract throughout life suggests that synaptic connections are normally in equilibrium.

To what extent is this equilibrium a dynamic one? The possibility that synapses are turning over continually in the absence of any experimental manipulation has been raised several times over the years (see, for example, Barker and Ip 1966; Tuffery 1971). This idea, however, has not found general acceptance. A number of recent studies have now added significantly to the evidence for this point (Mallart et al. 1980; **Wernig, Pécot-Dechavassine,** and **Stöver 1980a**,b, 1981; Wernig et al. 1981; Haimann et al. 1981). In part, this work takes advantage of anatomical techniques that highlight the detailed geometry of both the pre- and postsynaptic elements at the frog neuromuscular junction. Using these methods, fine presynaptic terminals unopposed by a postsynaptic element are often found; these are interpreted as recently formed nerve sprouts that have not yet induced postsynaptic specializations. Conversely, postsynaptic specializations unopposed by presynaptic terminals are also observed; these are interpreted as sites recently vacated by nerve terminals undergoing local regression. Since both configurations are present in normal adult muscle, some degree of synaptic turnover, at least at this level of the nervous system, may occur continually. Some caution about normal turnover will still be warranted, however, until the phenomenon can be observed directly and its presence in other parts of the nervous system evaluated.

In summary, the synaptic connections established during development probably represent an initial balance that must be actively maintained and that can be altered to some degree throughout life. We have not attempted to review the very large literature on learning, particularly changes in synaptic function that have been associated with behavioral changes, but they are obviously relevant to the topics discussed here. It is attractive to suppose that the persistent malleability of synaptic connections is complementary to changes in the efficacy of individual synapses. Both phenomena would allow the nervous system to profit from experience.

References

Barker, D. and M.C. Ip. 1966. Sprouting and degeneration of mammalian motor axons in normal and de-afferented skeletal muscle. *Proc. R. Soc. Lond. B 163:* 538–554.

Brenner, H.R. and E.W. Johnson. 1976. Physiological and morphological effects of post-ganglionic axotomy on presynaptic nerve terminals. *J. Physiol. 260:* 143–158.

Brown, M.C. and R. Ironton. 1977. Motor neurone sprouting induced by prolonged tetrodotoxin block of nerve action potentials. *Nature 265:* 459–461.

Brown, M.C., R.L. Holland, and W.G. Hopkins. 1981. Motor nerve sprouting. *Annu. Rev. Neurosci. 4:* 17–42.

Brown, M.C., R.L. Holland, and R. Ironton. 1978. Degenerating nerve products affect innervated muscle fibres. *Nature 275:* 652–654.

Cotman, C.W. and J.V. Nadler. 1978. Reactive synaptogenesis in the hippocampus. In *Neuronal plasticity* (ed. C.W. Cotman), pp. 227–271. Raven Press, New York.

Diamond, J. and P.C. Jackson. 1980. Regeneration and collateral sprouting of peripheral nerves. In *Nerve repair and regeneration. Its clinical and experimental basis* (ed. D.L. Jewett and H.R. McCarroll), pp. 115–129. Mosby, St. Louis.

Diamond, J., E. Cooper, C. Turner, and L. Macintyre. 1976. Trophic regulation of nerve sprouting. *Science 193:* 371–377.

Duchen, L.W. and S.J. Strich. 1968. Changes in the pattern of motor innervation of skeletal muscle in the mouse after local injection of clostridium botulinum toxin. *Q. J. Exp. Physiol. 53:* 84–89.

Edds, M.V. 1953. Collateral nerve regeneration. *Q. Rev. Biol. 28:* 260–276.

Haimann, C., A. Mallart, J. Tomas i Ferre, and N.F. Zilber-Gachelin. 1981. Patterns of motor innervation in the pectoral muscle of adult *Xenopus laevis:* Evidence for possible synaptic remodelling. *J. Physiol. 310:* 241–256.

Hoffman, H. 1951. A study of the factors influencing innervation of muscles by implanted nerves. *Aust. J. Exp. Biol. Med. Sci. 29:* 289–307.

Jackson, P.C. and J. Diamond. 1981. Regenerating axons reclaim sensory targets from collateral nerve sprouts. *Science 214:* 926–928.

Jones, R. and G. Vrbová. 1974. Two factors responsible for the development of denervation hypersensitivity. *J. Physiol. 236:* 517–538.

Levi-Montalcini, R. and P.U. Angeletti. 1968. Nerve growth factor. *Physiol. Rev. 48:* 534–569.

Macintyre, L. and J. Diamond. 1981. Domains and mechanosensory fields in salamander skin. *Proc. R. Soc. Lond. B 211:* 471–499.

Mallart, A., D. Angaut-Petit, N.F. Zilber-Gachelin, J. Tomas i Ferre, and C. Haimann. 1980. Synaptic efficacy and turnover of endings in pauci-innervated muscle fibres of *Xenopus laevis. INSERM Symp. 13:* 213–223.

Matthews, M.R. and V.H. Nelson. 1975. Detachment of structurally intact nerve endings from chromatolytic neurones of the rat superior cervical ganglion during depression of synaptic transmission induced by post-ganglionic axotomy. *J. Physiol. 245:* 91–135.

Njå, A. and D. Purves. 1978. The effects of nerve growth factor and its antiserum on synapses in the superior cervical ganglion of the guinea-pig. *J. Physiol. 277:* 53–75.

Purves, D. 1975. Functional and structural changes in mammalian sympathetic neurones following interruption of their axons. *J. Physiol. 252:* 429–463.

———. 1976. Functional and structural changes in mammalian sympathetic neurones following colchicine application to post-ganglionic nerves. *J. Physiol. 259:* 159–175.

———. 1977. The formation and maintenance of synaptic connections. In *Function and formation of neural systems* (ed. G.S. Stent), pp. 21–49. Dahlem Konferenzen, Berlin.

Purves, D. and A. Njå. 1978. Trophic maintenance of synaptic connections in autonomic ganglia. In *Neuronal plasticity* (ed. C.W. Cotman), pp. 27–49. Raven Press, New York.

Raisman, G. and P.H. Field. 1973. A quantitative investigation of the development of collateral reinnervation after partial deafferentation of the septal nuclei. *Brain Res. 50:* 241–264.

Roper, S. and C.-P. Ko. 1978. Synaptic remodeling in the partially denervated parasympathetic ganglion in the heart of the frog. In *Neuronal plasticity* (ed. C.W. Cotman), pp. 1–25. Raven Press, New York.

Schneider, G.E. 1973. Early lesions of the superior colliculus: Factors affecting the formation of abnormal retinal projections. *Brain Behav. Evol. 8:* 73–109.

Tsukahara, N. 1981. Synaptic plasticity in the mammalian central nervous system. *Annu. Rev. Neurosci. 4:* 351–379.

Tuffery, A.R. 1971. Growth and degeneration of motor end-plates in normal cat hind limb muscles. *J. Anat. 110:* 221–247.

Watson, W.E. 1974. Cellular responses to axotomy and to related procedures. *Br. Med. Bull. 30:* 112–115.

Wernig, A., A.P. Anzil, and A. Bieser. 1981. Light and electron microscopic identification of a nerve sprout in muscle of normal adult frog. *Neurosci. Lett. 21:* 261–266.

Wernig, A., M. Pécot-Dechavassine, and H. Stöver. 1980a. Sprouting and regression of the nerve at the frog neuromuscular junction in normal conditions and after prolonged paralysis with curare. *J. Neurocytol.* 9: 277–303.

———. 1980b. Signs of nerve regression and sprouting in the frog neuromuscular synapse. *INSERM Symp.* 13: 225–238.

(Reprinted from Nature, Vol. 265, No. 5593, pp. 459–461, February 3, 1977)

© *Macmillan Journals Ltd., 1977*

Motor neurone sprouting induced by prolonged tetrodotoxin block of nerve action potentials

PERIPHERAL axons retain into adult life the ability to grow, and do so either if they themselves are cut or if neighbouring tissues are denervated (collateral sprouting[1]). Collateral sprouting also occurs in botulinum toxin poisoning[2], motor end plate disease of mice[3] and myasthenia gravis of man[4]. Muscle inactivity is common to these otherwise different conditions. We have therefore investigated whether inactivity in a muscle, produced by a local nerve block, will give rise to collateral sprouting. By paralysing motor nerves for a few days with a local application of tetrodotoxin (TTX) we have found that motor nerve terminals in the affected muscles do grow collateral sprouts. We conclude that muscle inactivity results in a sprouting stimulus to nerves.

TTX was used because it is a specific blocker of Na^+ conductance in nerve[5] and does not interfere with axoplasmic transport[6,7]. This is important because Diamond et al.[8,9] believe that interference with axoplasmic flow can lead to sprouting. Adult mice, male and female (20–30 g), were anaesthetised with ether, the right sciatic nerve was exposed and a hollow cylindrical cuff of Silastoseal B (Midland Silicones) was placed carefully around the nerve. Cuffs were 1.5–3 mm long, 2 mm in diameter with a 1-mm diameter hollow core. They were made as described by Lavoie et al.[6], except that the quantities of TTX and NaCl were different. In the first experiments the cuffs contained approximately 1 μg of TTX and 3 mg of NaCl. These paralysed for 24–48 h and two or three had to be used to give sufficient paralysis. In later experiments the cuffs contained about 5 μg of TTX and 0.5 mg of NaCl, and before insertion they were sprayed inside and out with poly tetra-fluoroethylene (PTFE, DMC Industrial Aerosols, No. 889RB). This delayed release of TTX and allowed larger doses to be given, thus prolonging paralysis, but often the paralysis was not as profound as with the other type of cuff. Control animals were mice with cuffs containing no TTX and mice with TTX-containing cuffs which paralysed for only 1 or 2 d; some of these were coated with PTFE,

others were not. The ineffective cuffs were left *in situ* for a further 3 or 4 d to bring the period when the cuffs were present up to that for animals where paralysis lasted for 3.5–7 d. Paralysis was checked twice a day by observing the movement and stance of the mice and by picking them up by the tail to see if their toes spread normally. Paralysis was not always complete but provided it was marked it was counted as successful. Different cuffs of a given batch did not necessarily paralyse to the same extent. We attributed this to the difficulty of mixing the small quantities of TTX, NaCl and silicone rubber into a uniform paste, so that different amounts of TTX were probably present.

Animals were used for the acute experiment within 24 h of the disappearance or marked diminution of paralysis. The peroneus tertius and solar muscles together with their nerves were dissected out of the right and left leg and studied *in vitro* at room temperature (normally 20 °C), perfused continuously with well oxygenated fluid of the following composition: 150 mM NaCl, 5 mM KCl, 1 mM MgCl₂, 5 mM CaCl₂, 1.24 mM HEPES, pH 7.4, 16.5 M glucose. Maximum isometric twitch and tetanic (50 per s) tension was recorded on stimulation of the nerve below the block. These tensions were compared with that evoked by direct stimulation of the muscle fibres (stimulus applied by two bright silver wires on either side of the muscle). The direct stimulus intensity was turned up gradually and usually maximum tension was produced by 10-V, 100-μs pulses. A 20-V, 300-μs pulse was then used to check that all the muscle fibres were being stimulated. If the direct and nerve-evoked tensions were not identical, the muscle was discarded as some axons had presumably been killed. This occurred on four out of 13 occasions in peroneus tertius, but not at all in 13 soleus muscles. When the two tensions were identical, a further check for absence of denervation was to grade the stimulus to the muscle nerve and, by sequentially bringing in motor units of different threshold, to count them. The number counted in this way in the experimental soleus and peroneus tertius was then compared with the figure for normal muscles from the opposite leg. When the direct tension equalled the nerve evoked tension, the unit numbers counted in this way were the same on the normal and experimental sides. The mean unit number for peroneus tertius was 11 and for soleus 21. The

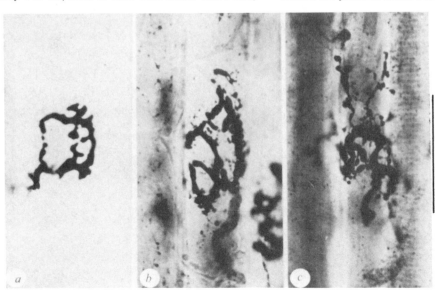

Fig. 1 Photomicrographs of mouse soleus end-plates stained with zinc odide and osmium tetroxide[7] from: *a*, a control animal in which a nonparalysing cuff was present for 5 d; *b*, paralysis for 3.5d; *c*, paralysis for 5 d. The calibration bar on the right is 50 μm.

muscles were then curarised and end plate potentials were recorded with conventional 10 MΩ glass micropipettes. We sometimes had to use up to five times the normal dose ($5 \times 0.5\ \mu g\ ml^{-1}$) of d-tubocurarine to block transmission in the experimental muscles. The recording of end plate potentials enabled us to check first that all fibres were innervated and second, by grading the stimulus to the nerve, whether as a result of sprouting any fibres had become polyneuronally innervated. Twenty to fifty fibres were examined in each muscle. Finally the preparations were stained for 5–6 h in a 4 : 1 solution of zinc iodide and osmium tetroxide[10], washed in water, teased with forceps and scissors into fine bundles, dehydrated, cleared in xylol and mounted in Permount.

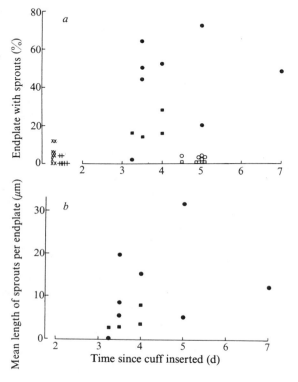

Fig. 2 *a*, Percentage of endplates with ultraterminal sprouts; *b*, mean length of sprouts per endplate (see text); ●, paralysed soleus; ■, paralysed peroneus tertius; ○, control soleus; □, control peroneus tertius; ×, normal soleus; +, normal peroneus tertius.

Provided paralysis had lasted for 3.5 d or longer the histology showed fine ultraterminal sprouts extending from the motor nerve terminals. In some cases the fine branches were very short (Fig. 1*b*) and in others extensive outgrowths could be seen (Fig. 1*c*). The soleus endplates sprouted more vigorously than those in peroneus tertius which usually had only a single large sprout. This is in agreement with results from sprouting induced by botulinum toxin[11]. Five control animals with non-paralysing cuffs had normal endplates (Fig. 1*a*). To obtain an objective figure for the degree of sprouting, we measured for 50 endplates in each muscle, first the length, in the long axis of the muscle fibre, of the nerve terminal which is densely stained by zinc iodide and osmium tetroxide, and second in those endplates with sprouts the length of endplate plus the furthest sprout extensions in both directions along the muscle fibre. Sprout

length was taken as the difference between these two measurements. The percentage of endplates with sprouts in each experiment is shown in Fig. 2*a*, for paralysed, cuffed but not paralysed, and for normal muscles. Figure 2*b* shows, for each experimental muscle, the extent of sprouting (μm per endplate) obtained by dividing the total length of sprouts measured for that muscle by the number of endplates measured. For the control muscles the figure is near zero. As described by Barker and Ip[12], a small amount of sprouting is seen in normal muscles.

Even in muscles with much sprouting some endplates appeared quite normal. Our test for paralysis was not very sophisticated and it seems likely that not all the motor units were blocked for all the time, and it may also be that within one muscle the latent period before sprouting starts differs between motor units, as it does between units in different muscles[11]. Less than 2% of the fibres were found to be polyneuronally innervated by our physiological test. As a similarly very small proportion of normal mouse soleus fibres is polyneuronally innervated, it seems that the blocking times we have achieved are not long enough for sprouts to form functional endings on other fibres in significant numbers. If we can achieve longer blocks in future it will be interesting to see if they do and what their fate will be when paralysis wears off. In both normal and experimental muscles we failed to record endplate potentials in about 3% of fibres impaled.

These results show, in agreement with others[6,7] that TTX can be used to paralyse without killing nerves, and as control animals with cuffs showed no more than normal sprouting[12] any interference of the cuff *per se* with axoplasmic transport was not enough to cause sprouting. We therefore conclude that a few days inactivity of muscle gives rise to a sprouting stimulus. The work of Lomo[13,14] *et al.* has shown that inactivity induced by a local anaesthetic nerve block causes changes in the muscle membrane similar to those of denervation and this result has been confirmed by using TTX block[6,7]. The denervation changes can be prevented by direct stimulation of the muscle[13,14]. We have found (unpublished observations with G. M. Goodwin) that induction of sprouting by botulinum toxin can be prevented by direct stimulation of the muscle. Inflammation also causes muscle membrane hypersensitivity and can cause nerve sprouting[15]. It seems that sprouting is induced by a stimulus from the muscle which may be present normally to a small degree, but is greatly increased in various conditions; for example during prolonged inactivity or inflammation. Whether the stimulus is a diffusible chemical, or a change in the surface of tissues surrounding the nerve terminals is unknown.

M. C. Brown
R. Ironton

University Laboratory of Physiology,
Parks Road,
Oxford OX1 3PT, UK

Received October 8; accepted December 16, 1976.

1 Edds, MacV., *Q. Rev. Biol.*, **28**, 260–276 (1953).
2 Duchen, L. W., and Strich, S. J., *Q. J. exp. Physiol.*, **53**, 84–89 (1968).
3 Duchen, L. W., and Stefani, E., *J. Physiol., Lond.*, **212**, 535–548 (1971).
4 Brownell, B., Oppenheimer, D. R., and Spalding, J. M. R., *J. Neurol. Neurosurg. Psychiat.*, **35**, 311–322 (1972).
5 Hille, B., *Prog. Biophys.*, **21**, 1–32 (1970).
6 Lavoie, P.-A., Collier, B., and Tenenhouse, A., *Nature*, **260**, 349–350 (1976).
7 Pestronk, A., Drachman, D. B., and Griffin, J. W., *Nature*, **260**, 352–353 (1976).
8 Aguilar, C. F., Bisby, M. A., Cooper, E., and Diamond, J., *J. Physiol., Lond.*, **234**, 449–464 (1973).
9 Diamond, J., Cooper, E., Turner, C., and Macintyre, L., *Science*, **193**, 371–377 (1976).
10 Akert, K., and Sandri, C., *Brain Res.*, **7**, 286–295 (1968).
11 Duchen, L. W., *J. Neurol. Neurosurg. Psychiat.*, **33**, 40–54 (1970).
12 Barker, D., and Ip, M. C., *Proc. R. Soc., Lond.*, **B163**, 538–554 (1966).
13 Lømo, T., and Rosenthal, J., *J. Physiol., Lond.*, **221**, 493–513 (1972).
14 Lømo, T., and Westgaard, R. H., *J. Physiol., Lond.*, **252**, 603–626 (1975).
15 Jones, R., and Tuffery, A. R., *J. Physiol., Lond.*, **232**, 13–15P (1973).

Reprinted from Science, Vol. 193, pp. 371–377. 1976

Trophic Regulation of Nerve Sprouting

Neuron-target interactions and spatial relations control sensory nerve fields in salamander skin.

J. Diamond, E. Cooper, C. Turner,* Lynn Macintyre

Studies on developing nervous systems have revealed that nerve cells can change their shape by sprouting axonal branches and reabsorbing old ones. The physiological connections which these branches make with their target cells are the basis for the establishment of circuitry in the nervous system. In studying nerve sprouting, we need to consider both the stimulus for its initiation and the way it is controlled. This control applies to the area over which endings are distributed and to the density of the endings within it. These two parameters, density

and area, define the terminal field of a nerve. The control of sprouting then is a principal means of determining how nerve fields develop. This development could be regulated entirely by a rigid genetic program intrinsic to either the target tissue or the nerve, but a potentially more interesting mechanism would have a competence to respond to internal and external environmental demands. If so, then the dynamic regulation of terminal fields, including sprouting and possibly regression of endings, may be a normal feature of both central and peripher-

al neurons, even in the mature organism. This article deals with investigations of the regulation of terminal fields in a readily accessible peripheral system. It appears that an interaction between the nerve and the target tissue controls the density of the endings, while the area of a terminal field is more determined by spatial relations.

Sprouting During Development

In his observations on the genesis of epithelial innervation, Ramón y Cajal detected an important influence from the target tissue (*1*). He observed that the incoming fibers often grow relatively long distances to reach the epithelial tissues, but only after arriving at them do the nerves start sprouting collateral branches, each growing to a territory devoid of nerves. This sprouting eventually stops, and Ramón y Cajal noted the absence both of any vast aneuritic spaces and of any excessive collection of nerve fibers. He suggested that there are growth-pro-

Dr. Diamond is a member of the M.R.C. Group in Developmental Neurobiology, Department of Neurosciences, McMaster University, 1200 Main Street West, Hamilton, Ontario, Canada L8S 4J9. Dr. Cooper and Dr. Turner are postdoctoral trainees and Lynn Macintyre is a predoctoral trainee, supported by the Medical Research Council of Canada.

371

moting influences emanating from the target tissue, and that these influences ultimately become neutralized in some way by factors released from the nerves themselves. Speidel's visual observations on the living nerves growing into the transparent tail of the tadpole directly supported Ramón y Cajal's suggestion (2). In addition, he noticed that some of the collateral branches produced by the cutaneous nerves sprouted inappropriately into deep tissues. These were subjected to continual remodeling; some would suddenly change their direction, sometimes first retracting for variable distances, to establish connections with the skin successfully, while others eventually stopped elongating and degenerated completely.

The studies of Speidel and Ramón y Cajal revealed that collateral sprouting during development occurs almost entirely in the vicinity of the end organ. A later study by Fitzgerald on the primary innervation of the epidermis of the pig's snout indicated more convincingly the source of the sprouting stimulus (3). In this organ the number of dermal axons present at birth remains constant, but they continually sprout branches which penetrate to the epidermal ridges. Fitzgerald observed that the number of these endings increased in direct proportion to the increase in number of epidermal ridges after birth, suggesting that it is indeed the epidermis which provides the stimulus for the dermal axons to sprout.

Sprouting After Partial Denervation

Nerve sprouting occurs not only during primary development but also during maturity. There is evidence which suggests the possibility that both peripheral and central nerve endings may not be static, but that new endings may be forming as others degenerate (4). However, the most striking demonstration of the ability of mature nerves to sprout is that which occurs when adjacent ones are cut; this "denervation sprouting" occurs in virtually all nerves, certainly in those of vertebrates. Speidel demonstrated this phenomenon by directly observing intact axons 3 days after sectioning one of the nearby cutaneous nerves of the tadpole tail. Weddell, Guttmann, and Gutmann (5), using behavioral and histological techniques, reported similar evidence for collateral sprouting of sensory nerves in the rabbit. Collateral reinnervation of partially denervated skeletal muscle has been quantitatively demonstrated, both histologically as well as functionally, by numerous workers, in-

cluding Edds, Weiss, Hoffmann, and Van Harreveld (see 6). In studying the autonomic nervous system of cats, Murray and Thompson (7) detected sprouting of preganglionic fibers after section of adjacent ones supplying the superior cervical ganglion. This work has been confirmed and extended (8). In man, the recovery of function after section of certain peripheral nerves and during some degenerative nerve conditions is best explained by collateral sprouting of the remaining fibers (9).

Although often more difficult to demonstrate, axonal sprouting occurs also in the mature central nervous system (CNS) of both mammals and lower vertebrates (10). The first clear demonstration of its occurrence in mature mammals was in the well-known experiments of Liu and Chambers (11). They sectioned all but one of the dorsal roots on the left side in the cat and, by histological techniques, showed that after 6 months the spinal ramifications of the remaining root extended further up and down the cord than did those of the corresponding root on the opposite side. In a comparable study on the rat, Goodman and Horel (12) demonstrated the sprouting of retinal projections in some visual nuclei after they were partially denervated by section of the visual cortical efferent fibers. Both of these pioneering studies were based on light microscopy and did not indicate whether new synapses formed. That collateral sprouts can form synapses was convincingly shown by Raisman (13), who studied the septal nuclei with the electron microscope; he showed that after lesions of the medial forebrain bundle, fimbrial fibers (which normally end on dendrites of septal cells) sprouted to form new synapses on some of the vacated sites on the somata of the cells. Although morphologically they looked normal, it was not possible to show whether these new synapses were functional. The occurrence of collateral sprouting in the mammalian CNS is now well established (14). Recent studies suggest that new collateral sprouts in the hippocampus and in the red nucleus do indeed make functional contacts (15).

Sprouting Without Denervation

The exact cause of "denervation sprouting" has always been a mystery. When nerves are cut, either in the central or peripheral nervous system, the part distal to the cell body degenerates and is removed by phagocytic activity involving a variety of other cell types. On the assumption that these nonneural

cellular responses are triggered by products of nerve degeneration, it has long been thought that the stimulus for the nearby intact axons to sprout was of similar origin, even though attempts to obtain direct evidence for this have been unsuccessful (16).

A most striking example of adult nerve sprouting without nerve degeneration is that of Olsen and Malmfors (17), who showed that a piece of iris which had been deprived of its nerves 3 months earlier, when transplanted into the anterior chamber of the eye evokes collateral branching from the intact sympathetic nerves of the host. Some influence from the target tissue [perhaps nerve growth factor (18)] is clearly implicated, as Olsen and Malmfors suggested. The observations by Duchen and Strich (19) of sprouting of motor axons treated with doses of botulinum toxin, which prevented the release of acetylcholine but did not visibly cause nerve degeneration, do not support the "products of degeneration" hypothesis. More recently Aguilar, Bisby, Cooper, and Diamond (20) provided evidence suggesting that factors in living axons regulate nerve sprouting. In these experiments one of the three nerves to the hind limb of the salamander was briefly (30 minutes) exposed to a concentration of colchicine that interrupted fast axoplasmic transport, without noticeably interfering with the ability of the nerves to signal sensory information or drive muscles. After the colchicine treatment the peripheral fields of the two adjacent untreated nerves to the limb enlarged in area, as they did in experiments in which the nerve was sectioned rather than treated with colchicine (21).

In order to exclude the possibility that a scattered degeneration of some of the terminals of the colchicine-treated nerve may have occurred, we have now investigated the density of the mechanosensory endings in addition to the area over which they spread. To measure density, we recorded the mechanical stimulus required to evoke an afferent impulse at each of a large number of points on the skin, and made an appropriate analysis of the distribution of the thresholds. This analysis (22) gives the density of the touch receptors, and the method provides a very sensitive measure of receptor function. The validity of the analysis has now been shown by a direct correlation of physiologically identified "touch spots" with morphologically demonstrated sensory terminal processes; each mechanoreceptor is associated with a single Merkel cell (23). When an appropriate dose of colchicine was used, the number of mechanosensory endings of the treated nerve was unchanged at a time when the adjacent nerves sprouted (Fig. 1B). From 5 to 6 days after nerve section the mechanical threshold needed to evoke an action potential rose markedly, and total insensitivity developed a day later, even though the axons usually were able to respond normally to electrical excitation. The results demonstrate that the effects of the colchicine were not due to nerve degeneration (24). Nor did the drug cause sprouting by a direct action on the skin; after tritium-labeled colchicine was used to treat the nerve, the small amount of systemically distributed label was always equal in the skin of both hind limbs, although the sprouting was on one side only (24). We conclude therefore that colchicine was effective in initiating sprouting in untreated nerves because of its interference with axonal transport in the treated ones.

Hypothesis for Sprouting

Aguilar *et al*. (20) proposed the following hypothesis to explain nerve sprouting. The target tissue continually manufactures a substance that stimulates nerves to sprout, and this effect is neutralized in some way by the release of neural factors which are carried to the endings by neuronal transport. This mechanism represents a negative feedback control system to regulate the density of nerve endings at the target. This hypothesis also explains "denervation-sprouting." As a consequence of the elimination from cut nerves of the neural factors, the preexisting balance between them and the target-tissue growth-promoting substances is disturbed. The intact nerves then sprout until the new nerve terminals can release enough of the neutralizing factors to restore the original equilibrium. Consistent with this hypothesis is our finding that for every ending lost by nerve section, a new one appears from the adjacent nerves; that is, sprouting ceases when the original number of endings is restored (Fig. 1A). At least one implication of this hypothesis is that it accounts for the local acquisition of territory by nerve endings (and even individual nerves) during primary development, since each ending releases factors that hinder other endings from sprouting into its own immediate region [see (1)]. In the salamander skin a finding consistent with this hypothesis is that each mechanosensory nerve axon acquires an area of skin which it virtually "owns"; there is a mosaic of axonal receptive fields with only slight overlapping (22).

Spatial Relations and Sprouting

It is largely accepted that nerve fields are spatially organized, some overlapping, others not. If, as we have indicated, the production of terminal fields involves sprouting whose density is regulated by the mechanisms described above, then there must be some territorial control of these mechanisms. This control could be achieved by an appropriate proximity between a nerve and its prospective target tissue at the correct time during embryonic development. We further investigated our model of nerve sprouting by asking whether there are territorial controls of nerve sprouting in the mature organism. From the results we might hope to learn something of the extent to which the apportioning of territory during development is permanent, and whether it could be subject to continual remodeling during the life of the animal.

We mapped the mechanosensory field areas in the hind limbs of salamanders by brushing the skin and recording the evoked afferent impulses. The three segmental nerves that supply the limb have precisely defined fields, which, although they vary from animal to animal, are symmetrical between the two hind limbs.

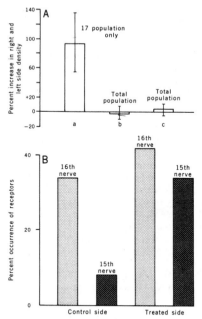

The 16th nerve innervates most of the dorsal surface. When this nerve is cut or treated with colchicine, the fields of nerves 15 and 17 enlarge, reaching a maximum in 8 to 12 days (Fig. 2, A and C). This enlargement, however, continues only until the two fields meet; they never overlap. In many animals the fields of nerves 15 and 17 already have a common frontier between them (Fig. 2B), and in these cases there is no area enlargement when nerve 16 is cut, although nerves 15 and 17 do sprout *within* their own fields (Fig. 1A). To investigate the possibility that a competitive situation exists here, whereby nerves actively exclude each other from their own territory, two nerves to the limb were cut, either 15 and 16, or 16 and 17.

Surprisingly, neither of the nerves 15 and 17 takes over the other's territory during the normal period when sprouting occurs, and, since the territory was totally denervated, the result could not be due to competition between the two nerves. One possible explanation, that there is a mechanical barrier to sprouting between the 15th and 17th fields (25), was excluded by a fortuitous finding. The 16th nerve has two branches, the anterior (16A) and posterior (16P), which join respectively the 15th and 17th nerve

Fig. 1. (A) Quantitative sprouting after partial denervation. We measured the percent occurrence (the density) of the low-threshold touch spots (22) in a region of skin shared by the 16th and 17th nerves, and compared the values between right and left limbs. In the normal animal there is a high degree of symmetry between the two sides, that is, the total number of receptors is the same and so is their distribution among the spinal nerves which supply the corresponding regions of skin. Column a refers to a group of animals in which the right 16th nerve had been sectioned 3 weeks previously and shows the percent difference between right and left for the 17th nerve touch-receptor population only. Normally there is no difference. The increase in 17th nerve receptors is clearly seen. Column b shows, for the same group of animals, that there is no right-left difference when the total receptor population is compared (on the treated side there was only a 17th nerve innervation, but on the control side there was a shared 16th and 17th nerve supply). Column c shows the absence of a right-left difference in total population of touch receptors in a control group of animals, with 16th and 17th nerves intact on both sides. There is no significant difference between columns b and c; this indicates that the increase in 17th nerve receptors on the right side of the experimental group had quantitatively made up the loss due to 16th nerve section (vertical bars = S.E.M.). (B) Sprouting after colchicine treatment of adjacent nerve. Results from a single animal show touch-receptor density in a region of skin shared by the 15th and 16th nerves. In this animal the number of touch receptors associated with the 15th nerve was only a small proportion of the total. There was no loss in the population of receptors supplied by the right colchicine-treated 16th nerve, compared to the left (the increase is within the normal variation). However, on the right side the 15th nerve supplied a significantly increased population of receptors.

trunks (Fig. 2A); the frontier between the two 16 subfields is also that up to which 15 and 17 will grow. We found that, in many animals, when we cut nerves 15 plus 16A or nerves 17 plus 16P, the remaining branch of 16 invaded the denervated region beyond the frontier; however, nerves 15 and 17 stopped at it. We conclude then that there is no mechanical barrier to sprouting across the boundary region. Over significantly longer periods (1½ to 3 months), which we are examining, nerve 17 displays a clear capacity to make a limited incursion into the area of nerve 15 in the distal part of the limb although 15 has never invaded the nerve 17 area.

Another possibility to explain the apparent restriction in sprouting is that the nerves were close to an upper limit of field area that they could supply by sprouting. We excluded this by cutting all the nerves in the leg except for one 17th nerve branch, which supplied a region of skin adjacent to the boundary; extensive sprouting of this branch occurred, but only within the permitted zone—the 17th nerve field.

Location of Territorial Control

In the absence of a mechanical barrier to sprouting, of competition between the nerves, or of an inadequate capacity to enlarge their territories sufficiently, we considered the possibility that the skin stimulus to sprout is specific to each

area. To test the possibility of specificity of the sprouting stimulus, skin rotation experiments were performed. Areas of hind limb skin (up to 100 mm²) were rotated 180°, and their reinnervation patterns were studied (Fig. 3). The results were unexpected, since the ingrowing 15th nerve fibers created a new frontier, which was coincident with the position on the limb of the original 15–17 one, as though no skin rotation had occurred at all, and showed no preference for their original skin. This result was not simply dependent on the presence and location of the surviving central nerve stumps beneath the rotated skin flap. In some experiments in which the limb was partially denervated in addition to rotation of the skin (for example, by section of nerves 17 and 16P), the uncut branch of the 16th nerve (16A) was observed to grow across the rotated implant, as it often does in normal unrotated skin. However, the 15th nerve in most animals was confined to the newly created frontier even when this frontier straddled a region that was originally part of the 15th nerve's territory (Fig. 3). Nerve 17 tended to spread more or less indiscriminately over the transplant along with the corresponding (posterior) branch of the 16th nerve. Probably all of the fibers that invaded the transplant were those cut at the border of the excised piece of skin, and thus were regenerating. We conclude that the tendency for nerve 17 to "break out" of its territory, normally requiring both a longer time to be ex-

pressed and appearing primarily in the distal part of the limb, is enhanced when the nerve is regenerating. This is in contrast to the more rigorous containment of nerve 15 within its territory. Differences between regenerating and sprouting intact nerves are discussed below.

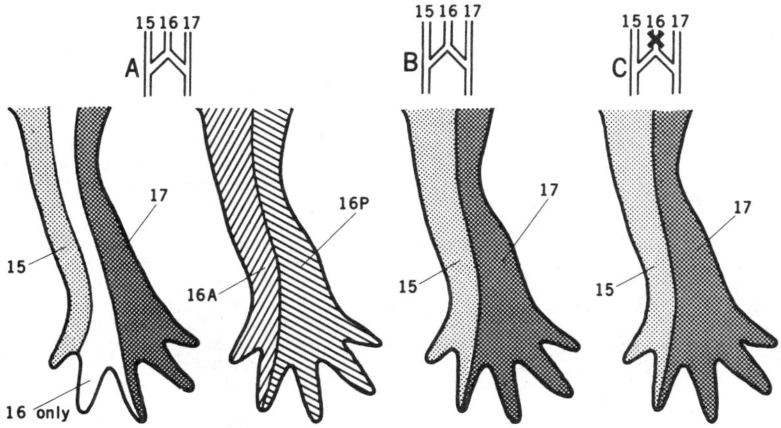

In summary, nerve 15 refuses to sprout into skin normally supplied by nerve 17 when that skin is in situ, and yet invades it when it is transplanted into the original territory of nerve 15, but only up to the line that defines the limit of that territory on the surface of the limb. Moreover, the 15th nerve is apparently unable to invade even a sector of its own skin, which occupies a position beyond that line. The 17th nerve initially is governed by similar territorial limitations. It becomes less so in the distal part of the limb with the passage of time, or when it is regenerating. Finally, nerves 16A and 16P are able to cross the frontier more readily than either nerve 15 or 17.

In interpreting the above findings, we must first abandon *skin* fields as defining nerve territory and instead substitute a territory defined with reference to some coordinate system, which must relate to the body. We refer to this coordinate system as "body space." For the 15th nerve especially, the body space rigorously determines where the nerve will sprout, that is, where its nerve field occurs. Second, nerves seem capable of sprouting functional endings nonselectively, even into "foreign" skin, provided that skin is within the body-space territory of the nerve. Third, and important in its implications, the stringency with which the nerve field is governed by or complies with this body-space territorial limitation, is variable. There may be a time dependency, in that the intact 17th nerve conformed to the body-space control only for about 1 month, and the 15th nerve for as long as we have followed it (at least 4 months). Finally, our results indicate that nerves which do "break out" of their body space to invade adjacent denervated skin do so more readily in the distal, rather than proximal, region of the limb.

Sprouting of Regenerating Nerves

According to our hypothesis for nerve sprouting, the prior occupancy of skin by a nerve will have neutralized the sprouting stimulus. Therefore, under normal conditions there is no tendency for invasion by adjacent nerves. However, such invasion may occur when the occupying nerve is cut, or when its neuronally transported factors are reduced by

Fig. 2. Nerve territories in dorsal skin of salamander hind limb. (A) Control limb in which fields of nerves 15 and 17 do not meet. The two subfields of nerve 16, 16A and 16P, are shown separately for clarity; the whole of this skin was supplied by the 16th nerve, which overlapped with the other two nerves as shown. (B) Control limb in which fields of nerves 15 and 17 meet. (C) Experimental limb in which nerve 16 has been cut, showing enlargement of the fields of nerves 15 and 17, which, in the control limb, were as shown in (A); they now meet at the common border between 16A and 16P. The fields of nerves 15 and 17 of a limb similarly treated, whose fields are shown in (B), were unchanged in area, although the *density* of their endings increased (see text). For convenience, in this and subsequent figures the control and experimental limbs are represented with the same anteroposterior orientation.

SCIENCE, VOL. 193

colchicine. Invasion by adjacent nerves, however, depends on how rigorously the body-space limitations are imposed and possibly on how long the now excessive skin stimulus is permitted to be available. Regenerating nerves, in contrast, appear to have special qualities. When we cut all three nerves and redirected the regenerating fibers of nerve 15 into the distal stump of the cut 16th nerve (while preventing regeneration of 16 and 17), we found that they were apparently guided to "foreign" skin and formed mechanosensory endings in it which functioned quite normally. A similar finding has recently been reported (26). Moreover, the redirected 15th nerve fibers showed no apparent preference for the 16A branch (which would have guided them to their original territory) but freely entered both divisions of nerve 16.

In the example shown (Fig. 4, A and B), the innervation pattern was relatively uncommon in that the posterior branch of the 16th nerve failed to supply the most lateral strip of limb skin, which therefore received only 17th nerve fibers. The regenerating 15th nerve fibers filled both 16A and 16P fields, although the latter overlapped with the field of nerve 17. However, they did not invade the strip previously occupied by nerve 17 only. It seems, therefore, that, outside the limits of the presumed mechanical guidance provided by the degenerating trunk of nerve 16, the body-space territorial limitation applied. While they are actively regenerating, therefore, nerves may be guided into normally alien territory (see 27).

Simultaneous collateral sprouting and regeneration. A nice example that distinguishes between the territorial containment of the sprouting of intact nerves, in contrast to that of regenerating ones, was obtained in the following kind of experiment. The 15th and 16th dorsal root ganglia were removed, and all the nerves to the limb were cut except for one branch of the 17th. This branch sprouted up to the border between the 15th and 17th territories, and stopped there. However, the skin field of nerve 15 did eventually become completely innervated by the regenerating fibers from the other cut branches of the 17th nerve; these fibers had grown up, around, and into the denervated stump of 16A, which guided them downward into the skin territory of 16A and 15 (28).

There is another reason for believing that there are differences between the sprouting of intact and of regenerating nerves. In winter we found that salamander nerves frequently will not sprout col-

laterals at all after the cutting of adjacent nerves, although the distal portions of the cut nerves always underwent the usual Wallerian degeneration. However, the cut nerves always regenerate quite normally to produce new functional endings in skin and muscle. It seems that regenerating nerves are not under the control of the sprouting stimulus from the target tissue, but more likely respond to some innate "drive" that is triggered in an all-or-nothing fashion by nerve section; given mechanical guidance they are not specially sensitive to the foreignness of the body region invaded. Our findings with regenerating nerves suggest that they may not always provide an appropriate model of the development of normal innervation (see 29). In contrast to regenerating nerves, normal intact nerves sprout in a graded manner, dependent on the balance between the peripheral stimulus (which may be reduced in salamanders during winter) and the neuronally transported factors; they are also to a greater or lesser extent governed by limitations imposed by their body space (see above).

We also investigated the question of whether nerves regenerating along with a limb newly growing after complete amputation in the adult animal would form normal fields. When one spinal nerve was given an opportunity to innervate the blastema in advance of the other two (30), all three spinal nerves overlapped everywhere in the limb (Fig. 4D). However, when all three nerves were allowed to regenerate simultaneously, there was some restoration of the normal pattern of innervation. We are further investigating the extent to which territorial limitations become expressed in this type of situation.

Discussion

As to general conclusions that may be made from these results, of most importance is the indication that there exists throughout life a means of continuous regulation of nerve fields. This regulation involves an interaction between the effects of "sprouting-stimuli" produced in or near the target tissue, and of factors brought to the periphery by neuronal transport. During development there is evidence that an initial "overshoot" in sprouting occurs at muscle, followed by a regression of endings to achieve an appropriate pattern of innervation (31). An ideal control system should be able both to increase and to decrease the density of nerve endings. The mechanism that regulates sprouting, however, is subject to limitations imposed on the nerves by their occupancy of territories in body space. These determine the extent to which nerves will or will not enlarge the areas of their terminal fields. The ability of nerves to "break out" of their territories varies, possibly, with the position of the origin of the nerves along the neuraxis, with the time over which they are exposed to the sprouting stimulus, and with the distance from the central axis of the body. The establishment of distinct body territories occurs presumably during primary development by as yet unknown mechanisms and could involve chemical gradients (32, 33). Perhaps the territories we have suggested as being defined in body space are analogous to the compartments discovered in *Drosophila* (34), whose possible role in controlling shape and size was discussed by Crick and Lawrence (35). The imposing of spatial character on a nerve fiber population could require the participation of the peri-

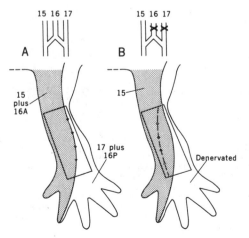

Fig. 3. Effects of rotating skin areas on nerve fields. (A) and (B) refer to an experiment in which the rectangle of skin shown in limb (A) was rotated 180° in limb (B). The unshaded area in the control limb (A) is the field of nerves 16P and 17. The 15th field is shaded. In the experimental limb both the 16th and 17th nerves had been cut at the time of skin rotation. The unshaded area shows the denervated region of skin. The dashed line in the skin rectangle of limb (B) shows the original boundary between the 15th and 17th fields in the skin before rotation. (This was also the boundary between fields of 16A and 16P; see Fig. 2.) After sprouting and invasion of the rotated skin flap, the new 15 boundary established in limb (B) skin is in the identical position in body space to that in the control limb (A).

neurium or some analogous structural component in the CNS; such an involvement of nonneural cells may confer on these a role well beyond that of metabolic or mechanical support.

Our findings are of interest in relation to the results of other experiments which suggest that skin can, at an early enough stage of development, apparently provide information about its location in the body to the incoming nerve, which is then used to construct appropriate reflex circuitry in the spinal cord (36). Possibly the body space influence on the nerve we describe is that which confers regional specificity on the skin too. If so, then the spatial influence, while it directly controls the areas of nerve fields at the level of the peripheral target, may affect the central connections of the nerve mostly by this indirect means. In the experiments quoted above, if respecification of rotated skin occurred, it took too long a time for its result to be effective in the CNS. What is clear is that a regional character of skin does not affect the peripheral fields of the incoming nerves (36), but only their central reflex connections.

The mechanisms involved in the interactions between neuron and target, along with the existence of spatial influences on sprouting, help us to understand a variety of related phenomena involving the terminal nerve sprouting of normal nerves as well as that of denervation sprouting. The sprouting found by Olsen and Malmfors (17) into the iris transplant in the anterior chamber of the eye clearly indicates a target stimulus. The sprouting of motor nerves treated with botulinum toxin (19) would also be explained if, in addition to release of acetylcholine, release of the postulated neural factors was also blocked by the toxin. Another phenomenon that becomes understandable is the way in which the density of endings apparently remains constant during the growth of an organ or tissues (3), suggesting that a peripheral stimulus is involved in the initiation of sprouting (1, 18, 37).

Neural mechanisms of the sort we propose should have their counterparts in the CNS; there is evidence, for example, that spatial gradients may control nerve fields in the visual system (33, 38). Hubel, Wiesel, and Le Vay found that the cortical projections of the lateral geniculate neurons connected to one eye enlarged their territories in layer IV at the expense of adjacent territories associated with the other eye, after monocular deprivation earlier in life either by eye removal (39) or by lid suture (40). These changes presumably reflect a sprouting of one set of terminals and very likely either an arrest of growth or a regression (or both) of the other set; such changes could be related to a reduced neuronal transport in the deprived axons (see 41). There is evidence (20) that axons treated with colchicine are not themselves able to respond to the sprouting stimulus, as if this ability too were dependent on neuronal transport. In any event, our hypothesis explains why a failure of one neural input to establish or maintain its normal territory could result in an unusual enlargement of the territory of an adjacent input, provided the latter's exclusion by body space territorial limitations is not absolute.

Our speculations do not exclude the possibility either of the operation of specific target influences that can guide nerves to make preferential connections (37), or of the establishment of territorial limitations which apply over circumscribed three-dimensional spaces such as a segment of spinal cord, a limb, or even a single neuron (42). What we are emphasizing is the potential importance in the mature nervous system of the dynamic regulation of the density of terminal fields, whose areas are also subject to territorial limitations. While the skin is a simple model there is no reason why the principle should not apply to any target. We now have some evidence that the influence of body space in governing nerve fields may be an attribute also of the muscle fields of the nerves we have investigated, in addition to those in the skin. Presumably, synaptic fields on neurons represent an analogous system.

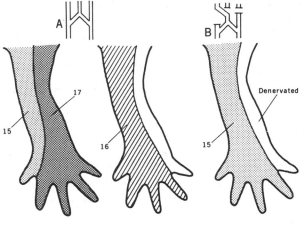

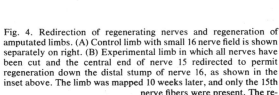

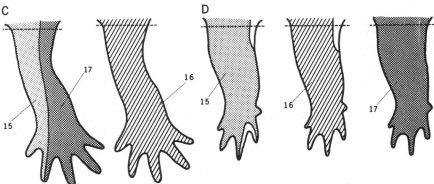

Fig. 4. Redirection of regenerating nerves and regeneration of amputated limbs. (A) Control limb with small 16 nerve field is shown separately on right. (B) Experimental limb in which all nerves have been cut and the central end of nerve 15 redirected to permit regeneration down the distal stump of nerve 16, as shown in the inset above. The limb was mapped 10 weeks later, and only the 15th nerve fibers were present. The region originally supplied by nerve 17 only was not invaded by the regenerated 15 nerve fibers. (C) and (D) Compare the 15, 16, and 17 nerve fields respectively in a control limb and in a limb which had regenerated for 4 months after amputation at the level shown by the horizontal dashed line. For clarity the 16th field is shown separately in the control, and all three fields are shown separately in the regenerate. In this experiment the 17th nerve regenerated ahead of the other two (30). Note that except for two very small regions, all three nerves overlapped in the regenerated limb.

376

Conclusion

1) Our hypothesis, that the density of endings in a given nerve field is regulated by the interaction of sprouting factors continually manufactured by the target tissue, with neutralizing (antisprouting) agents carried to the nerve endings by neuronal transport, has been strengthened by quantitative studies on the mechanosensory innervation of salamander skin.

2) After we partially interrupted fast axoplasmic transport in one nerve by colchicine application, its terminal field was invaded by sprouting fibers from neighboring axons, even though its own endings might be unchanged in number, distribution, and sensory threshold.

3) This mechanism to regulate sprouting is observed in the mature animal. Its operation, involving either provision of extra sprouting factor or reduced neuronal transport, can explain various developmental and experimental situations in peripheral and central nervous systems (such as partial denervation), in which collateral nerve sprouting occurs (43).

4) The area of a given nerve field (the extent of target territory over which the nerve endings occur) is susceptible to a spatial control that is not located in the target itself, but relates to the coordinate system provided by the body. Nerves will normally sprout only within their "body space" territory, which is presumably allotted to them during primary development. Some cutaneous mechanosensory nerves of the salamander, for example, will invade apparently "foreign" skin only if it is relocated in their appropriate body space, and will not usually sprout even into their own original skin if the skin lies beyond the defined boundary of their territory. This boundary however is not a mechanical barrier to sprouting. Other nerves, exposed long enough to the sprouting stimulus provided by adjacent denervated skin, can break out of their body space territory to a limited extent, especially when these particular nerves are regenerating.

5) The stimulus that initiates regeneration in a cut nerve is different from that causing collateral sprouting of intact nerves at a target tissue. Regenerating fibers seem to have "central drive" and can ignore the limitations imposed by the body space control of territory. When guided by degenerating nerve trunks, regenerating axons of a nerve will readily innervate alien territory whose border is not crossed by the collateral sprouts of intact fibers of the same nerve. In newly regenerating salamander limbs, nerves are less rigorously governed by this spatial control of territory.

6) It seems that both mechanisms, the local neuron-target interaction that regulates the density of endings within a field, and the more generalized body space control that serves to limit the permitted area of the terminal field, could conceivably be involved in adjustments of neural circuitry throughout the life of the organism.

References and Notes

1. S. Ramón y Cajal, *Trab. Lab. Invest. Biol. Univ. Madrid* **17**, 181 (1919); in *Studies on Vertebrate Neurogenesis*, L. Guth, Transl. (Thomas, Springfield, Ill., 1960), pp. 149–200.
2. C. C. Speidel, *Am. J. Anat.* **52**, 1 (1933); *J. Comp. Neurol.* **61**, 1 (1935); *Biol. Bull. (Woods Hole, Mass.)* **68**, 140 (1935); *Harvey Lect.* **36**, 126 (1941).
3. J. T. Fitzgerald, *J. Anat.* **95**, 495 (1961).
4. D. Barker and M. C. Ip, *Proc. R. Soc. London Ser. B* **163**, 538 (1966); A. R. Tuffery, *J. Anat.* **110**, 221 (1971); C. Sotelo and S.L. Palay, *Lab. Invest.* **25**, 653 (1971).
5. G. Weddell, L. Guttmann, E. Guttmann, *J. Neurol. Neurosurg. Psychiatry* **4**, 206 (1941).
6. M. V. Edds, *Q. Rev. Biol.* **28**, 260 (1953).
7. J. G. Murray and J. W. Thompson, *J. Physiol. (London)* **135**, 133 (1957).
8. L. Guth and J. J. Bernstein, *Exp. Neurol.* **4**, 59 (1961); T. H. Williams, J. Jew, S. L. Palay, *ibid.* **39**, 181 (1973). See also K. Courtney and S. Roper, *Nature (London)* **259**, 317 (1976); S. Roper, *ibid.* **261**, 148 (1976).
9. C. Coers and A. L. Woolf, *The Innervation of Muscle; A Biopsy Study* (Blackwell Scientific, Oxford, 1959); W. K. Livingstone, *J. Neurosurg.* **4**, 140 (1947).
10. L. Guth and F. Windle, *Exp. Neurol. Suppl.* **5**, 1 (1970).
11. C. N. Liu and W. W. Chambers, *Arch. Neurol. (Chicago)* **79**, 46 (1958).
12. D. C. Goodman and J. A. Horel, *J. Comp. Neurol.* **127**, 71 (1966).
13. G. Raisman, *Brain Res.* **14**, 25 (1969).
14. R. Y. Moore, in *Plasticity and Recovery of Function in the Central Nervous System*, D. G. Stein, J. J. Rosen, N. Butters, Eds. (Academic Press, New York, 1974), pp. 111–128.
15. O. Steward, C. W. Cotman, G. Lynch, *Exp. Brain Res.* **18**, 396 (1973); N. Tsukahara, H. Hultborn, F. Murakami, Y. Fujito, *J. Neurophysiol.* **38**, 1359 (1975).
16. P. Weiss, *J. Exp. Neurol.* **68**, 393 (1934); ——— and A. C. Taylor, *J. Exp. Zool.* **95**, 233 (1944); but see H. Hoffman, *Aust. J. Exp. Biol. Med. Sci.* **30**, 541 (1952).
17. L. Olsen and T. Malmfors, *Acta Physiol. Scand. Suppl.* **348**, 1 (1970).
18. R. Levi-Montalcini and P. V. Angeletti, *Physiol. Rev.* **48**, 534 (1968); E. Zaimis, Ed., *Nerve Growth Factor and Its Antiserum* (Athlone, London, 1972); K. Stoeckel and H. Thoenen, *Brain Res.* **85**, 337 (1975).
19. L. W. Duchen and S. J. Strich, *J. Exp. Physiol.* **53**, 84 (1968).
20. C. E. Aguilar, M. A. Bisby, E. Cooper, J. Diamond, *J. Physiol. (London)* **234**, 449 (1973).
21. This increase in the area of the adjacent nerve fields was not due to the unmasking of previously "silent" endings [D. T. Cass, T. J. Sutton, R. F. Mark, *Nature (London)* **243**, 201 (1973); S. A. Scott, *Science* **189**, 644 (1975)]. We have applied localized electrical stimulation with a fine probe which selectively activates single mechanosensory axons, and shown that no electrically excitable axons exist outside their mapped areas.
22. E. Cooper and J. Diamond, in preparation.
23. ———, R. Leslie, A. Parducz, C. Turner, *J. Physiol. (London)* **256**, 117 (1976).
24. E. Cooper, J. Diamond, C. Turner, in preparation.
25. We had not obtained evidence either by light or electron microscopy that the regions of the skin at the edges of the cutaneous spinal nerve fields differ from elsewhere in the limb.
26. B. T. Johnson, J. E. Schrameck, R. F. Mark, *Proc. R. Soc. London Ser. B* **190**, 59 (1975).
27. R. W. Sperry, in *Handbook of Experimental Psychology*, S. S. Stevens, Ed. (Wiley, New York, 1951), chap. 7, pp. 236–280; A. F. W. Hughes, Ed., *Aspects of Neural Ontogeny* (Academic Press, New York, 1968), pp. 1–249.
28. The regenerating 17th fibers that grew up and around to join the 16th nerve trunk originated from the 17th nerve trunk. We recorded the total mechanosensory 17th nerve input from that trunk. The whole dorsal skin was found to be innervated by the 17th nerve fibers. When the 16A branch was recut, all the innervation from the 16A and 15th fields disappeared, leaving only the unchanged mechanosensory input from the 17th nerve field. Thus, the 16A trunk was the route taken by the 17th nerve axons which supplied the "alien" 16A and 15th nerve field. It was then necessary to test whether these were regenerating 17th nerve fibers of the cut branches or aberrant sprouts from the uncut ones of the intact 17th nerve branch. This was done by an occlusion experiment. We electrically stimulated the 16A trunk and the intact 17th nerve branch, and recorded the compound action potentials (CAP) from the main 17th nerve trunk. Simultaneous stimulation through both pairs of electrodes gave a CAP which exactly equaled the sum of the individual CAP's obtained from stimulation of each pair of electrodes alone. This result meant that the fibers of the uncut 17th nerve branch were not responsible for branches that had grown up and around into the 16th nerve trunk.
29. M. Constantine-Paton and R. R. Capranica, *Science* **189**, 480 (1975).
30. To achieve this both nerves 15 and 16 were cut and tied, leaving nerve 17 free to innervate the blastema. Eventually nerves 15 and 16 regenerated around their ligatures and also innervated the regenerating limb.
31. P. A. Redfern, *J. Physiol. (London)* **209**, 701 (1970); J. Bagust, D. M. Lewis, R. A. Westerman, *ibid.* **229**, 241 (1973); M. R. Bennett and A. G. Pettigrew, *ibid.* **241**, 547 (1974); M. C. Brown, J. K. S. Jansen, D. Van Essen, *Acta Physiol. Scand.* **95**, 3A (1975).
32. R. Sperry, in *Organogenesis*, R. L. De Haan and H. Ursprung, Eds. (Holt, Rinehart & Winston, New York, 1965), pp. 161–186.
33. M. Jacobson, *Developmental Neurobiology* (Holt, Rinehart & Winston, New York, 1970).
34. A. Garcia-Bellido, *Ciba Found. Symp.* **29**, 161 (1975).
35. F. H. C. Crick and P. A. Lawrence, *Science* **189**, 340 (1975).
36. N. Miner, *J. Comp. Neurol.* **105**, 161 (1956); M. Jacobson and R. E. Baker, *ibid.* **137**, 121 (1969); J. H. Sklar and R. K. Hunt, *Proc. Natl. Acad. Sci. U.S.A.* **70**, 3684 (1973).
37. M. D. Coughlin, *Dev. Biol.* **43**, 140 (1975).
38. M. Gaze, *The Formation of Nerve Connections* (Academic Press, London, 1970).
39. T. N. Wiesel and D. H. Hubel, *Soc. Neurosci. Abstr.* **740**, 478 (1974).
40. D. H. Hubel, T. N. Wiesel, S. Le Vay, personal communication.
41. B. Grafstein, M. Murray, N. Ingoglia, *Brain Res.* **44**, 37 (1972).
42. S. M. Crain and E. R. Peterson, *Science* **188**, 275 (1975).
43. There are other possibilities than those specifically outlined in our hypothesis of nerve sprouting which our evidence does not preclude. For example, neuronally transported materials may act intracellularly to limit uptake of the sprouting factors into the nerve endings. Alternatively, the target tissue factors may be continually taken up and retrogradely transported to act at the cell body (18). There is a similarity between our hypothesis and the first of these two alternatives in that both involve two agents, one produced by the target tissue, the other by the nerve. Our hypothesis, however, proposes that the neural factor is released from the nerve endings. The second alternative involves only a target factor. However, it does require the assumptions that the retrograde transport of this factor is blocked by colchicine, and that this leads to a damming up of the factor sufficiently to limit its uptake at the nerve endings and so cause a buildup in the target tissue.
* Present address: Department of Physiology, Queen's University, Kingston, Ontario K7L 3N6.

Journal of Neurocytology **9**, 277–303 (1980)

Sprouting and regression of the nerve at the frog neuromuscular junction in normal conditions and after prolonged paralysis with curare

A. WERNIG[1], M. PÉCOT-DECHAVASSINE[2] and H. STÖVER[1]

[1]*Max-Planck-Institut für Psychiatrie, Kraepelinstraße 2, 8000 München 40, West Germany*
[2]*Equipe de Recherche du CNRS No. 160, Laboratoire de Cytologie, Université Pierre et Marie Curie, 7, Quai St. Bernard, Paris, France*

Received 18 January 1979; revised 26 July and 20 September 1979; accepted 26 September 1979

Summary

A light microscopical, histochemical and electron microscopical investigation of the frog neuromuscular junction has been performed on muscles from animals in different functional states of activity.

The combined staining of axon terminals and cholinesterase (ChE) allows a precise description of the nerve terminal arborization and its synaptic contacts. Most terminal arborizations form long continuous contacts with the muscle cell. Distinguishable from these are nerve branches (usually of small diameter) or distal endings of branches with one or several small and isolated contacts. It is assumed that these are sprouts with newly-formed synaptic sites. Other sprouts end without apparent synaptic contact. At the ultrastructural level, nerve sprouts growing into empty, well-differentiated synaptic gutters or inducing the formation of new synaptic sites were observed.

In other sites, ChE is apparently located at postsynaptic gutters with no nerve present. Similarly, in the electron microscope, well-differentiated synaptic gutters lacking any nerve or Schwann cell elements were observed. In addition, synaptic gutters only partially occupied by the nerve were frequently seen. These features have been interpreted as signs of regression of the nerve terminals.

Nerve regression and sprouting were found in animals chronically paralysed with curare over several weeks as well as in untreated frogs (winter and summer frogs, laboratory frogs, fed and unfed). When quantitatively evaluating the occurrence of presumed features of nerve sprouting and nerve regression, differences were found between different experimental groups. From this it is concluded that, in addition to developmental changes, the degree of nerve sprouting and regression is controlled by external factors such as muscle activity and seasonal variations.

Signs of sprouting and nerve regression can be simultaneously present in a single synapse. It appears that the frog neuromuscular synapse is not a static structure, but is in a state of permanent remodelling.

Introduction

Sprouts from the distal part of the axon of motor neurons, including the nerve terminal, have been described in a variety of conditions such as experimental partial denervation (Edds, 1953; Haimann et al., 1976; Brown & Ironton, 1978; Thompson, 1978) or pathological partial denervation due to a progressive loss of motor neurons in poliomyelitis and other diseases (for details, see Bowden & Duchen, 1976). Nerve sprouting has also been observed after blockade of transmitter release by botulinum toxin and tetanus toxin (Duchen & Strich, 1968; Watson, 1969; Duchen, 1970, 1971; Duchen & Tonge, 1973; Brown et al., 1977; Pestronk & Drachman, 1978) and after blockade of electrical activity of the nerve by tetrodotoxin (Brown & Ironton, 1977a; Pestronk & Drachman, 1978). From these observations, it is rather clear that sprouting from the peripheral motor neuron is a common reaction of the nerve cell in response to a variety of factors. It is of interest to note that in all cases the activity of a portion or all of the muscle is blocked (see Discussion).

The original purpose of this investigation was to study the functional characteristics and morphological appearance of the frog neuromuscular junction after prolonged paralysis of synaptic transmission by curare. Prolonged curarization produces denervation-like changes in the muscle fibre as interpreted from the development of extrasynaptic receptors for ACh (Berg & Hall, 1975; Wernig & Stöver, 1977). It was of special interest to see whether the motor neuron would also react to this kind of paralysis in which transmitter release is not directly impaired. However, when we found that the signs of nerve sprouting and regression were not absent in preparations obtained from animals which were considered to be normal and, thus, control animals, the need for a quantitative measure of these features became pressing. In the course of this work, then, the neuromuscular junctions were investigated in frogs selected from groups which included winter frogs, summer frogs and frogs kept in the laboratory for a long time with and without feeding. Light microscopical, electron microscopical and electrophysiological methods were employed.

The results have already been presented in preliminary form (Pécot-Dechavassine & Wernig, 1978; Wernig & Stöver, 1979).

Methods

Animals and treatment with curare
Experiments were performed on frogs (*Rana temporaria*) freshly caught or kept in the laboratory over longer periods of time. '*Summer frogs*' were obtained in August (mean temperature 16° C) and '*winter frogs*' in January (mean temperature 0° C); the acute experiments were performed within a few days after the animals had been brought to the laboratory. '*Laboratory frogs*' and

'*starving lean frogs*' had been kept under laboratory conditions for several months; the first group was fed on meal worms twice a week, the latter was starved. Curarization of frogs used for the histochemical investigations was started in January.

To paralyse frogs, doses of 0.1 ml of Curarin-Asta (containing 3 mg D-tubocurarine/ml) were injected into the dorsal lymph sacs. Frogs treated with curare were kept in small lucite containers in which 5–10 animals were placed on moist tissue paper. Twice a day the animals were bathed in cold tap water and the papers replaced. The animals were kept in these containers at room temperature each day from about 9 a.m. to 6 p.m. and at 4° C during the night. During the day, the animals were frequently checked for signs of muscular activity and curare was applied whenever necessary. With this experimental method, animals were paralysed most of the time. During day time (at room temperature), there were short periods in which individual animals were not paralysed; on average this might amount to a few hours (probably less than 5 h) per week per animal. At 4° C activity of animals was reduced even when the level of curarization was not sufficient for a total block.

Once a week, animals were force fed small pieces of liver or meal worms. The animals displayed fluid retention in the lymph system ('oedema') which appeared to be related to the depth of the curare blockade and was thus probably due to blockade of the lymph hearts. Mortality of animals thus treated was low (around 15%); death occurred more frequently in the first few days after beginning the treatment than thereafter. When curarization was started in summer, mortality was considerably higher; the difference might be due to different contributions of skin and lung respiration to the gas exchange in summer and winter (see Müller, 1976).

Electrophysiological investigation

Isolated nerve–muscle preparations were pinned out in lucite chambers and bathed in normal Ringer. Square pulses of 0.2–1 ms duration were applied to the nerve through platinum wires. Conventional recording techniques using potassium chloride (3 M)-filled glass micropipettes were employed to record spontaneous and evoked endplate potentials.

Histochemical procedures

The following method was developed especially to evaluate the exact relation between the nerve terminal arborizations and the synaptic area on the postsynaptic cell. For the latter, the staining method for ChE described by Karnovsky & Roots (1964) was found to be especially valuable since in combination with axon stain it allows a distinction between postsynaptic gutters occupied or unoccupied by presynaptic elements (Figs. 3–6, see also Letinsky *et al.*, 1976). Silver impregnation of the nerve terminal arborizations was performed by adapting Bodian's (1936) method for mammals.

Cutaneus pectoris muscles removed from the animals were carefully pinned out in normal Ringer. It was important to stretch the muscle such that most muscle fibres were under stretch. The following solutions were applied consecutively (Pécot-Dechavassine *et al.*, 1979):

(1) 1% neutralized formalin in normal Ringer for 3 min; stirring of the fluid several times (Pasteur pipette).
(2) Solution for ChE staining (Karnovsky & Roots, 1964) for 7–15 min (until strong deposit is visible), stirring of solution; brief rinsing with normal Ringer.
(3) 5% neutralized formalin in deionized water for 20 min.
(4) 80% ethyl alcohol for at least 60 min.
(5) 0.5–1% aqueous Protargol (Winthrop Lab.) solution for at least 12 h at 37° C.
(6) Reduction for 3–15 min with a fresh solution containing 0.25 g hydroquinone, 0.31 g sodium sulphite (anhydrous), deionized water to 100 ml.

Preparations were kept in deionized water until mounted. Whole muscles cleaned of superficial connective tissue were then embedded in aqueous mounting medium.

Electron microscopical investigation

For electron microscopical investigation, muscles of the hind leg (m. rectus internus major and m. sartorius) were usually used; sometimes (when the muscle was not used for electrophysiology or histochemistry) m. cutaneus pectoris was also used (four frogs). Results from 14 frogs in which light microscopical and electron microscopical investigations were performed on muscles from the same animal are included here. Muscles were isolated in a chamber containing standard Ringer solution. Tetrodotoxin (TTX) (10^{-6} g/ml) was usually added 10 min before fixation in order to suppress the contractions provoked by the fixative. The Ringer solution was replaced successively by cacodylate buffer (0.1 M, pH 7.4) with sucrose (0.2 M) for 2 min and then by the fixative solution (2.5% glutaraldehyde in 0.1 M cacodylate buffer) for 2 h. Pieces were taken from the superficial region of the muscles. They were postfixed for 2 h in 2% oxmium tetroxide in cacodylate buffer, dehydrated in graded alcohols and embedded in Araldite. Thin sections (60–100 nm) were stained with saturated uranyl acetate and with lead citrate. Several sections from each block were examined so that structures were seen at various levels.

Muscles from 25 curarized frogs (2–17 weeks) and from 13 untreated frogs (starving, winter and laboratory frogs) were examined by electron microscopy.

Quantitative measurements of morphological features

All quantitative measurements in the light microscope were performed on cutaneous pectoris muscles. Only superficial synapses which could clearly be attributed to a single muscle fibre were evaluated. Usually, 20 synapses were evaluated per muscle and results from the two cutaneous pectoris muscles of an animal were averaged. The average sarcomere length per muscle (stained preparation) ranged from 2.5 to 3.4 μm and was 3.0 μm on average (12 muscles); all measurements were made by counting the number of sarcomeres times 3.0 μm. Only animals with a rump-nose length of 6.0 to 6.5 cm were included in the evaluation.

In the ultrastructural investigation, a quantitative estimation of the relative frequency of occurrence of 'usual' synaptic sites, on the one hand, and of 'unusual' synaptic sites, on the other hand, was performed on transverse sections of muscles from treated and untreated animals. 'Unusual' synaptic sites were classified in three main categories: *empty gutters, partially occupied gutters* and *features of nerve sprouting* (described below). There is some overlap in the quantitative evaluation presented in Table 2 since sprouts into abandoned gutters were classified under features of nerve sprouting *and* partially-occupied or empty gutter (when the sprout was not in contact with the muscle fibre membrane). Synaptic gutters with a juxta-synaptic area wider than 500 nm were considered as 'unusual' and called *'partially occupied gutters'*.

Two kinds of estimation were made from transverse sections for comparing the size of the synaptic gutters and their relative occupation by the nerve terminals in curarized and untreated frogs. (1) The total *width* of gutters and the width of the gutter occupied by the nerve were estimated on micrographs by measuring the direct distance between the two edges of the differentiated synaptic gutters and the two points where the synaptic clefts open (that is, measuring the diameter of the synaptic gutter covered by the nerve terminal and its Schwann cell). The width of the synaptic gutter measured by this method is directly comparable to the apparent diameter observed in light microscopy. (2) The circumference of the entire differentiated postsynaptic membrane of the gutter and the circumference covered by the nerve was estimated.

The degree of occupation of the gutter was consequently expressed either by the percentage of the width of the occupied gutter relative to the width of the synaptic gutter or by the percentage of the circumference of the postsynaptic membrane occupied by the nerve relative to the entire circumference of the postsynaptic membrane of the primary gutter. Significance of differences were estimated by Student's *t*-test.

The mean diameter of the nerve fibres was estimated from the half sum of two measures made at right angles.

Results

Usual features of the 'normal' neuromuscular junction

Here we shall summarize those morphological and ultrastructural characteristics of frog neuromuscular junctions which are especially relevant to the present investigation (for detailed descriptions of the frog neuromuscular synapse, see Couteaux, 1960; Birks *et al.*, 1960).

Close to the muscle fibre, motor axons often give rise to two (Fig. 1) or more branches which contact the muscle fibre. Frequently branches which seem to originate from different axons are also present. Terminal branches on the muscle fibre bifurcate and usually follow the long axis of the muscle fibre, sometimes in opposite directions. The degree of branching differs from one muscle fibre to another; those with small diameters often have simpler synapses than those with larger diameters.

Fig. 1 shows an endplate after a combined silver and ChE stain. Although ChE is present throughout the gutter, with this method the ChE reaction product develops only at the edges of the synaptic gutter, thus giving rise to the typical double lines. This appearance is typical for a gutter occupied by the axon (middle line) and its accompanying Schwann cell. When presynaptic elements are missing (see below) ChE stains throughout the gutter. Usually most or all terminal branches of the axon are followed by the continuous dark double line of the ChE reaction product, indicating that a large part of the terminal arborization is in contact with the muscle fibre. At bifurcations (arrows in Fig. 1) the double line is frequently missing.

At the ultrastructural level (Fig. 2) the axon terminals lie in a depression of the muscle membrane called the synaptic gutter. The area of postsynaptic membrane in contact with the terminal is characteristically differentiated from the adjacent membrane by infoldings and by the presence of electron-opaque material immediately beneath it and of subneural filaments (F, Fig. 2). Each terminal branch usually occupies the whole length of the synaptic gutter and laterally it covers all of the differentiated postsynaptic area. However, an uncovered 'juxta-synaptic area' (with an average width of 100 nm on either side of the synaptic cleft) was observed quite frequently (see also Couteaux & Pécot-Dechavassine, 1968).

The characteristic ultrastructural constituents of nerve terminals are mainly synaptic vesicles, glycogen granules, mitochondria, neurofilaments and a few microtubules (Fig. 2). Sections through the preterminal axon (Fig. 19) contain mainly

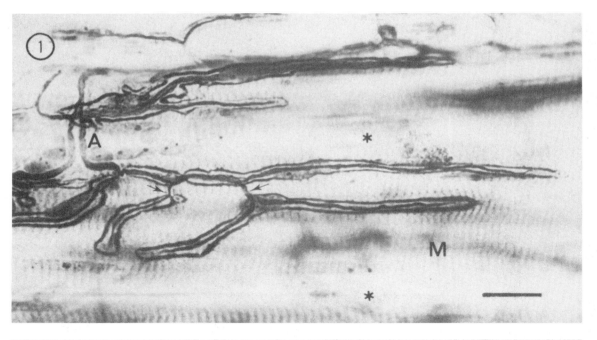

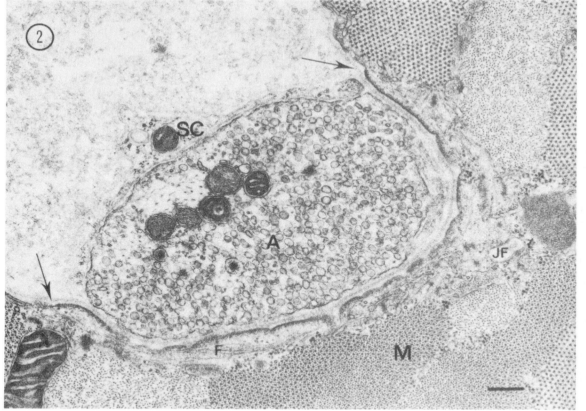

neurofilaments and microtubules; a few vesicles are sometimes present. In this region the axon, which is not yet in contact with the muscle fibre, is enclosed in several layers of Schwann cell processes whereas, in the terminal region, the Schwann cell mainly covers the outer surface of the nerve ending.

Features of regression and sprouting of nerve terminals
When evaluating the appearance of endplates in more detail, important additional features were found at both the light microscopic and at the electron microscopic level. These features were observed in all the different animal groups examined including frogs chronically paralysed with curare for different periods of time as well as untreated animals.

Signs of regression
Apparently because of diffusion barriers, usually only the ChE located at the edges of the synaptic cleft is stained. Where the synaptic gutter is not occupied by a presynaptic element, the ChE reaction product develops throughout the gutter and is more or less homogeneously distributed along the length of the synaptic gutter (Figs. 3–6). Since the nerve is absent, we will define such a ChE reaction product as a *ChE remnant*. Different appearances of such *ChE remnants* were observed at different synapses within the same muscle and in different preparations. In Fig. 3 the ChE reaction product is arranged in a palisade-like manner which probably reflects the arrangement of the postsynaptic infoldings. The position of *ChE remnants* within a synapse is usually at the very distal end and sometimes at the proximal end of a synaptic contact; less frequently a whole branch may be devoid of an axon (Fig. 6, arrow). The length of the *ChE remnant* per synapse ranges from a few to 100 micrometres or more (about 130 μm in Fig. 4). It is suggested that these sites are abandoned parts of the synaptic gutter which were previously occupied by an axon, although light microscopical observations cannot exclude the possibility that the enzyme is located at sites to which the nerve terminal is destined to grow. However,

---

Figs. 1–23. Abbreviations: A, axon; BL, basal lamina; ChER, cholinesterase remnants; F, filaments; Fu, furrows; JF, junctional fold; M, muscle fibre; S, sprout; SC, Schwann cell; Sy, synapse.

Fig. 1. 'Normal' endplates in frog cutaneous pectoris muscle after combined staining of axons (A) and ChE. All light microscopic pictures were taken from muscles mounted *in toto*. At arrows ChE is missing. Borders of the muscle fibre are indicated by the asterisks. Untreated *summer frog*. Scale bar: 20 μm.

Fig. 2. Electron micrograph of a 'normal' neuromuscular junction (transverse section). The arrows indicate the lateral edges of the differentiated postsynaptic area which is characterized by junctional folds, electron-opaque material beneath the muscle membrane and subneural filaments. *Laboratory frog*. Scale bar: 0.2 μm.

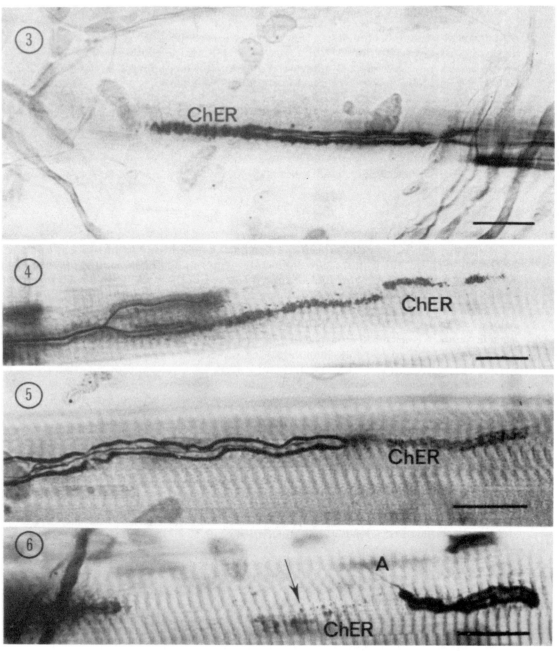

Figs. 3–6. *ChE remnants* of different length and appearance. Note the palisade-like arrangement of the reaction product in Fig. 3. A whole nerve branch seems to be missing in the synapse visible in Fig. 6 (arrow). Untreated *summer frogs*. Scale bars: 20 μm.

Table 1. Average sizes of nerve terminals and synaptic gutters in normally and partially occupied gutters (from transverse EM sections).

	No. of samples	Mean diameter of nerve terminals (μm)	Total synaptic gutter A (μm)	Part of the synaptic gutter occupied by the nerve B (μm)	% occupation from ratio B/A
Width measurement					
Normally occupied gutters ('normal' frogs)	20	1.72* ±0.36	2.80 ±0.63	2.43 ±0.49	88
Partially occupied gutters (curarized frogs)	30	1.21 ±0.38	3.90 ±0.77	1.46 ±0.49	37
Measurement of circumference of the postsynaptic membrane					
Normally occupied gutters ('normal' frogs)	20		3.71 ±0.76	3.30 ±0.76	88
Partially occupied gutters (curarized frogs)	30		4.83 ±0.99	1.80 ±0.55	38

*Mean ± standard deviation.

evidence in favour of the first interpretation comes from the electron microscopical observations in which certain well-differentiated postsynaptic gutters (with characteristic infoldings of the postsynaptic membrane) were seen to be devoid of any nervous elements (Fig. 7). *Empty gutters* are usually filled with collagen fibrils and devoid of Schwann cell elements. Some of these gutters have enlarged and flattened folds and appear more degenerate than others. In Figs. 8 and 9 the synaptic gutters are only partially occupied by nerve terminals ('partially occupied gutters') but otherwise show the same structural differentiation as normal neuromuscular junctions. In *partially occupied gutters* the juxta-synaptic area, previously found to extend on average about 100 nm on either side of the synaptic cleft, is now much larger (more than 500 nm). At individual synaptic sites the width of the uncovered juxta-synaptic area was found to be as much as 2000 nm on each side (Figs. 8, 9). The differentiated postsynaptic membrane often exhibits furrows which are especially deep in the juxta-synaptic area (Figs. 8, 9); similar furrows have been found when the sarcoplasmic membrane is in a state of remodelling especially during the dedifferentiation of the synaptic gutter which occurs after denervation (Verma, 1977).

The mean occupation of a gutter by the nerve terminal, as determined by the ratio total circumference: nerve-occupied circumference of the synaptic gutter, was 37% in a series of 30 samples of *partially occupied gutters* (see Methods) (Table 1). The lowest percentage of the series was 23%. The discrepancy between the sizes of nerve and gutter could be due both to a reduced nerve terminal size and a widening of the synaptic gutter. In considering these possibilities the average nerve terminal diameter in *partially occupied gutters* (1.21 μm) was significantly smaller ($P<0.001$, Student's *t*-test) than that in normal synaptic sites (1.72 μm) (Table 1). However, the mean width of the *partially occupied gutters* and, surprisingly, even the total circumference of the differentiated postsynaptic membrane delimiting the primary gutter in transverse sections were significantly ($P<0.001$) *larger* than at normal synaptic sites (Table 1). *Partially occupied gutters* may be early signs of nerve regression or alternatively late signs of nerve regrowth (see Discussion).

In the light microscope, an intermediate stage between normally innervated and abandoned synaptic gutters is apparent at some synapses (see Fig. 23). Occasionally at the most distal parts of synaptic contacts the ChE reaction product may still be arranged in the typical double line or as a ring, whereas stained axonal elements may be missing. It is possible that these sites are still occupied by the nerve which lacks argyrophilic elements at these points. Alternatively, these sites could be occupied by parts of the Schwann cell after withdrawal or, more likely, before ingrowth of the nerve. (See Discussion.)

Signs of nerve sprouting

In contrast to branches with apparently continuous synaptic contact (as judged from the ChE double lines) nerve branches with only one or a few small ring-like arrangements of the ChE reaction product have been observed (Figs. 11–17). It is assumed that these branches are sprouts with newly-formed synaptic contacts. Less frequently, branches end without apparent synaptic contact (Fig. 10); occasionally a light deposit of ChE reaction product is apparent at the tip of such nerve endings. The apparent diameter of the presumed sprouts is usually considerably smaller than the diameter of the parent branches (for example, Fig. 17). Often the enzyme activity at such rings is less than at other parts of the synapse. In Fig. 12 (arrow) a bridge of less intense ChE activity seems to connect a site with a continuous double line to a ChE ring. These observations suggest that ChE rings are early signs of synapse formation. It is not known at present whether synaptic transmission occurs at these sites and is absent at sites where ChE apparently is not present; since ChE seems to

---

Fig. 7. Electron micrograph (transverse section) of an abandoned synaptic gutter (*empty gutter*). The old postsynaptic area is still characteristically differentiated. The gutter is mostly filled with collagen fibrils; two small processes (possibly from a Schwann cell) are present (arrow). *Curarized frog* (5 weeks). Scale bar: 0.5 μm.

Figs. 8 and 9. Electron micrographs of *partially occupied gutters* (transverse sections). The edges of the well-differentiated gutters are indicated by arrows. The coefficient of occupation by the nerve (see text) is 32% in both cases. The postsynaptic membrane shows furrows. *Curarized frogs* (15 weeks). Scale bars: 0.5 μm.

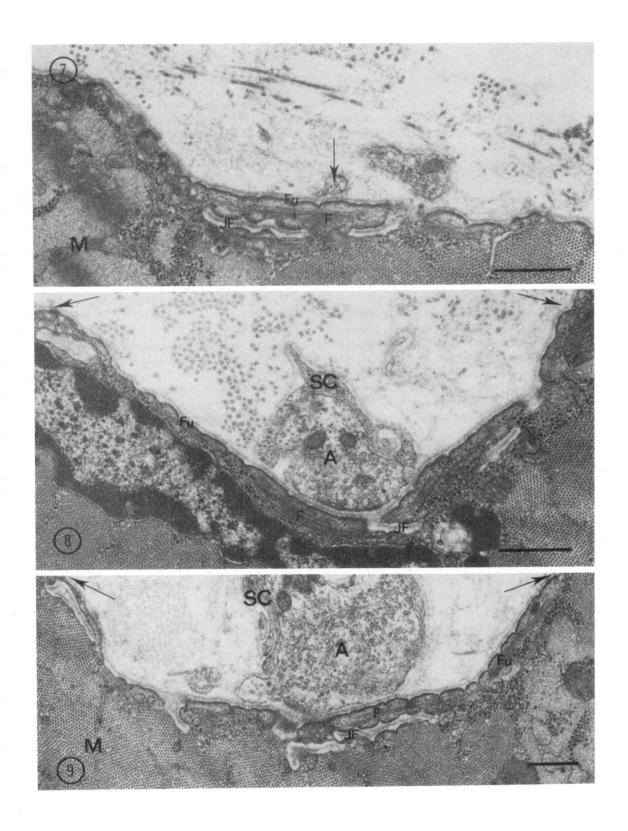

661

appear some time after contact is established (Lømo & Slater, 1976), lack of ChE does not necessarily mean that functional nerve muscle contact is absent.

Judging from the location and the number of ChE rings per branch and the origin of the nerve branches the following different classes of sprouts were defined.

Sprouts without apparent synaptic contact. These structures are thin nerve branches which at their distal end are not associated with an obvious ChE reaction product (Fig. 10). The location of the branch point on the parent axon was not taken into consideration. However, it seems to occur equally frequently from the axon and from the endplate.

When a single ChE ring (diameter < 15 μm) was present sprouts from the endplate were distinguished from sprouts from the axon according to the origin of the branch bearing it. *Sprouts from the endplate* originate from within the complex of the synapse (Figs. 11–13). Their length was usually short (Figs. 11, 12) and rarely as long as in Fig. 13. Occasionally such sprouts can leave one muscle fibre to form contact on a neighbouring fibre.

Sprouts from the axon are branches of the parent axon outside the immediate complex of the synapse, that is, proximally from the first synaptic contact of a 'main' nerve branch (a nerve branch which itself branches off an axon at some distance from the muscle cell), regardless of whether the branch originates a short distance before the first synaptic contact of a main branch (for example, Fig. 14) or from any axon at any distance from the synapse under investigation. Thus, branches probably originating from nodes of Ranvier as well as branches within the terminal arborization of an axon are included. Since myelin sheaths of axons are not revealed by the present staining procedure the usual classification of sprouts (for example, Barker & Ip, 1966) could not be used.

Jumping fibres are thin nerve branches accompanied by several small ChE rings, each with a diameter of < 15 μm and spaced at more or less regular intervals (Figs. 15–17). Such branches can originate within a synapse as the continuation of a branch (Fig. 15) or as a side branch. Branches can also originate from the pre-terminal axon. Occasionally, the nerve makes an obvious departure from the surface of the muscle fibre between two synaptic sites (Fig. 16, star), whereas in other cases the nerve seems to remain on the muscle fibre surface between contacts (Fig. 17). The length

---

Fig. 10. *Sprouts without apparent contact.* Two nerve sprouts (S) leave the synapse and terminate without apparent association with ChE. *Curarized frog* (15 weeks). Scale bar: 50 μm.

Figs. 11–13. *Sprouts from the endplate* (S). Thin nerve branches terminate at a ringlike arrangement of the ChE reaction product. In Fig. 12 light deposits of ChE are visible between the ChE ring and the main synaptic contact (arrow). A rather complex synapse with several ringlike or elongated ChE arrangements is visible in Fig. 13; also a long sprout (S) with a single small contact is present. *Summer frogs* (Figs. 11, 12), *curarized frog* (15 weeks) (Fig. 13). Scale bars: 10 μm (Figs. 11, 12); 20 μm (Fig. 13).

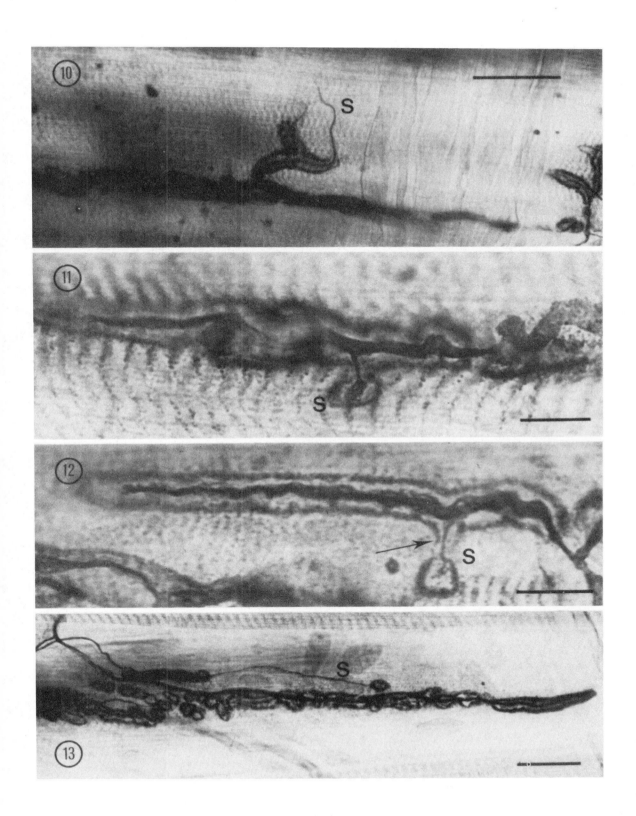

663

of these sprouts ranges from a few to more than a few hundred micrometers, and thus the sprout may constitute from a small fraction up to a major fraction of the total synapse length. Also the number of ChE rings per sprout varies considerably, ranging from two to about ten or twenty. In some branches, larger rings may alternate with smaller ones. If a ChE ring with a diameter larger than 15 μm was interposed in a row of ChE circles < 15 μm, only the part distal to this circle was counted as a *jumping fibre*. Thus branches with small and isolated contacts along their length and a longer (> 15 μm) contact at their distal end are also excluded. From this it is obvious that *jumping fibres* as defined here merely represent a fraction of the nerve branches with discontinuous synaptic contacts.

The notion that formation of new synaptic contacts occurs in adult muscles is strongly supported by ultrastructural observations. Small terminal profiles can be seen in close contact with muscle fibre membrane which lacks typical features of postsynaptic differentiation. The synaptic membrane shows furrows delimiting areas of high electron opacity (Fig. 18). Folds of the sarcoplasmic membrane are either rudimentary or absent, and the subneural filaments are discontinuous. These features are characteristic of developing synapses (Couteaux, 1975). At the ultrastructural level still other features of sprouting are visible. Very thin axons surrounded by several Schwann cell layers were frequently observed close to or inside empty synaptic gutters. In Fig. 19 such a nerve profile is located in a highly differentiated gutter. In Fig. 20 a small nerve sprout is completely surrounded by the Schwann cell which separates it from the postsynaptic membrane; the presence of a fold suggests that this is an old gutter. At other places, a small nerve sprout occupies an empty part of a gutter already partially occupied by a 'mature' nerve ending. It appears, therefore, that newly-formed axonal sprouts are able to re-occupy empty synaptic gutters which evidently had been previously abandoned.

In the ultrastructural investigation, some atrophy of the muscle fibre was observed in *curarized frogs* and in *starving lean frogs*. Longitudinal wrinklings of the muscle fibre membrane parallel to the fibre axis and folds of dissociated basal lamina were observed (Figs. 20, 21). Similar pictures have been observed in denervated muscles (Birks *et al.*, 1959). Despite muscle fibre atrophy, many synaptic sites appeared normal. Fig. 21 shows a normal synaptic site on a very atrophied muscle of a *starving lean frog*. Similarly, synaptic sites of normal appearance are present in muscles of frogs paralysed for long periods (11 weeks in Fig. 22).

Fig. 14. *Sprout from the axon* (S). The branching (arrow) occurs proximal to the first synaptic contact (Sy, not in focus) of the main branch. *Curarized frog* (2 weeks). Scale bar: 15 μm.

Figs. 15–17. Different *jumping fibres*. In Fig. 16, a *jumping fibre* is in contact with a small diameter (about 15 μm) muscle cell; borders of the muscle cell are not visible in the picture. Arrows point to nerve processes. Untreated *summer frogs*. Scale bars: 20 μm (Fig. 15), 10 μm (Figs. 16, 17).

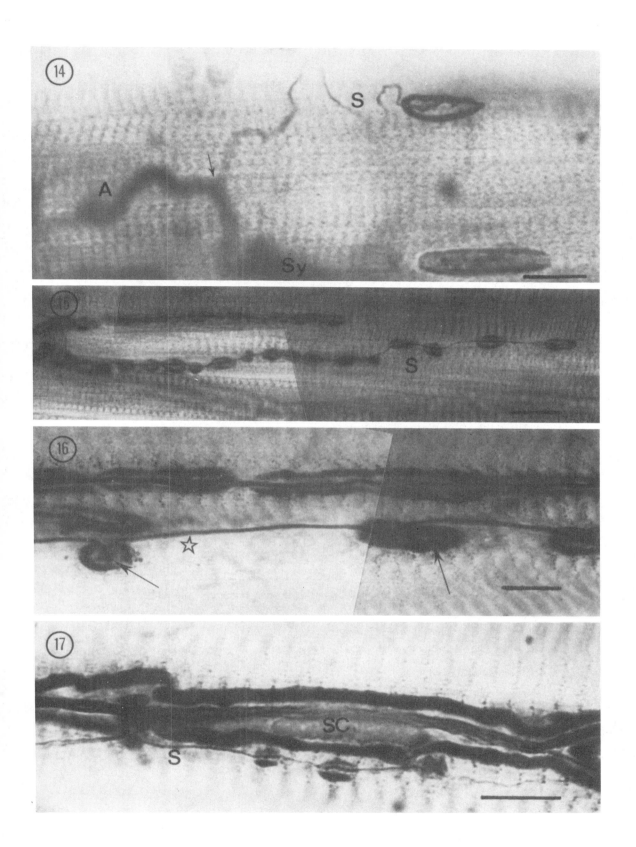

It is important to stress that for any of the animal groups studied, normal as well as unusual junctional sites could be seen in a single transverse section of a muscle fibre. Similarly in the light microscopical investigation, signs of nerve sprouting, nerve regression and normal synaptic contacts were observed on the same muscle fibre.

Quantitative estimation of 'unusual' synaptic features in curarized and untreated frogs
The original purpose of this study was to investigate the influence of prolonged muscle paralysis on the appearance of the neuromuscular junction. Therefore, animals were compared after different periods of curarization. Curarization was performed on freshly caught winter frogs. In addition, untreated animals taken from the natural environment when in a state of low activity (*winter frogs*) and higher activity (*summer frogs*) were used, as well as frogs kept under laboratory conditions (*laboratory frogs*). Since some of the curarized frogs used for the ultrastructural investigations were not fed during treatment the influence of muscle atrophy caused by starvation was studied (*starving lean frogs*). In some cases light and electron microscopic investigations were performed on muscles taken from the same animal. In some experimental groups only light or electron microscopic investigations were performed.

Muscles taken from curarized animals contracted upon stimulation of the nerve after soaking preparations in normal Ringer. Using intracellular microelectrodes amplitude histograms of spontaneous m.e.p.p.s. with overall bell-shaped distributions were observed. The mean m.e.p.p. amplitude in single fibres ranged from 0.51–1.9 mV (mean 0.95 ± 0.37 mV, 13 fibres in six muscles measured in normal Ringer solution), which is comparable to, and certainly not smaller than, the range in normal muscles. In magnesium-block, synchronized release of transmitter was found upon nerve stimulation resulting in endplate potentials of normal risetime (about 1 ms measured at the endplate) in all fibres impaled (210 fibres in muscles from 11 animals). No attempt was made to quantify evoked transmitter release. It can be concluded from these results that mechanisms of synaptic transmission are

---

Fig. 18. A differentiated axon terminal displays an active zone (ZA) opposite a rudimentary postsynaptic fold. The postsynaptic membrane is scalloped. Areas of dense material are present beneath between the furrows. The subneural filaments are discontinuous. All these features characterize newly-formed synaptic sites. *Curarized frog* (15 weeks). Scale bar: 0.2 μm.

Fig. 19. A small *preterminal* nerve sprout (S) is surrounded by several layers of Schwann cell, and lies close to a specialized gutter. This aspect suggests that the nerve sprout is re-occupying a previously abandoned gutter. *Curarized frog* (5 weeks). Scale bar: 0.5 μm.

Fig. 20. A small nerve sprout is enclosed in Schwann cell processes which are in contact with a differentiated postsynaptic membrane (which displays a junctional fold). Note the folds of the dissociated muscle basal lamina, typical of muscle fibre atrophy. *Curarized frog* (11 weeks). Scale bar: 0.5 μm.

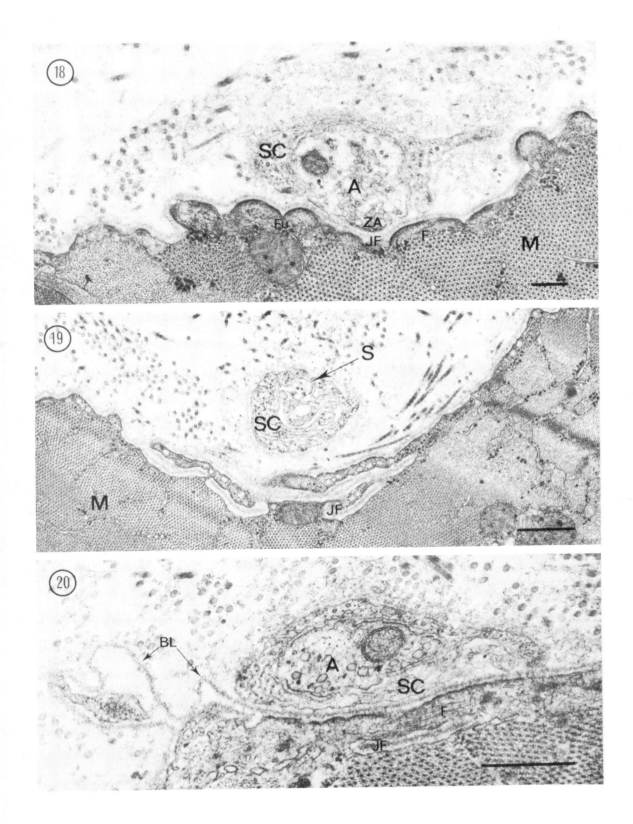

667

Table 2. Quantitative distribution of signs of nerve regression and nerve sprouting from light microscopic investigations. The mean number of synapses (in average percentage of synapses per muscle) showing a parameter, the mean length of *ChE remnants* and *jumping fibres*, and the mean number of *sprouts from the endplate* in synapses which show this parameter are indicated.

	Untreated frogs		Curarized frogs		
	Summer frogs	*Winter frogs*	*1–3 weeks*	*4–7 weeks*	*8–16 weeks*
No. of frogs	7 11*	4 7*	7	4	6
No. of synapses	226 400*	120 221*	214	140	199
ChE remnants					
Percentage	56.6 ±12.2	16.3 ± 7.6	15.3 ±11.4	43.3 ±18.7	41.2 ±11.6
Length (μm)	42.1 ±16.5	15.2 ± 6.5	26.6 ±14.8	46.7 ±24.1	47.3 ±13.0
Sprouts without apparent contact					
Percentage	0.7 ±1.1	5.1 ±1.5	4.9 ±3.6	11.3 ± 3.7	13.4 ± 7.9
Sprouts from the endplate					
Percentage	19.5 ± 8.7	39.8 ±12.3	46.0 ±16.9	69.3 ±18.6	58.2 ± 6.7
No.	1.3 ± 0.2	2.1 ± 0.5	2.2 ± 0.4	2.8 ± 0.3	2.9 ± 0.7
Sprouts from the axon					
Percentage	8.3 ±4.4	11.1 ± 3.4	18.2 ± 7.8	18.5 ±10.0	22.5 ± 6.7
Jumping fibres					
Percentage	26.7 ± 9.3	25.0 ± 9.1	22.0 ± 8.8	31.0 ± 5.7	53.0 ± 11.0
Length (μm)	123.0 ± 25.2	109.0 ± 38.2	133.0 ± 42.5	141.0 ± 26.2	140.0 ± 28.3

*Sprouts from the endplate and jumping fibres were evaluated from the larger numbers of frogs and synapses.

not drastically impaired after prolonged treatment with curare though finer changes would not have been detected with the methods employed.

Table 2 indicates the results obtained from the light microscopical evaluation of features of nerve regression and nerve sprouting as defined above. Despite a large scatter present within groups some differences between groups are apparent. Probably the most striking differences are present between untreated *summer* and

Table 3. Quantitative distribution of 'usual' and 'unusual' synaptic sites from electron microscopic investigations on untreated and curarized frogs.

	Untreated frogs			Curarized frogs		
	Laboratory frogs	Starving lean frogs	Winter frogs	5–6 weeks	7–10 weeks	11–15 weeks
No. of frogs	5	3	4	4	4	3
No. of explored synaptic sites	89	120	156	178	168	155
'Usual' features						
'Usual' synaptic sites (%)	93	86	76	57	44	54
'Unusual' features						
Partially occupied gutters (%)	6	10	13	30	43	38
Empty gutters (%)	1	3	5	11	8	6
Nerve sprouting (%)	1*	3	6	6	9	4
	(0)	(1)	(6)	(2)	(5)	(2)

*The percentage of occurrence of three kinds of synaptic sites (normally and partially occupied and empty gutters) was calculated relative to the others from the total number of explored synaptic sites. The percentage of nerve sprouts lying in or close to a differentiated postsynaptic gutter was independently evaluated from the total number of synaptic sites; this percentage comprises both features of nerve sprouts forming new synaptic sites (cf. Fig. 18) and nerve sprouts approaching a partially occupied or empty gutter (cf. Fig. 19). The numbers in brackets represent the percentage of newly-formed synaptic sites.

winter frogs. In *winter frogs* there are significantly more *sprouts from the endplate* ($P <$ 0.0025 for both parameters, Mann–Whitney test) and more *sprouts without apparent contact* ($P < 0.01$) while there are fewer and smaller *ChE remnants* ($P < 0.01$ for both parameters). On average as many as 50% of the synapses in *summer frogs* are associated with *ChE remnants* and about 40% of the synapses in *winter frogs* have *sprouts from the endplate*. In *curarized frogs* features of sprouting are generally more frequent than in untreated *winter frogs* but there is only a slight trend for an increase with time of paralysis (see Discussion). At the same time the occurrence of *ChE remnants* increases. *Jumping fibres* remain constant for most experimental groups but appear to occur more frequently after longer periods of curarization (see Discussion). The total length of the individual *jumping fibres* ranged from 45 to 460 μm.

Table 3 shows the results from the ultrastructural investigation. The relative occurrences of 'usual' junctional sites and 'unusual' junctional sites (*partially occupied gutters, empty gutters* and features of nerve sprouting) in different experimental animal groups are presented. 'Unusual' features are present in any of the studied series, although clear differences do exist between different animal groups. 'Unusual' features are more frequent in *curarized muscles*: they are present in almost 50% of the explored junctional sites. No clear increase in the number of 'unusual' junctional sites was found from 5 to 15 weeks of paralysis. In the three groups of frogs not

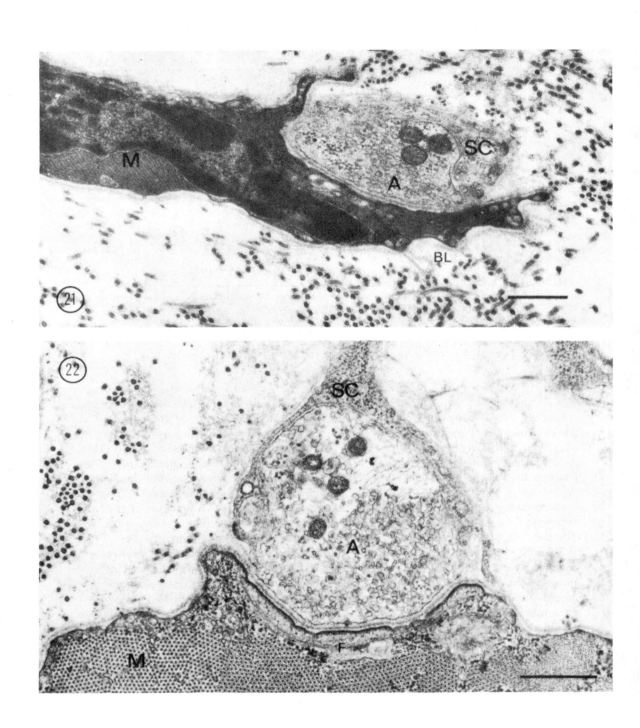

670

curarized, the frequency of occurrence of 'unusual' junctional sites is lower; among these they are more frequent in *starving lean frogs* (14%) and in *winter frogs* (24%) than in *laboratory frogs* (7%). *Summer frogs* were not used in this comparison.

Discussion

The 'normal' frog neuromuscular junction

Signs of both nerve regression and sprouting were found by both light and electron microscopy. By light microscopy the striking feature of nerve regression is the presence of *ChE remnants* as part of an otherwise normal-looking synapse. Since it is known that ChE may persist at abandoned synaptic sites for several months after denervation (Pécot-Dechavassine, 1968; Landmesser, 1972) the different intensity and appearance of the ChE reaction product observed probably reflect different time periods following regression of the nerve terminal from such sites. This hypothesis is suggested by the presence of *ChE remnants* of different intensity and appearance within the same muscle. In this context it should be noted that the quantitative evaluation of the occurrence of *ChE remnants* in different muscles depends to some degree on the quality of the staining which can never be identical for all muscles.

The observation that *ChE remnants* are usually located in distal portions of the nerve terminal arborizations suggests that the tips of nerve terminals can retract. The absence of Schwann cell elements in *empty gutters* indicates that the nerve terminals have not been removed by a degenerative process as observed after nerve section (Birks *et al.*, 1960; Letinsky *et al.*, 1976; Verma & Pécot-Dechavassine, 1977). In the latter case, there is an initial engulfment and phagocytosis of the nerve terminal by the Schwann cell, which subsequently replaces the terminal before occupying the whole synaptic gutter. Except for one of the interpretations given above in connection with Fig. 23 (where there is an absence of stained axonal elements at typically stained junctional sites), there is no evidence for a dissociation of nerve and Schwann cell. It appears, therefore, that the regression of axon terminals and Schwann cells usually occurs concomitantly.

Since the nerve diameter in *partially occupied gutters* is smaller than normal (Table 1) one can imagine that the nerve terminals shrink, retract and progressively withdraw from the synaptic gutters. The flattening of the *partially occupied gutters* could occur

---

Fig. 21. Electron micrograph (transverse section) of a neuromuscular synapse of a *starving lean frog*. The muscle fibre is atrophied and the basal lamina is dissociated from the muscle fibre membrane at some places. The axon terminal, otherwise quite normal, lies in a synaptic gutter located at the extremity of a muscle fibre extension. Scale bar: 0.5 μm.

Fig. 22. Transverse section through a neuromuscular synapse of normal appearance (*curarized frog*, 15 weeks). As in Fig. 2, the axon terminal covers almost all the differentiated postsynaptic area. Scale bar: 0.5 μm.

during retraction of the nerve as a consequence of a 'partial denervation'. Similar features appear after denervation by nerve section (Verma, 1977) and are apparently due to the progressive unfolding of the postsynaptic membrane. Also the increase in the circumference of the differentiated postsynaptic membrane found here could be related to this unfolding. On the other hand it is likely that some of the thinner axon profiles originated from former sprouts which had re-occupied *empty gutters*. We could not distinguish between these two categories in our ultrastructural studies. In the results from curarized frogs there is indirect evidence that *partially occupied gutters* resulted predominantly from synapse regression. If *partially occupied gutters* were mostly re-occupied gutters, *empty gutters* developing simultaneously at an initial stage during treatment would be expected while *partially occupied gutters* were still missing. Such a stage, however, was not observed. By electron microscopy, the proportion of *partially occupied gutters* was higher than the percentage of *empty gutters* during the whole treatment and by light microscopy *ChE remnants* were less frequent after 1–3 weeks of curarization than after 4–15 weeks. Thus it is probable that *partially occupied gutters* are (at least in *curarized frogs*) early signs of regression. We cannot distinguish the relative proportion of *partially occupied gutters* which are due to nerve regression as opposed to regeneration in the other categories of frogs.

The marked longitudinal extent of the terminal branches in the frog neuromuscular junction complicates the light microscopical identification of sprouts. The most striking but less frequent signs of sprouting are nerve terminals which apparently are not accompanied by ChE. It is possible that ChE gradually develops about these nerve endings after the nerve has been present for some time, as suggested by the presence of ChE rings of light to dark staining intensity.

Jumping fibres might develop from a long nerve branch with a single distal ChE ring by subsequent formation of several small and isolated contacts (ChE rings) proximally from the first contact. Alternatively sprouts with a single ChE ring might extend distally to form one or more additional small contacts. Maturation of *jumping fibres* into branches with continuous synaptic contacts probably occurs by enlargement and confluence of the small and isolated synaptic sites (see above). The frequency and length of the *jumping fibres* is difficult to evaluate if the rate of the presumed maturation process is different from the rate of production of the *jumping fibres* themselves. Such rates could even be different for different animal groups. It is unlikely that the isolated small rings of ChE are steps in a regressive development of the synapse, for example, after fractionation of the usual continuous synaptic contacts. In this case one should find *ChE remnants* regularly present near rings of ChE which, however, is not the case (but see Fig. 23a).

Thus it appears that regenerative and regressive events occur simultaneously in a muscle and even within an individual synapse while other parts of the synapse look normal. This suggests that the endplates are in a state of permanent remodelling. Nerve terminals successively leave and re-occupy the synaptic gutters and nerve sprouts form new junctional sites. The existence of remodelling is further supported

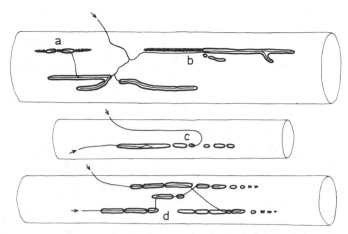

Fig. 23. Camera lucida drawing showing three different synapses in which re-occupation of previously abandoned gutters has apparently occurred. At (a) a sprout (*jumping fibre*) from the neighbouring branch forms two small synaptic contacts (rings of ChE reaction product) at a site with *ChE remnants*. *ChE remnants* in proximal prolongation of a normally innervated part of the synapse (b); it was rare to find a nerve branch in the close vicinity of *ChE remnants*. It is not clear from the picture whether part of the nerve branch has recently detached from the synaptic gutter or has failed to re-occupy a previously abandoned gutter. Also shown are sites apparently occupied by some elements (presumably Schwann cells which lead the axons) but devoid of stained nerve elements (also in c and d). In (c) and (d) nerve branches abruptly change direction to reach synaptic gutters which, judging from their location, were probably connected in a different way before. The features shown in (a) and (b) were in reality located at different synapses. The observations depicted in (a), (c) and (d) were made in muscles curarized for two weeks, in (b) in a muscle curarized for 15 weeks.

by the occurrence of certain complex synapses which give the impression of a partly wrong 're-wiring' (Fig. 23c, d).

'Unusual' features of the neuromuscular synapse in different animal groups
Identical signs of nerve sprouting and nerve regression have been found in all animal groups studied. Two different interpretations are conceivable. (1) It is possible that sprouting and regression occur independently at different periods during the lifetime. (2) Sprouting and regression are physiological reactions, not at all, or not exclusively, related to development; they occur through the whole life span of the animal and are controlled by external factors.

From current experiments (Wernig, unpublished observations), it appears that, in frogs (*Rana temporaria*) with a rump–nose length of 5, 6 and 7 cm, the average synapse length (measured from the most proximal synaptic contact of a branch and including those parts of a branch not accompanied by ChE) is roughly 400, 600 and over 800 μm. Although it is not clear how reliably the size of an animal is related to its age (a large dependence of animal size and weight in the course of ontogenesis of *Xenopus laevis* on food supply, temperature and population density under laboratory conditions has indeed been observed, H. Müller, personal communication), it appears that in the frog, growth in length of the animal continues non-linearly throughout life (H. Müller, personal communication), and it is likely that the enlargement of synapses occurs by means of sprouting. Tuffery (1971) has claimed that an increase in the complexity of synapses due to sprouting occurs in the course of development of mammalian muscle. The quantitative differences in occurrence of signs of nerve sprouting and regression in frogs of different animal groups but equal body length on the other hand, show that their frequency of occurrence is modulated by external factors.

The results obtained from the animal groups used in the present study do not allow conclusions about the rates of nerve sprouting and regression or the nature of the mechanisms responsible for them. Also, the effects of prolonged curarization might be better appreciated by comparison with different control groups (for example, freshly caught winter frogs which are given the same temperature treatment). It appears, however, that the frequency of occurrence of sprouting and regression can change over a period of about six months (when comparing untreated *summer* and *winter frogs*) and is obviously controlled by seasonal factors (for example, differences in activity of the animal, in food uptake, temperature and hormonal state).

Nerve sprouting is also observed after different types of presynaptic blockade in mammalian muscles (Duchen & Strich, 1968; Duchen, 1970, 1971; Duchen & Tonge, 1973; Brown & Ironton, 1977a; Brown et al., 1977; Pestronk & Drachman, 1978). On the other hand direct stimulation of muscles after total or partial denervation (Lømo & Rosenthal, 1972; Brown & Ironton, 1977b; Lømo & Slater, 1978) or after presynaptic blockade (Brown et al., 1977) prevents nerve sprouting (and the occurrence of extrasynaptic ACh receptors). From studies on cell cultures of chick embryo it is known that the formation of new synapses can occur in the presence of ACh receptor-blocking drugs such as curare (Crain & Peterson, 1971; Cohen, 1972; Freeman et al., 1976). The blockade of muscle activity in chick embryo by curare (for example, Srihari & Vrbová, 1978) also seems to delay or suppress the reduction of multiple innervation in embryonic muscle. These results can be interpreted to mean that nerve sprouting, synapse formation and elimination of multiple innervation can be induced by different factors which are related to muscle activity.

Similarly, from the present results it appears that nerve sprouting is inversely related to muscle activity, since it is more frequent in *winter* and *curarized frogs* than in *summer* and *laboratory frogs*. Signs of nerve regression, on the other hand, develop during periods of low activity (*curarized frogs*) but are infrequent in untreated *winter frogs* and frequent in *summer frogs*. It is possible that different mechanisms cause nerve regression in the different animal groups.

In conclusion, our results suggest that frog neuromuscular synapses are permanently undergoing remodelling. A process of remodelling has also been assumed to occur in mammals (Barker & Ip, 1966; Tuffery, 1971; Ip, 1974). Letinsky *et al.* (1976) concluded from some of their observations that 'some ongoing morphological changes may occur normally at the frog neuromuscular junction'. Young (1952) suggested that in the synapse there is simultaneous growth and degeneration. Our results further suggest that in the frog the intensity of remodelling of neuromuscular synapses is modulated by external factors such as seasonal factors and muscle activity.

Acknowledgement

Brigitte Wernig performed much of the histochemical work. Professor R. Couteaux and Professor G. Kreutzberg were helpful in many discussions. The work was supported by a Twinning Grant from the European Training Programme in Brain and Behaviour Research (ETP).

References

BARKER, D. & IP, M. C. (1966) Sprouting and degeneration of mammalian motor axons in normal and deafferentated skeletal muscle. *Proceedings of the Royal Society of London, Series B* **163**, 538–54.

BERG, D. K. & HALL, Z. W. (1975) Increased extrajunctional acetylcholine sensitivity produced by chronic post-synaptic neuromuscular blockade. *Journal of Physiology* **244**, 659–76.

BIRKS, R., HUXLEY, H. E. & KATZ, B. (1960) The fine structure of the neuromuscular junction of the frog. *Journal of Physiology* **150**, 134–44.

BIRKS, R., KATZ, B. & MILEDI, R. (1959) Dissociation of the 'surface membrane complex' in atrophic muscle fibres. *Nature* **184**, 1507–8.

BIRKS, R., KATZ, B. & MILEDI, R. (1960) Physiological and structural changes at the amphibian myoneural junction in the course of nerve degeneration. *Journal of Physiology* **150**, 145–68.

BODIAN, D. (1936) A new method for staining nerve fibres and nerve endings in mounted paraffin sections. *Anatomical Record* **65**, 89–97.

BOWDEN, R. E. M. & DUCHEN, L. W. (1976) The anatomy and pathology of the neuromuscular junction. In *Neuromuscular Junction* (edited by ZAIMIS, E.), pp. 23–29. Berlin, Heidelberg, New York: Springer-Verlag.

BROWN, M. C., GOODWIN, G. M. & IRONTON, R. (1977) Prevention of motor nerve sprouting in botulinum toxin poisoned mouse soleus muscles by direct stimulation of the muscle. *Journal of Physiology* **267**, 42–3P.

BROWN, M. C. & IRONTON, R. (1977a) Motor neuron sprouting induced by prolonged tetrodotoxin block of nerve action potentials. *Nature* **265**, 459–61.

BROWN, M. C. & IRONTON, R. (1977b) Suppression of motor nerve terminal sprouting in partially denervated mouse muscles. *Journal of Physiology* **272**, 70–1P.

BROWN, M. C. & IRONTON, R. (1978) Sprouting and regression of neuromuscular synapses in partially denervated mammalian muscles. *Journal of Physiology* **278**, 325–48.

COHEN, M. W. (1972) The development of neuromuscular connexions in the presence of d-tubocurarine. *Brain Research* **41**, 457–63.

COUTEAUX, R. (1960) Motor end-plate structure. In *Structure and Function of Muscle* (edited by BOURNE, G. H.), pp. 337–380. New York: Academic Press.

COUTEAUX, R. (1975) Facteurs de la différenciation des 'zones actives' des membranes présynaptiques. *Comptes rendus des Séances de l'Académie des Sciences (D)* **280**, 299–301.

COUTEAUX, R. & PÉCOT-DECHAVASSINE, M. (1968) Particularités structurales du sarcoplasme sous-neural. *Comptes rendus des Séances de l'Académie des Sciences (D)* **266**, 8–10.

CRAIN, S. M. & PETERSON, E. M. (1971) Development of paired explants of foetal spinal cord and adult skeletal muscle during chronic exposure to curare and hemicholinium. *In vitro* **6**, 373–81.

DUCHEN, L. W. (1970) Changes in motor innervation and cholinesterase localization induced by botulinum toxin in skeletal muscle of the mouse: differences between fast and slow muscles. *Journal of Neurology, Neurosurgery and Psychiatry* **33**, 40–54.

DUCHEN, L. W. (1971) An electron microscopic study of the changes induced by botulinum toxin in the motor end-plates of slow and fast skeletal muscle fibres of the mouse. *Journal of the Neurological Sciences* **14**, 47–60.

DUCHEN, L. W. & STRICH, S. J. (1968) The effects of botulinum toxin on the pattern of innervation of skeletal muscle in the mouse. *Quarterly Journal of Experimental Physiology* **53**, 84–9.

DUCHEN, L. W. & TONGE, D. A. (1973) The effects of tetanus toxin on neuromuscular transmission and on the morphology of motor endplates in slow and fast skeletal muscle of the mouse. *Journal of Physiology* **228**, 157–72.

EDDS, M. V. (1953) Collateral nerve regeneration. *Quarterly Review of Biology* **28**, 260–76.

FREEMAN, S. S., ENGEL, A. G. & DRACHMAN, D. B. (1976) Experimental acetylcholine blockade of the neuromuscular junction. Effects on end-plate and muscle fibre ultrastructure. *Annals of the New York Academy of Sciences* **266**, 46–59.

HAIMANN, C., MALLART, A. & ZILBER-GACHELIN, N. F. (1976) Competition between motor nerves in the establishment of neuromuscular junctions in striated muscles of *Xenopus laevis*. *Neuroscience Letters* **2**, 15–20.

IP, M. C. (1974) Some morphological features of the myoneural junction in certain normal muscles of the rat. *Anatomical Record* **180**, 605–16.

KARNOVSKY, M. J. & ROOTS, L. (1964) A 'direct-coloring' thiocholine method for cholinesterases. *Journal of Histochemistry and Cytochemistry* **12**, 219–21.

LANDMESSER, L. (1972) Pharmacological properties, cholinesterase activity and anatomy of nerve-muscle junctions in vagus-innervated frog sartorius. *Journal of Physiology* **220**, 243–56.

LETINSKY, M. S., FISCHBECK, K. H. & McMAHAN, U. J. (1976) Precision of reinnervation of original postsynaptic sites in frog muscle after a nerve crush. *Journal of Neurocytology* **5**, 691–718.

LØMO, T. & ROSENTHAL, J. (1972) Control of ACh sensitivity by muscle activity in the rat. *Journal of Physiology* **221**, 493–513.

LØMO, T. & SLATER, C. R. (1976) Control of neuromuscular formation. In *Gif Lectures in Neurobiology on 'Synaptogenesis'* (edited by TAUC, L.), pp. 9–30. Jouy en Josas.

LØMO, T. & SLATER, C. R. (1978) Control of acetylcholine sensitivity and synapse formation by muscle activity. *Journal of Physiology* **275**, 391–402.

MÜLLER, H. K. (1976) The frog as an experimental animal. In *Frog Neurobiology* (edited by LLINAS, R. and PRECHT, W.), pp. 1023–1039. Berlin, Heidelberg, New York: Springer-Verlag.

PÉCOT-DECHAVASSINE, M. (1968) Evolution de l'activité des cholinestérases et de leur capacité fonctionnelle au niveau des jonctions neuromusculaires et musculotendineuses de la grenouille après section du nerf moteur. *Archives internationales de Pharmacodynamie et de Therapie* **176**, 118–33.

PÉCOT-DECHAVASSINE, M. & WERNIG, A. (1978) The effect of longtime treatment with curare on the frog neuromuscular synapse. *Neuroscience Letters* Suppl. **1**, S39.

PÉCOT-DECHAVASSINE, M., WERNIG, A. & STÖVER, H. (1979) A combined silver and cholinesterase method for studying exact relations between the pre- and postsynaptic elements at the frog neuromuscular junction. *Stain Technology* **54**, 25–8.

PESTRONK, A. & DRACHMAN, D. B. (1978) Motor nerve sprouting and acetylcholine receptors. *Science* **199**, 1223–5.

SRIHARI, T. & VRBOVÁ, G. (1978) The role of muscle activity in the differentiation of neuromuscular junctions in slow and fast chick muscles. *Journal of Neurocytology* **7**, 529–40.

THOMPSON, W. (1978) Reinnervation of partially denervated rat soleus muscle. *Acta physiologica scandinavica* **103**, 81–91.

TUFFERY, A. R. (1971) Growth and degeneration of motor end-plates in normal cat hind limb muscles. *Journal of Anatomy* **110**, 221–47.

VERMA, V. (1977) *Modifications ultrastructurales et physiologiques de la jonction neuromusculaire après section du nerf moteur*. Thèse d'Université. Paris.

VERMA, V. & PÉCOT-DECHAVASSINE, M. (1977) A comparative study of physiological and structural changes at the myoneural junction in two species of frog after transection of the motor nerve. *Cell and Tissue Research* **185**, 451–64.

WATSON, W. E. (1969) The response of motoneurones to intramuscular injections of botulinum toxin. *Journal of Physiology* **202**, 611–30.

WERNIG, A. & STÖVER, H. (1977) Extrajunctional ACh receptors and the formation of foreign nerve synapses after curare and botulinum toxin. *Pflügers Archiv* Suppl. **368**, R32.

WERNIG, A. & STÖVER, H. (1979) Sprouting and regression of the nerve at the neuromuscular junction. *Pflügers Archiv* Suppl. **379**, R38.

YOUNG, J. Z. (1952) Growth and plasticity in the nervous system. *Proceedings of the Royal Society of London, Series B* **139**, 18–37.

Section 13
Development of Behavior

Marler, P. and S. Peters. 1977. Selective vocal learning in a sparrow. *Science* 198: 519–521.

Nottebohm, F. and A.P. Arnold. 1976. Sexual dimorphism in vocal control areas of the songbird brain. *Science* 194: 211–213.

DeVoogd, T.J. and F. Nottebohm. 1981. Sex differences in dendritic morphology of a song control nucleus in the canary: A quantitative Golgi study. *J. Comp. Neurol.* 196: 309–316.

Perhaps the ultimate expression of the developmental principles outlined in previous sections is animal behavior. Understanding the development of behavior in terms of underlying neuronal events has progressed rapidly in the last few decades, largely because neurobiologists have taken advantage of a wealth of psychological and ethological information about vertebrate behavior. In the work discussed in this section, the advantages of studying sexually dimorphic behaviors and their control by hormones is highlighted.

The ontogeny of birdsong provides a good example of the recent synthesis of ethology and cellular neurobiology. Birdsong consists of stereotyped calls and more complex sounds that, for each species, constitute a characteristic song; males in reproductive condition sing, whereas females typically do not. The systematic investigation of birdsong began with Thorpe's work in the 1950s (see Thorpe 1961; Nottebohm 1970). Thorpe showed that song is actually learned from conspecifics during a limited "critical period" in early life (Thorpe 1958; Marler and Tamura 1964; **Marler** and **Peters 1977**). In zebra finches, for example, song learning is restricted to about the first 80 days after hatching (Immelmann 1969); canaries, however, can learn a new song repertoire in successive years (Nottebohm and Nottebohm 1978). Vocal learning apparently occurs by modification of the vocal output until the auditory feedback it generates matches a previously acquired model (Konishi 1965; Marler and Peters 1977).

What is the neural basis of the ability to sing? A good correlation exists between singing and the size of the telencephalic vocal control areas of the songbird brain. These areas are much larger in males than in females (**Nottebohm** and **Arnold 1976**) and, within the same species, they are larger in males with more complex song repertoires than in males with simple repertoires (Nottebohm et al. 1981). The sexual dimorphism of these nuclei is accounted for both by different numbers of neurons and different neuronal morphologies (Gurney and Konishi 1980; **DeVoogd** and **Nottebohm 1981**; Gurney 1981).

As might be expected, the sexual dimorphism of the vocal control pathways has a hormonal basis. If testosterone is given during the development of the female zebra finch, the size of these brain areas is increased. Administration of the hormone to mature females that were treated as chicks will then elicit song (Gurney and Konishi 1980). The early "masculinizing" effect of testosterone is due mainly to the action of one of its metabolites, estradiol. Thus, the effect of hormones on the brain pathways for vocal control in birds is apparently both to "organize" and to "activate" this behavior. That is, the hormone influences the differentiation of specific nuclei and triggers song production in the adult.

Recently, an even more striking plasticity has been discovered in the canary brain: The size of telencephalic vocal control nuclei in adult males changes seasonally, in parallel with testosterone levels. These nuclei are larger in the spring, when the birds are in full song, and smaller in the fall (Nottebohm 1981). The question has been raised whether these size changes also involve the making and breaking of synaptic connections and whether such changes in connectivity could be the basis for learning a new song each year. Since neurons in these vocal areas bind gonadal hormones (Arnold et al. 1976; Arnold and Saltiel 1979), the swelling and shrinking of these nuclei may result from direct actions of testosterone or its metabolites. Because there is a sex-dependent differential uptake of hormone by cells in some of the sexually dimorphic nuclei of the zebra finch brain, it has also been suggested that the early "organizational" effect of testosterone is achieved by modulating the prevalence of cytoplasmic hormone receptors (Arnold and Saltiel 1979).

The neural basis of sexually dimorphic behavior is also being studied in mammals. Lordosis behavior in female rats (a posture that is adopted for coitus) is thought to be controlled in part by neurons in the preoptic area and the hypothalamus (see McEwen 1978, 1981). Raisman and Field (1973) described sexual dimorphism in the types of synapses in the preoptic area of adult rats. This difference is sensitive to androgens in the early postnatal period, since exposure of young female rats to testosterone abolishes the dimorphism. Subsequent study of the preoptic area has also uncovered differences in neuronal number and morphology and in the overall volume of the sexually dimorphic regions (Greenough et al. 1977; Harlan et al. 1979; Gorski et al. 1980). Furthermore, the overall volume of the dimorphic area is also androgen-sensitive during a critical period in early postnatal life (Gorski 1979; Gorski et al. 1980). Hormones probably act directly on the neurons of interest, since estradiol and testosterone stimulate outgrowth of neurites in explants from the relevant regions of the preoptic nucleus and hypothalamus (Toran-Allerand 1976, 1980).

Finally, sexual dimorphism has also been described in the visual and olfactory systems of some invertebrates. For example, male flies display courtship and chasing behaviors not usually seen in females. In the region of the brain most concerned with the chasing behavior, the male *Musca* has two retinotopic columns of neurons and two giant tangential cells not found in the female (Hausen and Strausfeld 1980; Strausfeld 1980). With respect to olfaction, many species of insects have sexually dimorphic antennae. In the moth, for instance, the male antennae are larger and are specialized for detection and orientation towards a pheromone released by the female. In the part of the brain concerned with olfaction, the male has another specialized area (the macroglomerular complex) believed to be responsible for processing the pheromone signal (Boeckh et al. 1977; Hildebrand et al. 1980). Projecting into the macroglomerular complex are the dendrites of a set of male-specific neurons that are excited when the antennae are stimulated by the pheromone (Boeckh et al. 1977; Hildebrand et al. 1980; Matsumoto and Hildebrand 1981).

How do these sex-specific properties of the invertebrate brain arise? Unlike birds and mammals, insects generally do not have a system of sex hormones that acts during development (although they are certainly subject to other hormones that act systemically). In at least some insects the primary sensory neurons appear to influence the development of central neurons directly. This interaction has been studied in moth brains innervated by neurons from implanted male or female antennae. The transplants showed that both the physiological and morphological properties of the sexually dimorphic central neurons are dictated by the gender of the antennal neurons that innervate them (Schneiderman et al. 1980).

In summary, studies of the development of behavior and of the neural components underlying it have made remarkable progress. Because this work deals directly with behavior, it may offer unique insights into difficult areas such as the basis of learning and memory.

References

Arnold, A.P. and A. Saltiel. 1979. Sexual difference in pattern of hormone accumulation in the brain of a songbird. *Science 205:* 702–705.

Arnold, A.P., F. Nottebohm, and D.W. Pfaff. 1976. Hormone concentrating cells in vocal control and other areas of the brain of the zebra finch *(Poephila guttata). J. Comp. Neurol. 165:* 487–512.

Boeckh, J., V. Boeckh, and A. Kuhn. 1977. Further data on the topography and physiology of central olfactory neurons in insects. *Olfaction Taste Proc. Int. Symp. 6:* 315–321.

DeVoogd, T.J. and F. Nottebohm. 1981. Sex differences in dendritic morphology of a song control nucleus in the canary: A quantitative Golgi study. *J. Comp. Neurol. 196:* 309–316.

Gorski, R.A. 1979. Long-term hormonal modulation of neuronal structure and function. In *The neurosciences fourth study program* (ed. F.O. Schmidt and F.G. Worden), pp. 969–982. MIT Press, Cambridge, Massachusetts.

Gorski, R.A., L.D. Jacobson, J.E. Shryne, and V. Csernus. 1980. The influence of neonatal gonadectomy and androgens on the sexually dimorphic nucleus of the preoptic area. *Soc. Neurosci. 6:* 381. *(Abstr.)*

Greenough, W.T., C.S. Carter, C. Steerman, and T.J. DeVoogd. 1977. Sex differences in dendritic patterns in hamster preoptic area. *Brain Res. 126:* 63–72.

Gurney, M.E. 1981. Hormonal control of cell form and number in the zebra finch song system. *J. Neurosci. 1:* 658–673.

Gurney, M.E. and M. Konishi. 1980. Hormone-induced sexual differentiation of brain and behavior in zebra finches. *Science 208:* 1380–1383.

Harlan, R.E., J.H. Gordon, and R.A. Gorski. 1979. Sexual differentiation of the brain: Implication for neuroscience. *Annu. Rev. Neurosci. 4:* 31–71.

Hausen, K. and N.J. Strausfeld. 1980. Sexually dimorphic interneuron arrangements in the fly visual system. *Proc. R. Soc. Lond. B 208:* 57–71.

Hildebrand, J.G., S.G. Matsumoto, S.M. Camazine, L.P. Tolbert, S. Blank, H. Ferguson, and V. Ecker. 1980. Organization and physiology of antennal centres in the brain of the moth *Manduca sexta.* In *Insect neurobiology and pesticide action* (ed. F.E. Rickett), pp. 375–382. Society of Chemical Industries, London.

Immelmann, K. 1969. Song development in the zebra finch and other estrildid finches. In *Bird vocalizations* (ed. R.A. Hinde), pp. 61. Cambridge University Press, New York.

Konishi, M. 1965. The role of auditory feedback in the control of vocalization in the white-crowned sparrow. *Z. Tierpsychol. 22:* 770–783.

Marler, P. and S. Peters. 1977. Selective vocal learning in a sparrow. *Science 198:* 519–521.

Marler, P. and M. Tamura. 1964. Culturally transmitted patterns of vocal behavior in sparrows. *Science 146:* 1483–1486.

Matsumoto, S.G. and J.G. Hildebrand. 1981. Olfactory mechanisms in the moth *Manduca sexta:* Response characteristics and morphology of central neurones in antennal lobes. *Proc. R. Soc. Lond. B 213:* 249–277.

McEwen, B.S. 1978. Steroid hormone interactions with the brain: Cellular and molecular aspects. *Annu. Rev. Neurosci. 4:* 1–30.

———. 1981. Neural gonadal steroid actions. *Science 211:* 1303–1311.

Nottebohm, F. 1970. Ontogeny of birdsong. *Science 167:* 950–956.

———. 1981. A brain for all seasons: Cyclical anatomical changes in song control nuclei of the canary brain. *Science 214:* 1368–1370.

Nottebohm, F. and A.P. Arnold. 1976. Sexual dimorphism in vocal control areas of the songbird brain. *Science 194:* 211–213.

Nottebohm, F. and M. Nottebohm. 1978. Relationship between song repertoire and age in the canary, *Serinus canarius. Z. Tierpsychol. 46:* 298–305.

Nottebohm, F., S. Kasparian, and C. Pandazis. 1981. Brain space for a learned task. *Brain Res. 213:* 99–109.

Raisman, G. and P.M. Field. 1973. Sexual dimorphism in the neuropil of the preoptic area of the rat and its dependence on neonatal androgen. *Brain Res. 54:* 1–29.

Schneiderman, A., S. Matsumoto, and J. Hildebrand. 1980. Role of afferents in development of male-specific components in antennal lobes of *Manduca sexta. Am. Zool. 20:* 944.

Strausfeld, N.J. 1980. Male and female visual neurones in dipterous insects. *Nature 283:* 381–383.

Thorpe, W.H. 1958. The learning of song patterns by birds, with special reference to the song of the chaffinch *(Fringella coelebs). Ibis 100:* 535–570.

———. 1961. *Bird song: The biology of vocal communication and expression in birds.* Cambridge University Press, New York.

Toran-Allerand, C.D. 1976. Sex steroids and the development of the newborn mouse hypothalamus and preoptic area *in vitro:* Implications for sexual differentiation. *Brain Res. 106:* 407–412.

———. 1980. Sex steroids and the development of the newborn mouse hypothalamus and preoptic area *in vitro.* II. Morphological correlates and hormonal specificity. *Brain Res. 189:* 413–427.

Reprinted from Science, Vol. 198, pp. 519–521. 1977
© 1977 AAAS

Selective Vocal Learning in a Sparrow

Abstract. *Male swamp sparrows learn their songs; they fail to learn songs of the sympatric song sparrow. Syllables from tape recordings of both species of sparrow were spliced into an array of swamp sparrow–like and song sparrow–like temporal patterns. Swamp sparrows learned only those songs made of swamp sparrow syllables. They did so irrespective of whether the temporal pattern was swamp sparrow–like or song sparrow–like. Selectivity was retained by birds reared in total isolation from adult conspecific sounds.*

It is a long-standing premise of classical learning theory that any sensory stimulus can be attached through learning to any arbitrarily chosen response. Biological approaches to animal learning have called several assumptions of learning theory into question, including the principle of equipotentiality (*1*). Vocal learning is widespread in birds, and all oscine songbirds studied to date show some degree of song abnormality when reared in social isolation (*2*). A feature of

683

Table 1. Design plan for the "artificial" training songs each about 2 seconds in duration. The ten artificial songs of one set of training songs were created from 16 different song sparrow syllables. Another set was created of the same song patterns, but with 16 different swamp sparrow syllables. Examples of the patterns marked with asterisks are shown in Fig. 1. Each complete set of 20 artificial songs was supplemented by two additional fully synthetic songs, modeled after natural song and swamp sparrow songs created on the Pattern Playback Speech Synthesizer (Haskins Laboratories, New Haven, Conn.), making 22 songs per set in all. Five complete sets were created, all based on the same set of 32 different syllable types, but with each syllable type placed in a different pattern in each of the five sets. A given bird heard one set only, thus experiencing 32 natural syllable types, 16 of each species.

Overall pattern	Song type	Tempo	Syllable types (No.)
Swamp sparrow–like (one-part)	A	Steady, fast	1
	B	Steady, slow*	1
	C	Accelerated*	1
	D	Decelerated	1
Song sparrow–like (two-part)	E	Fast/slow*	2
	F	Slow/fast	2
	G	Decelerated/slow	2
	H	Decelerated/fast*	2
	I	Accelerated/slow	2
	J	Accelerated/fast	2

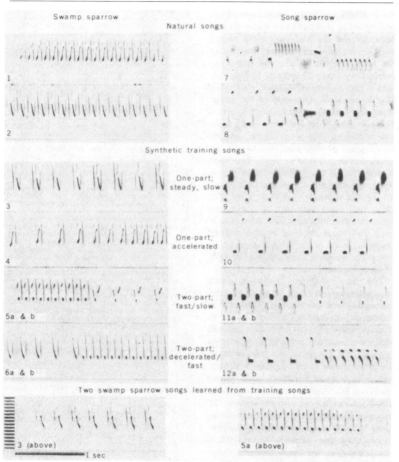

Fig. 1. Sound spectrograms of natural song sparrow and swamp sparrow songs and artificial training songs. Natural songs are shown at the top. Syllables from these and others were assembled in synthetic songs, some created from swamp sparrow syllables (for example, 3 to 6), some from song sparrow syllables (for example, 9 to 12), some in "swamp sparrow–like" patterns (for example, 3 and 9), some in "song sparrow–like" patterns (for example, 4, 5, 6, 10, 11, and 12); syllables from songs 1 and 2 can be seen in songs 3 and 4, syllables from song 8 in songs 10 and 11. Pattern B (see Table 1) is illustrated in songs 3 and 9, C in songs 4 and 10, E in songs 5 and 11, and H in songs 6 and 12. At the bottom are two songs of male swamp sparrows copied from training songs 3 and 5. A 1-second time marker is given at the bottom left, with a 500-hertz interval frequency scale.

the song-learning process in some, though not all, bird species is its selectivity, which is such that a male presented with a natural choice of songs to copy will selectively learn conspecific models (3). We present here a new example of selective vocal learning with evidence on some of the acoustical features on which the choice is based.

Song and swamp sparrows are closely related North American members of the genus *Melospiza*. The normal songs of males of the two species, although similar in duration, are very different in temporal organization (Fig. 1). The swamp sparrow song is simple, consisting of "a slow trill of similar slurred liquid notes." That of the song sparrow is complex, with several distinct parts, consisting "of many short notes and a trill near the end" (4). Within different, relatively stable, species-specific overall patterns, both species exhibit a great deal of individual variability in the acoustic structure of song syllables. Swamp sparrows engage in vocal learning, and songs of socially isolated males are significantly abnormal, with simpler syllables and fewer component parts than usual (5). Although their preferred microhabitats differ, the two species live within earshot of one another in the study area in Dutchess County, New York. Preliminary study revealed no evidence that the two species learn one another's songs in nature.

Our aim was to present male swamp sparrows with swamp and song sparrow songs to see whether selective learning occurs, and if so, to specify some of the acoustic parameters involved. We expected the major differences in overall temporal patterning of songs of the two species to provide the basis for any selective learning that might take place. In order to test this hypothesis, series of artificial songs were created. Distinctively different sound elements or syllables were edited out from tape recordings of normal local songs of both species. These were spliced together in a variety of simple temporal patterns, chosen to provide variants on some of the organization features by which normal songs of the two species differ (Table 1). "Swamp sparrow–like" patterns included sequences of identical syllables at various steady rates; "song sparrow–like" patterns included variable intervals between syllables (accelerating, decelerating) and a two-part structure. Song sparrows sometimes use two-part, never one-part, songs. Although three or more parts often occur in song sparrow songs (for example, Fig. 1, parts 7 and 8), we hypothesized that the contrast between one- and two-part patterns would suffice for the discrimination. Each set of ten song types (Table 1, A to J) was created in duplicate, once with 16 different swamp sparrow syllables and again with 16 different song sparrow syllables. Each syllable type was used only once in a set. These types were sufficiently distinct so that if imitation occurred we could determine from which temporal patterns they had been selected (Fig. 1). Two additional songs were created on the Haskins Laboratories speech synthesizer (see legend, Table 1), which were not learned and will not be mentioned further in this report. These 22 "artificial" songs were presented in song bouts at characteristic singing rates for these species. Each subject heard all 22 songs (6).

Anticipating the possibility that particular associations of syllable type and temporal pattern might influence the birds' choice, we prepared five sets of training tapes from the same 32-syllable types of the two species, but with each pattern assembled from a different syllable type in each set. A given bird heard only one of these five sets.

In the first experiment eight male swamp sparrows between 3 and 10 days of age were taken from wild nests and reared by hand with female siblings in small groups in acoustically shielded chambers. During rearing they could also hear song sparrows of a similar age present in the same chambers until the end of the song training period. A single set of tapes was presented to each group of subjects in varying order twice a day—morning and evening. Training continued for 30 days, when the sparrows were between 20 and 50 days old. We know that this included the sensitive period for vocal learning in this species (5). As with other songbirds, such as the white-crowned sparrow (3), male swamp sparrows learn to sing from memory. They came into song some months after training, while on an approximately normal photoperiod. The group of eight males produced 19 syllable types. As in nature, each male sang several songs, ranging from one to three types. We compared these syllables with the models experienced earlier in life, and judged 12 of the 19 to be close copies (see Fig. 1, bottom). These 12 represented eight different swamp sparrow syllables presented as models; no song sparrow models were copied. Thus the male swamp sparrows exhibited extremely selective vocal learning, accepting only conspecific syllables for imitation, and rejecting song sparrow syllables even when presented in swamp sparrow–like patterns.

The choice was clearly made at the level of components from which the song is constructed, and not the overall pattern of the song. Thus four of the 12 examples of learned syllables were extracted from one-part song (the normal swamp sparrow pattern) and eight from two-part models, which are closer to the song sparrow pattern. Five of the accepted models came from series with a steady rate (the normal swamp sparrow pattern) and seven from accelerated or decelerated series. Syllables presented in two-part models, or with variable rates, were usually transposed into one-part patterns, with a steady rate, typical of normal swamp sparrow song.

In order to explore further the developmental basis of this predisposition to learn songs selectively, swamp sparrows were reared under foster parents. Eggs were transferred early in incubation from wild nests to nests of canaries in the laboratory, and the nestlings were reared with the aid of supplementary feeding by the experimenter. Six males were exposed from 20 to 50 days of age to synthetic song patterns like those used in the first experiment. One-half of the songs were made from normal swamp sparrow syllables; the other half from song sparrow syllables that were either normal (two males) or subjected to a 13 percent upward transposition in frequency (four males) (7). Of ten syllable types developed, six matched the models closely—all swamp sparrow syllables. Thus it is clear that song syllables of these two sparrows are not equivalent stimuli as a basis for vocal learning by the swamp sparrow, even with subjects reared in complete isolation from all adult sounds of their species.

The many parallels between avian song learning and the development of the perception and production of speech in human infants lend added significance to these results (8). In particular, recent studies of auditory perception in infants suggest that young of our own species are predisposed to be responsive to particular aspects of speech sounds before speaking (9), just as some young songbirds are responsive to species-specific features of song before they themselves come into full song. Such perceptual predispositions are valuable as biological constraints on the vocal learning process, serving to focus the young organism's attention on an appropriate set of sounds and on particular features that they exhibit (10). The birds are guided to a set of conspecific models, thus reducing the potential hazards of learning the song of another species. Human infants stand to benefit (i) from being encouraged to attend closely to sounds of speech; (ii) from guidance, in embarking on the perceptual analysis of speech sounds, in the extraction of particular meaningful features from the multitude of cues of varying reliability that speech presents; and (iii) from the possession of mechanisms that can steer the processes of later vocal development from babbling to mature speech by auditory feedback, much as a bird passes from subsong to the fully crystallized patterns of adult song.

PETER MARLER
SUSAN PETERS
Rockefeller University Field Research Center, Millbrook, New York 12545

References and Notes

1. M. E. P. Seligman and J. L. Hager, *Biological Boundaries of Learning* (Appleton-Century-Crofts, New York, 1972); S. J. Shettleworth, in *Advances in the Study of Behavior*, D. S. Lehrman, R. A. Hinde, E. Shaw, Eds. (Academic Press, New York, 1972), pp. 1–68; R. A. Hinde and J. Stevenson-Hinde, *Constraints on Learning* (Academic Press, New York, 1973).
2. M. Konishi and F. Nottebohm, in *Bird Vocalizations: Their Relation to Current Problems in Biology and Psychology*, R. A. Hinde, Ed. (Cambridge Univ. Press, London, 1969), pp. 29–48; P. Marler and P. Mundinger, in *Ontogeny of Vertebrate Behavior*, M. Moltz, Ed. (Academic Press, New York, 1971), pp. 389–450; F. Nottebohm, in *Avian Biology*, D. S. Farner and J. R. Kind, Eds. (Academic Press, New York, 1975), vol. 5, pp. 287–332; W. H. Thorpe, *Bird Song: Biology of Vocal Communication and Expression in Birds* (Cambridge Univ. Press, London, 1971).
3. W. H. Thorpe, *Ibis* **100**, 535 (1958); P. Marler and M. Tamura, *Science* **146**, 1483 (1964); P. Marler, *J. Comp. Physiol. Psychol.* **71**, 1 (1970).
4. J. A. Mulligan, in *Proceedings of the 13th International Ornithology Congress* (1963), p. 272; C. S. Robbins, B. Bruun, H. S. Zim, *Birds of North America* (Golden, New York, 1966).
5. D. K. Kroodsma, P. Marler, S. Peters, in preparation.
6. Each song type was presented in a bout of 16 repetitions (= 2.5 minutes; that is, within the range of normal bout lengths for both species). Bouts of the song types making up a set were sequenced in random order and dubbed onto three "training" tapes, eight song types on one tape, seven on each of the other two. Three tapes comprising one set were played in random order, each morning and evening during the 30-day training period, beginning when the sparrows were 17 to 23 days old.
7. A tendency for song sparrow syllables to be pitched 13 percent lower than those of swamp sparrows although overlapping greatly in range, was the basis for this transposition.
8. P. Marler, *Am. Sci.* **58**, 669 (1970); in *The Role of Speech in Language*, J. F. Kavanagh and J. E. Cutting, Eds. (MIT Press, Cambridge, Mass., 1975), pp. 11–37.
9. P. D. Eimas, *Percept. Psychophys.* **16**, 513 (1974); in *Infant Perception: from Sensation to Cognition*, L. B. Cohen and P. Salapatek, Eds. (Academic Press, New York, 1975), vol. 2, pp. 193–231; _____, E. R. Siqueland, P. Jusczyk, J. Vigorito, *Science* **171**, 303 (1971); R. Eilers and F. Minifie, *J. Speech Hear. Res.* **18**, 158 (1975); R. Lasky, A. Syrdal-Lasky, R. Klein, *J. Exp. Child Psychol.* **20**, 215 (1975); L. A. Streeter, *Nature (London)* **259**, 39 (1975); P. A. Morse, *J. Exp. Child Psychol.* **14**, 477 (1972); P. K. Kuhl, in *Hearing and Davis: Essays Honoring Hallowell Davis*, S. K. Hirsh, D. H. Eldridge, I. J. Hirsh, S. R. Silverman, Eds. (Washington Univ. Press, St. Louis, 1976), pp. 265–280.
10. P. Marler, in *Recognition of Complex Acoustic Signals*, T. H. Bullock, Ed. (Dahlem Konferenzen, Berlin, 1977).
11. We are deeply indebted to R. Dooling, M. Konishi, D. Kroodsma, and F. Nottebohm for help and advice in design and conduct of experiments and in manuscript preparation. D. Baylis prepared the synthetic songs. Research was supported by NIMH grant MH 14651.

17 March 1977; revised 15 June 1977

Reprinted from Science, Vol. 194, pp. 211–213. 1976
© 1976 AAAS

Sexual Dimorphism in Vocal Control Areas
of the Songbird Brain

Abstract. *In canaries and zebra finches, three vocal control areas in the brain are strikingly larger in males than in females. A fourth, area X of the lobus parolfactorius, is well developed in males of both species, less well developed in female canaries, and absent or not recognizable in female zebra finches. These size differences correlate well with differences in singing behavior. Males of both species learn song by reference to auditory information, and females do not normally sing. Exogenous testosterone induces singing in female canaries but not in female zebra finches. This is believed to be the first report of such gross sexual dimorphism in a vertebrate brain.*

In many species of animals, males and females exhibit different patterns of behavior, especially in contexts related to courtship and reproduction (*1*). Recent evidence suggests that structural differences in male and female central nervous systems may contribute to these differences in behavior (*2*). We have discovered a striking sexual dimorphism in song control areas of the brain of the canary (*Serinus canarius*) and the zebra finch (*Poephila guttata*), which can be related to behavioral differences between the two sexes.

Adult male canaries have a complex song repertoire learned by reference to auditory information (*3, 4*). Female canaries do not normally sing, although they will produce a song similar to that of the males when administered testosterone (*5, 6*); the song, however, is considerably less varied than that of males (*6*). Female canaries also produce a variety of other calls (*7*), and, as in the case of other carduelines (*8*), some of these calls may be learned.

Male zebra finches have a single song type, which, as in the canary, is devel-

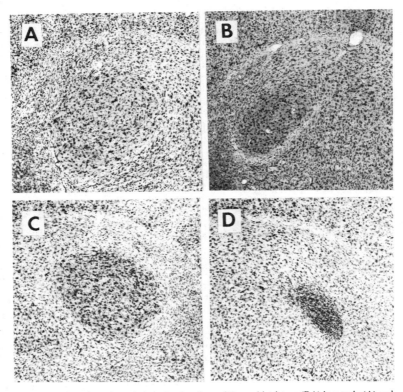

Fig. 1. Frontal sections through the robust nucleus of the archistriatum (RA) in a male (A) and female canary (B) and a male (C) and female zebra finch (D). The canary photographs are from the left hemisphere, and those of zebra finch are from the right. For each of the four birds shown, the rostro-caudal level corresponds to the largest area of RA seen in this plane of section. The relatively unstained eyebrow-shaped structure is the lamina archistriatalis dorsalis, which separates the neostriatum (dorsal) from the archistriatum (ventral). The prominent ellipsoidal nucleus is RA. Cresyl violet–stained sections, 50 μm thick (×42).

686

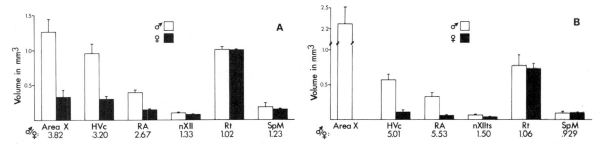

Fig. 2. The volumes occupied by four neural regions associated with vocal behavior (area X, HVc, RA, and nXII) and by two regions not associated with vocalization (Rt and SpM) in male and female canaries (A) and zebra finches (B). Each bar represents the mean of the total (right plus left) volumes of each area sampled (18, 26), and the vertical line above the bar is the standard deviation of the individual values. The ratio of the male to the female mean is given for each region.

oped by reference to auditory information (9). Female zebra finches do not sing even when testosterone propionate is implanted when they are adults (10). The vocal repertoire of female zebra finches is otherwise small, consisting of contact and enticement notes produced in a variety of circumstances (11). Because of this simplicity, the calls may develop normally in the absence of auditory models.

Five adult male canaries, five adult female canaries, six adult male zebra finches, and seven adult female zebra finches (12) were anesthetized and then perfused with saline followed by 10 percent formalin in physiological saline. The brains were removed, blocked, fixed, embedded, and sectioned; the sections were mounted on glass slides (13, 14). All brains were weighed before being embedded (15). Serial sections cut at 10 to 50 μm were mounted, stained with cresyl violet for cell bodies or silver stain (Fink-Schneider) (14) for unmyelinated nerve fibers, and viewed under the light microscope. The volume of certain brain structures was measured as follows. A microprojector (Bausch and Lomb) projected magnified ($\times 53$) images of cresyl violet–stained sections on drawing paper. A perimeter was then drawn around the regions of interest, and the area enclosed was measured with a polar planimeter. These areas were then multiplied by the thickness of the sections, and the resulting volume was corrected for the frequency of sampling (for example, multiplied by 2 if every other section was measured). The sum of all such products for a given brain region was an estimate of its volume.

We made drawings of four cytoarchitectonically distinct brain structures: (i) area X of the lobus parolfactorius (LPO), (ii) the hyperstriatum ventrale, pars caudale (HVc), (iii) the robust nucleus of the archistriatum (RA) (Fig. 1), and (iv) the hypoglossal nucleus of the medulla (nXII) (16). Nottebohm et al. (4) have described these structures in the canary and presented anatomical and behavioral evidence that they are part of the vocal control system of the canary brain. The brain of the male zebra finch includes areas that are similar to these four regions in position and cytoarchitecture; we thus presume that they have a similar role in vocalization (17, 18). We also drew and estimated the volume of two thalamic brain structures not related to vocal control, the nucleus rotundus (Rt) and the nucleus spiriformis medialis (SpM), which were chosen because of their discrete boundaries (19).

In both the canary and the zebra finch, the four vocal control areas are markedly larger in males than in females ($P < .02$, two-tailed t-test) (Figs. 1 and 2). These differences are highly significant. That there were no such differences in the volume estimates of the two structures not related to vocal control or in total brain weight ($P > .2$) (15) suggests that the differences are specific to song areas and related to a sexual difference in vocal behavior. This conclusion is also supported by the observation that the sexual differences in volume are more marked in zebra finches than in canaries, as would be expected from the total absence of song in female zebra finches.

In zebra finches, we detected no differences between the right and left sides of any of the four vocal and two nonvocal areas. Similarly, there was no systematic difference between the volumes of the right and left area X, HVc, RA, Rt, and SpM in canaries. This result is intriguing in light of the marked left hemispheric dominance for vocal control described for this species (4, 20). There was significant difference between the volumes of the right and the left hypoglossal nuclei of canaries (21). The larger size of the left side in all ten male and female canaries may be related to the left hypoglossal

dominance for song control in this species (22).

The size ratio of male to female canary brain areas increases as one goes from the hypoglossal nucleus to RA, HVc, and area X, that is, as one goes to structures further removed from the motoneurons innervating the syringeal musculature (23). This graded series of ratios suggests that the "higher" (that is, further removed) neural regions in this system are involved in some aspect of vocal performance in males that is specifically absent or underrepresented in females. It may be that the higher centers are responsible for a disproportionately large share of the neural operations controlling vocal learning and size of vocal repertoire; therefore, in females, who normally do not sing, these areas should be less well represented. The zebra finch brain departs from this pattern in that the volume ratio of male to female brains is somewhat smaller in HVc than in RA (Fig. 2), and area X is not recognizable in the female.

In both male and female canaries, area X contains larger cell clusters than the surrounding LPO; perhaps as a result, cresyl violet stains area X darker than the surrounding tissue (4). In Fink-Schneider stains of unmyelinated fibers, area X is discriminable from the rest of LPO because it contains a rich mesh of fibers, some of which are projections from HVc (24). Area X in male zebra finches is similar in these respects [see also (19)]. However, in the corresponding area of the female zebra finch brain area X is not recognizable, which suggests that it is grossly modified or absent. We have assumed it to be absent (Fig. 2). It is not clear how the disproportionately large size of area X in the male zebra finch compared with that of the canary might relate to differences in behavior.

From the extent of the sexual differences in the volumes of the vocal areas, we infer that sexual differences are not confined to cell size alone (Fig. 1). The density of cell packing and the amount of neuropil in RA and HVc also differ between males and females (25). Males, with a greater commitment to vocal learning, also have more neuropil. The sexual dimorphism in vocal areas of these two songbird species may be related to the fact that, whereas males of both species learn their song by reference to auditory information, females do not normally sing.

FERNANDO NOTTEBOHM
ARTHUR P. ARNOLD*

*Field Research Center,
Rockefeller University,
Millbrook, New York 12545*

References and Notes

1. N. Tinbergen, *The Study of Instinct* (Oxford Univ. Press, Toronto, 1951); W. C. Young, in *Sex and Internal Secretions*, W. C. Young, Ed. (Williams & Wilkins, Baltimore, ed. 3, 1961), vol. 2, p. 1139.
2. G. Raisman and P. M. Field, *Science* 173, 731 (1971); *Brain Res.* 54, 1 (1973); D. W. Pfaff, *J. Endocrinol.* 36, 415 (1966); G. Dörner and J. Staudt, *Neuroendocrinology* 3, 136 (1968); F. R. Calaresu and J. L. Henry, *Science* 173, 343 (1971); J. L. Henry and F. R. Calaresu, *J. Comp. Neurol.* 144, 205 (1972); G. A. Bubenik and G. M. Brown, *Experientia* 29, 619 (1973).
3. P. Marler and M. S. Waser, *J. Comp. Physiol. Psychol.*, in press; M. S. Waser and P. Marler, *ibid.*, in press; P. Marler *et al.*, *Proc. Natl. Acad. Sci. U.S.A.* 70, 1393 (1973).
4. F. Nottebohm, T. M. Stokes, C. M. Leonard, *J. Comp. Neurol.* 165, 457 (1976).
5. S. L. Leonard, *Proc. Soc. Exp. Biol. Med.* 41, 229 (1939); H. H. Shoemaker, *ibid.*, p. 299; E. H. Herrick and J. O. Harris, *Science* 125, 1299 (1957).
6. F. M. Baldwin, H. S. Goldin, M. Metfessel, *Proc. Soc. Exp. Biol. Med.* 44, 373 (1940).
7. J. A. Mulligan and K. C. Olsen, in *Bird Vocalizations*, R. A. Hinde, Ed. (Cambridge Univ. Press, London, 1969), p. 165.
8. P. Mundinger, *Science* 168, 480 (1970).
9. K. Immelmann, in *Bird Vocalizations*, R. A. Hinde, Ed. (Cambridge Univ. Press, London, 1969), p. 61.
10. On occasion an intact adult female that has had a pellet of testosterone propionate implanted will produce a repetitive vocalization not otherwise heard from members of this species. The manner of delivery of such a sound is reminiscent of song but its physical characteristics differ greatly from normal song [A. P. Arnold, thesis, Rockefeller University (1974)].
11. K. Immelmann, *Zool. Jahrb. Abt. Allg. Zool. Physiol.* 90, 1 (1962).
12. Wasserschlager canaries of our own inbred stock ranged in age from 19 to 34 months old. All but two of the zebra finches were descendants of a single pair of domesticated birds and were between 29 and 56 months (usually 29 to 31 months) old.
13. T. M. Stokes, C. M. Leonard, F. Nottebohm, *J. Comp. Neurol.* 156, 337 (1974). The method was modified in some cases. All canary brains were embedded in gelatin albumin and stained with cresyl violet. They were sectioned serially at 25 or 50 μm, and drawings were made of neuronal regions in single sections at intervals of 100 and 125 μm. All drawings of canary brains were made without prior knowledge of the sex of the animal. Of the zebra finch brains, five male and six female brains were embedded in gelatin albumin, sectioned serially at 25 or 50 μm, and stained with cresyl violet. Drawings were made from sections taken at intervals of 50 to 100 μm. One male and one female zebra finch brain were embedded in paraffin, sectioned serially at 10 μm, and stained with cresyl violet. Of the gelatin albumin–embedded brains of zebra finches, one male and one female brain were sectioned serially at 25, 50, 25, 50 μm, etc., and the 25-μm sections were stained for unmyelinated fibers by the Fink-Schneider method (14).
14. G. E. Schneider, *Science* 163, 895 (1969).
15. Canary brains were weighed after being fixed in sucrose-formalin, and zebra finch brains were weighed after being fixed in formalin. There was no statistical difference between the two sexes of either species in brain weights (two-tailed t-test, P > .2). Means and standard deviations of brain weights were 0.74 ± 0.09 g (male canary), 0.68 ± 0.05 g (female canary), 0.53 ± 0.04 g (male zebra finch), and 0.51 ± 0.04 g (female zebra finch).
16. In the case of the motor nucleus of the hypoglossus (nXII), the volume of the entire nucleus was measured in the canaries. It includes an anterior portion innervating the tongue, and a caudal portion (tracheosyringeal portion, nXIIts), which is composed of the motoneurons innervating the vocal organ (syrinx). In the zebra finches, only the volume of nXIIts was measured. This was possible because in each of five males and females, the tracheosyringeal branch of the hypoglossus had been cut unilaterally (three male-female pairs on the left, two on the right) 7 to 9 days before the birds were killed. Under this procedure, the ipsilateral syringeal motoneurons of nXIIts become chromatolytic and swell and serve as a guideline for the limits of nXIIts on the nonchromatolytic side. Since the swelling also enlarges the volume of nXIIts, the values presented in Fig. 2 are derived from twice the volume of the nonchromatolytic side of nXIIts for each zebra finch. In both species the perimeter drawn around the motor nucleus circumscribed all of the motoneuron cell bodies but not the neuropil that surrounds the motor nucleus.
17. The motor nucleus nXIIts innervates the syrinx in both canaries and zebra finches (4, 19).
18. A. Arnold, F. Nottebohm, D. W. Pfaff, *J. Comp. Neurol.* 165, 487 (1976).
19. In the pigeon, Rt is part of the tectofugal visual pathway [H. J. Karten and A. M. Revzin, *Brain Res.* 2, 368 (1966); A. M. Revzin and H. J. Karten, *ibid.* 3, 264 (1966–1967)], and SpM receives input from the telencephalon and projects to the cerebellum [H. J. Karten and T. E. Finger, *ibid.* 102, 335 (1976)].
20. F. Nottebohm, in *Lateralization in the Nervous System*, S. R. Harnad *et al.*, Eds. (Academic Press, New York, in press).
21. In females, the mean volume of nXII on the right was 0.0332 ± 0.0021 mm³ (mean ± standard deviation), compared with 0.0436 ± 0.0053 mm³ on the left (two-tailed t-test, P < .001). In males, the volume was 0.0495 ± 0.0074 mm³ on the right and 0.0526 ± 0.0075 mm³ on the left (P < .02). Since neurons on one side of nXIIts were swollen and chromatolytic in the zebra finches (16), we could not assess any possible differences in volume between the sides of the brain in that species.
22. F. Nottebohm and M. Nottebohm, *J. Comp. Physiol.* 108, 171 (1976).
23. The syringeal musculature is larger in male canaries and zebra finches than in females; we have not calculated the male/female ratio of syringeal muscle volume.
24. Observations (4) are of male canaries. As in males, area X of female canaries also receives a discrete fiber projection from the ipsilateral HVc (F. Nottebohm, unpublished observations).
25. F. Nottebohm, in preparation; A. P. Arnold, in preparation.
26. In Fig. 2, N = 5 for measurements on canaries, and N = 4 to 7 for zebra finches.
27. We thank C. M. Leonard and P. Marler for discussion of our results and Y. Holland for technical assistance. Supported by NIMH grant 18343 to F.N. A.P.A. was a NIMH postdoctoral fellow (No. 00559).
* Present address: Department of Psychology, University of California, Los Angeles 90024.

28 May 1976

THE JOURNAL OF COMPARATIVE NEUROLOGY 196:309–316 (1981)

Sex Differences in Dendritic Morphology of a Song Control Nucleus in the Canary: A Quantitative Golgi Study

TIMOTHY J. DeVOOGD AND FERNANDO NOTTEBOHM
Field Research Center, Rockefeller University, Millbrook, New York 12545

Abstract   Singing in the canary is a learned male behavior controlled predominantly by nuclei in the left hemisphere (Nottebohm and Nottebohm, '76; Nottebohm et al., '76; Nottebohm, '77). These nuclei are several times larger in males than in females (Nottebohm and Arnold, '76). One of the telencephalic song control nuclei, robustus archistriatalis (RA), was examined in Golgi-stained tissue sections from the left and right hemispheres of male and female canaries. At least four cell classes were present in each sex. One of these cell classes was further studied with a variety of quantitative techniques. No hemispheric differences were seen in either sex. However, dendrites from male cells tend to branch and end further from the cell body than do dendrites from female cells. This difference is seen most clearly when serial sections are used to reconstruct the entire dendritic tree.

Singing is a sexually dimorphic behavior in canaries. Males develop very complex songs as part of courtship. These songs are learned by reference to auditory information (Marler and Waser, '77; Waser and Marler, '77). Females sing rarely if at all. Recently, several brain nuclei have been described which, if damaged, cause marked song deterioration. One of these, nucleus robustus archistriatalis (RA) of the caudal telencephalon, has been likened to layer five of the mammalian motor cortex because of its widespread projections to mesencephalon, medulla, and spinal cord (Nottebohm et al., '76). This nucleus appears substantially larger in Nissl-stained sections from male canaries than in those from females (Nottebohm and Arnold, '76). No previous work has described the morphology of cells within the canary RA or the relationship of the dendritic fields of these cells to the difference in overall nuclear size between the sexes.

In addition, we brought to this study a second intent. Unilateral lesions at various levels of the vocal control pathway of the canary brain indicate that the left side is dominant for singing (Nottebohm and Nottebohm, '76; Nottebohm et al., '76; Nottebohm, '77). The present study is a first step in trying to understand whether this dominant-subordinate relationship is accompanied by quantifiable anatomical differences between neurons in vocal control nuclei of the two sides of the brain.

METHODS

Subjects

Nine male and 11 female canaries in reproductive condition were used. The males were about 8 months old and fully in song. The females were between 8 and 13 months old. These birds came from a close-bred colony of Wasserschlager canaries kept at Rockefeller University since 1967. All birds were perfused with 4% paraformaldehyde; their brains were removed and stained with a rapid Golgi technique (Lund, '73), embedded in celloidin, and sectioned at 100 μm. RA proved to be well demarcated in both males and females by dense axonal branching within and at the margins of the nucleus (see Fig. 1). From the initial group, five female brains and five male brains had well-stained cells within RA and were used in further analyses.

Procedure

RA was scanned in all the brains. Cells were categorized according to position within the nucleus, spine density, and dendritic conformation. One cell class was chosen for further quantitative study.

Quantification

All neuronal quantification was done using a computer-microscope system modeled after those of Wann and Greenough (Wann et al., '73;

DeVoogd et al., in press). A Zeiss stage with stepping motors and a stepping motor attached to the microscope fine focus drive were interfaced with a PDP 11/10 minicomputer. An operator at the microscope then directs stage movement in any direction. Ocular crosshairs are superimposed over dendrites which are then signaled by the operator with a keypad. The computer cumulates the number of steps moved by the stepping motors between key presses, and thus the computer can acquire and store coordinates of points along the dendrites. Dendrites which were shortened by sectioning were noted. Following transmission of points characterizing a cell's dendritic field within a section, segments that had been interrupted at the section edges were completed from adjacent sections. This procedure involved manually positioning the microscope at the approximate site where continuing dendrites would be expected in RA on an adjacent tissue section. This region is then compared to a graphics terminal display of attenuated dendrites. When the dendrites are found in the tissue which match the position and the orientation of the display, they are edited into the data set. Stained cells in RA were sufficiently separated so that sectioned dendrites from all the cells in this sample could be followed unambiguously.

Since RA does not fill a large volume and not very many cells stained in each nucleus, it was important that all well-stained cells be used in the quantified analyses. Occasionally, well-stained cells were seen in sections in which the background in RA was darkly stained. These sections were detached from their slides and coverslips by soaking them in xylene. They were then remounted between two coverslips. The data acquisition program was modified so that dendritic coordinate information could be entered from either side of these sections after registering one site from both perspectives. This procedure allowed accurate mapping of dendrites at all depths of these dark sections. All sections were rechecked after computer mapping. Three cells were found which appeared better classified as members of other cell classes and one cell was found which had been mapped twice. These were not included in the statistical analyses.

Data from 30 male and 30 female cells were then analyzed in several ways. Mean dendritic branch length and number were derived at each order of branching. A Sholl analysis was performed in which the computer calculated the number of intersections of the dendrites with spheres of different radii centered on the cell body (Sholl, '56; DeVoogd et al., in press).

This analysis preserves the neuronal geometry and thus measures the Cartesian dispersion of dendrites away from the cell body. A second kind of Sholl analysis was also used in which all dendrites are first remapped by the computer to appear perfectly straight and oriented radially away from the cell body. This radial Sholl analysis is a measure of the number of potential synaptic inputs at different effective transmission distances from the spike initiating zone.

Since we mapped cells from locations throughout RA, we were concerned that neuronal morphology, and hence statistical measures describing the dendritic tree, might be affected if the experimental groups differed in cell position within RA. Cells were subdivided according to whether their somas were located centrally, intermediately between center and periphery, or peripherally within the nucleus.

In addition to male-female comparisons, cells of both sexes were subdivided according to whether they were from the left or right hemisphere. All measures derived from these neurons were compared statistically using two-factor analysis of variance.

RESULTS

At least four types of cells are found within RA. All cell types occurred in both hemispheres of both sexes. These four cell types are (1) small nonspiny neurons (Fig. 2a); (2) spiny neurons at the margin of RA, tightly enmeshed in the marginal fiber plexus (Fig. 2b); (3) moderately spiny neurons with fine, radially oriented dendrites (Fig. 2c); and (4) neurons with thick, sinuous, very spiny dendrites (Fig. 3).

The fourth type was the one most frequently stained and was therefore chosen for quantitative analysis. Although fewer type-four female cells than male cells were located centrally in RA, cell position did not relate systematically to either Sholl analysis dispersion or total dendritic length, so that cell position was ignored for the rest of our quantification. The Sholl analysis of type-four cells (Fig. 4) indicates that many of the dendrites tend to be located further from the cell body in cells from males than in cells from females. The median of the distribution—i.e., the radial distance from the cell at which there are equal numbers of intersections proximally and distally—occurs at 84.1 μm from the cell body for male cells and 68.5 μm for female cells (p < 0.001). No significant difference was seen between left and right sides in either sex. The radial Sholl analysis (Fig. 5) shows a similar pattern. Dendrites are concentrated at nearer conduction distances from the cell body in female cells than in male cells. Here

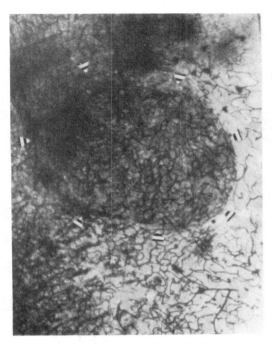

Fig. 1. RA as seen in a Golgi-stained 100 μm coronal section. Increased axonal staining within and at the margins of this nucleus (arrowheads) allow it to be easily distinguished from surrounding tissue.

too, the cell samples from the right and left hemispheres produce very similar profiles.

Dendrites were classified by branch order from the cell body to the terminals. The length of dendrite between two contiguous branching points is called a "segment." These segments were then analyzed according to number, length, and distance at the end of the segment from the cell body. These data are given in Table 1. Mean numbers of segments are alike between males and females at all branching orders. Total numbers of segments per cell did not differ significantly between sexes. Segments from male cells tend to be longer than those in female cells, but at no branch order is this difference significant. Segments from branch orders 1–5 end about 20% closer to the cell body in females than in males; segments from branch order 6 end 11% closer to the cell body in females than in males. In addition, terminal segments regardless of their order end 17% closer to the cell body in female cells. The summed length of all dendrites averaged 1838 μm for female cells and 2085 μm for male cells, a difference of about 12% (p < 0.001). As is shown in Table 1, cells from the left and right

hemispheres of both sexes are remarkably similar in number and size of dendritic segments at each branching order.

The coordinate points representing these cells were plotted in two dimensions from several perspectives. These plots showed that the dendrite tree of each cell maps an elipsoidal space. The cell body is near the center of this space except when the cell occurs near a boundary of the nucleus, in which case the dendrites exiting the cell body near the boundary quickly turn toward the center of the nucleus (see Fig. 6). The volume of this space was estimated by averaging the three-dimensional coordinates of each terminal dendritic tip so as to obtain a volume center. The distances from this volume center to each tip were averaged to obtain a mean volume radius. When these mean radii were treated as the radii of spheres, male and female cells emcompassed volumes of 0.0075 mm^3 and 0.0043 mm^3 respectively (p < 0.001). Here too there is no significant difference between cells from the right and left hemispheres in either sex.

DISCUSSION

RA is a moderately large, heterogeneous nucleus. It contains a variety of cell types; four which are easily distinguished in Golgi preparations are described above. In the present study, all cell types were observed in both sexes. A sample of one type, consisting of large, very spiny cells, was examined in detail. The principal difference in dendritic morphology between male and female cells is that male cells have longer branches. The overall difference in total dendritic length between male and female cells is about 12%. This difference translates into a 1.75:1 (male:female) difference in the volume encompassed by the dendrites. Thus, male cells are potentially in contact with nearly twice as large a tissue volume as are female cells. This pattern of differences can be clearly seen in the profiles of a male cell and a female cell chosen because they possess near-median Sholl values (Fig. 7).

This volume difference is smaller than the overall difference reported in the volume of RA. RA in 1-year-old canaries is 2.96 times larger in males than in females (N = 10 for each sex. Nissl stain; Nottebohm, Kasparian, and Pandazis, in press). In addition to dendritic volume, the male-female difference in RA size could be due to differences in afferent fibers, cell number, or cell size.

No significant differences are seen between cells from the right and left hemispheres in

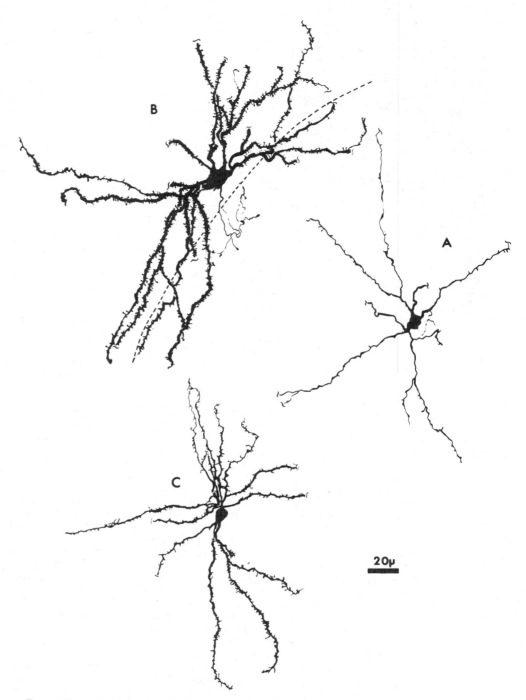

Fig. 2. Camera lucida tracings of cells representative of three of the cell classes within RA. Cells of the sort shown in Figure 2A have fine dendrites with few if any spines. Cells of the sort shown in Figure 2B are very spiny and are found exclusively at the margin of RA. Cells of the sort shown in Figure 2C have fine, radially oriented dendrites and are moderately spiny.

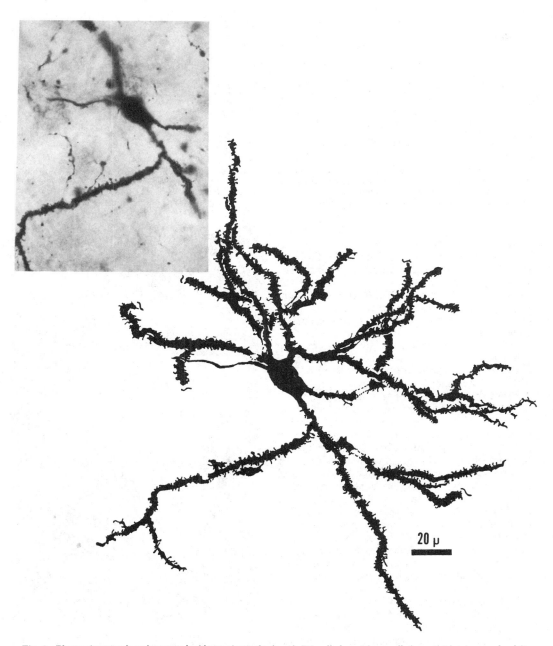

Fig. 3   Photomicrograph and camera lucida tracings of a fourth RA cell class. These cells have thick, sinuous dendrites densely covered with spines. Cells of this sort were used for quantitative analyses.

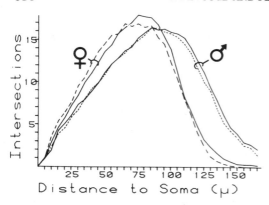

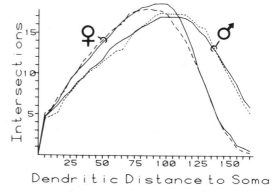

Fig. 4. Sholl analysis of type-four cells. Dendrite-sphere intersections were derived with concentric spheres 5 μm apart. Cells from the left hemispheres are shown with dashed lines, cells from the right hemispheres with solid lines.

Fig. 5. Radial Sholl analysis of type-four cells. For this analysis the computer altered the cellular coordinate data so that the dendrites appeared perfectly straight and oriented radially away from the cell body. A Sholl analysis was then run with spheres separated by 5 μm as in Figure 4.

either males or females, and these microanatomical similarities are in line with gross observations, indicating an absence of consistent volume differences between right and left RA (Nottebohm and Arnold, '76; Nottebohm et al., in press). Our microanatomical data are sufficiently uniform that this lack does not appear to be a sampling problem but rather evidence that the left hemispheric dominance for song production results from right-left asymmetries arising at a different anatomical level or in a different manner.

From the viewpoint of the techniques used, our study suggests that an accurate picture of neuronal morphology and geometry is possible with far fewer cells than deemed necessary in previous investigations. This result may be due to reductions in the distortion introduced by random dendritic deletions due to the use of single sections. In fact, our data indicate that the pattern of differences between groups may be distorted by the use of incomplete cells. The total dendritic field (summed segment lengths) of male and female cells, for example, does not differ when only the dendrites from the tissue section containing the soma are analyzed (Fig. 8). This distortion probably results from the tendency for the dendritic mass of the female cells to be concentrated closer to the cell body than the dendritic mass of the male cells. On average, a substantially larger proportion of the dendritic field of female than male cells is contained within the Golgi-stained section of the soma, as is shown in Figure 7. Thus, although big intergroup differences can be recognized in cells using single sections or even

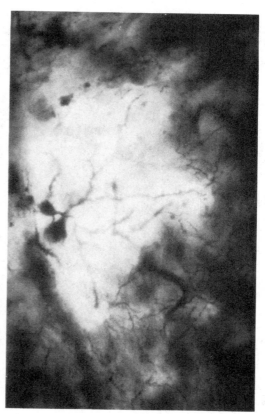

Fig. 6. A type-four cell found at the periphery of RA. Dendrites were followed using multiple exposures with spot illumination (method learned from E.M. Glazer, personal communication). Immediately below the cell body is a capillary cut in cross section. There is a tendency for dendrites whose primary segments are oriented toward the center of RA to have larger trees than other dendrites. Dendrites approaching the edge of RA turn back toward the center. In spite of these stereological differences, the total dendritic length for such peripheral cells does not differ from centrally located ones.

	Branch order							
	1	2	3	4	5	6	7	All orders
Left male cells N = 15								
Mean number of branches	4.40	8.27	11.47	10.53	4.13	1.33	0.40	40.53
Mean branch length (μm)	29.03	56.49	55.66	55.04	41.73	40.1	55.83	50.83
Mean distance from segment end to soma	37.3	79.5	103.0	115.6	122.7	111.6	139.1	122.60*
Right male cells N = 15								
Mean number of branches	4.47	8.53	12.53	8.67	3.6	0.93	0.13	38.87
Mean branch length (μm)	30.88	55.42	64.62	54.99	44.93	38.07	112.5	54.27
Mean distance from segment end to soma	39.6	79.4	110.7	118.8	120.6	119.4	165.1	127.05*
Left female cells N = 13								
Mean number of branches	4.77	9.23	11.85	8.46	4.00	0.62		38.92
Mean branch length (μm)	26.27	50.49	53.43	48.29	40.52	37.63		46.71
Mean distance from segment end to soma	32.9	68.6	88.9	94.7	99.6	100.6		102.69*
Right female cells N = 17								
Mean number of branches	4.47	8.47	12.00	8.59	4.47	0.82		38.82
Mean branch length (μm)	26.86	45.97	54.46	54.90	44.00	31.86		47.85
Mean distance from segment end to soma	34.1	66.2	89.3	96.1	105.1	104.6		105.87*

*Only terminal segments are included here.

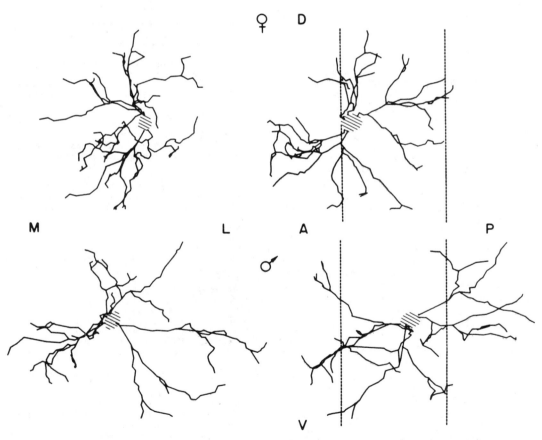

Fig. 7.   Computer-generated plots of a cell from a male and a cell from a female, each shown in two perspectives. These particular cells were chosen since total dendritic length and median Sholl value for each of them was close to the mean male and female values. The dashed lines indicate section boundaries. Using data from single sections results in ignoring a higher proportion of the dendrites of male cells, thus obscuring sex differences. All branch segments were included in this study, including those from adjacent tissue sections.

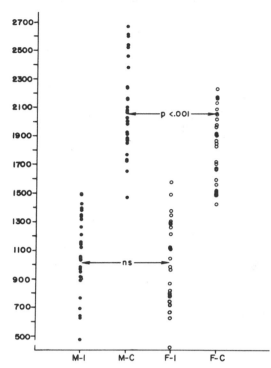

Fig. 8. Total dendritic length (μm) for each male and female cell present in the one tissue section containing the cell body (M-1, F-1) and which was present when the neurons were completed from adjacent sections (M-C, F-C). One (1) and C stand for single section and complete dendritic reconstructions, respectively.

using camera lucida analysis (DeVoogd et al., in press), computer-aided quantification of all dendritic branches by integration of contiguous sections appears more sensitive, and thus to be the method of choice for measuring differences of unknown magnitude.

It may seem puzzling that macroanatomical and microanatomical differences in vocal control nuclei are so noticeable between the sexes, while anatomical differences between the right and left sides remain so elusive. However, there are reasons to believe that the same principles of space or network economy need not apply to the two situations. Normally female canaries sing little if at all. By contrast, vocal control nuclei in the right hemisphere of male canaries do play a role in singing, as determined by lesion studies, even if this role is less dramatic than that of the left side (Nottebohm et al., '76; Nottebohm, '77). Moreover, whereas female canaries induced to sing by testosterone therapy produce abnormally small song repertoires (Baldwin et al., '40; Nottebohm, '80), male ca-

naries with an induced reversal of dominance produce fairly normal song repertoires (Nottebohm, '77). This suggests that whereas song control pathways are deficient in females, in males the right hemisphere's song control pathways are, potentially, as competent as their left counterparts. Our microanatomical observations are in line with this interpretation.

ACKNOWLEDGMENTS

We are grateful to Susan Kasparian and Constantine Pandazis for assistance in the histology, to Charles Petersen for the design of the computer-microscope interface, and to Robert Schor for facilitating our adaptation to a different computer system. D.B. Kelley and J. Paton read the manuscript and made helpful suggestions. This research was supported by PHS grants F32 NS05911 to T.D.V., 5R01 MH18343 to F.N., and by Rockefeller Foundation grant RF 70095 for Research in Reproductive Biology.

LITERATURE CITED

Baldwin, F.M., H.S. Goldin, and M. Metfessel (1940) Effects of testosterone propionate on female roller canaries under complete song isolation. Proc. Soc. Exp. Biol. Med. 44:373–375.

DeVoogd, T.J., F.F. Chang, M.K. Floeter, M.J. Jencius, and W.T. Greenough (in press) Distortions induced in neuronal quantification by using camera lucida analysis: Comparisons using a semiautomated data acquisition system. J. Neurosci. Methods.

Lund, J.S. (1973) Organization of neurons in the visual cortex, area 17, of the monkey (Macaca mulatta). J. Comp. Neurol. 159:305–334.

Marler, P., and M.S. Waser (1977) Role of auditory feedback in canary song development. J. Comp. Physiol. Psychol. 91:8–16.

Nottebohm, F. (1977) Asymmetries in neural control of vocalization in the canary. In S.R. Harnad, R.W. Doty, L. Goldstein, J. Jaynes, and G. Krauthamer (eds): Lateralization in the Nervous System. New York: Academic Press, pp. 23–44.

Nottebohm, F. (1980) Testosterone triggers growth of brain vocal control nuclei in adult female canaries. Brain Res. 189:429–436.

Nottebohm, F., and A.P. Arnold (1976) Sexual dimorphism in vocal control areas of the songbird brain. Science 194:211–213.

Nottebohm, F., S. Kasparian, and C. Pandazis (in press) Brain space for a learned task. Brain Res.

Nottebohm, F., and M.E. Nottebohm (1976) Left hypoglossal dominance in the control of canary and white-crowned sparrow song. J. Comp. Physiol. Series A 108:171–192.

Nottebohm, F., T.M. Stokes, and C.M. Leonard (1976) Central control of song in the canary, Serinus canarius. J. Comp. Neurol. 165:457–486.

Sholl, D.A. (1956) The Organization of the Cerebral Cortex. New York: Methuen.

Wann, D.F., T.A. Woolsey, M.L. Dierker, and W.M. Cowan (1973) An on-line digital-computer system for the semiautomatic analysis of Golgi-impregnated neurons. IEEE Trans. Biomed. Eng. 20:233–247.

Waser, M.S., and P. Marler (1977) Song learning in canaries. J. Comp. Physiol. Psychol. 91:1–7.

Afterword

From the papers reprinted in this collection and the introductions to them, what general points emerge?

Certainly the recurrence of a few basic themes in a variety of contexts is striking. As Hamburger makes clear in his paper reprinted in Section 1, the observations and theories of the late 19th and early 20th centuries set the stage for much of modern developmental neurobiology. It was during this period that biologists first turned their attention to the systematic restriction of a cell's potential during development, to reciprocal trophic interactions between neurons and their targets, to competition between neurons, and to the specificity of connections in the nervous system. Since these major themes, which still pervade neuroscience, were established early on, what has modern work contributed? First, each of these themes has evolved dramatically under the influence of subsequent observations. For example, Ramón y Cajal's largely speculative concept of neurotrophism is now set in a Darwinian framework in which cells compete during development for essential factors provided by their intended partners in neuronal function. Second, modern biologists have dissected cellular interactions in development at a much finer level, and it is now clear that both macromolecular signals and neural activity are important mediators of trophic effects. Neural activity influences the distribution of receptors, determination of transmitter choice, induction of a variety of enzymes, and competition for innervation of targets. At the same time, biochemists are purifying factors which control neruonal survival and growth, receptor clustering, axon outgrowth, glial proliferation, formation of synaptic specializations, cell migration, determination of transmitter choice, and aggregation of specific cell types. It has also been found that diffusible hormones act on specific neuronal populations to control neuron size, dendritic morphology, and transmitter phenotype. The fact that cellular interactions can be understood at this level of detail has obviously altered the rather general and sometimes philosophical tone that characterized much earlier work on these same themes.

It is perhaps worth pointing out some areas that seem likely to provide further insight into developmental issues in the immediate future. One of these is the emerging concept that a general scheme of positional information plays a crucial role not only in morphogenesis but possibly in several aspects of neural development such as cell migration, axon guidance, and perhaps synapse formation. The fascinating work on the compartmental development of insects seems likely to have profound significance for the development of the vertebrate nervous system as well. Similarly, the general theme of competition, which for several decades has flourished in the context of neuronal death, is just beginning to be applied to connections between cells, their specificities, and the regulation of convergence. Clearly, understanding the intimate details of competitive interactions between axons vying for innervation of the same targets provides an opportunity to elevate the idea of neuronal competition to a new level of understanding. Especially attractive is the promise of basic links between the idea of neurotrophism, the importance of neuronal activity, and knowledge about how synaptic connections are formed and maintained. Finally, perhaps at the heart of the matter, recent advances in molecular biology and genetics promise, and in some instances are beginning to deliver, insight into the way in which gene expression is controlled during development. Obviously, most major questions in developmental neurobiology are still open ones. Perhaps it is just this unfinished quality that makes this such an exciting and attractive field at present.

Reference Index

Italics indicate where full reference can be found; **boldface** type designates where author's article in this volume is located.